ANTIBIOTIC AND CHEMOTHERAPY:
Anti-infective agents and their use in therapy

All preparation and dosage information in Part II prepared by Sue Burton

For Churchill Livingstone

Commissioning Editor: Gavin Smith
Copy Editor: Julie Gorman
Indexer: Hilary Tarrant
Project Controller: Sarah Lowe
Text Design: Andrew Jones
Cover Design: Jeannette Jacobs

SEVENTH EDITION

Antibiotic and chemotherapy:

Anti-infective agents and their use in therapy

EDITED BY

Francis O'Grady
CBE TD MD MSc FRCP FRCPathHon FFPM
Foundation Professor of Microbiology Emeritus, University of Nottingham, Medical School, Queen's Medical Centre, Nottingham, UK

Harold P. Lambert
MA MD FRCP FRCPath FFPHM HonFCPCH
Emeritus Professor of Microbial Diseases, St George's Hospital Medical School; Consulting Physician, St George's Hospital; Visiting Professor, London School of Hygiene and Tropical Medicine, London, UK

Roger G. Finch
FRCP FRCPath FFPM
Professor of Infectious Diseases, Division of Microbiology and Infectious Diseases, Department of Clinical Laboratory Sciences, University of Nottingham and the Nottingham City Hospital NHS Trust, Nottingham, UK

David Greenwood
BSc PhD DSc FRCPath
Professor of Antimicrobial Science, Division of Microbiology and Infectious Diseases, Department of Clinical Laboratory Sciences, University Hospital, Queen's Medical Centre, Nottingham, UK

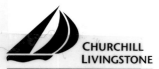
CHURCHILL LIVINGSTONE

NEW YORK EDINBURGH LONDON MADRID MELBOURNE SAN FRANCISCO TOKYO 1997

CHURCHILL LIVINGSTONE
Medical Division of Pearson Professional Limited

Distributed in the United States of America by Churchill Livingstone Inc.,
650 Avenue of the Americas, New York, N.Y. 10011, and by associated
companies, branches and representatives throughout the world.

First edition 1963
Second edition 1968
Third edition 1971
Fourth edition 1973
Fifth edition 1981
Sixth edition 1992
Seventh edition 1997

ISBN 0 443 05255 7

While great care has been taken to ensure the accuracy of the book's
content when it went to press, neither the authors nor the publishers can be
responsible for the accuracy and completeness of the information. If there is
any doubt, the manufacturer's current literature or other suitable reference
should be consulted.

British Library Cataloguing in Publication Data
A catalogue record for this book is available from the British Library.

Library of Congress Cataloging in Publication Data
A catalog record for this book is available from the Library of Congress.

Produced by Longman Singapore Publishers (Pte) Ltd
Printed in Singapore

Preface

Successive editions of this book record the astonishing progress of antimicrobial chemotherapy, charting the huge developments in its scope and complexity over three decades. The first edition, published in 1963 and covering the subject fully, was a small volume of 366 pages. Now, 32 years later, three times that number of pages and perhaps ten times the number of words are needed to do justice to our subject.

For five editions, over the best part of 20 years, the whole of this book was written by two, then three, authors. The sixth edition, published only four years ago, marked a radical change. We continued to write the bulk of the book ourselves but, in recognition of the growing complexity of the subject, no fewer than 16 additional authors contributed chapters on their specialist subjects.

With this edition, that process is complete. We have been joined by Professor Roger Finch and Professor David Greenwood as editors and the book is transformed into a full multi-author text in which 60 contributors provide authoritative and expert guidance on every aspect of our subject.

We have made two other major changes. First, a new introductory Part I has been added which deals with general issues underlying antimicrobial chemotherapy, such as modes of action, pharmacokinetics, interactions with other drugs and microbial resistance, and principles underlying their successful therapeutic use, like the role of the laboratory and antibiotic policies. In the second major change, the tentative references made in previous editions to antiprotozoal and anthelminthic agents have been expanded and systematized with the addition of completely new chapters devoted to those agents and the infections which they cause. Otherwise, the division made in all previous editions between a section (now Part II) on the agents and a section (now Part III) on treatment has been maintained. In Part II, the reader will find for each group of agents an introductory review describing the general properties and uses of the group. There follow individual accounts of each agent in the group giving all relevant details of antimicrobial activity, resistance, pharmacokinetics and clinical use. As in the past, we have confined ourselves to agents currently used in various parts of the world to treat human infections, but refer to a few antimicrobials which are used in animals, or are still in development, or have been withdrawn, when these throw light on the group as a whole.

In Part III, dealing with the treatment of particular infections, we have relented to some extent on our previous policy of confining ourselves strictly to antimicrobial treatment, and have included, where relevant, material about other aspects of management. Marking their growing importance, we have expanded into individual new chapters a number of topics covered only briefly in previous editions. These include abdominal and other surgical infections; infections associated with neutropenia and transplants; infections in intensive care patients; infections associated with implanted devices; HIV and AIDS; hepatitis; bone and joint infections and fungal infections.

It is a pleasure to thank Timothy Horne, Gavin Smith, Sarah Lowe and their colleagues at Churchill Livingstone, for their encouragement and support throughout the gestation of this 7th edition.

1996

Francis O'Grady
Harold Lambert

Preface

This book is mainly about antibiotics, but embraces the sulphonamides and other synthetic drugs employed in the chemotherapy of the microbic infections of temperate climates. That of malaria and most other protozoal infections, helminthiasis and malignant disease is excluded. The first part describes the properties of antibiotics and other drugs, with emphasis on their degree of activity against different bacterial species. The large body of detailed information on this presented in a series of tables, some of it hitherto unpublished, provides one essential basis for rational prescribing, since the first requirement of any drug is an adequate and preferably high degree of activity against the species responsible for the infection.

The second part is concerned with chemotherapy in its practical aspects, in infections which are classified by systems. As professional bacteriologists who have had no clinical responsibilities for many years we are fully conscious of our temerity in invading the sphere of therapeutics. Nevertheless each of us has been so frequently consulted by clinical colleagues about the treatment of individual patients that we can claim a knowledge of this subject in its practical as well as theoretical aspects, and feel justified in writing of what we have learned. The treatment we describe is solely that directed against the microbe. We are well aware that other kinds of treatment, quite outside our sphere, are sometimes an important element in success, and moreover that circumstances may exist, again beyond our ken, which can modify the usual indications for chemotherapy. The clinician must be the ultimate judge: our aim has been to provide him with as much factual information as possible, and accounts of the results achieved by previous competent observers. We believe that this information may be found useful at all levels in the profession; to both junior and senior members of hospital staffs and to consultants as well as general practitioners. We trust also that laboratory workers may find the book helpful.

We are indebted to many colleagues for advice, mainly on clinical matters, among whom we would particularly mention Miss J. Allen, FPS, Professor J. W. Crofton, Mr H. G. Dixon, Dr S. C. Gold, Dr D. A. Mitchison, Dr C. S. Nicol, Professor J. G. Scadding, Mr W. H. Stephenson and Dr J. P. M. Tizard. They have not actually read our text, and should not be held responsible for the views expressed, or for any errors. Our special thanks are due to Miss Pamela M. Waterworth, who has served both of us as a research assistant. She performed most of the experiments on which our original observations are based: among those hitherto unpublished are numerous data in Tables XI and XXII, and the findings illustrated in Figures 6 and 9. Some of her other contributions to the subject are referred to in the text. We are also indebted to her for advice about Chapter XXVII and for preparing the index.

1963

M.B.
L.P.G.

Contributors

Stephen Ash FRCP MBBS BSc
Consultant Physician, Ealing Hospital Trust, London, UK

A P Ball MB ChB FRCPEdin
Senior Lecturer, Department of Microbiology, St Andrew's University, Scotland, UK

Roger Bayston MMedSci MSc PhD DipClinMed MIBiol FRCPath
University Research Fellow, Department of Microbiological Infectious Diseases, University of Nottingham; Clinical Microbiologist, City Hospital, Nottingham, UK

Anthony J Bron BSc MB BS FRCOphth DO
Professor and Head of Department of Ophthalmology, University of Oxford, Nuffield Laboratory of Ophthalmology, Oxford, UK

E M Brown BSc DipBact MSc MB BCh FRCPath
Consultant Medical Microbiologist, Frenchay Hospital, Bristol, UK

André Bryskier MD
Head of Clinical Pharmacology Anti-infectives, Department of Microbiology, Hoechst–Marion–Roussel, Romainville, France

Sue Burton BPharm MRPharmS
Formerly Principal Pharmaceutical Advisor at Lambeth, Southwark and Lewisham Health Authority, London, UK

Karen Bush PhD
Director of Microbial Biochemistry, Astra Research Centre Boston, Cambridge, Massachusetts, USA

Jean-Paul Butzler MD PhD
Professor and Chair, Department of Clinical Microbiology, University Hospitals St. Pierre, Brugmann and Queen Fabiola, Brussels, Belgium

Mark W Casewell MRCP FRCPath BSc MD
Professor of Medical Microbiology, Dulwich Public Health Laboratory and Medical Microbiology, King's College School of Medicine and Dentistry, London, UK

Peter L Chiodini PhD FRCP
Consultant Parasitologist, The Hospital for Tropical Diseases, London; Honorary Senior Lecturer, The London School of Hygiene and Tropical Medicine, London, UK

Jonathan Cohen MSc MB FRCP FRCPath
Head, Department of Infectious Diseases, Royal Postgraduate Medical School, Hammersmith Hospital, London, UK

G C Cook MD DSc(Lond) FRCP FRACP FLS
Physician, Hospital for Tropical Diseases; Lecturer, London School of Hygiene and Tropical Medicine London, UK

Rodney Cove-Smith MA MB BChir MD FRCP
Consultant Nephrologist, South Cleveland Hospital, Middlesborough, Cleveland, UK

Simon L Croft BSc PhD
Senior Lecturer, Department of Medical Parasitology, London School of Hygiene and Tropical Medicine, London, UK

P F D'Arcy OBE BPharm PhD DSc FRPharmS FRSC
Emeritus Professor of Pharmacy, The Queen's University of Belfast, Belfast, Northern Ireland, UK

Peter G Davey MD FRCP
Reader in Clinical Pharmacology and Infectious Diseases, Ninewells Hospital and Medical School, Dundee, Scotland, UK

Robert N Davidson MD FRCP DTM&H
Senior Lecturer and Consultant, Department of Infection and Tropical Medicine, Northwick Park Hospital, Harrow, UK

D A Denham BSc MSc PhD DSc
Reader, London School of Hygiene and Tropical Medicine, London, UK

David W Denning FRCP MRCPath DCH
Senior Lecturer and Honorary Consultant in Infectious Diseases, North Manchester General and Hope Hospital, University of Manchester, Manchester, UK

David T Durack MB DPhil FRCP FRACP FACP
Consulting Professor of Medicine, Duke University, Durham, North Carolina; Worldwide Medical Director, Becton Dickinson Microbiology Systems, Baltimore, Maryland, USA

David I Edwards PhD CChem FRSC MRCPath
Professor and Head, Department of Life Sciences, Chemotherapy Research Unit, University of East London, London, UK

A M Elliot MD MRCP DTM&H
Senior Lecturer, Department of Clinical Sciences, London School of Hygiene and Tropical Medicine, London, UK

M J G Farthing MD FRCP
Professor of Gastroenterology, Department of Gastroenterology, St Bartholomew's and the Royal London School of Medicine and Dentistry, London, UK

Robert J Fass MD MS FACP
Professor of Internal Medicine and Medical Microbiology and Immunology, and Director, Division of Infectious Diseases, The Ohio State University Medical Center, Columbus, Ohio, USA

David Felmingham BSc MSc
Formerly Top Grade Clinical Scientist (Microbiology), University College Hospital, London, UK

Roger G Finch FRCP FRCPath FFPM
Professor of Infectious Diseases, Division of Microbiology and Infectious Diseases, Department of Clinical Laboratory Sciences, University of Nottingham and the Nottingham City Hospital NHS Trust, Nottingham, UK

G L French MD FRCPath FRCPA
Professor of Microbiology, Department of Microbiology, St Thomas's Hospital, London, UK

Curtis G Gemmell BSc PhD FRCPath
Reader and Head of Department, Department of Bacteriology, University of Glasgow Medical School, Royal Infirmary, Glasgow, Scotland, UK

John Grange MD MSc
Reader in Clinical Microbiology, Department of Microbiology, Imperial College of Science, Technology and Medicine, National Heart and Lung Institute, London, UK

David Greenwood BSc PhD DSc FRCPath
Professor of Antimicrobial Science, Division of Microbiology and Infectious Diseases, Department of Clinical Laboratory Sciences, University Hospital, Queen's Medical Centre, Nottingham, UK

J P Griffin BSc PhD MB BS FRCP FRCPath FFPM
Honorary Consultant, Clinical Pharmacology, Lister Hospital, Stevenage; Chairman, John Griffin Associates Ltd; Formerly Director, ABPI, Whitehall, London; Formerly Professional Head, Medicines Division, Department of Health, London, UK

J M T Hamilton-Miller PhD DSc FRCPath
Professor of Medical Microbiology, Royal Free Hospital School of Medicine; Honorary Clinical Scientist, Royal Free Hampstead NHS Trust, London, UK

D T D Hughes BSc BM BCh FRCP
Consultant Physician, Department of Thoracic Medicine, The Royal London Hospital, London, UK

Ian Hutchinson BPharms MRPharmS
Senior Pharmacist, Department of Drug Information, City Hospital NHS Trust, Nottingham, UK

Paul Kelly MRCP
Research Fellow, Digestive Diseases Research Centre, St Bartholomew's and Royal London Hospitals Medical School, London, UK

C C Kibbler MA MRCP MRCPath
Consultant in Medical Microbiology, Royal Free Hospital, London, UK

Neil R Kitteringham BSc(Hons) PhD
Senior Lecturer, Department of Pharmacology and Therapeutics, University of Liverpool, Liverpool, UK

Harold P Lambert MA MD FRCP FRCPath FFPHM HonFCPCH
Emeritus Professor of Microbial Diseases, St George's Hospital Medical School; Consulting Physician, St George's Hospital; Visiting Professor, London School of Hygiene and Tropical Medicine, London, UK

Giancarlo Lancini
Lepetit Research Centre, Gerenzano, Italy

Janice Main FRCP(Edin & London)
Senior Lecturer in Infectious Diseases and Medicine, Department of Medicine, Imperial College School of Medicine, St Mary's Hospital, London, UK

A R O Miller MA MB FRCP(Ed) FRCP DTM&H
Consultant Physician, Kidderminster General Hospital; Honorary Senior Lecturer in Infection, University of Birmingham, Birmingham, UK

D Nathwani FRCP(Ed) DTM&H
Consultant Physician, Dundee Teaching Hospitals NHS Trust, King's Cross Hospital, Dundee, Scotland, UK

Karl G Nicholson MD FRCP FRCPath
Senior Lecturer in Infectious and Tropical Diseases, Leicester Royal Infirmary, Leicester, UK

Francis O'Grady CBE TD MD MSc FRCP FRCPathHon FFPM
Foundation Professor of Microbiology Emeritus, University of Nottingham, Medical School, Queen's Medical Centre, Nottingham, UK

Francesco Parenti
Marion Merrell Dow Europe AG, Thalwil, Switzerland

B Kevin Park BSc(Hons) PhD FRCP(Hon)
Wellcome Principal Research Fellow, Department of Pharmacology and Therapeutics, University of Liverpool, Liverpool, UK

Jean-Claude Pechere
Department of Genetics and Microbiology, University of Geneva Medical School, Geneva, Switzerland

Tim Peto BM BCh DPhil FRCP
Reader in Medicine, University of Oxford; Consultant Physician in Infectious Diseases, John Radcliffe Hospital, Oxford, UK

Ian Phillips MD FRCPath FRCP MFPHM
Emeritus Professor of Microbiology, Department of Microbiology, UMDS, St Thomas's Hospital, London, UK

S Ragnor Norrby MD PhD
Professor and Head, Department of Infectious Diseases, Lund University Hospital, Lund, Sweden

D S Reeves MD FRCPath
Honorary Professor of Medical Microbiology, Medical Microbiology Department, University of Bristol; Consultant Medical Microbiologist, Southmead Hospital, Bristol, UK

David V Seal MD FRCOphth FRCPath
Senior Lecturer in Ocular Infectious Diseases, Tennent Institute of Ophthalmology, University of Glasgow, Glasgow, Scotland, UK

Kevin P Shannon BSc PhD FRCPath
Lecturer, Department of Microbiology, UMDS, St Thomas's Hospital, London, UK

David C Shanson MB BS FRCPath
Consultant Microbiologist, JS Pathology and Unilabs, London: Formerly Senior Lecturer and Honorary Consultant in Medical Microbiology at Charing Cross and Westminster Medical School, London, UK

F Smaill MB ChB FRACP FRCPC
Associate Professor, Department of Microbiology and Medicine, McMaster University, Hamilton, Ontario, Canada

R Sutherland DSc
Consultant Microbiologist, Dorking, UK

Eric W Taylor MBBS FRCS
Consultant Surgeon and Medical Director, Vale of Leven Hospital, Alexandria, Scotland, UK

M G Thomas MB ChB MD FRACP
Senior Lecturer in Infectious Diseases, Department of Molecular Medicine, University of Auckland, Auckland, New Zealand

Howard C Thomas BSc PhD FRCP FRCPath
Professor of Medicine, Department of Medicine, Imperial College School of Medicine, St Mary's Hospital, London, UK

David W Warnock BSc PhD FRCPath
Consultant Clinical Scientist, Public Health Laboratory, University of Bristol; Honorary Senior Clinical Lecturer in Medical Mycology, University of Bristol, Bristol, UK

N J White DSc MD FRCP
Director, Wellcome-Mahidol University Oxford Tropical Medicine Research Programme, Faculty of Tropical Medicine, Bangkok, Thailand; Wellcome Trust Clinical Research Unit, Centre for Tropical Diseases, Ho Chi Minh City, Vietnam

M H Wilcox BMedSci BM BS MD MRCPath
Senior Lecturer, Department of Microbiology, University of Leeds; Honorary Consultant, The General Infirmary, Leeds, UK

Richard Wise MD FRCPath
Professor and Consultant in Medical Microbiology, City Hospital Trust and University of Birmingham, Birmingham, UK

Contents

General aspects

Historical introduction

D. Greenwood

The first part of this chapter was included as an introduction to editions 2–5 of this book. It was written by Professor L. P. Garrod, co-author of the first five editions. Garrod, after serving as a surgeon probationer in the Navy during the 1914–18 war, had then qualified and practised clinical medicine before specializing in bacteriology, later achieving world recognition as the foremost authority on antimicrobial chemotherapy. He had witnessed, and studied profoundly, the whole development of modern chemotherapy.

The evolution of antimicrobic drugs

No one recently qualified even with the liveliest imagination, can picture the ravages of bacterial infection which continued until rather less than 40 years ago. To take only two examples, lobar pneumonia was a common cause of death even in young and vigorous patients, and puerperal septicaemia and other forms of acute streptoccocal sepsis had a high mortality, little affected by any treatment then available. One purpose of this introduction is therefore to place the subject of this book in historical perspective.

This subject is chemotherapy, which may be defined as the administration of a substance with a systemic antimicrobic action. Some would confine the term to synthetic drugs, and the distinction is recognized in the title of this book, but since some all-embracing term is needed, this one might with advantage be understood also to include substances of natural origin. Several antibiotics can now be synthesized, and it would be ludicrous if their use should qualify for description as chemotherapy only because they happened to be prepared in this way. The essence of the term is that the effect must be systemic, the substance being absorbed, whether from the alimentary tract or a site of injection, and reaching the infected area by way of the blood stream. 'Local chemotherapy' is in this sense a contradiction in terms: any application to a surface, even of something capable of exerting a systemic effect, is better described as antisepsis.

THE THREE ERAS OF CHEMOTHERAPY

There are three distinct periods in the history of this subject. In the first, which is of great antiquity, the only substances capable of curing an infection by systemic action were natural plant products. The second was the era of synthesis, and in the third we return to natural plant products, although from plants of a much lower order, the moulds and bacteria forming antibiotics.

1. *Alkaloids.* This era may be dated from 1619, since it is from this year that the first record is derived of the successful treatment of malaria with an extract of cinchona bark, the patient being the wife of the Spanish governor of Peru.* Another South American discovery was the efficacy of ipecacuanha root in amoebic dysentery. Until the early years of this century these extracts, and in more recent times the alkaloids, quinine and emetine, derived from them, provided the only curative chemotherapy known.

2. *Synthetic compounds.* Therapeutic progress in this field, which initially and for many years after was due almost entirely to research in Germany, dates from the discovery of salvarsan by Ehrlich in 1909. His successors produced germanin for trypanosomiasis and other drugs effective in protozoal infections. A common view at that time was that protozoa were susceptible to chemotherapeutic attack, but that bacteria were not: the treponemata, which had been

---

* Garrod was mistaken in perpetuating this legend, which is now discounted by medical historians.

shown to be susceptible to organic arsenicals, are no ordinary bacteria, and were regarded as a class apart.

The belief that bacteria are by nature insusceptible to any drug which is not also prohibitively toxic to the human body was finally destroyed by the discovery of Prontosil. This, the forerunner of the sulphonamides, was again a product of German research, and its discovery was publicly announced in 1935. All the work with which this book is concerned is subsequent to this year: it saw the beginning of the effective treatment of bacterial infections.

Progress in the synthesis of antimicrobic drugs has continued to the present day. Apart from many new sulphonamides, perhaps the most notable additions have been the synthetic compounds used in the treatment of tuberculosis.

3. *Antibiotics.* The therapeutic revolution produced by the sulphonamides, which included the conquest of haemolytic streptococcal and pneumococcal infections and of gonorrhoea and cerebrospinal fever, was still in progress and even causing some bewilderment when the first report appeared of a study which was to have even wider consequences. This was not the discovery of penicillin – that had been made by Fleming in 1929 – but the demonstration by Florey and his colleagues that it was a chemotherapeutic agent of unexampled potency. The first announcement of this, made in 1940, was the beginning of the antibiotic era, and the unimagined developments from it are still in progress. We little knew at the time that penicillin, besides providing a remedy for infections insusceptible to sulphonamide treatment, was also a necessary second line of defence against those fully susceptible to it. During the early 1940s, resistance to sulphonamides appeared successively in gonococci, haemolytic streptococci and pneumococci: nearly 20 years later it has appeared also in meningoccoci. But for the advent of the antibiotics, all the benefits stemming from Domagk's discovery might by now have been lost, and bacterial infections have regained their pre-1935 prevalence and mortality.

The earlier history of two of these discoveries calls for further description.

Sulphonamides

Prontosil, or sulphonamido-chrysoidin, was first synthesized by Klarer & Mietzsch in 1932, and was one of a series of azo dyes examined by Domagk for possible effects on haemolytic streptococcal infection. When a curative effect in mice had been demonstrated, cautious trials in erysipelas and other human infections were undertaken, and not until the evidence afforded by these was conclusive did the discoverers make their announcement. Domagk (1935) published the original claims, and the same information was communicated by Hörlein (1935) to a notable meeting in London.

These claims, which initially concerned only the treatment of haemolytic streptococcal infections, were soon confirmed in other countries, and one of the most notable early studies was that of Colebrook & Kenny (1936) in England, who demonstrated the efficacy of the drug in puerperal fever. This infection had until then been taking a steady toll of about 1000 young lives per annum in England and Wales, despite every effort to prevent it by hygiene measures and futile efforts to overcome it by serotherapy. The immediate effect of the adoption of this treatment can be seen in Figure 1.1: a steep fall in mortality began in 1935, and continued, as the treatment became universal and better understood, and as more potent sulphonamides were introduced, until the present-day low level had almost been reached *before penicillin became generally available.* The effect of penicillin between 1945 and 1950 is perhaps more evident on incidence: its widespread use tends completely to banish haemolytic streptococci from the environment. The apparent rise in incidence after 1950 is due to the redefinition of puerperal pyrexia as any rise of temperature to 38°C, whereas previously the term was only applied when the temperature was maintained for 24 h or recurred. Needless to say, fever so defined is frequently not of uterine origin.

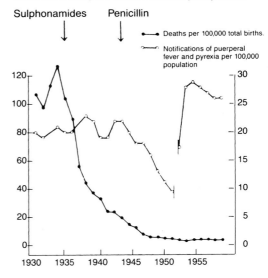

Infection during childbirth and the puerpenum

Fig. 1.1 *Puerperal pyrexia. Deaths per 100 000 total births and incidence per 100 000 population in England and Wales, 1930–1957. N.B. The apparent rise in incidence in 1950 is due to the fact that the definition of puerperal pyrexia was changed in this year (see text).*

(Reproduced with permission from Barber 1960 Journal of Obstetrics and Gynaecology 67: 727 by kind permission of the editor.)

Prontosil had no antibacterial action in vitro, and it was soon suggested by workers in Paris (Tréfouel et al 1935) that it owed its activity to the liberation from it in the body of *p*-aminobenzene sulphonamide (sulphanilamide); that this compound is so formed was subsequently proved by Fuller (1937). Sulphanilamide had a demonstrable inhibitory action on streptococci in vitro, much dependent on the medium and particularly on the size of the inoculum, facts which are readily understandable in the light of modern knowledge. This explanation of the therapeutic action of prontosil was hotly contested by Domagk. It must be remembered that it relegated the chrysoidin component to an inert role, whereas the affinity of dyes for bacteria had been a basis of German research since the time of Ehrlich, and was the doctrine underlying the choice of this series of compounds for examination. German workers also took the attitude that there must be something mysterious about the action of a true chemotherapeutic agent: an effect easily demonstrable in a test tube by any tyro was too banal altogether to explain it. Finally, they felt justifiable resentment that sulphanilamide, as a compound which had been described many years earlier, could be freely manufactured by anyone.

Every enterprising pharmaceutical house in the world was soon making this drug, and at one time it was on the market under at least 70 different proprietary names. What was more important, chemists were soon busy modifying the molecule to improve its performance. Early advances so secured were of two kinds, the first being higher activity against a wider range of bacteria: sulphapyridine (M and B 693), discovered in 1938, was the greatest single advance, since it was the first drug to be effective in pneumococcal pneumonia. The next stage, the introduction of sulpha-thiazole and sulphadiazine, while retaining and enhancing antibacterial activity, eliminated the frequent nausea and cyanosis caused by earlier drugs. Further developments, mainly in the direction of altered pharmacokinetic properties, have continued to the present day and are described in Chapter 1 [*now Ch. 34*].

ANTIBIOTICS

'Out of the earth shall come thy salvation.'

S. A. Waksman

Definition

Of many definitions of the term antibiotic which have been proposed, the narrower seem preferable. It is true that the word 'antibiosis' was coined by Vuillemin in 1889 to denote antagonism between living creatures in general, but the noun 'antibiotic' was first used by Waksman in 1942 (Waksman & Lechevalier 1962), which gives him a right to re-define it, and definition confines it to substances produced by micro-organisms antagonistic to the growth or life of others in high dilution (the last clause being necessary to exclude such metabolic products as organic acids, hydrogen peroxide and alcohol). To define an antibiotic simply as an antibacterial substance from a living source would embrace gastric juice, antibodies and lysozyme from man, essential oils and alkaloids from plants, and such oddities as the substance in the faeces of blowfly larvae which exerts an antiseptic effect in wounds. All substances known as antibiotics which are in clinical use and capable of exerting systemic effect are in fact products of micro-organisms.

Early history

The study of intermicrobic antagonism is almost as old as microbiology itself: several instances of it were described, one by Pasteur himself, in the seventies of the last century. Therapeutic applications followed, some employing actual living cultures, others extracts of bacteria or moulds which had been found active. One of the best known products was an extract of *Pseudomonas aeruginosa*, first used as a local application by Czech workers, Honl & Bukovsky, in 1899: this was commercially available as 'pyocyanase' on the continent for many years. Other investigators used extracts of species of *Penicillium* and *Aspergillus* which probably or certainly contained antibiotics, but in too low a concentration to exert more than a local and transient effect. Florey (1945) gave a revealing account of these early developments in a lecture with the intriguing title 'The Use of Micro-organisms as Therapeutic Agents': this was amplified in a later publication (Florey 1949).

The systemic search, by an ingenious method, for an organism which could attack pyogenic cocci, conducted by Dubos (1939) in New York, led to the discovery of tyrothricin (gramicidin + tyrocidine), formed by *Bacillus brevis*, a substance which, although too toxic for systemic use in man, had in fact a systemic curative effect in mice. This work exerted a strong influence in inducing Florey and his colleagues to embark on a study of naturally formed antibacterial substances, and penicillin was the second on their list.

Penicillin

The present antibiotic era may be said to date from 1940, when the first account of the properties of an extract of cultures of *Penicillium notatum* appeared from Oxford (Chain et al 1940): a fuller account followed, with impressive clinical evidence (Abraham et al 1941). It had been necessary to find means of extracting a very labile substance from culture fluids, to examine its action on a wide range of bacteria, to examine its toxicity by a variety of methods, to establish a unit of its activity, to study its distribution and excretion when administered to animals, and finally to prove its systemic efficacy in mouse infections. There then remained the gigantic task, seemingly impossible except on a factory scale, of producing in the School of Pathology at Oxford enough of a substance, which was known to be excreted with unexampled rapidity, for the treatment of human disease. One means of maintaining supplies was extraction from the patients' urine and re-administration.

It was several years before penicillin was fully purified, its structure ascertained, and its large-scale commercial production achieved. That this was of necessity first entrusted to manufacturers in the USA gave them a lead in a highly profitable industry which was not to be overtaken for many years.

Later antibiotics

The dates of discovery and sources of the principal antibiotics are given chronologically in Table 1.1. This is far from being a complete list, but subsequently discovered antibiotics have been closely related to others already known, such as aminoglycosides and macrolides. A few, including penicillin, were chance discoveries, but 'stretching out suppliant Petri dishes' (Florey 1945) in the hope of catching a new antibiotic-producing organism was not to lead anywhere. Most further discoveries resulted from soil surveys, a process from which a large annual outlay might or might not be repaid a hundred-fold, a gamble against much longer odds than most oil prospecting. Soil contains a profuse and very mixed flora varying with climate, vegetation, mineral content and other factors, and is a medium in which antibiotic formation may well play a part in the competition for nutriment. A soil survey consists of obtaining samples from as many and as varied sources as possible, cultivating them on plates, subcultivating all colonies of promising organisms such as actinomycetes and examining each for antibacterial activity. Alternatively the primary plate culture may be inoculated by spraying or by agar layering with suitable bacteria, the growth of which may then be seen to be inhibited in a zone surrounding some of the original colonies. This is only a beginning: many thousands of successive colonies so examined are found to form an antibiotic already known or useless by reason of toxicity.

Antibiotics have been derived from some odd sources other than soil. Although the original strain of *P. notatum* apparently floated into Fleming's laboratory at St. Mary's from one on another floor of the building in which moulds were being studied, that of *Penicillium chrysogenum* now used for penicillin production was derived from a mouldy Canteloupe melon in the market at Peoria, Illinois. Perhaps the strangest derivation was that of helenine, an antibiotic with some antiviral activity, isolated by Shope (1953) from *Penicillium funiculosum* growing on 'the isinglass cover of a photograph of my wife, Helen, on Guam, near the end of the

Table 1.1 *Date of discovery and source of natural antibiotics*

Name	Date of discovery	Microbe
Penicillin	1929–40	*Penicillium notatum*
Tyrothricin { Gramicidin Tyrocidine }	1939	*Bacillus brevis*
Griseofluvin	1939	*Penicillium griseofulvum Dierckx*
	1945	*Penicillium janczewski*
Streptomycin	1944	*Streptomyces griseus*
Bacitracin	1945	*Bacillus licheniformis*
Chloramphenicol	1947	*Streptomyces venezuelae*
Polymyxin	1947	*Bacillus polymyxa*
Framycetin	1947–53	*Streptomyces lavendulae*
Chlortetracycline	1948	*Streptomyces aureofaciens*
Cephalosporin C, N and P	1948	*Cephalosporium sp.*
Neomycin	1949	*Streptomyces fradiae*
Oxytetracycline	1950	*Streptomyces rimosus*
Nystatin	1950	*Streptomyces noursei*
Erythromycin	1952	*Streptomyces erythreus*
Oleandomycin	1954	*Streptomyces antibioticus*
Spiramycin	1954	*Streptomyces ambofaciens*
Novobiocin	1955	*Streptomyces spheroides Streptomyces niveus*
Cycloserine	1955	*Streptomyces orchidaceus Streptomyces gaeryphalus*
Vancomycin	1956	*Streptomyces orientalis*
Rifamycin	1957	*Streptomyces mediterranei*
Kanamycin	1957	*Streptomyces kanamyceticus*
Nebramycins	1958	*Streptomyces tenebraeus*
Paromomycin	1959	*Streptomyces rimosus*
Fusidic acid	1960	*Fusidium coccineum*
Spectinomycin	1961–62	*Streptomyces flavopersicus*
Lincomycin	1962	*Streptomyces lincolnensis*
Gentamicin	1963	*Micromonospora purpurea*
Josamycin	1964	*Streptomyces narvonensis var. josamyceticus*
Tobramycin	1968	*Streptomyces tenebraeus*
Ribostamycin	1970	*Streptomyces ribosidificus*
Butirosin	1970	*Bacillus circulans*
Sissomicin	1970	*Micromonospora myosensis*
Rosaramicin	1972	*Micromonospora rosaria*

war in 1945'. He proceeds to explain that he chose the name because it was non-descriptive, non-committal and not pre-empted, 'but largely out of recognition of the good taste shown by the mould . . . in locating on the picture of my wife'.

Those antibiotics out of thousands now discovered which have qualified for therapeutic use are described in chapters which follow.

FUTURE PROSPECTS

All successful chemotherapeutic agents have certain properties in common. They must exert an antimicrobic action, whether inhibitory or lethal, in high dilution, and in the complex chemical environment which they encounter in the body. Secondly, since they are brought into contact with every tissue in the body, they must so far as possible be without harmful effect on the function of any organ. To these two essential qualities may be added others which are highly desirable, although sometimes lacking in useful drugs: stability, free solubility, a slow rate of excretion, and diffusibility into remote areas.

If a drug is toxic to bacteria but not to mammalian cells the probability is that it interferes with some structure or function peculiar to bacteria. When the mode of action of sulphanilamide was elucidated by Woods and Fildes, and the theory was put forward of bacterial inhibition by metabolite analogues, the way seemed open for devising further antibacterial drugs on a rational basis. Immense subsequent advances in knowledge of the anatomy, chemical composition and metabolism of the bacterial cell should have encouraged such hopes still further. This new knowledge has been helpful in explaining what drugs do to bacteria, but not in devising new ones. Discoveries have continued to result only from random trials, purely empirical in the antibiotic field, although sometimes based on reasonable theoretical expectation in the synthetic.

Not only is the action of any new drug on individual bacteria still unpredictable on a theoretical basis, but so are its effects on the body itself. Most of the toxic effects of antibiotics have come to light only after extensive use, and even now no one can explain their affinity for some of the organs attacked. Some new observations in this field have contributed something to the present climate of suspicion about new drugs generally, which is insisting on far more searching tests of toxicity, and delaying the release of drugs for therapeutic use, particularly in the USA.

The present scope of chemotherapy

Successive discoveries have added to the list of infections amenable to chemotherapy until nothing remains altogether untouched except the viruses. On the other hand, however, some of the drugs which it is necessary to use are far from ideal, whether because of toxicity or of unsatisfactory pharmacokinetic properties, and some forms of treatment are consequently less often successful than others. Moreover, microbic resistance is a constant threat to the future usefulness of almost any drug. It seems unlikely that any totally new antibiotic remains to be discovered, since those of recent origin have similar properties to others already known. It therefore will be wise to husband our resources, and employ them in such a way as to preserve

them. The problems of drug resistance and policies for preventing it are discussed in Chapters 13 and 14 [*now Chs. 3 and 12*].

Adaptation of existing drugs

A line of advance other than the discovery of new drugs is the adaptation of old ones. An outstanding example of what can be achieved in this way is presented by the sulphonamides. Similar attention has naturally been directed to the antibiotics, with fruitful results of two different kinds. One is simply an alteration for the better in pharmacokinetic properties. Thus procaine penicillin, because less soluble, is longer acting than potassium penicillin: the esterification of macrolides improves absorption: chloramphenicol palmitate is palatable, and other variants so produced are more stable, more soluble and less irritant. Secondly, synthetic modification may also enhance antimicrobic properties. Sometimes both types of change can be achieved together; thus rifampicin is not only well absorbed after oral administration, whereas rifamycin, from which it is derived, is not, but antibacterially much more active. The most varied achievements of these kinds have been among the penicillins, overcoming to varying degrees three defects in benzylpenicillin, its susceptibility to destruction by gastric acid and by staphylococcal penicillinase, and the relative insusceptibility to it of many species of Gram-negative bacilli. Similar developments have provided many new derivatives of cephalosporin C, although the majority differ from their prototypes much less than the penicillins.

One effect of these developments, of which it may seem captious to complain, is that a quite bewildering variety of products is now available for the same purposes. There are still many sulphonamides, about 10 tetracyclines, more than 20 semi-synthetic penicillins, and a rapidly extending list of cephalosporins, and a confident choice between them for any given purpose is one which few prescribers are qualified to make – indeed no one may be, since there is often no significant difference between the effects to be expected. Manufacturers whose costly research laboratories have produced some new derivative with a marginal advantage over others are entitled to make the most of their discovery. But if an antibiotic in a new form has a substantial advantage over that from which it was derived and no countervailing disadvantages, could not its predecessor sometimes simply be dropped? This rarely seems to happen, and there are doubtless good reasons for it, but the only foreseeable opportunity for simplifying the prescriber's choice has thus been missed.

References

Abraham E P, Chain E, Fletcher C M et al 1941 *Lancet* ii: 177–189

Chain E, Florey H W, Gardner A D et al 1940 *Lancet* ii: 226–228

Colebrook L, Kenny M 1936 *Lancet* i: 1279–1286

Domagk G 1935 *Deutsche Medizinische Wochenschrift* 61: 250–253

Dubos R J 1939 *Journal of Experimental Medicine* 70: 1–10

Florey H W 1945 *British Medical Journal* 2: 635–642

Florey H W 1949 Antibiotics. Oxford University Press, London, ch 1

Fuller A T 1937 *Lancet* i: 194–198

Honl J, Bukovsky J 1899 Zentralblatt für Bakteriologie, Parasitenkunde, Infektionskrankheiten und Hygiene, Abteilung I 26: 305 (see Florey 1949)

Hörlein H 1935 *Proceedings of the Royal Society of Medicine* 29: 313–324

Shope R E 1953 *Journal of Experimental Medicine* 97: 601–626

Tréfouël J, Tréfouël J, Nitti F, Bovet D 1935 *Comptes Rendus des Séances de la Société de Biologie et de ses Filiales (Paris)* 120: 756–758

Waksman S A, Lechevalier H A 1962 The Actinomycetes. Baillière, London, vol 3

Professor Garrod died while the 5th edition was in preparation in 1979, but had already completed his contribution to the book. He has summarized the development of antimicrobial chemotherapy so well, and with such characteristic lucidity, that to add anything seems superfluous. The following is a brief summary of developments that have occurred since about 1975.

At the time of Garrod's death, penicillins and cephalosporins were still in the ascendancy: apart from the aminoglycoside, amikacin, the latest advances in antimicrobial therapy to reach the formulary in the late 1970s were the antipseudomonal penicillins, azlocillin, mezlocillin and piperacillin, the amidinopenicillin, mecillinam, and the β-lactamase-stable cephalosporins, cefuroxime and cefoxitin. The latter compounds emerged in response to the growing importance of enterobacterial β-lactamases, which were the subject of intense scrutiny around this time (see, e.g., Richmond & Sykes 1973). Cefoxitin is an example of a cephamycin, a semi-synthetic derivative of a naturally occurring cephalosporin that owes its β-lactamase stability to a methoxy substitution on the β-lactam ring. Discovery of other novel, enzyme-resistant, β-lactam molecules elaborated by micro-organisms, including clavams, carbapenems and monobactams (see Ch. 16) were to follow, reminding us that Mother Nature still has some antimicrobial surprises up her copious sleeves.

The other solution to the β-lactamase problem,

cefuroxime, was achieved by adding a sterically protective methoximino group to the cephalosporin side-chain. The appearance of this compound, first described in 1976 (O'Callaghan et al 1976), was soon followed by the synthesis of cefotaxime (Heymès et al 1977) a methoximino-cephalosporin that was not only β-lactamase stable, but also possessed much enhanced intrinsic activity. The early 1980s were dominated by the appearance of several variations on the cefotaxime theme (ceftizoxime, ceftriaxone, cefmenoxime, ceftazidime and the oxa-cephem, latamoxef), to provide a group of compounds that arguably represents the high point in a continuing development of cephalosporins from 1964, when cephaloridine and cephalothin were first introduced.

Antibacterial agents 1987–1995

Antibacterial agents released on the UK market in 3-year periods since 1987 are listed in Table 1.2. It is notable that

Table 1.2 *Antibacterial agents introduced on the UK market 1987–1995*

Agent	Type
1987–1989	
Aztreonam	Monobactam
Cefuroxime axetil	Oral cephalosporin
Ciprofloxacin	Fluoroquinolone
Enoxacin*	Fluoroquinolone
Imipenem	Carbapenem
Mupirocin	Monic acid (topical)
Temocillin	Penicillin
Ticarcillin + clavulanate†	Penicillin/β-lactamase inhibitor combination
1990-1992	
Azithromycin	Macrolide (azalide)
Cefixime	Oral cephalosporin
Cefodizime	Parenteral cephalosporin
Clarithromycin	Macrolide
Norfloxacin	Fluoroquinolone
Ofloxacin	Fluoroquinolone
Sulbactam (+ ampicillin)	β-Lactamase inhibitor
Tazobactam (+ piperacillin)	β-Lactamase inhibitor
Teicoplanin	Glycopeptide
Temafloxacin*	Fluoroquinolone
1993–1995	
Cefpodoxime	Oral cephalosporin
Ceftibuten	Oral cephalosporin
Ceftriaxone	Parenteral cephalosporin
Fosfomycin trometamol	Phosphonic acid
Rifabutin	Rifamycin (antimycobacterial)

* Later withdrawn.
† A new combination of older compounds.

half the compounds that have been licensed during that time are β-lactam derivatives. Moreover, only one of these, temocillin, is a penicillin, although several older penicillins have been relaunched in fixed-dose combinations with β-lactamase inhibitors. A steady trickle of new cephalosporins continues to appear, with an emphasis on orally-absorbed compounds that exhibit stability to enterobacterial and other β-lactamases.

Among non-β-lactam compounds that appeared in the 1980s, most interest has centred on quinolones and macrolides. The quinolone group of antibacterial agents enjoyed a renaissance when it was realized that fluorinated, piperazine-substituted derivatives exhibited much enhanced potency and a broader spectrum of activity than earlier congeners (see Ch. 32). Other quinolones with further improved properties are poised to appear, but enthusiasm has been muted to some extent by the rapid demise of temafloxacin, which had to be withdrawn soon after it was launched in 1992 because of unacceptable toxicity. Several new macrolides were described during the 1980s and two representatives of this antibiotic family, azithromycin and clarithromycin, both of which claim pharmacological advantages over erythromycin (see Ch. 27), reached the UK market in 1991.

An array of β-lactam antibiotics, aminoglycosides, quinolones and macrolides that are not available in the UK have been marketed in various countries around the world, but few examples of other types of antibacterial agent have appeared. Only four have been licensed for use in Britain in the last 9 years: mupirocin (Ch. 28), teicoplanin (Ch. 24), rifabutin (Ch. 33) and fosfomycin trometamol (Ch. 22). Of these compounds, just one, the topical agent mupirocin, is truly novel in structure.

Meanwhile, old agents are judged redundant almost as fast as new ones appear. Many sulphonamides and other drugs have been withdrawn over the years, and at least nine β-lactam antibiotics (carfecillin, cephaloridine, cephalothin, ciclacillin, latamoxef, methicillin, mezlocillin, penamecillin and phenethicillin) have been deleted from the British National Formulary since 1990.

Antifungal, antiviral and antiparasitic agents

In addition to the continued development of antibacterial agents, the search for drugs in other therapeutic categories has also met with some success (Table 1.3). Most notable has been development of several new antifungal and antiviral compounds, stimulated by the increased importance of fungal and viral pathogens in immunosuppressed patients, including those with acquired

Table 1.3 *Non-antibacterial agents introduced on the UK market 1987–1995*

Agent	Type	Category
Albendazole	Benzimidazole	Anthelminthic
Amorolfine	Phenylmorpholine	Antifungal (topical)
Didanosine	Nucleoside analogue	Antiviral
Famciclovir	Nucleoside analogue	Antiviral
Fluconazole	Triazole	Antifungal
Foscarnet	Phosphonoformate	Antiviral
Ganciclovir	Nucleoside analogue	Antiviral
Halofantrine	Phenanthrenemethanol	Antimalarial
Itraconazole	Triazole	Antifungal
Mefloquine	Quinolinemethanol	Antimalarial
Terbinafine	Allylamine	Antifungal
Tribavirin*	Nucleoside analogue	Antiviral
Valaciclovir	Nucleoside analogue	Antiviral
Zidovudine	Nucleoside analogue	Antiviral

* Known as ribavirin outside the UK.

immune deficiency syndrome (AIDS). Many of these new drugs are variations on older themes: for example, antifungal azoles and antiviral nucleoside analogues. Numerous ingenious approaches to the HIV problem have been proposed and several innovative antiviral agents are presently under investigation. Novel antifungal agents include the interesting new allylamine antifungal agent, terbinafine (Ch. 60).

Among new compounds that have been introduced in the USA and elsewhere are the diaminopyrimidine, trimetrexate, and the hyroxynaphthoquinone, atovaquone, which were approved by the US Food and Drug Administration in 1992 and 1993, respectively, for use in *Pneumocystis carinii* pneumonia. Atovaquone was originally developed as an antimalarial agent. Although early trials were disappointing, interest has been revived by the demonstration of synergy with proguanil.

The most serious effects of parasitic infections are borne by the economically poorer countries of the Third World, and research into agents for the treatment of parasitic disease of humans has always received low priority. Nevertheless, some useful new antimalarial compounds have eventually found their way into therapeutic use. These include mefloquine and halofantrine, which originally emerged in the early 1980s from the extensive antimalarial research programme undertaken by the Walter Reed Army Institute of Research in Washington. Derivatives of artemisinin, the active principle of the Chinese herbal remedy qinghaosu, are also now in use, especially in parts of the Far East. These developments have been slow, but are nonetheless welcome in view of the inexorable spread of chloroquine resistance in *Plasmodium falciparum* which continues unabated (see Ch. 62). The only noteworthy development among new drugs for the treatment of other protozoan diseases is eflornithine (difluoromethylornithine), which provides a long-awaited alternative to arsenicals in trypanosomiasis. Eflornithine has been dubbed the 'resurrection drug' in West Africa because of its effect in the late stages of sleeping sickness (Anonymous 1991), but unfortunately it appears ineffective in the East African form of the disease.

On the anthelminthic front we now, amazingly, have three agents – albendazole, praziquantel and ivermectin – which between them cover nearly all the important causes of intestinal and systemic worm infections (see Chs. 38, 63 and 64). Most anthelminthic compounds enter the human anti-infective formulary by the veterinary route, underlying the melancholy fact that animal husbandry is of relatively greater economic importance than the well-being of the approximately 1.5 billion people who harbour parasitic worms.

occasional reality among seriously ill patients in high-dependency units where there is intense selective pressure created by widespread use of potent, broad-spectrum agents. On a global scale, multiple drug resistance in a number of different organisms, including those that cause typhoid fever, tuberculosis and malaria, is an unsolved problem. These are life-threatening infections for which treatment options are limited, even when fully sensitive organisms are involved.

Science, with a little help from Lady Luck, has provided us with formidable resources for the treatment of infectious disease during the last 60 years. Garrod, surveying the scope of chemotherapy in 1979, warned of the threat of microbial resistance and the need to husband our resources. That threat and that need have not diminished. The challenge for the future is to preserve the precious assets that we have acquired by sensible regulation of the availability of antimicrobial drugs in countries in which controls are presently inadequate and by informed and cautious prescribing everywhere.

The scope of antimicrobial chemotherapy at the end of the 20th century

Hundreds of new antibacterial agents have been described in the world literature during the last 25 years. There have been many false dawns, but relatively few compounds have survived the stages of development and licensing to reach the pharmacist's shelf. The commercial reality behind this is plain: it has been estimated in the USA that the process of bringing a new drug to market presently takes about 12 years and costs in excess of $350 million (about £225 million); only about a third of the drugs that are launched yield a profit (Billstein 1994). Given this, and the already crowded market for antibacterial drugs, it is not surprising that anti-infective research in the pharmaceutical houses is being scaled down or turned to the potentially more lucrative fields of antifungal and antiviral drugs. Meanwhile, resistance continues to increase inexorably (Cohen 1992, Kunin 1993). Although most bacterial infection remains amenable to therapy with common, well-established drugs, the prospect of untreatable infection is already becoming an

References

Anonymous 1991 New drug for trypanosomiasis. *Lancet* 337: 42

Billstein S A 1994 How the pharmaceutical industry brings an antibiotic drug to market in the United States. *Antimicrobial Agents and Chemotherapy* 38: 2679–2682

Cohen M L 1992 Epidemiology of drug resistance: implications for a post-antimicrobial era. *Science* 257: 1050–1055

Heymès R, Lutz A, Schrinner E 1977 Experimental evaluation of HR756, a new cephalosporin derivative: pre-clinical study. *Infection* 5: 259–260

Kunin C M 1993 Resistance to antimicrobial agents – a worldwide calamity. *Annals of Internal Medicine* 118: 557–561

O'Callaghan C H, Sykes R B, Ryan D M et al 1976 Cefuroxime: a new cephalosporin antibiotic. *Journal of Antibiotics* 29: 29–33

Richmond M H, Sykes R B 1973 The β-lactamases of Gram-negative bacteria and their possible physiological role. In: Rose A H, Tempest D W (eds) Advances in microbial physiology. Academic Press, London, vol 9, p 31–88

Modes of action

D. Greenwood

Introduction

At the basis of all antimicrobial chemotherapy lies the concept of selective toxicity. The necessary selectivity can be achieved in several ways: vulnerable targets within the microbe may be absent from the cells of the host or, alternatively, the analogous targets within the host cells may be sufficiently different, or at least sufficiently inaccessible, for selective attack to be possible. With agents like the polymyxins, the organic arsenicals used in trypanosomiasis, the antifungal polyenes and many antiviral compounds, the gap between toxicity to the microbe and to the host is small, but in most cases antimicrobial agents are able to exploit fundamental differences in structure and function within the microbial cell, and host toxicity generally results from unexpected secondary effects.

Antibacterial agents

The minute size and capacity for very rapid multiplication of bacteria ensures that they are structurally and metabolically very different from mammalian cells and, in theory, there are numerous ways in which bacteria can be selectively killed or disabled. In the event, it turns out that only the bacterial cell wall is structurally unique; other subcellular structures, including the cytoplasmic membrane, ribosomes and DNA, are built on the same pattern as those of mammalian cells, although, fortunately, sufficient differences in construction and organization do exist at these sites to make exploitation of the selective toxicity principle feasible.

Antibacterial agents have been discovered – rarely designed – that attack each of these vulnerable sites; the most successful compounds seem to be those that interfere

with the construction of the bacterial cell wall, the synthesis of protein, or the replication and transcription of DNA. Relatively few clinically useful agents act at the level of the cell membrane or by interfering with specific metabolic processes of the bacterial cell (Table 2.1).

Unless the target is located on the outside of the bacterial cell, antimicrobial agents must be able to penetrate to the site of action. Access through the cytoplasmic membrane is usually achieved by simple diffusion or (as, for example, with aminoglycosides and tetracyclines) by active transport. In the case of Gram-negative organisms the antibiotic must also negotiate an outer membrane, consisting of a

Table 2.1 Sites of action of antibacterial agents

Site	Agent	Principal target
Cell wall	Penicillins	Transpeptidase
	Cephalosporins	Transpeptidase
	Bacitracin	Isoprenylphosphate
	Glycopeptides	Acyl-D-alanyl-D-alanine
	Cycloserine	Alanine racemase/synthetase
	Fosfomycin	Pyruvyl transferase
Ribosome	Chloramphenicol	Peptidyl transferase
	Macrolides	Translocation
	Lincosamides	?Peptidyl transferase
	Fusidic acid	Elongation factor G
	Tetracyclines	Ribosomal A site
	Aminoglycosides	Initiation complex/translation
Nucleic acid	Quinolones	DNA gyrase (α subunit)
	Novobiocin	DNA gyrase (β subunit)
	Rifampicin	RNA polymerase
	5-Nitroimidazoles	DNA strands
	Nitrofurans	DNA strands
Cell membrane	Polymyxins	Phospholipids
	Ionophores	Ion transport
Folate synthesis	Sulphonamides	Pteroate synthetase
	Diaminopyrimidines	Dihydrofolate reductase

characteristic lipopolysaccharide–lipoprotein complex, which is responsible for preventing many antibiotics from reaching an otherwise sensitive intracellular target. This lipophilic outer membrane contains aqueous transmembrane channels (porins) which selectively allow passage of hydrophilic molecules depending on their molecular size and ionic charge. Many antibacterial agents use porins to gain access to Gram-negative organisms, although other pathways are also used (Hancock & Bellido 1992).

INHIBITORS OF BACTERIAL CELL WALL SYNTHESIS

Penicillins, cephalosporins and other β-lactam agents, as well as fosfomycin, cycloserine, bacitracin and the glycopeptides vancomycin and teicoplanin, selectively inhibit different stages in the construction of the peptidoglycan (syn.: murein; mucopeptide) that forms the rigid, shape-

maintaining layer of all medically-important bacteria except mycoplasmas. The peptidoglycan layer of all bacterial cells is basically similar, although important differences exist between Gram-positive and Gram-negative organisms (Fig. 2.1). In both types of organism the basic macromolecular chain consists of *N*-acetylglucosamine alternating with its lactyl ether, *N*-acetylmuramic acid. Each muramic acid unit carries a pentapeptide, the third amino acid of which is L-lysine in most Gram-positive cocci and *meso*-diaminopimelic acid in Gram-negative bacilli. The cell wall is given its rigidity by cross-links between this amino acid and the penultimate amino acid (which is always D-alanine) of adjacent chains, with loss of the terminal amino acid (also D-alanine) (Fig. 2.1). Gram-negative bacilli have a very thin peptidoglycan layer which is loosely cross-linked; Gram-positive cocci, in contrast, possess a very thick peptidoglycan coat which is tightly cross-linked through interpeptide bridges. The walls of Gram-positive bacteria also differ in containing considerable amounts of polymeric

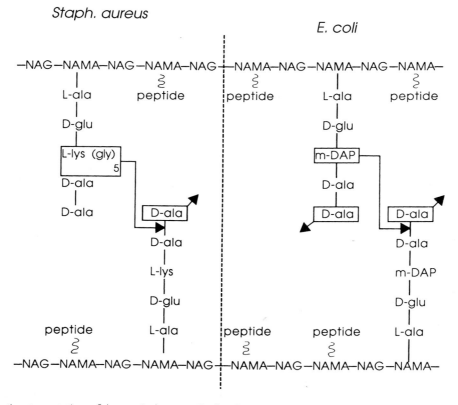

Fig. 2.1 *Schematic representations of the terminal stages of cell wall synthesis in Gram-positive (*Staphylococcus aureus*) and Gram-negative (*Escherichia coli*) bacteria. See text for explanation. Arrows indicate formation of cross-links, with loss of terminal D-alanine; in Gram-negative bacilli many D-alanine residues are not involved in cross-linking and are removed by D-alanine carboxypeptidase. NAG, N-acetylglucosamine; NAMA, N-acetylmuramic acid; ala, alanine; glu, glutamic acid; lys, lysine; gly, glycine; m-DAP, meso-diaminopimelic acid.*

sugar alcohol phosphates (teichoic and teichuronic acids), while Gram-negative bacteria possess an external membrane-like envelope as described above.

The process by which the peptidoglycan is assembled is summarized in Fig. 2.2. The basic building block consists of an *N*-acetylglucosamine-*N*-acetylmuramylpentapeptide with an additional bridging chain in Gram-positive cocci (Fig. 2.1). *N*-Acetylmuramic acid is derived from *N*-acetyl-glucosamine by the addition of a lactic acid substituent derived from phosphoenolpyruvate; this reaction is blocked by fosfomycin, which inactivates the pyruvyl transferase enzyme involved. The first three amino acids of the pentapeptide chain of muramic acid are added sequentially, but the terminal D-alanyl-D-alanine is added as a unit. To form this unit the natural form of the amino acid, L-alanine,

must first be racemized to D-alanine and two molecules are then joined together by D-alanine synthetase. Both of these reactions are blocked by the antibiotic cycloserine, which is a structural analogue of D-alanine.

Once the muramylpentapeptide is formed in the cell cytoplasm, an *N*-acetylglucosamine unit is added, together with any amino acids needed for the interpeptide bridge of Gram-positive organisms. It is then passed to a lipid carrier molecule which transfers the whole unit across the cell membrane to be added to the growing end of the peptidoglycan macromolecule. Addition of the new building block is prevented by vancomycin, which binds to the acyl-D-alanyl-D-alanine tail of the muramylpentapeptide. The related glycopeptide, teicoplanin, almost certainly acts in the same way (Parenti 1986). Because these glycopeptides

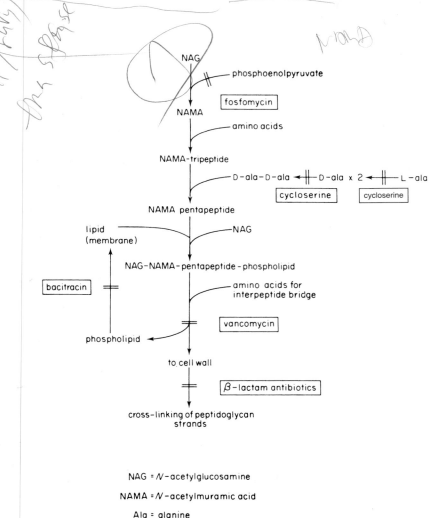

Fig. 2.2 *Simplified scheme of bacterial cell wall synthesis, showing the sites of action of cell wall active antibiotics. (Reproduced with permission from Greenwood D 1995 Antimicrobial chemotherapy, 3rd edn. Oxford University Press, Oxford.)*

are large polar molecules they are unable to penetrate the outer membrane of Gram-negative organisms, and this explains their restricted spectrum of activity.

The lipid carrier involved in transporting the cell wall building block across the membrane has been characterized as a C_{55} isoprenyl phosphate. The lipid acquires an additional phosphate group in the transport process and must be dephosphorylated in order to regenerate the native compound for another round of transfer. The cyclic peptide antibiotic bacitracin binds to the isoprenylpyrophosphate and prevents this dephosphorylation. Unfortunately, analogous reactions in eukaryotic cells are also inhibited by bacitracin, and this may be the basis of the toxicity of the compound.

Mode of action of β-lactam antibiotics

The final cross-linking reaction that gives the bacterial cell wall its characteristic rigidity was pinpointed many years ago as the primary target of penicillin and other β-lactam agents. These compounds were postulated to inhibit formation of the transpeptide bond by virtue of their structural resemblance to the terminal D-alanyl-D-alanine that participates in the transpeptidation reaction. This knowledge had to be reconciled with the various concentration-dependent morphological responses that Gram-negative bacilli were known to undergo on exposure to penicillin and other β-lactam compounds: filamentation (caused by inhibition of division rather than growth of the bacteria) at low concentrations, and the formation of osmotically-fragile spheroplasts (peptidoglycan-deficient forms that have lost their bacillary shape) at high concentrations.

At first it was possible to postulate that these concentration-dependent effects were due to partial and complete inhibition of transpeptidase by low and high concentrations of antibiotic. However, the validity of this view was thrown into doubt when it was realized that the oral cephalosporin, cephalexin, caused the filamentation response over an extremely wide range of concentrations, and the amidinopenicillin, mecillinam, elicited a completely novel series of morphological events. This suggested that two effects of β-lactam antibiotics could be dissociated, and this was given added weight when it was further shown that the combined effect of cephalexin and mecillinam was to evoke the 'typical' spheroplast response in *Escherichia coli* that neither agent could induce when acting alone. It was subsequently shown that isolated membranes of bacteria contain a number of proteins which are able to bind penicillin and other β-lactam antibiotics. These penicillin-binding proteins (PBPs) are numbered in descending order of their molecular weight according to their separation by polyacrylamide gel electrophoresis. The number found in bacterial cells varies from species to species: *Esch. coli* has

at least seven and *Staphylococcus aureus* four. Cephalexin (and some other β-lactam agents, including cephradine, temocillin and the monobactam, aztreonam, that predominantly induce filamentation in Gram-negative bacilli) binds to PBP3; similarly, mecillinam binds exclusively to PBP2. Most β-lactam antibiotics, when present in sufficient concentration, bind to both these sites and to others (PBP1a and PBP1b) which participate in the rapidly lytic response of Gram-negative bacilli to many penicillins and cephalosporins. The carbapenem, imipenem, binds preferentially to PBP2, but also binds to PBP1. However, the related compound, meropenem, also appears to bind strongly to PBP3 (Kitzis et al 1989).

The low molecular weight PBPs (4, 5 and 6) of *Esch. coli* are carboxypeptidases which may operate to control the extent of cross-linking in the cell wall. Mutants lacking these enzymes have been shown to grow normally and they have thus been ruled out as targets for the inhibitory or lethal actions of β-lactam antibiotics. The PBPs with higher molecular weights (PBPs 1a, 1b, 2 and 3) possess transpeptidase activity, and it seems that these PBPs represent different forms of the transpeptidase enzyme necessary to arrange the complicated architecture of the cylindrical or spherical bacterial cell during growth, septation and division.

The nature of the lethal event

In Gram-negative bacilli, the bactericidal effect of β-lactam antibiotics can be quantitatively prevented by providing sufficient osmotic protection. In these circumstances the bacteria survive as spheroplasts which readily revert to the bacillary shape on removal of the antibiotic. It thus seems clear that cell death in Gram-negative bacilli is a direct consequence of osmotic lysis of cells deprived of the protective peptidoglycan coat.

The nature of the lethal event in Gram-positive cocci appears to be different. Since these bacteria possess a much thicker, tougher peptidoglycan layer than that present in the Gram-negative cell wall, much greater damage has to be inflicted before death of the cell ensues. However, one of the first events that occurs on exposure of Gram-positive cocci to β-lactam antibiotics is a release of lipoteichoic acid, an event which appears to trigger a suicide response of autolytic dismantling of the peptidoglycan.

Non-lethal effects of β-lactam antibiotics

Although β-lactam antibiotics are conventionally classified as bactericidal agents, various factors can mitigate the bactericidal effect. One consequence of the osmotic basis of lethality in Gram-negative bacilli is that those bacteria, notably *Proteus* and *Haemophilus influenzae*, that exhibit a naturally low intracellular osmolality, are much less susceptible to osmotic lysis than, for example, *Esch. coli*. Some species, such as *Pseudomonas aeruginosa*, respond to therapeutically achievable levels of active β-lactam agents by the formation of filaments rather than spheroplasts and are killed only slowly. Imipenem and meropenem are atypical in this respect in that they induce the formation of spheroplasts in *Ps. aeruginosa* and rapidly kill the organisms. β-Lactam antibiotics such as cephalexin and mecillinam (and low concentrations of most other β-lactam agents) that do not induce spheroplast formation are only slowly bactericidal to susceptible Gram-negative rods.

Eagle effect

For many, but not all, strains of Gram-positive cocci, an optimal bactericidal concentration of β-lactam antibiotics can be identified above which the killing effect is reduced, sometimes very strikingly. The basis of this optimal dosage effect, known after its discoverer as the 'Eagle phenomenon', has never been satisfactorily explained. A plausible hypothesis is that the lethal event is triggered by low concentrations of the antibiotic as a consequence of binding to one particular target protein; binding at higher concentrations to other targets (PBPs) stops the bacterial cell from growing and this antagonizes the lethal effect, which requires continued cell growth.

Persisters

A culture of bacteria exposed to β-lactam antibiotics is not completely killed; even on prolonged exposure to an optimal bactericidal concentration about 1 in 10^5 bacteria usually survive. These 'persisters' have not acquired resistance, since most of their immediate progeny are killed on re-exposure to antibiotic, just as the parent culture is. How persisters arise is not known, but clearly they are bacteria caught in a particular metabolic state which prevents the β-lactam drug from achieving its lethal effect. In this sense, spheroplasts of Gram-negative bacilli represent one form of persister, but the term is usually reserved for bacteria (both Gram-positive and Gram-negative) that survive in a morphologically normal form. Persisters may be cells in which the peptidoglycan coat exists transiently as a complete covalently-linked macromolecule. In order to grow, a cell in this state has to use autolytic enzymes to create holes in the peptidoglycan where new cell wall building blocks can be added. If β-lactam antibiotics inhibit such enzymes, then these cells would be trapped in a state in which they could not grow (and therefore could not be killed) until the antibiotic is removed.

Tolerance

In some Gram-positive cocci there may be a marked dissociation between the concentrations of β-lactam agents (and vancomycin) required to achieve a bacteristatic and a

bactericidal effect. The organisms are not 'resistant' since they remain fully susceptible to the inhibitory activity of the antibiotic, although the bactericidal effect is reduced. Defective autolysins remain the most likely explanation of the effect which has some similarities to the persister phenomenon (Handwerger & Tomasz 1985).

INHIBITORS OF BACTERIAL PROTEIN SYNTHESIS

The amazing process by which the genetic message in DNA is translated into large and unique protein molecules is one of the wonders of the subcellular world. The fundamental process is universal and in prokaryotic, as in eukaryotic cells, the workbench is the ribosome, composed of two distinct subunits, each a complex of ribosomal RNA (rRNA) and numerous proteins. However, bacterial ribosomes are open to selective attack since they differ from their mammalian counterparts in both protein and RNA content; indeed they can be readily distinguished in the ultracentrifuge: bacterial ribosomes exhibit a sedimentation coefficient of 70S (composed of 30S and 50S subunits), whereas mammalian ribosomes display a coefficient of 80S (composed of 40S and 60S subunits).

In the first stage of bacterial protein synthesis, messenger RNA (mRNA), transcribed from the appropriate region of DNA, binds to the smaller ribosomal subunit and attracts *N*-formylmethionyl transfer RNA (fMet-tRNA) to the initiator codon AUG. The larger subunit is then added to form a complete initiation complex. The site occupied by the fMet-tRNA is called the P (peptidyl donor) site; adjacent to it is the A (aminoacyl acceptor) site aligned with the next trinucleotide codon of the mRNA. Transfer RNA (tRNA) bearing the appropriate anticodon, and its specific amino acid, enters the A site, and an enzyme known as peptidyl transferase joins *N*-formylmethionine to the new amino acid with loss of the tRNA in the P site; the first peptide bond of the protein has been formed. The next step is a translocation event which moves the remaining tRNA with its dipeptide to the P site and concomitantly aligns the next triplet codon of mRNA with the now vacant A site. The appropriate aminoacyl-tRNA enters the A site and the transfer process and subsequent translocation are repeated. In this way, the peptide chain is built up in precise fashion, faithful to the original DNA blueprint, until a so-called 'nonsense' codon is encountered on the mRNA that signals chain termination and release of the peptide chain. The mRNA is disengaged from the ribosome, which dissociates into its two subunits ready to form a new initiation complex. Within the bacterial cells, many ribosomes are engaged in protein synthesis during active growth, and a single strand of mRNA may interact with many ribosomes along its length to form a polysome.

Many antibiotics interfere with the process of protein synthesis. Some, like puromycin, which is an analogue of the aminoacyl tail of charged tRNA and causes premature chain termination, act on bacterial and mammalian ribosomes alike and are therefore unsuitable for systemic use in man. Therapeutically useful inhibitors of protein synthesis include chloramphenicol, tetracyclines, fusidic acid, macrolides, lincosamides and aminoglycosides.

Chloramphenicol

The molecular target for chloramphenicol has been identified as the peptidyl transferase enzyme that links amino acids in the growing peptide chain. The effect of the antibiotic is thus to freeze the process of chain elongation, and bacterial growth is brought to an abrupt halt. The process is completely reversible, and chloramphenicol is fundamentally a bacteristatic agent. The binding of chloramphenicol to the 50S subunit of 70S ribosomes is highly specific. The basis for the rare, but fatal, marrow aplasia associated with this compound is not therefore a generalized effect on mammalian protein synthesis, although mitochondrial ribosomes, which are similar to those of bacteria, may be involved.

Tetracyclines

Antibiotics of the tetracycline group are actively transported into bacterial cells and attach to 30S ribosomal subunits in such a manner as to prevent binding of aminoacyl-tRNA. Because the P site is always occupied by peptidyl-tRNA or deacylated tRNA, it is the A site, awaiting the incoming aminoacyl-tRNA, that is primarily affected by tetracyclines (Chopra et al 1992). Interference with the binding of tRNA effectively halts chain elongation and, like chloramphenicol, these antibiotics are predominantly bacteristatic.

Tetracyclines also penetrate into mammalian cells (indeed the effect on chlamydia depends on this) and can interfere with protein synthesis on eukaryotic ribosomes. Fortunately, cytoplasmic ribosomes are not affected at the concentrations achieved during therapy, although mitochondrial ribosomes are. The selective toxicity of tetracyclines thus presents something of a puzzle, the solution to which is presumably that these antibiotics are not actively concentrated by mitochondria as they are by bacteria and concentrations reached are insufficient to deplete respiratory chain enzymes (Chopra et al 1992).

Fusidic acid

Fusidic acid is unusual among inhibitors of protein synthesis in that it does not bind directly to the ribosome. The compound forms a stable complex with an elongation factor (EF-G) involved in translocation and with guanosine triphosphate (GTP), which provides energy for the translocation process. One round of translocation occurs,

with hydrolysis of GTP, but the fusidic acid–EF–G–GDP–ribosome complex blocks further chain elongation, leaving peptidyl-tRNA in the P site.

Although protein synthesis in Gram-negative bacilli and, indeed, mammalian cells is susceptible to fusidic acid, the antibiotic penetrates poorly into these cells and the spectrum of action is virtually restricted to Gram-positive bacteria, notably staphylococci; in this organism inhibition of protein synthesis leads to cell death, apparently by a secondary effect on the cell wall.

Macrolides, lincosamides, streptogramins

These antibiotic groups are structurally very different, but bind to closely related sites on the 50S ribosome of bacteria. One consequence of this is that staphylococci exhibiting inducible resistance to erythromycin, which is caused by methylation of certain adenine residues in the rRNA, also become resistant to other macrolides, lincosamides and streptogramin B in the presence of erythromycin (p. 383).

The detailed mode of action of these antibiotics has not yet been definitively worked out, but all the compounds affect the early stages of protein synthesis; ribosomes, bearing short peptides, remain unaffected until the message has been read completely and free ribosomes generated. Thus erythromycin (and the aminocyclitol antibiotic, spectinomycin) binds almost exclusively to free ribosomes and brings protein synthesis to a halt after formation of the initiation complex, probably by interfering with the first translocation reaction (Tai & Davis 1985). The precise mechanism of action of lincosamides is even less clear, but they appear to interfere indirectly with the peptidyl transferase reaction, possibly by blocking the P site.

The streptogramins, which are composed of two interacting components (p. 416), probably occupy adjacent sites on the ribosome and may achieve their bactericidal effect by causing an irreversible constriction of the channel through which newly formed polypeptides are released (Aumercier et al 1992).

Aminoglycosides

Most of the large volume of literature on the mode of action of aminoglycosides is devoted to the investigation of streptomycin. Other members of this antibiotic family are assumed to act in a similar manner, but the effect is clearly not identical, since gentamicin and other deoxystreptamine containing aminoglycosides bind at more than one site on the ribosome, whereas streptomycin binds in a 1 : 1 ratio at a unique site. This may explain the fact that single-step resistance to high concentrations of streptomycin, which has been characterized as a change in a specific protein of the 30S ribosomal subunit, does not extend to other aminoglycosides.

Elucidation of the mode of action of streptomycin has been complicated by the need to reconcile a variety of enigmatic observations. Thus, it has been known for many years that low concentrations of streptomycin and other aminoglycosides can cause misreading of mRNA on the ribosome while, paradoxically, halting protein synthesis completely by interfering with the formation of functional initiation complexes. Moreover, inhibition of protein synthesis by aminoglycosides leads not just to bacteriostasis, as with, for example, tetracycline or chloramphenicol, but to rapid cell death. Several other phenomena must be embraced by any comprehensive theory of aminoglycoside action: the fact that susceptible bacteria (but not those with resistant ribosomes) quickly become leaky to small molecules on exposure to the drug, apparently because of an effect on the cell membrane; the occurrence of mutations that render the bacterial cell dependent on streptomycin for growth; and the observation that susceptibility is dominant over resistance in merozygotes that are diploid for the two allelic forms.

A well-lit path through this maze has not yet been definitively charted, but the situation is slowly becoming clearer. It now appears that streptomycin and other aminoglycosides exert a differential effect depending on whether the ribosome is engaged in the formation of the initiation complex, or in the process of chain elongation (Tai & Davis 1985). This suggests a plausible explanation for the two effects of aminoglycosides on initiation and misreading: in the presence of a sufficiently high concentration of drug, protein synthesis is completely halted once the mRNA is run off, since reinitiation is blocked; under these circumstances there is little or no opportunity for misreading to occur. However, at concentrations at which only a proportion of the ribosomes can be blocked at initiation, some protein synthesis will take place and the opportunity for misreading will be provided. These differential effects appear to be a consequence of binding to a single ribosomal site, perhaps because the less drastic effect of misreading arises by virtue of imperfect binding of the aminoglycoside in the crowded microenvironment of a ribosome actively engaged in protein synthesis.

The dominance of susceptibility over resistance has been tentatively explained by the fact that the non-functional initiation complexes formed in the presence of aminoglycosides are unstable, so that the ribosomes continuously dissociate from mRNA and recycle in an inoperative form. These crippled ribosomes (of which there are twice as many as there are resistant ones in merozygotes) are hence continuously made reavailable to sequester newly-formed mRNA and prevent the resistant ribosomes from maintaining a supply of the polypeptides that the cell needs (Tai & Davis 1985).

The effects of aminoglycosides on membrane permeability, and the potent bactericidal activity of these compounds remain enigmatic. However, recent speculation has returned to earlier theories that the two phenomena are related (Davis 1988). In bacteria, as in mammalian cells, some of the ribosomes (presumably those engaged in transmembrane protein transfer) may be membrane bound; moreover, aminoglycosides are taken up by bacteria via an active transport process that is dependent on protein synthesis. The possibility therefore exists that site specific uptake of the drug at ribosomal attachment sites and subsequent binding to the ribosome–membrane complex, may, in some way, lead to membrane leakiness and cell death (Davis 1987).

INHIBITORS OF NUCLEIC ACID SYNTHESIS

Many compounds are known which intercalate between base pairs of the double helix, or otherwise interact with DNA, and a number of these have, in fact, found a use in cancer chemotherapy. However, since the structure of DNA is universal, compounds that bind directly to the double helix are generally highly toxic to mammalian cells and only a few compounds that interfere with DNA-associated enzymic processes exhibit sufficient selectivity for use as antibacterial agents. These compounds include antibacterial quinolones, novobiocin and rifampicin. Diaminopyrimidines, sulphonamides, 5-nitroimidazoles and (probably) nitrofurans also act indirectly on DNA synthesis and will be considered under this heading.

Quinolones

The DNA of the circular chromosome of bacteria is more than 1 mm long, and solving the problem of packaging this enormous macromolecule into a microscopic cell, while making adequate arrangements for transcription and replication, has necessitated some considerable ingenuity on the part of the microbe (Smith 1985). The solution has been to condense the DNA down and to twist it into a 'supercoiled' state – a process which is aided by the natural strain imposed on a covalently-closed double helix. The twists are introduced in the opposite sense to those of the double helix itself and the molecule is said to be negatively supercoiled. The process involves precisely regulated nicking and resealing of the DNA strands, and the enzyme that accomplishes this remarkable feat is called DNA gyrase. The enzyme is a tetramer composed of two pairs of α and β subunits. It is clear that it is the α subunit of DNA gyrase that is the primary target of the action of nalidixic acid and other quinolones (Hooper & Wolfson 1988), although much remains to be learned about the precise interaction and its consequences (Hooper 1993). Curiously, novobiocin, which displays an exactly opposite spectrum of activity to that of nalidixic acid, acts in a complementary fashion by binding specifically to the β subunit of DNA gyrase.

Inhibition of DNA gyrase by quinolones rapidly causes death of the bacterial cell but, paradoxically, the bactericidal effect is reduced as the drug concentration is raised. This effect has been attributed to inhibition of RNA synthesis at high concentration of drug.

Rifampicin

Rifampicin and other compounds of the ansamycin group specifically inhibit DNA-dependent RNA polymerase; that is, they prevent the transcription of RNA species from the DNA template. Rifampicin is an extremely efficient inhibitor of the bacterial enzyme, but fortunately eukaryotic RNA polymerase is not affected. RNA polymerase consists of a core enzyme made up of four polypeptide subunits. Experiments in which subunits from resistant and sensitive bacteria were dissociated and reconstituted have identified the α subunit as the one to which rifampicin specifically binds. However, isolated α subunit does not bind rifampicin, so presumably the precise configuration in which it is locked in the core enzyme is important.

Sulphonamides and diaminopyrimidines

These agents act at separate stages in the pathway of folic acid synthesis and thus act indirectly on DNA synthesis, since the active form of the co-enzyme, tetrahydrofolic acid, serves as intermediate in the transfer of methyl, formyl and other single carbon fragments, in the biosynthesis of purine nucleotides and thymidylic acid, as well as of some amino acids.

Sulphonamides are analogues of p-aminobenzoic acid and inhibit the condensation of this compound with dihydropteroic acid in the early stages of folic acid synthesis. Most bacteria need to synthesize folic acid and cannot utilize exogenous sources of the vitamin. Mammalian cells, in contrast, require preformed folate and this is the basis of the selective action of sulphonamides. The antileprotic sulphone, dapsone, and the antituberculous drug, p-aminosalicylic acid, act in a similar way.

Diaminopyrimidines act later in the pathway of folate synthesis. These compounds, which include the antiprotozoal agent pyrimethamine, the antipneumocystis agent trimetrexate, the anticancer drug methotrexate, and the antibacterial compounds trimethoprim and tetroxoprim, inhibit dihydrofolate reductase, the enzyme which reduces dihydrofolate to the active tetrahydrofolate form. In most of the reactions in which tetrahydrofolate takes part, the co-enzyme remains unchanged. However, in the biosynthesis of thymidylic acid, tetrahydrofolate acts as hydrogen donor as well as a methyl group carrier and is thus oxidized to dihydrofolic acid in the process. Dihydrofolate reductase is therefore a rather crucial enzyme in recycling tetrahydrofolate, and diaminopyrimidines act relatively quickly to halt bacterial growth. Sulphonamides, in contrast, cut off the supply of folic acid at source and act slowly, since the existing folate pool can satisfy the needs of the cell for several generations.

The selective toxicity of diaminopyrimidines comes about because of differential affinity of these compounds for dihydrofolate reductase from various sources. Thus trimethoprim has a vastly greater affinity for the bacterial enzyme than for its mammalian counterpart; pyrimethamine, exhibits a particularly high affinity for the plasmodial version of the enzyme; and, in keeping with its anticancer activity, methotrexate has high affinity for the enzyme found in mammalian cells.

5-Nitroimidazoles

The most intensively investigated compound in this group is metronidazole, but other 5-nitroimidazoles are thought to act in a similar manner. The spectrum of activity of metronidazole is restricted to anaerobic and certain microaerophilic bacteria, and to some protozoa such as *Trichomonas vaginalis*, *Giardia lamblia* and *Entamoeba histolytica*. The common link between these organisms is that they all exhibit anaerobic metabolism, and it is now known that it is a form of the drug in which the nitro group is reduced that actually achieves the antimicrobial effect. This reduced form (which is unstable and has thus not been isolated) is generated intracellularly only at the very low redox values achieved by anaerobic organisms. The lethal event has not been definitively characterized, but the target of the reduced drug appears to be DNA, which undergoes strand breakage in the presence of metronidazole (Edwards 1993). The basis for activity against microaerophilic species such as *Helicobacter pylori* and *Gardnerella vaginalis* remains speculative.

Nitrofurans

As with nitroimidazoles, the reduction of the nitro group of nitrofurantoin and other nitrofurans is a pre-requisite for antibacterial activity. Bacteria with appropriate nitro-reductases act on nitrofurans to produce a highly reactive electrophilic intermediate and this is postulated to affect DNA as the reduced intermediates of nitroimidazoles do. Other evidence suggests that the reduced nitrofurans bind to bacterial ribosomes and prevent protein synthesis (McOsker & Fitzpatrick 1994); inducible enzyme synthesis seems to be particularly susceptible. An effect on DNA has the virtue of explaining the known mutagenicity of these compounds in vitro and any revised mechanism relating to inhibition of protein synthesis needs to be reconciled with this property.

AGENTS AFFECTING MEMBRANE PERMEABILITY

Two of the earliest antibiotics, gramicidin and tyrocidine (the components of the tyrothricin complex discovered in 1939 by Dubos) (p. 4), act on the bacterial cell membrane. Unfortunately, antibacterial agents acting at this site do not discriminate between bacterial and mammalian membranes, although the fungal cell membrane has proved more amenable (see below).

The only membrane active antibacterial agents to be administered systemically in human medicine are polymyxin B and the closely related compound colistin (polymyxin E). The polymyxins appear to act like cationic detergents; they disrupt the cytoplasmic membrane of the cell, probably by attacking the exposed phosphate groups of the membrane phospholipid. They also have an effect on the external membrane of Gram-negative bacilli, which might explain their preferential action on these organisms. The end result is leakage of cytoplasmic contents and death of the cell. Various factors, including growth phase and incubation temperature, alter the balance of fatty acids within the bacterial cell membrane, and this can concomitantly affect the response to polymyxins (Gilleland et al 1984).

Gramicidin A (which, unlike gramicidin S, is a linear polypeptide) and macrotetralides such as monensin, which has been widely used in veterinary medicine, interfere with membrane permeability by folding themselves into an open helical structure, stabilized by hydrogen bonds, which forms a hydrophobic complex with the cell membrane. The helical configuration provides a transmembrane channel through which potassium and certain other cations can selectively pass. Compounds that act in this manner are called ionophores. Depsipeptides such as valinomycin also act as ionophores, but the mechanism is slightly different: rather than forming membrane channels, the depsipeptides selectively transport ions through the lipid core of the cell membrane by trapping them in a protective hydrophobic envelope which shuttles across the membrane.

Naturally-occurring antimicrobial peptides, such as the cecropins, magainins and defensins, as well as the lanthionine-containing antibiotics, disrupt cell membranes, sometimes in a selective manner; some of these peptides appear to form aggregates with ionophoric properties (Boman et al 1994).

Antifungal agents

In view of the scarcity of antibacterial agents acting on the cytoplasmic membrane, it is perhaps surprising to find that the most successful groups of antifungal agents – the polyenes, azoles, and allylamines – all achieve their effects in this way (Elewski 1993).

Polyenes

These compounds bind only to membranes containing sterols, and ergosterol, the predominant sterol of fungal membranes, appears to be particularly susceptible. The effect of the binding of polyenes is to make the membrane leaky by a mechanism that might be analogous to that of the antibacterial ionophores. Since bacterial cell membranes (except those of mycoplasmas) do not contain sterols, they are unaffected by polyenes, even in high concentration; unfortunately, this immunity does not extend to sterol-containing mammalian cells, and polyenes consequently exhibit a low therapeutic index.

Azoles

The selective activity of the antifungal azoles is also dependent on the presence of ergosterol in the fungal cell membrane. These compounds block the synthesis of ergosterol, probably by interfering with the demethylation of lanosterol, a precursor of ergosterol and cholesterol (Borgers 1985). However, cholesterol synthesis seems to be considerably less sensitive to inhibition.

Antifungal azole derivatives are predominantly fungistatic, but some compounds, notably miconazole and clotrimazole, kill fungi at concentrations higher than those which merely inhibit growth, apparently by causing direct membrane damage. Other, less well characterized effects of azoles on fungal respiration have also been described (Fromtling 1988).

Allylamines

The antifungal allylamine derivatives, terbinafine and naftifine, inhibit squalene epoxidase, an enzyme involved in the biosynthesis of ergosterol (Stütz 1990). The fungicidal effect may be due to accumulation of squalene rather than a deficiency of ergosterol. In *Candida albicans* the effect is fungistatic and the yeast form is less susceptible than is mycelial growth. In this species there is less accumulation of squalene than in dermatophytes, and ergosterol deficiency may be the limiting factor (Ryder 1989).

Flucytosine

The spectrum of activity of flucytosine (5-fluorocytosine) is virtually restricted to yeasts. In these fungi flucytosine is transported into the cell by a cytosine permease; a cytosine deaminase then converts flucytosine to 5-fluorouracil, which is incorporated into RNA in place of uracil, leading to the formation of abnormal proteins. There is also an effect on DNA synthesis through inhibition of thymidylate synthetase (Odds 1988).

Griseofulvin

The antidermatophyte antibiotic griseofulvin probably interferes in some way with the microtubules of the mitotic spindle, but the mechanism of action and the basis of its selective toxicity remain to be elucidated.

Antiprotozoal agents

Protozoa, like fungi, are eukaryotic cells and it might be expected that it would be difficult to find agents selectively active against them. In terms of the restricted number of antiprotozoal agents available, this expectation has certainly been fulfilled, but it is curious that two of the most successful of ancient herbal remedies, cinchona bark (quinine) and ipecacuanha (emetine), should be directed against protozoa; the Chinese antimalarial, qinghaosu (artemisinin), in which much recent interest has been shown, could be added to the list.

In some cases, the actions of antiprotozoal drugs overlap with, or are analogous to, those seen with the antibacterial and antifungal agents already discussed. Thus, the activity of 5-nitroimidazoles, such as metronidazole, extends to those protozoa which exhibit an essentially anaerobic metabolism; the antimalarial agents pyrimethamine and proguanil, like trimethoprim, inhibit dihydrofolate reductase (see above); some polyenes and antifungal imidazoles display sufficient activity against *Leishmania* and certain other protozoa for them to have received attention as potential therapeutic agents.

Antimalarial agents

Quinine and the various quinoline antimalarials that have been developed subsequently were once thought to achieve their effect by intercalation with plasmodial DNA after concentration in parasitized erythrocytes. However, these effects occur only at concentrations in excess of those achieved in vivo; moreover, a non-specific effect on DNA does not explain the selective action of these compounds at precise points in the plasmodial life cycle, or the differential activity of antimalarial quinolines.

Clarification of the precise mode of action of these compounds proved elusive, although an effect on the formation of malarial pigment was suspected, since forms of malaria parasite that did not make pigment were resistant to antimalarial quinolines (Foote & Cowman 1994). Malarial pigment consists of granules of polymerized haem (ferriprotoporphyrin IX) which is produced from the red cell haemoglobin in the food vacuole of the parasites.

Ferriprotoporphyrin IX is a toxic metabolite that must be rendered innocuous by polymerization if the parasite is to survive. It now seems likely that quinine, chloroquine and related compounds act primarily by inhibiting haem polymerase (Slater & Cerami 1992), thus preventing detoxification of the metabolite.

8-Aminoquinolines, like primaquine, which exhibit selective activity against liver-stage parasites at therapeutically useful concentrations, act in a different way, possibly by inhibiting mitochondrial enzyme systems after undergoing hepatic metabolism. However, the precise mechanism of action is unknown.

Artemisinin, the active principle of the Chinese herbal remedy qinghaosu, has several effects on malaria parasites, but the activity of the compound appears to be due chiefly to the reactivity of the endoperoxide bridge which is cleaved in the presence of haem or free iron within the parasitized red cell to form a short-lived, but highly reactive, free radical. This intermediate irreversibly alkylates malarial proteins (Meshnick 1994; Meshnick et al 1996).

The hydroxynaphthoquinone, atovaquone, which exhibits antimalarial and antipneumocystis activity, is an electron transport inhibitor which causes depletion of the ATP pool. The primary effect is on the iron flavoprotein dihydro-orotate dehydrogenase, an essential enzyme in the production of pyrimidines. Mammalian cells are able to avoid undue toxicity by use of preformed pyrimidines (Artymowicz & James 1993). Dihydro-orotate dehydrogenase from *Plasmodium falciparum* is inhibited by concentrations of atovaquone that are very much lower than those needed to inhibit the pneumocystis enzyme, raising the possibility that the antimicrobial consequences might differ in the two organisms (Ittarat et al 1995).

Antitrypanosomal and antileishmanial agents

Arsenical and antimonial compounds, which are still the mainstay of treatment of trypanosomal and leishmanial infections, poison the cell by an effect on glucose catabolism, thus cutting off the energy supply. In protozoa of the trypanosome family, the primary sites of glycolysis are specialized glycosomes, and this may aid the selective toxicity of arsenicals and antimonials, which nevertheless remain quite toxic to the host (Peters 1985).

Eflornithine (difluoromethylornithine) is a selective inhibitor of ornithine decarboxylase and achieves its effect by depleting the biosynthesis of polyamines, such as putrescine and spermidine (McCann et al 1986). The corresponding mammalian enzyme has a much shorter half-life than its trypanosomal counterpart, and this may account for the apparent selectivity of action. The reason for the preferential activity against *Trypanosoma brucei gambiense*, rather than the related *rhodesiense* form has not been elucidated.

Anthelminthic agents

Just as the cell wall of bacteria is a prime target for selective agents and the cell membrane is peculiarly vulnerable in fungi, so the neuromuscular system appears to be the Achilles' heel of parasitic worms. Despite the fact that present understanding of the neurobiology of helminths is extremely meagre, a considerable number of anthelminthic agents have been shown to work by paralysing the neuromusculature in various ways. Such compounds include piperazine, praziquantel, levamisole, pyrantel pamoate, ivermectin, metriphonate and dichlorovos (Fisher & Mrozik 1992, Geary et al 1992, Rosenblatt 1992). Praziquantel induces schistosomes to disengage from their intravascular attachment site and migrate to the liver, but there is also a profound effect on schistosome metabolism and disruption of the tegument, causing exposure of parasite antigens. All these effects appear to be referable to alterations in calcium homeostasis (Day et al 1992).

A notable exception to the general rule that anthelminthic agents act on the neuromuscular systems of worms is provided by the benzimidazole derivatives, including mebendazole and albendazole. These broad-spectrum anthelminthic drugs seem to have at least two effects on adult worms and larvae: inhibition of the uptake of the chief energy source, glucose; and binding to tubulin, the structural protein of microtubules. There is some evidence that the related compound thiabendazole may inhibit fumarate reductase in mitochondria.

Antiviral agents

The prospects for the development of selectively toxic antiviral agents were long thought to be poor, since the life cycle of the virus is so closely bound to normal cellular processes. However, closer scrutiny of the relationship of the virus to the cell reveals several points at which the viral cycle might be interrupted (Crumpacker 1989). These include: adsorption to and penetration of the cell; uncoating of the viral nucleic acid; the various stages of nucleic acid replication; assembly of the new viral particles; and, if the cell is not destroyed, export of the virions.

Nucleoside analogues

In the event, it is the process of viral replication (which is extremely rapid relative to most mammalian cells) that has proved to be the most vulnerable point of attack, and most clinically useful antiviral agents are nucleoside analogues. Among these, only acyclovir (acycloguanosine) and penciclovir (the active product of the oral agent famciclovir)

exhibit a genuine selectivity. In order to achieve their antiviral effect, nucleoside analogues have to be converted within the cell to the triphosphate derivative. In the case of acyclovir and penciclovir the initial phosphorylation, yielding acyclovir or penciclovir monophosphate, is accomplished by a thymidine kinase coded for by the virus itself. The corresponding cellular thymidine kinase phosphorylates these compounds very inefficiently and consequently only cells harbouring the virus are affected. Moreover, the triphosphates of acyclovir and penciclovir inhibit viral DNA polymerase more efficiently than the cellular enzyme and this is another feature of their selective activity. As well as inhibiting viral DNA polymerase, acyclovir and penciclovir triphosphates are incorporated into the growing DNA chain and cause premature termination of DNA synthesis.

Other nucleoside analogues, including the anti-human immunodeficiency virus (HIV) agents zidovudine, didanosine and zalcitabine, and the anti-cytomegalovirus agent ganciclovir, act in a non-specific manner because they are phosphorylated by cellular enzymes. The anti-HIV compounds are thought to act primarily to inhibit reverse transcriptase activity by causing premature chain termination during the transcription of DNA from the single-stranded RNA template. Similarly, ganciclovir acts as a chain terminator and DNA polymerase inhibitor during the transcription of cytomegalovirus DNA. Since these compounds lack a hydroxyl group on the deoxyribose ring, they are unable to form phosphodiester linkages in the DNA chain (Lipsky 1993). Tribavirin, in contrast, allows DNA synthesis to occur, but prevents the formation of viral proteins, probably by interfering with capping of viral mRNA (Hall 1987). In vitro, tribavirin antagonizes the action of zidovudine, probably by feedback inhibition of thymidine kinase so that the zidovudine is not phosphorylated (Vogt et al 1987).

An alternative tactic to disable HIV is to inhibit the enzyme that cleaves the polypeptide precursor of several essential viral proteins (Debouck 1992). Such protease inhibitors include saquinavir and ritonavir which are now in therapeutic use.

Phosphonic acid derivatives

The simple phosphonoformate salt foscarnet and its close analogue phosphonoacetic acid inhibit DNA polymerase activity of herpes viruses by preventing pyrophosphate exchange (Crumpacker 1992). The action is selective in that the corresponding mammalian polymerase is much less susceptible to inhibition. Activity of foscarnet against HIV seems to be due to a different mechanism. Like the nucleoside analogues, it inhibits reverse transcriptase activity of retroviruses, but it binds to the enzyme at a site distinct from that of the nucleoside triphosphates. The effect is non-competitive and reversible.

Amantadine

The anti-influenza A compound amantadine (and its close relative rimantadine) appears to act at the stage of viral uptake by preventing membrane fusion; these compounds also interfere with virus disassembly. Both effects may be due to specific interaction of the drugs with a membrane-associated protein of the virus (Hay et al 1985; Skehel 1992).

Further information

Detailed information on the mode of action of anti-infective agents can be found in the following sources:

Campbell W C, Few R S (eds) 1986 Chemotherapy of parasitic disease. Plenum, New York

Franklin T J, Snow G A 1989 Biochemistry of antimicrobial action, 4th edn. Chapman & Hall, London

Gale E F, Cundliffe E, Reynolds P E, Richmond M H, Waring M J 1981 The molecular basis of antibiotic action, 2nd edn. Wiley, Chichester

Greenwood D, O'Grady F (eds) 1985 The scientific basis of antimicrobial chemotherapy. Cambridge University Press, Cambridge

James D H, Gilles H M 1985 Human antiparasitic drugs: Pharmacology and usage. Wiley, Chichester

Pratt W B, Fekety R 1986 The antimicrobial drugs. Oxford University Press, Oxford

Russell A D, Chopra I 1996 Understanding antibacterial action and resistance, 2nd edn. Ellis Horwood, London

References

Artymowicz R J, James V E 1993 Atovaquone: a new antipneumocystis agent. Clinical Pharmacy 12: 563–569

Aumercier M, Bouhallab S, Capmau M-L, Le Goffic F 1992 RP 59500: a proposed mechanism for its bactericidal activity. Journal of Antimicrobial Chemotherapy 30 (suppl A): 9–14

Boman H G, Marsh J, Góode J A (eds) 1994 Antimicrobial peptides. Ciba Foundation Symposium 186. Wiley, Chichester

Borgers M 1985 Antifungal azole derivatives. In: Greenwood D, O'Grady F (eds) The scientific basis of antimicrobial chemotherapy. Cambridge University Press, Cambridge, p 133–153

Chopra I, Hawkey P M, Hinton M 1992 Tetracyclines, molecular and clinical aspects. Journal of Antimicrobial Chemotherapy 29: 245–277

Crumpacker C S 1989 Molecular targets of antiviral therapy. New England Journal of Medicine 321: 163–172

Crumpacker C S 1992 Mechanism of action of foscarnet against viral polymerases. American Journal of Medicine 92 (suppl 2A): 2A-35–2A-75

Davis B D 1987 Mechanism of bactericidal action of aminoglycosides. Microbiological Reviews 51: 341–350

Davis B D 1988 The lethal action of aminoglycosides. Journal of Antimicrobial Chemotherapy 22: 1–3

Day T A, Bennett J L, Pax R A 1992 Praziquantel: the enigmatic antiparasitic. Parasitology Today 8: 342–344

Debouck C 1992 The HIV-1 protease as a therapeutic target for AIDS. AIDS Research and Human Retroviruses 8: 153–164

Edwards D I 1993 Nitroimidazole drugs – action and resistance mechanisms. I. Mechanisms of action. Journal of Antimicrobial Chemotherapy 31: 9–20

Elewski B E 1993 Mechanisms of action of systemic antifungal agents. Journal of the American Academy of Dermatology 28: S28–S34

Fisher M H, Mrozik H 1992 The chemistry and pharmacology of avermectins. Annual Review of Pharmacology and Toxicology 32: 537–553

Foote S J, Cowman A F 1994 The mode of action and the mechanism of resistance to antimalarial drugs. Acta Tropica 56: 157–171

Fromtling R A 1988 Overview of medically important antifungal azole derivatives. Clinical Microbiology Reviews 1: 187–217

Geary T G, Klein R D, Vanover L, Bowman J W, Thompson D P 1992 The nervous systems of helminths as targets for drugs. Journal of Parasitology 78: 215–230

Gilleland H E, Champlin F R, Conrad R S 1984 Chemical alterations in cell envelopes of Pseudomonas aeruginosa upon exposure to polymyxin: a possible mechanism to explain adaptive resistance to polymyxin. Canadian Journal of Microbiology 20: 869–873

Hall C B 1987 Ribavirin. In: Peterson P K, Verhoef J (eds) The antimicrobial agents annual – 2. Elsevier, Amsterdam, p 351–362

Hancock R E W, Bellido F 1992 Antibiotic uptake: unusual results for unusual molecules. Journal of Antimicrobial Chemotherapy 29: 235–239

Handwerger S, Tomasz A 1985 Antibiotic tolerance among clinical isolates of bacteria. Reviews of Infectious Diseases 7: 368–386

Hay A J, Wolstenholme A J, Skehel J J, Smith M H 1985 The molecular basis of the specific anti-influenza action of amantadine. EMBO Journal 4: 3021–3024

Hooper D C 1993 Quinolone mode of action – new aspects. *Drugs* 45 (suppl 3): 8–14

Hooper D C, Wolfson J S 1988 Mode of action of the quinolone antimicrobial agents. *Reviews of Infectious Diseases* 10 (suppl 1): S14–S21

Ittarat I, Asawamahasakada W, Bartlett M S, Smith J W, Meshnick S R 1995 Effects of atovaquone and other inhibitors on *Pneumocystis carinii* dihydroorotate dehydrogenase. *Antimicrobial Agents and Chemotherapy* 39: 325–328

Kitzis M D, Acar J F, Gutmann L 1989 Antibacterial activity of meropenem against Gram-negative bacteria with a permeability defect and against staphylococci. *Journal of Antimicrobial Chemotherapy* 24 (suppl A): 125–132

Lipsky J J 1993 Zalcitabine and didanosine. *Lancet* 341: 30–32

McCann P P, Bacchi C J, Clarkson A B et al 1986 Inhibition of polyamine biosynthesis by α-difluoromethylornithine in African trypanosomes and *Pneumocystis carinii* as a basis for chemotherapy: biochemical and clinical aspects. *American Journal of Tropical Medicine and Hygiene* 35: 1153–1156

McOsker C C, Fitzpatrick P M 1994 Nitrofurantoin: mechanism of action and implications for resistance development in common uropathogens. *Journal of Antimicrobial Chemotherapy* 33 (suppl A): 23–30

Meshnick S R 1994 The mode of action of antimalarial endoperoxides. *Transactions of the Royal Society of Tropical Medicine and Hygiene* 88 (suppl 1): 31–32

Meshnick S R, Taylor T E, Kamchonwongpaison S 1996 Artemisinin and the antimalarial endoperoxides: from herbal remedy to targeted chemotherapy. *Microbiological Reviews* 60: 301–315

Odds F C 1988 *Candida* and candidosis. Baillière Tindall, London, p 305–306

Parenti F 1986 Structure and mechanism of action of teicoplanin. *Journal of Hospital Infection* 7 (suppl A): 79–83

Peters W 1985 Antiprotozoal agents. In: Greenwood D, O'Grady F (eds) The scientific basis of antimicrobial chemotherapy. Cambridge University Press, Cambridge, p 95–132

Rosenblatt J E 1992 Antiparasitic agents. *Mayo Clinic Proceedings* 67: 276–287

Ryder N S 1989 The mode of action of terbinafine. *Clinical and Experimental Dermatology* 14: 98–100

Skehel J J 1992 Amantadine blocks the channel. *Nature* 358: 110–111

Slater A F G, Cerami A 1992 Inhibition by chloroquine of a novel haem polymerase enzyme activity in malaria trophozoites. *Nature* 355: 167–169

Smith J T 1985 The 4-quinolone antibacterials. In: Greenwood D, O'Grady F (eds) The scientific basis of antimicrobial chemotherapy. Cambridge University Press, Cambridge, p 69–94

Stütz A 1990 Allylamine derivatives – inhibitors of fungal squalene epoxidase. In: Borowski E, Shugar D (eds) Molecular aspects of chemotherapy. Pergamon, New York, p 205–213

Tai P C, Davis B D 1985 The actions of antibiotics on the ribosome. In: Greenwood D, O'Grady F (eds) The scientific basis of antimicrobial chemotherapy. Cambridge University Press, Cambridge, p 41–68

Vogt M W, Hartshorn K L, Furman P A et al 1987 Ribavirin antagonizes the effect of azidothymidine on HIV replication. *Science* 235: 1376–1379

3

Resistance

G. L. French and I. Phillips

Definition of resistance

MICROBIOLOGICAL RESISTANCE

Fleming described the phenomenon of resistance very clearly, if qualitatively, in initial tests of the antibacterial activity of penicillin: streptococci and staphylococci were sensitive, while Gram-negative bacilli such as *Escherichia coli*, were resistant. This is an example of *inherent* or *intrinsic resistance*, which defines the spectrum of an antibiotic. The spectrum may be narrow for agents such as benzylpenicillin or vancomycin (active against most Gram-positive organisms), colistin (active against most Gram-negatives), or metronidazole (active only against anaerobes); or broad, for a wide variety of agents such as tetracycline or chloramphenicol, which are active against most species of bacteria.

When quantitative measurements of antimicrobial susceptibility are made (e.g. by determining minimum inhibitory concentrations (MICs) of an antibiotic), some species are clearly less sensitive than others (Fig. 3.1). Furthermore, there is a range of susceptibilities within a species, and some isolates of either sensitive or resistant

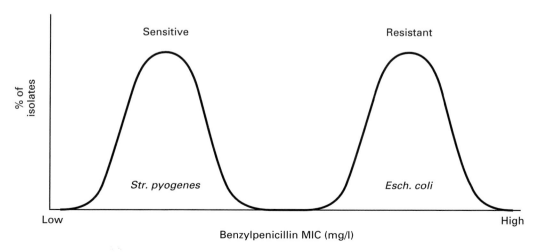

Fig. 3.1 *Example of distribution of the MIC of benzylpenicillin for isolates of a sensitive organism (*Streptococcus pyogenes*) and a resistant organism (*Escherichia coli*)*

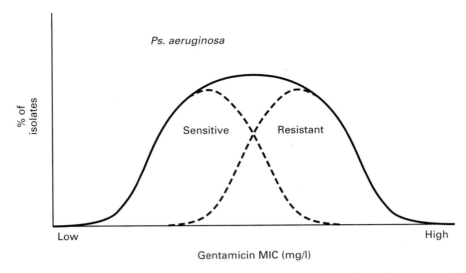

Fig. 3.2 *Distribution of the MIC of gentamicin for sensitive and resistant strains of* Pseudomonas aeruginosa.

species may prove to be more sensitive than normal: such strains are more familiar in the experimental than the diagnostic laboratory and are usually referred to as 'hypersensitive'.

Some strains of species that are normally inherently sensitive to an antibiotic may later *acquire* resistance to the drug. This phenomenon commonly arises when populations of bacteria have grown in the presence of the antibiotic. In some cases it is easily observable in vitro. For example, a culture of a strain of *Staphylococcus aureus* will contain individual organisms that are resistant to fusidic acid or rifampicin that grow out in the presence of appropriate concentrations of the antibiotic; the same phenomenon may occur in individual patients treated with these agents for staphylococcal infection. On the other hand, it may occur among clinical bacterial isolates on a demographic scale when the antibiotics are used extensively to treat large numbers of patients: this occurs to a greater or lesser degree with virtually all antibiotics in clinical use.

The range of 'sensitive' and 'resistant' isolates of a given species may overlap (Fig. 3.2). In such cases most sensitive isolates can be distinguished from most resistant ones, but for the range of overlap it will be necessary to demonstrate that some isolates have a resistance mechanism (see below) not present in others. A rational definition of a microbiologically resistant isolate or species is thus one that possesses one or more identifiable resistance mechanisms, the major problem being the greater difficulty of detecting the mechanism rather than its effect in vitro.

CLINICAL RESISTANCE

Clinical resistance is more complex than microbiological resistance, since it relates to the probability of a response to antimicrobial therapy. Clinically, a sensitive isolate is one that is likely to respond to therapy with the agent tested and a resistant isolate is one that will not. Between the two are isolates of intermediate or indeterminate susceptibility, over which range a positive clinical response is increasingly unlikely (Fig. 3.3). In practice, the dividing lines imposed by breakpoints may not be so clear, since populations may again coalesce.

Unfortunately, definitions that relate clinical response and microbiological susceptibility are less useful than might be expected because of the many confounding factors that may be present in patients. These range from relative inaccessibility of the infection to the antibiotic, the results of surgical intervention and the many varieties of altered immunity, to ignorance of the true infective agent and straightforward sampling or testing error. In infections in which there is a clear relationship between clinical success and in vitro susceptibility, such as gonorrhoea and to a lesser extent meningitis, typhoid fever and even urinary tract infection, clinical trial would distinguish sensitive from resistant strains, if it were not generally unethical to conduct such trials. In practice, much of the evidence on efficacy is gained from patients treated empirically, from whom organisms are subsequently tested for antimicrobial susceptibility. Until recently even this evidence has not been

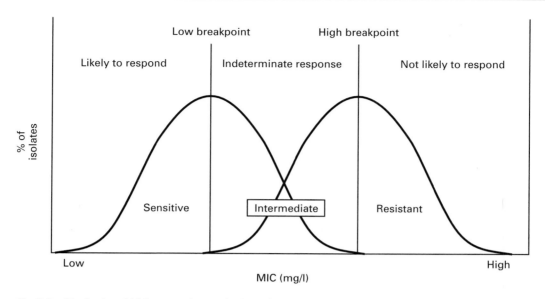

Fig. 3.3 *Distribution of MICs among bacterial isolates that are sensitive, intermediate or resistant to an antibiotic.*

required for antibiotic registration by regulatory agencies, and has been difficult to obtain outside pharmaceutical companies.

From an early stage in the development of antibacterial agents it became clear that a knowledge of antibiotic pharmacokinetics could be used to bolster the inadequate information gained from clinical use. It is assumed that if an antibiotic reaches a concentration at the site of infection higher than the MIC for the infecting agent, the infection is likely to respond – at least to the extent possible in the presence of the other confounding factors discussed above. Clearly, the antibiotic must be free to act at the site, and not, for example, bound to protein and thus neutralized. Assays of antibiotics in sites of infection are complex both theoretically and practically (see p. 137); serum assays are much more straightforward, and have been widely used as a proxy, even though it is realized that there may again be confounding factors arising from differences in distribution. For most antibiotics, this proxy has reasonable validity, but for some agents such as quinolones (Ch. 32) and newer macrolides such as azithromycin (Ch. 27), serum concentrations are considerably lower than those at the presumed site of infection.

Different national groups have used different pharmacokinetic parameters in their correlations with pharmacodynamic characteristics. For example, the relevant serum concentration has variously been taken as the 'peak' concentration (itself theoretical rather than actual), the concentration midway between dosage, or various summations of concentrations under the concentration–time curve. The method evolved by a working party of the British Society for Antimicrobial Chemotherapy (Report 1991) may be used as an example. In this formula the breakpoint concentration – that is the inhibitory concentration that separates sensitive from resistant strains – is defined as:

$$\text{Breakpoint} = \frac{C_{max}f}{te} \times s$$

where C_{max} is the theoretical peak serum concentration following a standard dose (obtained from pharmacological literature); e is a factor by which C_{max} should exceed the breakpoint MIC (usually taken to be 4, an arbitrary figure derived from work on endocarditis); t is a half-life factor (2.0 for half-lives of <1 h, 1.0 for 1–3 h and 0.5 for > 3 h); f is a serum binding factor (1.0 for < 70%, 0.5 for 70–90% and 0.2 for >90%); and s is the shift needed for optimum laboratory reproducibility, or to allow for organisms that have MICs in the sensitive range but which have recognized resistance mechanisms.

The formula has been criticized as applying mathematics to uncertainty, but it produces breakpoint concentrations that are close to those conventionally used in most parts of Europe. Furthermore, the formula can be easily adapted – for example to take account of the high local concentrations achieved by many quinolones. It is also possible to evolve low and high breakpoints to define strains of intermediate susceptibility.

The Working Party of the European Society of Clinical Microbiology and Infectious Diseases has taken a similar approach (Phillips 1991) but has not used a strict formula in determining tentative breakpoints for a small number of new agents. The approach of the National Committee for Clinical Laboratory Standards (NCCLS) in the USA has been based on wide consultation, and includes strong input from the antibiotic manufacturers. Their discussions usually lead to higher breakpoints, particularly for β-lactam antibiotics, than those used in Europe.

To many who work in this field, a consensus on breakpoints seems desirable, since it is clearly confusing for a given strain to be labelled sensitive (or susceptible) in the USA and in countries in which the Kirby–Bauer technique (p. 138) is used (including several in southern Europe) and resistant in others including much of northern Europe. Such discrepancies make it necessary to assess the literature on resistance with great attention to detail, and especially to compare results for control strains.

Mechanisms of resistance

For an antimicrobial agent to be effective against a given microorganism, three conditions must normally be met: a vital target susceptible to a low concentration of the antibiotic must exist in the microorganism; the antibiotic must penetrate the bacterial surface and reach the target in sufficient quantity; and the antibiotic must not be inactivated or extruded before binding to the target.

There are thus four main mechanisms by which bacteria may circumvent the actions of antimicrobial agents:

- Specific enzymes may inactivate or modify the drug before or after it enters the bacterial cell;
- The bacterial cell envelope may be modified so that it becomes less permeable to the antibiotic;
- The drug may be actively expelled from the cell; or
- The target may be modified so that it binds less avidly with the antibiotic.

However, these resistance mechanisms do not exist in isolation, and two or more distinct mechanisms may interact to determine the actual level of resistance of a microorganism to an antibiotic.

RESISTANCE RESULTING FROM THE PRODUCTION OF DRUG-MODIFYING ENZYMES

β-Lactamases

The most important mechanism of resistance to β-lactam antibiotics is the production of specific enzymes (β-lactamases). These enzymes bind to β-lactam antibiotics usually via active serine sites, and the cyclic amide bonds of the β-lactam rings are hydrolysed by the serine hydroxyl group. The open ring forms of β-lactams cannot bind to their target sites and thus have no antimicrobial activity (Fig. 3.4). The ester linkage of the residual β-lactamase acylenzyme complex is usually readily hydrolysed by water, regenerating the active enzyme. Among Gram-positive cocci, the only β-lactamase of major clinical significance is staphylococcal β-lactamase, which rapidly hydrolyses benzylpenicillin, ampicillin, carbenicillin and related compounds, but is much less active against the anti-staphylococcal penicillins and most cephalosporins. Among Gram-negative bacilli the situation is more complex, and isoelectric focusing has shown that these organisms produce many different β-lactamases with different spectra of activity. Many anaerobic bacteria also produce β-lactamases, and this is the major mechanism of β-lactam antibiotic resistance in this group.

The classification and properties of β-lactamases are described more fully in Chapter 16.

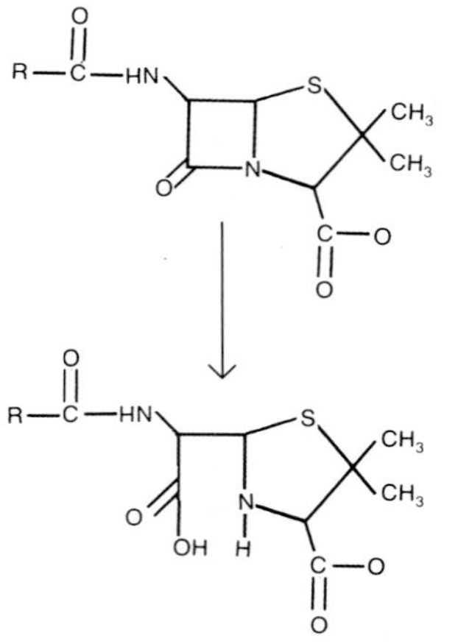

Fig. 3.4 *Hydrolysis of penicillin by β-lactamase, which yields the corresponding penicilloic acid.*

Aminoglycoside-modifying enzymes

Much of the resistance to aminoglycoside antibiotics observed in clinical isolates of Gram-negative bacilli and Gram-positive cocci is due to transferable plasmid-mediated enzymes that modify the amino groups or hydroxyl groups of the aminoglycoside molecule (see Ch. 13). The modified antibiotic molecules are unable to bind to the target protein in the ribosome. The genes encoding these enzymes are often transposable and in some cases have now transferred to the chromosome. These enzymes include many different types of acetyltransferases, phosphotransferases and nucleotidyl transferases which vary greatly in their spectrum of activity and in the degree to which they inactivate different aminoglycosides (p. 166). The newer amino-glycosides have been designed so that their three-dimensional structures prevent them from binding with many of these modifying enzymes, and organisms resistant to one of the aminoglycosides by an enzymatic mechanism may thus remain susceptible to another. However, in recent years there has been a tendency for multiply drug-resistant pathogens to acquire multiple modifying enzymes, rendering them resistant to all or most of the available amino-glycosides.

Chloramphenicol acetyltransferase

The major mechanism of acquired resistance to chloramphenicol in both Gram-positive and Gram-negative species is the production of a chloramphenicol acetyltrans-ferase which converts the drug to either the monoacetate or diacetate (Shaw 1984). These derivatives are unable to bind to the bacterial 50S ribosomal subunit and thus cannot perform the function of normal chloramphenicol which is to inhibit peptidyl transferase activity. There are several different types of chloramphenicol acetyltransferases produced by different bacterial species, and the enzymes are usually inducible. The gene is usually encoded on a plasmid, but may transpose to the chromosome. Surprisingly, in view of the very limited use of chloram-phenicol, resistance is not uncommon, even in *Esch. coli*, although it is most frequently seen in organisms that are also multiply resistant to other agents.

Location of drug-inactivating enzymes

In Gram-positive bacteria, β-lactam antibiotics enter the cell easily because of the permeable cell wall, and β-lactamase is released freely from the cell. In *Staph. aureus*, resistance to benzylpenicillin is usually caused by the release of β-lactamase into the extracellular environment where it reduces the concentration of drug in the vicinity of the organism. Under optimal conditions, one molecule of this potent enzyme can destroy 100 000 molecules of benzylpenicillin per minute. Resistance of *Staph. aureus* to benzylpenicillin is thus a population phenomenon: a large inoculum of organisms is much more resistant than a small one. Furthermore, staphylococcal penicillinase is an inducible enzyme: up to 300 times more penicillinase is produced in the presence of penicillin than in its absence.

In Gram-negative bacteria the outer membrane retards entry of penicillins and cephalosporins into the cell. The β-lactamase needs only to inactivate molecules of drug that penetrate the cell wall, since drug remaining in the extracellular environment is harmless to the cell. In these organisms the β-lactamase is retained within the periplasmic space between the cytoplasmic membrane and the cell wall. Each cell is thus responsible for its own protection – a more efficient mechanism than the external excretion of β-lactamase seen in Gram-positive bacteria. Enzymes are often produced constitutively (i.e. even when the antibiotic is not present) and a small inoculum of bacteria may be almost as resistant as a large one.

A similar functional organization is exhibited by the aminoglycoside-modifying enzymes. These enzymes are located at the surface of the cytoplasmic membrane and only those molecules of aminoglycoside that are in the process of being transported across the membrane are modified.

RESISTANCE RESULTING FROM ALTERATIONS TO THE PERMEABILITY OF THE BACTERIAL CELL ENVELOPE

The bacterial cell envelope consists of an outer slime layer, a cell wall and a cytoplasmic membrane. This structure allows the passage of bacterial nutrients and excreted products, while acting as a barrier to harmful substances such as antibiotics.

The slime layer (or capsule) is composed mainly of carbohydrate; it is often associated with virulence, but is highly variable and is probably not a major barrier to the passage of antibiotics.

The Gram-positive cell wall is relatively thick but simple in structure, being made up of a network of cross-linked peptidoglycan complexed with teichoic and teichuronic acids (Fig. 3.5). It is readily permeable to most antibiotics.

The cell wall of Gram-negative bacteria (Figs 3.6, 3.7) is generally thinner but more complex, comprising an outer membrane of lipopolysaccharide, protein and phospholipid, attached to a thin layer of peptidoglycan. The lipopolysac-charide molecules cover the surface of the cell, with their hydrophilic portions pointing outwards. Their inner lipophilic regions interact with the fatty acid chains of the phospholipid monolayer of the inner surface of the outer membrane and are stabilized by divalent cation bridges. The phospholipid and lipopolysaccharide of the outer membrane form a classic lipid bilayer which acts as a barrier to both

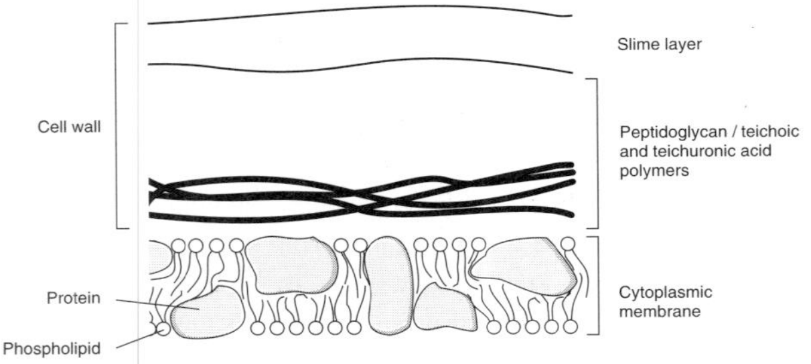

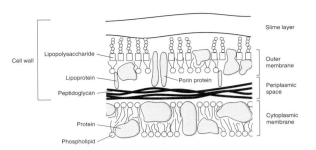

Fig. 3.5 *Diagrammatic representation of the Gram-positive cell envelope. (Reprinted with permission from Russel A D, Quesnel L B, eds, Antibiotics: assessment of antimicrobial activity and resistance. The Society for Applied Bacteriology Technical Series no. 18, London: Academic Press, p. 62.)*

Fig. 3.6 *Diagrammatic representation of the Gram-negative cell envelope. The periplasmic space contains the peptidoglycan and some enzymes. (Reprinted with permission from Russel A D, Quesnel L B, eds, Antibiotics: assessment of antimicrobial activity and resistance. The Society for Applied Bacteriology Technical Series no. 18, London: Academic Press, p. 62.)*

hydrophobic and hydrophilic drug molecules. Natural permeability varies among different Gram-negative species and generally correlates with innate resistance. For example, the cell walls of *Neisseria* species and *Haemophilus influenzae* are more permeable than that of *Esch. coli*, while the walls of *Pseudomonas aeruginosa* and indole-positive *Proteus* spp. are markedly less permeable. However, changes in the cell wall may result in changes in natural antimicrobial sensitivity.

Hydrophobic antibiotics can enter the Gram-negative cell by direct solubilization through the lipid layer of the outer membrane, but the closely packed lipopolysaccharide molecules which cover the membrane may physically block this pathway. Rough mutants, which are relatively deficient in lipopolysaccharide, are more permeable and thus more sensitive to many antibiotics. In contrast, other changes in surface lipopolysaccharides may increase permeability resistance. This mechanism is involved in some aminoglycoside resistance in *Ps. aeruginosa*, and in resistance to the relatively lipophilic tetracycline, minocycline, but few isolates have been investigated. Resistance to nalidixic acid may result from alterations in surface lipopolysaccharide, but this does not affect susceptibility to the more hydrophilic fluoroquinolones such as ciprofloxacin.

However, most antibiotics are hydrophilic and pass through the outer membrane of Gram-negative cells via water-filled channels created by membrane proteins called porins (Figs 3.6, 3.7) (Nikaido 1993). The ease with which an antibiotic passes through these channels depends on its size and physicochemical structure. Some antimicrobial resistance in Gram-negative bacteria is due to reduced drug entry caused by decreased amounts of specific porin proteins, especially OmpF (Nikaido 1989). This mechanism may affect several antibiotic classes of drug simultaneously, producing a broad spectrum of resistance to hydrophilic drugs such as chloramphenicol, trimethoprim, tetracycline and quinolones, as well as the β-lactam compounds. The resistance is usually low level because entry is impeded rather than completely prevented, and clinically significant resistance is usually seen only when other resistance mechanisms are also active. However, chloramphenicol and tetracycline can select mutants that show high-level resistance to a broad spectrum of hydrophilic drugs, mediated by a reduction in OmpF, increased efflux of chloramphenicol and tetracycline, and other, incompletely defined, mechanisms (Cohen et al 1988). This phenomenon of multiple antibiotic resistance (MAR) results from pleiotropic mutations in the *mar*RAB operon which is normally regulated and derepressed by chloramphenicol and tetracycline.

The target molecules of antibiotics that inhibit cell wall synthesis, such as the β-lactam antibiotics and the glycopeptides, are located outside the cytoplasmic membrane, and it is not necessary for these drugs to pass through this membrane to exert their effect. Most other antibiotics must cross the membrane to reach their sites of action. The cytoplasmic membrane is freely permeable to lipophilic agents such as minocycline, chloramphenicol, trimethoprim, fluoroquinolones and rifampicin, but poses a significant barrier to non-lipophilic agents such as most tetracyclines, aminoglycosides, erythromycin, clindamycin

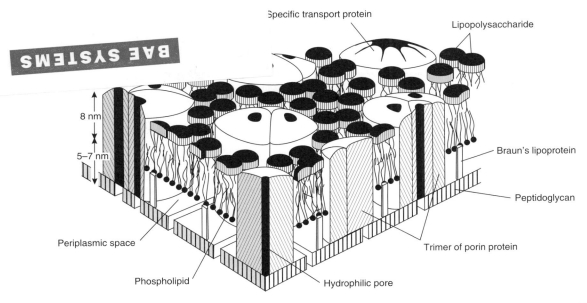

Fig. 3.7 *A tentative structure of the Gram-negative cell wall (adapted from Nikaido H, Nakae T 1979 Advances in Microbial Physiology 20: 163). The oligosaccharide chains extending from the lipopolysaccharide into the external environment are omitted for visual clarity.*

and the sulphonamides. These drugs are actively transported across the membrane by carrier proteins, and some resistances have been associated with various changes in the cytoplasmic membrane proteins, but these mechanisms have not been widely studied (Nikaido 1989).

Resistance due to drug efflux

Tetracycline resistance can be due to a number of mechanisms, and is associated with the production of a variety of inducible proteins (Chopra & Howe 1978). Although tetracycline resistance may result from reduced membrane permeability, failure of the drug to bind properly to 30S rRNA, or because of interference by inducible proteins, it is more commonly caused by active extrusion of the drug from the bacterial cell (Levy 1992). Rapid efflux of tetracycline from resistant bacteria is associated with the production of a family of inner membrane proteins called Tet, which may be constitutive or inducible (McMurray et al 1980). Minocycline is not usually extruded by these proteins. This form of tetracycline resistance is usually encoded on transferable plasmids, but may also be chromosomal. Increased extrusion of tetracycline, but by another mechanism, may result from mutations of the chromosomal *mar*RAB operon.

Although quinolone resistance is usually due to mutations in the target DNA gyrase molecule (see below), some low-level resistance in Gram-negative bacteria – often associated with *mar* mutations – can be caused by efflux mechanisms. A gene responsible for efflux-dependent quinolone resistance in *Staph. aureus* (*norA*) has been sequenced, and the gene product shows many similarities to the Tet proteins (Levy 1989). Some resistance to other antibiotics, and to a variety of disinfectants and heavy metals, are now known to be caused by increased efflux, and it is likely that this mechanism of resistance is more widespread than previously thought (Levy 1989).

RESISTANCE DUE TO ALTERATIONS IN TARGET MOLECULES

Alterations to penicillin-binding proteins (PBPs)

These are proteins associated with the bacterial cell envelope that bind penicillin and are the target sites for β-lactam antibiotics. Each bacterial cell has several PBPs, which vary with the species. PBPs appear to be enzymes such as transpeptidases, carboxypeptidases and endopeptidases, and are required for cell wall synthesis and alteration during growth. Some, but not all, PBPs are essential for cell survival. PBPs are related to β-lactamases, which also bind β-lactam antibiotics. However, unlike β-lactamases, PBPs form stable complexes with β-lactams and are themselves inactivated. β-Lactam antibiotics thus inactivate PBPs, preventing proper cell growth and division, and producing cell-wall defects that lead to death by osmolysis. Alterations in PBPs, leading to decreased binding affinity with β-lactam antibiotics, are important causes of β-lactam resistance in a number of species, most commonly Gram-positive bacteria.

Penicillin-resistant strains of *Streptococcus pneumoniae* produce one or more altered PBPs that have reduced ability to bind penicillin. Step-wise acquisition of multiple changes in the genes encoding these PBPs produce various levels of penicillin resistance (Markiewicz & Tomasz 1989). The genetic sequences encoding normal PBPs in sensitive strains of *Str. pneumoniae* are highly conserved; the genes in resistant strains are said to be 'mosaics' since they consist of blocks of conserved sequences interspersed with blocks of variant sequences. As more variant blocks are introduced into the mosaic, the more penicillin resistant the recipient strain tends to become. These gene sequences have probably been derived by transformation from oral streptococcal species such as *Streptococcus mitis*, although the donors may themselves be phenotypically penicillin-sensitive and do not produce low-affinity PBPs (Dowson et al 1993). Although many penicillin-resistant isolates are sensitive to newer β-lactams such as cefotaxime, some strains have appeared that are resistant to these drugs by the production of simultaneous changes in PBP1a and PBP2x (Muñoz et al 1992).

Methicillin resistance in *Staph. aureus* is caused by an acquired chromosomal gene (*mecA*) which results in the synthesis of a new methicillin-inducible penicillin-binding protein (PBP2a or PBP2'), with decreased affinity for methicillin and other β-lactam agents (Chambers & Hackbarth 1992). The same gene and mechanism is seen in methicillin-resistant strains of coagulase-negative staphylococci (Ubukata et al 1990). The *mecA* gene is located on a transposon that may have spread between the species.

Other species showing β-lactam resistance due to altered PBPs include β-lactamase-negative strains of penicillin-resistant *Neisseria gonorrhoeae*, penicillin-resistant *Neisseria meningitidis* and ampicillin-resistant *H. influenzae*. The genes encoding altered PBPs in both *Neisseria* species appear to be mosaics, and the variant genetic blocks may have been derived from *Neisseria flavescens*. The relative penicillin resistance of enterococci is due to the normal production of PBPs with low binding affinity. The acquisition of other PBPs is responsible for higher levels of penicillin and ampicillin resistance often seen in *Enterococcus faecium*.

Other altered targets

Aminoglycoside resistance

Aminoglycoside resistance may be produced by alterations in specific ribosomal binding proteins, although this is uncommon in clinical isolates. Clinically important examples of this mechanism include high-level resistance to streptomycin in *Mycobacterium tuberculosis* and high-level resistance to streptomycin or gentamicin in some strains of enterococci, in which the combination of penicillin plus streptomycin or gentamicin fails to produce the usual synergistic bactericidal effect.

Quinolone resistance

The main target for quinolones is the A subunit of bacterial DNA gyrase. Mutations of the gene *gyrA*, which encodes this subunit, produce broad-spectrum resistance to all members of the quinolone group. Alterations of the gyrase B subunit have been derived mainly in the laboratory: they produce low-level resistance and are uncommon in nature. Organisms that are highly sensitive to quinolones, such as the enterobacteria, do not show clinically significant resistance to the newer quinolones unless there are at least two mutations in the *gyrA* gene. In contrast, organisms that are naturally rather less sensitive, such as *Campylobacter jejuni*, *Ps. aeruginosa* and *Staph. aureus*, may develop significant resistance after only a single mutation. As a result, resistance to quinolones has emerged relatively quickly in these latter three organisms, while acquired resistance is still uncommon in other species.

MLS resistance

The most common type of acquired resistance to erythromycin and clindamycin (and other macrolides and lincosamides) is seen in streptococci, enterococci and staphylococci and is called macrolide–lincosamide–streptogramin (MLS) resistance. This is due to the production of enzymes that methylate specific adenine residues in 23S rRNA, resulting in reduced ribosomal binding of macrolides and lincosamides (Weisblum 1985). Low concentrations of erythromycin induce resistance to all the macrolides and lincosamides (so-called 'dissociated' resistance), but some strains may produce the methylase constitutively. The genes encoding the resistance are plasmid borne and associated with transposons. Increased use of macrolides may encourage further spread of MLS resistance in *Staph. aureus*, group A β-haemolytic streptococci and pneumococci.

Rifampicin resistance

Rifampicin resistance is commonly the result of a mutation which alters the β-subunit of RNA polymerase, reducing its binding affinity for rifampicin. Mutation usually produces high-level resistance in a single step, but intermediate resistance is sometimes seen. Mutational resistance occurs relatively frequently, and for this reason rifampicin is combined with other agents for the treatment of tuberculosis. Meningococcal carriers have usually been treated with rifampicin alone, and this has resulted in the emergence of rifampicin resistance in many strains of *N. meningitidis*.

Mupirocin resistance

Mupirocin (pseudomonic acid), is widely used for topical treatment of Gram-positive skin infections and the clearance of nasal carriers of methicillin-sensitive and methicillin-resistant *Staph. aureus*. It acts by inhibiting bacterial isoleucyl-tRNA synthetase, and resistance is mediated by the production of modified enzymes. Isolates showing low-level resistance have a single chromosomally-encoded modified synthetase, while those with high-level resistance also have a second enzyme encoded on a plasmid that can transfer to other strains (Cookson 1990, Gilbart et al 1993).

Sulphonamide and trimethoprim resistance

Acquired sulphonamide resistance is usually due to the production of an altered dihydropteroate synthetase that has reduced affinity for sulphonamides, but not for *p*-aminobenzoic acid. Resistance is encoded on transferable plasmids and associated with transposons. Trimethoprim resistance occurs much less commonly. It is usually due to plasmid-mediated synthesis of new dihydrofolate reductases, which are much less susceptible to trimethoprim than the natural ones. The resistance genes are again associated with transposons.

Fusidic acid resistance

Fusidic acid acts by inhibiting protein synthesis by interfering with ribosome translation (Tanaka et al 1968). Chromosomal mutation to fusidic acid resistance results from an alteration of the target molecule, elongation factor G, causing reduced affinity for fusidic acid. This occurs at high frequency in *Staph. aureus* in vitro, and therefore it is often recommended that fusidic acid should not be used alone to treat staphylococcal infections.

Glycopeptide resistance

Most clinically important Gram-positive bacteria are naturally sensitive to the glycopeptides vancomycin and teicoplanin, and until recently resistance has been extremely rare. However, at least three different resistance phenotypes are now recognized (Reynolds 1992, Arthur & Courvalin 1993):

1. VanA, high-level transferable resistance to both vancomycin and teicoplanin, associated with the production of a 38–40 kDa membrane protein; this is usually seen in *Ent. faecium*, sometimes in *Enterococcus faecalis* and rarely in *Enterococcus avium*.
2. VanB, inducible low-level resistance, usually to vancomycin alone, which in some strains is transferable, associated with a 39.5 kDa membrane protein; also seen in enterococci.

3. VanC, constitutive low-level vancomycin resistance, seen in some strains of *Enterococcus gallinarum*. *Enterococcus casseliflavus* appears to have intrinsic low-level resistance unrelated to the other phenotypes.

The VanA phenotype of high-level resistance to both vancomycin and teicoplanin is encoded on a transposon, usually located on transferable plasmids of about 30 MDa, but also transposing to the chromosome. VanA resistance has been seen so far only in clinical isolates of enterococci, most frequently in *Ent. faecium*. The *vanA* gene encodes an abnormal D-alanine:D-alanine ligase that results in the replacement of the normal D-alanine:D-alanine termini of peptidoglycan precursors by D-alanine:D-lactate, which cannot bind glycopeptides. *vanA* has been transferred in vitro to other Gram-positive bacteria, including *Staph. aureus* (Noble et al 1992), but it has not yet passed to other genera in vivo. Low-level resistance (the VanB and VanC phenotypes) usually involves only one of the glycopeptides, and is usually encoded on the chromosome. This type of resistance is probably also due to the production of an altered bacterial ligase.

Failure to metabolize the drug to the active form

Both metronidazole and nitrofurantoin must be converted to an active form within the bacterium before they can have effect. Resistance to them arises if the pathogen cannot effect this conversion. Aerobic organisms cannot reduce metronidazole to its active form and are therefore inherently resistant, but resistance in anaerobic organisms is very uncommon. The few resistant strains of *Bacteroides fragilis* that have been investigated have reduced levels of pyruvate dehydrogenase, the enzyme necessary for the reduction of metronidazole to the active intermediate. In *Helicobacter pylori*, metronidazole resistance may be due to the failure of resistant strains to achieve a sufficiently low internal redox potential during micro-aerophilic growth to reduce the drug to the active form (Cederbrant et al 1992).

Nitrofurantoin must be reduced to an active intermediate by NADH- or NADPH-linked reductases. One of these enzymes acts aerobically and another anaerobically. Although laboratory mutants can be obtained that lack the aerobic reductase, they remain susceptible to nitrofurans under anaerobic conditions. Naturally occurring resistance to nitrofurans is uncommon, since such strains must lose more than one reductase to become resistant.

Genetic basis of resistance

INHERENT RESISTANCE

Resistance of bacteria to antimicrobial agents may be

inherent or acquired. Inherent (or innate) resistance to some antibiotics is the natural resistance possessed by most strains of a bacterial species and is part of their genetic make-up, encoded on the chromosome. Inherent multiple resistance is characteristic of free-living organisms, which may have evolved because of exposure to natural antibiotics in the environment. These organisms have low virulence, but their multiple resistance allows them to produce opportunistic infections in hospital environments. An example of a free-living opportunistic pathogen with a high degree of inherent resistance is *Ps. aeruginosa*. From before the beginning of the antibiotic era, virtually all strains of this organism were already resistant to many antibiotics that subsequently became available.

Mutational resistance

Acquired resistance may be due either to mutations affecting genes on the bacterial chromosome or to acquisition of genes conferring resistance upon a previously sensitive micro-organism. Mutations usually involve deletion, substitution, or addition of one or a few base pairs, causing substitution of one or a few amino acids in a crucial (target) peptide. This usually results in a gene product with reduced or absent ability to bind the antibiotic. Examples are high-level resistance to streptomycin seen in *M. tuberculosis* and *Ent. faecalis*, caused by a mutation affecting the specific streptomycin-binding protein of the 30S subunit of the ribosome. Other clinically important examples of mutational resistance are: rifampicin resistance in *M. tuberculosis* caused by mutations in RNA polymerase; broad-spectrum aminoglycoside resistance in *Ps. aeruginosa* due to altered cell membrane permeability; and fluoroquinolone resistance in *Esch. coli* resulting from alterations in DNA gyrase.

TRANSFERABLE RESISTANCE

Plasmids

These are independently replicating molecules of DNA that can exist outside the bacterial chromosome. 'R-plasmids' carry one or more markers for drug resistance. This type of resistance is due to a dominant gene, usually one resulting in production of a drug-inactivating or drug-modifying enzyme.

Plasmids are transmissible by conjugation, transduction via bacteriophage, or transformation (uptake of naked DNA). The acquisition of resistance by transduction is rare in nature (the most important example in pathogenic bacteria is the transfer of penicillinase production by *Staph. aureus*). Transformation of resistance factors is relatively uncommon. Only a few bacterial species are readily transformable

during at least part of their life cycle and are said to be naturally competent. These organisms, which include *Bacillus subtilis, Str. pneumoniae, H. influenzae,* and *Staphylococcus, Helicobacter, Acinetobacter, Neisseria* and *Moraxella* spp., show extensive genetic variation resulting from natural transformation. They may also acquire chromosomally-encoded antimicrobial resistance. For example, some strains of methicillin-resistant *Staph. aureus,* and penicillin- or ampicillin-resistant *Str. pneumoniae, H. influenzae* and *N. gonorrhoeae,* may have acquired genes for the production of altered PBPs by transformation from related non-pathogenic species.

Conjugation is the most common method of resistance transfer in clinically important bacteria. Conjugative plasmids, which are capable of self-transmission to other bacterial hosts, are common in Gram-negative enteric bacilli and are relatively large (25–150 MDa); non-conjugative plasmids, common in Gram-positive cocci, *H. influenzae, N. gonorrhoeae* and *Bact. fragilis,* are usually small (1–10 MDa). Conjugative plasmids can sometimes separate into a plasmid carrying the resistance genes and one carrying the transfer genes (resistance transfer factor (RTF)). Non-conjugative plasmids can transfer to other bacteria if they are mobilized by other conjugative plasmids (or RTFs) present in the same cell, or by transduction or transformation. Large plasmids are usually present at one or two copies per cell, and their replication is closely linked to replication of the bacterial chromosome. Small plasmids may be present at more than 30 copies per cell, and their distribution to progeny during cell division is ensured by the large number present. Plasmids tend to have a restricted host range: for example, those from Gram-negative bacteria cannot generally transfer to or maintain themselves in Gram-positive organisms, and vice versa.

Transposons

These are discrete sequences of DNA, capable of translocation from one replicon (plasmid or chromosome) to another – hence the epithet 'jumping gene'. They may encode genes for resistance to a wide variety of antibiotics, as well as many other metabolic properties. They are circular segments of double-stranded DNA, 4–25 kb in length, and usually consist of a functional central region flanked by long terminal repeats, usually inverted repeats. Complex transposons also carry genes for the transposition enzymes transposase and resolvase and their repressors. They need not share extensive regions of homology with the replicon into which they insert, as is required in classical genetic recombination. Depending upon the transposon involved, they may transpose into a replicon randomly or into favoured sites, and they may insert at only a few or at many different places. Transposons are responsible for much of the diversity observed among plasmids, and play a major role in the evolution and dissemination of antibiotic resistance among bacteria, especially in the hospital environment.

The emergence of resistance

In the early 1940s, when sulphonamides and penicillin first came into widespread clinical usage, the common serious bacterial infections presenting in hospitals were due to the pneumococcus, the β-haemolytic streptococcus and penicillin-susceptible strains of *Staph. aureus*. Very few antibiotic-resistant strains of these organisms were encountered and few physicians anticipated that resistance to antimicrobial agents would become a serious medical problem.

However, the explosion in antibiotic usage world-wide was followed by the appearance of clinical infection with organisms resistant to the agents in common use (Finland et al 1959). Indeed, whenever new drugs have been introduced to combat resistant bacteria, this has been followed – sooner or later – by the appearance of yet more resistant infections. This is because antimicrobial therapy tends to select resistant bacteria that survive and spread in environments where antibiotic use is concentrated, whether in individual patients, hospitals or special areas such as farms. The organisms that survive are either inherently resistant species or strains of sensitive species that have acquired resistance to the drugs in use. The rapid emergence of acquired resistance in previously sensitive species is facilitated by transfer of genetic resistance determinants on plasmids. The origin of these transferable resistance factors is unclear, but they were present in organisms isolated before the antibiotic era, and in the normal flora of man and animals never exposed to antibiotics.

Increasing antibiotic usage is thus generally associated with increasing antibiotic resistance (McGowan 1983), a relationship often referred to as 'antibiotic pressure'. A decline in antibiotic usage is often followed by a fall in resistance rates; this may be because acquired resistance does not confer an advantage on a pathogen in the absence of antibiotic pressure and the maintenance of resistance mechanisms is costly in terms of energy. However, the relationship between use and resistance is complex and neither inevitable nor linear. For example, opportunistic hospital infection is often caused by inherently multiply resistant free-living organisms that may cause equipment-related infections even in the absence of antibiotic pressure. Furthermore, some centres see few resistant pathogens despite average antibiotic usage, and sometimes resistance rates decline for no apparent reason.

MULTIPLE DRUG RESISTANCE

Organisms that are resistant to several commonly used antibiotics are often referred to as multiply-drug resistant (MDR) pathogens. This term has not been properly defined, but implies that the degree of multiple resistance presents therapeutic problems. The magnitude of multiple drug resistance may be exaggerated: there is a publication bias that encourages reporting of resistant rather than sensitive strains (McGowan 1983); multiple resistance is more common (and more publicized) in hospitals than in the community, in tertiary referral centres than in district hospitals, and in intensive care units than in general wards; and some clusters of multiresistant organisms represent transient local outbreaks of single MDR strains rather than a general trend. Nevertheless, despite these caveats, MDR pathogens appear to be increasing in frequency throughout the world. A very few clinical isolates (some enterococci, mycobacteria and non-fermenting Gram-negative bacteria) are now resistant to all available antimicrobial agents. The possibility that such strains will become increasingly common, and that other fully resistant species will soon emerge, has led to some authorities to warn of 'the end of the antibiotic era' (Cohen 1992, Neu 1992, Kunin 1993).

DEVELOPMENT OF RESISTANCE IN STAPHYLOCOCCI AND THE EMERGENCE OF MULTIRESISTANT GRAM-NEGATIVE BACTERIA

Penicillin was introduced in the late 1940s, and by 1950 penicillinase-producing strains of *Staph. aureus* had become a major cause of serious infection in hospital patients. This problem remained unsolved until development of the penicillinase-resistant penicillins in the 1960s. Following the successful control of antibiotic-resistant staphylococcal infections, the aerobic enteric Gram-negative bacilli (*Esch. coli* and its relatives) emerged as important pathogens. These organisms were significantly more resistant to available antimicrobial agents than those prevalent at the beginning of the antibiotic era. Antibiotics effective against these Gram-negative species were introduced – including ampicillin, carbenicillin, the early cephalosporins and aminoglycosides – but resistance to them eventually began to appear and MDR Gram-negative bacteria became the main therapeutic problem of hospital-acquired infection during the 1970s and 1980s. Further research and development by the pharmaceutical industry produced new drugs active against these organisms, including new aminoglycosides, extended-spectrum β-lactams, β-lactam/β-lactamase-inhibitor combinations and the fluoroquinolones. As a result, we now have effective drugs for most Gram-negative bacterial infections, and although MDR Gram-negative strains still occur, they are not, at present, the problem they once were. Instead, MDR Gram-positive bacteria have emerged as a major therapeutic problem in the 1990s.

THE EMERGENCE OF MULTIRESISTANT GRAM-POSITIVE BACTERIA

Since the 1960s, a wide range of antimicrobials has been available for the treatment of Gram-positive bacteria, including (either alone or in combination) the penicillins, cephalosporins, aminoglycosides, glycopeptides, tetra-cyclines, macrolides, lincosamines, trimethoprim, sulphon-amides and chloramphenicol. Because of this wide range of effective agents, there was little research into new drugs for these organisms. However, opportunistic Gram-positive species resistant to many – and in a few cases all – of these drugs have emerged as major pathogens in the last 10 years. This may have been because the widespread use of cephalosporins, aminoglycosides and quinolones for Gram-negative infections has selected out Gram-positive species inherently resistant to these agents. In addition, some Gram-positive organisms have flourished in hospital environments because they can colonize the increasingly common plastic catheters and prostheses, and because – like the MDR Gram-negative organisms before them – they have a special ability to acquire and disseminate multiple resistance genes.

M. tuberculosis is another Gram-positive bacterium that has recently emerged as an important MDR pathogen. *M. tuberculosis* has always had the ability to rapidly develop mutational resistance to the common antituberculous drugs, and multidrug regimens are employed to prevent this. The emergence of multiply-resistant strains of *M. tuberculosis* has probably been due mainly to the failure of patients to take their drugs or complete treatment courses, followed by uncontrolled spread to others.

Some current problems with resistance

STAPHYLOCOCCUS AUREUS

Most strains (approximately 90%) of *Staph. aureus* – whether isolated in hospital or in the community – now produce β-lactamase and are resistant to penicillin and ampicillin. This type of resistance is plasmid mediated, resulting from bacteriophage transduction, and is often associated with resistance to erythromycin and other agents. During the 1950s, large epidemics of hospital infection were caused by 'the hospital staphylococcus', a virulent strain of *Staph. aureus* resistant to penicillin, tetracycline, erythromycin, chloramphenicol and other drugs. After the introduction of the penicillinase-stable methicillin (followed later by cloxacillin and flucloxacillin), the incidence of hospital infection with multiply-resistant staphylococci gradually declined during the 1960s and 1970s (Shanson 1981). Although strains of methicillin-resistant *Staph. aureus* (MRSA) were seen as early as 1961, it was not until the late 1970s that MRSA emerged as a major pathogen of hospital infection throughout the world (Haley et al 1982, Keane & Cafferky 1984, Cookson & Phillips 1988). MRSA are resistant to methicillin and other penicillinase-stable β-lactams by the production of an altered penicillin-binding protein PBP2a (p. 30). Although MRSA may appear sensitive to some β-lactams in vitro, they are resistant to clinical treatment with these agents and should be regarded as resistant to all β-lactams. Methicillin resistance is often expressed by only a proportion of cells in a clonal population, a phenomenon called 'heteroresistance'. In this situation special conditions, such as a high salt content in the culture medium or a lowered incubation temperature, are required to detect the resistance during in vitro testing (Report 1990).

The chromosomal region encoding the *mecA* gene contains a number of insertion sites. These permit the accumulation of multiple chromosomal resistances to other classes of antibiotics such as erythromycin, fusidic acid, rifampicin, streptomycin, sulphonamides and tetracycline. In addition, MRSA may acquire other resistances encoded on plasmids, including β-lactamase production and resistance to trimethoprim and the aminoglycosides. Aminoglycoside resistance in *Staph. aureus* is mediated by a bifunctional protein with both aminoglycoside acetyltransferase and phosphotransferase activities and is encoded by a transposon. MRSA now often exhibit chromosomally encoded gentamicin resistance resulting from genetic transposition from a plasmid.

Following the rapid emergence of resistance to quinolones (Schaefler 1989), many strains of MRSA remain sensitive only to the glycopeptides, vancomycin and teicoplanin. MRSA have become a major problem of multiply drug-resistant hospital infection in the 1990s, analogous to 'the hospital staphylococcus' of the 1950s. If MRSA were to acquire vancomycin resistance from enterococci (this has been produced in vitro but has not yet been seen in vivo), serious, untreatable staphylococcal infection would result.

COAGULASE-NEGATIVE STAPHYLOCOCCI

These organisms are important causes of nosocomial infections associated with prosthetic devices. In the community, people are normally colonized by relatively sensitive strains of *Staph. epidermidis*; after admission to hospital and treatment with antibiotics, patients often become colonized with more resistant strains of *Staph. epidermidis* or with inherently more resistant species such as *Staph. haemolyticus*. About half the coagulase-negative staphylococci isolated in hospitals show multiple antibiotic resistance, including resistance to methicillin (and other β-lactams), gentamicin and, to a lesser extent, quinolones. In some hospitals 2% or more of clinical isolates show the VanB phenotype of glycopeptide resistance (low-level, inducible, usually non-transferable, teicoplanin resistance) (Goldstein et al 1990), and this may be even more common in *Staph. haemolyticus*. Resistance in coagulase-negative staphylococci appears to be increasing, and multiresistant strains may act as a reservoir of resistance genes that can be transferred to *Staph. aureus* (Archer 1988). In addition, since MDR strains of coagulase-negative staphylococci are being isolated with increasing frequency from clinical specimens, they have stimulated the use of glycopeptides. These infections often do not require antibiotic therapy, and the unnecessary use of vancomycin for these organisms may be one factor in the emergence of glycopeptide resistance.

CORYNEFORM BACTERIA

Coryneform bacteria behave in many ways like the coagulase-negative staphylococci: they are normal skin commensals that are usually relatively antibiotic sensitive; after admission to hospital, patients often become colonized with more resistant strains and species, and these multiresistant types may go on to cause opportunistic infections, especially in association with plastic prostheses and catheters. The JK group of coryneform bacteria (now called *Corynebacterium jeikeium* after the initials of their discoverers Johnson and Kaye) are inherently resistant to many common antibiotics, and often sensitive only to vancomycin. They cause opportunistic infections in compromised patients, especially those with haematological and other malignancies.

STREPTOCOCCUS PNEUMONIAE

Str. pneumoniae frequently acquires resistance to tetracycline, and sometimes to sulphonamides, erythromycin, lincomycin or chloramphenicol (Klugman 1990). Pneumococci are normally relatively resistant to aminoglycosides (MICs of streptomycin about 8 mg/l), but some strains show high-level resistance (MIC >2 000 mg/l). Penicillin resistance was first reported in 1967 from Papua New Guinea, and since then has been seen with increasing frequency in many countries of the world (Klugman 1990,

Allen 1991). The MIC of penicillin for sensitive strains of pneumococci is <0.01 mg/l; the first penicillin-resistant isolates showed 'low-level' resistance with MICs of up to 1.0 mg/l, but in 1977 pneumococci were isolated in South Africa showing 'high-level' resistance with penicillin MICs of >1 mg/l. This resistance may not be detected by routine sensitivity-testing methods, and for disc testing a 1 μg oxacillin disc is recommended. High-level penicillin resistance has so far been confined to a small number of serotypes, whereas low-level resistance is now found in nearly all the common serotypes. There is a wide geographical variation in the prevalence of penicillin-resistant pneumococci, but there is evidence of international spread of resistant strains. In some countries only a few per cent of pneumococcal isolates show low-level penicillin resistance and high-level resistance is rare; however, in Hungary, Spain, South Africa and Israel, 40% or more of isolates have low-level resistance and 15% of isolates in Spain and 36% in Hungary are high-level resistant (Table 3.1). It is likely that the world-wide prevalence of penicillin- and multiple-antibiotic resistant pneumococci will continue to increase.

Respiratory infections with strains of pneumococci showing low-level penicillin resistance can be treated with high doses of penicillin. Meningitis and infections with high-level resistant strains have been successfully treated with vancomycin or third generation cephalosporins such as cefotaxime. Unfortunately cefotaxime-resistant strains have now appeared, although they remain uncommon (Johnson et al 1995, Lonks & Medeiros 1995). MICs of cefotaxime for sensitive pneumococci are <0.01 mg/l; for isolates with low-level penicillin resistance the MICs of cefotaxime are 0.125–0.25 mg/l, and for those with high-level penicillin resistance

Table 3.1 *Prevalence of antimicrobial resistance (%) in* Streptococcus pneumoniae *isolates from different countries.*

Country	Year	Penicillin		Erythromycin	Chloramphenicol
		All	High-level		
Hungary	1989	59	36	49	26
Spain	1989	44	15	10	41
Romania	1990	25	–	6	6
France	1990	12	6	29	12
UK	1990	2	?	8	–
Belgium	1988	1	–	12	2
Finland	1989	0	0	3	–
S. Africa	1991	45	4	4	9
Israel	1992	39	4	<5	<5
USA	1992	7	1	6	1

they are 0.2–2.0 mg/l. Increasing cefotaxime resistance is associated with acquisition of PBPs 2X or 1A, and fully resistant isolates have both these PBPs (Muñoz et al 1992).

ENTEROCOCCI

The enterococci are typically sensitive to ampicillin or amoxycillin, but are intrinsically relatively resistant to penicillin and other β-lactams such as cloxacillin, the cephalosporins and the carbapenems. They are also usually resistant to trimethoprim and the sulphonamides, the quinolones, low levels of aminoglycosides and low levels of clindamycin. However, these organisms have a remarkable ability to acquire new resistances to ampicillin, amoxycillin and other drugs used against Gram-positive bacteria, including chloramphenicol, erythromycin, tetracycline, high levels of aminoglycosides and clindamycin, and, now, high levels of vancomycin and teicoplanin (Murray 1990).

Ent. faecalis is the most common enterococcal species to be isolated from human faeces and from clinical specimens, but *Ent. faecium* is increasing in frequency as a human pathogen. *Ent. faecium* is inherently more resistant to penicillin and ampicillin than *Ent. faecalis*, and hospital isolates tend to show increasing high-level resistance. High-level ampicillin resistance is probably due to changes in affinity of the enterococcal penicillin-binding proteins, and contributes to the growing importance of *Ent. faecium* as a nosocomial pathogen. Transferable β-lactamase-mediated ampicillin resistance has been reported in *Ent. faecalis* (Murray 1990) but, although such strains have caused several large hospital outbreaks, they are generally very uncommon in clinical material.

The enterococci (particularly *Ent. faecium*) are thus now frequently multiply drug resistant, often showing high-level resistance to ampicillin, the aminoglycosides and the glycopeptides, and some strains are now resistant to virtually all available antimicrobial agents. Because of this, and because they may carry transferable glycopeptide resistance, these organisms are among the most important and problematic multidrug resistant pathogens of the 1990s.

HAEMOPHILUS INFLUENZAE

Ampicillin resistance due to plasmid-mediated β-lactamase production was first noted in 1972, and is now widespread. In the USA about 17% of isolates were β-lactamase producers in 1990, and in the UK repeated surveys have shown a rise in the prevalence of such isolates from 2% in 1976 to about 9% in 1990 (Table 3.2). More recently, non β-lactamase mediated ampicillin resistance has been identified, associated with changes in penicillin-binding proteins, but this form of ampicillin resistance remains

Table 3.2 *Percentage antimicrobial resistances of isolates of H. influenzae in various surveys.*

	UK			USA	Australia
	1976	1981	1990	1990	1988–90
Ampicillin					
β-lactamase –ve strains	2	6	9	17	16
β-lactamase +ve strains	2	0.5	5	<1	0
Co-trimoxazole	<1	2	5	<1	5
Tetracycline	3	3	5	2	4
Chloramphenicol	<1	1	–	0	2
Erythromycin	–	–	87	99	–
Cefaclor	–	–	5	1	6
Cefuroxime	–	–	–	<1	–

uncommon. Chloramphenicol resistance has emerged in a number of countries, but the frequency is usually low (Table 3.2). However, an explosive increase in resistant *H. influenzae* was seen in Barcelona, Spain, during 1981–84, with ampicillin resistance in 60% of strains isolated from patients with meningitis, chloramphenicol resistance in 66%, and resistance to both agents in 57% (Needham 1989). *H. influenzae* is intrinsically resistant to erythromycin, but most isolates remain sensitive to cefaclor and, even more so, to cefuroxime.

NEISSERIA GONORRHOEAE

Low-level resistance to benzylpenicillin (MIC 0.1–2 mg/l) has been increasing in strains of *N. gonorrhoeae* for several decades, and is now very common. This type of resistance is due to mutational alterations in the penicillin-binding proteins and to impermeability. Since 1976, a high-level plasmid mediated type of resistance to penicillin, caused by production of β-lactamase, appeared in South-East Asia and West Africa, and spread to Western countries (Phillips 1976, Elwell et al 1977). These penicillinase-producing strains of *N. gonorrhoeae* remain common in many developing countries, but account for only a few per cent of gonococcal isolates in the West (Schwarcz et al 1990). The emergence of plasmid-mediated high-level resistance to tetracycline has caused additional problems where this group of drugs is used for the treatment of dual infection with gonococci and chlamydia. In the USA, 17% of strains have chromosomally mediated resistance to tetracycline and 2% show high-level plasmid-mediated resistance (Schwarcz et al 1990). Spectinomycin resistance remains rare. Resistance to fluorinated quinolones is beginning to emerge in the UK, the USA and elsewhere (Turner et al 1990, Gransden et al 1990, Anonymous 1994).

NEISSERIA MENINGITIDIS

The emergence of sulphonamide resistance in *N. meningitidis* during the early 1960s greatly limited the value of sulphonamides for treatment. Since then, two developments in drug resistance of potential clinical importance have emerged. Firstly, up to 10% of carriers treated with rifampicin are subsequently found to harbour rifampicin-resistant meningococci in the nasopharynx, and such strains have occasionally caused invasive disease. Because of this, an oral quinolone (usually ciprofloxacin) is becoming widely used for the eradication of throat carriage in adults. This is not a licensed indication for children because of theoretical toxicity, but has been so used by some physicians. The second, and equally disturbing development, is that of decreased susceptibility to penicillin. The MIC of penicillin for meningococci is usually <0.08 mg/l, and this may be increased in moderately resistant isolates up to 0.5 mg/l. These strains have been reported especially from Spain (Saez-Nieto & Campos 1988) but also in other countries, including the UK (Sutcliffe et al 1988). None was found in Spain until 1985, but by 1987 7% and by 1987–89 20% of isolates showed some reduced susceptibility to penicillin. The strains are not β-lactamase producers, and resistance is probably due to alterations in PBPs, possibly caused by genetic transformation from other *Neisseria* species (Saez-Nieto et al 1990).

ENTEROBACTERIA

For the past 20 years the prevalence of resistance to commonly used antibiotics has been steadily increasing in nosocomial isolates of enterobacteria, especially in large teaching hospitals. Many strains are now susceptible only to newer β-lactams and the aminoglycosides. Much of the problem is due to the wide distribution in hospitals of plasmids and transposons encoding multiple drug resistance and their dissemination among many different enterobacterial species.

Escherichia coli

Esch. coli is naturally sensitive to ampicillin and amoxycillin. Acquired resistance conferred by a plasmid-encoded TEM-1 β-lactamase was first described in 1965, and this has spread so extensively throughout the world that 40–60% of both hospital and community strains are now resistant by this mechanism. Other plasmid-encoded β-lactamases are sometimes seen in *Esch. coli*, but about 90% of resistant strains produce TEM-1. These resistant organisms are usually sensitive to co-amoxiclav, the combination of amoxycillin with the β-lactamase inhibitor clavulanic acid;

however, up to 30% of resistant isolates may be resistant to the combination because of hyperproduction of TEM-1 β-lactamase. Apart from β-lactamase production, *Esch. coli*, which is primarily an endogenous pathogen, usually remains sensitive to the aminoglycosides, cephalosporins and quinolones, although sporadic multiresistant strains are sometimes seen.

Klebsiella, Enterobacter and *Serratia* spp.

These organisms are inherently resistant to ampicillin, and *Enterobacter* and *Serratia* spp. are resistant to older cephalosporins. They all have the ability to cause hospital outbreaks of opportunistic infection, and they often exchange plasmid-borne resistances. *Klebsiella pneumoniae* is the most common nosocomial pathogen of the three, and appears to have the greatest ability to receive and disseminate resistance factors. The ampicillin resistance of *K. pneumoniae* is usually mediated by SHV-1 β-lactamase which may be encoded on either the plasmid or the chromosome. In the 1970s, klebsiellae carrying plasmid-borne aminoglycoside resistance often caused large outbreaks of hospital infection and sometimes disseminated their resistances to *Enterobacter, Serratia* and other enterobacterial species. These outbreaks became uncommon when the newer cephalosporins and aminoglycosides became available. Recently, however, klebsiellae have appeared that have plasmid-borne resistance to third-generation cephalosporins and, usually, to all the presently available aminoglycosides. The cephalosporin resistance results from the production of extended-spectrum β-lactamases derived from small mutations to TEM-1, TEM-2 or SHV-1 genes (see Ch. 16). These organisms can cause large hospital outbreaks and can disseminate their resistances to other enterobacteria. Although these extended-spectrum enzymes can be inhibited by clavulanic acid, and thus are theoretically susceptible to co-amoxiclav and other β-lactam–β-lactamase-inhibitor combinations, some are hyperproducers of the β-lactamase and resistant to this therapy. Some strains are also resistant to quinolones. These new klebsiellae (and their *Serratia* and *Enterobacter* relatives) can produce serious infection in the compromised; since some of them are susceptible only to carbapenems among presently available antimicrobials, they represent a worrying threat for the 1990s.

Shigella, Salmonella and *Campylobacter* spp.

Shigellae were among the first organisms to be shown to harbour transferable antibiotic resistance factors. Throughout the world, but especially in developing countries, rates of antibiotic resistance and multiple resistance in salmonellae have shown an inexorable increase. Nowadays, about 80% of isolates are resistant to at least one of the standard antimicrobials, and 30% or more to two. In developing countries 30–70% of isolates are resistant to ampicillin, chloramphenicol, tetracycline or co-trimoxazole, with more resistance being seen in *Shigella dysenteriae* and *Shigella flexneri* than *Shigella sonnei*. In developed countries rates of resistance are higher in patients with a history of travel abroad. Resistance to co-trimoxazole and nalidixic acid has increased dramatically in recent years (Bennish et al 1992, Gascon et al 1994), but most isolates remain susceptible to fluoroquinolones.

A similar pattern of increasing resistance and multiple resistance has been seen in animal strains of salmonellae. Although the subject has stimulated considerable debate, there is strong evidence that antibiotics used in animal husbandry have contributed to antibiotic resistance in human isolates (Little et al 1986, DuPont & Steele 1987). In Britain, multiple resistance in *Salmonella typhimurium* doubled in human isolates between 1981 and 1990 and quadrupled in bovine isolates. In contrast, multiple resistance was uncommon in *Salmonella enteritidis*, which is usually derived from poultry in which there is less use of antibiotics in feeds than in cattle (Threlfall et al 1993). Aminoglycoside resistance appeared in British isolates of salmonellae after 1983 following the veterinary treatment of calves with the related drug apramycin (Threlfall et al 1986), and both in the UK and the USA, evidence is now emerging that the veterinary use of quinolones is stimulating the emergence of quinolone-resistant isolates of salmonellae (Griggs et al 1994, Lee et al 1994). The extended-spectrum β-lactamases that have emerged in klebsiellae, and other commensal enterobacteria have recently appeared in some salmonella strains, possibly as a result of plasmid transfer in the human gut (Issack et al 1995).

In contrast to the multiple resistance seen in animal strains of Salmonellae, *Salmonella typhi* has generally remained antibiotic sensitive – further support for the theory that much of the resistance in animal salmonellae has resulted from the selective pressure of antibiotics in animal husbandry. However, resistant and multiply resistant strains of *Salm. typhi* (especially those showing ampicillin and chloramphenicol resistance) have appeared sporadically and in localized outbreaks in various parts of the world.

Campylobacter spp. have also shown increasing antimicrobial resistance, and again some of this resistance may be related to the veterinary use of antibiotics. Although there is considerable geographic variation, macrolide resistance in *Camp. jejuni* appears to have remained stable in recent years, at less than 5% (Sanchez et al 1994, Reina et al 1994). In contrast, the proportion of isolates resistant to quinolones has increased dramatically over the last 10 years (from 0% to 30%), probably as a result of the addition of quinolones to chicken feed (Endtz et al 1991, Sanchez et al 1994, Reina et al 1994).

PSEUDOMONAS AERUGINOSA

Ps. aeruginosa is inherently resistant to most β-lactam antibiotics, tetracyclines, chloramphenicol, sulphonamides and nalidixic acid, and acquired resistance to other antibiotics is common. Two types of aminoglycoside resistance are seen: high-level, plasmid-mediated resistance to one or two aminoglycosides, due to the production of aminoglycoside-modifying enzymes (p. 166), is often observed during nosocomial outbreaks; and a more common form of resistance in sporadic isolates is broad-spectrum resistance to all the aminoglycosides, due to a reduction in the permeability of the cell envelope. This type of resistance may appear during treatment with any aminoglycoside. Resistance to ceftazidime and other antipseudomonal cephalosporins by mutation to constitutive production of chromosomal β-lactamase (p. 203) may also occur during treatment. Resistance to imipenem is also seen, but this usually arises by changes in membrane permeability. Finally, quinolone resistance – due to mutations in DNA gyrase, decreases in membrane permeability, or both – has also emerged relatively rapidly.

ACINETOBACTER SPP.

Acinetobacters are free-living non-fermenting organisms that often colonize human skin and cause opportunistic infections. The most frequently isolated acinetobacter, and one most likely to acquire multiple antibiotic resistance, is *Acinetobacter baumannii*, formerly known as *Acinetobacter calcoaceticus* var. *anitratus*. In the early 1970s, acinetobacters were usually sensitive to many common antimicrobial agents, such as gentamicin and the cephalosporins. Nowadays, many hospital strains are resistant to most available agents, including the aminoglycosides and older and newer cephalosporins, and some have developed resistance to the quinolones and carbapenems. The mechanisms and genetics of resistance in this species are complex, but they involve several plasmid-borne β-lactamases and aminoglycoside-modifying enzymes, as well as alterations in membrane permeability and penicillin-binding proteins. The acquisition of these multiple mechanisms may be due to the fact that this group of organisms is physiologically competent and can acquire DNA by transformation in vivo.

OTHER NON-FERMENTING ORGANISMS

A number of other non-fermenting organisms have recently emerged as important nosocomial pathogens. These organisms are inherently resistant to many of the antimicrobial agents used for infection with Gram-negative organisms, including the aminoglycosides and newer cephalosporins, and often have the ability to acquire further resistance to quinolones and carbapenems. Because of this, and despite their relatively low virulence, they are seen with increasing frequency in areas of high antibiotic usage such as intensive care units. *Burkholderia cepacia* (formerly known as *Pseudomonas cepacia* or *Pseudomonas multivorans*) is inherently resistant to the aminoglycosides and most β-lactam antibiotics, but sensitive to co-trimoxazole and chloramphenicol. However, additional acquired multiple resistance is becoming more common in this species. *Achromobacter xylosoxidans* is characteristically sensitive to co-trimoxazole, ceftazidime and ciprofloxacin, but resistant to aminoglycosides. *Stenotrophomonas maltophilia* (formerly known as *Xanthomonas maltophilia* or *Ps. maltophilia*) is often resistant to all the aminoglycosides and to imipenem, although it is characteristically sensitive to co-trimoxazole and tetracyclines. It has considerable ability to develop further multiple resistance by several mechanisms, including decrease in outer membrane permeability and the production of inducible broad-spectrum β-lactamases.

MYCOBACTERIUM TUBERCULOSIS

M. tuberculosis has limited susceptibility to standard antimicrobial agents, but can be treated by combinations of antituberculous drugs, of which the common first-line agents are rifampicin, isoniazid, ethambutol and streptomycin (see Ch. 37). *M. tuberculosis* develops resistance to these agents spontaneously (primary resistance) or after exposure to them (secondary resistance). Resistance mechanisms for different classes of antituberculous drugs are genetically unrelated, and resistance is thought usually to be the result of spontaneous chromosomal mutations. Mutational resistance occurs at the rate of about 1 in 10^8 for rifampicin, 1 in 10^8 to 1 in 10^9 for isoniazid, 1 in 10^6 for ethambutol and 1 in 10^5 for streptomycin. Since a cavitating lung lesion contains up to 10^9 organisms, mutational resistance appears quite frequently when these drugs are used singly for treatment, but is uncommon if three or more are used simultaneously.

For many years, resistance to antituberculous therapy was not a clinical problem, but recently there have been increasing reports of multiply-drug-resistant tuberculosis (MDR-TB) causing treatment failure, although the numbers of such cases is still extremely small. MDR-TB implies resistance to at least two of the first-line antituberculous drugs, usually rifampicin and isoniazid. These two drugs are essential for most initial or short-course treatment regimens, and strains of *M. tuberculosis* resistant to them soon develop resistance to other drugs also. Patients with MDR-TB thus fail to respond to standard therapy and disseminate resistant strains to their contacts (including health care workers), both before and after the resistance is discovered. Mortality rates in MDR-TB are high in all patients, but especially so in those infected with human immunodeficiency virus (HIV), which is a common association in hospital outbreaks.

There are several reasons for the appearance of MDR-TB in the West. The main factor is probably failure of patients to comply with their treatment regimens, resulting in inadequate therapy and the emergence of resistant mutants. Factors that contribute to this situation include: deterioration of public-health services directed towards control of tuberculosis; inadequate training of health-care workers in the diagnosis, treatment and control of tuberculosis; laboratory delays in the detection and sensitivity testing of *M. tuberculosis*; addition of single drugs to failing treatment regimens; an increase in the number of individuals at high-risk of acquiring and disseminating tuberculosis, including those infected with HIV, the poor and the homeless; and increasing migration of people from areas where tuberculosis is common (Snider & Roper 1992, Jacobs 1994). The single most important factor in the prevention of further emergence of MDR-TB is probably the reintroduction of supervised observed therapy.

After many years of neglect, recent research has begun to unravel the molecular basis of antimicrobial resistance in mycobacteria (Zhang & Young 1994). Rifampicin resistance in *M. tuberculosis* is usually the result of mutations in the *rpoB* gene that encodes the β subunit of RNA polymerase, the target molecule for rifampicin. In other mycobacteria, rifampicin resistance may be more frequently due to alterations in cell wall permeability or to altered efflux mechanisms. The action of isoniazid against *M. tuberculosis* is not completely understood but may involve multiple mechanisms, including transport and activation of the drug by mechanisms involving catalase–peroxidase, pigment precursors, NAD and peroxide; generation of reactive oxygen radicals; interference of mycolic acid metabolism; and reaction with mycobacterial proteins, specifically tyrosine residues (Jacobs 1994). Clearly, several mechanisms might be involved in decreased susceptibility to isoniazid. One appears to be mutation or deletion of the *katG* gene that encodes catalase–peroxidase activity (Zhang et al 1992), and another appears to be changes to the *inhA* gene which is probably involved in mycolic acid synthesis (Banerjee et al 1994). High-level fluoroquinolone and streptomycin resistances in *M. tuberculosis* appear to be caused by a similar mechanism to those seen in other species, namely mutations in the *gyrA* gene encoding the A subunit of bacterial DNA polymerase (Takiff et al 1994) and the *rpsL* (or *strA*) encoding the S12 ribosomal protein respectively (Zhang & Young 1994). Mechanisms of resistance to other antituberculous agents have yet to be elucidated.

Prevention and control

The genetic mechanisms that confer antibiotic resistance on bacteria must have existed long before the antibiotic era. It is inconceivable that the spontaneous mutations giving rise to resistant variants found constantly in modern bacterial populations did not exist then, and that resistant populations were not selected out, for example in the intensively competitive environment of the soil, inhabited by a multitude of antibiotic-producing fungi and bacteria. Other resistance genes betray a more distant origin in genes responsible for normal cellular functions such as cell-wall synthesis: an example is the complex regulation of inducible β-lactamases in certain enterobacteria (Toumanen et al 1991). Unfortunately, direct evidence of the existence of genetic and biochemical mechanisms before the 1940s is virtually impossible to obtain since there are no representative collections of bacteria from that time. However, Fleming had no difficulty in obtaining Gram-negative organisms resistant to penicillin in 1929, and β-lactamase has been identified in a strain of *Esch. coli* isolated in 1940. Similarly, resistance plasmids have been isolated from organisms isolated in the 1940s. The existence of elements that would later carry more and more resistance determinants can be confidently assumed.

Whatever the origins of resistance genes, there has clearly been a major increase in their prevalence during the past 40 years. It is generally held that this can be closely correlated with the use of antibiotics in man and animals, and it is clear that with the introduction of each new agent, resistance has eventually emerged to every one of them.

The phenomenon is common to hospitals, which have seen the emergence of a range of multiply-drug resistant pathogens, to the community at large, where respiratory and gut pathogens have become resistant to often freely available antibiotics, and to animal husbandry, where the use of antibiotics for growth promotion and for mass therapy has promoted resistance in salmonella and campylobacter. It is difficult to refute Spanish evidence that penicillin resistance in pneumococci has increased as the national use of β-lactam antibiotics has increased – and, conversely, that chloramphenicol resistance in pneumococci has declined as a direct result of the much diminished use of that drug.

The use of antibiotics is not the only feature common to hospitals, farms and even sections of the outside community, that encourages the spread of antibiotic resistance. Equally important is the opportunity for organisms to spread. The control of hospital infection is crucial to the control of the spread of antibiotic-resistant organisms.

The modern hospital is a model site for the evolution and dissemination of drug resistance. Here, usage of antibiotics is much more concentrated than in the community, and

opportunities for cross-infection are abundant. Most new drugs are first given in hospitals, and almost all injectable agents are administered to hospital patients. Topical antibiotics are particularly likely to select for resistance, and the emergence of gentamicin-resistant *Ps. aeruginosa* and fusidic-acid- or mupirocin-resistant *Staph. aureus* has often followed heavy topical use of gentamicin in burns and fusidic acid or mupirocin in dermatological patients respectively. Multiple drug resistance can be encouraged even by the use of a single agent, since this may select for plasmids conferring resistance to multiple antibiotics. Hospital patients and staff may become colonized with resistant bacteria, especially in the faeces or on the skin, and disseminate these organisms both within the hospital and into the community. To control the development and spread of antibiotic resistance it is therefore essential to reduce unnecessary antibiotic usage within hospitals and to prevent cross-infection with multiply-drug-resistant pathogens.

Although it is widely accepted that the control of antibiotic prescribing is essential for the control of antibiotic resistance, antibiotic misuse is common. Studies have suggested that up to 70% of treatment courses are 'unnecessary' or 'inappropriate', therapy is often unnecessarily prolonged and prophylaxis is often inappropriate or given at the wrong time. Physicians are often poorly informed about the use of antibiotics and may obtain most of their information from pharmaceutical companies. Educational programmes on good prescribing are needed both in medical schools and in postgraduate programmes.

Several other strategies have been used to improve antibiotic usage in hospitals (Report 1994). These include the setting up of authoritative committees (usually formulary committees) representing clinicians (including consultants in infectious diseases), microbiologists, clinical pharmacologists, pharmacists and managers to control antibiotic use (see Ch. 12). They should publish guidelines on the rational use of antibiotics for treatment and prophylaxis and policies for the restriction on antibiotic usage within their hospital. These policies should take into account the current resistance patterns of local bacterial isolates and should be designed to reduce the emergence of yet more resistant organisms. Of equal importance is the need to minimize costs and avoid confusion, especially among junior staff who are often responsible for writing the majority of antibiotic prescriptions in a hospital. The pronouncements of these committees are often reinforced by selective reporting of sensitivity results by the laboratory, by selective stocking of approved drugs by the pharmacy, and by audit of actual usage. Dosage and duration of treatment should also be controlled.

For the first time in 20 years we are facing the threat of untreatable bacterial infection. Strains of enterococci, mycobacteria and non-fermenting Gram-negative bacilli resistant to all currently available agents are already circulating. In the next decade there will almost certainly be further dissemination of plasmids encoding resistance for glycopeptides, aminoglycosides, expanded-spectrum cephalosporins and carbapenems, more frequent occurrence of enzyme hyperproduction and increasing mutational resistance to penicillins and quinolones. This may result in the emergence of other fully resistant species, including staphylococci, streptococci, pneumococci, corynebacteria and enterobacteria. Although new antimicrobial agents will continue to be developed, albeit currently at a reduced rate, it is likely that resistance to these also will eventually appear. It seems clear that judicious use of antimicrobial agents in man and animals, and strict control of cross-infection, is essential to combat the emergence of such potentially devastating pathogens.

References

Allen K D 1991 Penicillin-resistant pneumococci. *Journal of Hospital Infection* 17: 3–13

Anonymous 1994 From the Centers for Disease Control and Prevention. Decreased susceptibility of *Neisseria gonorrhoeae* to fluoroquinolones – Ohio and Hawaii, 1992–1994 *Journal of the American Medical Association* 271: 1733–1734

Arthur M, Courvalin P 1993 Genetics and mechanisms of glycopeptide resistance in enterococci. *Antimicrobial Agents and Chemotherapy* 37: 1563–1571

Archer G L 1982 Molecular epidemiology of multiresistant *Staphylococcus epidermidis*. *Journal of Antimicrobial Chemotherapy* 21 (suppl C): 133–138

Banerjee A, Dubnau E, Quemard A et al 1994 *inhA*, a gene encoding a target for isoniazid and ethionamide in *Mycobacterium tuberculosis*. *Science* 263: 227–230

Bennish M L, Salam M A, Hossain M A et al 1992 Antimicrobial resistance of *Shigella* isolates in Bangladesh, 1983–1990: increasing frequency of strains multiply resistant to ampicillin, trimethoprim–sulfamethoxazole and nalidixic acid. *Clinics in Infectious Diseases* 14: 1055–1060

Cederbrant G, Kahlmeter G, Ljungh A 1992 Proposed mechanism for metronidazole resistance in *Helicobacter pylori*. *Journal of Antimicrobial Chemotherapy* 29: 115–120

Chambers H F, Hackbarth C J 1992 Methicillin-resistant *Staphylococcus aureus*: genetics and mechanism of resistance. In: Cafferkey MT (ed) *Methicillin-resistant Staphylococcus aureus*. Marcel Dekker, New York, p 21–35

Chopra I, Howe T G B 1978 Bacterial resistance to the tetracyclines. *Microbiological Reviews* 42: 707–724

Cohen M L 1992 Epidemiology of drug resistance: implications for a post-antimicrobial era. *Science* 257: 1050–1055

Cohen S P, McMurry L M, Levy S B 1988 MarA locus causes decreased expression of OmpF porin in multiple-antibiotic-resistant (Mar) mutants of *Escherichia coli*. *Journal of Bacteriology* 170: 5416–5422

Cookson B 1990 Mupirocin resistance in staphylococci. *Journal of Antimicrobial Chemotherapy* 25: 497–503

Cookson B, Phillips I 1988 Epidemic methicillin-resistant *Staphylococcus aureus*. *Journal of Antimicrobial Chemotherapy* 21 (suppl C): 57–65

Dowson C G, Coffey T J, Kell C, Whiley R A 1993 Evolution of penicillin resistance in *Streptococcus pneumoniae*; the role of *Streptococcus mitis* in the formation of a low affinity PBP2B in *S. pneumoniae*. *Molecular Microbiology* 9: 635–643

DuPont H L, Steele J H 1987 Use of antimicrobial agents in animal feeds: implications for human health. *Reviews of Infectious Diseases* 9: 447–460

Elwell L P, Roberts M, Mayer L W, Falkow S 1977 Plasmid-mediated beta-lactamase production in *Neisseria gonorrhoeae*. *Antimicrobial Agents and Chemotherapy* 11: 528–533

Endtz H P, Rujis G J, van Klingeren B, Jansen W H, van der Reyden T, Mouton R P 1991 Quinolone resistance in campylobacter isolated from man and poultry following the introduction of fluoroquinolones in veterinary medicine. *Journal of Antimicrobial Chemotherapy* 27: 199–208

Finland M, Jones W F, Barnes M W 1959 Occurrence of serious bacterial infections since the introduction of antibacterial agents. *Journal of the American Medical Association* 170: 2188–2197

Gascon V J, Abdalla S, Gomez J et al 1994 Antimicrobial resistance of Shigella isolates causing traveler's diarrhea. *Antimicrobial Agents and Chemotherapy* 38: 2668–2670

Gilbart J, Perry C R, Slocombe B 1993 High-level mupirocin resistance in *Staphylococcus aureus*: evidence for two distinct isoleucyl-tRNA synthetases. *Antimicrobial Agents and Chemotherapy* 37: 32–38

Goldstein F W, Coutrot A, Seiffer A, Acar J F 1990 Percentages and distributions of vancomycin-resistant strains among coagulase-negative staphylococci. *Antimicrobial Agents and Chemotherapy* 34: 899–900

Gransden W R, Warren C A, Phillips I, Hodges M, Barlow D 1990 Decreased susceptibility of *Neisseria gonorrhoeae* to ciprofloxacin. *Lancet* 335: 165

Griggs D J, Hall M C, Yin Y F, Piddock L J 1994 Quinolone resistance in veterinary isolates of salmonellae. *Journal of Antimicrobial Chemotherapy* 33: 1173–1189

Haley R W, Hightower A W, Khabbaz R F et al 1982 The emergence of methicillin-resistant *Staphylococcus aureus* infections in United States hospitals. *Annals of Internal Medicine* 97: 297–308

Issack M I, Shannon K P, Qureshi S A, French G L 1995 Extended-spectrum β-lactamase in *Salmonella* spp. *Journal of Hospital Infection* 30: 319–321

Jacobs R F 1994 Multiple-drug-resistant tuberculosis. *Clinics in Infectious Disease* 19: 1–10

Johnson A P, Speller D C E, Patel B C 1995 Sensitivity to cefotaxime of pneumococci isolated in the UK. *Journal of Antimicrobial Chemotherapy* 35: 443–444

Keane C T, Cafferkey M T 1984 Re-emergence of methicillin-resistant *Staphylococcus aureus* causing severe infection. *Journal of Infection* 9: 6–16

Klugman K P 1990 Pneumococcal resistance to antibiotics. *Clinical Microbiology Reviews* 3: 171–196

Kunin C M 1993 Resistance to antimicrobial drugs – a worldwide calamity. *Annals of Internal Medicine* 118: 557–561

Lee L A, Puhr N D, Maloney E K, Bean N H, Tauxe R V 1994 Increase in antimicrobial-resistant salmonella infections in the United States, 1989–1990. *Journal of Infectious Diseases* 170: 128–134

Levy S B 1989 Evolution and spread of tetracycline resistance determinants. *Journal of Antimicrobial Chemotherapy* 24: 1–3

Levy S B 1992 Active efflux mechanisms for antimicrobial resistance. *Antimicrobial Agents and Chemotherapy* 36: 695–703

Little T W, Sojka W J, Wray C 1986 Consequences of emergence of resistant bacteria from the use of antibacterials in animal husbandry. *Scandinavian Journal of Infectious Diseases* 49: 124–128

Lonks J R, Medeiros A A 1995 The growing threat of antibiotic-resistant *Streptococcus pneumoniae*. *Medical Clinics of North America* 79: 523–535

Markiewicz Z, Tomasz A 1989 Variation in penicillin-binding protein patterns of penicillin-resistant clinical isolates of pneumococci. *Journal of Clinical Microbiology* 27: 405–410

McGowan J E 1983 Antimicrobial resistance in hospital organisms and its relation to antibiotic use. *Reviews of Infectious Diseases* 5: 1033–1048

McMurry L, Petrucci R E, Levy S B 1980 Active efflux of tetracycline encoded by four genetically different tetracycline resistance determinants in *Escherichia coli*. *Proceedings of the National Academy of Sciences USA* 24: 554–551

Murray B E 1990 The life and times of the enterococcus. *Clinical Microbiology Reviews* 3: 46–65

Muñoz R, Dowson C G, Daniels M et al 1992 Genetics of resistance to third-generation cephalosporins in clinical isolates of *Streptococcus pneumoniae*. *Molecular Microbiology* 6: 2461–2465

Needham C 1989 *Haemophilus influenzae*: antibiotic susceptibility. *Clinical Microbiology Reviews* 1: 218–227

Neu H C 1992 The crisis in antibiotic resistance. *Science* 257: 1064–1072

Nikaido H 1989 Outer membrane barrier as a mechanism of antimicrobial resistance. *Antimicrobial Agents and Chemotherapy* 33: 1831–1836

Nikaido H 1993 Transport across the bacterial outer membrane. *Journal of Bioenergetics and Biomembranes* 25: 581–589

Noble W C, Virani Z, Cree R G A 1992 Co-transfer of vancomycin and other resistance genes from *Enterococcus faecalis* NCTC 12201 to *Staphylococcus aureus*. *FEMS Microbiology Letters* 93: 195–198

Phillips I 1976 Beta-lactamase-producing, penicillin-resistant gonococcus. *Lancet* ii: 656–657

Phillips I 1991 Reports of the European study group on antibiotic breakpoints. *European Journal of Clinical Microbiology and Infectious Diseases* 10: 989–990

Reina J, Ros M J, Serra A 1994 Susceptibilities to 10 antimicrobial agents of 1,220 *Campylobacter* strains isolated from 1987 to 1993 from feces of pediatric patients. *Antimicrobial Agents and Chemotherapy* 38: 2917–2920

Report of a Combined Working Party of the Hospital Infection Society and British Society for Antimicrobial Chemotherapy 1990 Revised guidelines for the control of epidemic methicillin-resistant *Staphylococcus aureus*. *Journal of Hospital Infection* 16: 351–377

Report of a Working Party of the British Society for Antimicrobial Chemotherapy 1991 A guide to sensitivity testing. *Journal of Antimicrobial Chemotherapy* 27 (suppl D): 1–50

Report of a Working Party of the British Society for Antimicrobial Chemotherapy 1994 Hospital antibiotic control measures in the UK. *Journal of Antimicrobial Chemotherapy* 34: 21–42

Reynolds P E 1992 Glycopeptide resistance in Gram-positive bacteria. *Journal of Medical Microbiology* 36: 14–17

Saez-Nieto J A, Campos J 1988 Penicillin-resistant strains of *Neisseria meningitidis* in Spain. *Lancet* i: 1452–1453

Saez-Nieto J A, Lujan R, Martinez-Suarez J V et al 1990 *Neisseria lactamica* and *Neisseria polysaccharea* as possible sources of meningococcal β-lactam resistance by genetic transformation. *Antimicrobial Agents and Chemotherapy* 34: 2269–2272

Sanchez R, Fernandez-Baca V, Diaz M D, Munoz P, Rodriguez-Creixems M, Bouza E 1994 Evolution of susceptibilities of *Campylobacter* spp. to quinolones and macrolides. *Antimicrobial Agents and Chemotherapy* 38: 1879–1882

Schaefler S 1989 Methicillin-resistant strains of *Staphylococcus aureus* resistant to quinolones. *Journal of Clinical Microbiology* 27: 335–336

Schwarcz S K, Zenilman J M, Schnell D et al 1990 National surveillance of penicillin resistance in *Neisseria gonorrhoeae*. *Journal of the American Medical Association* 264: 1413–1417

Shanson D C 1981 Antibiotic resistance in *Staphylococcus aureus*. *Journal of Hospital Infection* 2: 11–36

Shaw W V 1984 Bacterial resistance to chloramphenicol. *British Medical Bulletin* 40: 36–41

Snider D E, Roper W L 1992 The new tuberculosis. *New England Journal of Medicine* 326: 703–705

Sutcliffe E M, Jones D M, El-Sheikh S, Percival A 1988 Penicillin-insensitive meningococci in the UK. *Lancet* i: 657–658

Takiff H E, Salazar L, Guerrero C et al 1994 Cloning and nucleotide sequence of *Mycobacterium tuberculosis gyrA* and *gyrB* genes and detection of quinolone resistance mutations. *Antimicrobial Agents and Chemotherapy* 38: 773–780

Tanaka K, Teraoka H, Tamaki M, Otaka E, Osawa S 1968 Erythromycin-resistant mutant of *Escherichia coli* with altered ribosomal protein component. *Science* 162: 576–678

Threlfall E J, Rowe B, Ferguson J L, Ward L R 1986 Characterization of plasmids conferring resistance to gentamicin and apramycin in strains of *Salmonella typhimurium* phage type 204c in Britain. *Journal of Hygiene* 97: 419–426

Threlfall E J, Rowe B, Ward L R 1993 A comparison of multiple drug resistance in salmonellas from humans and food animals in England and Wales, 1981 and 1990. *Epidemiology and Infection* 111: 189–197

Toumanen E, Lindquist S, Sande S et al 1991 Coordinate regulation of beta-lactamase induction and peptidoglycan composition by the *amp* operon. *Science* 251: 201–204

Turner A, Jephcott A E, Haji T C, Gupta P C 1990 Ciprofloxacin resistant *Neisseria gonorrhoeae* in the UK. *Genitourinary Medicine* 66: 43

Ubukata K, Nonoguchi R, Song M D, Matsuhashi M, Konno M 1990 Homology of *mecA* gene in methicillin-resistant *Staphylococcus haemolyticus* and *Staphylococcus simulans* to that of *Staphylococcus aureus*. *Antimicrobial Agents and Chemotherapy* 34: 170–172

Weisblum B 1995 Inducible resistance to macrolides, lincosamides and streptogramin type B antibiotics: the resistance phenomenon, its biological diversity, and structural elements that regulate expression – a review. *Journal of Antimicrobial Chemotherapy* 16 (suppl A): 63

Zhang Y, Heym B, Allen B, Young D, Cole S 1992 The catalase–peroxidase gene and isoniazid resistance of *Mycobacterium tuberculosis*. *Nature* 358: 591–593

Zhang Y, Young D 1994 Molecular genetics of drug resistance in *Mycobacterium tuberculosis*. *Journal of Antimicrobial Chemotherapy* 34: 313–319

Pharmacokinetics

N. R. Kitteringham and B. K. Park

Introduction

The physician considering the treatment of any disease with a chemical agent is faced with two crucial decisions: first, what is the correct drug to deal adequately with the condition as it is presented; and secondly, what is the most suitable regimen for the administration of the drug? With chemotherapeutic agents the initial diagnosis will often be straightforward – as our ability to identify accurately the pathogenic agent has improved, be it a bacterium, parasite or virus, so the physician's task in correctly ascribing the most suitable treatment has simplified. In contrast, the selection of the most appropriate dosage protocol may often be far from trivial, and an error or miscalculation in its design may have serious consequences. The basis of antimicrobial therapy being one of selective toxicity – and selectivity being, by definition, never absolute – such therapy carries with it a risk of host toxicity. In addition, our increasing awareness and understanding of resistance mechanisms has highlighted the responsibilities of the physician, not only towards his current patient, but also to those who may need treatment in the future. Not only must the correct balance be struck between the effective and the toxic concentration of the drug – its therapeutic 'window' – as is the sole objective with most drug therapy, but the use of antimicrobial agents also carries the requirement of exposing the causative bacterium, virus or fungus to sublethal concentrations for the minimum possible period during the treatment protocol. It is with regard to this latter aspect that a precise and detailed knowledge of the pharmacokinetics of antimicrobial and chemotherapeutic agents attains an even greater significance.

A further difference in the use of antimicrobial drugs and those used purely as corrective agents in the treatment of physiological abnormalities (e.g. antihypertensive, anticonvulsant and oral hypoglycaemic agents) is the need to consider their pharmacokinetics with respect to the microbe itself. It is of no benefit to develop an antibiotic with good oral availability, low host toxicity and a long duration in the body if it is incapable of penetrating the bacterial cell wall or is destroyed by a bacterial enzyme. Thus the better our understanding of the fundamental pharmacokinetics of a drug, both within the host and the microbe, the greater the possibility of designing a superior agent without prejudicing the original efficacy.

Having selected the drug most appropriate to the symptoms presented, the physician must decide on the dose, route, frequency and duration of its administration. The objective of defining a pharmacokinetic profile for a given drug is to facilitate these choices by providing a rational framework for drug dosage design, without resort to the empirical approach which was, by necessity the only option before pharmacokinetic data became readily available. In general terms, the 'correct' dosage regimen is one that alleviates the symptoms, without giving rise to a toxic response – in the special case of antimicrobial agents, however, avoidance of creating conditions favourable to the development of drug resistance should also be a prime consideration. Hence, topical application of antibiotics may appeal in the treatment of burn infections, but the benefit of this mode of application must be weighed against the increased risk of resistance which it also carries.

Thus the objectives to be applied during antimicrobial therapy are to maximize blood concentration, preferably several-fold higher than the minimum inhibitory concentration (MIC) for the particular agent, but to minimize both the risk of toxicity to the patient and of promoting microbial resistance. This concept is illustrated in Figure 4.1, which shows typical plasma concentration–time profiles for an antibiotic given orally at three different doses. The target range is denoted by the area between the MIC value (approximately 15 mg/l) for the bacterium being treated and the toxic concentration of the drug; this represents the

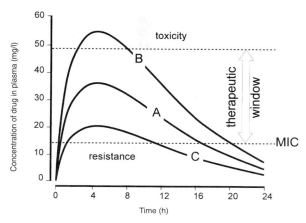

Fig. 4.1 *Plasma concentration–time curves for a hypothetical antibiotic given orally at three different doses (A–C) (see text).*

drug's therapeutic window. Ideally, the antibiotic concentration should reside within this range for as long as possible (exemplified by curve A). Curves B and C show the result of inappropriate dosage regimens; with B there is a danger of toxicity as the peak concentration enters the toxic range. Profile C demonstrates the joint dangers of underdosing, since the concentrations fall below MIC values and are thus ineffective, but in addition are sustained at subtherapeutic levels, favouring the development of resistance. Thus a knowledge of the drug's pharmacokinetic variables is essential in the accurate design of dosage regimens.

The field of antibiotic and chemotherapy covers an enormous number of disparate pharmacological agents and the extent of our knowledge of their pharmacokinetics is equally variable. In some instances the compounds are among the best studied and characterized with respect to their kinetic properties (the penicillins, dapsone and isoniazid would fall into this category), while others are still prescribed with the most rudimentary knowledge of how they will be handled by the body, as is the case with many anticancer agents. It is not the purpose of this chapter to provide a comprehensive description of the pharmacokinetics associated with all chemotherapeutic agents – such detailed information is contained within the monographs on individual agents. Rather, the aim is to outline the basic principles of pharmacokinetics and to draw on such specific examples as serve to emphasize the singular importance of pharmacokinetics in the field of antibiotic and chemotherapy.

Route of administration

There are many possible routes by which drugs are administered in the treatment of bacterial, viral or parasitic infections. Table 4.1 lists the various routes with a limited number of examples of the preparations and types of agent that appertain to each. The unrivalled ability of pathogenic microbes to colonize every possible site within the human body dictates that the ingenuity required to deliver the appropriate therapy at the correct site be equally

Table 4.1 *Routes of administration of antimicrobial agents*

Route	Site	Preparations	Examples
Topical	Eye	Ointment, drops	Chloramphenicol, tetracycline, gentamicin
	Skin	Ointment, creams, lotions, liniments, powders	Chloramphenicol, neomycin, tetracycline, gentamicin
Inhalation		Aerosols, inhalers	Gentamicin, carbenicillin
Oral		Solutions, suspensions, tablets, capsules, powders	Penicillin
Subcutaneous		Solutions	Rarely used in antimicrobial therapy
Intravenous		Solutions	Frequently used route where rapid achievement of high plasma levels are indicated. Penicillins, clindamycin, erythromycin and many other antibiotics
Intramuscular		Solutions, suspensions	Widely used for depot injections to provide slow release. Penicillins, suramin, pentamidine
Intraperitoneal		Solutions	Cephalosporins, vancomycin
Intrathecal	Lumbar	Solutions	Gentamicin, vancomycin
Intraventricular	Brain	Solutions	Amphotericin B, gentamicin
Intravitreal	Eye	Solutions	Ampicillin
Periocular	Eye	Solutions	Penicillin, neomycin
Rectal		Suppositories	Polymixin B
Vaginal		Creams, tablets, pessaries	Clotrimazole, econazole

imaginative. Consequently, antimicrobial therapy probably encompasses the widest variety of different routes of administration in medicine today. Nevertheless, by far the most common modes of dosing are the *oral, intravenous* and *intramuscular* routes. Use of other routes is generally restricted to infections at sites with poor blood supply (e.g. *topical* application to the eye) or where exceptionally high local concentrations are required. The latter is exemplified in the complicated treatment of neonatal meningitis where *intrathecal* or, in some instances *intraventricular* injections of antibiotics may be required. *Intraperitoneal* administration of antibiotics, such as vancomycin, has been used in the control of peritonitis. The *inhalation* route has limited application in antimicrobial therapy, an exception being the difficult treatment of respiratory tract infection in cystic fibrosis sufferers where long-term use of gentamicin and carbenicillin has been shown to be effective. In general, however, the factors that will dictate the choice of route are a combination of the physicochemical properties of the drug and the clinical demands of the infection itself.

Although oral administration will usually be the preferred route, with respect to convenience and expense, in the case of antibiotics and other antimicrobial agents this route is frequently unattractive because of their low or variable oral bioavailability. In addition, the extremely high plasma concentrations of antibiotics frequently required to achieve their MIC values towards certain Gram-negative bacteria may often only be achieved by direct administration close to their site of action. A further factor of particular importance to antimicrobial therapy is the avoidance of conditions favourable to the development of resistance. This consideration may also influence the choice of the most appropriate route of administration, since delayed-release preparations or other methods of dosing that favour steady-state blood concentrations, such as intravenous infusion or deep intramuscular injection, are less likely to leave the pathogens exposed to sublethal drug concentrations (conditions that promote resistance) than are bolus-dosing procedures.

The routes of administration described above, and in Table 4.1, may conveniently be divided into those in which the drug is given directly into the circulation, the *intravascular* routes (intravenous and intra-arterial administration), and those in which the drug must cross membrane barriers in order to gain access to the circulation, the *extravascular* routes (e.g. oral, intramuscular and rectal).

Basic pharmacokinetic principles

The pharmacokinetics of a drug describe the rates of the

various processes, such as absorption, distribution, metabolism and excretion (ADME) which define the blood or tissue concentration of the drug at any time point (Fig. 4.2). Ideally, it is the concentration of the drug at its site of action, for example, in the aqueous medium bathing the microbial target, which should be known; this is rarely a practicable objective. Consequently, the favoured practice is to measure concentrations at an accessible site, usually plasma, and by building up a kinetic profile within that tissue, to extrapolate to another, less accessible site. The influence of the various processes of absorption, distribution, metabolism and elimination on the pharmacokinetic profile will be considered in relation to the use of chemotherapeutic agents. Although a comprehensive description of the mathematics of pharmacokinetic modelling is outside the scope of this chapter, in order to understand the physiological processes that determine the ADME of a drug, it is necessary to consider the *drug concentration–time curve* and to describe some of the parameters and relationships that derive from such curves under various conditions. Consequently, the next section describes some important pharmacokinetic models and the concepts upon which they are based. This is followed by a detailed description of the processes of absorption, distribution, metabolism and elimination as they apply specifically to antimicrobial agents.

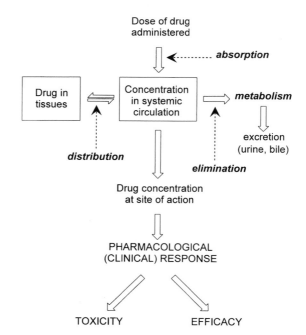

Fig. 4.2 *The influence of pharmacokinetic factors (absorption, distribution, metabolism and elimination) on the pharmacodynamics and toxicity of drugs.*

Pharmacokinetic models

Several of the parameters used in the following description of ADME are the product of a rigorous mathematical treatment of the theoretical behaviour of small chemicals in a biological environment. For example, the ability to estimate the hypothetical plasma concentration of a drug at time zero, $C_{(0)}$*, relies on the pharmacokinetics of the drug conforming to a prescribed pattern, in other words that it fits to a predefined pharmacokinetic model, since the true $C_{(0)}$ cannot be measured. Compartmental modelling, in which the body is visualized as a collection of homogeneous compartments, formed the basis of theoretical pharmaco-kinetics until the mid-1970s when a more physiological approach, based on clearance concepts, was developed by Benet, Wilkinson and others (Tozer 1981). For the purposes of a clinically orientated, practically based discussion of antimicrobial pharmacokinetics such as this, a comprehensive mathematical description of pharmacokinetic modelling is unwarranted. Nevertheless, the derivation of several pharmacokinetic parameters requires the employment, whether consciously or otherwise, of at least an elementary theoretical analysis, and thus a brief description of such systems is required.

Intravenous administration

Figure 4.3 shows the simplest pharmacokinetic situation in which a drug, given intravenously, distributes into a single homogeneous compartment and is eliminated directly from that compartment under linear conditions. In this case, a plot of plasma concentration against time (Fig. 4.4a) will show an exponential fall, such that the rate of elimination decreases with concentration. A plot of log(plasma concentration) against time (Fig. 4.4b), however, will be linear and the values of $C_{(0)}$ and the half-life, $t_{1/2}$, can be

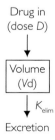

Drug in
(dose D)

Volume
(Vd)

K_{elim}

Excretion

Fig. 4.3 *The one-compartment model.*

*The abbreviations used for pharmacokinetic parameters in this chapter conform as closely as possible to the guidelines suggested by the American College of Clinical Pharmacology as modified by Aronson et al (1988).

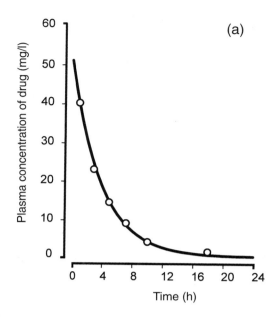

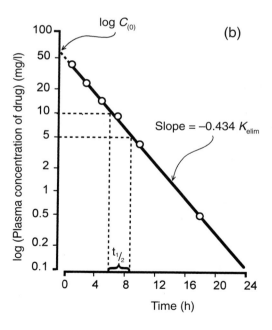

Fig. 4.4 *(a) Plasma concentration–time curve for an antibiotic given intravenously. The concentration falls exponentially such that the rate of elimination is directly proportional to the concentration. (b) A log(plasma concentration) versus time plot gives a straight line, indicating that the pharmacokinetics are described by the one-compartment model shown in Fig. 4.3.*

estimated directly as the intercept on the ordinate axis and the time taken for the plasma concentration to fall by 50%, respectively. The rate constant for elimination (K_{elim}) is then simply related to the slope of the line

$$\text{Slope} = \ln 2. \, K_{elim} = -0.434 \, . \, K_{elim}$$

and

$$t_{1/2} = \frac{0.693}{K_{elim}}$$

The calculation of half-lives and volumes of distribution quoted in the literature for most drugs are based on this model. However, in almost all cases at least two compartments are required to describe adequately the pharmacokinetic profile of a drug, since distribution is rarely confined to the circulation, and diffusion of drug to its equilibrium state will take a finite time; a period known as the *distribution phase*. Generally this will occur relatively rapidly and will thus be missed if blood sampling times are not sufficiently close to the injection time. Under these circumstances the half-life determined will only represent the elimination phase and should more accurately be described as the *elimination half life*, $t_{1/2,elim}$.

In practical terms, for most antimicrobial therapy, parameters such as the distribution half-life and the volume of the central compartment, which can be determined using a multicompartmental approach, are of theoretical interest only; thus, where the plasma concentrations may be described adequately by a one-compartment analysis, a more sophisticated treatment is unwarranted. However, many drugs do not conveniently fit with this model and a second, tissue compartment must be added, into which drug can distribute, but cannot be eliminated (Fig. 4.5). For a two-compartment model such as this a plot of log(plasma concentration) versus time gives a non-linear relationship. In this case it is important to be able to distinguish the elimination of the drug from the background distribution and thus 'dissect out' a value for the elimination half-life. This is achieved by the *method of residuals* as indicated in Figure 4.6. This method also allows a steady-state value of V_d ($V_{d,ss}$)

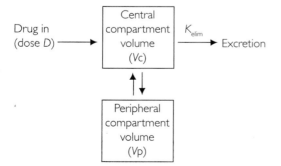

Fig. 4.5 The two-compartment model.

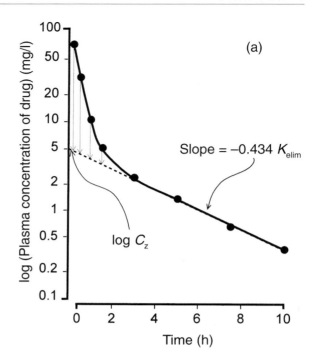

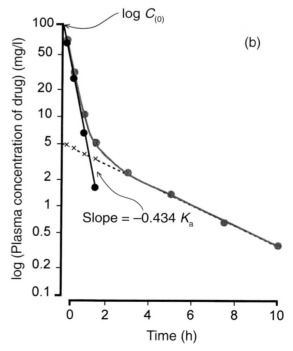

Fig. 4.6 The method of residuals. (a) Plot of log(plasma concentration) vs time for an antibiotic given intravenously and conforming to a two-compartment model. (b) Plot of the residual values representing the distribution phase. (K_d).

to be calculated since the apparent $C_{(0)}$ at equilibrium may be extrapolated from the terminal log-linear portion of the graph.

Oral administration

Although intravascular administration is widely used in antimicrobial therapy, by far the most common method of administration is via the oral route which, as with all extravascular routes, results in an additional absorption phase. The simplest way to model the kinetics of a drug following oral administration is to represent the absorption phase as an additional compartment (Fig. 4.7), from which drug can gain access to the central compartment at a rate determined by the *absorption constant, K_a*. Figure 4.8 shows how this alters the concentration–time profile, compared

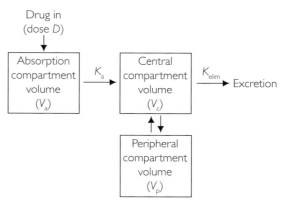

Fig. 4.7 *Modification of the two-compartment model to accommodate an absorption phase.*

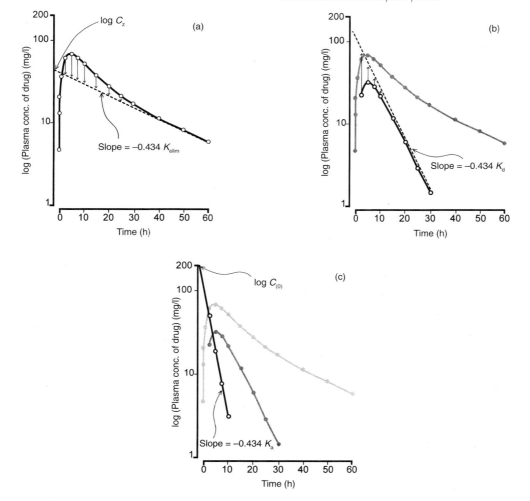

Fig. 4.8 *The method of residuals after oral administration. (a) Plot of log(plasma concentration) versus time for an antibiotic given orally and conforming to a two-compartment model. (b) Plot of the residual values representing a combination of the absorption and distribution phases. (c) Plot of another set of residual concentrations.*

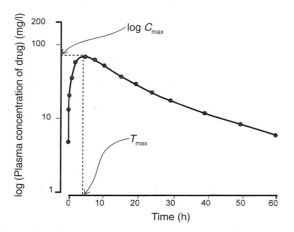

Fig. 4.9 *Plasma concentration–time curve following oral administration, indicating the values of* C_{max} *and* T_{max}.

immediately accessible to the practising clinician. The central core of these methods is the parameter clearance (CL) which may be obtained from the area under the concentration–time curve (AUC), calculated from the plasma concentration–time curve using the trapezoidal rule without resort to the assumptions upon which compartmental analyses are based. Calculation of AUC then allows the use of the simple relationship

$$CL = \frac{Dose}{AUC}$$

to estimate clearance, an extremely powerful parameter for describing the kinetics of a drug. The clearance of a drug is defined as the *volume of plasma or blood from which drug is entirely removed per unit time*, and thus it has the same units as flow. Its advantage over half-life as a descriptor of drug elimination is its independence of the volume of distribution. The equation:

$$t_{1/2} = \frac{0.693 \times V_d}{CL}$$

indicates the hybrid nature of half-life which can be altered by a change in either V_d or CL. Moreover, as in some disease states where a decrease in elimination can be accompanied by an increase in V_d (e.g. through a change in protein binding), such opposing influences on CL and V_d may leave the half-life unaltered whilst the concentration of the drug at its site of action is markedly different from the non-disease state.

The apparently simple relationship dose/AUC gives a value for total body clearance; however, this parameter is in fact the sum of several different clearance processes, such as renal clearance (CL_R), and clearance by other organs (e.g. hepatic clearance, CL_H). Another important parameter is *intrinsic clearance* (Cl_{int}), which is the *maximum clearance possible by an organ if blood flow is not limiting*, and may be used to link in vitro and in vivo elimination data as the ratio of the Michaelis–Menten parameters, V_{max}/K_m, gives an estimate of intrinsic clearance. It is important to note that the clearance calculated after oral administration will be influenced by the drug's bioavailability, *F* (see below), since the true CL is only obtained when the AUC is calculated following intravenous administration ($AUC_{i.v.}$) and $AUC_{oral} = F.AUC_{i.v.}$. Consequently, the value of CL obtained from the equation dose/AUC_{oral} is referred to as the *apparent oral clearance*.

with intravenous dosing, and indicates how the method of residuals can again be used to obtain K_a. Figure 4.8a shows the original log(plasma concentration) versus time curve, which becomes linear as absorption and distribution are completed, allowing the final elimination phase to be back-extrapolated to provide the equilibrium plasma concentration, C_z. Plotting the residuals between the original data and this extrapolated line gives a second curve (Fig. 4.8b), which again becomes linear as distribution outlasts absorption. Repeating the residual procedure gives a third line (Fig. 4.8c), the slope of which is proportional to the absorption rate constant. Two further parameters that may be derived following extravascular administration, and that are commonly cited with respect to antimicrobial agents, are the maximum plasma concentration, C_{max}, and the time taken to achieve that concentration, T_{max}. As is readily appreciated from Figure 4.9, these parameters are very simply obtained from the plasma-concentration curve, and again they assume greater importance in the field of antimicrobial therapy where it is of paramount importance that the C_{max} value falls within the therapeutic window. Appendix 4.1 gives C_{max} and T_{max} values for some of the commonly used antimicrobial agents related to a typical oral dose.

Model independent methods

In the wake of the classical pharmacokinetic modellers followed a school of physiological pharmacokineticists who attempted to describe the behaviour of a drug in terms of the actual functions of the body rather than hypothetical interconnecting boxes. Although there are limitations and complexities inherent to this approach, it has led to the development of concepts and parameters which are more

Renal clearance

Renal clearance is calculated from the rate of urine formation and the ratio of the concentrations of the drug in urine, $[drug]_u$, and in plasma, $[drug]_p$, according to the relationship

$$CL_R = \frac{[drug]_u}{[drug]_p} \times \text{Urine flow rate}$$

This value may then be usefully compared with the glomerular filtration rate (GFR) to give the ratio:

$$\text{Clearance ratio} = \frac{CL_R}{GFR}$$

A ratio greater than unity indicates that tubular secretion has occurred. Equally, values less than 1 suggest a degree of tubular reabsorption. For drugs whose elimination is exclusively via urinary excretion, such as the amino-glycosides and many of the cephalosporins, their renal clearance is directly proportional to the elimination rate constant, and this relationship may be used to estimate the volume of distribution of the drug:

$$K_{elim} = \frac{CL_R}{V_d}$$

Repeated administration and continuous infusion

Most drugs used to treat microbial infections are given more than once during a dosage regimen; it is therefore important to understand how the kinetics of a drug change with repeated administration. This will ensure that the correct interval between dosage and, if necessary, any alteration in size of dose can be made to maintain efficacy but diminish the possibility of toxicity and resistance occurring.

If, upon repeated administration, the drug from the previous dose is not completely cleared before the next dose is administered, drug will accumulate in the body until the rate of elimination equals the rate of excretion. In this case a plot of plasma concentrations against time will appear as shown in Figure 4.10.

At this time, the drug plasma concentration reaches an equilibrium, or steady-state concentration, the value of which can be calculated from a knowledge of the half-life, bioavailability (if given orally) and volume of distribution of the drug. Thus the steady-state concentration

$$C_{ss} = 1.44 \times \frac{t_{1/2} \cdot F \cdot \text{Dose}}{V_d \cdot i}$$

where i is the time interval between dosing. In practice, the rule of thumb that steady state is achieved within three half-lives of the drug is a reasonable working approximation. A second dosage strategy that is frequently applicable, particularly with antibiotics, is the *continuous intravenous infusion*. This procedure has effectively the same result as repeated administrations; however, a smooth increase in plasma concentration is obtained, without the peaks and troughs associated with discrete dosage regimens. Where very rapid attainment of steady state is required, in severe

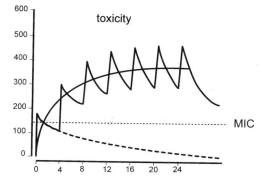

Fig. 4.10 *Multiple dosing and continuous infusion of a drug by intravenous administration. Equivalent doses given every 4 h results in the typical 'peak and trough' profile which eventually oscillates about the steady state value when the rate of elimination is equal to the rate of administration. Typically, this is achieved after 3–4 half-lives of the drug. The value of an optimized repeated dosing schedule is highlighted by the maintenance of both peak and trough concentrations within the therapeutic window. In contrast, the profile of a single intravenous dose (broken line and shaded area) remains within the sub-MIC range for most of the duration, with the associated risk of promoting resistance. The infusion curve (full line) gives a smooth increase to steady state.*

infections or if the drug has an inordinately long half-life, it is customary to give a loading dose followed by a maintenance infusion. Usually the loading dose will be two to three times the size of the maintenance dose.

Absorption

Although the term 'absorption' is used loosely to describe the process whereby a drug gains entry to the circulation, it applies only in situations in which the drug must cross a plasma membrane. Thus the choice of route of administration will determine whether or not an absorption phase occurs.

Extravascular administration

For all extravascular routes, absorption is a prerequisite for antimicrobial activity, assuming that the drug has not been administered directly to the site of infection, as is the case with some antifungal agents. For absorption to occur the drug must be in solution, and consequently the choice of *enteral* (sublingual, oral or rectal) rather than *parenteral* administration will be dictated largely by the physico-chemical properties of the drug under the various conditions that it experiences during its passage through the gastrointestinal tract.

For a drug to pass through the lipid bilayer that constitutes the plasma membranes of all cells it must be un-ionized and, preferably, strongly lipophilic. The degree of ionization will be influenced by the ambient pH and will be determined by the pK_a of the drug according to the Henderson–Hasselbach equation.

For an acidic drug:

$$pK_a - pH = \frac{\log [\text{un-ionized}]}{\log [\text{ionized}]}$$

For a basic drug:

$$pH - pK_a = \frac{\log [\text{un-ionized}]}{\log [\text{ionized}]}$$

Put into words, these relationships tell us that the drug's pK_a is equivalent to the pH at which half of it is in the ionized state and half in the un-ionized, lipophilic state. The effect of altering the pH above or below the pK_a of the drug will depend on whether the compound is acidic or basic. For example, a weakly acidic drug such as benzylpenicillin (pK_a 2.8) would be 50% ionized at pH 2.8, but this degree of ionization would rise rapidly as the pH rose, such that at pH 3.8 only 5% is un-ionized and at pH 4.8 only 0.5%. Thus small variations in the pH within the stomach, which is normally at around pH 3.0, will have a profound effect on the degree of ionization, and consequently on the proportion of the drug that is free to pass through lipid membranes. For weakly basic drugs the reverse situation applies, such that as the pH rises, so the fraction of the drug in the un-ionized state will increase. In theory, these considerations suggest that absorption from the stomach would be favoured by weak acids, whereas the almost neutral conditions found in the upper gastro-intestinal tract might only be amenable to the absorption of more basic compounds. In practice this is only partly true. The conditions experienced by a chemical during its passage through the gastro-intestinal (GI) tract are not those of static equilibria. The extensive blood supply to these organs ensures that drug is rapidly removed from the vicinity, thereby maintaining a permanent concentration gradient which favours absorption of any un-ionized drug, regardless of how small a fraction of the whole this represents. This fact, coupled with the uniquely fashioned architecture of the small intestine, whose microvilli present an enormous surface area across which absorption can occur (1000 times greater than that of the stomach) make this organ the predominant site of absorption for virtually all orally administered drugs. Drugs which are not suitable for oral administration – unless their intended site of action is within the gut lumen itself – include both strongly acid or basic drugs with pK_a values that are so low or high, respectively, that ionization is virtually total at any pH encountered within the GI tract. Appendix 4.2 gives pK_a values for some of the more commonly prescribed antimicrobial agents.

Bioavailability

The bioavailability, *F*, of a drug is defined as the *fraction of the administered dose that is absorbed intact*. The precise pharmacokinetic derivation of the term is shown below. Clearly a drug that has low lipophilicity or is charged at the pH values encountered in the GI tract will display low or even negligible bioavailability and there are several drugs which fall into this category among the commonly used antibiotics. The monobactam antibiotics and the polycationic aminoglycosides are examples of drugs whose oral availability is less than 1%. Where oral administration is clearly inappropriate for a particular agent, an alternative, albeit less convenient, route can be adopted. A situation that presents more of a problem to the clinician is inconsistent and unpredictable absorption, since ineffective plasma levels may result. There are several reasons for low bioavailability of lipophilic drugs that would otherwise be well absorbed. The principal cause is lack of stability within the GI tract. The chemical alteration of an antimicrobial drug may occur in the GI tract by one of three mechanisms. First, it may be intrinsically unstable at the various pH values within the gut lumen; examples being the penicillins and other β-lactam antibiotics which are subject to acid hydrolysis in the stomach. Secondly, it may undergo enzyme-mediated biotransformation, either by host enzymes, such as trypsin, or by enzymes present in the gut microflora. Thirdly, an interaction may occur with a co-administered drug or a food component. The well-documented example of tetracycline serves to illustrate this mechanism. Low bioavailability has been shown when either milk or antacids are taken with tetracyclines, and this phenomenon is caused by complexation of the antibiotic with Ca^{2+} or Al^{3+} ions originating in the milk or antacid, respectively (see p. 105).

Other factors that can alter the extent of bioavailability are the sheer size of the molecule and the presence of food in the intestine. Neomycin, a compound with a molecular weight of over 700 kDa, is so slowly absorbed because of its size that the normal 2–4 h passage time through the small intestine is insufficient for complete absorption. The influence of food is less predictable. In many cases the increased blood flow and gut motility caused by ingestion of food will enhance absorption. However, in general, the presence of food will impair absorption through a combination of complexation with food constituents, reduced access of drug to the site of absorption and delayed gastric emptying.

Poor and erratic absorption have both therapeutic and cost implications. Consequently, several methods have been employed in an effort to minimize such problems. These include enteric coating of tablets of compounds that are unstable in the stomach, to allow them to pass securely into the small intestine before being released. An obvious problem with this approach is the variable rate of gastric emptying which may delay release of the drug by several hours and thus disrupt the predicted dosage schedule. More complex slow-release preparations have also been developed to overcome the problem of poor and erratic absorption, but with these there is the danger of too rapid release, resulting in potentially toxic plasma drug concentrations (Pratt & Taylor 1990).

More successful has been the chemical modification of a drug to produce a compound with similar pharmacology but enhanced oral stability. This has been achieved in the case of penicillin with the various analogues, such as phenoxymethylpenicillin (penicillin V), which are active orally although their activity is slightly different from benzylpenicillin itself. Another approach is to produce a *pro-drug*, which lacks intrinsic activity but is chemically 'programmed' to release the active species once it has safely

negotiated the perils of the GI tract. Benzathine penicillin exemplifies the principle of prodrug design and clinical use.

Enzymatic transformation of drugs given orally is not restricted to the lumen of the GI tract. It can also occur in the epithelial cells of the gastric mucosa, in the blood draining from the mesentery into the hepatic portal vein or, and in particular, in the liver (see below) before reaching the systemic circulation (Fig. 4.11). Reduced bioavailability due to one of these mechanisms is referred to as the *first-pass effect* and is probably the largest source of 'lost' pharmacological activity for orally active drugs. Table 4.2 shows the percentage first-pass elimination for some commonly used antimicrobial agents.

A strategy for avoiding the hepatic first-pass effect has been to administer drugs with low bioavailability at the extremes of the GI tract. Sublingual administration results

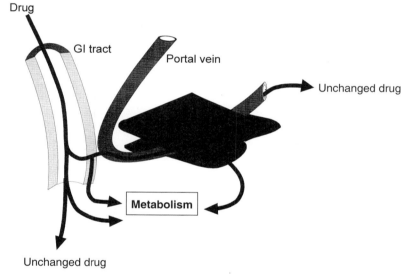

Fig. 4.11   *Schematic diagram illustrating the anatomical relationship between the liver and the gastrointestinal tract. Drug entering the gastrointestinal tract is absorbed either from the stomach or from the small intestine, and passes via the mesenteric blood supply into the hepatic portal vein. Thus orally administered drug must pass through the liver, the principal site of drug metabolism, before gaining access to the systemic circulation. Consequently, drugs that readily undergo hepatic metabolism may be substantially cleared during this first pass through the liver. In addition, metabolism may occur in the lumen or in the wall of the GI tract.*

Table 4.2   *Pharmacokinetic parameters for some commonly used antimicrobial agents. (Data collated from various sources, principally Dollery et al 1991)*

Agent	Oral availability (%)	First pass (%)	Half-life, $t_{1/2}$ (h)	Volume of distribution (l/kg)	Protein binding (%)
Aminoglycosides					
Amikacin	Negligible	NA	2.2–2.5	0.2–0.3	<10
Gentamicin	Negligible	NA	2.3	0.3	<5
Kanamycin	Poor	NA	1–4	0.2	25
Neomycin	<5	NA	2	0.3	20
Streptomycin	0–40	0	2.4–9	1.4	33
Tobramycin	Poor	NA	2.3	0.3	10

Table 4.2 *Cont'd*

Agent	Oral availability (%)	First pass (%)	Half-life, $t_{1/2}$ (h)	Volume of distribution (l/kg)	Protein binding (%)
Antifungal agents					
Amphotericin B	Negligible	NA	24–48	4	90–97
Fluconazole	>90	<5	30	0.6	11
Flucytosine	100	<20	3	1	4
Griseofulvin	Variable	NA	9.5–21	1.3	NA
Itraconazole	>85	NA	20	10.7	99
Ketoconazole	Variable	High	6–10	0.4	99
Miconazole	20	NA	24	20	91–93
Terbinafine	80	NA	11–17	14	99
Anthelmintics					
Diethylcarbamazine	>90	NA	10	1.5–5	Negligible
Mebendazole	5–10	80	1.4–5.3	1–1.2	95
Oxamniquine	Good	NA	1–1.3	NA	NA
Praziquantel	>90	High	1.5	NA	80
Antimycobacterial agents					
Clofazimine	20–85	NA	250	NA	NA
Dapsone	>90	NA	27	NA	50
Ethambutol	80	NA	10–15	4	10–40
Isoniazid	~100	Variable	0.5–2 (>6.5*)	0.6–0.8	Negligible
Pyrazinamide	Extensive	NA	10–24	NA	50
Antiprotozoal agents					
Amodiaquine	High	Extensive	5.2	NA	Extensive
Chloroquine	100	NA	30–60 days	200	50–70
Mefloquine	75–80	Negligible	15–37 days	16–25	>95
Pyrimethamine	Good	NA	85	3	87
Quinine	>80	<10	8.7	1.5	70–90
Suramin	Very poor	NA	36–60 days	0.3–1.2	99.7
Antiviral agents					
Acyclovir	13–21	0	1.5–6.3	NA	9.2
Amantadine	>90	0	11.8	10.4	65
Ganciclovir	NA	NA	3.6	1	<2
Idoxuridine	Negligible	NA	30	NA	0
Zidovudine	>90	25–40	1	1.6	34–38
β-Lactams					
Aztreonam	1	NA	1.7	0.2	56
Clavulanic acid	75	NA	1	NA	30
Cephalosporins					
Cefaclor	NA	NA	48 min	0.4	25
Cefamandole	100	NA	0.5–1.5	0.3	65–74
Cefixime	60	NA	3	0.1	70
Cefotaxime	Negligible	NA	1.3	NA	40
Cefotetan	NA	NA	2.8–4	0.1–0.2	88
Cefoxitin	Nil	NA	1	0.1–0.2	65–80
Cefuroxime	NA	NA	1.2	NA	6–15
Cephalexin	80–100	0	1	0.2	65
Cephalothin	NA	NA	0.6	0.3	<10
Cephradine	Good	0	2–3	0.3	53
Chloramphenicol					
Chloramphenicol	80–90	Negligible	5	0.2–2	97
Fusidanes					
Fusidic acid	100	0	9	0.15	97
Macrolides					
Erythromycin	NA	NA	1–1.5	0.75	73–93
Spiramycin	Variable	NA	3–7	5.5	15

Table 4.2 Cont'd

Agent	Oral availability (%)	First pass (%)	Half-life, $t_{1/2}$ (h)	Volume of distribution (l/kg)	Protein binding (%)
Nitrofurans					
Nitrofurantoin	95	Negligible	0.75	0.6	60–77
Penicillins					
Amoxycillin	90	Negligible	1	0.3	20
Ampicillin	30–40	Negligible	1–2	0.4	20
Azlocillin	0	NA	1	0.2	28
Benzyl penicillin	2–30	NA	0.8	0.50	50
Carbenicillin	0	NA	1–1.5	0.2	50
Cloxacillin	40–70	Negligible	0.5–1	0.1–0.2	94
Flucloxacillin	>80	NA	0.5–1.5	0.1–0.3	95
Mecillinam	<10	NA	1	0.2–0.4	5–10
Peptides					
Polymixin B	Negligible	NA	6	NA	Low
Vancomycin	Very low	NA	5–11	0.6	50
Quinolones					
Cinoxacin	95	NA	1.5	0.2	63
Ciprofloxacin	50–84	NA	3–4	2.9	30
Enoxacin	NA	NA	5–7	2.5–3	35–51
Nalidixic acid	>90	Minimal	1.5	0.4	93
Norfloxacin	50–80	NA	3	2.5–3.1	15
Rifamycins					
Rifampicin	Extensive	<10	3.4	1	60–80
Sulphonamides					
Sulphadiazine	100	13–38	10	0.4	20–55
Sulphadimidine	>95	NA	1.5 (5.5*)	0.6	90
Sulphamethoxazole	100	NA	7–12	0.2	65
Sulphasalazine	20–30	70–80	6	NA	95–99
Sulphinpyrazone	90–100	NA	6	0.6	98–99
Tetracyclines					
Doxycycline	93	NA	20	1–2	82–93
Oxytetracycline	60	Negligible	9.2	NA	27–35
Tetracycline	Variable	0	8.5	1.3	36–50

NA, data not available.
*Value in patients phenotyped as slow acetylators.

in the drug gaining access directly to the superior vena cava, whilst rectal use of suppositories also avoids the liver, since the middle and lower haemorrhoidal veins, which supply the rectum, drain directly into the inferior vena cava. However, neither route produces reproducible availability profiles, and thus both are of little applicability in antimicrobial therapy.

Distribution

The manner in which a drug distributes throughout the body tissues, following entry to the systemic circulation, is controlled by the same characteristics that determine its absorption from the site of administration. Lipophilic, non-polar compounds, which pass readily through plasma membranes, will have the potential to diffuse throughout the body, while more hydrophilic, highly polar or charged compounds will be restricted to extracellular sites and denied access to deep tissue compartments. Thus, in theory, the simple biophysics of diffusion can be used to predict the disposition of a drug away from its port of entry. In practice, other factors need to be considered, in particular the affinity of the drug for various endogenous macromolecules, notably the proteins (both soluble and cellular) in blood. Mathematically, the volume available to a drug for distribution (volume of distribution) is described by the relationship between dose and plasma concentration, such that

$$V_d = \frac{\text{Dose}}{C_{(0)}}$$

where V_d is the volume of distribution and $C_{(0)}$ is the concentration in plasma at time zero. Normally the value of V_d for a given drug will be recorded as litres per kilogram (this will only apply when the units of dose and $C_{(0)}$ are mass per kilogram and mass per litre, respectively). It is important to note that a drug's true volume of distribution would be almost impossible to determine and that the value obtained using the above equation is an *apparent* volume, for the following reasons: (1) the concentration $C_{(0)}$ at time zero is fictive and cannot be measured directly, but is derived by extrapolation from plasma concentrations measured at subsequent time points; and (2) it is implicit in the above equation that the concentration throughout the body is uniform and equivalent, at all time points, to the concentration in the sampled body fluid, normally plasma.

Since there are very few drugs whose distribution is not influenced by interactions with proteins or other macromolecules, a V_d value should be regarded, at best, as an approximation of the drug's true distribution; in other cases the apparent V_d will bear no relation to the actual physiological distribution of a drug, and can be used only to deduce other aspects of its pharmacokinetic profile, such as an extremely high degree of plasma protein binding ($V_d < 0.06$ l/kg, the plasma volume), or extensive distribution throughout a tissue compartment ($V_d > 0.55$ l/kg, the volume of total body water). The physiological volume of extracellular fluid is approximately 0.2 l/kg; therefore, drugs whose lipophilicity is not sufficient to allow diffusion through plasma membranes will be restricted to a volume equivalent to or less than this value. As can be seen from Table 4.2, the apparent volumes of distribution of antimicrobial agents vary widely. Although none is so low as to represent complete retention within the plasma, some of the penicillins and most of the cephalosporins have V_d values of less than 0.5 l/kg, due predominantly to their high level of plasma protein binding. Other classes of antimicrobial agents are less homogeneous with respect to their V_d values; for example, the antifungal agents for which factors other than the extent of protein binding must dictate their distribution. At the opposite end of the spectrum fall the antiprotozoal agents (a structurally diverse group of compounds) whose V_d values range from under 1.0 l/kg (e.g. suramin, a drug almost exclusively bound to plasma albumin) (Karbwang & Harinasuta 1992), through to values that exceed 100 l/kg (as seen with chloroquine) which represent some of the highest apparent V_d values seen for any group of agents. Such grossly unphysiological apparent V_d values can only reflect a high degree of tissue sequestration, and this is reinforced by the inordinately long plasma half-lives seen with these drugs which, in the case of chloroquine, can exceed 30 days (Edwards et al 1988).

Plasma protein binding

The proteins contained in the plasma not only play an essential role in maintaining the osmolality of the blood but, in addition, act as transporters for a variety of endogenous compounds, including vitamin C, steroids, bilirubin and several metal ions. As such, they possess structures amenable to the binding of ligands, and consequently it is no surprise that most drugs are, to some extent, found associated with plasma proteins in the circulation. Albumin is generally the most significant of the plasma proteins where drug binding is considered, although other proteins can be equally important in the case of specific drugs. Albumin carries an overall negative charge, and would therefore be expected to bind basic drugs preferentially. Although it is involved in the binding of a wide range of such drugs, this generally involves low-affinity, high-capacity binding. In contrast, binding of acidic drugs may be of extremely high affinity, though the number of binding sites is usually low. Lipophilic compounds are also readily accepted by albumin due to the presence of a large number of lipophilic amino acid side-chains on the molecule. Thus albumin may be regarded as a fairly universal ligand-carrier system and this is reflected in the high fractional binding values shown by many of the drugs listed in Table 4.2. In addition to albumin, the plasma contains at least 100 different proteins, some in quite high concentrations; however, the contribution made by these proteins to the overall binding is largely unknown. A major exception to this is the globulin α_1-acid glycoprotein, which has been shown to have important binding sites for basic drugs. Within the antimicrobial field, drugs for which α_1-acid glycoprotein binding has been shown to be a major factor include erythromycin and quinidine.

With respect to drug disposition, there is no doubt that plasma protein binding is a major determinant of the distribution of a drug. Frequently, compounds show a far higher affinity for albumin than for any other tissue proteins, and consequently the pharmacological effect achieved – usually regarded as a function of the *unbound* drug concentration – will be heavily influenced by the extent to which the drug is retained within the central compartment. It might be expected, therefore, that displacement of drug from its plasma protein binding sites would result in toxicological sequelae for drugs with a narrow therapeutic index. In practice, predicting the effect of altered protein binding is a complex procedure and depends on several drug specific variables (Katzung 1995). Primary amongst these is whether the clearance of the drug is *restricted* by its binding to plasma proteins, such that only free drug is eliminated, or whether the drug is stripped from its binding sites as it passes through the liver (*non-restrictive* elimination). For a full description of the effects of altered

Table 4.3 *Effect of plasma protein binding on drug pharmacokinetics: comparison of the likely effects of decreased binding to plasma proteins on the main pharmacokinetic parameters of drugs that are cleared by restrictive or non-restrictive elimination (Adapted from Lindup 1987)*

Elimination	AUC	CL	V_d	$t_{1/2}$
Restrictive	↓	↑	↑	↓
Non-restrictive	↔	↔	↑	↑

plasma binding on drug pharmacokinetics the reader is referred to Rowland & Tozer (1989). Suffice to say here that an increased pharmacological effect is not always a predictable outcome of binding displacement, and where there is a possibility of a drug–drug interaction at the level of protein binding no alteration of dosage should be implemented without a clear understanding of the pharmacokinetic profiles of both drugs. Table 4.3 summarizes the likely effects of decreased binding on the pharmacokinetics of drugs that show restrictive (or flow-dependent) and non-restrictive (flow-independent) extraction by the liver.

The number of drug–drug interactions resulting in enhanced pharmacological effect or toxicity is probably greatly overstated and, upon closer examination, usually result from a change in some other function such as metabolism or renal elimination which, coupled with the change in binding, produces the observed interaction. Nevertheless, such multiple effects often go hand in hand, since binding interactions with proteins are·involved in the processes of renal secretion and drug metabolism, as well as plasma binding. In addition, several disease states may cause a change in plasma proteins, including renal, hepatic and inflammatory conditions, and again these are often associated with alterations in other aspects of drug handling, such as metabolism and excretion. Thus, although a change in plasma binding is rarely the major factor in determining the pharmacokinetic profile of a drug, when coupled with alterations in other physiological processes, it may make a significant contribution in defining the ultimate pharmacological effect.

Metabolism

Metabolism, more precisely referred to as *biotransformation*, is an all-embracing term used to describe the various processes, resulting in the chemical alteration of a drug, used by the body to promote its excretion. The two major routes of excretion, biliary and renal, both show preferences with respect to the physicochemical properties

of the compounds eliminated via these pathways. For biliary excretion, the size of the molecule is a predominant factor, and thus metabolism frequently results in a conjugated product with a molecular weight over twice that of the original drug. For urinary excretion, the most important route quantitatively, water solubility, is paramount as lipid soluble compounds will be readily reabsorbed from the kidney tubules following glomerular filtration. Since most drugs are fairly lipophilic, to allow oral administration (see above), it is not surprising that only a small number of drugs are eliminated renally without first undergoing some form of metabolic change. Thus, the major role of drug metabolism is to decrease the lipophilicity of drugs by producing either a charged or a highly polar derivative of the parent compound. The formation of a charged, usually acidic, product has the added advantage that it may act as a substrate for tubular secretion, and thus clearance of such compounds can exceed even the glomerular filtration rate.

Drug metabolism can occur in multiple sites and organs within the body, including the gut wall, blood, kidney, lung, skin and even brain; in addition, many microbes themselves have a rudimentary drug metabolizing capacity, and this is particularly pronounced in certain of the bacteria that colonize the intestinal tract. However, by far the most significant site of drug metabolism is the liver. The anatomical location of the liver between the hepatic portal vein and the rest of the systemic circulation places it ideally to act as the body's guardian, protecting it from the accumulation of potentially toxic or bioactive xenobiotics.

Drug metabolism can be divided into two processes, referred to as pha*se* I and *phase* II (Fig. 4.12) and, although not absolute, it is convenient to think of biotransformation as occurring by these two successive stages. Phase I metabolism comprises mainly oxidation, but also encompasses reduction and hydrolysis. The structural changes involved are generally small and, although an increase in polarity is normally involved, the main function of phase I is to generate functional groups that can participate in phase II reactions. Consequently, phase II is exclusively associated with the addition of an endogenous molecular group to the drug which has been functionalized during phase I, to produce a conjugate. This molecular group

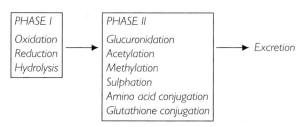

Fig. 4.12 *Classification of human drug metabolism.*

may be as small as a methyl group or a large as a tripeptide and almost always involves an increase in both size and polarity;* in addition, charged compounds are frequently produced. The process of conjugation involves the transfer of a molecular group from a chemically labile conjugating agent and is mediated by one of a large family of enzymes known as transferases. Quantitatively, the most important phase II metabolic pathway in man is glucuronidation, which involves the transfer of the large residue (glucuronic acid) from the activated donor (*uridine diphosphoglucuronic acid (UDPGA)*) to the drug by means of the enzyme glucuronyl transferase. However, sulphation, acetylation, amino acid conjugation and glutathione conjugation are also major pathways in their own right, and contribute to the metabolic profiles of many chemotherapeutic agents.

The enzymes involved in phase I metabolism are also many and varied; however, in contrast to phase II, the significance of the majority of these enzymes is dwarfed by that of a single family of enzymes referred to collectively as cytochrome P450. This group of enzymes reside in the endoplasmic reticulum of most cells and are thus referred to as microsomal enzymes; their principal location, however, is in the parenchymal cells of the liver where they constitute about 1% of the total cellular protein. Their ability both to oxidize or to reduce almost any small lipophilic molecule is only partly explained by the existence of multiple isozymic forms which constitute the family (Nelson et al 1993); equally important is the fact that the individual enzymes are among the least selective, in terms of substrate specificity, that exist in the human body. Although most reactions at a fundamental level involve an identical mechanism, whereby a single atom of oxygen is transferred from molecular oxygen to the drug, there are numerous different chemical reactions that ensue (Koymans et al 1993) including oxidations (such as hydroxylation, both aliphatic and aromatic, dealkylation, deamination, direct oxidation of nitrogen or sulphur atoms, epoxide formation and dehalogenation) as well as the reductions of azo and nitro groups. The use of molecular biology techniques has now confirmed the existence of over 200 cytochrome P450 isozymes throughout the animal kingdom (Nelson et al 1993) and more than 30 of these have been cloned from man. The major human forms are shown in Table 4.4 along with model substrates and inhibitors for each; the pie chart shows the relative amounts of each of the major isozymes found in human liver. The

Table 4.4 *The family structure of human cytochromes P450. Each of the major drug metabolizing families (CYP1 to CYP3) are listed with their subfamilies, denoted by a capital letter, and individual isozymes, signified by a final arabic numeral. Families are defined as being < 40% similar with respect to their amino acid primary sequence, subfamilies <70% similar and individual isozymes must have an identical structure within the bounds of normal random mutation. The relative proportions of each of the major isoforms in human liver is shown in this pie chart:*

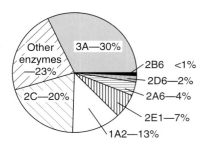

Enzyme	Substrates	Characteristics
CYP1A1	Caffeine	*Inducers:* cigarette smoke, omeprazole
CYP1A2	PAH, aromatic amines	*Inhibitor:* enoxacin
CYP2A6 CYP2C8-10	Coumarin Tolbutamide, (S)-warfarin, phenytoin	*Inducers:* phenobarbitone, rifampicin *Inhibitor:* sulphaphenazole
CYP2D6	Debrisoquine	*Inducers:* not inducible; genetic polymorphism *Inhibitor:* quinidine
CYP2E1	Ethanol, benzene, nitrosamines	
CYP3A3-6	Cyclosporin, oestrogens, nifedipine, cortisol, carbamazepine	*Inducers:* phenobarbitone, rifampicin, carbamazepine, phenytoin *Inhibitors:* ketoconazole, cimetidine

* An important exception to this general rule, in the field of antibacterial therapy, is the acetylation of sulphonamides. Acetylation is the favoured phase II mechanism for primary amines and sulphonamide groups but, unlike the products of most other conjugation reactions, the metabolites are often less soluble than the parent compounds. The kidney toxicity associated with some of the earlier sulphonamides has been attributed to crystallization of their acetylated conjugates within the kidney tubules.

existence of multiple forms was in fact well established before the advent of gene cloning, because certain individuals were shown to have a deficiency in a few specific metabolic pathways, whilst other pathways were identical to those found in the population as a whole. Intense investigation of this phenomenon revealed that the cause was a relatively common (5–10%) absence of a particular isoform of cytochrome P450, known as CYP2D6, due to a series of unrelated genetic aberrations within the individuals (Gonzalez & Meyer 1991). The significance of this discovery has not been lost on either the pharmaceutical companies or the regulatory authorities, and it is now considered of prime importance to determine the contribution, if any, of CYP2D6 to the overall metabolism of a new compound, since it is a reasonable assumption that the risk of toxicity may be elevated in those with the poor metabolizer phenotype (Brosen & Gram 1989).

Although cytochrome P450 is quantitatively the major phase I enzyme system, it is by no means exclusively responsible for the initial metabolism of antimicrobial agents. Several other enzymes are capable of oxidizing xenobiotics, including monoamine oxidase, alcohol and aldehyde dehydrogenases, xanthine oxidase (see Fig. 4.15) and amine oxidase (also known as Zeigler's enzyme). Also of particular importance to antibiotic agents are the hydrolytic enzymes, which are widely distributed in various tissues throughout the body, especially blood. A second location of importance for enzymes that carry out hydrolysis is the GI tract where the microflora may be responsible for the release of the parent compound from its glucuronide or sulphate conjugate following excretion in the bile. The hydrolysis of these phase II products is mediated by the enzymes β-glucuronidase and sulphatase, respectively. This may result in reabsorption of the deconjugated compound, a process known as *enterohepatic circulation*, which may radically increase the effective half-life of the affected drug. Hydrolysis may also play an important role in preventing the toxicity of drug metabolites, as exemplified by the enzyme epoxide hydrolase. This ubiquitous enzyme converts epoxide products of cyctochrome P450 oxidation into their corresponding dihydrodiol (see terbinafine in Figure 4.13 for an example of epoxidation and subsequent hydrolysis to the dihydrodiol) (Jensen 1989). Since epoxides are highly reactive species that have been implicated in the toxicity of many drugs and environmental pollutants, particularly carcinogenicity (Gonzalez & Gelboin 1994), epoxide hydrolysis may be viewed as a true detoxication pathway (Guenthner 1990).

Within the group of drugs that comprise antibiotics and other chemotherapeutic agents, almost all pathways of drug metabolism are represented, from the relatively common hydroxylation, deethylation and glucuronidation reactions, to the more obscure epoxidation and *N*-oxidations. As a conjugation reaction, acetylation is well represented, for example with dapsone, isoniazid and particularly among the sulphonamides. The importance of this route is amplified by the polymorphic nature of *N*-acetyl transferase which is found at very low levels in about 50% of the population. Dosage regimens may have to be closely monitored with drugs metabolized predominantly by this enzyme, as cases

of toxicity have been linked to an inability to acetylate certain drugs (Price Evans 1993).

As well as displaying multifarious metabolic reactions, antibiotics are unusual for the number of drugs which undergo little or no metabolism. This includes all the aminoglycosides, most cephalosporins and a large number of the older penicillins. A few related examples of phase I metabolic pathways that are found amongst antimicrobial agents are given in Figure 4.13 to demonstrate the diversity of enzymes and reactions that can occur. Figure 4.14 shows representative examples of pertinent phase II reactions. In each case the pathway shown may not represent the sole or even the major pathway; in contrast, Figure 4.15 shows the complete metabolic scheme for sulphasalazine, and highlights the importance of gut flora as well as the hepatic drug metabolizing enzymes in converting the parent compound into readily excretable products.

FACTORS AFFECTING DRUG METABOLISM

For the physician administering antimicrobial drugs, the main issue is not how the drug is metabolized but what factors or circumstances are likely to change the degree or extent of metabolism with the associated risk of low efficacy or toxicity. Most changes in drug metabolism may be attributed to one of two mechanisms: enzyme induction or enzyme inhibition.

Enzyme induction

Induction of drug metabolizing enzymes results in enhanced biotransformation of compounds that are substrates for the enzymes and is caused by an increase in the de novo synthesis of the enzyme apoprotein. It can be brought about either by the drug substrate itself (autoinduction) or by a variety of non-specific inducers that increase the metabolism of a large number of other compounds (heteroinduction). The best known example of the latter type is the barbiturates, such as phenobarbitone. The enzymes that have received the most attention with respect to induction and its consequences are the cytochrome P450 family, but many other enzymes involved in drug metabolism, including glucuronyl transferase, glutathione transferase and epoxide hydrolase, are susceptible to certain inducers, often iden- tical to those that increase cytochrome P450, such as phenobarbitone. Curiously, some other drug metabolizing enzymes, particularly cytosolic ones such as alcohol dehydrogenase, appear resistant to induction, and even some forms of cytochrome P450, notably CYP2D6, equally do not respond. The mechanisms involved in enzyme induction are complex and largely outside the scope of this chapter. Most involve transcriptional activation of nuclear DNA, either directly or via a cytosolic interaction with a

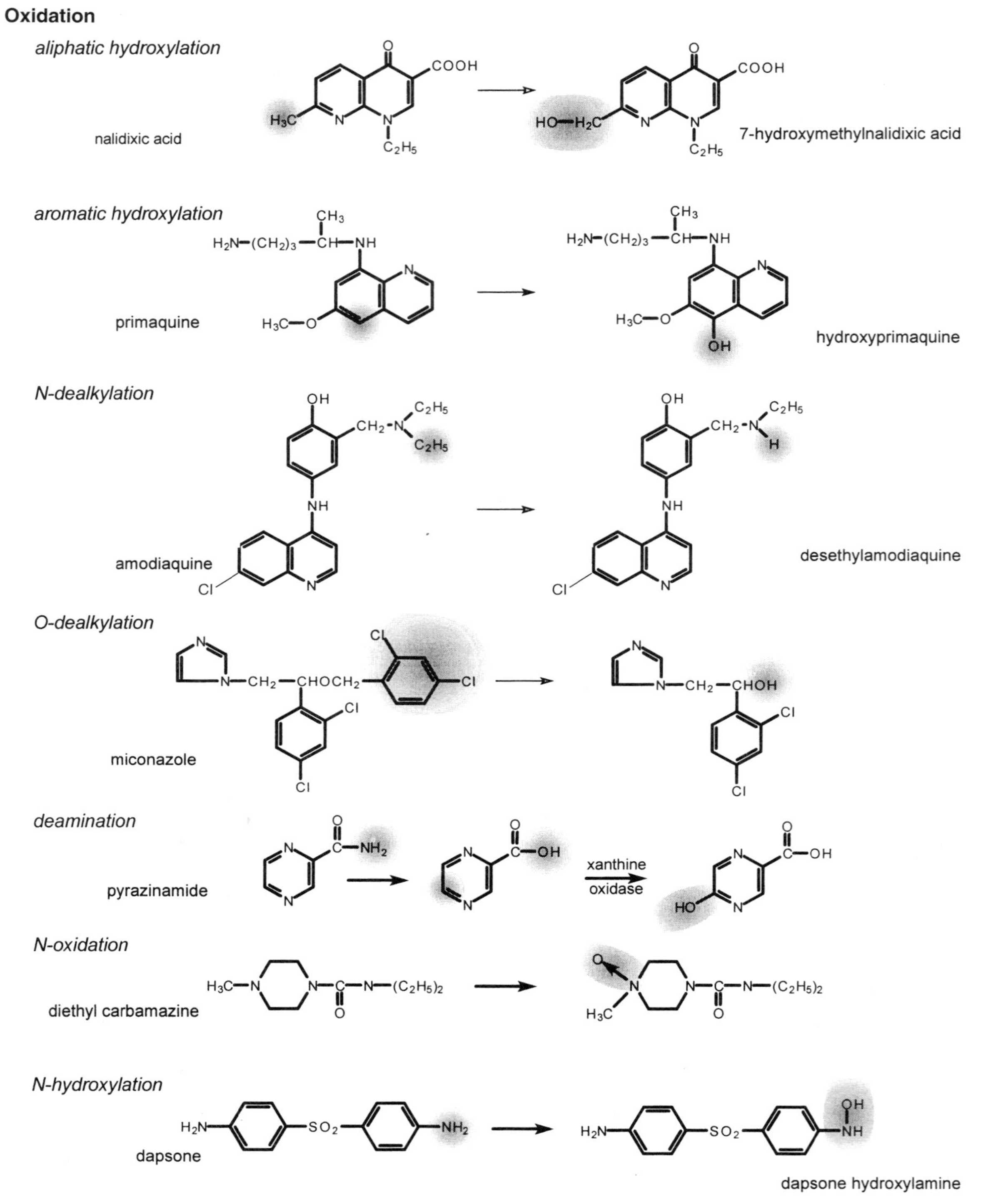

Oxidation

aliphatic hydroxylation

nalidixic acid

7-hydroxymethylnalidixic acid

aromatic hydroxylation

primaquine

hydroxyprimaquine

N-dealkylation

amodiaquine

desethylamodiaquine

O-dealkylation

miconazole

deamination

pyrazinamide

xanthine oxidase

N-oxidation

diethyl carbamazine

N-hydroxylation

dapsone

dapsone hydroxylamine

Fig. 4.13 *Phase I metabolic pathways of some commonly used antimicrobial agents. Selected examples demonstrating the variety and complexity of drug biotransformations seen with these classes of agents. Inclusion in the scheme does not imply that the given pathway is the sole, or even the major, route of metabolism for that drug.*

Reduction

nitro reduction

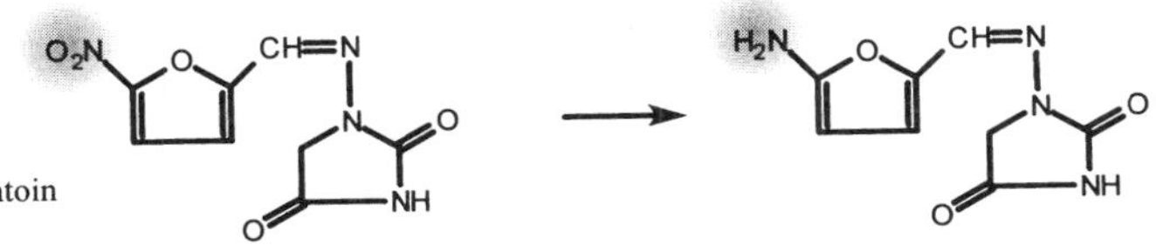

nitrofurantoin → aminofurantoin

keto reduction

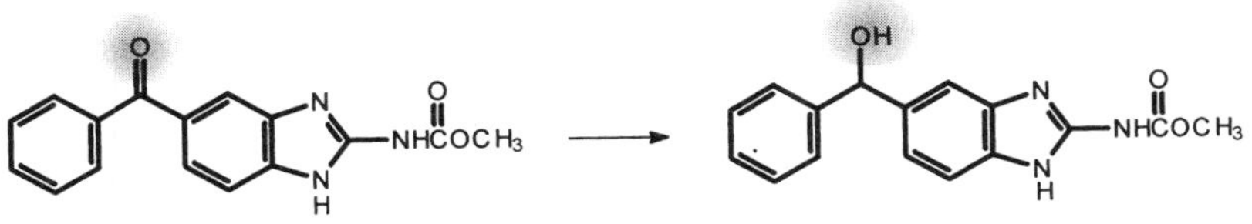

mebendazole

Hydrolysis

ester hydrolysis

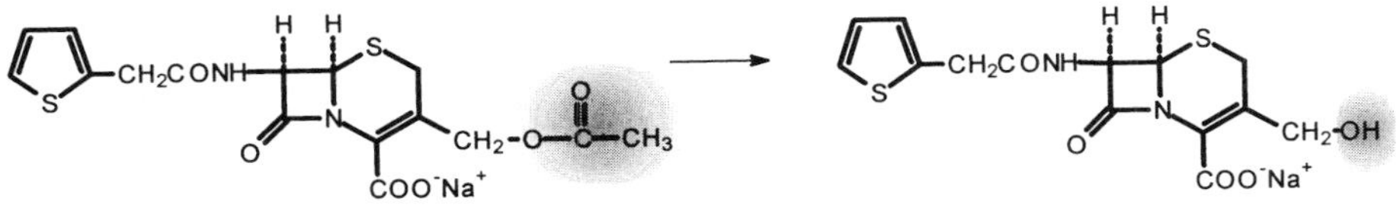

amide hydrolysis

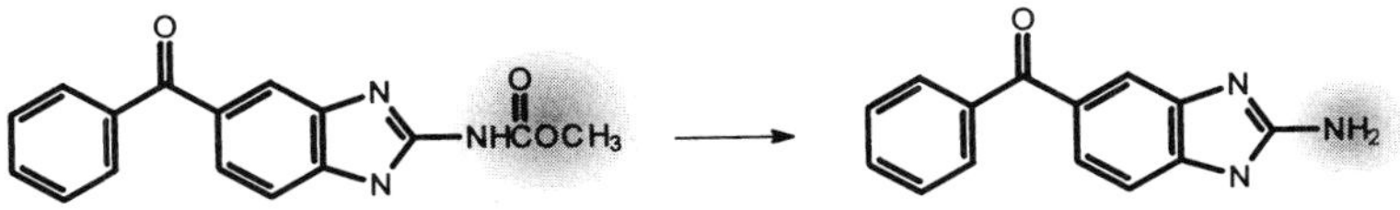

mebendazole

epoxide hydrolysis

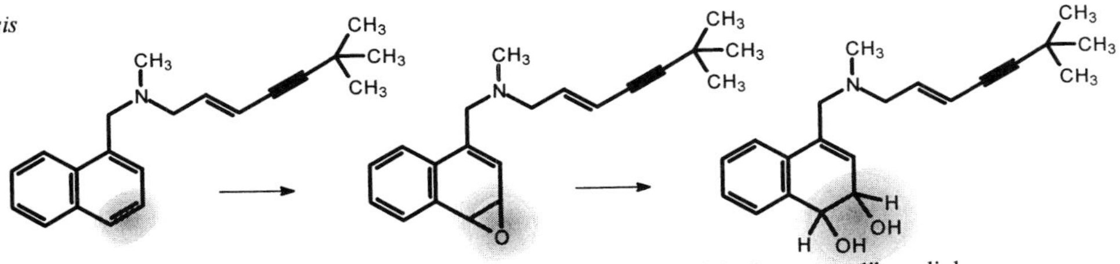

terbinafine → terbinafine epoxide → terbinafine *trans*-dihyrodiol

β-lactam hydrolysis

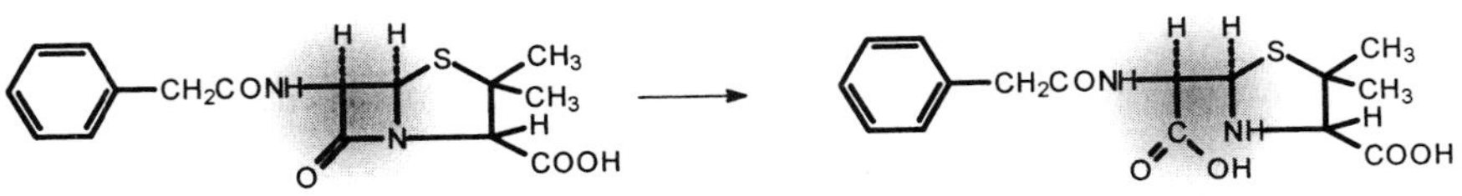

benzylpenicillin → penicilloic acid

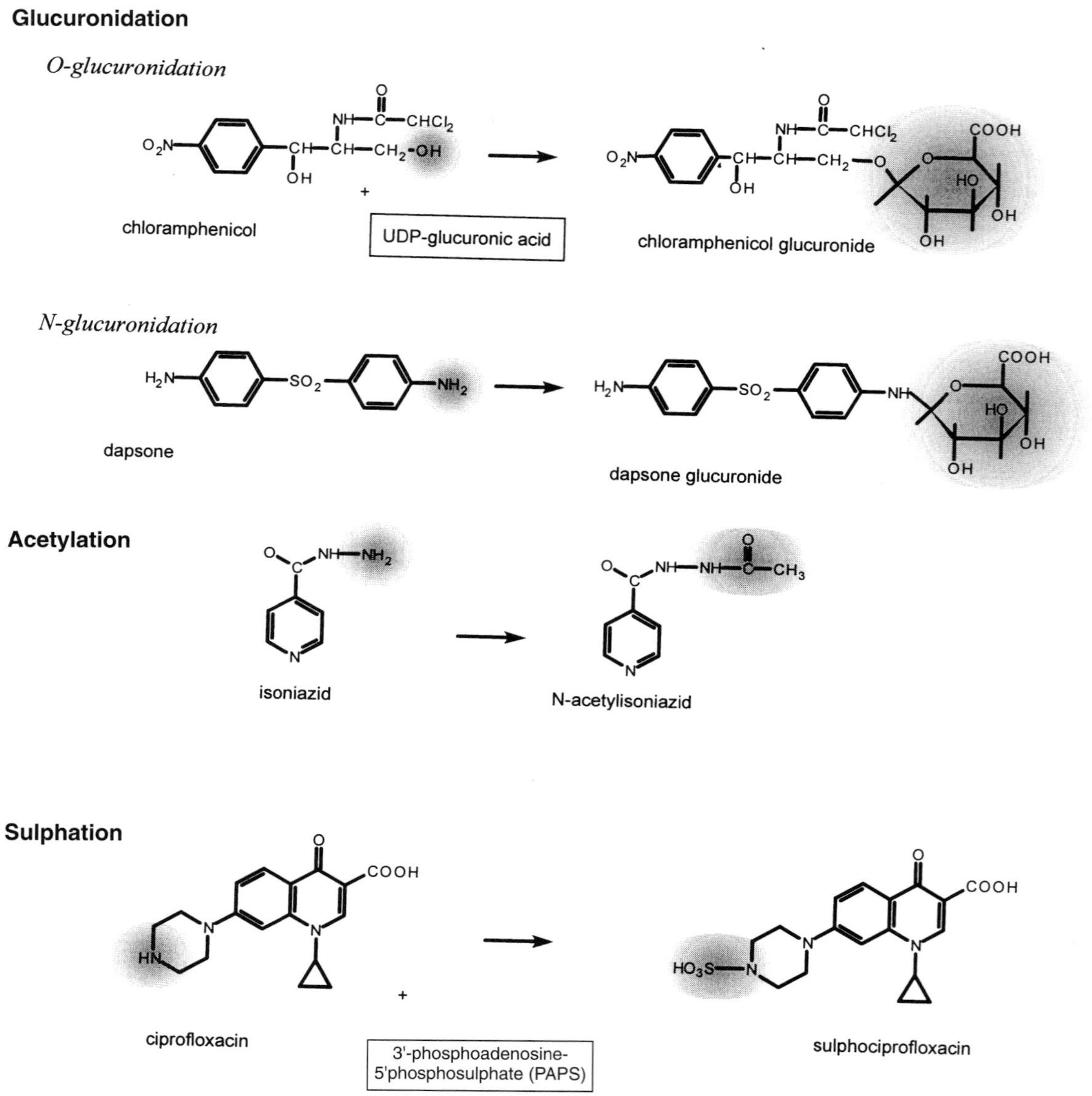

Glucuronidation

O-glucuronidation

chloramphenicol

UDP-glucuronic acid

chloramphenicol glucuronide

N-glucuronidation

dapsone

dapsone glucuronide

Acetylation

isoniazid

N-acetylisoniazid

Sulphation

ciprofloxacin

3'-phosphoadenosine-
5'phosphosulphate (PAPS)

sulphociprofloxacin

Fig. 4.14 *Phase II metabolism of commonly used antimicrobial agents. Selected examples to demonstrate the variety and complexity of drug biotransformations seen with this class of agents. Inclusion in this scheme does not imply that the given pathway is the sole, or even the major, route of metabolism for that drug.*

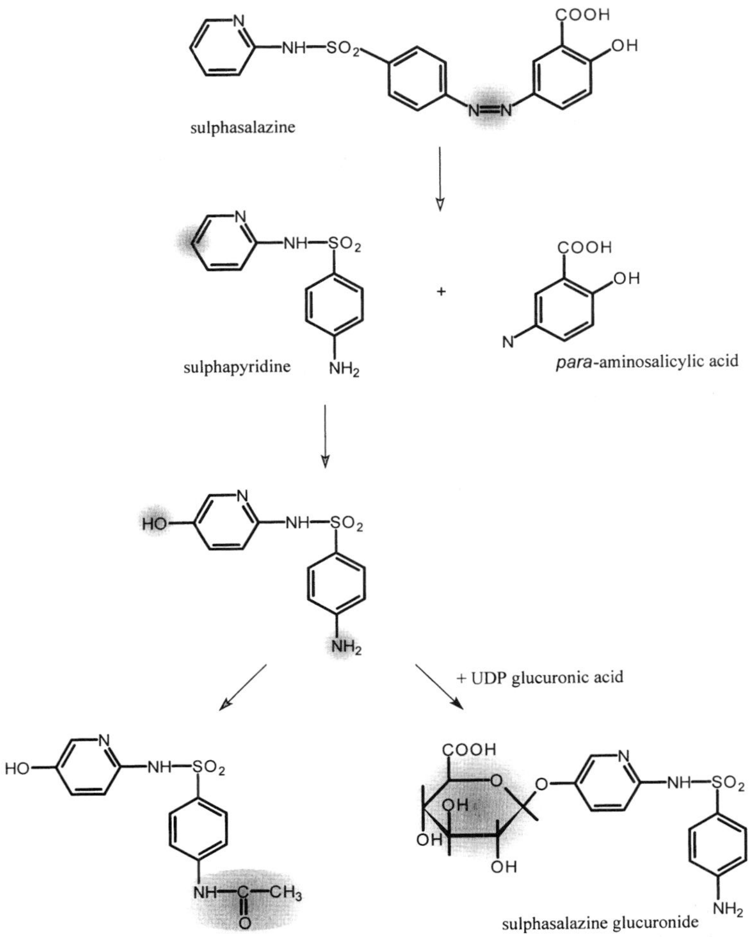

Fig. 4.15 *Metabolism of sulphasalazine. The scheme uses the drug sulphasalazine to illustrate the sequential pathways of intestinal flora, phase I and phase II processes. Azo reduction occurs mainly in the gastro-intestinal tract and results in the release of sulphapyridine and p-aminosalicylic acid. The former compound then undergoes functionalization by the phase I enzyme, cytochrome P450, to leave a free primary hydroxyl target for the enzyme glucuronyl transferase, resulting in a glucuronide conjugate. In addition, the free primary amino group on sulphapyridine provides a target for a second phase II process.*

receptor which then activates the gene, as in the case of the polyaromatic hydrocarbons (Hankinson 1991, Watson & Hankinson 1992, Poland & Bradfield 1992). The mechanism for the classical inducer phenobarbitone still remains to be elucidated, but may involve binding to the cytochrome P450 protein itself. Despite considerable searching, no specific cytosolic receptor has so far been identified for the barbiturates (Waxman & Azaroff 1992). Other mechanisms, such as stabilization of mRNA and stabilization of the translated protein itself, seen with CYP2E1 have also been proposed (Gonzalez et al 1991). The clinical significance of enzyme induction may be quite profound, and is of particular concern in the field of antimicrobial therapy where increased drug biotransformation may leave the patient exposed to subtherapeutic plasma levels, thereby jeopardizing effective treatment and establishing conditions favourable for resistance to develop.

In general, antibiotics and other chemotherapeutic agents include few agents which are themselves noted for their inducing ability; important exceptions being the macrolides and rifamycins. Several of the macrolides, including both erythromycin and troleandomycin, have long been known to cause an increase in the activity of the glucocorticoid-responsive cytochromes P450, in both animals and man (Babany et al 1988). Rifampicin is probably the most potent inducer of human isozymes of cytochrome P450, particularly the major human form, CYP3A (Park & Kitteringham 1989, 1990). Consequently, combination therapies involving rifampicin, rifabutin or other rifamycins should be monitored carefully to ensure that MIC values are exceeded (Venkatesan 1992).

Enzyme inhibition

Although enzyme induction is a major consideration in drug efficacy assessments from the aspect of a drug's toxicity, a more worrying phenomenon is enzyme inhibition. A far wider variety of drugs are inhibitors of cytochrome P450 and other metabolizing enzymes than are inducers, particularly within the spectrum of chemotherapeutic agents. Reported interactions between antimicrobial drugs as a result of one agent inhibiting the metabolism of another are too numerous to list here – for a comprehensive review see Gillum et al (1993). A potent group of P450 inhibitors worthy of particular emphasis are the azole antifungal agents, typified by ketoconazole. It is no surprise that these drugs are human cytochrome P450 inhibitors, since their mode of action is directed against a fungal form of the same enzyme (Breckenridge 1992). Nevertheless, caution must be shown when prescribing these agents along with other drugs with a narrow therapeutic window, as the catalogue of serious clinical interactions associated with these azole derivatives is ever lengthening. As with induction, the inhibition of cytochrome P450 is achieved via several different

mechanisms (Murray 1992). These range from the classical competitive inhibitors, through to the so-called suicide inhibitors, which are themselves substrates for cytochrome P450 but form a covalent complex with the haemoprotein upon activation (Ortiz-de-Montellano 1988). Chloramphenicol is an example of a competitive inhibitor, although it shows elements of suicide inhibition also (Ortiz-de-Montellano 1988), as too is the anticancer agent ellipticine, which is specific for the CYP1A subfamily of cytochrome P450 (Gibson & Skett 1994). In contrast, dapsone, isoniazid and sulphanilamide are all examples of drugs that form irreversible complexes with cytochrome P450, having first undergone activation by the same enzyme. The macrolides, particularly troleandomycin, are potent inhibitors of CYP3A isoforms, though their mechanism is complicated by their dual ability both to induce and inhibit these enzymes (Ortiz-de-Montellano 1988).

Several other pharmacokinetic drug interactions with antimicrobials are well documented, for example the complexation with antacids that results in reduced absorption of tetracyclines (see p. 105). In addition, there are the beneficial and intentional interactions employed in antibiotic therapy to enhance the effective bioavailability of certain agents. Widely applied examples of this type include the co-administration of inhibitors of β-lactamases alongside antibiotics that contain this structural moiety (see p. 320) and the reduced tubular secretion of antibiotics by probenecid. Nevertheless, it is true to say that the greatest number of interactions are disadvantageous and result from altered metabolism of one agent by another; these interactions should certainly be considered when combined therapy is indicated.

Excretion

As stated above, the two major routes of excretion, both for drugs themselves and their metabolites, are in urine and faeces. Other routes, such as in expired air and sweat, are important for some agents (e.g. volatile anaesthetics and alcohol), but have little significance in the field of antimicrobial therapy.

Renal excretion

The extent to which a drug is excreted in the urine is dictated by three processes: the extent to which it is filtered in the glomerulus, the extent to which it is actively secreted into the kidney tubules and the degree to which it is reabsorbed from the tubules. The three processes will in turn be influenced by the physicochemical properties of the drug, the degree to which the drug is protein bound in the circulation and internal or external factors that can alter renal processes, such as disease, urine pH and other drugs that compete for transport mechanisms. Consequently, it is difficult to state precisely the rate or extent of urinary clearance for a given compound. However, estimations can be made based on certain general principles. First, a drug, or metabolite, that is un-ionized at physiological pH will be a suitable substrate for tubular secretion. Two independent and non-specific transport systems exist, one for anions, the other for negatively charged ions; usually the affinity of charged species for these systems exceeds their affinity for plasma proteins and so the extent of binding within the plasma will not affect tubular secretion. Particularly with respect to antibiotic therapy, active tubular secretion is a significant route of elimination in chemotherapy. Appendix 4.3 gives a few examples of some acidic antimicrobial agents subject to tubular secretion.

From a therapeutic standpoint, the importance of tubular secretion in antibiotic therapy nowadays is the avoidance of potentially toxic interactions caused by competition for the same transport process (p. 98). In previous times, positive use of such interactions was made by the co-administration of carinamide or probenicid with penicillins and cephalosporins to delay the excretion of costly therapeutic agents. Such an approach is rarely used now, except where the maintenance of extremely high plasma antibiotic levels is called for. In contrast, it is important to avoid the co-administration of drugs such as probenicid, to treat gout, alongside agents such as aminosalicylic acid and nalidixic acid, which may precipitate toxic reactions, or with agents whose therapeutic efficacy may be compromised, such as nitrofurantoin for the treatment of urinary tract infection.

Unlike tubular secretion, the glomerular filtration of drugs and metabolites may be profoundly influenced by the extent of plasma protein binding. Thus factors such as disease (which can alter plasma protein concentration) and displacement from binding sites by other drugs, must be taken into account when predicting the clearance of a drug whose elimination is rate limited by its filtration in the glomerulus. For such drugs the effect of renal disease, with associated uraemia, may have profound effects on the elimination rate, an example being streptomycin whose normal plasma half-life of 2.5 h may be extended up to 50-fold when blood urea nitrogen concentrations exceed 1 mg/ml. Extreme caution must be exercised when treating oliguric or anuric patients with antibiotics (see Ch. 5). Where renal elimination is known, or suspected to be, the predominant route, plasma monitoring may be warranted, and indeed this is recommended for streptomycin and similarly cleared compounds (colistin, gentamicin, kanamicin and vancomycin) to avoid possible toxic consequences of high plasma concentrations. The use of some other antibiotics should be avoided completely because of their known renal toxicity which may exacerbate the patient's

original condition; such agents include chloramphenicol, cephalothin and the tetracyclines.

The final process involved in the renal excretion of drugs is their reabsorption into plasma as they pass through the loop of Henle and the distal tubules. Reabsorption of water during this process will invariably result in an increase in the concentration gradient, favouring reabsorption of the drug. However, the extent to which reabsorption will occur is determined by the lipophilicity of the drug, since only the un-ionized form will be free to diffuse through the tubular epithelial membrane; active reabsorption is a minor mechanism of no significance in antimicrobial drug therapy. In turn, the ionization of the drug will be influenced greatly by the pH of the urine, and consequently urine pH may have a profound effect on urinary clearance. This is exemplified by nalidixic acid, nitrofurantoin and streptomycin, the excretion of all of which in urine is markedly exacerbated if the urine is alkalinized with sodium bicarbonate. As a general rule, one should anticipate a change in drug clearance, if the urinary pH changes, for an acidic drug whose pK_a lies between 3 and 8.

References

Aronson J K, Dengler H J, Dettli L, Follath F 1988 Standardization of symbols in clinical pharmacology. *European Journal of Clinical Pharmacology* 35: 1–7

Babany G, Larrey D, Pessayre D 1988 Macrolide antibiotics as inducers and inhibitors of cytochrome P-450 in experimental animals and man. In: Gibson G G (ed) Progress in drug metabolism. Taylor & Francis, London, p 61–98

Breckenridge A 1992 Clinical significance of interactions with antifungal agents. British Journal of Dermatology 126 (suppl 39): 19–22

Brosen K, Gram L F 1989 Clinical significance of the sparteine/debrisoquine oxidation polymorphism. *European Journal of Clinical Pharmacology* 36: 537–547

Dollery C T, Boobis A R, Burley D et al 1991 Therapeutic drugs. Churchill Livingstone, Edinburgh

Edwards I G, Looareesuwa S, Davies A, Wattanagoon Y, Phillips R E, Warrell D A 1988 Pharmacokinetics of chloroquine in Thais: plasma and red-cell concentrations following an intravenous infusion to healthy subjects and patients with *Plasmodium vivax* malaria. *British Journal of Clinical Pharmacology* 25: 477–485

Gibson G G, Skett P 1994 Introduction to drug metabolism, 2nd edn. Blackie Academic and Professional, London

Gillum J G, Israel D S, Polk R E 1993 Pharmacokinetic drug-interactions with antimicrobial agents. *Clinical Pharmacokinetics* 25: 450–482

Gonzalez F J, Gelboin H V 1994 Role of human cytochromes P450 in the metabolic activation of chemical carcinogens and toxins. *Drug Metabolism Reviews* 26: 165–183

Gonzalez F, Meyer U A 1991 Molecular genetics of the debrisoquin–sparteine polymorphism. *Clinical Pharmacology and Therapeutics* 50: 233–238

Gonzalez F J, Ueno T, Umeno M, Song B J, Veech R L, Gelboin H V 1991 Microsomal ethanol oxidizing system – transcriptional and posttranscriptional regulation of cytochrome-P450, cyp2e1. *Alcohol and Alcoholism* 97–101

Guenthner T M 1990 Epoxide hydrolases. In: Mulder G J (ed) Conjugation reactions in drug metabolism: an integrated approach. Taylor & Francis, London, p 365–404

Hankinson O 1991 Genetic and molecular analysis of the Ah receptor and cyp 1A1 gene expression. *Biochimie* 73: 61–66

Jensen J C 1989 Pharmacokinetics of Lamisil in humans. *Journal of Dermatological Treatment* 1 (suppl 2): 15–18

Karbwang J, Harinasuta T 1992 Chemotherapy of malaria in Southeast Asia. Ruamtasana, Bangkok

Katzung B G 1995 Basic and clinical pharmacology, 6th edn. Appleton and Lange, Connecticut

Koymans L M H, Donne-Op den Kelder G M, Koppele T E, Vermeulen N P E 1993 Cytochromes P450: their active-site structure and mechanism of oxidation. *Drug Metabolism Reviews* 25: 325–387

Lindup W E 1987 Plasma protein binding of drugs. Some basic and clinical aspects. In: Bridges J W, Chasseaud L F, Gibson G G (eds) Progress in drug metabolism. Taylor & Francis, London

Murray M 1992 P450 enzymes: inhibition mechanisms, genetic regulation and effects of liver disease. *Clinical Pharmacokinetics* 23: 132–146

Nelson D R, Kamataki T, Waxman D J et al 1993 The P450 superfamily – update on new sequences, gene-mapping, accession numbers, early trivial names of enzymes, and nomenclature. *DNA and Cell Biology* 12: 1–51

Ortiz-de-Montellano P R 1988 Suicide substrates for drug metabolizing enzymes: mechanisms and biological consequences. In: Gibson G G (ed) Progress in drug metabolism. Taylor & Francis, London, p 99–148

Park B K, Kitteringham N R 1989 Relevance of and means of assessing induction and inhibition of drug metabolism in man. In: Gibson G G (ed) Progress in drug metabolism. Taylor & Francis, London, p 1–60

Park B K, Kitteringham N R 1990 Assessment of enzyme induction and enzyme inhibition in humans: toxicological implications. *Xenobiotica* 20: 1171–1185

Poland A, Bradfield C 1992 A brief review of the Ah locus. *Tohoku Journal of Experimental Medicine* 168: 83–87

Pratt W B, Taylor P 1990 Principles of drug action. The basis of pharmacology, 3rd edn. Churchill Livingstone, New York

Price Evans D A 1993 Genetic factors in drug therapy. Clinical and molecular pharmacogenetics. Cambridge University Press, Cambridge

Rowland M, Tozer T N 1989 Clinical pharmacokinetics: concepts and applications, 2nd edn. Lea & Febiger, Philadelphia

Tozer T N 1981 Concepts basic to pharmacokinetics. *Pharmacology and Therapeutics* 12: 109–132

Venkatesan K 1992 Pharmacokinetic drug interactions with rifampicin. *Clinical Pharmacokinetics* 22: 47–65

Watson A J, Hankinson O 1992 Dioxin- and Ah receptor-dependent protein binding to xenobiotic responsive elements and G-rich DNA studied by in vivo foot printing *Journal of Biological Chemistry* 266: 6874–6878

Waxman D J, Azaroff L 1992 Phenobarbital induction of cytochrome P-450 gene expression. *Biochemical Journal* 281: 577–592

Appendix 4.1 Peak plasma concentrations (C_{max}) and time to peak (T_{max}) for some commonly used antibiotics and antimicrobial agents (Data collated from various sources, principally Dollery et al 1991).

Agent	Route	Dose (mg)	C_{max} (mg/l)	T_{max} (h)
Aminoglycosides				
Amikacin	i.m.	500	20	1
Gentamicin	i.m.	80	4–12	0.5–2
Kanamycin	i.m.	500	25–30	1–1.5
Neomycin	i.m.	500	20	1
Streptomycin	i.m.	500	25–50	0.5–1.5

Appendix 4.1 *Cont'd*

Agent	Route	Dose (mg)	C_{max} (mg/l)	T_{max} (h)
Antifungal agents				
Fluconazole	Oral	50	1 – 1.2	2 – 4
Itraconazole	Oral	100	0.1 – 0.2	2 – 4
Ketoconazole	Oral	400	5 – 6	2 – 4
Terbinafine	Oral	250	0.8	2
Anthelmintics				
Albendazole	Oral	400	0.1 – 0.4	2 – 4
Diethylcarbamazine	Oral	50	0.1 – 0.15	1 – 2
Metronidazole	Oral	500	14	1 – 3
Antimycobacterial agents				
p-Amino salicylic acid	Oral	4000	7 – 8	1 – 2
Dapsone	Oral	100	2	3 – 6
Ethambutol	Oral	25 mg/kg	5	2 – 4
Isoniazid	Oral	12.5 mg/kg	10 – 15	1 – 2
Pyrazinamide	Oral	1500	30	2
Antiprotozoal agents				
Mefloquine	Oral	750	0.6 – 1.5	10 – 18
Antiviral agents				
Amantadine	Oral	200	0.4 – 0.9	4 – 6
Rimantadine	Oral	100	0.4 – 0.5	–
Zidovudine	Oral	100	–	0.5
Cephalosporins				
Cefaclor	Oral	250	6 – 7	50 min
Cefamandole	i.m.	500	13 – 15	0.75 – 1
Cefazolin	i.m.	500	35	1
Cefixime	Oral	400	4 – 5.5	4
Cefotaxime	i.m.	500	10	–
Cefoxitin	i.m.	500	11	20 min
Cefuroxime	i.m.	500	18 – 25	0.5
Cephalexin	Oral	500	9	–
Cephalothin	i.m.	500	6 – 8	0.5 – 1
Cephradine	Oral	500	18 – 20	1
Chloramphenicol				
Chloramphenicol	Oral	500	10 – 13	1 – 2
Thiamphenicol	Oral	500	3 – 6	2
Fusidanes				
Fusidic acid	Oral	500	31	4 – 8
Macrolides				
Erythromycin	Oral	500	0.9 – 1.4	2 – 4
Oleandomycin	Oral	500	0.8	–
Penicillins				
Amoxycillin	Oral	125	2.7	2
Ampicillin	Oral	500	0.6 – 6	2
Benzathine penicillin	i.m.	1.2 MU	0.1	1 week
Benzyl penicillin	i.m.	1 MU	2	Few minutes
Carbenicillin	i.m.	1000	20 – 30	0.5 – 1
Cloxacillin	Oral	500	8	1
Flucloxacillin	Oral	500	15	0.5 – 1
Methicillin	i.m.	1000	17	0.5
Pivampicillin	Oral	700	10	1 – 2
Temocillin	i.m.	500	48	
Peptides				
Polymixin B sulphate	i.m.	50	1 – 8	–
Quinolones				
Cinoxacin	Oral	500	15	1 – 3
Ciprofloxacin	Oral	1000	5.9	0.5 – 2
Nalidixic acid	Oral	1000	25	–
Norfloxacin	Oral	400	1.4 – 1.6	1 – 2

Appendix 4.1 *Cont'd*

Agent	Route	Dose (mg)	C_{max} (mg/l)	T_{max} (h)
Rifamycins				
Rifampicin	Oral	600	14 – 16	–
Sulphonamides	Oral	200	100	2 – 4
Tetracyclines				
Doxycycline	Oral	100–200	1.7 – 5.7	2 – 3.5
Oxytetracycline	Oral	500	3 – 4	–
Tetracycline	Oral	500	4 – 5	–

Appendix 4.2 pK_a *values for some commonly used antimicrobial agents.**

Agent	Functional group type	
	Cation forming	Anion forming
Aminoglycosides		
Amikacin	8.1	
Kanamycin		7.2
Antifungal agents		
Amphotericin B	5.7	10
Itraconazole		3–4
Miconazole		6.7
Anthelmintics		
Diethylcarbamazine		7.7
Piperazine		4.2
Antimycobacterial agents		
Dapsone		1.3, 2.5
·Isoniazid		1.8, 3.5, 9.5
Pyrazinamide		0.5
Antiprotozoal agents		
Chloroquine		8.4, 10.8
Mefloquine		8.6
Pentamidine		11.4
Pyrimethamine		7.3
Quinine		4.1, 8.5
Antiviral agents		
Acyclovir	2.3	9.3
Amantadine		10.4
Zidovudine		9.7
Cephalosporins		
Cefaclor		8.0
Cefamandole	2.5	
Cefixime	2–2.5	
Cefotaxime	3.8	
Cefotetan	2.1, 3.3	
Cefoxitin	3.5	
Cefuroxime	2.5	7.3
Cephalexin	5.3	
Cephalothin	2.2	
Cephazolin	2.1	
Cephradine	2.6	7.3
Fusidanes		
Fusidic acid	5.4	
Macrolides		
Erythromycin		8.8
Spiramycin		8
Nitrofurans		
Nitrofurantoin	7.0	

Appendix 4.2 *Cont'd*

Agent	Functional group type	
	Cation forming	Anion forming
Penicillins		
Amoxycillin	2.4, 7.4	9.6
Ampicillin	2.7	7.2
Benzylpenicillin	2.8	
Carbenicillin	2.6, 3.3	
Cloxacillin	2.7	
Mecillinam	3.4	
Peptides		
Polymixin B		8.9
Quinolones		
Cinoxacin	4.7	
Ciprofloxacin	6	8.8
Nalidixic acid	6.7	8.8
Norfloxacin	6.3	
Rifamycins		
Rifampicin	1.7	7.9
Sulphonamides		
Sulphadiazine		6.4
Sulphadimidine		7.4
Sulphamethoxazole		5.7
Sulphasalazine	2.4, 8.3	11.0
Tetracyclines		
Tetracycline	3.3, 7.7	9.7

*The pK_a is given for basic (cation forming) and acidic (anion forming) functional groups. In some instances more than one pK_a value is shown, indicating the presence of more than one ionizable group.

Appendix 4.3 *Tubular secretion. Some examples of acidic antimicrobial agents whose excretion involves direct transport-mediated secretion into the proximal kidney tubule. Several products of phase II metabolism are also excellent substrates for tubular secretion.*

Drug	Metabolites
Aminosalicylic acid	Glucuronide conjugates
Most cephalosporins:	Amino acid conjugates
Cephalordine	
Cephalothin	
Cephalexin	
Cefamandole	
Nalidixic acid	
Nitrofurantoin	
Penicillins:	
Amoxycillin	
Ampicillin	
Azlocillin	
Benzyl penicillin	
Carbenicillin	
Cloxacillin	
Rifampicin	
Sulphonamides:	
Sulphathiazole	
Sulphamethizole	
Sulphinpyrazone	

Antibiotics in renal failure

R. Cove-Smith

Introduction

The kidney provides the final common pathway for the excretion of most drugs and their metabolites and is subjected to high concentrations of potentially toxic substances. As a result, many groups of drugs can cause renal damage, especially in the presence of pre-existing renal disease.

In renal failure, drug pharmacokinetics are altered in several ways, so that doses must be carefully regulated to provide adequate therapeutic levels without provoking toxic effects. With the increasing availability of facilities for renal dialysis and transplantation, many doctors now face the challenge of providing safe and effective therapy for renal failure patients. The proliferation of new drugs and their diverse actions makes prescribing for patients with renal disease both difficult and hazardous.

This chapter considers the ways in which drug metabolism and excretion are altered in renal disease, and provides guidelines for prescribing antibiotics in patients with renal failure, including those on dialysis. A later section deals with individual antibiotics and the problems of nephrotoxicity.

Choice of an antibiotic

An important factor to consider in choosing an antibiotic is its mode of elimination. Treating a urinary tract infection in an elderly patient with impaired renal function may appear simple, but antibiotics such as nalidixic acid and nitrofurantoin may not reach the urine in adequate bactericidal doses; instead, plasma levels are increased and toxicity may result. At the other extreme is the seriously ill

patient in the intensive therapy unit, with septicaemia and cardiorespiratory problems, whose renal function is deteriorating. Renal dialysis may be contemplated and the choice of a suitable antibiotic regimen requires close consultation and cooperation between the physician, the microbiologist and the nephrologist.

The risk of toxicity is greatest with drugs such as the aminoglycosides, which are excreted entirely by the kidney and have a narrow gap between therapeutic and toxic levels. Penicillins and cephalosporins, which are also excreted mainly by the kidney, are generally less toxic, and the high plasma and tissue levels achieved in the presence of renal failure may be beneficial. Other groups, such as the macrolides, are largely eliminated by non-renal mechanisms and require no dosage modification. Continuous and careful monitoring is essential in these ill patients to ensure therapeutic success without serious toxicity.

DRUG METABOLISM IN RENAL FAILURE

When prescribing antibiotics for patients with renal disease it is important to understand the ways in which the pharmacokinetics of the drug may be altered. The most important factor is the degree of reduction in glomerular filtration and tubular transport, but changes may also occur in gastro-intestinal absorption, protein binding, volume of distribution, cardiac and hepatic function and receptor sensitivity. If the drug is excreted primarily by the kidney the plasma level will be increased, but there may also be an alteration in the ratio of the parent drug to its metabolites, some of which may be microbiologically active. Other metabolites may accumulate and lead to unsuspected toxicity.

Absorption

Nausea and vomiting are common features of uraemia and

may be increased by some antibiotics, especially the tetracyclines, which should be avoided in renal failure. Few data are available concerning the absorption of antibiotics in renal failure, but an increase in gastric pH has been described (Anderson et al 1976). Antacids and phosphate binders may impede gastrointestinal absorption of some drugs.

Absorption of antibiotics from intramuscular sites is impaired in the presence of oedema or reduced peripheral perfusion. The intravenous route is preferable.

Protein binding

Most drugs circulate in the blood bound to plasma proteins. Only the free portion of the drug is pharmacologically active. In renal failure the protein binding of several antimicrobial agents is reduced. These include the organic acids such as sulphonamides, penicillin and cloxacillin; organic bases such as trimethoprim are unaffected. Reduced protein binding is chiefly due to an inhibitor which is present in uraemic plasma (Depner & Gulyassy 1980). Hypoproteinaemic states, which may occur in septicaemic patients or those with heavy proteinuria, may also lead to increased levels of free drug.

Elimination half-life

After a single dose the plasma concentration of most antibiotics reaches a peak and then declines exponentially at a rate characteristic of that particular drug. The elimination half-life provides a useful general measure of its duration of action. A steady state is generally achieved after four or five doses. In renal failure the elimination half-life of many drugs is increased, so that the time taken to reach a steady state, although still four or five half-lives, is prolonged. The degree to which the half-life is prolonged offers a useful guide to dosage in renal failure.

The half-life of many antimicrobial agents has been estimated for different degrees of renal failure, and dosage formulae, nomograms and computer programs exist to determine the doses of potentially toxic drugs such as the aminoglycosides. These provide only a rough guide and should always be accompanied by the measurement of plasma levels to avoid toxicity. In renal failure 'peak' and 'trough' levels may be considerably increased and the antibiotics must be given less frequently and in a lower dose.

RENAL EXCRETION

Only a few antibiotics are sufficiently water soluble to be excreted unchanged by the kidney. Drugs that are excreted largely unchanged by the kidney include the following:

- acyclovir
- aminoglycosides
- cephalosporins
- ethambutol
- flucytosine
- penicillins
- tetracycline.

Most drugs are lipid soluble and must be converted in the liver to water-soluble metabolites.

The kidney excretes drugs and their metabolites by glomerular and tubular mechanisms. The rate of elimination of a drug by the kidney depends on the plasma concentration, the molecular size, the glomerular filtration rate (GFR), tubular handling and the degree of protein binding. Only the non-protein-bound moiety of the drug passes through the glomerular filter to enter the tubular lumen. This topic is discussed in more detail in Chapter 4.

Clearance of a drug depends on the rate of filtration at the glomerulus and the degree of tubular secretion or reabsorption. Both the GFR and tubular transport are impaired in renal disease. Some tubular systems are disproportionately affected in diseases affecting the renal medulla, such as chronic pyelonephritis, analgesic nephropathy and polycystic kidney disease, but it is unclear how this affects the renal handling of drugs (Marsh 1983).

In practice, modification of drug dosage in renal failure is related to the GFR, since loss of glomerular function is the major factor limiting the renal excretion of drugs and metabolites.

DOSAGE MODIFICATION IN RENAL FAILURE

The aim of dosage modification in renal failure should be to maintain the same drug levels in the body as would exist under conditions of normal renal function. This can be achieved by reducing the dose or increasing the dosing interval, or a combination of the two.

A number of formulae have been devised for calculating the size of dose and the dosing interval for patients with renal failure, but these are only a guide. They assume that drug excretion is linearly related to creatinine clearance, that absorption, distribution, hepatic function and protein binding are normal in renal failure, and that any metabolites are non-toxic. It is preferable, therefore, to monitor drug levels and modify the dose accordingly, especially if potentially toxic drugs are used.

With antimicrobial agents the aim must be to produce adequate therapeutic levels without provoking toxic effects. For a bactericidal but toxic antibiotic such as gentamicin, intermittent administration should be designed to achieve high peaks and low troughs; however, as the elimination half-life is greatly prolonged in renal failure (36–48 h), long intervals between doses result in a blood concentration below the bacterial minimum inhibitory concentration (MIC) for a large part of the time. In end-stage renal disease a combination of a reduced dose and an increased dosing interval provides the most satisfactory approach, combined with frequent measurement of plasma levels.

For drugs which are relatively non-toxic, such as the penicillins, the dose is usually unchanged, but the dosing interval is increased in severe renal failure to allow for the prolonged half-life.

MONITORING PLASMA LEVELS

Measurement of plasma levels is recommended for a number of antimicrobials when given to patients with renal impairment. These include the aminoglycosides, ethambutol, isoniazid, vancomycin and flucytosine.

For aminoglycosides and vancomycin it is normal practice to take peak and trough levels. Trough levels are taken immediately before the next dose; peak levels should be taken 1 h after administration. It was previously suggested that peak levels be taken at 15–45 min after intravenous administration, and 1 h after intramuscular administration, but there are theoretical and practical reasons why 1 h post-dose measurements are preferable in all cases (Reeves & Paton 1987). The distribution phase of the plasma levels is complete by 1 h and plasma levels more closely reflect tissue levels (Fig. 5.1).

The post-dose sample for vancomycin concentration is conveniently taken at the end of the 1 h infusion; where the infusion lasts more than 1 h, a post-infusion level should be taken. Post-infusion levels are also suitable for flucytosine. The sample should be taken from a remote limb and not that used for the infusion.

Close cooperation with the microbiologist will ensure that the timing and quantity of the sample are satisfactory and that the results are available promptly, so that decisions on dosing can be made before the next dose is due. The frequency of monitoring will depend on the state and renal function of the patient and the potential toxicity of the antimicrobial prescribed. In patients with changing renal function, aminoglycosides should be monitored daily. In patients with stable renal function, thrice weekly measurements are usually sufficient.

Prescribing for patients with renal failure

Patients on dialysis

When antimicrobial agents are prescribed for patients on dialysis the dosage regimen must be modified to ensure adequate therapeutic levels. Haemodialysis and peritoneal dialysis generally remove drugs at different rates. Clearance of a drug by haemodialysis depends on the molecular size and configuration, the degree of protein binding, the size of the dialyser and the flow rate through the membrane. Only the non-protein-bound moiety is available for dialysis. In peritoneal dialysis flow rates are slow (5–10 ml/min) and clearance is generally less efficient. Some indication of the effect of dialysis is given in Tables 5.1–5.8, but for detailed information the reader is referred to specialized articles (Manuel et al 1983, Matzke & Keane 1986).

Even among the antibiotics there is great variation in dialysance. Aminoglycosides are generally well dialysed, the plasma concentration falling by 50% after 6–8 h of haemodialysis. Doses should be given after dialysis, with measurement of peak and trough plasma levels; the trough level should be taken after dialysis. Other antibiotics are not significantly removed by any form of dialysis; these include cloxacillin, clindamycin, vancomycin and amphotericin. Dosing regimens should be as for patients with severe renal failure.

It is important to remember that plasma creatinine levels will be misleading in patients on dialysis, and it should be assumed that the patient has severe renal failure (GFR < 5 ml/min).

In acute renal failure, haemodialysis may be required daily for 3–4 h to remove uraemic toxins and fluid, to correct electrolyte imbalance and to allow satisfactory feeding regimens. Administration of antibiotics daily after dialysis will often provide adequate therapeutic levels.

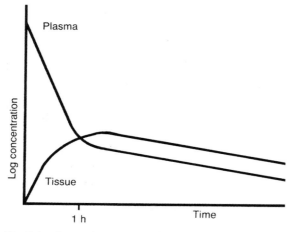

Fig. 5.1 *Curves demonstrating theoretical plasma and tissue levels of a drug given by intravenous bolus. Equilibration of plasma and tissue levels occur at about 1 h.*

An alternative therapy now widely used in intensive therapy units is continuous haemofiltration – either arteriovenous (CAVH) or venovenous (CVVH). Many antibiotics will be removed by haemofiltration and it is therefore sensible to discontinue the procedure for a few hours each day to administer antibiotics and other medication. This will allow therapeutic levels to be achieved. Little modification is required for patients with chronic renal failure on maintenance haemodialysis, which is usually performed for 3–6 h two or three times a week. On dialysis days doses should be given after dialysis.

Dialysis patients tend to have poor immune responses. Infections may arise from the access site and are due to skin organisms, mainly staphylococci; they usually respond to flucloxacillin. In the case of an indwelling dialysis catheter infection (usually a subclavian line) a single dose of vancomycin (500 mg) into the catheter will eliminate the infection. Unusual opportunist infections, including fungi, are sometimes encountered. Any infection in a dialysis patient is potentially serious and must be treated vigorously (see p. 649).

An important use of antibiotics is in the peritoneal infection associated with continuous ambulatory peritoneal dialysis (CAPD). More than 50% of cases are associated with staphylococcal infection (Gokal et al 1982) and respond to intraperitoneal antibiotics. Treatment of CAPD peritonitis is discussed in detail in Chapter 45.

Details of the fate of drugs in peritoneal dialysis are beyond the scope of this chapter, but a good account is given by Manuel et al (1983).

Guidelines in renal failure

In the accompanying tables guidelines are provided for the modification of drug dosage with various degrees of renal impairment. For most antibiotics the initial loading dose will be similar to that for patients without renal disease and produces a suitable drug concentration which can then be maintained by the dosage adjustments recommended. The tables provide guidelines only; further modification of dosage may be required for individual patients. In seriously ill patients with renal failure and septicaemia further problems arise. Absorption from the injection site may be variable, the volume of distribution may be changing with renal function and the presence of oedema may affect drug availability. Serum albumin levels are often low, and accurate assessment of renal function may be difficult. For this reason the patient must be monitored carefully for clinical efficacy and evidence of toxicity.

The guidelines for prescribing for patients with renal failure are as follows:

- Only use antibiotics in renal failure if a definite indication is present
- Choose an agent with minimal nephrotoxic effects

- Use plasma levels to adjust the dose wherever possible
- Use recommended dosage regimens for renal failure
- Avoid prolonged courses of potentially nephrotoxic drugs
- Avoid potentially nephrotoxic combinations
- Monitor the patient carefully for clinical efficacy and signs of toxicity.

The data in Tables 5.1–5.8 are derived from many sources, including Bennett (1986), Brater (1994), original reports and drug data sheets. Information about haemodialysis (HD) and peritoneal dialysis (PD) is not available for every drug. 'Yes' indicates significant removal, so that in dialysis patients a dosage supplement is required to ensure adequate therapeutic levels.

PENICILLINS (Table 5.1)

Penicillins are widely used in patients with renal failure because of their excellent safety profile. Most penicillins are eliminated by glomerular filtration and secretion in the proximal tubule. In renal failure the elimination half-life is prolonged, apart from the isoxazolyl penicillins (cloxacillin, flucloxacillin, oxacillin and nafcillin) which have significant biliary excretion. The high plasma levels seen in renal failure may be beneficial, since toxicity is minimal and only occurs with extremely high doses. Little or no dosage reduction is required, except in virtually anephric patients, since many members of the group have some non-renal excretion. For those penicillins which are excreted unchanged the dose interval should be increased when the GFR is less than 5–10 ml/min. In the presence of combined hepatic and renal failure the half-life of all penicillins is increased and doses should be reduced.

The effect of dialysis is variable. The isoxazolyl penicillins are not removed by either haemodialysis or peritoneal dialysis. Most other penicillins are significantly removed by haemodialysis, but to varying degrees. For those agents removed by haemodialysis a supplementary dose is recommended after dialysis – usually one-half or one-third of the normal dose. Removal by peritoneal dialysis is generally poor.

The antipseudomonal penicillins appear to be safe in renal failure. Azlocillin follows first-order kinetics and in anuric patients the half-life is increased to 4 h (Whelton et al 1983). Dosing nomograms are available for renal failure patients. Mezlocillin is unusual in having non-linear kinetics and monitoring of plasma levels is recommended if the GFR is less than 20 ml/min (Aronoff 1982, Bergan 1983). Azlocillin, mezlocillin, carbenicillin and ticarcillin all affect platelet function and can prolong the bleeding time. This effect is dose related and may cause problems in uraemia: haemorrhagic colitis has been described with azlocillin in a patient with renal failure.

Table 5.1 *Penicillins.*

Drug	Metabolism and excretion	Normal dose interval (h)	Dose interval in renal failure (h)			Removal by dialysis		Toxic effects and comments
			GFR > 50 ml/min	GFR 10–50 ml/min	GFR < 10 ml/min	HD	PD	
Benzylpenicillin	75–90% excreted unchanged; slight hepatic excretion	8	8	8–12	12–16	Partial (5–20%)	Poor	Sodium salt may cause sodium load. Avoid potassium salt in renal failure
Cloxacillin Flucloxacillin	40–70% excreted unchanged; significant hepatic excretion	6	6	6	6	No	No	
Methicillin	65% excreted unchanged; slight hepatic excretion	4	4	4	8–12	No	No	Interstitial nephritis
Ampicillin Amoxycillin	50–90% excreted unchanged; some hepatic excretion	6 8	6 8	6–12 8–12	12–16 12–16	Yes Yes	Poor Poor	Give 1/3 normal dose after dialysis
Mecillinam	50–60% excreted unchanged; significant hepatic excretion	8	8	8	12*	Yes	Poor	*Halve dose if GFR < 25 ml/min
Azlocillin	50–60% excreted unchanged; 15–30% hepatic excretion	8	8	8	12*	Yes	Poor	*Halve dose if GFR < 25 ml/min; 1/4 dose if GFR < 10 ml/min. Monitor plasma levels. Give 1/2 normal dose after dialysis
Mezlocillin	70% excreted unchanged; 30% hepatic excretion	6–8	6–8	8	12	Yes	Poor	Monitor plasma levels
Piperacillin	70–80% excreted unchanged	6	6	8	12	Yes	Poor	Reduce dose if GFR < 20 ml/min. Give supplementary dose (1 g) after dialysis
Ticarcillin	70–80% excreted unchanged	4–6	6–12	12–24	24–48	Yes	Poor	May interact with aminoglycosides. May be ineffective for urinary tract infections if GFR < 20 ml/min. Measure serum levels. Significant sodium load
Carbenicillin	60% excreted unchanged; significant hepatic excretion	4–6	6–12	12–24	24–48	Yes	Poor	May interact with aminoglycosides. May be ineffective for urinary tract infections if GFR < 20 ml/min. Significant sodium load
Temocillin	75% excreted unchanged	12	12	24	48	Yes	Poor	May interact with aminoglycosides. Give supplementary dose (1 g) after dialysis. Significant sodium load

HD, haemodialysis; PD, peritoneal dialysis.

Synergy has been demonstrated between the antipseudomonal penicillins and the aminoglycosides in subjects with normal kidneys, but there have been reports of mutual inactivation if these two drugs are mixed in the same infusion fluid (Wallace & Chan 1985). Similar inactivation may occur in severe renal failure, when the two agents persist for long periods in the plasma (Thompson et al 1982).

Renal side-effects

When penicillins are given in very high doses electrolyte disturbance can occur. Sodium salts are commonly used in the UK and can provide a significant sodium load. Carbenicillin and ticarcillin, for example, contain 5.4 mmol of sodium per gram, so that with a full dose of 30 g daily the patient will receive 160 mmol sodium per day. In the USA potassium salts are also used and cardiac arrest has been attributed to rapid infusion. Sodium concentrations of commonly prescribed injectable antibiotics have been listed by Baron et al (1984).

Important renal side-effects of penicillins include hypokalaemic alkalosis and interstitial nephritis. The penicillin moiety itself may act as a non-re-absorbable anion within the tubular lumen which increases the negativity of the distal tubular fluid. Passive excretion of potassium and hydrogen ions can cause a hypokalaemic alkalosis. This has been described with benzylpenicillin, carbenicillin and ticarcillin.

Nephrotoxicity due to penicillins has two main forms. An allergic angiitis, similar to Henoch–Schönlein purpura, has been described, accompanied by fever, abdominal pains and vasculitic lesions. Urinalysis reveals proteinuria, haematuria, white cells and casts, and renal biopsy has shown changes similar to polyarteritis nodosa, with vascular changes and acute focal glomerulonephritis. Fatalities have occurred.

A second pattern is acute interstitial nephritis. This was initially reported with methicillin, but has been described with other penicillins, including benzylpenicillin, ampicillin, carbenicillin, nafcillin and oxacillin. It appears to be more common after prolonged therapy in relatively high doses, and the features suggest a delayed hypersensitivity reaction. Renal function declines and the patient has fever, eosinophilia and a rash. Urinalysis typically shows haematuria, but white cells, proteinuria and casts may be present. Most patients recover rapidly on withdrawal of the drug, but fatal renal failure has occurred. Renal biopsy shows patchy tubular damage with interstitial oedema and accumulation of monocytes, eosinophils and plasma cells. Glomeruli are normal. Immunoglobulins have been demonstrated which are specific for the penicilloyl hapten in both glomerular and tubular basement membranes. It appears that penicillin acts as a hapten and binds directly to renal tissue. The process usually remits on withdrawal of the drug, but in severe cases corticosteroids may hasten recovery.

CEPHALOSPORINS (Table 5.2)

Cephalosporins are excreted mainly via the kidneys, but some members of the group have significant non-renal excretion. Cefotaxime, for example, is metabolized to a desacetyl metabolite which has significant antimicrobial activity. Little dosage modification is therefore required in renal failure (Wise & Wright 1981). The elimination half-life of most other cephalosporins is increased in renal failure. Dosing intervals should be increased when the GFR is less than 20 ml/min, and dose reduction may also be required. Care is needed with cefoxitin, which can interfere with creatinine estimation.

The main concern with the early cephalosporins was renal toxicity, but this is less of a problem with second- and third-generation drugs. Cephaloridine is now rarely used in clinical practice, but has been studied extensively in animals as a model of cephalosporin nephrotoxicity. It produces necrosis of the proximal tubule in animals and man which is dose related. Nephrotoxicity is enhanced by concurrent administration of aminoglycosides or loop diuretics.

Cephalothin can also potentiate renal damage caused by aminoglycosides, especially if given in high doses. Histology shows acute tubular necrosis, interstitial oedema and a mononuclear cell infiltrate. Glomeruli are normal. Similar appearances have been described in animals. Cephalothin is largely excreted unchanged by the renal tubule, but 30–40% is transformed to the biologically less active desacetyl metabolite. Cephalothin may exacerbate acute interstitial nephritis induced by methicillin or nafcillin and should probably be avoided in patients with reduced renal function.

At present there is no evidence that the newer cephalosporins are nephrotoxic, even when administered together with aminoglycosides or loop diuretics, although proximal tubular necrosis has been described in animals with cefazolin. Nevertheless, potentially toxic combinations must be used with caution, especially in dehydrated patients with evidence of renal damage. The data sheets of the newer agents include sensible recommendations about dosage reduction in renal failure, which should be followed carefully.

Psychotic reactions have been described when cephalosporins are given to patients with renal failure (Vincken 1984). The drugs implicated include cephaloridine, cephalothin, cephalexin and cefuroxime. Confusion and encephalopathy have been reported with ceftazidime (Jackson & Berkovic 1992).

Table 5.2 *Cephalosporins*

Drug	Major route of excretion	Normal dose interval (h)	Dose interval in renal failure (h)			Removal by dialysis		Toxic effects and comments
			GFR > 50 ml/min	GFR 10–50 ml/min	GFR < 10 ml/min	HD	PD	
Cephalexin	80–95% unchanged	6	6	6	6–12	Yes	Yes	Usual dose for urinary infections
Cephradine	86% unchanged	6	6	6–9	9–12	Yes	Poor	
Cephazolin	60–90% unchanged	8	8	12	24–48	Yes	Poor	Ineffective for urinary infections if GFR < 10 ml/min
Cefamandole	75% unchanged	4–6	6	6–9	9–12	Yes	Poor	
Cefoxitin	90% unchanged	6–8	8	8–12	24	Yes	Poor	Interferes with creatinine estimation
Cefuroxime	85% unchanged	8	8	12	24	Yes	Poor	Psychotic reactions described in renal failure. Useful in CAPD
Cefotaxime	50% renal; 50% hepatic	8–12	12	12	12*	Yes	Poor	*Halve dose if GFR < 5 ml/min. Desacetyl derivative
Cefaclor	54% renal; significant hepatic	8	8	8	8*	Yes	Poor	*Reduce dose. Chemically unstable
Ceftizoxime	90% unchanged	8	8	8–12	12–24	Yes	Yes	
Cefsulodin	90% unchanged	6–8	6–8	8–12	12*	Yes	Poor	*Reduce dose if GFR < 10 ml/min
Ceftazidime	88% unchanged	12	12–24	24	48*	Yes	Poor	*Halve dose if GFR < 50 ml/min; $1/4$ dose if GFR < 15 ml/min
Latamoxef	88% unchanged	8	8	12	12–24*	Yes	Poor	*Reduce dose if GFR < 10 ml/min
Cefixime	40% unchanged	12–24	12–24	24	24	No	No	Reduce dose if GFR < 50 ml/min
Ceftriaxone	40–65%	24	24	24	24	No	No	Limit dose to 2 g if GFR < 10 ml/min. No dose supplement needed after dialysis. Measure plasma levels

HD, haemodialysis; PD, peritoneal dialysis.

Sodium bicarbonate is added to some injectable cephalosporins, but the sodium load is rarely a problem in renal failure. Maximum daily sodium load varies from 7 to 48 mmol/day (Baron et al 1984).

Haemodialysis for 6–8 h removes 30–50% of most cephalosporins, but peritoneal dialysis only removes 10–30%. Exceptions are cephalexin and ceftizoxime, which are well cleared by peritoneal dialysis (Manuel et al 1983).

OTHER β-LACTAMS (Table 5.3)

Aztreonam

Aztreonam is a monolactam active against many Gram-negative organisms, including *Pseudomonas* species. It has to be administered parenterally and has been recommended for treatment of urinary, prostatic and gynaecological infections, as well as life-threatening systemic infections. In

Table 5.3 β–Lactams

Drug	Major route of excretion	Normal dose interval (h)	Dosing interval in renal failure (h)			Removal by dialysis		Toxic effects and comments
			GFR > 50 ml/min	GFR 10–50 ml/min	GFR < 10 ml/min	HD	PD	
Aztreonam	Renal	8	8	8 $^1/_2$ dose	8 $^1/_4$ dose	Yes	No	
Clavulanate	Renal	6–8	6–8	8–12	12–24	Yes	?	Gastro-intestinal disturbance
Imipenem (+ Cilastatin)	Renal	6	6	6–8 $^1/_2$ dose	12 $^1/_2$ dose	Yes	No	Pharmacokinetics of two components differ in renal failure. Seizures reported
Meropenem	Renal	6–8	12	12*	24	Yes	?	*Halve dose if GFR < 25 ml/min

HD, haemodialysis; PD, peritoneal dialysis.

healthy subjects, 60–70% of a single dose is recovered from the urine by 8 h and renal excretion is complete by 12 h. In renal failure the normal dose interval should be maintained, but the dose should be reduced if the creatinine clearance is less than 30 ml/min.

Clavulanic acid

Clavulanic acid is a β-lactamase inhibitor with little anti-bacterial activity when used alone. It has been combined with amoxycillin or ticarcillin to counteract the effect of β-lactamase and extend the spectrum of activity. The pharmacokinetics of the two components are similar. Clavulanate is about 20% protein bound and is excreted by the kidney.

Imipenem

Imipenem is a parenteral β-lactam with broad-spectrum activity against Gram-negative and Gram-positive organisms. Unlike penicillins and cephalosporins, it is recognized and extensively metabolized by a human renal brush-border enzyme, dehydropeptidase-1. In order to prevent this inactivation, imipenem is administered together with cilastatin, an enzyme inhibitor (Calandra et al 1988a).

The pharmacokinetics of the two components are well matched in normal renal function, but cilastatin has different characteristics in renal failure. In severe renal failure the half-life of imipenem is 3.4 h, while that for cilastatin is 16 h. Furthermore, imipenem/cilastatin has substantial neurotoxicity. Seizures have been reported in up to 2% of patients, and renal impairment appears to be one of the risk factors (Calandra et al 1988b). Seizures are commoner in elderly or debilitated patients and those with head injury or

epilepsy. Concomitant therapy with ganciclovir, theophylline or cyclosporin may increase the risk of seizures (Job & Dretler 1990, Steurer et al 1991). Imipenem/cilastatin is readily removed by haemodialysis and haemofiltration, but not by CAPD.

Meropenem

Meropenem is a recently introduced carbapenem which is relatively stable to human dehydropeptidase-1 and does not require the addition of a tubular entry blocker. Studies in animals and man suggest a low potential for nephrotoxicity (Christensson et al 1992). Clearance of meropenem is linearly related to GFR and doses should be reduced in patients with renal impairment. Non-renal clearance is normally 20% but increases to 50% when the GFR falls below 30 ml/min. Protein binding is negligible (2%).

Meropenem and its main metabolite are readily removed by haemodialysis and an additional dose (half the normal dose) is recommended following dialysis (Leroy et al 1992). No information is yet available about clearance by peritoneal dialysis. The incidence of seizures appears to be lower with meropenem than with imipenem/cilastatin (Del Favero 1994).

AMINOGLYCOSIDES (Table 5.4)

The problem of aminoglycoside nephrotoxicity and ototoxicity is now well recognized, but despite the availability of facilities for measuring plasma levels, renal and auditory damage still occurs. All aminoglycosides have a relatively

Table 5.4 *Aminoglycosides and tetracyclines*

Drug	Major route of excretion (h)	Normal dose interval	Dose intervals in renal failure (h)			Removal by dialysis		Toxic effects and comments
			GFR > 50 ml/min	GFR 10–50 ml/min	GFR < 10 ml/min	HD	PD	
*Aminoglycosides**								All members of the group are nephrotoxic and ototoxic. Use nomogram and adjust dose according to plasma levels
Amikacin	Renal	8–12	12–18	24–36	36–48	Yes	No	
Gentamicin	Renal	8	8–12	12–24	24–48	Yes	No	
Netilmicin	Renal	8	8–12	12–24	24–48	Yes	No	? Less nephrotoxic and ototoxic than other aminoglycosides
Streptomycin	Renal	12	24	24–72	72–96	Yes	No	
Tobramycin	Renal	8	8–12	12–24	24–48	Yes	No	Interaction with carbenicillin and latamoxef
Tetracyclines								
Tetracycline Oxytetracycline	Renal and hepatic	6–8	8–12	12–24	Avoid	No	No	Members of group have anti-anabolic effect, raise blood urea and cause acidosis
Minocycline	Hepatic	12	12	18–24	Avoid	No	No	Acute interstitial nephritis. High Incidence of vestibular toxicity
Doxycycline	Renal (hepatic and GI tract)	12	12	12–24	18–24	No	No	Does not cause rise in blood urea. Drug of choice in this group if indicated, but ineffective for urinary tract infection if GFR < 20 ml/min. Increases plasma cyclosporin levels

GI, gastro-intestinal; HD, haemodialysis; PD, peritoneal dialysis.
* Aminoglycosides are now sometimes administered using a 24 hourly dosing schedule.

narrow margin of safety, with toxic levels close to the therapeutic range. They are often prescribed for seriously ill patients with septicaemia and impaired renal function, and particular care is needed if renal function is changing rapidly.

The plasma concentration is largely dependent on renal function. Most aminoglycosides are excreted almost entirely by glomerular filtration, with a clearance of 80–90 ml/min. In patients with normal renal function the elimination half-life is 2–3 h, but in end-stage renal disease this is prolonged to 50–80 h.

The prevalence of nephrotoxicity is difficult to assess, but several series have reported a frequency of 2–10% (Hou et al 1983). Moore et al (1984) have shown that advanced age, liver disease and high plasma aminoglycoside levels are significant risk factors for nephrotoxicity. The same group of workers (Sawyers et al 1986) demonstrated that duration of therapy is an important risk factor; they have developed a predictive model, based on a bedside scoring system. A good account of renal damage due to aminoglycosides is given by Kaloyanides & Pastoriza-Munoz (1980) and Humes (1988). In patients with renal failure it is always worth considering a less toxic antimicrobial. If an aminoglycoside is the only choice then a short course should be prescribed, with careful monitoring of plasma levels and renal function.

Comparative studies suggest little difference in the nephrotoxicity of the newer aminoglycosides (Meyer 1986). The nephrotoxicity of gentamicin and tobramycin appears to be similar (Smith et al 1980), and both agents are widely used. Netilmicin has found favour because it appears to be less nephrotoxic and ototoxic than other aminoglycosides (Bergeron et al 1983, Lerner et al 1983). Although relatively expensive, it has proved useful in patients with renal disease and in the treatment of CAPD peritonitis (Gokal et al 1982).

Neomycin is the most toxic of the aminoglycosides in terms of renal and auditory damage, and is now largely restricted to topical use. Streptomycin is the least nephrotoxic, with a toxic level about 20 times the therapeutic dose; ototoxicity is, however, a common problem.

In the kidney aminoglycosides bind to renal cortical tissue and cause proximal tubular necrosis. Concentrations in the renal cortex may reach 10 times that in the plasma. Enzymuria may be an early sign of damage. Renal toxicity is increased by dehydration, sodium depletion, the use of loop diuretics or concurrent administration of certain cephalosporins (cephaloridine and cephalothin). Enhanced toxicity has also been described with methoxyflurane anaesthesia. If the aminoglycoside is withdrawn early the tubular damage is usually reversible. There are no data to suggest enhanced nephrotoxicity with the newer cephalosporins, but combination of these two groups of antibiotics should be used with great care in patients with renal impairment.

A number of authors have suggested guidelines for prescribing aminoglycosides to patients with renal disease (Davey et al 1983), including nomograms and computer programs. Gentamicin is the most widely used aminoglycoside in clinical practice and has been studied extensively. The initial loading dose is calculated according to the patient's weight, age and renal function (using the plasma creatinine). The dosing interval should be increased and the dose of aminoglycoside reduced according to the degree of renal failure, with subsequent doses being adjusted with reference to frequent plasma levels.

It has recently been suggested that once-daily dosing may reduce the risk of aminoglycoside toxicity. This is based on the premise that nephrotoxicity and ototoxicity are less likely with high but transient peak levels, followed by longer and lower trough levels (Nordstrom et al 1990). Giving the total recommended daily requirement as a single dose has found favour with microbiologists and is probably preferable to more frequent dosing (Gilbert 1991). It is likely to reduce the incidence of aminoglycoside nephrotoxicity.

Most aminoglycosides are poorly protein bound and readily removed by haemodialysis. In patients on daily haemodialysis, trough levels should be taken immediately after dialysis; the recommended dose should then be given and plasma levels checked 1 h later. The importance of frequent measurements of plasma levels and close cooperation with the laboratory cannot be overemphasized. Removal by peritoneal dialysis is relatively inefficient.

TETRACYCLINES (Table 5.4)

Tetracyclines are best avoided in renal failure. They reduce protein anabolism and cause a rise in blood urea; they have an irritant effect on the gastric mucosa, causing nausea and vomiting. In renal failure symptoms of uraemia may be increased; vomiting and diarrhoea lead to dehydration and further deterioration in renal function. The problems are potentiated by diuretics.

Doxycycline is the one member of the group which is probably safe in patients with renal impairment. It has significant non-renal elimination, via the bowel lumen, and the elimination half-life is unchanged in renal failure. Even in severe renal disease plasma drug levels do not rise and renal function is unaffected. Tetracyclines are poorly dialysed.

Other renal side-effects

Outdated tetracyclines have caused a distal tubular Fanconi syndrome due to the formation of anhydro-4-epitetracycline. Since citric acid was removed from the formulation, this has not been a problem.

Demethylchlortetracycline can produce nephrogenic diabetes insipidus. It has been used to treat the syndrome of inappropriate antidiuretic hormone secretion, but care must be taken to avoid dehydration and the development of acute renal failure.

Acute interstitial nephritis has been reported with minocycline. Although excretion of minocycline is not delayed in renal failure, deterioration in renal function can occur.

SULPHONAMIDES (Table 5.5)

Sulphonamides undergo hepatic acetylation and conjugation; metabolites and free drug are then excreted by the kidney. The metabolites are generally more hydrophilic than the parent drug and are reabsorbed to a lesser extent in the renal tubules. Individual drugs are filtered, re-absorbed and secreted to different degrees according to their characteristics. Elimination half-life varies greatly, from 2.5 to 150 h. Solubility in the urine depends on the drug

Table 5.5 *Miscellaneous antibacterial agents*

Drug	Major route of excretion	Normal dose interval (h)	Dose intervals in renal failure (h)			Removal by dialysis		Toxic effects and comments
			GFR > 50 ml/min	GFR 10–50 ml/min	GFR < 10 ml/min	HD	PD	
Sulphonamides	Hepatic	6–8	6–8	6–8	6–8	Yes	No	Crystalluria may occur; maintain good hydration. Measure plasma levels in severe renal failure
Trimethoprim	Renal	12	12	18	24 ½ dose	Yes	No	May cause temporary and reversible rise in plasma creatinine levels. Often effective in urinary infection, even with low GFR. Safe in renal failure, but measure plasma levels if GFR < 10 ml/min
Sulphonamide/ trimethoprim combinations	Hepatic/ renal	12	12	18	24 ½ dose	Yes	No	Individual components handled differently in renal failure
Ciprofloxacin	Renal	Systemic infection: 12 UTI: 12	12 12 ½ dose	12 12 ½ dose	12 ½ dose 12 ½ dose	No	No	Significant tubular secretion. Active metabolites in urine
Nalidixic acid	Renal (hepatic)	6	6	6	Avoid	?	?	Unsuitable for use in renal failure. Metabolites accumulate
Norfloxacin	Hepatic/ renal	12	12	24*	24	No	?	Some active metabolites. *Halve dose if GFR < 20 ml/min
Ofloxacin	Renal (hepatic)	12–24	12–24*	24*	24	No	No	*Halve dose if GFR < 50 ml/min; ¼ dose if GFR < 20 ml/min. Interstitial nephritis reported
Nitrofurantoin	Renal	8	8	Avoid	Avoid	Yes	?	Ineffective if GFR < 30 ml/min. High risk of peripheral neuropathy in renal failure due to metabolites
Metronidazole	GI and hepatic	8	8	8	8–12	Yes	Yes	Drug and hydroxy metabolite readily removed by HD. Give ½ dose after dialysis
Tinidazole	Hepatic (renal)	24	24	24	24	Yes	?	Give ½ dose after haemodialysis
Vancomycin	Renal	24	24–72	72–240	240	No	No	Ototoxic. Measure plasma levels

Table 5.5 *Cont'd*

Drug	Major route of excretion	Normal dose interval (h)	Dose intervals in renal failure (h)			Removal by dialysis		Toxic effects and comments
			GFR > 50 ml/min	GFR 10–50 ml/min	GFR < 10 ml/min	HD	PD	
Teicoplanin	Renal	24	24–72	72–120	120–240	No	No	
Chloramphenicol	Hepatic (renal)	6	6	6	6	Yes	No	Ineffective for UTI if GFR < 40 ml/min
Clindamycin	Hepatic (renal)	6–8	6–8	6–8	6–8	No	No	Pseudomembranous colitis
Lincomycin	Hepatic (renal)	6	6	12	24*	No	No	Pseudomembranous colitis. *Reduce dose if GFR < 10 ml/min
Erythromycin	Hepatic	6	6	6	6	No	No	? Ototoxic in renal failure
Clarithromycin	Hepatic (renal)	12	12	12*	12*	No	No	*Halve dose if GFR < 20 ml/min
Azithromycin	Hepatic (renal)	24	24	24	24	No	?	

GI, gastrointestinal; HD, haemodialysis; PD, peritoneal dialysis; UTI, urinary tract infection.

concentration, urinary pH and the intrinsic solubility of the individual sulphonamide. Early sulphonamides tended to crystallize in the urine, causing crystalluria, tubular damage and obstructive uropathy. This is rare with modern drugs, but can still occur, especially in dehydrated patients with pre-existing renal disease who are given relatively insoluble agents.

Other renal effects include: acute interstitial nephritis; a syndrome resembling serum sickness; and a hypersensitivity angiitis similar to polyarteritis nodosa. Nephrotic syndrome has been described due to immune-complex glomerulo-nephritis. It is presumed that these are allergic reactions in which the drug acts as a hapten and stimulates antibody production. In patients with glucose-6-phosphate dehydro-genase deficiency, sulphonamides may cause haemolysis, resulting in haemoglobinuria and acute renal failure.

In view of their potential nephrotoxicity, sulphonamides should be used with caution in patients with impaired renal function. Short-acting, soluble agents should be used, and the dose reduced if the GFR is less than 25 ml/min. Hydration must be well maintained. If sulphonamides are given for more than a few days, plasma levels should be measured. The shorter acting drugs are readily dialysed.

TRIMETHOPRIM

Trimethoprim was originally introduced in combination with a sulphonamide, but in terms of the renal handling of the two components this was somewhat illogical. Trimethoprim is a weak base and excretion increases as the pH falls and non-ionic back-diffusion is reduced; sulphamethoxazole, by contrast, is a weak acid and is best excreted in an alkaline urine. Furthermore, in renal failure the elimination half-lives of the two components alter to different degrees, thus changing the concentration ratio in blood and tissues (Reeves 1982). Metabolites of sulphamethoxazole undergo in vivo hydrolysis back to the parent drug. On bacteriological, pharmacological and clinical grounds there seems little advantage of sulphonamide/trimethoprim combinations over trimethoprim alone, especially in renal failure.

Trimethoprim is excreted mainly by the kidney, with an elimination half-life of 10–12 h in normal subjects. In renal failure the half-life may be prolonged 2–3 times and a reduction in the frequency of dosage is recommended. Urinary concentration remains satisfactory even with quite severely impaired renal function, but the danger of toxicity increases because of accumulation in the plasma. Anorexia and gastrointestinal side-effects may cause problems. The haematological side-effects can be countered by giving folinic acid.

Initial reports suggested that impaired renal function seen with co-trimoxazole might be due to the trimethoprim component, but subsequent studies showed no significant deterioration in GFR. Trimethoprim appears to inhibit the tubular secretion of creatinine (Sandberg & Trollfors 1986) both in normal subjects and in those with renal damage, but the effect is transient and reversible. Cotrimoxazole and trimethoprim appear relatively safe in renal failure, provided the dose is adjusted according to the degree of renal impairment. In patients with a GFR between 10 and 25 ml/min the dose should be reduced after 3 days of treatment. If the GFR is less than 10 ml/min the dose should be halved and blood levels monitored.

4-QUINOLONES AND FLUOROQUINOLONE (Table 5.5)

Nalidixic acid

Nalidixic acid was formerly widely used in the treatment of urinary tract infections. It should be avoided in renal failure, since very little free drug reaches the urine and toxicity is increased. Nalidixic acid undergoes rapid metabolism to the hydroxyacid, which has significant microbiological activity. In mild renal impairment, urinary levels can be increased by administration of alkali, which reduces tubular reabsorption.

Cinoxacin

Cinoxacin is similar to, but less protein bound than, nalidixic acid. Fifty per cent is excreted unchanged in the urine and it has been used successfully to treat patients with impaired renal function.

Ciprofloxacin

Ciprofloxacin has aroused particular interest as the first orally-active broad-spectrum antimicrobial against *Pseudomonas aeruginosa*. There is also a parenteral preparation, and ciprofloxacin has bactericidal activity against a wide range of Gram-positive and Gram-negative organisms.

In healthy individuals, 60–70% of the drug is eliminated by the renal route and there is significant tubular secretion. In renal impairment, there is increased hepatic clearance and some drug is secreted through the bowel wall (Roberts & Williams 1989), but total clearance is still reduced (Nix & Schentag 1988). There is no obvious accumulation of toxic metabolites, but crystalluria has been described in a few patients. Hydration should be well maintained. Interstitial nephritis has been reported (Rippelmeyer & Synhavsky 1988), and is believed to be due to allergic mechanisms.

Ciprofloxacin can safely be used to treat both urinary tract infections and systemic infections in patients with moderately impaired renal function. In severe renal impairment, urinary concentration is significantly reduced.

Webb et al (1986) recommend an 8-hourly regimen for the treatment of urinary tract infection in patients with a creatinine clearance of 30 ml/min or less. For the treatment of systemic infections dosage adjustment is not required until the creatinine clearance falls below 20 ml/min.

Norfloxacin

Norfloxacin was the first fluorinated quinolone. Some 30–40% is excreted unchanged in the urine, but the metabolites also have some antimicrobial activity. It increases plasma levels of cyclosporin if given concurrently. The dose should be reduced in severe renal failure.

Ofloxacin

Ofloxacin is excreted largely unchanged (70–98%) and doses should be reduced in renal impairment. Interstitial nephritis has been reported.

Pefloxacin

Pefloxacin is metabolized largely by the liver. Interest was aroused when it was found to reduce urinary protein excretion in some patients with nephrotic syndrome. The mechanism is uncertain.

The fluoroquinolones can cause sleeplessness, psychotic reactions and seizures, possibly through an effect on γ-aminobutyric acid A receptors (Halliwell et al 1993). These reactions may be commoner in patients with renal impairment.

NITROFURANTOIN

Nitrofurantoin is rapidly excreted in the urine of normal subjects by glomerular filtration and tubular secretion. In alkaline urine, one-third of the dose is reabsorbed in the distal tubule by non-ionic back-diffusion. In renal failure inadequate concentrations of nitrofurantoin reach the urine and rapid breakdown of the drug leads to the accumulation of toxic metabolites which cause peripheral neuropathy. This may not be reversible. Nitrofurantoin is contraindicated in patients with moderate or severe renal failure.

METRONIDAZOLE

Metronidazole is metabolized in the liver by oxidation and conjugation. Of the two major metabolites the hydroxy form accounts for up to 30% of the plasma concentration. A total of 60–75% of the drug is excreted in the urine, two-thirds unchanged and the rest as metabolites and glucuronides. Some of the drug may be eliminated by the gut.

In renal failure non-renal excretion remains unaltered, but the hydroxymetabolite accumulates in the plasma. No dosage adjustment is therefore required.

Both the unchanged drug and the hydroxymetabolite are readily removed by haemodialysis (Somogyi et al 1984, Bergan & Thorsteinsson 1986). A further dose is recommended following dialysis.

No modification is required in patients on peritoneal dialysis and adequate peritoneal concentrations of metronidazole are achieved after oral dosing (Bush et al 1983).

Tinidazole

Tinidazole is excreted mainly in the urine, and to a lesser extent in the faeces. Pharmacokinetics are not significantly altered in renal failure and no dosage modification is required. It is only 12% protein bound and is readily dialysed. Half the prescribed dose should be given as a supplementary dose after haemodialysis.

SODIUM FUSIDATE

Sodium fusidate is excreted mainly in the bile, and no dosage modification is required in renal failure. Removal by haemodialysis is poor.

LINCOSAMIDES (Table 5.5)

Clindamycin

Clindamycin is metabolized in the liver, and the elimination rate is not significantly prolonged in renal failure. Doses of clindamycin should be limited to 300 mg 8-hourly in severe renal disease.

Lincomycin

The half-life of lincomycin is prolonged in renal failure, and the dose should be reduced if the GFR is less than 15 ml/min. Lincomycin and clindamycin must be used with care because of the hazards of antibiotic-associated (pseudomembranous) colitis. Removal of lincosamides by dialysis is negligible.

MACROLIDES (Table 5.5)

Erythromycin, clarithromycin and azithromycin

This group of drugs is metabolized in the liver, and no dose modification is required in patients with renal failure. There is a risk of ototoxicity with erythromycin in severe renal

failure and the dose should be limited to 1.5 g/day. Erythromycin increases plasma levels of cyclosporin.

Both clarithromycin and its principal metabolite 14-hydroxyclarithromycin have antimicrobial activity and 20–30% is excreted by the kidney. The half-life is prolonged in renal failure and the dose should be reduced to 250 mg/day when the GFR is less than 20 ml/min.

Azithromycin requires no dosage adjustment in mild renal impairment. No information is available about the effect of dialysis, but the other macrolides are not significantly dialysed.

PEPTIDES

Bacitracin, polymyxin B and colistin

This group of drugs is highly nephrotoxic and should be avoided in renal failure. They bind to cell membranes and are excreted predominantly by the kidneys. They have been superseded by the aminoglycosides and are now reserved mainly for topical use. Removal of polymyxin and colistin is significant by haemodialysis, but poor with peritoneal dialysis.

CHLORAMPHENICOL

Chloramphenicol is conjugated in the liver and about 60% protein bound. Its metabolites are excreted in the kidney; they are largely inactive and are not believed to be nephrotoxic. Chloramphenicol is rarely used in patients with renal failure. It is readily removed by haemodialysis, but not by peritoneal dialysis.

VANCOMYCIN

Vancomycin is a glycopeptide antibiotic, which is eliminated almost entirely by the kidney with an elimination half-life of 6–8 h in the normal subject. In renal failure the half-life becomes enormously prolonged, reaching 4–6 days. Thus in a subject with normal renal function the recommended dose is 1 g 12-hourly; in the anephric patient a suitable dose would be 1 g every 7–10 days. With lesser degrees of renal failure a nomogram can be used (Moellering et al 1981). Clearance of vancomycin is linearly related to creatinine clearance. Plasma levels should be measured where possible and should be kept below 50 mg/l. Brown & Mauro (1988) have issued dosing guidelines for patients with renal impairment.

Nephrotoxicity was a problem with early impure preparations of vancomycin, but is now uncommon. A modest but reversible rise in serum creatinine levels occurs even in normal individuals (Gudmundsson & Jensen 1989). The main side-effect is deafness. Great care must be taken if the patient is, or has been, receiving aminoglycosides, since the toxic side-effects may be additive.

Vancomycin is becoming increasingly used for the treatment of peritoneal infection in patients on CAPD. It is not significantly removed from the serum by either haemodialysis or peritoneal dialysis. It is, however, readily removed by high flow haemofiltration (Rawer & Seim 1989). Renal function does not deteriorate in patients given vancomycin after renal transplantation.

Other glycopeptides, such as teicoplanin, are currently being studied. Teicoplanin has similar pharmacokinetics to vancomycin, but can be administered intramuscularly. It is 90% protein bound and dosage regimens are similar to those for vancomycin.

ANTIMYCOBACTERIAL AGENTS (Table 5.6)

Cycloserine, *p*-aminosalicylic acid (PAS) and ethambutol are

excreted mainly by the kidney. Levels accumulate in renal failure and may lead to toxic effects. If treatment is required with these agents for patients with impaired renal function, plasma levels should be monitored. Cycloserine and PAS are best avoided if possible.

The elimination of isoniazid may be prolonged in renal failure, but plasma levels depend more on acetylator status. Dosing in renal failure should be carefully monitored by means of plasma levels. Isoniazid is one of the drugs which more commonly causes the lupus erythematosus syndrome, but renal involvement rarely occurs. It is readily dialysed.

Rifampicin undergoes hepatic metabolism and is 65–80% protein bound. Clearance is somewhat reduced in renal failure, but little dosage modification is required. In severe renal failure it is excreted entirely in the bile. Its main renal side-effect is interstitial nephritis, which may occasionally cause acute renal failure. The risk of nephritis seems to be increased if repeated, intermittent doses are given. Histology has shown tubulo-interstitial nephritis, interstitial fibrosis and tubular necrosis. Immunofluorescence is generally negative, but glomerular lesions and heavy proteinuria have been reported (Neugarten et al 1983).

Table 5.6 *Antimycobacterial agents*

Drug	Major route of excretion	Normal dose interval (h)	Dose intervals in renal failure (h)			Removal by dialysis		Toxic effects and comments
			GFR > 50 ml/min	GFR 10–50 ml/min	GFR < 10 ml/min	HD	PD	
Cycloserine	Renal	12	12	12*	Avoid	No	No	*1/2 dose. Measure plasma levels; aim to keep them < 30 mg/l. CNS toxicity
Isoniazid	Hepatic	24	24	24	24	Yes	Yes	Genetic variation in acetylation. Peripheral neuropathy. LE syndrome
Ethambutol	Renal	24	24	24–36	48	Yes	Yes	Visual damage (optic neuritis), dose related. Measure plasma levels
Rifampicin	Hepatic	24	24	24	24	No	No	Hepatotoxic. Interstitial nephritis reported. Rarely, acute renal failure. Reduces plasma cyclosporin levels
Pyrazinamide	Hepatic	24	24	24	24	Yes	Yes	Uric acid excretion diminished. Risk of gout

CNS, central nervous system; HD, haemodialysis; LE, lupus erythematosus; PD, peritoneal dialysis.

Rifampicin has been used successfully in treating CAPD peritonitis. Care is needed in renal transplant patients as it reduces plasma cyclosporin levels due to its liver enzyme-inducing properties.

ANTIFUNGAL AGENTS (Table 5.7)

Amphotericin

Amphotericin is an antibiotic with a high incidence of toxicity, including gastrointestinal symptoms, thrombophlebitis, pyrexia, hypokalaemia and renal damage. As with other drugs used for systemic mycoses, it often has to be given to patients with debilitating illness, in whom renal function may already be impaired. Its distribution and fate remain uncertain; only 3% is unchanged in the urine. It is 90% protein bound and is not dialysable. Amphotericin binds extensively to tissues; it is still detectable in liver, kidney and spleen one year after discontinuation of therapy (Janknegt et al 1993). It has been suggested that its high affinity for cholesterol in the mammalian cell wall may contribute to its nephrotoxicity (Fromtling 1993).

Table 5.7 *Antifungal agents*

Drug	Major route of excretion	Normal dose interval (h)	Dose intervals in renal failure (h)			Removal by dialysis		Toxic effects and comments
			GFR > 50 ml/min	GFR 10–50 ml/min	GFR < 10 ml/min	HD	PD	
Amphotericin	Non-renal	24	24	24	36	No	No	Nephrotoxic, especially with dehydration; causes glomerular and tubular damage, resulting in hypokalaemia and renal tubular acidosis. Measure plasma levels
Flucytosine	Renal	6	6	12–24	24–48	Yes	Yes	Bone marrow suppression and hepatic dysfunction commoner in uraemic patients. Measure plasma levels
Miconazole	Hepatic (renal)	8	8	8	8*	No	No	May cause hyponatraemia. *Reduce dose
Ketoconazole	Hepatic	12–24	12–24	12–24	12–24	No	No	Increases plasma cyclosporin levels
Fluconazole	Renal	24	24	48 or ¹/₂ dose	72 or ¹/₄ dose	Yes	Yes	Increases plasma cyclosporin levels. Give ¹/₂ dose after haemodialysis. Useful in fungal CAPD peritonitis
Itraconazole	Hepatic	24	24	24	24	No	No	Increases plasma cyclosporin levels. Peripheral neuropathy reported. Measure plasma levels

CAPD, continuous ambulatory peritoneal dialysis; HD, haemodialysis; PD, peritoneal dialysis.
CNS, central nervous system; HD, haemodialysis; LE, lupus erythematosus; PD, peritoneal dialysis.

Virtually all patients given amphotericin develop renal changes. The mechanism involves renal vasoconstriction, followed by damage to the glomeruli and tubules. Renal damage is worse in elderly and dehydrated patients, and is probably dose related. Permanent renal damage can occur, particularly with cumulative doses greater than 5 g. Early tubular damage is associated with increased excretion of uric acid and severe tubular loss of potassium. Hypokalaemia may develop rapidly, and serum electrolytes must be monitored frequently. Impaired acidification of the urine also occurs. Histology shows tubular necrosis and calcification. Nephrocalcinosis may develop later. Attempts have been made to reduce nephrotoxicity with mannitol, but the evidence suggests that this is ineffective. During therapy the GFR may fall to 40% of normal and recovery is often incomplete. Doses should therefore be kept to a minimum and regular checks made on the plasma creatinine and potassium levels.

Since amphotericin is excreted slowly, patients requiring a high dosage (1.5 mg/kg) can be given doses on alternate days in an attempt to reduce nephrotoxicity.

In renal failure, protein binding of amphotericin is reduced, but the concentration of the free drug is not altered. This must be considered when measuring plasma levels. The dose should be reduced when the GFR is less than 10 ml/min.

A recently developed colloidal dispersion formulation of amphotericin appears to be less nephrotoxic, with reduced binding to kidney tissue in animal studies (Fielding et al 1992). Further studies of this preparation are required in man.

Although synergy has been reported between amphotericin and flucytosine, some studies suggest that amphotericin may enhance toxicity of flucytosine by increasing its cellular uptake and reducing its renal excretion.

Flucytosine

Flucytosine is excreted largely unchanged by the kidneys and accumulates in renal failure. Nephrotoxicity is not a problem, but bone-marrow suppression and hepatic dysfunction are commoner in uraemic patients. Dosing intervals should be extended in renal failure. If the GFR is less than 10 ml/min, plasma levels should be closely monitored, aiming to keep levels between 25 and 50 mg/ml. If flucytosine infusion is used, levels should be measured at least 30 min after the end of the infusion. In renal failure allowance must be made for the high chloride content of the infusion solution (138 mmol/l). Flucytosine is readily removed by haemodialysis and peritoneal dialysis.

Miconazole

Miconazole is 98% protein bound. Some unchanged drug is excreted in the bowel, but most of the dose is rapidly metabolized in the liver and excreted via the kidney. Plasma levels are elevated in renal failure and the volume of distribution is reduced, but dosage modification is unnecessary until the GFR is less than 20 ml/min. There is no evidence of nephrotoxicity, but with intravenous infusion hyponatraemia may occur, together with a fall in haemoglobin and haematocrit. No supplementary dose is required after dialysis.

Ketoconazole

Ketoconazole is well absorbed from the gastro-intestinal tract and is extensively bound to plasma proteins. No dosage modification is required in renal failure. When given together with cyclosporin, for example in renal transplant recipients, blood levels of cyclosporin are increased; careful monitoring of cyclosporin blood levels is advisable.

Fluconazole

A total of 75–80% of fluconazole is excreted unchanged in the urine. For single-dose therapy no modification is required in renal failure. If a longer course is required in moderate or severe renal failure, it is suggested that the normal dose be given for the first 2 days; thereafter the dosing interval and/or daily dose should be modified according to the GFR (see Table 5.7) (Grant & Clissold 1990).

Fluconazole is readily removed by dialysis (50% of the dose in 3 h) and half the prescribed dose should be given after a dialysis session. It is also removed by peritoneal dialysis, but can be used to treat fungal peritonitis, both intraperitoneally and systemically. Bioavailability after intraperitoneal instillation is 87% (Brater 1994). In common with other azoles, fluconazole increases plasma cyclosporin levels in patients with renal transplants.

Itraconazole

Itraconazole is predominantly metabolized in the liver to a large number of metabolites which are excreted in the urine. Gastro-intestinal absorption may be reduced in renal failure, but no dosage modification is required. It is 99.8% bound to plasma proteins and is not dialysed. Peripheral neuropathy has been reported following long-term therapy, and doses must be reduced in hepatic disease. It increases plasma cyclosporin concentrations.

Griseofulvin

Griseofulvin is metabolized by the liver and no dosage modification is required in renal failure.

ANTIPROTOZOAL AND ANTHELMINTIC AGENTS

Most agents used to treat or prevent tropical diseases are metabolized in the liver and little modification is required except in severe renal impairment or in combined hepatic and renal disease. A brief review of the use of these agents in patients with renal impairment is given below.

ANTIMALARIALS

Chloroquine

Chloroquine has a monodesethyl metabolite with similar activity to chloroquine itself; the didesethyl metabolite is cardiotoxic and neuromyopathic. A total of 55% of chloroquine is excreted unchanged in the urine. For prophylactic use no modification is required in renal disease (300 mg once a week).

For treatment of malaria, the dose should be modified according to the GFR. Half the normal dose should be given if the GFR is 10–50 ml/min and quarter of the normal dose if the GFR is less than 10 ml/min. Negligible amounts are removed by haemodialysis and no supplementary dose is necessary.

Quinine

No change in dose is required in chronic renal failure. Indeed quinine sulphate is used to treat or prevent muscle cramps in renal failure patients. A total of 20% of a dose is excreted unchanged, and removal by dialysis is negligible. In acute renal failure induced by malaria the dose should be reduced by 30–50% (White 1985).

Mefloquine

Mefloquine is metabolized in the liver, and only 5–13% is excreted unchanged. No dosage modification is required in renal failure.

Primaquine

Primaquine is also metabolized in the liver, and normal doses should be given in renal failure.

Pyrimethamine/sulphadoxine

Mainly used for prophylaxis of *Plasmodium falciparum* malaria, given once a week. Both components have a long half-life of several days and are eliminated via the kidneys. Both are highly protein bound and no modification of dose is required in renal failure, but the mixture should not be continued for long periods in severe renal failure; it is also used to treat *P. falciparum* malaria in areas of chloroquine resistance. High blood levels are obtained after a single dose. If repeat doses are indicated, a high fluid intake should be maintained. Forced diuresis has been recommended for the treatment of overdosage, and alkalinization of the urine will increase excretion of the sulphadoxine component.

Proguanil

Proguanil is partly eliminated by the kidneys and the dose should be halved if the GFR is less than 10 ml/min.

ANTHELMINTICS

Mebendazole

Mebendazole is metabolized in the liver, is highly protein bound and is not dialysed (Allgayer et al 1984). No dosage modification is required in renal failure.

Thiabendazole

Thiabendazole is also metabolized in the liver. The parent drug and 5-hydroxymetabolite do not accumulate in renal failure, but the potentially toxic glucuronide and sulphate metabolites do. Central nervous system and gastro-intestinal disturbances may occur in patients with renal impairment, and the dose should be reduced to 25 mg/kg body weight daily. Haemodialysis produces very little clearance, but some removal is achieved by haemoperfusion. Crystalluria and haematuria have been described, and some patients excrete a metabolite in the urine with a characteristic asparagus-like odour.

Diethylcarbamazine

Diethylcarbamazine (for *Wucheria bancroftii* filariasis) is cleared by the kidneys. Renal excretion is reduced in alkaline urine and the dose should be reduced in patients with renal impairment (Adjepon-Yamoah et al 1982).

Praziquantel and ozamniquone

Praziquantel and ozamniquone, used to treat schistosomiasis, are metabolized in the liver and no dose modification is required in renal failure.

OTHER AGENTS

Benzidazole and nifurtimox

Benzidazole and nifurtimox, used in Chagas' disease, are metabolized in the liver and no dose modification is required in renal failure.

Suramin

Suramin (for trypanosomiasis) is almost 100% protein bound, has a very long half-life (44–54 days) and is not dialysed. It can cause haematuria and proteinuria.

Pentamidine

Pentamidine has considerable tissue-binding capacity and the drug is excreted in the urine over long periods. Particular care should be taken in treating patients with renal and hepatic disease.

Pentamidine is nephrotoxic, even after nebulized therapy (Miller et al 1989). After intravenous therapy, renal function must be carefully monitored and treatment stopped if the serum creatinine rises rapidly. Hypocalcaemia and profound hypotension may also occur.

In severe renal failure (GFR < 10 ml/min) the dose should be modified. In life-threatening *Pneumocystis carinii* pneumonia, 4 mg/kg body weight should be given daily for 7–10 days, and then on alternate days for a further week. In less severe cases, alternate-day therapy for 14 days will reduce the risk of nephrotoxicity.

ANTIVIRAL AGENTS

Acyclovir

Acyclovir is widely used in immunosuppressed patients, such as those who have received a renal transplant, to treat herpes zoster virus. It is also given to prevent cytomegalovirus (CMV) infection in CMV-antibody-negative recipients given a CMV-positive kidney. Treatment is usually continued for 3 months. A total of 75–80% of the drug is excreted unchanged and some tubular secretion occurs. Doses should be reduced in renal failure according to the GFR (Table 5.8). Transient renal impairment has been described, but severe renal impairment is rare. Adequate hydration is required to prevent renal precipitation of the drug. For intravenous therapy dosing is based on the body weight. Haemodialysis removes approximately 60% of the dose, and a supplementary dose (half the prescribed dose) should be given after dialysis. No additional dosing is required in CAPD patients

Table 5.8 *Dosing for intravenous acyclovir and ganciclovir*

Drug	GFR (ml/min)	Dose (ml/min)	Dosing interval (h)
Acyclovir	25–50	5–10	12
	10–25	5–10	24
	< 10	$1/_2$ dose	24
Ganciclovir	25–50	5	12
	10–25	2.5	24
	< 10	1.25	24

For oral acyclovir little modification is required until the GFR falls below 10 ml/min. For herpes simplex infections a dose of 200 mg twice daily is recommended. For varicella-zoster infections 800 mg 8-hourly is adequate if the GFR is 10–25 ml/min, or 800 mg 12-hourly if the GFR is less than 10 ml/min.

Neurological and psychiatric disturbances have been described in renal failure patients given high doses of acyclovir and ganciclovir, causing headache, confusion, sleeplessness, tremor and psychosis (Thomson et al 1985, Gill & Burgess 1990).

Ganciclovir

Ganciclovir is indicated for CMV infections in immuno-compromised patients, such as those with renal transplants. It is excreted unchanged and is only slightly protein bound. In renal failure the dose should be modified according to the body weight and GFR (Table 5.8). About 10–14% of patients develop neutropenia and thrombocytopenia. Neutropenia is particularly common in the second week of therapy. Haemodialysis removes 50% of the drug and a supplementary dose (half the prescribed dose) should be given after dialysis.

Famciclovir

Famciclovir has recently been introduced for varicella-zoster infections. It is predominantly excreted by the kidney and doses should be reduced in renal failure in relation to the GFR.

References

Adjepon-Yamoah K K, Edwards G, Breckenridge A M, Orme M L E Ward S A 1982 The effects of renal disease on the pharmacokinetics of diethylcarbamazine in man. *British Journal of Clinical Pharmacology* 13: 829–834

Allgayer H, Zahringer J, Bach P, Bircher J 1984 Lack of effect of haemodialysis on mebendazole kinetics: studies in a patient with echinococciosis and renal failure. *European Journal of Clinical Pharmacology* 27: 243–245

Aronoff G R 1982 Mezlocillin elimination in patients with impaired renal function. *Journal of Antimicrobial Chemotherapy* 9: S77–S79

Baron D N, Hamilton-Miller J M T, Brumfitt W 1984 Sodium content of injectable β-lactam antibiotics. *Lancet* i: 1113–1114

Bennett W M 1986 Drugs and renal disease, 2nd edn. Edinburgh, Churchill Livingstone

Bergan T 1983 Review of the pharmacokinetics of mezlocillin. *Journal of Antimicrobial Chemotherapy* 11: S1–S16

Bergan T, Thorsteinsson S B 1986 Pharmacokinetics of metronidazole and its metabolites in reduced renal function. *Chemotherapy* 32: 305–318

Bergeron M G, Lessard C, Ronald A, Stiver G, van Rooyen C E, Chadwick P 1983 Three to eight weeks of therapy with netilmicin: toxicity in normal and diabetic patients. *Journal of Antimicrobial Chemotherapy* 12: 245–248

Brater D C 1994 Pocket manual of drug use in clinical medicine, 6th edn. Improved Therapeutics, Indianapolis

Brown D L, Mauro L S 1988 Vancomycin dosing chart for use in patients with renal impairment. *American Journal of Kidney Diseases* 11: 15–19

Bush A, Holt J E, Sankey C M, Kaye C M, Gabriel R 1983 Penetration of metronidazole into continuous ambulatory peritoneal dialysate. *Peritoneal Dialysis Bulletin* 3: 176–177

Calandra G B, Ricci F M, Wang C, Brown K R 1988a The efficacy results and safety profile of imipenem/cilastatin from the clinical research trials. *Journal of Clinical Pharmacology* 28: 120–127

Calandra G B, Lydick E, Weiss L, Guess H 1988b Factors predisposing to seizures in seriously ill infected patients receiving antibiotics: experience with imipenem/cilastatin. *American Journal of Medicine* 84: 911–918

Christensson B A, Nilsson-Ehle I, Hutchinson M, Haworth S J, Oqvist B, Norrby S R 1992 Pharmacokinetics of meropenem in subjects with various degrees of renal impairment. *Antimicrobial Agents and Chemotherapy* 36 (7): 1532–1537

Davey P G, Geddes A M, Gonda I, Harpur E S, Scott D K 1983 Clinical experience with a method for adjusting gentamicin dose from measured drug clearance. *Journal of Antimicrobial Chemotherapy* 12: 613–622

Del Favero A 1994 Clinically important aspects of carbapenem safety. *Current Opinion in Infectious Diseases* 7 (suppl 1): S38–S42

Depner T A, Gulyassy P F 1980 Plasma protein binding in uremia: extraction and characterisation of an inhibitor. *Kidney International* 18: 86–94

Fielding R M, Singer A W, Wang L H, Babbar S, Guo L S S 1992 Relationship of pharmacokinetics and drug distribution in tissues to increased safety of amphotericin B colloidal dispersion in dogs. *Antimicrobial Agents and Chemotherapy* 36: 299–307

Fromtling R A 1993 Amphotericin B cholesteryl sulfate complex. *Drugs of the Future* 18: 303–306

Gilbert D N 1991 Once daily aminoglycoside therapy. *Antimicrobial Agents and Chemotherapy* 35: 399–406

Gill M J, Burgess E 1990 Neurotoxicity of acyclovir in end-stage renal disease. *Journal of Antimicrobial Chemotherapy* 25: 300–301

Gokal R, Ramos J M, Francis D M A et al 1982 Peritonitis in continuous ambulatory peritoneal dialysis. *Lancet* ii: 1388–1391

Grant S M, Clissold S P 1990 Fluconazole: a review of its pharmacodynamic and pharmacokinetic properties and therapeutic potential in superficial and systemic mycoses. *Drugs* 39: 877–916

Gudmundsson G H, Jensen L J 1989 Vancomycin and nephrotoxicity. *Lancet* i: 625

Halliwell R F, Davey P G, Lambert J J 1993 Antagonism of GABA A receptors by 4-quinolones. *Journal of Antimicrobial Chemotherapy* 31: 457–462

Hou S H, Bashinsky D A, Wish J B, Cohen J J, Harrington J T 1983 Hospital acquired renal insufficiency. A prospective study. *American Journal of Medicine* 74: 243–251

Humes H D 1988 Aminoglycoside nephrotoxocity. *Kidney International* 33: 900–911

Jackson G D, Berkovic S L 1992 Ceftazidime encephalopathy: absence states and toxic hallucinations. *Journal of Neurology, Neurosurgery and Psychiatry* 55: 33–34

Janknegt R, de Marie S, Bakker-Woudenberg I A J M, Crommelin D J A 1992 Liposomal and lipid formulations of amphotericin B. *Clinical Pharmacokinetics* 23: 279–291

Job L M, Dretler R H 1990 Seizure activity with imipenem therapy: incidence and risk factors. *Annals of Pharmacotherapy* 24: 467–469

Kaloyanides G J, Pastoriza-Munoz E 1980 Aminoglycoside nephrotoxicity. *Kidney International* 18: 571–582

Lerner A M, Reyes M P, Cone L A et al 1983 Randomised controlled trial of the comparative efficacy, auditory toxicity and nephrotoxicity of tobramycin and netilmicin. *Lancet* i: 1123–1125

Leroy A, Fillastre J P, Etienne I, Borsa-Lebas F, Humbert G 1992 Pharmacokinetics of meropenem in subjects with renal insufficiency. *European Journal of Pharmacology* 45 (5): 535–538

Manuel M A, Paton T W, Cornish W R 1983 Drugs and peritoneal dialysis. *Peritoneal Dialysis Bulletin* 3: 117–125

Marsh F P 1983 Drugs and the kidney. In: Weatherall D J, Ledingham J G G, Warrell D A (eds) Oxford textbook of medicine. Oxford University Press, Oxford, pp 18.107–18.110

Matzke G R, Keane W F 1986 The use of antibiotics in patients with renal insufficiency. In: Peterson P K, Verhoef J (eds) Antimicrobial agents annual J. Elsevier, Amsterdam, pp 472–488

Meyer R D 1986 Risk factors and comparisons of clinical nephrotoxicity of aminoglycosides. *American Journal of Medicine* 80 (suppl 6B): 119–125

Miller R F, Delany S, Semple S J G 1989 Acute renal failure after nebulised pentamidine. *Lancet* i: 1271–1272

Moellering R C, Krogstad D J, Greenblatt D J 1981 Vancomycin therapy in patients with impaired renal function: a nomogram for dosage. *Annals of Internal Medicine* 94: 343–346

Moore R D, Smith C R, Lipsky J J, Mellits E D, Lietman P S 1984 Risk factors for nephrotoxicity in patients treated with aminoglycosides. *Annals of Internal Medicine* 100: 352–357

Neugarten J, Gallo G R, Baldwin D S 1983 Rifampicin-induced nephrotic syndrome and acute interstitial nephritis. *American Journal of Nephrology* 3: 38–42

Nilsson-Ehle I, Ursing B, Nilsson-Ehle P 1981 Liquid chromatographic assay for metronidazole and tinidazole: pharmacokinetic and metabolic studies in human subjects. *Antimicrobial Agents and Chemotherapy* 19: 754–760

Nix D E, Schentag J J 1988 The quinolones: an overview and comparative appraisal of their pharmacokinetics and pharmacodynamics. *Journal of Clinical Pharmacology* 28: 169–178

Nordstrom L, Ringberg H, Cronberg S, Tjernstrom O, Walder M 1990 Does administration of an aminoglycoside in a single daily dose affect its efficacy and toxicity? *Journal of Antimicrobial Chemotherapy* 25: 159–173

Rawer P, Seim K E 1989 Elimination of vancomycin during haemofiltration. *European Journal of Clinical Microbiology and Infectious Diseases* 8: 529–531

Reeves D 1982 Sulphonamides and trimethoprim. In: Geddes A M (ed) Good antimicrobial prescribing. *Lancet*, London, pp 63–74

Reeves D, Paton J 1987 Antimicrobial agents for intensive care patients with renal failure. *Care of the Critically Ill* 3: 100–104

Rippelmeyer D J, Synhavsky A 1988 Ciprofloxacin and allergic interstitial nephritis. *Annals of Internal Medicine* 109: 170

Roberts D E, Williams J D 1989 Ciprofloxacin in renal failure. *Antimicrobial Agents and Chemotherapy* 23: 820–823

Sandberg T, Trollfors B 1986 Effect of trimethoprim on serum creatinine in patients with acute cystitis. *Journal of Antimicrobial Chemotherapy* 17: 123–124

Sawyers C L, Moore R D, Lerner S A, Smith C R 1986 A model for predicting nephrotoxicity in patients treated with aminoglycosides. *Journal of Infectious Diseases* 153: 1062–1068

Smith C R, Lipsky J J, Laskin O L et al 1980 Double-blind comparison of the nephrotoxicity of gentamicin and tobramycin. *New England Journal of Medicine* 302: 1106–1109

Somogyi A A, Kong C B, Gurr F W, Sabto J, Spicer W J, McLean A J 1984 Metronidazole pharmacokinetics in patients with acute renal failure. *Journal of Antimicrobial Chemotherapy* 13: 183–189

Steurer B C, Konigsreiner A, Willert J, Margreiter R 1991 Increased risk of central nervous toxicity in patients treated with cyclosporin and imipenem/cilastatin. *Nephron* 58: 362–364

Thompson M I B, Russo M E, Saxon B J, Atkin-Thor E, Matsen J M 1982 Gentamicin inactivation by piperacillin or carbenicillin in patients with end-stage renal disease. *Antimicrobial Agents and Chemotherapy* 21: 268–273

Thomson C R, Goodship T H J, Rodger R C S 1985 Psychiatric side-effects of acyclovir in patients with chronic renal failure. *Lancet* ii: 385–386

Vincken W 1984 Psychotic reactions to cefuroxime described in patients with renal failure. *Lancet* i: 965

Wallace S M, Chan L Y 1985 In vitro interaction of aminoglycosides with beta-lactam penicillins. *Antimicrobial Agents and Chemotherapy* 28: 274–281

Webb D B, Roberts D E, Williams J D, Asscher A W 1986 Pharmacokinetics of ciprofloxacin in healthy volunteers and patients with impaired kidney function. *Journal of Antimicrobial Chemotherapy* 18 (suppl D): 83–87

Whelton A, Stout R L, Delgado F A 1983 Azlocillin kinetics during extracorporeal haemodialysis and peritoneal dialysis. *Journal of Antimicrobial Chemotherapy* 11: S89–S95

White N J 1985 Clinical pharmacokinetics of antimalarial drugs. *Clinical Pharmacokinetics* 10: 187–215

Wise R, Wright N 1981 Cefotaxime metabolism and renal function. *Lancet* i: 1106–1107

Drug interactions involving antimicrobial agents

J. P. Griffin and P. F. D'Arcy

Basic mechanisms

Drug interactions can occur inside or outside the body. They can occur before administration when drugs are added in vitro to an intravenous drip, or they can have origins in a tablet or capsule when one component of the formulation (e.g. an excipient) alters the subsequent bioavailability of the active drug. They can occur in the intestine before absorption when a drug or food component modifies the absorption characteristics of another drug. They can occur after absorption either from drug competition for protein-binding sites in the plasma and tissues, or from drug competition at binding sites or antagonism at receptor sites in the tissues at which they arrive.

Interactions may modify the degradation of a drug by inducing or inhibiting metabolic enzyme systems, especially those associated with liver microsomes. They may intervene

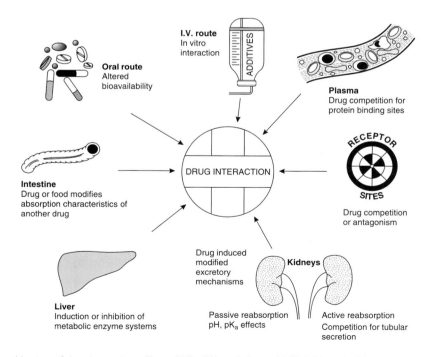

Fig. 6.1   *The possible sites of drug interactions. (From Griffin, D'Arcy & Speirs 1988 A Manual of Adverse Drug Interactions, John Wright, London.)*

in the excretory processes of the drug in the kidney tubules; indeed, there is no phase from formulation to elimination where drug interactions are excluded.

The many possible sites of drug interactions are shown in Figure 6.1; this illustrates clearly the extent of the problem which, in this present context, is discussed under the following main headings: drug interactions in vitro; drug interactions at the absorption site; drug interactions at plasma, tissue and receptor-binding sites; drug interactions and drug-metabolizing enzymes; and drug interactions in excretory mechanisms. It should be borne in mind that an interaction between two drugs can occur at more than one site.

Drug interactions in vitro

There are four problem areas that for the purpose of this chapter have been regarded as drug interactions occurring in vitro:

- excipients in medicinal formulations
- additives to intravenous fluids
- drug–container interactions (mainly drug–plastics interactions)
- drug–contact lens interactions.

EXCIPIENTS

Excipients have generally been considered to be inert, pharmacologically inactive and non-toxic, in contrast to active drugs. This may have been so in the past, but excipients in modern formulations cannot automatically be regarded as inactive. They are not necessarily free from toxicity in all persons and they can enter into interactions which influence the bioavailability of the active drug substance in the formulation. A review by D'Arcy (1990) has publicized such problems with formulation excipients.

An example of this first category is the impaired intestinal absorption of rifampicin when combined with *p*-aminosalicylic acid (PAS). This was first noticed in the early 1970s and was originally thought to be a drug–drug interaction. Later it was shown to be due to the reduced absorption of rifampicin caused by the bentonite used as an excipient in the PAS granules. A further example is bacitracin, which is slowly inactivated in bases of topical preparations containing stearlyl alcohol, cholesterol, polyoxyethylene derivatives and sodium lauryl sulphate, and is rapidly inactivated in bases containing water, macrogols, propylene glycol, glycerol, cetylpyridinium chloride, benzalkonium chloride, icthammol, phenol and tannic acid. The absorption rate, but not the extent of absorption, of clindamycin in healthy subjects is markedly reduced by a kaolin–pectin suspension.

Other examples of antimicrobials entering into this type of interaction in vivo are hard to find and probably equally difficult to substantiate, although there is much in vitro evidence available. Such interactions may well occur with generic preparations where the active drug is the same as the proprietary preparation, although the formulation will be different in terms of the content and nature of the excipients. The bioavailability of the active drug may be different in the two formulations, as may its safety spectrum.

ADDITIVES TO INTRAVENOUS FLUIDS

This second category is by far the most important in relation to in vitro interactions. The number of incompatibilities that have been recorded between various drugs added indiscriminately to intravenous fluids is legion. The result of the interactions may be inactivation of one or both of the therapeutic substances added to the fluid, an altered therapeutic response or the combination may be toxic. Table 6.1 lists a number of the common incompatibilities that occur involving antimicrobial substances in combination with other drugs in intravenous fluids. The list is illustrative and not comprehensive, but the principles laid down below should be followed. Comprehensive details on antimicrobial interactions in intravenous fluids are given in the individual monographs of the 30th edition of *Martindale, The Extra Pharmacopoeia* (Reynolds 1993).

We recommend that before any drug is added to any intravenous fluid container the following questions should be asked:

- Is it necessary that the drug be given in this way?
- Is the stability of the particular drug in the selected infusion fluid firmly established?
- If multiple additives are intended, is the stability in the selected infusion fluid of each drug, both separately and together, firmly established?
- Will the drug(s) have the intended therapeutic effect if given in high dilution over a period of hours?
- Since many drugs decompose slowly in infusion fluids, will the interval between drug addition and use be kept to a minimum?

As a further general principle, it is undesirable to add drugs to blood, plasma or amino acid solutions. Intravenous drug(s) are best given by the injection site provided in the giving set.

CONTAINER INTERACTIONS

Knowledge about drug interactions with plastics is still at the elementary stage, despite the long use of plastic containers and syringes. A number of drugs may exhibit

Table 6.1 *Antimicrobials in intravenous fluids: common incompatibilities with other drug substances in vitro (From Griffin, D'Arcy & Speirs 1988 A Manual of Adverse Drug Interactions, John Wright, London.)*

Antimicrobial	Interacting drugs
Ampicillin	Adrenaline, amino acids, Aminosol Vitrium, atropine, calcium chloride, calcium gluconate, chloramphenicol, chlorpromazine, chlortetracycline, dopamine, erythromycin, gentamicin, hydralazine, hydrocortisone, kanamycin, lincomycin, metaraminol, noradrenaline, novobiocin, oxytetracycline, pentobarbitone, phenobarbitone, polymyxin B, prochlorperazine, protein hydrolysates, streptomycin, sulphafurazole, suxamethonium tetracycline, thiopentone, B group vitamins, vitamin C
Benzylpenicillin	Amphotericin, cephalothin, chlorpromazine, erythromycin, hydroxyzine, lincomycin, metaraminol, noradrenaline, oxytetracycline, phenytoin, prochlorperazine, promazine, promethazine, tetracycline, thiopentone, vancomycin, B group vitamins, vitamin C
Carbenicillin	Amikacin, amphotericin, chloramphenicol, erythromycin, gentamicin, hydrocortisone, kanamycin, lincomycin, oxytetracycline, phenytoin, promethazine, streptomycin, sympathomimetic amines, tetracycline, tobramycin, B group vitamins, vitamin C. Solutions of carbenicillin sodium should be protected from light
Cephaloridine (change all infusion fluids containing cephaloridine after 6 h)	Erythromycin, oxytetracycline, phenylephrine, polymyxin B, tetracycline, all barbiturates (10–15% loss of cephaloridine potency in 6 h), all bacteriostatic antibiotics (reduced activity)
Chloramphenicol	Benzyl alcohol, erythromycin (gluceptate and lactobionate), hydrocortisone, hydroxyzine, novobiocin, oxytetracycline, phenytoin, polymyxin B, prochlorperazine, promethazine, sulphadiazine, tetracycline, tripelennamine, vancomycin
Ciprofloxacin	Infusion has pH 3.9–4.5 and is incompatible with injections chemically or physically unstable at this pH range. Reported incompatibility with aminophylline, amoxycillin, amoxycillin with potassium clavulanate, clindamycin, flucloxacillin, heparin sodium
Cloxacillin	Alevaire (tyloxapol 0.125% solution for nebulization), chlorpromazine, erythromycin, gentamicin, oxytetracycline, polymyxin B, tetracycline, vitamin C. Some loss of potency has been reported with colistin sulphomethate and kanamycin. Do not add to lactate solutions or to carbohydrate solutions with pH < 4. Acetic acid, acetate ions, bicarbonate, dihydrogen and monohydrogen phosphate ions, citric acid, and dihydrogen and monohydrogen citrate ions can catalyse the degradation of cloxacillin
Colistin sulphomethate	Cephaloridine, cephalothin, chlortetracycline, erythromycin, hydrocortisone, hydroxyzine, kanamycin, methicillin, tetracycline. Solutions of colistin sulphomethate sodium should be protected from light
Erythromycin ethylsuccinate	Ampicillin, cloxacillin
Erythromycin gluceptate	Amikacin, carbenicillin, cephaloridine, cephalothin, cephazolin, chloramphenicol, colistin sulphomethate, heparin, novobiocin, pentobarbitone, phenobarbitone, phenytoin, protein hydrolysate, quinalbarbitone, streptomycin, tetracycline, thiopentone, vitamin B complex, sodium chloride solutions
Erythromycin lactobionate	Acidic substances, aminophylline, ampicillin, carbenicillin, cephalothin, chloramphenicol, cloxacillin, colistin sulphomethate, gentamicin, heparin, hydrocortisone, metaraminol, protein hydrolysate, tetracycline, thiopentone, vitamin B complex, vitamin C
Gentamicin	Amphotericin, cephalothin, chloramphenicol, erythromycin, heparin, soluble sulphonamides, all penicillins (loss of gentamicin activity), streptomycin or kanamycin (increased toxicity), ticarcillin (inactivates gentamicin)
Lincomycin	Ampicillin, benzylpenicillin, carbenicillin, erythromycin, novobiocin, phenytoin, soluble sulphonamides
Methicillin (may precipitate in dextrose solution, change infusion fluid every 8 h or sooner if cloudy)	Adrenaline, amiphenazole, atropine sulphate, calcium chloride, canrenoate potassium, cephalothin, chloramphenicol, chlorpromazine, chlortetracycline, codeine, colistin sulphomethate, dextrose and saline infusion fluids, erythromycin, gentamicin, hydrocortisone, kanamycin, levallorphan, levorphanol, lincomycin, metaraminol, methadone, methohexitone, morphine salts, neomycin, novobiocin, oxytetracycline, pentobarbitone, pethidine, polymyxin B, prochlorperazine, promazine, promethazine, protein hydrolysates, sodium bicarbonate, streptomycin, sulphadiazine, sulphafurazole, suxamethonium, tetracycline, thiopentone, vancomycin, B group vitamins, vitamin C
Nafcillin	Aminophylline, chlortetracycline, gentamicin, hydrocortisone, oxytetracycline, polymyxin B, sympathomimetic amines, tetracycline, B group vitamins, vitamin C
Nitrofurantoin	Amikacin, ammonium chloride injection, amphotericin, insulin, kanamycin, lactated Ringer's injection, metaraminol, narcotic salts, noradrenaline, polymyxin B, procaine, prochlorperazine, promethazine, protein hydrolysates, streptomycin, tetracycline, vancomycin

Table 6.1 *Cont'd*

Antimicrobial	Interacting drugs
Novobiocin (incompatible with dextrose solutions and lactated Ringer's solution)	Adrenaline, calcium gluconate, chloramphenicol, corticotrophin, dimenhydrinate, erythromycin, heparin, hydrocortisone, insulin, oxytetracycline, procaine, protein hydrolysate, streptomycin, tetracycline, vancomycin, Parentrovite
Oxytetracycline	Alkalis, amikacin (depending on diluent), aminophylline, amphotericin, ampicillin, soluble barbiturates, benzylpenicillin, calcium chloride, calcium gluceptate, calcium gluconate, carbenicillin sodium, cefapirin, cephaloridine, cephalothin, cephazolin, chloramphenicol, cloxacillin, erythromycin salts, heparin, hydrocortisone, hydroxyzine, iron dextran injection, lactated Ringer's injection, metaraminol, methicillin, methylprednisolone, novobiocin, oxacillin, phenytoin, prochlorperazine, promethazine, protein hydrolysate, sodium bicarbonate, sodium lactate, sulphadiazine, sulphafurazole, suxamethonium, thiopentone, B group vitamins. Solutions of oxytetracycline hydrochloride should be protected from light
Polymyxin B	Amphotericin, ampicillin, cefapirin, cephalothin, cephazolin, chloramphenicol, chlorothiazide, chlortetracycline, cloxacillin, heparin, nitrofurantoin, prednisolone, tetracycline. Solutions of polymyxin B sulphate should be protected from light
Sulphonamides: Sulphadiazine sod. Sulphadimidine sod. (Incompatible with dextrose and fructose solutions)	Acid electrolytes, amiphenazole, chloramphenicol, chlorpromazine, gentamicin, hydralazine, insulin, iron dextran, kanamycin, lincomycin, metaraminol, methicillin, methyldopate, narcotic salts, noradrenaline, procaine, prochlorperazine, promazine, promethazine, streptomycin, tetracyclines, vancomycin, Parentrovite
Tetracycline	Amphotericin, ampicillin, amylobarbitone, benzylpenicillin, carbenicillin, cephalothin, chloramphenicol, chlorothiazide, cloxacillin, dimenhydrinate, erythromycin, heparin, hydrocortisone (cortisol), methicillin, methohexitone, methyldopate, nitrofurantoin, novobiocin, pentobarbitone, phenobarbitone, phenytoin, polymyxin B, quinalbarbitone, riboflavine, sodium bicarbonate, sulphadiazine, sulphafurazole, thiopentone, warfarin. Protect solutions from light. (Nitrofurantoin sodium and tetracycline hydrochloride are compatible in sodium chloride injection)
Vancomycin	Incompatible in infusion fluids with methicillin, ticarcillin, penicillin G

clinically significant adsorption onto plastic materials. In addition, some drugs alter the physical characteristics of plastic materials. Such interactions, although more common with plastics, can also occur with glass. Chloroquine, for example, is almost totally bound to soda glass. This is most important in laboratory work where large decreases in the concentration of chloroquine can lead to the false assumption of *Plasmodium falciparum* resistance to chloroquine.

Generally, this type of interaction has not proved troublesome with antimicrobial agents; D'Arcy (1983) has reviewed drug interactions with medicinal plastics.

INTERACTIONS WITH SOFT CONTACT LENSES

A number of drugs which are secreted from the lachrymal glands in the tears can lead to discoloration of soft contact lenses. Rifampicin can lead to a permanent pink discoloration of the lenses. Adrenaline hydrochloride and epinephryl borate eye drops can lead to adrenochrome being deposited in the lenses, giving a dense brown spotted discoloration. Sulphasalazine can cause an irreversible yellow/green staining of certain types of soft lens.

Drug interactions at the absorption site

DRUG INTERACTIONS IN THE INTESTINE

To reach the bloodstream from the alimentary tract, a drug must cross the intestinal epithelium, basement membrane and capillary epithelium. For most drugs the most important process of absorption is that of passive diffusion; no energy is required, it is not saturable and the transfer is directly proportional to the concentration gradient and to the lipid–water partition coefficient of the drug. However, there are a number of inter-related factors that can complicate efficient drug absorption: the passive diffusion may be pH dependent; some drugs and foodstuffs delay gastric emptying and thus may slow the absorption of other drugs taken at the same time; and the drug may interact with specific cations in the bowel to produce non-absorbable complexes. Drugs may quite specifically reduce the intestinal absorption of each other, and dietary components may influence drug absorption or, conversely, have their own absorption influenced by drugs.

The reverse is also evident: some drugs are better absorbed with food; this increased absorption has been attributed to a number of mechanisms, including delayed stomach emptying time, permitting greater dissolution of the drug, improved dispersion, reduced protein binding and increased splanchnic blood flow. Food increases splanchnic blood flow and hence enhances drug absorption. For example, the absorption of cefuroxime axetil is enhanced by the presence of food, as is that of nitrofurantoin, griseofulvin, itraconazole, ketoconazole and clofazimine, if taken immediately after food.

It is recommended that nitrofurantoin be given with food to avoid gastric irritation; fortuitously, its bioavailability is increased by 20–400% in the presence of food or milk, probably by delayed stomach emptying allowing greater dissolution of the drug. Griseofulvin is absorbed faster in the presence of a fatty meal and serum levels are double those of the fasting state (Fig. 6.2). Absorption of capsules of the antifungal agent itraconazole is enhanced by administration immediately after breakfast. Absorption of the related ketoconazole increases with decreasing stomach pH and, although some recommend administration after a meal, conflicting results have been reported from bioavailability studies.

In some circumstances, the absorption of the drug may result in a high percentage of the drug being rendered inactive by metabolic transformation as it passes through the intestinal wall; an example of this is the sulphation of a number of β-sympathomimetic bronchodilators. In other circumstances, for example with pro-drug forms of the penicillins (bacampicillin, hetacillin, metampicillin, pivampicillin, talampicillin), conversion to the active substance may occur during transit through the intestinal wall. The metabolic processes taking place in the gut wall may offer a site for drug interaction to take place.

pH AND IONIC INTERACTIONS IN THE INTESTINE

The bioavailability of tetracyclines is reduced in patients being treated with H_2 antagonists. Investigation has shown that this is an effect on the dissolution of the solid dose form, since the absorption of tetracycline from syrups was not affected. The reduction in the bioavailability from the solid dose form was as high as 30–40%.

The presence of food in the gut induces changes in pH, and food-induced reduction of the absorption of, for example, erythromycin may depend on gastric acidity. Food has an adverse effect on the absorption of lincomycin, cloxacillin and minocycline. The absorption of tetracyclines is reduced by the formation of insoluble chelates in the gut in the presence of milky and other foods containing bivalent and trivalent metal ions (e.g. calcium, magnesium, aluminium, iron), and serum levels of oral tetracycline may be decreased by more than 50% if they are taken with ferrous sulphate, aluminium hydroxide or milk (Figs 6.3 and 6.4). The intestinal absorption of quinolone antibacterials is reduced by the concomitant intake of iron preparations. The aluminium content of the ulcer-healing drug sucralfate and concomitant treatment with aluminium or magnesium-containing laxatives or preparations containing zinc also reduce the absorption of quinolones.

DRUG–DRUG ABSORPTION REACTIONS

Barbiturates can reduce the intestinal absorption of a number of drugs. The absorption of griseofulvin is impaired by phenobarbitone, independent of any enzyme induction by the barbiturate which could have affected the metabolism of the antifungal.

NON-SPECIFIC EFFECTS OF MEALS

As already mentioned, the absorption of drugs may be reduced, delayed or enhanced by concurrent food intake. These effects are essentially due to either delayed gastric emptying or dilution of the drug in the gut contents. Gastric emptying time may be delayed by hot meals, high fat content and high-viscosity solutions. In general, fatty meals delay gastric emptying times to a greater extent than either

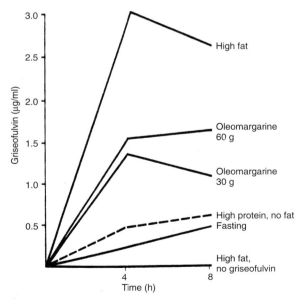

Fig. 6.2 *Effects of different types of food intake on serum griseofulvin concentrations following a 1 g oral dose of the drug. (After Crounse R G 1961 Journal of Investigative Dermatology 37: 529–533.) (From Griffin, D'Arcy & Speirs 1988 A Manual of Adverse Drug Interactions, John Wright, London.)*

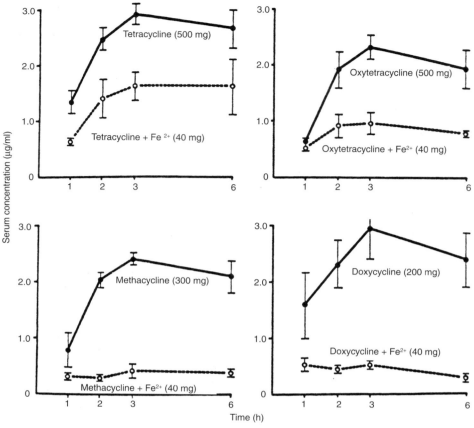

Fig. 6.3 *The effect of concomitant administration of iron tablets on the serum concentrations of tetracyclines; both drugs given orally. (After Neuvonen P J et al 1970 British Medical Journal 4: 532–534.) (From Griffin, D'Arcy & Speirs 1988 A Manual of Adverse Drug Interactions, John Wright, London.)*

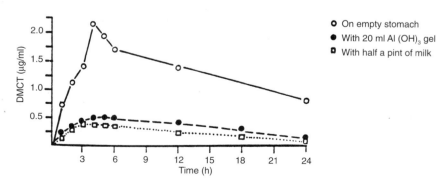

Fig. 6.4 *Effect of co-administration of aluminium hydroxide or half a pint of milk on the serum concentration of demethylchlortetracycline (DMCT) after a single oral dose of 300 mg of the drug. (After Levy G 1970 In: Sprowls J B (ed) Prescription pharmacy, 2nd edn. J B Lippincott, Philadelphia, p 70, 75, 80.) (From Griffin, D'Arcy & Speirs 1988 A Manual of Adverse Drug Interactions, John Wright, London.)*

protein-rich or carbohydrate-rich meals. Delayed absorption of drugs brought about by food does not always imply that a lesser amount of drug is absorbed, but rather that the time for a drug to reach peak blood levels after a single dose is lengthened; this may have clinical advantage.

The influence of food on the absorption of antimicrobial substances has been studied extensively by Welling & Tse (1982) and the information in Tables 6.2 and 6.3 is adapted from their work. With some exceptions, the absorption of

Table 6.2 *Influence of food on the absorption of antimicrobial agents**

Agent	Form
Absorption may be reduced	
Amoxycillin	Capsules, suspension
Ampicillin	Capsules
Cephalexin	Capsules, suspension
Demethylchlortetracycline	Capsules
Doxycycline	Capsules (absorption slightly reduced)
Isoniazid	Tablets
Methacycline	Capsules
Nafcillin	Tablets
Oxytetracycline	Capsules
Penicillin G	Suspension, tablets
Penicillin V (K)	Capsules, suspension, tablets
Penicillin V (Ca)	Tablets
Penicillin V (acid)	Tablets
Phenethicillin	Capsules, tablets
Phenylmercaptomethyl penicillin	Capsules
Pivampicillin	Capsules
Rifampicin	Formulation not indicated
Tetracycline	Capsule
Absorption may be delayed	
Cefaclor	Capsules, suspension
Cephalexin	Capsules
Cephradine	Capsules
Metronidazole	Tablets
Sulfasymazine	Formulation not indicated
Sulfisoxazole	Formulation not indicated
Sulphadiazine	Solution
Sulphadimethoxine	Formulation not indicated
Sulphamethoxypyridazine	Formulation not indicated
Sulphanilamide	Suspension
Absorption may be increased	
Alafosfin	Capsules
Griseofulvin	Formulation not indicated
Hetacillin	Capsules (absorption slightly increased)
Nitrofurantoin	Capsules, tablets
Sulphamethoxydiazine	Tablets
Absorption generally unaffected	
Amoxycillin	Capsules
Ampicillin	Suspension
Penicillin V (acid)	Tablets
Spiramycin	Tablets
Sulphasomidine	Tablets

* Modified from Welling & Tse (1982), where reference citations to these individual interaction reports are given.

Table 6.3 *Influence of food on the absorption of erythromycin products**

Product type	Effect on absorption
Capsules	Reduced
Tablets	Reduced
Coated tablets	Delayed, reduced or unaffected
Estolate suspension	Unaffected
Ethylcarbamate suspension	Unaffected
Ethylsuccinate coated tablets	Increased
Ethylsuccinate film tablets	Delayed
Ethylsuccinate suspension	Increased or unaffected
Stearate coated tablets	Reduced or increased

* Modified from Welling & Tse (1982), where reference citations to these individual interaction reports are given.

most penicillins, cephalosporins and tetracyclines and some erythromycin products is markedly reduced by food. Thus, in order to obtain maximum circulating blood levels for a given dose and to maintain reproducible drug levels between doses, as a general rule antibiotics should be administered at least 1 h (and longer, if possible) before meals.

SPECIFIC INTERACTIONS BETWEEN DIETARY COMPONENTS AND DRUG ABSORPTION

There is a minority of drugs for which the precise nature of the concomitant diet is important. A classic example is that of griseofulvin, which is lipid soluble and shows increased absorption and higher plasma concentrations when given with a meal of high fat content (see Fig. 6.2).

The absorption of the anthelmintic, tetrachloroethylene, which is lipid soluble, is enhanced when the diet is rich in fat, or alcohol is taken concomitantly. This effect is undesirable on two counts. Firstly, the hookworm (*Ankylostoma* or *Necator*), against which the drug is used, matures in the intestine and a local effect rather than a systemic effect is desired. Secondly, tetrachloroethylene is hepatotoxic and nephrotoxic and its absorption by the human host should be kept to a minimum.

DRUG INTERACTIONS AFFECTING INTESTINAL METABOLIC MECHANISMS

Drug interactions affecting drug metabolism by the intestinal mucosa can, theoretically, be classified as being due to either enzyme induction, enzyme inhibition or competition for conjugation mechanisms. The only potentially clinically significant drug interactions to occur at this level are those related to competition for sulphation and glucuronation and those due to enzyme inhibition. Also of importance is the interaction between antibiotics and combined-type oral contraceptives. Contraceptive steroids are normally well absorbed from the gastrointestinal tract, but are susceptible to a high first-pass effect in the liver (60% with ethinyl-oestradiol) where they are metabolized to form sulphate and glucuronide conjugates. Oestrogen conjugates are excreted in bile where they are hydrolysed by bacteria in the lower gut to release unchanged oestrogens which are reabsorbed into the portal circulation, a process called 'enterohepatic circulation'. Antibiotics interfere with the intestinal flora involved in the enterohepatic circulation of the low-level oestrogens and negate their contraceptive action. This inter-action has been reviewed by, for example, D'Arcy (1986) and Back & Orme (1990).

DRUG-INDUCED MALABSORPTION AND VITAMIN DEPLETION

Many drugs are known to evoke vitamin deficiency states; for example, isoniazid, hydrallazine and penicillamine are antagonistic to vitamin B_6, anticonvulsants cause folate and vitamin D deficiency, and vitamin B_{12} deficiency may occur after prolonged treatment with the antidiabetic, metformin. Of specific interest in this review, vitamin K depletion can occur in the presence of antibiotics which interfere with the gastro-intestinal flora. This is not usually of any clinical significance unless the patient has low dietary vitamin K levels and is concurrently being treated with oral anticoag-ulants, a combination which could result in enhancement of anticoagulation. Foods rich in vitamin K are also capable of altering the prothrombin time and reducing the effects of anticoagulation.

Cytotoxic agents such as methotrexate can poison all metabolic processes in the gut which are involved in active absorption.

GASTRO-INTESTINAL DISEASE AND DRUG ABSORPTION

Various diseases of the gastro-intestinal tract affect the absorption of a wide range of drugs, including antimicrobial agents (Table 6.4). Drug absorption in patients with gastro-intestinal disease is variable and unpredictable and depends on the severity of the disease process at any given time.

The lack of predictability of the bioavailability of a drug is increased if the drug is subjected to metabolic change in the gut wall. For example, if the drug undergoes sulphonation or glucuronation, or if it is activated by esterases in the gut wall during the absorption process, then the gastro-intestinal disease may greatly affect bioavailability. For example, it is at these sites that the penicillin pro-drugs (bacampicillin, hetacillin, metampicillin, pivampicillin, talampicillin) undergo metabolic change to active penicillins. Gastro-intestinal disease may reduce their absorption.

Table 6.4 *Effect of gastro-intestinal disease on absorption of antimicrobial agents**

Disease	Drugs
Drug absorption increased	
Crohn's disease	Clindamycin, co-trimoxazole, erythromycin
Coeliac disease	Cephalexin, clindamycin, co-trimoxazole, erythromycin ethylsuccinate, ethinyloestradiol, PAS, sodium fusidate
Postgastrectomy	Cephalexin, PAS, phenoxymethylpenicillin
Drug absorption reduced	
Achlorhydria	Phenoxymethylpenicillin, tetracycline
Coeliac disease	Amoxycillin, phenoxymethylpenicillin, pivampicillin, rifampicin
Cystic fibrosis	Azidocillin, cephalexin, dicloxacillin
Diarrhoea	Rapid transit times can upset the absorption of many drugs, particularly those in delayed-release formulations
Pancreatitis	Phenoxymethylpenicillin
Postgastrectomy	Ethambutol, ethionamide, sulphafurazole

PAS, *p*-aminosalicylic acid.
* After Parsons & David (1980).

Drug interactions at plasma, tissue and receptor binding sites

Drug absorption is favoured when a drug is highly bound to plasma proteins, since the concentration gradient of free drug between the absorption site (usually the gut) and the bloodstream is maintained.

Once absorbed, drugs are distributed by the blood to the various tissues of the body, many being bound to the plasma proteins, particularly albumin. Important changes in drug distribution can arise from competition between drugs for protein-binding sites in plasma or tissues; certain groups of drugs seem to share a limited number of common binding sites, and one drug can displace another, sometimes with dramatic consequences.

An important example of this type of interaction is that involving warfarin: normally 98% of warfarin is bound to albumin so that only the unbound 2% of the total drug in the plasma is biologically active. If another drug (e.g. nalidixic acid) competes for the same plasma albumin-binding sites and marginally reduces the binding of warfarin from, say, 98% to 96%, then this effectively doubles the concentration of pharmacologically active warfarin. This has roughly the same effect on the prothrombin time as doubling the administered dose of the anticoagulant.

A number of antimicrobial substances enter into drug–drug interactions by virtue of displacement of a less strongly bound substance from plasma proteins. For example, sulphonamides displace tolbutamide and other sulphony-lurea hypoglycaemic agents, and thus potentiate their glucose lowering action. Phenylbutazone, which is more strongly protein bound than sulphonamides, can displace sulphonamides from plasma proteins, leading to higher plasma levels of unbound sulphonamide and increased antibacterial action. Sulphonamides can displace metho-trexate from plasma protein binding, and thus increase the risk of methotrexate toxicity.

Generally, there are few examples of antimicrobial substances causing drug interactions of clinical significance by displacement of other drugs from protein binding. In fact, Griffin et al (1988) were of the view that the importance of this type of interaction had been 'overestimated and over-stated especially since it was largely based on in vitro data'.

Drugs may also be displaced from specific protein-binding sites in tissues; for example, the sulphonylurea hypogly-caemics displace insulin from protein-binding sites in the pancreas, plasma and elsewhere, and this may indeed be the basic mechanism of their hypoglycaemic action. Tissue binding sites do not seem to be of great importance in interactions involving antimicrobial agents.

Drug may interact by antagonizing each other at the same receptor site (competitive antagonism) or at separate but physiologically related sites (physiological antagonism). There are also specific instances where a drug may interact with its own metabolite at a common receptor.

Examples are not numerous with antimicrobials, although ticarcillin has been shown to inactivate gentamicin in vivo by a physicochemical mechanism, tobramycin is inactivated by ticarcillin in vivo and simultaneous treatment with gentamicin and carbenicillin has been shown to cause a profound fall in gentamicin plasma levels in patients with severe renal impairment.

Drug interactions and drug-metabolizing enzymes

Many of the interactions between drugs are due to drug-metabolizing enzymes, particularly where the P450 enzyme system in the liver is affected by the previous administration of other drugs. The simplest example of this is where pre-treatment with a drug increases the activity of the enzyme system responsible for metabolizing that drug. This is known as 'enzyme induction'.

The major problem, however, arises when one drug cross-stimulates or inhibits the metabolism of another drug. As to how these augmenting actions arise is a matter of contention and biochemical discussion (see Schenkman & Greim 1993), but it has been suggested that they are due to the synthesis of enzyme protein being stimulated by polycyclic hydro-carbons and drugs. Support for this view is given by the observation that this induction of increased cytochrome P450 and microsomal enzyme activity is completely pre-vented by introducing the amino-acid antagonist ethionine into the system. This prevents the incorporation of methio-nine and glycine into liver protein.

ANTIMICROBIALS AS ENZYME INDUCERS

The liver microsomal hydroxylating system is centred on the cytochrome, named from its characteristic absorption spectrum, cytochrome P450. The microsomal hydroxylating system appears to be a family of enzymes capable of acting upon a number of different substrates. A number of apparently different reactions other than hydroxylation (e.g. phenytoin, debrisoquine) are catalysed by the cytochrome-P450-dependent system; such transformations include de-amination (e.g. amphetamine), dealkylation (e.g. morphine, azathioprine), sulphoxidation (e.g. chlorpromazine, phenyl-butazone), desulphuration (e.g. thiopentone) and dehalo-genation (e.g. DDT (dichlorodiphenyltrichloroethane), halogenated anaesthetics). From this lack of specificity arises the ability of a single inducing agent to stimulate the metabolism of a host of other drugs and also of one drug to inhibit the metabolism of another structurally unrelated drug.

Smoking, pesticides, alcohol and many drugs will act as enzyme inducers, as will many antimicrobial agents if used at a constant dosage for long periods of time; it is this effect that may be the prime cause of their own inadequate levels in the blood. This problem has particular relevance in, for example, the long-term treatment of tuberculosis: rifampicin administered constantly at 600 mg/day for 7 days gave significantly lower blood levels on the seventh day than it did on the first day of treatment.

Rifampicin has been shown to increase the rate of metabolism of a whole range of drugs, including oral contraceptives. The therapeutic action of all these agents is significantly reduced.

Other antimicrobial substances that can cause enzyme induction include griseofulvin, which can negate oral contra-ceptive action, and isoniazid, which seems to affect selectively the metabolism of only one or two agents, e.g. cyclosporin. Some examples of enzyme-induced interactions involving antimicrobials are shown in Table 6.5.

ANTIMICROBIALS AS ENZYME INHIBITORS

The slowing or inhibition of the metabolism of one drug by another is well documented and there are many examples of antimicrobials causing an increase in both the duration and the intensity of the effect of other agents. Antimicrobials

Table 6.5 *Interactions involving antimicrobial agents with enzyme inducer properties*

Antimicrobial agent	Drugs
Drug activity decreased by increased metabolism	
Ampicillin	Oral contraceptives (other mechanisms may be also involved)
Griseofulvin	Coumarin anticoagulants
	Oral contraceptives
Isoniazid	Cyclosporin
Rifampicin	Anticonvulsants
	Chloramphenicol
	Cimetidine
	Corticosteroids
	Coumarin anticoagulants
	Cyclosporin
	Dapsone
	Disopyramide
	Haloperidol
	Itroconazole
	Ketoconazole
	Methadone
	Mexiletine
	Oral contraceptives
	Quinidine
	Sulphonylurea hypoglycaemics
	Theophylline
	Thyroxine
Tetracyclines	Oral contraceptives (other mechanisms may also be involved)
Drug activity increased by decreased metabolism	
Chloramphenicol	Coumarin anticoagulants
	Paracetamol
	Phenytoin
	Sulphonylurea hypoglycaemics
Erythromycin	Carbamazepine
	Cyclosporin
	Theophylline
	Warfarin
Ketoconazole	Cyclosporin
Latamoxef disodium	Cyclosporin
Metronidazole	Warfarin
Quinolones	Cyclosporin
	Nicoumalone
	Theophylline
	Warfarin
Sulphonamides	Sulphonylurea hypoglycaemics

causing enzyme inhibition include chloramphenicol, erythromycin, the quinolones and triacetyloleandomycin. Conversely, interactions have been reported where antimicrobial action is reduced by the enzyme inhibiting properties of other agents. Table 6.5 lists some drug interactions due to enzyme inhibition involving antimicrobials. The P450 enzyme systems are not the only enzyme systems inhibited; thus, for example, the prolonged administration of furazolidone causes a cumulative inhibition of monoamine oxidase and has produced hypersensitivity to tyramine and amphetamine in patients.

Drug interactions in excretory mechanisms

Since most drugs pass through and are eliminated by the kidneys, this is obviously a fruitful site for drug interactions to occur. Drugs may undergo passive re-absorption or active secretion in the kidneys and, since the elimination of many drugs is markedly dependent upon urinary pH, it is not surprising that one drug may alter the excretion pattern of another by its influence on the pH of the renal environment.

Competition among drugs for a common renal secretory pathway is another way by which drug excretion can be disproportionately affected by changes in the glomerular filtration rate. If two drugs secreted by the same pathway are given together, the renal clearance of each will be less than if it had been given alone.

PASSIVE RE-ABSORPTION

A non-protein-bound drug is filtered at the glomerulus and is progressively concentrated as water is reabsorbed during its passage down the nephron. A concentration gradient is therefore established, and if the drug is lipid soluble and able to permeate the tubular epithelium it will be passively re-absorbed back into the systemic circulation.

Many drugs are weak electrolytes, and passive reabsorption can occur only in the non-ionized lipid soluble form; the degree of ionization is determined by the pH of the renal environment so that changes in the pH of the tubular fluid must influence the re-absorption or excretion of the drug.

Drugs which are weak bases (e.g. amitriptyline, the amphetamines, antihistamines, chloroquine, imipramine, mecamylamine, mepacrine, morphine, pethidine, procaine) are excreted more rapidly in urine of low pH and more slowly at high pH. Conversely, weak acids (e.g. nalidixic acid, nitrofurantoin, phenobarbitone, salicylic acid, streptomycin and some sulphonamides) are excreted more rapidly at high urinary pH and more slowly at low pH. Thus, in summary, acidic urine favours the ionization of alkaline drugs (and vice versa) so that re-absorption is reduced and renal excretion is increased.

These effects are only of clinical significance if the pK_a value (dissociation constant) of the drug is in the range of about 7.5–10.5 for bases and 3.0–7.5 for acids, and if a significant proportion of the drug is normally excreted unchanged in the urine. However, the influence of urinary pH does not seem to be particularly well documented insofar as drug interactions are concerned, although urinary pH has for long been a factor of importance in the treatment of drug overdosage, in the diagnosis of addiction to drugs and in drug misuse in sport. Elimination of potentially toxic drugs, for example salicylates and barbiturates, may be accelerated by appropriate adjustment of urinary pH, i.e. forced alkaline diuresis.

Foods and food supplements, antacids and mineral-containing laxatives can affect the urinary excretion of drugs. Thus the use of large doses of vitamin C (up to 5 g/day) taken prophylactically against the common cold may alter urinary pH sufficiently to influence renal elimination and therefore the clinical response of alkaline drugs. Acid fruit juices and squashes may reduce the efficacy of the antimalarials quinine and chloroquine.

ACTIVE SECRETION

Many acidic drugs and drug metabolites are actively secreted by the proximal tubular active transport mechanism, and interactions may arise from competition for this system. Drugs actively secreted include acetazolamide, chlorpropamide, hippuric acid, indomethacin, penicillins, phenolsulphonphthalein, phenylbutazone, probenecid, salicylic acid, sulphinpyrazone, sulphonamides, sulphonic acids, thiazide diuretics and many drug metabolites. Thus the plasma half-life of benzylpenicillin may be prolonged not only by probenecid but also by aspirin, phenylbutazone, sulphonamides, indomethacin, thiazide diuretics, frusemide and ethacrynic acid.

Probenecid was extremely useful in the early days of penicillin when the combination raised and prolonged penicillin plasma levels (Fig. 6.5). It is still useful in that inhibition of the urinary excretion of penicillin and some cephalosporins has been used as a device to increase the biliary excretion of these agents, thereby raising the antibiotic concentrations in the biliary tract. This has been used to improve the efficacy of antibiotic treatment of chole-

cystitis. Several workers have reported that the level of cephalexin in the bile was raised when probenecid was given concurrently. Probenecid has also been shown to reduce the excretion of quinolones and increase their side-effects.

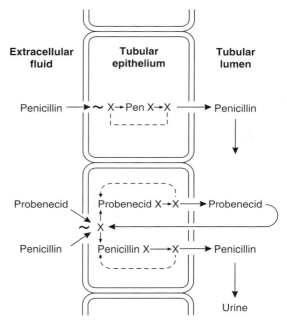

Fig. 6.5 *Interaction between probenecid and penicillin in the renal tubule. It has been suggested that the excretion of penicillin is slowed down by the competition of probenecid for the hypothetical carrier X. The recycling of probenecid causes penicillin to be retained in the body. (From Griffin, D'Arcy & Speirs 1988 A Manual of Adverse Drug Interactions, John Wright, London.)*

Further information

Association of the British Pharmaceutical Industry 1995 The data sheet compendium 1995–1996. DataPharm, London

Griffin J P, D'Arcy P F 1997 A manual of adverse drug interactions, 5th edn. Elsevier, Amsterdam (in press)

References

Back D J, Orme M L E 1990 Pharmacokinetic drug interactions with oral contraceptives. *Clinical Pharmacokinetics* 18: 472–484

Crounse R G 1961 Human pharmacology of griseofulvin: the effect of fat intake on gastrointestinal absorption. *Journal of Investigative Dermatology* 37: 529–533

D'Arcy P F 1983 Drug interactions with medicinal plastics. *Drug Intelligence and Clinical Pharmacy* 17: 726–731

D'Arcy P F 1986 Drug interactions with oral contraceptives. *Drug Intelligence and Clinical Pharmacy* 20: 353–362

D'Arcy P F 1990 Adverse reactions to excipients in pharmaceutical formulations. In: Florence A T, Salole E G (eds) Formulation factors in adverse reactions. John Wright (Butterworth), London, p 1–22

Griffin J P, D'Arcy P F, Speirs C J 1988 A Manual of Adverse Drug Interactions, 4th edn. John Wright (Butterworth), London, p 45–46

Levy G 1970 Biopharmaceutical considerations in dosage form design and evaluation. In: Sprowls J B (ed) Prescription pharmacy, 2nd edn. J B Lippincott, Philadelphia, p 70, 75, 80

Reynolds J E F (ed) 1993 Martindale, The extra pharmacopoeia, 30th edn. Pharmaceutical Press, London, p 79–224

Neuvonen P J, Gothoni G, Hackman R, Af. Björksten K 1970 Interference of iron with the absorption of tetracyclines in man. *British Medical Journal* 4: 532–534

Parsons R L, David J A 1980 Gastrointestinal disease and drug absorption. In: Prescott L F, Nimmo W S (eds) Drug absorption. ADIS Press, Australasia, p 262–277

Schenkman J B, Greim H (eds) 1993 Cytochrome P450. Springer-Verlag, Berlin

Welling P G, Tse F L S 1982 The influence of food on the absorption of antimicrobial agents. *Journal of Antimicrobial Chemotherapy* 9: 7–27

Drug interaction tables

The following tables do not cover interactions that might occur in vitro. It is recommended that before any anti-infective agents are added to intravenous transfusion fluids, the following questions should all be answered in the affirmative:

- Is it necessary that the drug be given in this way?
- Is the stability of the particular drug in the selected infusion fluid firmly established?
- If multiple additives are intended, is the stability in the selected infusion fluid of each drug in the presence of the others firmly established?
- Will the drug(s) have the intended therapeutic effect if given in high dilution over a period of hours?
- Since many drugs decompose slowly in infusion fluids, will the interval between drug addition and use of the fluid be short?

Unless all these questions are answered 'yes', then the anti-infective agents should be given intramuscularly or intravenously via the injection site provided in the giving set.

Therapeutic class of interacting agent	Effect of co-administration
Bi(s)phosphates Disodium etidronate Disodium parmidronate Disodium clodronate	Can lead to severe hypocalcaemia. Aminoglycosides and bi(s)phosphonates can induce hypocalcaemia by different mechanisms; these effects can be additive
Cholinergic agents Neostigmine Physostigmine Distigmine bromide Pyridostigmine bromide	Can antagonize the effects of cholinergic agents
Cytotoxics Cisplatin	Can increase risk of both nephrotoxicity and ototoxicity
Diuretics Ethacrynic acid Frusemide	Can increase risk of ototoxicity
Muscle relaxants	Can potentiate effects of non-depolarizing muscle relaxants such as tubocurarine

1 Aminoglycosides

The major adverse effects of this group of antibiotics are nephrotoxicity and ototoxicity. The risk of ototoxicity is enhanced if two aminoglycoside antibiotics are co-administered; the risk of nephrotoxicity is increased if an aminoglycoside antibiotic is administered with a polymyxin such as colistin or systemic antifungal agents such as amphotericin B or the glycopeptide antibiotics, vancomycin or teicoplanin

2 Cephalosporins

As a group, the cephalosporins do not create major problems, but individual compounds have some specific interactions

Therapeutic class of interacting agent	Effect of co-administration
Alcohol	Cephamandole, cefoperazone and latamoxef can lead to antabuse-like effects

Anticoagulants	Cephamandole, other cephalosporins and latamoxef can enhance anticoagulant effect of warfarin and nicoumalone
Colistin	Cephalosporins are alleged to increase risk of renal damage
Probenecid	Can increase the plasma levels of most cephalosporins due to reduced renal clearance

5 Fusidic acid

Although fusidic acid has been shown to displace bilirubin from plasma binding, which could be relevant with respect of displacement of other drugs from plasma binding, no interactions of clinical relevance have been reported

3 Chloramphenicol

The drug interactions referred to below refer to systemic use of chloramphenicol and not to use of ophthalmic preparations

Therapeutic class of interacting agent	Effect of co-administration
Anticoagulants (warfarin, nicoumalone, phenindione)	Decreases vitamin K production by intestinal bacteria and directly inhibits the metabolism of coumarin anticoagulants in the liver with enhanced anticoagulant effect
Antidiabetic agents (sulphonylureas)	2 g/day for 10 days results in a 3-fold increase in the half-life of tolbutamide and other sulphonylurea derivatives. Profound hypoglycaemia can ensue
Antiepileptic agents (carbamazepine, phenobarbitone, phenytoin)	Can reduce chloramphenicol plasma levels due to enzyme-inducing effects of phenobarbitone, or increase plasma levels of both chloramphenicol and phenytoin due to phenytoin competition for chloramphenicol hepatic binding sites and chloramphenicol inhibition of phenytoin hepatic metabolism. Blood dyscrasias may result

6 Glycopeptide antibiotics

Both vancomycin and teicoplanin have been reported to show ototoxicity and vancomycin can cause nephrotoxicity and renal failure

Therapeutic class of interacting agent	Effect of co-administration
Anaesthetic agents	Has been associated with erythema, histamine-like flushing and anaphylactoid reactions

7 Imidazoles

Therapeutic class of interacting agent	Effect of co-administration
Alcohol	With metronidazole results in pronounced antabuse effect
Antacids	Can reduce absorption of imidazoles
Anticoagulants	May enhance anticoagulant effect of nicoumalone and warfarin due to inhibition of metabolism
Antiepileptic	Metronidazole inhibits metabolism of phenytoin and increases plasma levels. Phenobarbitone accelerates metabolism of metronidazole. Phenytoin or phenobarbitone accelerate metabolism of ketoconazole
Cytotoxics	Metronidazole inhibits the metabolism of fluorouracil. Ketoconazole inhibits metabolism of cyclosporin
Disulfiram	Imidazoles inhibit disulfiram hepatic metabolism; psychotic reactions reported
Lithium	Imidazoles may increase lithium toxicity
H_2 antagonists	H_2 antagonists, also omeprazole, and sucralfate with imidazoles reduce imidazole absorption

4 Clindamycin

Therapeutic class of interacting agent	Effect of co-administration
Cholinergics (neostigmine, pyridostigmine)	Antagonizes the effect of neostigmine
Muscle relaxants	Potentiates the effect of non-depolarizing muscle relaxants such as tubocurarine and fazidinium bromide

8 Macrolides

The most significant interactions of macrolide antibiotics with other therapeutic substances is due to their ability to inhibit the hepatic metabolism of other substances

Therapeutic class of interacting agent	Effect of co-administration
Analgesics	Erythromycin increases plasma concentration of alfentanil
Antacids	Reduces absorption of azithromycin from gut
Antiarrhythmics (disopyramide)	Erythromycin increases plasma concentration of disopyramide
Anticoagulants (warfarin, nicoumalone)	Macrolides enhance anticoagulant effect of nicoumalone and warfarin due to inhibition of metabolism
Antihistamines (astemizole, terfenidine)	Macrolides inhibit the metabolism of the non-sedating antihistamines, astemizole and terfenidine. This can lead to overdosage and cardiotoxicity in the form of ventricular arrhythmias, including torsades de pointes
Antiepileptics (carbamazepine)	Clarithromycin and erythromycin inhibit the metabolism of carbamazepine and enhance its potential for side-effects
Benzodiazepines (midazolam)	Erythromycin inhibits the metabolism of midazolam and increases the plasma level significantly
Cardiac glycosides (digoxin)	Erythromycin inhibits the metabolism of digoxin and can precipitate digoxin toxicity. This is probably a general property of macrolide antibiotics
Cyclosporin	Erythromycin inhibits the hepatic metabolism of cyclosporin and increases risk of renal damage
Ergotamine	Erythromycin inhibits the metabolism of ergotomine with clinical ergotism
Dopaminergics (bromocriptine)	Erythromycin inhibits bromocriptine metabolism
Xanthines (Theophylline)	Clarithromycin and erythromycin inhibit the hepatic metabolism of theophylline and increase the risk of toxicity

9 Nitrofurans

Therapeutic class of interacting agent	Effect of co-administration
4-Quinolones (nalidixic acid)	Nitrofurantoin inhibits the antibacterial action of nalidixic acid. The concomitant use of these two agents in urinary tract infections should be avoided
Uricosurics (probenecid)	Reduces renal clearance of nitrofurantoin and therefore increases its risk of toxicity

10 Penicillins

Very few interactions between penicillins and other medication are clinically significant

Therapeutic class of interacting agent	Effect of co-administration
Antacids	Reduce absorption of pivampicillin
Allopurinol	With ampicillin or amoxycillin reported to double or quadruple, respectively, the incidence of rashes
Anticoagulants	With broad spectrum penicillins can potentiate the effect of anticoagulants by reducing vitamin K synthesis by bowel flora
Cytotoxics (methotrexate)	With penicillins can reduce the excretion of methotrexate and therefore increase the risk of toxicity
Guar gum	Reduces the absorption of phenoxy-methylpenicillin
Muscle relaxants	Azlocillin increases the effect of non-depolarizing muscle relaxants such as tubocurarine
Probenecid	Reduces the renal excretion of penicillin
Oral contraceptives	With ampicillin in women who develop antibiotic-associated diarrhoea can lead to malabsorption of oestrogen and progestogen components of oral contraceptives and pregnancy

11 Polymyxins

Interactions are largely as for aminoglycoside antibiotics

Therapeutic class of interacting agent	Effect of co-administration
Muscle relaxants	Enhance neuromuscular blocking effect of non-depolarizing muscle relaxants (e.g. tubocurarine, fazidinium bromide). This effect is enhanced by K^+ depletion or low ionized serum Ca^{2+}. Cholinergic agents are of little value in reversing this prolongation of action

12 4-Quinolones

Antibacterial quinolones enter into interactions because they chelate with cations such as calcium, magnesium, iron, aluminium and zinc, reducing their absorption. 4-Quinolones inhibit hepatic metabolism

Therapeutic class of interacting agent	Effect of co-administration
Analgesics/non-steroidal anti-inflammatory drugs (NSAIDS)	With 4-quinolones may increase the risk of convulsions. The mechanism of this interaction is not known
Antacids containing aluminium, bismuth, calcium, magnesium cations; Iron and zinc salts; Milk and dairy products; Anti-ulcer agents (sucralfate)	Reduce absorption of 4-quinolones by forming poorly soluble cation complexes. This effect involves: iron given for anaemia; dairy products, all of which contain Ca^{2+} cations; and sucralfate which releases aluminium cations in the stomach
Anticoagulants (warfarin, nicoumalone)	Ciprofloxacin, nalidixic acid and ofloxacin can slow the hepatic metabolism of warfarin and nicoumalone, with enhanced anticoagulant effect
Antidiabetic agents	4-Quinolones can impair the hepatic metabolism of sulphonylurea antidiabetic agents, with enhanced hypoglycaemic effect
Probenecid	Reduces the renal excretion of cinoxacin and nalidixic acid
Xanthines	4-Quinolones reduce the hepatic clearance of xanthines such as theophylline and caffeine and increase the risk of toxicity

13 Sulphonamides

Interactions of sulphonamides with other therapeutic agents hinges on: their antifolate actions; their ability to displace other drugs from plasma binding sites; and the inhibition of a number of metabolic processes

Therapeutic class of interacting agent	Effect of co-administration
Anaesthetics (thiopentone)	Sulphonamides increase effect of thiopentone
Anticoagulants (nicoumalone, warfarin)	Sulphonamides reduce vitamin K synthesis by intestinal flora and displace coumarin anticoagulants from plasma protein binding sites, potentiating the anticoagulant effect
Antidiabetic agents (sulphonylureas)	Sulphonamides inhibit the carboxylation of tolbutamide and displace tolbutamide and chlorpropamide from plasma protein binding sites, enhancing hypoglycaemic action
Antiepileptic agents (phenytoin)	Sulphonamides increase the plasma concentration of phenytoin, antifolate effect and phenytoin toxicity
Cyclosporin	Increases risk of nephrotoxicity
Cytotoxics (methotrexate)	Sulphonamides displace methotrexate from plasma protein binding sites, increasing its toxicity and antifolate action

Local anaesthetics (amethocaine, benzocaine, butacaine, procaine)	Sulphonamides impair antibacterial activity: local anaesthetics which are derivatives of p-aminobenzoic acid are hydrolysed in the body to p-aminobenzoic acid, a sulphonamide competitor

14 Tetracyclines

The absorption of tetracyclines is reduced by divalent and trivalent cations (e.g. aluminium, bismuth, calcium, iron, magnesium, zinc) with which tetracyclines form non-absorbable complexes; cations are also present in certain excipients used in other pharmaceuticals and calcium is present in all milk and dairy products

Therapeutic class of interacting agent	Effect of co-administration
Antiulcer drug (sucralfate)	Leads to impaired tetracycline absorption through sucralfate release of aluminium cations in the stomach
Cimetidine	Cimetidine (1000 mg/day for 3 days) reduces the absorption of tetracyclines
Anticoagulants	Tetracyclines reduce plasma prothrombin activity by impairing prothrombin utilization, but decrease vitamin K production by intestinal bacteria potentiating anticoagulant activity
Anticonvulsants (carbamazepine, phenobarbitone, phenytoin)	Enzyme-inducing antiepileptic agents approximately halve the plasma half-life of doxycycline
Retinoids	Increase the incidence of benign intracranial hypertension; the mechanism in unknown

15 Trimethoprim

Therapeutic class of interacting agent	Effect of co-administration
Antiarrhythmics (procainamide)	Trimethoprim increases plasma concentrations of procainamide
Anticoagulants (nicoumalone, warfarin)	Trimethoprim enhances effects of nicoumalone and warfarin
Antidiabetics (sulphonylureas)	Trimethoprim increases hypoglycaemic effect of sulphonylureas
Antiepileptics (phenytoin) Antimalarials (pyrimethamine) Cytotoxics (pyrimethamine)	Trimethoprim enhances antifolate effects of phenytoin, pyrimethamine and methotrexate

16 Antituberculous Agents

Most interactions relate to increased metabolic breakdown induced by rifampicin

Therapeutic class of interacting agent	Effect of co-administration
Rifampicin *Anticoagulants* *(coumarins)* *Antidepressants* *(tricyclics)* *Antiepileptics* *(phenytoin)* *Antibacterials and antifungals* *(imidazoles)* *Antipsychotics* *(haloperidol)* *Benzodiazepines* *Beta-adrenergic blockers* *Calcium channel blockers* *(diltiazam, verapamil and nifedipine)* *Cardiac glycosides* *(digitoxin only)* *Corticosteroids, oestrogens, progestogens* *(oral contraceptives)* *Cyclosporin* *H_2 blockers* *(cimetidine)* *Theophylline* *Thyroxine*	Rifampicin accelerates metabolism of all these drugs and reduces their efficacy
Capreomycin *Antibiotics* *(Colistin)*	Capreomycin increases risk of nephrotoxicity
Aminoglycosides *(Vancomycin)*	Capreomycin increases risk of nephrotoxicity and ototoxicity
Cytotoxics *(Cisplatin)*	Capreomycin increases risk of nephrotoxicity and ototoxicity

Isoniazid

There is increased risk of isoniazid toxicity in patients who are slow acetylators. This pharmacogenetic dysmorphism is also relevant in manifestation of interactions. Most interactions are due to isoniazid-induced metabolic inhibition, which is greater in slow acetylators

Antacids, absorbants	Reduce absorption of isoniazid
Antibiotics *(cycloserine)*	Isoniazid inhibits cycloserine metabolism and increases CNS toxicity
Antiepileptics *(carbamazepine, ethosuxamide, phenytoin)*	Isoniazid inhibits hepatic metabolism of these antiepileptics and increases risk of toxicity
Benzodiazepines *(diazepan)*	Isoniazid inhibits metabolism of diazepine
Xanthines *(theophylline)*	Isoniazid increases plasma levels of theophylline

Cycloserine

Antibiotics *(isoniazid)*	Inhibits hepatic metabolism, increasing cycloserine plasma levels and CNS toxicity
Antiepileptics *(phenytoin)*	Cycloserine increases plasma concentration of phenytoin, with increased risk of toxicity

Other antituberculous agents

Antacids	Reduce absorption of ethambutol, by forming cation complexes
Uricosurics *(probenecid)*	Probenecid reduces renal clearance of pyrazinamide

17 Antifungal agents

Amphoterecin

Antibiotics *(aminoglycosides)*	Amphoterecin increases risk of ototoxicity and nephrotoxicity
Cyclosporin	Amphoterecin increases risk of nephrotoxicity

Fluocytosine

Antibiotics *(rifampicin)*	Increases metabolism of fluocytosine and reduces efficacy
Anticoagulants *(nicoumalone, warfarin)*	Fluocytosine increases anticoagulant effect
Antidiabetic agents *(sulphonylureas)*	Fluocytosine potentiates hypoglycaemia effect
Antiepileptics	Fluocytosine inhibits metabolism of phenytoin with increased risk of toxicity
Cyclosporin	Fluocytosine inhibits metabolism of cyclosporin, with increased risk of nephrotoxicity
Theophylline	Fluocytosine inhibits metabolism of theophylline

Griseofulvin

Anticoagulants *(nicoumalone, warfarin)* *Cyclosporin* *Oral contraceptives*	Griseofulvin-induced metabolism increases efficacy of these drugs

18 Antiviral agents

Therapeutic class of interacting agent	Effect of co-administration
Aminoglycosides	Renal toxicity of aminoglycosides enhanced by foscarnet
β-Lactam antibiotics	Ganciclovir with imipen and cilastatin may result in generalized seizures

Pentamidine isethionate	Foscarnet with pentamidine may result in renal impairment and symptomatic hypo-calcaemia (Trousseau and Chvostek's signs)
Probenecid	Probenecid reduces the renal elimination of ganciclovir and increases the mean half-life and area under the plasma concentration curve of systemically administered acyclovir
Various	Zidovudine may enhance toxicity of any agent which is potentially nephrotoxic, including pentamidine, dapsone, amphotericin fluocytosine, ganciclovir, interferon, vincristine, vinblastine and doxorubin

7

Toxicity

A. P. Ball

Introduction

Antibacterial agents are thought of, with some justification, as being amongst the safest of all drugs. A Danish study noted that, although 8% of hospital admissions were caused by adverse reactions to drugs, only 7.5% of this total related to antibiotic therapy and, of these, approximately one-third comprised reactions to nitrofurantoin (Hallas et al 1992). Serious idiosyncratic reactions are exceptionally rare, and dose-related problems are largely preventable either by anticipation (e.g. chloramphenicol toxicity in neonates) or by therapeutic drug monitoring (e.g. aminoglycosides and vancomycin). Nevertheless, serious untoward reactions can occur following licensure, despite an apparently satisfactory adverse drug reaction (ADR) profile during extensive premarketing trials. The morbidity which followed temafloxacin-induced haemolytic anaemia with uraemia syndrome and which led to the rapid withdrawal of the product within months of its launch is a recent example (Blum et al 1994). In many cases, prelicensing investigation identifies specific ADRs and development of potentially useful products is halted or abandoned, as recently befell several phototoxic fluoroquinolones. However, antibacterial agents may be available for many years before accumulating evidence focuses attention on a previously unappreciated problem, for example flucloxacillin-induced hepatotoxicity (Fairley et al 1993), or highlights the true incidence of a problem such as the excess of deaths occurring in the elderly as a result of co-trimoxazole-induced Stevens–Johnson syndrome and aplasia (Ball 1986). Specific disease groups may be at increased risk of certain ADRs, for example the high incidence of co-trimoxazole hypersensitivity reactions in patients with autoimmune deficiency syndrome (AIDS) (Carr et al 1993). Co-administration of certain antibiotics may increase the risk of toxicity, for example aminoglycosides and vancomycin (Goetz & Sayers 1993).

Structure–activity studies of newly synthesized antibacterials can predict ADR profiles. Thus cephalosporins with the N-methylthiotetrazole side-chain are now avoided because of their association with bleeding (Lipsky 1988). Equally, 8-halogenated fluoroquinolones will, in the future, be closely scrutinized for phototoxicity (Domagala 1994). Such investigations will be mandatory during the initial structure–activity evaluation of future compounds as pharmaceutical companies can ill afford the wasted development costs associated with delayed discovery of a predictable ADR at the clinical stage of evaluation.

This chapter will focus on the mechanisms and incidence of antibiotic toxicity, toxic effects on particular organs and the effect of organ failure on toxicity, the safety of individual agents and groups of antibiotics in pregnancy, prevention of toxicity by therapeutic monitoring and other manoevres, and methods of assessment of ADR profiles before and after licensing.

ADRs and the gastro-intestinal system

UPPER GASTRO-INTESTINAL INTOLERANCE

Many antibiotics cause mild to moderate nausea and abdominal discomfort following oral administration. These include the β-lactams, fluoroquinolones, tetracyclines, fusidic acid and, notably, the macrolides. Erythromycin and its metabolites have significant stimulatory effects on motilin production and hence gastro-intestinal motility (Pilot & Qin 1988), resulting in upper abdominal pain, nausea and vomiting in up to 16% of patients, and withdrawal from therapy in up to 5% (Hughes & Cunliffe 1987). Acid stable macrolides, such as clarithromycin and azithromycin, reduce the incidence of such effects by 50% or more, and less than 2% of patients withdraw from therapy (Hopkins 1991, Wood 1991).

ANTIBIOTICS AND DIARRHOEA

Diarrhoea associated with antibiotic therapy may either relate to colonization and overgrowth of *Clostridium difficile* with subsequent toxin production, leading ultimately to pseudomembranous colitis (PMC), or to other mechanisms. *Cl. difficile* is implicated in up to 25% of all cases of antibiotic diarrhoea, in 50%–70% of those in whom inflammatory change is demonstrated by endoscopy, and in virtually all cases of PMC (Bartlett 1992). Alternative mechanisms of antibiotic-associated diarrhoea include overgrowth of *Candida* spp. or enterotoxin producing *Staphylococcus aureus*, direct toxic effects, such as those produced by neomycin and tetracyclines, and induction of malabsorption. The incidence of diarrhoea with oral agents, such as the broad-spectrum penicillins and cephalosporins, is related to the completeness or otherwise of absorption in the small bowel. For parenteral agents, biliary excretion is an important factor. Thus, diarrhoea is more common with cefoperazone than with other agents (Meyers 1985).

CL. DIFFICILE INDUCED DIARRHOEA

Virtually all antibiotics and some other drugs with antibacterial activity (e.g. methotrexate) are capable of producing pseudomembranous colitis. However, whilst it is classically linked to clindamycin (Tedesco et al 1974), broad-spectrum penicillins and cephalosporins are quantitatively most likely to be associated with development of this disease (Larson 1982). Antibiotic diarrhoea due to clindamycin occurs in 10–25% of patients, whilst ampicillin causes diarrhoea in 5–10% (Bartlett 1992). Clindamycin appears to induce toxin production by *Cl. difficile* and associated diarrhoea is much less common with tetracyclines, metronidazole, sulphonamides, quinolones, co-trimoxazole and aminoglycosides. There is a significant problem of hospital cross-infection of other patients by *Cl. difficile* who may then become symptomatic after antibiotic therapy (McFarland et al 1989).

The diagnosis of PMC is suggested by fluid diarrhoea accompanying or following antibiotic therapy (up to 6 weeks later), associated with fever, abdominal pain and leucocytosis. It is confirmed by demonstration of *Cl. difficile* and its toxin in stools, characteristic macroscopic appearances of bowel mucosa on sigmoidoscopy and the pathognomonic histopathological 'summit' lesion (Leading Article 1977).

Treatment for proven symptomatic disease is both supportive and specific. In severe cases, intravenous fluids, corticosteroids and blood transfusion may be required. The use of opioid and other antiperistaltic agents may precipitate toxic megacolon and is contraindicated. Eradicative therapy using oral vancomycin for 10–14 days is the treatment of choice (Tedesco et al 1978). It usually produces symptomatic improvement within 36 h, but relapse may occur in up to 40% of patients. Doses of oral vancomycin (125–500 mg, 6 hourly) have been advocated. Metronidazole by mouth is a significantly cheaper alternative which, although many prefer to continue with vancomycin, appears to give equivalent results (Teasley et al 1983).

Hepatic reactions

Antibiotics may cause the full range of potential hepatic adverse reactions (Westphal et al 1994). These include direct cytotoxicity (isoniazid), hypersensitivity effects both local (β-lactams) and generalized (p-aminosalicylate), cholestatic syndromes (macrolides, fusidate), chronic active hepatitis (nitrofurantoin) and fatty change (tetracyclines). The hepatic metabolites of certain agents may be more potentially toxic or immunogenic than the parent compound, for example isoniazid hydrazine derivatives, the production of which may be enhanced by rifampicin. Co-administration of these agents requires careful monitoring in patients with slow acetylator status (Westphal et al 1994).

Penicillins, notably oxacillin derivatives and acylureido-penicillins in high dosage, are well recognized to cause hepatitic or mixed cholestatic reactions (Parry & Neu 1982, Parry 1987). However, others may be available for prolonged periods before potential hepatotoxicity comes to light, for example the rare cholestatic syndromes reported with co-amoxiclav (Reddy et al 1989). Flucloxacillin-associated jaundice, which may persist for months, is most common amongst the elderly and after prolonged therapy (Fairley et al 1993). Cephalosporins are very common causes of mild elevations of the transaminases, but are rare causes of jaundice (Westphal et al 1994). However, derivatives with N-methylthiotetrazole side-chains, such as cefamandole and cefoperazone, are associated with hypoprothrombinaemia due to metabolic liver disturbance (Lipsky 1988).

Various erythromycin derivatives, notably but not exclusively the estolate, cause elevations of transaminase and alkaline phosphatase enzymes in up to 15% of cases treated for 10 days or more (Braun 1969, Elias 1982). Jaundice follows in less than 2%. The reaction is a cholestatic hepatitis (Lunzer et al 1975), which is reversible on discontinuation, and has an immunological basis. Associated eosinophilia is common (Westphal et al 1994). Fusidic acid therapy is also commonly accompanied by hepatic reactions, which again are largely benign and reversible. Intravenous therapy is associated with jaundice in 17–48% of patients, but the incidence with oral therapy is much lower at 6–13% (Eykyn 1990). Lincosamides, such as clindamycin, may cause biochemical 'transaminitis', but the relationship to hepatotoxicity is unclear.

Rifampicin is most likely to cause liver injury when combined with isoniazid (Westphal et al 1994). Used alone, it rarely causes significant hepatic reactions (Elias 1982). Elevation of serum transaminases and transient hyperbilirubinaemia may occur during the initial phase of therapy (Newman et al 1974, Sanders 1976). Neither alone contraindicate further therapy. Intermittent therapy has been associated with hepato-renal failure (Rothwell & Richmond 1974).

Tetracyclines may precipitate acute fatty degeneration, usually in association with intravenous therapy, high doses and pregnancy. However, routine doses can cause severe, potentially fatal reactions in young people with chronic renal failure in whom they are contraindicated (Phillips et al 1974).

Sulphonamides cause mixed liver injury, characterized by necrosis and cholestasis of varying severity, in 0.6% of patients, but up to 10% may exhibit benign transaminase elevations (Westphal et al 1994). Co-trimoxazole is also a common cause of subclinical hepatotoxicity, causing 6% of cases of drug-associated hepatitis in one series (Berg & Daniel 1987). The frequency is substantially higher in AIDS patients (Wofsy 1987).

Nitrofurantoin may cause both acute and chronic liver damage (Penn & Griffin 1982), including an immunologically mediated syndrome of liver injury, pulmonary fibrosis and autoantibody (antinuclear and antimitochondrial) formation (Back et al 1974) and cirrhosis (Holmberg et al 1980). Fluoroquinolone therapy quite commonly causes elevation of the transaminases, but clinical jaundice is rare (Halkin 1988, Westphal et al 1994). Metronidazole may interfere with hepatic metabolism of ethanol (Gupta et al 1970), resulting in a disulfiram (antabuse) type reaction, but is otherwise free of hepatic reactions.

CEFTRIAXONE AND THE BILIARY SYSTEM

Reversible ceftriaxone-induced biliary pseudolithiasis, presenting with biliary colic or with radiographic or sonographic abnormalities has been described in both children and adults (Schaad et al 1988, Pigrau et al 1989). The long-term implications are unknown, although to date there is no evidence of subsequent biliary calculi.

ADRs affecting the blood and the cardiovascular system

APLASTIC ANAEMIA, GRANULOCYTOSIS AND NEUTROPENIA

Aplastic anaemia is classically associated with chloramphenicol. However, long-acting sulphonamides are now undoubtedly a commoner cause due to the widespread use of co-trimoxazole. In the mid-1980s, the UK Committee on Safety of Medicines issued a warning notice which detailed 85 deaths following co-trimoxazole therapy, of which 50 related to blood dyscrasias. Most of these deaths occurred as a result of agranulocytosis in the elderly, and withdrawal of the drug in this age group was suggested (Ball 1986). Initial clinical evaluation indicated that the overall incidence of haematological reactions to co-trimoxazole was 0.35% (Havas et al 1973), half of which comprised agranulocytosis and thrombocytopenia, and a quarter anaemias (Frisch 1973).

The haematological toxicity of chloramphenicol includes idiosyncratic aplastic anaemia, dose-related reversible neutropenia and thrombocytopenia and rarely, haemolytic anaemia. Fatal aplastic anaemia appears to occur in around 1 in 20 000 treatment courses (Wallerstein et al 1969), often presents some weeks after discontinuation of therapy and has a mortality of 50% or more (Davis & Rubin 1972). It may be more frequent in patients with co-existent liver disease, notably acute hepatitis, and has not been described in association with parenteral therapy. A separate, benign syndrome of reversible neutropenia occurs in 5–10% of patients who receive high doses, but does not progress to aplasia.

Neutropenia is a rare complication of therapy with the natural penicillins and oral broad-spectrum derivatives, but is significantly more common with isoxazolyl and other antistaphylococcal penicillins. Reversible, dose-related neutropenia is common with methicillin (Yow et al 1976). Minor neutropenia may occur in 1–2% of patients receiving parenteral cephalosporins (Meyers 1985) and has also been reported infrequently with metronidazole and vancomycin.

HAEMOLYTIC ANAEMIA

Haemolytic anaemia is a rare complication of therapy with penicillins and cephalosporins, sulphonamides, nitrofurantoin, naphthyridines and quinolones. Haemolysis during β-lactam therapy is related to a hapten type of mechanism: large doses of benzylpenicillin producing haemolysis secondary to the development of immunoglobulin G (IgG) antibodies to penicillin-coated red blood cells and a positive direct Coombs' test (Garraty & Petz 1975). A positive test also develops in 0.5–6% of patients receiving parenteral cephalosporins, but significant haemolysis is extremely rare (Meyers 1985). Antibody-mediated haemolysis may rarely complicate intermittent rifampicin regimens (Pujet et al 1974). For other agents, such as nitrofurantoin and sulphonamides, haemolysis can be predicted in patients with glucose-6-phosphate dehydrogenase deficiency.

The recent withdrawal of temafloxacin followed the development of haemolysis in 95 patients, associated in over half with renal impairment and hepatic dysfunction, and in a further third with evidence of coagulation defects (Blum et al 1994). Four development central nervous system (CNS) complications including convulsions, and two died. Analysis of these cases suggested an immune-complex-mediated phenomenon.

MEGALOBLASTIC ANAEMIA

Interference with human folate metabolism by co-trimoxazole is probably minimal, suggested changes in folate levels relating to interference with biological assays (Ball 1986). Trimethoprim and co-trimoxazole may interfere with response to haematinic therapy in patients with megaloblastic anaemias, and such processes constitute relative contraindications (Chanarin & England 1972, Leading Article 1973, Golde et al 1978).

THROMBOCYTOPENIA AND INTERFERENCE WITH COAGULATION

Thrombocytopenia may uncommonly be associated with β-lactam therapy. It occurs in less than 1% of patients receiving the majority of cephalosporins (Meyers 1985). Antibody-mediated thrombocytopenia may accompany rifampicin therapy (Poole et al 1971, Pujet et al 1974) and defective platelet function has been reported during high-dose therapy with extended-spectrum penicillins such as carbenicillin and ticarcillin (Brown et al 1975).

A high incidence of hypoprothrombinaemia has been reported amongst patients receiving therapy with cephalosporins possessing the *N*-methylthiotetrazole side-chain, including cefamandole, latamoxef (moxalactam), cefoperazone and cefotetan (Lipsky 1988). It is due to inhibition of the vitamin K dependent step in clotting factor synthesis, but does not occur in healthy individuals. Risk factors include renal failure (Manian et al 1990), malignancy, postoperative status and ileus, all of which have in common diminished hepatic stores of reduced glutathione (Lipsky 1988).

THROMBOPHLEBITIS

The incidence of thrombophlebitis associated with infusion of antibiotics varies from 1–2% with most β-lactams to 10% or more with erythromycin. Previous formulations of fusidic acid may cause severe thrombophlebitis, necessitating withdrawal from therapy (Portier 1990). Amongst cephalosporins, injection-site reactions appear commonest with cefotaxime, with an incidence of about 5% (Meyers 1985). Chemical irritation due to vancomycin is less common with currently available purified preparations.

ADRs and the lungs

In the 1960s–1970s, nitrofurans were the commonest causes of allergic pulmonary eosinophilia (Penn & Griffin 1982). Both acute and chronic interstitial pneumonitis are reported with nitrofurantoin, including a syndrome associated with liver damage and autoantibody formation (Back et al 1974). Sulphonamides are less frequent causes of pulmonary eosinophilia, but may also cause a lupus-like syndrome with lung involvement (Leading Article 1969a).

ADRs and the CNS

CONVULSIONS

In the absence of co-administration of theophylline or non-steroidal anti-inflammatory drugs (NSAIDs), convulsions associated with fluoroquinolone therapy are rare (Christ 1990, Paton & Reeves 1991). They may occur more commonly in patients with a history of epilepsy or previous cerebral damage, in whom such drugs are contraindicated. Convulsions have accompanied major overdoses of metronidazole (Kusumi et al 1980) and nalidixic acid.

β-LACTAM ENCEPHALOPATHY

Convulsions and coma may result from inadvertent overdose of intrathecal benzylpenicillin, and this route of administration is contraindicated. Such neurotoxicity is extremely unlikely to result from therapeutic intravenous doses. In the past, massive doses and co-administration of probenecid may have precipitated convulsions in associated with very high cerebrospinal fluid concentrations (Weinstein et al 1964, Lerner et al 1967). A similar form of encephalopathy may accompany high-dose intravenous and intrathecal cephalosporin therapy (Murdoch et al 1964,

Taylor et al 1981). Imipenem is also recognized to cause seizures, most commonly in those with pre-existing CNS damage, cerebral neoplasia and epilepsy, probably via antagonism of neuroinhibitory γ-aminobutyric acid (GABA) and benzodiazepine receptors in the brain (Leo & Ballow 1991, del Favero 1994) and in those with renal failure. Meropenem appears to be less epileptogenic (del Favero 1994).

OTOTOXICITY

Aminoglycoside ototoxicity is usually associated with prolonged or repeated courses of these drugs, relating to total dose and duration of therapy (McCormack & Jewesson 1992), although single high peak concentrations can have an effect on cochlear output (Wilson & Ramsden 1977). It is a predictable, dose-related phenomenon caused by direct toxic effects on the hair and supporting cells of the organ of Corti resulting in high tone deafness and on the vestibular cells resulting in dizziness and ataxia. However, although vestibular disturbance is the hallmark of ototoxicity of streptomycin and the later aminoglycosides, deafness may follow systemic treatment with neomycin, dihydro-streptomycin and kanamycin. As with nephrotoxicity, the ototoxic potential of the individual aminoglycosides varies.

Measurements of ototoxicity in clinical trials usually rely on serial audiometry and, using this technique, netilmicin has been suggested to be less ototoxic than tobramycin (Lerner et al 1983). However, although animal studies also suggested that tobramycin might improve upon gentamicin, no difference was found in man (Smith et al 1980). Once daily netilmicin regimens reduce ototoxicity compared with conventional therapy in both animals and man (Gilbert 1991, Pechere et al 1991). However, the availability of third-generation cephalosporins and fluoroquinolones should reduce reliance on aminoglycosides in patients at risk of ototoxicity. The elderly, those with pre-existing auditory loss or renal impairment, and those receiving other ototoxic agents, such as frusemide or ethacrynic acid (Manian et al 1990), are at increased risk.

When aminoglycosides must be used, frequent therapeutic monitoring is mandatory. For gentamicin, tobramycin and netilmicin administered at a dose of 5 mg/kg daily in conventional divided 8–12 hourly regimens, peak serum concentrations 1 h after administration should approximate to 5–10 mg/l and trough levels before the next dose should not exceed 2 mg/l. However, it would appear that no studies have specifically addressed the preventative effect of therapeutic monitoring on ototoxicity and the definitions of 'normal therapeutic ranges' have been challenged (McCormack & Jewesson 1992).

Rare cases of ototoxicity have been described following prolonged, high-dose erythromycin therapy and in patients with renal failure (Manian et al 1990). Vancomycin may occasionally cause reversible ototoxicity, presenting as high tone hearing loss or tinnitus, most often in association with high serum concentrations and in patients receiving other potentially ototoxic drugs (McHenry & Gavan 1983, Saunders 1994).

PERIPHERAL NEUROPATHY

Antibiotics are uncommon causes of peripheral neuropathy, which has been reported rarely with nitrofurantoin (Penn & Griffin 1982), metronidazole (Ingham et al 1975) and chloramphenicol. High dose isoniazid (>5 mg/kg daily) predictably causes reversible peripheral neuropathy, which is preventable by co-administration of pyridoxine (reviewed by Kucers & Bennett 1979). Partially reversible optic neuritis has, rarely, been reported with chloramphenicol therapy, usually after prolonged high dosage (Leading Article 1969b).

OTHER NEUROLOGICAL ADVERSE REACTIONS

Benign intracranial hypertension and a bulging fontanelle have been described with nalidixic acid and may follow therapy with later quinolones in infancy (Paton & Reeves 1991). Transient neuromuscular blockade may occur after aminoglycoside therapy, notably after intraperitoneal administration of earlier members of the group (Arcieri et al 1970), and has been reported in association with intravenous clindamycin.

PSYCHOLOGICAL REACTIONS: CONFUSION AND PSYCHOSES

Confusion, hallucinations and delirium have been described with naphthyridines and fluoroquinolones (Ball 1989, Paton & Reeves 1991). Postmarketing surveillance studies on ofloxacin have highlighted a small number of psychotic reactions, mostly in older patients, and perhaps related to drug accumulation (Jungst & Mohr 1987).

Hypersensitivity to antimicrobial agents

ANAPHYLACTIC AND OTHER SEVERE HYPERSENSITIVITY REACTIONS

Classical anaphylactic IgE-mediated reactions, including

angioneurotic oedema and lesser urticarial phenomena occur in less than 0.05% of penicillin-treated patients (Idsoe et al 1968, Austen 1974, Porter & Jick 1977, Sher 1983). The mortality may be 10% or more but, although penicillins are probably responsible for most drug-induced anaphylactic episodes, fatal anaphylaxis possibly occurs in less than 2 per 100 000 treatments (Sher 1983). These reactions are due in most cases to penicillin degradation products, including penicilloyl derivatives (the major antigenic determinants) and both penicillenic and penicilloic acids, but may also relate to high molecular weight polymers which form in solution (Fishman & Hewitt 1970). Attempts to test for, or to desensitize, penicillin-allergic patients with penicilloyl derivatives (polylysines and others) have largely been abandoned due to the risk of anaphylactic reactions to these products themselves. A history of significant penicillin hypersensitivity is a contraindication to the further use of any penicillin; alternative antibiotic classes are always available. However, the public perception of penicillin hypersensitivity is far greater than its absolute incidence. In a recent investigation of 132 patients with alleged hypersensitivity only 4 had a positive radioallergosorbent test (RAST) test and the remaining 128 were re-challenged orally without ill effects (Surtees et al 1991).

Severe generalized hypersensitivity reactions may also occur with other agents, including the cephalosporins (Meyers 1985), nitrofurantoin (Penn & Griffin 1982) and quinolones (Stricker et al 1988, Paton & Reeves 1991). A specific syndrome, mimicking anaphylaxis but also associated with CNS manifestations including convulsions and coma, may follow inadvertent intravenous administration of procaine penicillin, which should never be given by this route (Galpin et al 1974).

Rifampicin may cause such reactions or a 'flu-like' syndrome (Aquinas et al 1972, Pujet et al 1974), sometimes associated with renal impairment, hepatorenal syndrome, thrombocytopenia or haemolysis (Poole et al 1971, Rothwell & Richmond 1974, Girling 1977). These reactions are almost certainly immunologicaly mediated, occurring most frequently, if not exclusively, in patients receiving intermittent regimens or repeated treatment. Reactions are dose and blood-level related and antibodies to rifampicin, which are probably responsible for haemolysis and thrombocytopenia, are found in most cases (Pujet et al 1974).

HISTAMINE RELEASE REACTIONS

The 'red man' syndrome, characterized in most cases by flushing and itch and associated with administration of vancomycin, is thought to relate to histamine release from cutaneous mast cells (Wallace et al 1991). Severity ranges widely, but may extend to anaphylactoid reactions which include dyspnoea, chest pain and hypotension. The incidence is related both to dose and to rapidity of infusion. It may affect 80% receiving a 1 g dose over 60 min (Polk 1991). There is considerable and unpredictable variation in susceptibility and in the relationship between histamine release and the syndrome. Other mediators may be involved (O'Sullivan et al 1993), although antihistamine administration can prevent the reaction (Wallace et al 1991).

MACULOPAPULAR SKIN RASHES

Simple 'antibiotic' rashes are amongst the commonest manifestation of drug hypersensitivity and occur commonly with β-lactams, sulphonamide-containing agents, nitrofurantoin and, less frequently, with fluoroquinolones and other agents. Rashes are rare with macrolides and aminoglycosides.

Ampicillin shares with the natural penicillins the problem of hypersensitivity reactions and is the archetypal cause of 'penicillin' rash. The incidence of maculopapular rash in patients receiving ampicillin is approximately 7% (Collaborative Study Group 1973), but it is considerably less with benzylpenicillin. Some such reactions can be shown to be associated with a rising titre of IgM antibodies to penicilloyl derivatives (Levine et al 1966), but no immunological basis is evident in the majority.

Maculopapular skin eruptions occur in 1–2% of patients receiving parenteral cephalosporins (Meyers 1985). Up to 10% of patients who have previously developed a penicillin rash will do so on subsequent exposure to a cephalosporin (Dash 1975). Penicillin-allergic patients may possibly be given aztreonam safely: 134 penicillin-allergic patients were treated during clinical trials and only one had a possible IgE-mediated reaction (Brogden & Heel 1986).

Allergic reactions, predominantly skin rashes but also including anaphylaxis and angioneurotic oedema, account for 40% of nitrofurantoin-induced phenomena (Penn & Griffin 1982). Rashes occur in 3% of patients receiving co-trimoxazole (Jick 1982) and range from maculopapular eruptions to erythema multiforme and the Stevens–Johnson syndrome. Rashes are generally uncommon with macrolides but may occur with clindamycin (Geddes et al 1970).

SERUM-SICKNESS-TYPE REACTIONS

Whereas serum-sickness reactions may occur with β-lactam antibiotics and many other agents including sulphonamides, a high incidence of these reactions has been reported following the use of cefaclor. A recent review of the US Food and Drug Administration spontaneous reporting system comparing cefaclor with amoxycillin, cephalexin and co-trimoxazole confirmed this finding, noting 638 reports after cefaclor, 51 after co-trimoxazole, 28 after cephalexin and 10 after amoxycillin (Platt et al 1988). Prescription-adjusted data on serum sickness, arthritis and arthralgia for 5 years after marketing showed greatly increased frequencies with cefaclor. These types of reaction have also, rarely, been reported with fluoroquinolones.

ERYTHEMA MULTIFORME AND THE STEVENS–JOHNSON SYNDROME

In the 1960s, long-acting sulphonamides accounted for up to 30% of cases of severe erythema multiforme and the Stevens–Johnson syndrome and mortality approached 25% in fully developed disease (Rallison et al 1961, Beveridge et al 1964, O'Carrol et al 1966). A third of co-trimoxazole reactions affect the skin (Frisch 1973), and a warning from the UK Committee on Safety of Medicines noted 14 deaths from severe skin reactions (Ball 1986). Erythema multiforme is occasionally observed during penicillin and cephalosporin therapy and with a number of other agents.

PHOTOTOXICITY AND PHOTOSENSITIVITY

Originally described with nalidixic acid (Baes 1968), quinolone phototoxicity is a class effect, although the 8-halogenated derivatives (e.g. fleroxacin, sparfloxacin, lomefloxacin) and those with better skin penetration are more likely to produce it (Paton & Reeves 1991, Marutani et al 1993, Domagala 1994). Other antibacterials, notably tetracyclines, may cause photoreactions (Kaidbey & Klingman 1978).

ADVERSE SKIN REACTIONS IN PATIENTS WITH LYMPHOID DISORDERS

In diseases associated with lymphoid proliferation, notably Epstein–Barr virus-induced mononucleosis (Pullen et al 1967), cytomegaloviraemia and, to a lesser degree, chronic lymphatic leukaemia, administration of ampicillin is associated with a high incidence of maculopapular rash. Amoxycillin hypersensitivity rashes are also more frequently reported in AIDS patients (Battegay et al 1989).

Hypersensitivity rash associated with co-trimoxazole is one of the commonest forms of allergic response in those with AIDS, occurring in 18–69% of patients (Caumes et al 1994). It is particularly common in those with higher CD4/CD8 ratios and during short-course therapy (Carr et al 1993). It becomes less common as the disease progresses and is infrequent in those receiving steroid therapy (Caumes et al 1994).

DRUG FEVER

Drug fever is an important ADR which may lead to confusion as to the adequacy of therapy in controlling the infection. In the past it occurred most commonly with long-acting sulphonamides but may be associated with β-lactams, chloramphenicol, fluoroquinolones and other agents, especially after prolonged high-dose therapy as, for example, in endocarditis. A high incidence (32%) has recently been reported with ureidopenicillins in high dosage (Lang et al 1991).

Antibacterial agents and the musculo-skeletal system

EFFECTS ON BONE AND TEETH

Tetracycline therapy is contraindicated in children aged less than 7 years due to irreversible staining of both deciduous and permanent teeth, but in many cases multiple exposure is required to cause more than minor cosmetic problems. The problem has been reviewed extensively by Kucers & Bennett (1979). Administration to infants may cause temporary and reversible cessation of bone growth (Cohlan et al 1963).

EFFECTS ON MUSCLES

Nalidixic acid may cause myopathy and myalgia (Paton & Reeves 1991). Ciprofloxacin may have precipitated a myasthenic crisis at high dosage (Moore et al 1988). Polymyositis may be caused by penicillins (Hart 1984).

EFFECTS ON ARTICULAR CARTILAGE, OTHER JOINT TISSUES AND TENDONS

Chronic, high-dose administration of naphthyridine and quinolone antibacterials may cause cartilaginous erosions in the di-arthrodial, weight-bearing joints of juvenile members of a number of animal species, notably beagle dogs (Ball 1989, Paton & Reeves 1991). Nalidixic acid is most likely to cause this problem, but modern fluoroquinolones, including ciprofloxacin and ofloxacin, may induce cartilage damage in very high doses (Ingham et al 1977, Schluter 1987, Mayer 1987) and the phenomenon appears to be a class effect (Domagala 1994). Although no such reactions have been observed with fluoroquinolones or their progenitors in children (Schaad & Wedgwood 1992,

Nuutinen et al 1994), one case of destructive polyarthropathy was reported in a 17 year old who had received pefloxacin for 3 months (Chevalier et al 1992). Several reports associate pefloxacin and ofloxacin therapy with severe Achilles tendinitis and tendon rupture (Ribard et al 1992).

Arthralgia may occur as part of a serum-sickness reaction, of which penicillin is the most common cause, and isoniazid may cause arthralgia as part of the shoulder–hand syndrome (Hart 1984). Polyarteritis and a systemic lupus-like syndrome may be caused by penicillins, sulphonamides, tetracyclines and isoniazid.

ADRs and the kidneys

ADVERSE EFFECTS OF ANTIBACTERIAL AGENTS ON THE KIDNEY

The major mechanisms of renal damage by antibiotics are direct toxicity and immunologically mediated acute interstitial nephritis (Davey 1982). Although direct damage from crystalluria, previously a problem with sulphonamides, was anticipated with fluoroquinolones, it does not occur in acid human urine (Paton & Reeves 1991). Direct toxicity is typical of aminoglycosides, the original cephalosporins (cephaloridine and cephalothin) and amphotericin B, whereas penicillins, notably methicillin, are most likely to cause damage via immunological reactions (Appel 1980).

AMINOGLYCOSIDE NEPHROTOXICITY

All aminoglycosides are concentrated in renal tubular cells, but the degree of their individual accumulation is only poorly correlated with their potential for nephrotoxicity and idiosyncratic hypersensitivity probably also applies (Davey 1982). The aminoglycosides cause acute tubular dysfunction and release of proteins and enzymes, such as β_2-microglobulin and n-acetyl-β-glucuronidase (NAG), which indicate tubular damage. High dosage can result in acute tubular necrosis (Appel & Neu 1977a) but less severe degrees of renal tubular damage are reversible (Luft 1984). A meta-analysis of clinical studies recorded the average frequencies of aminoglycoside nephrotoxicity as being 13–14% for tobramycin and gentamicin and 8.7–9.4% for netilmicin and amikacin (Kahlmeter & Dahlager 1984). Animal studies also suggest that netilmicin might be less nephrotoxic than other aminoglycosides (Luft 1984), and when trials comparing aminoglycosides were analysed individually netilmicin appeared less nephrotoxic (6.6%) than either tobramycin or gentamicin (12.7–17.1%)

(Kahlmeter & Dahlager 1984). Other studies have suggested that both tobramycin (Smith et al 1980) and netilmicin (Lerner et al 1983) are less nephrotoxic than gentamicin. However, these differences may reflect the criteria used to detect nephrotoxicity, which differ between reports, and the populations studied. Advanced age, liver and renal disease, prolonged therapy and high serum concentrations are independant risk factors for nephrotoxicity (Davey 1982, Moore et al 1984).

Once-daily aminoglycoside administration has been under discussion for some years. Encouraged by animal studies, which suggested lesser toxicity than that associated with conventional therapy, studies in man have now shown once-daily therapy to offer equivalent efficacy, and some reports have confirmed a reduction in toxicity (Gilbert 1991, Pechere et al 1991, Parker & Davey, 1993). No differences were observed between individual aminoglycosides, for example, gentamicin and netilmicin, when administered in once-daily regimens (Prins et al 1994).

COMBINATIONS OF AMINOGLYCOSIDES AND OTHER DRUGS

The nephrotoxicity of aminoglycosides is enhanced by co-administration of certain other drugs, notably cephalothin (Appell & Neu 1977b). Caution is required during co-administration of aminoglycosides and later generation cephalosporins, although these agents are probably not intrinsically nephrotoxic. Meta-analysis suggests that the nephrotoxicity of either aminoglycosides or vancomycin is significantly increased by co-administration of the other (Goetz & Sayers 1993).

EFFECTS OF AMINOGLYCOSIDES ON CATION EXCRETION

Patients receiving cytotoxic chemotherapy for both leukaemias and solid tumours may develop hypomagnes-aemia, hypokalaemia and hypocalcaemia in association with aminoglycoside therapy, probably in association with tubular damage (Keating et al 1977, Davey et al 1985).

VANCOMYCIN

Reversible nephrotoxicity may effect up to 5% of patients receiving vancomycin, usually in those with previously impaired renal function (Manian et al 1990, Saunders 1994). It is most likely to occur during co-administration with aminoglycosides (Goetz & Sayers 1993).

β-LACTAM ANTIBIOTICS

Dose-related nephrotoxicity is characteristic of the first-generation cephalosporins, which are concentrated within proximal tubular cells of the kidney. Cephalosporin nephrotoxicity leads initially to excretion of casts and ultimately to tubular necrosis (Foord 1975, Appell & Neu 1977b). Unlike cephalothin, cephaloridine is not secreted into the tubule, which accounts for its greater potential for toxicity (Tune 1975). Although at least some of these reactions were potentiated or precipitated by co-administration of potent diuretics, such as frusemide and ethacrynic acid (Dodds & Foord 1970), neither compound should now be used. Second- and third-generation agents, such as cefuroxime, cefotaxime, cefoxitin and ceftazidime, are essentially free of nephrotoxicity.

Carbapenems have similar nephrotoxic potential to the original cephalosporins. Imipenem administered alone in animals may precipitate acute tubular necrosis, but this effect is blocked by co-administration of cilastatin, an inhibitor of renal tubular brush border dehydropeptidase (Birnbaum et al 1985, del Favero 1994). Meropenem, which is free of this effect, is administered alone.

CO-TRIMOXAZOLE

Co-trimoxazole should be avoided in patients with significant renal impairment. An original report described irreversible renal impairment in 13 of 16 affected patients (Kalowski et al 1973). Subsequent studies demonstrated no significant nephrotoxicity, either directly or by measurement of ethylenediaminetetraacetic acid (EDTA) clearance and β_2-microglobulin secretion, in either normal patients or those with renal failure receiving adjusted doses (Tasker et al 1975, Trollfors 1980). However, the constituents may accumulate and there are reports of acute interstitial nephritis.

FLUOROQUINOLONES

Although crystalluria has not proved a problem, interstitial nephritis and direct nephrotoxicity have rarely been reported with new fluoroquinolones (Paton & Reeves 1991).

EFFECTS OF RENAL FAILURE ON ADVERSE REACTIONS

Reduced elimination of antibiotics normally cleared by renal excretion may produce effects on the nervous system, coagulation, glucose metabolism and the blood, and may enhance inactivation of aminoglycosides by co-administered β-lactams (Manian et al 1990). The effects of renal impairment on the potential for ototoxicity and nephrotoxicity due to aminoglycosides and vancomycin are summarized above.

Neurotoxicity of penicillins, cephalosporins and imipenem, manifesting as seizures, is enhanced by renal impairment which leads to high serum free drug concentrations. The physiological effects of uraemia on the blood–brain barrier and in reducing plasma protein binding contribute. Ototoxicity of erythromycin, reversible and dose related, and vancomycin is enhanced by renal insufficiency and two cases of reversible cephalexin-induced vestibular dysfunction have been reported (Manian et al 1990). Renal failure is a predisposing factor for peripheral neuropathy due to nitrofurantoin and isoniazid (Felts et al 1971).

Therapy with high-dose benzylpenicillin, carbenicillin and *N*-methylthiotetrazole side-chain cephalosporins (e.g. cefoperazone) in renal failure may result in bleeding due variously to platelet dysfunction, increased antithrombin-III activity, prolonged prothrombin times and hypoprothrombinaemia (Andrassy et al 1976, Lipsky 1988).

DOSAGE MONITORING AND MODIFICATION IN RENAL FAILURE

Aminoglycosides
Therapeutic monitoring of peak and trough concentrations is advised for all aminoglycosides administered on a multiple daily basis (see p. 142). For once-daily dosing, it may be acceptable to monitor only the trough concentration, ensuring that it remains below 2 mg/l (Parker & Davey 1993). Others suggest an even more conservative 1 mg/l (MacGowan & Reeves 1994).

Vancomycin
Peak and trough vancomycin serum concentrations are routinely monitored during therapy such that peak and trough levels are maintained at around 25–30 and 5–10 mg/l, respectively. Nephrotoxicity and ototoxicity can be minimized or avoided by ensuring that peak serum concentrations do not exceed 40 mg/l. However, such toxicity is uncommon and various authorities have questioned the need for therapeutic monitoring (Moellering 1994, Saunders 1994). Peak level testing may be unnecessary: mean increases of 16.6 mg/l were demonstrated in patients receiving standard therapy (Saunders 1994), indicating that, providing trough levels did not exceed 15 mg/l, toxic accumulation could be avoided and savings could be made. Nevertheless, although some dispute the effect of renal impairment on vancomycin toxicity, patients with rapidly altering renal function, in whom nomogram and other predictive dosing regimens do not apply, should continue to

have both peak and trough levels monitored to reduce potential toxicity and ensure therapeutic efficacy. Others would suggest that teicoplanin, which does not routinely require serum-level monitoring and has been used safely in patients with a history of vancomycin toxicity, should be substituted in infections where therapeutic equivalence applies.

Potential role of antimicrobials in carcinogenesis

Various antimicrobials, notably nitroimidazoles (metronidazole) and quinolones, are mutagenic and potentially carcinogenic in the laboratory. The development of liver tumours in rats delayed the availability of metronidazole for some years in the USA, but a follow-up study of women who had originally received the drug for vaginal trichomoniasis revealed no excess of malignancy compared with controls (Beard et al 1979). Similarly, there has been no observed increase in frequency of cancer in patients receiving naphthyridines and quinolones over the past 25 years. Recent studies have suggested that 8-fluorinated quinolones could be photocarcinogenic in mice; the matter remains under investigation.

Antibiotic use in pregnancy

Two separate problems are posed by the use of antimicrobial agents in pregnancy: (1) those arising from an increase in incidence of ADRs in the mother (maternal considerations), and (2) those affecting the fetus. The overall incidence of ADRs in pregnant patients does not appear significantly different from that in other adults (Chow & Jewesson 1985). Later effects on the newborn may result from excretion of antibiotics in breast milk.

MATERNAL CONSIDERATIONS

Routine use of most antibiotics during pregnancy poses no unusual hazards for the mother. There are two exceptions: tetracyclines may cause acute liver failure with a high mortality and is therefore contraindicated (Greene 1976); and use of erythromycin estolate results in a higher than expected incidence of hepatotoxicity in late pregnancy (McCormack et al 1977).

ADVERSE EFFECTS ON THE FETUS

Major adverse effects of antimicrobials (embryotoxicity and teratogenesis) are most likely to occur during the early period of embryogenesis in the first trimester of pregnancy (Beeley 1981a). Such risks recede thereafter.

β-Lactam drugs, particularly the penicillins, have an excellent record of safety in pregnancy and may usually be used for all normal indications. No evidence for teratogenesis has been found (Heinonen et al 1977). Penicillins cross the placenta and enter breast milk in small quantities, usually less than 10–15% of simultaneous serum levels.

Aminoglycosides were used quite extensively in pregnancy for the management of Gram-negative infection; modern cephalosporins are now preferred. Although teratogenesis has not been observed, aminoglycosides penetrate fetal tissue, including the kidneys, and ototoxicity has been recorded with streptomycin (Assael et al 1982). Data on the related agents, vancomycin and teicoplanin, are lacking, but on first principles they should be avoided where possible.

Fluoroquinolones must be used with caution in pregnancy. They are mutagens, similarly to metronidazole, and although mutation rates in eucaryotic cells are not increased by these agents and they have no effects on human DNA polymerase and topoisomerases at levels which are achievable in man (Hussy et al 1986), they should be avoided except when potential therapeutic benefit outweighs what may be a theoretical risk. These agents cross the placenta and deliver high concentrations in breast milk.

Although the potential effects of metronidazole on mammalian DNA are well recognized (Beard et al 1979), this agent has been used for many years with apparent safety in pregnancy, causing no more problems in the mother than would normally be expected. No increased rates of birth defects or teratogenic effects have been observed (Morgan 1978, Chow & Jewesson 1985). Rifampicin may cause fetal malformations in animals, and use during human pregnancy has been associated with abnormalities such as hydrocephalus and limb defects, although a causal relationship has yet to be proven (Steen & Stainton Ellis 1977).

Tetracyclines are contraindicated in pregnancy, partly because of maternal risk, partly due to their ability to cause staining and dysplasia of teeth and bone (Beeley 1981b), and partly because of a rare potential association with limb defects. In premature neonates, tetracyclines markedly inhibit bone growth.

Sulphonamides and co-trimoxazole are contraindicated in late pregnancy; they may precipitate kernicterus in the newborn (Silverman et al 1956).

Antimalarials pose problems in pregnancy, as either experimental or human evidence for teratogenesis affects most classes of agents. Proguanil is safe for prophylaxis, but pyrimethamine–sulfadoxine (Fansidar) is not recommended and mefloquine is contraindicated (Cook 1992). Chloroquine, although potentially problematic (retinitis and ototoxicity), may be used where benefit outweighs risk, but resistance poses a greater hazard. Quinine has been used extensively for therapy of acute cases and remains the drug of choice.

Specific problems in neonates

AMINOGLYCOSIDES

The volumes of distribution of these agents are largest in low-birth-weight infants and decrease with postnatal age. Likewise, the half-lives correlate inversely with birthweight and postnatal age. Thus specific dosage adjustment is required for the neonatal period such that toxicity may be avoided. Recommendations are given by McCracken & Nelson (1977).

GREY SYNDROME

The grey syndrome of neonates (Burns et al 1959), caused by inhibition of mitochondrial electron transport in liver, myocardium and skeletal muscle, and manifesting as lethargy, hypotension, reduced tissue and peripheral perfusion, hypoxia and abdominal distension, is precipitated by excessive levels of chloramphenicol consequent upon reduced clearance of the drug in this age group. It is most common in premature, low-birth-weight infants in whom prolonged high serum concentrations reflect immaturity of glucuronyl transferase biotransformation and renal function.

However, chloramphenicol remains a very useful agent for management of bacterial meningitis, especially in developing countries, and serious toxicity is almost always due to excessive prescriptions or overdosage. Grey syndrome may be avoided by attention to dosage, which should not exceed 25 mg/kg in a single dose in infants aged 0–14 days (15–30 days if weighing under 2000 g), and monitoring of serum concentrations which should be maintained in the range 15–25 mg/l (McCracken & Nelson 1977, Mulhall et al 1983). Exchange transfusion and charcoal haemoperfusion may be effective in gross overdosage.

KERNICTERUS

Sulphonamides compete with bilirubin for albumin binding sites and may precipitate kernicterus in the newborn (Silverman et al 1956). Their use and that of co-trimoxazole is contraindicated. Other highly protein bound antibiotics might have similar effects, although data are lacking. Recent in vitro studies have suggested that ceftriaxone may displace bilirubin from binding sites, mandating caution if this agent is to be used in icteric neonates. However, no clinical evidence for hyperbilirubinaemia has been observed.

BREAST FEEDING

Antibiotics are excreted in breast milk to a remarkably variable degree. β-Lactams and aminoglycosides usually achieve concentrations less than 20% of maternal serum levels, whereas chloramphenicol, erythromycin and tetracyclines reach ratios of 50–75%. Some agents, notably sulphonamides and quinolones, may be concentrated in breast milk. All such agents can induce similar hypersensitivity reactions in the neonate (e.g. drug rashes) to those which may affect the mother, and may cause acute alterations in the neonatal bowel flora with resultant diarrhoea.

Postmarketing surveillance

Most new antimicrobial agents are licensed on the basis of treatment of 5000 or more patients, during the course of which most common ADRs are likely to come to light. However, low-frequency effects may not be detected and very seriously ill patients, who may react more severely or atypically, are rarely included. Equally, some novel drugs for very limited indications, such as lipid-complexed amphotericin B derivatives, are unlikely to generate a large database. Experience of agents developed in the 1950s–1960s was distinctly inferior compared to modern agents prior to marketing, and most problems surfaced thereafter. For nitrofurantoin, reporting to various national registration authorities resulted in confusing disparities between countries. Thus Swedish regulatory authorities received more ADR reports on nitrofurantoin than for any other single drug, particularly in respect of pulmonary eosinophilia and hepatic reactions (Holmberg et al 1980). In contrast, gastro-intestinal symptoms and peripheral neuropathy were relatively more common in the UK (Penn & Griffin 1982). A five-fold greater prescription rate in Sweden at the time of warning letters from the authorities in both countries may have influenced the reporting of ADRs, but it is clear that the findings from one country cannot necessarily be applied to another. The overwhelming predominance of Americans in the temafloxacin-induced haemolytic anaemia/uraemia syndrome cohort and its apparent absence in Europeans supports this view.

New drugs marketed in the last 5 years have been subject to intensive surveillance during their initial year of general use and for a prolonged period thereafter. The thalidomide debacle in the 1960s and the recent withdrawal of temafloxacin indicate that not all serious ADRs can be identified during premarketing assessment. Some form of effective postmarketing surveillance of new compounds is necessary, and analysis of acceptable risk may be required when potentially serious problems are detected (Davey & McDonald 1993). Postmarketing (phase IV) trials are unlikely to supply adequate information. They are usually undertaken for promotional purposes and often select patients who are unrepresentative of the general population. Spontaneous direct reporting of ADRs to registration authorities is also unreliable as it cannot estimate either absolute or relative risks in the absence of denominator information. Prescription event monitoring allows the collection of unselective data in defined patient cohorts and may allow a more accurate assessment of the ADR profile of specific agents (Inman et al 1993).

The withdrawal of temafloxacin is a good example of these systems in action. Postmarketing surveillance of quinolones showed that temafloxacin ADRs were unusual in comparison with those encountered during the initial launch phase of other modern quinolones (Davey & McDonald 1993). Prescription event monitoring of ciprofloxacin and other quinolones revealed no similarly related cases (Inman et al 1993). However, some patients exhibited hypoglycaemia and hepatic or renal damage from unrelated causes, requiring differentiation from drug-induced effects.

Antibiotics are, with notable exceptions, essentially safe drugs. They did not feature when 20 leading authorities were approached to list the 10 most important ADRs since the thalidomide disaster (Venning 1983). However, pseudomembranous colitis caused by lincosamides ranked eleventh, and when deaths in relation to general-practice prescriptions were analysed separately it ranked highest, isoniazid hepatotoxicity coming second. Therefore, unexpected drug reactions should always be considered when unusual events complicate therapy with familiar and trusted agents.

References

Andrassy K, Scherz M, Ritz E et al 1976 Penicillin-induced coagulation disorder. Lancet ii: 1039–1041

Appel G B 1980 A decade of penicillin related acute interstitial nephritis – more questions than answers. Clinical Nephrology 13: 151–154

Appel G B, Neu H C 1977a The nephrotoxicity of antimicrobial agents. New England Journal of Medicine 296: 722–728

Appel G B, Neu H C 1977b The nephrotoxicity of antimicrobial agents. New England Journal of Medicine 296: 633–670

Arcieri G M, Falco F G, Smith H M, Hobson L B 1970 Clinical research experience with gentamicin: incidence of adverse reactions. Medical Journal of Australia 1 (spec. suppl): 30

Assael B M, Parini R, Rusconi F 1982 Ototoxicity of aminoglycoside antibiotics in infants and children. Pediatric Infectious Disease Journal 1: 357–365

Austen K F 1974 Current concepts. Systemic anaphylaxis in the human being. New England Journal of Medicine 291: 661

Aquinas S M, Allan W G L, Horsfall P A L et al 1972 Adverse reactions to daily and intermittent rifampicin regimens for pulmonary tuberculosis in Hong Kong. British Medical Journal i: 765–771

Back O, Lundgren R, Wiman L-G 1974 Nitrofurantoin-induced pulmonary fibrosis and lupus syndrome. Lancet i: 930

Baes H 1968 Photosensitivity caused by nalidixic acid. Dermatologica 136: 61–64

Ball P 1986 Toxicity of sulphonamide–diaminopyrimidine combinations: implications for future use. Journal of Antimicrobial Chemotherapy 17: 694–696

Ball P 1989 Adverse reactions and interactions of fluoro-quinolones. Clinical and Investigative Medicine 12: 28–34

Bartlett J G 1992 Antibiotic associated diarrhoea. Clinical Infectious Diseases 15: 573–581

Battegay M, Opravil M, Wuthrich B, Luthy R 1989 Rash with amoxycillin–clavulanate therapy in HIV-infected patients [letter]. Lancet ii: 1100

Beard C M, Noller K L, O'Fallon M, Kurland L T, Dockerty M B 1979 Lack of evidence for cancer due to use of metronidazole. New England Journal of Medicine 301: 519–522

Beeley L 1981a Adverse effects of drugs in the first trimester of pregnancy. Clinical Obstetrics and Gynaecology 8: 261–273

Beeley L 1981b Adverse effects of drugs in later pregnancy. Clinical Obstetrics and Gynaecology 8: 275–289

Berg P A, Daniel P T 1987 Co-trimoxazole induced hepatic injury: an analysis of cases with hypersensitivity-like reactions. Infection 15 (suppl 5): S259–S264

Beveridge J, Harris M, Wise G, Stevens L 1964 Long acting sulphonamides associated with Stevens–Johnson syndrome. Lancet ii: 593

Birnbaum J, Kahan F M, Kropp H, Macdonald J S 1985 Carbapenems, a new class of beta-lactam antibiotics. American Journal of Medicine 78 (suppl A): 3–21

Blum M D, Graham D J, McCloskey C A 1994 Temafloxacin syndrome: review of 95 cases. *Clinical Infectious Diseases* 18: 946–950

Braun P 1969 Hepatotoxicity of erythromycin. *Journal of Infectious Diseases* 119: 300–306

Brogden R N, Heel R C 1986 Aztreonam: a review of its antibacterial activity, pharmacokinetic properties and therapeutic use. *Drugs* 31: 96–130

Brown C H, Natelson E A, Bradshaw M W, Alfrey C P, Williams W T 1975 Study of the effects of ticacillin on blood coagulation and platelet function. *Antimicrobial Agents and Chemotherapy* 7: 652

Burns L E, Hodgman J E, Cass A B 1959 Fatal circulatory collapse in premature infants receiving chloramphenicol. *New England Journal of Medicine* 261: 1318–1321

Carr A, Swanson C, Penny R, Cooper D A 1993 Clinical and laboratory markers of hypersensitivity to trimethoprim–sulfamethoxazole in patients with *Pneumocystis carinii* pneumonia and AIDS. *Journal of Infectious Diseases* 167: 180–185

Caumes E, Roudier C, Rogeaux O, Bricaire F, Gentilini M 1994 Effect of corticosteroids on the incidence of adverse cutaneous reactions to trimethoprim–sulfamethoxazole during treatment of AIDS-associated *Pneumocystis carinii* pneumonia. *Clinics in Infectious Disease* 18: 319–323

Chanarin I, England J M 1972 Toxicity of trimethoprim–sulphamethoxazole in patients with megaloblastic haemopoesis. *British Medical Journal* i: 651–653

Chevalier X, Albengress E, Voisin M C, Tillment J P, Larget-Piet B 1992 A case of destructive polyarthropathy in a 17-year-old youth following pefloxacin treatment. *Drug Safety* 7: 310–314

Chow A W, Jewesson P J 1985 Pharmacokinetics and safety of antimicrobial agents during pregnancy. *Reviews of Infectious Diseases* 7: 287–313

Christ W 1990 Central nervous system toxicity of quinolones: human and animal findings. *Journal of Antimicrobial Chemotherapy* 26 (suppl B): 219–225

Cohlan S Q, Bevelander G, Tiamsic T 1963 Growth inhibition of prematures receiving tetracycline. *American Review of Diseases in Childhood* 105: 453

Collaborative Study Group 1973 Prospective study of ampicillin rash. *British Medical Journal* i: 7–9

Cook G C 1992 Use of antiprotozoal and antihelminthic drugs during pregnancy: side effects and contra-indications. *Journal of Infection* 25: 1–9

Dash C H 1975 Penicillin allergy and the cephalosporins. *Journal of Antimicrobial Chemotherapy* 1 (suppl): 107–118

Davey P G 1982 Adverse effects of antibiotics – the kidney. In: Reeves D S, Geddes A M (eds) Recent advances in infection – 2. Churchill Livingstone, Edinburgh

Davey P G, McDonald T 1993 Postmarketing surveillance of quinolones, 1990 to 1992. *Drugs* 45 (suppl 3): 46–53

Davey P, Gozzard D, Goodall M, Leyland M J 1985 Hypomagnesaemia: an underdiagnosed interaction between gentamicin and cytotoxic chemotherapy for acute non-lymphoblastic leukaemia. *Journal of Antimicrobial Chemotherapy* 15: 623–628

Davis S, Rubin A D 1972 Treatment and prognosis in aplastic anaemia. *Lancet* i: 871

del Favero A 1994 Clinically important aspects of carbapenem safety. *Current Opinions in Infectious Disease* 7 (suppl 1): S38–S42

Dodds M G, Foord R D 1970 Enhancement by potent diuretics of renal tubular necrosis induced by cephaloridine. *British Journal of Pharmacology* 40: 227–236

Domagala J M 1994 Structure–activity and structure–side-effect relationships for the quinolone antibacterials. *Journal of Antimicrobial Chemotherapy* 33: 685–706

Elias E 1982 Adverse effects of antibiotics – the liver. In: Reeves D S, Geddes A M (eds) Recent advances in infection – 2. Churchill Livingstone, Edinburgh

Eykyn S J 1990 Staphylococcal bacteraemia and endocarditis and fusidic acid. *Journal of Antimicrobial Chemotherapy* 25 (suppl B): 33–38

Fairley C K, McNeil J J, Desmond P et al 1993 Risk factors for development of flucloxacillin associated jaundice. *British Medical Journal* 306: 233–235

Felts J H, Hayes D M, Gergen J A, Toole J F 1971 Neural, hematological and bacteriologic effects of nitrofurantoin in renal insufficiency. *American Journal of Medicine* 51: 331–339

Fishman L S, Hewitt W L 1970 The natural penicillins. *Medical Clinics of North America* 54: 1081–1099

Foord R D 1975 Cephaloridine, cephalothin and the kidney. *Journal of Antimicrobial Chemotherapy* 1: 119–133

Frisch J M 1973 Clinical experience with adverse reactions to trimethoprim–sulphamethoxazole. *Journal of Infectious Diseases* 128 (suppl): S607–S611

Galpin J E, Chow A W, Yoshikawa T T, Guze L B 1974 Pseudoanaphylactic reactions from inadvertent infusion of procaine penicillin G. *Annals of Internal Medicine* 81: 358

Garraty G, Petz L D 1975 Drug induced haemolytic anaemia. *American Journal of Medicine* 58: 398

Geddes A M, Bridgwater F A J, Williams D N, Oon J, Grimshaw G J 1970 Clinical and bacteriological studies with clindamycin. *British Medical Journal* 2: 703–704

Gilbert D N 1991 Once daily aminoglycoside therapy. *Antimicrobial Agents and Chemotherapy* 35: 399–405

Girling D J 1977 Adverse reactions to rifampicin in antituberculosis regimens. *Journal of Antimicrobial Chemotherapy* 3: 115–132

Goetz M B, Sayers J 1993 Nephrotoxicity of vancomycin and aminoglycoside therapy separately and in combination. *Journal of Antimicrobial Chemotherapy* 32: 325–334

Golde D W, Bersch M, Quan S G 1978 Trimethoprim and sulphamethoxazole inhibition of haematopoiesis in vitro. *British Journal of Haematology* 40: 363–367

Greene G 1976 Tetracycline in pregnancy. *New England Journal of Medicine* 295: 512–513

Gupta N K, Woodley C L, Fried R 1970 Effect of metronidazole on liver alcohol dehydrogenase. *Biochemistry and Pharmacology* 19: 2805–2808

Halkin H 1988 Adverse effects of the fluoroquinolones. *Reviews of Infectious Diseases* 10 (suppl 1): S258–S261

Hallas J, Gram L F, Grodum E et al 1992 Drug-related admissions to medical wards: a population based survey. *British Journal of Clinical Pharmacology* 33: 61–68

Hart F D 1984 Drug-induced arthritis and arthralgia. *Drugs* 28: 347–354

Havas L, Fernex M, Lennox-Smith I 1973 The clinical efficacy and tolerance of co-trimoxazole. *Clinical Trials Journal* 10: 81–86

Heinonen O P, Slone D, Shapiro S 1977 Antimicrobial and antiparasitic agents. Birth defects and drugs in pregnancy. Publishing Sciences Group, Littleton, MA, p 296–313

Holmberg L, Boman G, Bottinger L E, Eriksson B, Spross R 1980 Adverse reactions to nitrofurantoin: analysis of 921 reports. *American Journal of Medicine* 69: 733–738

Hopkins S 1991 Clinical toleration and safety of azithromycin. *American Journal of Medicine* 91 (suppl 3A): 40S–45S

Hughes B R, Cunliffe W J 1987 Erythromycin and gastrointestinal motility. *Lancet* i: 1340

Hussy P, Maass G, Tuemmler B, Grosse F, Schomberg U 1986 Effect of 4-quinolones and novobiocin on calf thymus DNA polymerase alpha primase complex, topoisomerases I and II and growth of mammalian lymphoblasts. *Antimicrobial Agents and Chemotherapy* 29: 1073–1078

Idsoe O, Guthe T, Wilcox R R, de Weck A L 1968 The nature and extent of penicillin side-reactions, with particular reference to fatalities from anaphylactic shock. *Bulletin of the World Health Organization* 38: 159

Ingham H R, Selkon J B, Hale J H 1975 Treatment with metronidazole of three patients with serious infections due to *Bacteroides fragilis. Journal of Antimicrobial Chemotherapy* 1: 235–242

Ingham B, Brentnall D W, Dale E A, McFadzean J A 1977 Arthropathy induced by antibacterial fused N-alkyl-4-pyridone-3-carboxylic acids. *Toxicology Letters* 1: 21–26

Inman W, Kubota K, Pearce G, Wilton L 1993 PEM report number 4. *Pharmacoepidemiol and Drug Safety* 2: 341–364

Jick H 1982 Adverse reactions to trimethoprim-sulfamthoxazole in hospitalised patients. *Reviews of Infectious Diseases* 4: 426–428

Jungst G, Mohr R 1987 Side effects of ofloxacin in clinical trials and post-marketing surveillance. *Drugs* 34 (suppl 1): 144–149

Kaidbey K H, Klingman A M 1978 Identification of systemic phototoxic drugs by human intradermal assay. *Journal of Investigative Dermatology (USA)* 70: 272–274

Kahlmeter G, Dahlager J I 1984 Aminoglycoside toxicity – a review of clinical studies published between 1975 and 1982. *Journal of Antimicrobial Chemotherapy* 13 (suppl A): 9–22

Kalowski S, Nanra R S, Mathew T H, Kincid-Smith P 1973 Deterioration in renal function in association with co-trimoxazole therapy. *Lancet* i: 394–397

Keating M, Sethi M, Bodey G, Samaan M 1977 Hypocalcaemia with hypoparathyroidism and renal tubular dysfunction associated with aminoglycoside therapy. *Cancer* 39: 1410–1414

Kucers A, Bennet N McK 1979 The use of antibiotics, 3rd edn. William Heinemann Medical, London

Kusumi R K, Plouffe J F, Wyatt R H 1980 Central nervous system toxicity associated with metronidazole therapy. *Annals of Internal Medicine* 93: 59

Lang R, Lishner M, Ravid M 1991 Adverse reactions to prolonged treatment with high doses of carbenicillin and ureidopenicillins. *Reviews of Infectious Diseases* 13: 68–72

Larson H E 1982 Adverse effects of antibiotics – the bowel. In: Reeves D S, Geddes A M (eds) Recent advances in infection – 2. Churchill Livingstone, Edinburgh

Leading Article 1969a Lung disease caused by drugs. *British Medical Journal* iii: 729

Leading Article 1969b Chloramphenicol blindness. *British Medical Journal* i: 1511

Leading Article 1973 Co-trimoxazole and blood. *Lancet* ii: 950

Leading Article 1977 Pseudomembranous enterocolitis. *Lancet* i: 839–840

Leo R J, Ballow C H 1991 Seizure activity associated with imipenem use: clinical case reports and review of the literature. *DICP Annals of Pharmacotherapy* 25: 351–354

Lerner A M, Reyes M P, Cone L A et al 1983 Randomised, controlled trial of the comparative efficacy, auditory toxicity, and nephrotoxicity of tobramycin and netilmicin. *Lancet* i: 1123–1126

Lerner P I, Smith H, Weinstein L 1967 Penicillin neurotoxicity. *Annals of the New York Academy of Sciences* 145: 310

Levine B B, Redmond A P, Fellner M J 1966 Penicillin allergy and the heterogeneous immune response of man to benzylpenicillin. *Journal of Clinical Investigations* 45: 1895–1906

Lipsky J J 1988 Antibiotic associated hypoprothrombinaemia. *Journal of Antimicrobial Chemotherapy* 21: 281–300

Luft F C 1984 Clinical significance of renal changes engendered by aminoglycosides in man. *Journal of Antimicrobial Chemotherapy* 13 (suppl A): 23–28

Lunzer M R, Huang S N, Ward K M, Sherlock S 1975 Jaundice due to erythromycin estolate. *Gastroenterology* 68: 1284–1291

McCormack J P, Jewesson P J 1992 A critical re-evaluation of the 'therapeutic range' of aminoglycosides. *Clinical Infectious Diseases* 14: 320–339

McCormack W M, George H, Donner A et al 1977 Hepatotoxicity of erythromycin estolate during pregnancy. *Antimicrobial Agents and Chemotherapy* 12: 630–635

McCracken G H, Nelson J D 1977 Antimicrobial therapy for newborns. Grune & Stratton, New York

MacFarland L V, Mulligan M E, Kwok R Y, Stamm W E 1989 Nosocomial acquisition of *Clostridium difficile* infection. *New England Journal of Medicine* 320: 204–210

MacGowan A P, Reeves D S 1994 Serum monitoring and practicalities of once daily aminoglycoside dosing. *Journal of Antimicrobial Chemotherapy* 33: 349–350

McHenry M C, Gavan T L 1983 Vancomycin. *Medical Clinics of North America* 30: 31–47

Manian F A, Stone W J, Alford R H 1990 Adverse antibiotic effects associated with renal insufficiency. *Reviews of Infectious Diseases* 12: 236–249

Marutani K, Matsumoto M, Otabe Y et al 1993 Reduced phototoxicity of a fluoroquinolone antibacterial agent with a methoxy group at the 8 position in mice irradiated with long-wavelength UV light. *Antimicrobial Agents and Chemotherapy* 37: 2217–2233

Mayer D G 1987 Overview of toxicological studies. *Drugs* 34 (suppl 1): 150–153

Meyers B R 1985 Comparative toxicities of third generation cephalosporins. *American Journal of Medicine* 79 (suppl 12A): 96–103

Moellering R C 1994 Editorial: monitoring serum vancomycin levels: climbing the mountain because it is there. *Clinics in Infectious Disease* 18: 544–546

Moore B, Safrani M, Keesey J 1988 Possible exacerbation of myasthenia gravis by ciprofloxacin. *Lancet* i: 882

Moore R D, Smith C R, Lipsky J J, Mellits E D, Lietman P S 1984 Risk factors for nephrotoxicity in patients treated with aminoglycosides. *Annals of Internal Medicine* 100: 352–357

Morgan I 1978 Metronidazole treatment in pregnancy. *International Journal of Gynaecology and Obstetrics* 15: 501–502

Mulhall A, de Louvois J, Hurley R 1983 Chloramphenicol toxicity in neonates: its incidence and prevention. *British Medical Journal* 287: 1424–1427

Murdoch J McC, Speirs C F, Geddes A M, Wallace E T 1964 Clinical trial of cephaloridine (ceporan), a new broad spectrum antibiotic derived from cephalosporin C. *British Medical Journal* ii: 1238–1240

Newman R, Doster B E, Murray F J, Woolpert S F 1974 Rifampicin in initial treatment of pulmonary tuberculosis. *American Review of Respiratory Disease* 109: 216–232

Nuutinen M, Turtinen J, Uhari M 1994 Growth and joint symptoms in children treated with nalidixic acid. *Pediatric Infectious Diseases Journal* 13: 798–800

O'Carrol O M, Bryan P A, Robinson R J 1966 Stevens–Johnson syndrome associated with long-acting sulphonamides. *Journal of American Medical Association* 195: 691–693

O'Sullivan T L, Ruffing M J, Lamo K C, Warbasse L H, Rybak M J 1993 Prospective evaluation of red man syndrome in patients receiving vancomycin. *Journal of Infectious Diseases* 168: 773–776

Parker S E, Davey P G 1993 Practicalities of once-daily aminoglycoside dosing. *Journal of Antimicrobial Chemotherapy* 31: 4–8

Parry M F 1987 The penicillins. *Medical Clinics of North America* 71: 1093–1112

Parry M F, Neu H C 1982 The safety and tolerance of mezlocillin. *Journal of Antimicrobial Chemotherapy* 9 (suppl A): 273–280

Paton D H, Reeves D S 1991 Clinical features and management of adverse effects of quinolone antibacterials. *Drug Safety* 6: 8–27

Pechere J C, Craig W A, Meunier F 1991 Once daily dosing of aminoglycoside: one step forward. *Journal of Antimicrobial Chemotherapy* 27 (suppl C): 149–152

Penn R G, Griffin J P 1982 Adverse reactions to nitrofurantoin in the United Kingdom, Sweden, and Holland. *British Medical Journal* 284: 1440–1442

Phillips M E, Eastwood J B, Curtis J R, Gower P E, de Wardener H E 1974 Tetracycline poisoning in renal failure. *British Medical Journal* 2: 149–151

Pigrau C, Pahissa A, Gropper S, Sureda D, Martinez Vazquez J M 1989 Ceftriaxone-associated biliary pseudolithiasis in adults. *Lancet* ii: 165

Pilot M A, Qin X Y 1988 Macrolides and gastrointestinal motility. *Journal of Antimicrobial Chemotherapy* 22 (suppl B): 201–206

Platt R, Dreis M W, Kennedy D L, Kuritsky J N 1988 Serum sickness-like reactions to amoxicillin, cefaclor, cephalexin and trimethoprim-sulphamethoxazole. *Journal of Infectious Diseases* 158: 474–477

Polk R E 1991 Anaphylactoid reactions to glycopeptide antibiotics. *Journal of Antimicrobial Chemotherapy* 27 (suppl B): 17–29

Poole G, Stradler P, Worlledge S 1971 Potentially serious side-effects of high-dose twice-weekly rifampicin. *Postgraduate Medical Journal* 47: 742–747

Porter J, Jick H 1977 Drug-induced anaphylaxis, convulsions, deafness and extra-pyramidal reactions. *Lancet* i: 587

Portier H 1990 A multicentre, open, clinical trial of a new intravenous formulation of fusidic acid in severe staphylococcal infection. *Journal of Antimicrobial Chemotherapy* 25 (suppl B): 39–44

Prins J M, Buller H R, Kuijper E J, Tange R A, Speelman P 1994 Once-daily gentamicin versus once-daily netilmicin in patients with serious infections – a randomised clinical trial. *Journal of Antimicrobial Chemotherapy* 33: 823–835

Pujet J C, Homberg J C, Decroix G 1974 Sensitivity to rifampicin: incidence, mechanism and prevention. *British Medical Journal* ii: 415–418

Pullen H, Wright N, Murdoch J McC 1967 Hypersensitivity reactions to antibacterial drugs in infectious mononucleosis. *Lancet* 2: 1176

Rallison M L, O'Brien J, Good R A 1961 Severe reactions to long-acting sulfonamides. *Paediatrics* 28: 908–917

Reddy K R, Brillant P, Schiff E R 1989 Amoxycillin–clavulanate potassium-associated cholestasis. *Gastroenterology* 96: 1135–1141

Ribard P, Audisio F, Kahn M F et al 1992 Seven Achilles tendinitis including 3 complicated by rupture during fluoroquinolone therapy. *Journal of Rheumatology* 19: 1479–1481

Rothwell D L, Richmond D E 1974 Hepatorenal failure with self-initiated rifampicin therapy. *British Medical Journal* ii: 481–482

Sanders W E 1976 Rifampicin. *Annals Internal Medicine* 85: 82–86

Saunders N J 1994 Why monitor peak vancomycin concentrations. *Lancet* 344: 1748–1750

Schaad U B 1992 The role of the new quinolones in paediatric practice. *Ped Infect Dis J* 11: 1047–1049

Schaad U B, Wedgwood J 1992 Lack of quinolone-induced arthropathy in children. *Journal of Antimicrobial Chemotherapy* 30: 414–416

Schaad U B, Wedgwood Crucko J, Tschaepeller H 1988 Reversible ceftriaxone-associated biliary pseudolithiasis in children. *Lancet* ii: 1411–1413

Schluter G 1987 Ciprofloxacin: review of potential toxicologic effects. *American Journal of Medicine* 82 (suppl 4A): 91–93

Sher T H 1983 Penicillin hypersensitivity – a review. *Pediatrics Clinic of North America* 30: 161–176

Silverman W A, Anderson D H, Blanc W A 1956 A difference in mortality and incidence of kernicterus among premature infants allotted to two prophylactic antibiotic regimens. *Pediatrics* 18: 614–624

Smith C R, Lipsky J J, Laskin O L et al 1980 Double blind comparison of the nephrotoxicity and auditory toxicity of gentamicin and tobramycin. *New England Journal of Medicine* 302: 1106–1109

Steen J S M, Stainton-Ellis D M 1977 Rifampicin in pregnancy. *Lancet* ii: 604–605

Stricker B H Ch, Slagboom G, Demaeseneer R, Slootmaekers V, Thijs I, Olsson S 1988 Anaphylactic reactions to cinoxacin. *British Medical Journal* 297: 1434–1435

Surtees S J, Stockton M G, Gietzen T W 1991 Allergy to penicillin: fable or fact. *British Medical Journal* 302: 1051–1052

Tasker P R W, MacGregor G A, Wardener de H E, Thomas R D, Jones N F 1975 Use of co-trimoxazole in chronic renal failure. *Lancet* i: 1216–1218

Taylor R, Arze R, Gokal R, Stoddart J C 1981 Cephaloridine encephalopathy. *British Medical Journal* ii: 409–410

Teasley D G, Gerding D N, Olson M M et al 1983 Prospective randomised trial of metronidazole versus vancomycin for *Clostridium-difficile*-associated diarrhoea and colitis. *Lancet* ii: 1043–1046

Tedesco F, Barton R W, Alpers D H 1974 Clindamycin associated colitis, a prospective study. *Annals of Internal Medicine* 81: 429–433

Tedesco F, Markham R, Gurwith M, Christie D, Bartlett J G 1978 Oral vancomycin for antibiotic-associated pseudo-membranous colitis. *Lancet* ii: 226–228

Trollfors B 1980 Quantitative studies on antibiotic nephro-toxicity. *Scandinavian Journal of Infectious Disease* (suppl 21)

Tune B M 1975 Relationship between the transport and toxicity of cephalosporins in the kidney. *Journal of Infectious Diseases* 132: 189

Venning G R 1983 Identification of adverse reactions to new drugs. I: What have been the important adverse reactions since thalidomide? *British Medical Journal* 286: 199–202

Wallace M R, Mascola J R, Oldfield E C 1991 The red man syndrome: incidence, aetiology and prophylaxis. *Journal of Infectious Diseases* 164: 1180–1185

Wallerstein R O, Condit P K, Kasper C K, Brown J W, Morrison F R 1969 Statewide study of chloramphenicol therapy and fatal aplastic anaemia. *Journal of the American Medical Association* 208: 2045

Weinstein L, Lerner P I, Chew W H 1964 Clinical and bacteriologic studies of the effect of 'massive' doses of penicillin G on infections caused by Gram-negative bacilli. *New England Journal of Medicine* 271: 525

Westphal J F, Vetter D, Brogard J M 1994 Hepatic side effects of antibiotics. *Journal of Antimicrobial Chemotherapy* 33: 387–401

Wilson P, Ramsden R T 1977 Immediate effects of tobramycin on human cochlea and correlation with serum tobramycin levels. *British Medical Journal* i: 259–261

Wofsy C B 1987 Use of trimethoprim–sulfamethoxazole in the treatment of *Pneumocystics carinii* pneumonitis in patients with acquired immunodeficiency syndrome. *Reviews of Infectious Diseases* 9 (suppl 2): S184–S191

Wood M J 1991 The tolerance and toxicity of clarithromycin. *Journal of Hospital Infection* 19 (suppl A): 39–46

Yow M D, Taber L H, Barrett F F et al 1976 A ten year assessment of methicillin-associated side effects. *Pediatrics* 58: 329

Antibiotics and the immune system

C. G. Gemmell

Introduction

Assessment of antimicrobial action in vitro may not reflect therapeutic success or failure, since much depends on the patient's cellular and humoral defence mechanisms. The host immune system has evolved a variety of mechanisms to counteract attack by pathogenic micro-organisms, and the micro-organisms themselves have developed a variety of mechanisms to circumvent such defences. Indeed, in the immunocompromised host, normally innocuous bacterial invaders can cause disease. In such patients it is important that the correct choice of antibiotic is made to subdue the pathogen and allow some restoration of the host's normal immunological responsiveness.

The possible role of antibiotics as immunomodulators may be valuable in agents used for infection in immuno-compromised patients, including those suffering from cancer, diabetes mellitus, cystic fibrosis, trauma, burns, viral and parasitic diseases as well as the newborn and the elderly. The new approach that antibiotics with 'add on value' as stimulators of the host's immune system (Ritts 1990) might bring to the management of such patients warrants deeper investigation. Although biological effects seen in vitro may or may not take place in vivo, and vice versa, certain desirable properties of antibiotics as biological response modifiers may be defined:

- They should not depress natural defence mechanisms involving phagocytic cells and lymphocytes
- They should increase the bactericidal activity of such cells or potentiate humoral effects
- They should decrease the virulence of bacteria and/or increase their susceptibility to natural bactericidal mechanisms
- They should be able to restore immunocompetence to immunocompromised hosts.

Both old and new drugs may exhibit activity of these kinds, either in vitro or in vivo. Most studies have been directed towards the professional phagocytes of the host's immune system, namely polymorphonuclear leucocytes (PMNL), monocytes and macrophages. Much less is known about drug-induced modulation of lymphocyte function.

Professional phagocytes have the innate ability to migrate towards, attach to and ingest bacterial pathogens, usually in the presence of a serum opsonin such as complement or specific antibody. Once ingestion occurs, the continued viability of the intracellular particles is dependent upon whether the bacterium possesses cell-wall-associated or soluble components which can inhibit the oxygen-dependent or oxygen-independent killing mechanisms of the phagocyte. Many bacterial species can survive in an intracellular milieu for variable lengths of time, and any immunomodulatory activity of an antibiotic might assist in eradication of the pathogen.

Direct Action of Antibiotics on Professional Phagocytes

Several stages of phagocyte function can be measured in the laboratory and the effect of various concentrations of antibiotics on chemotaxis, phagocytic ingestion, induction of the respiratory burst (chemiluminescence) and cidal activity have been tested (Yourtree & Root 1982). However, the methods chosen by investigators have varied considerably and results should be assessed carefully before definitive conclusions are drawn.

Chemotaxis

Therapeutic concentrations of most β-lactam antibiotics as well as clindamycin and rifampicin have no effect on chemotaxis. The tetracyclines, on the other hand, inhibit cell movement at supratherapeutic levels, and some macrolides (erythromycin, clarithromycin and roxithromycin) are stimulatory.

The effect of aminoglycosides on chemotaxis is less clear. In general, chemotaxis is unchanged, but gentamicin may decrease PMNL chemotaxis.

Ingestion

Antibiotics also influence the ability of phagocytic cells to ingest bacteria, and it is clear that several cephalosporins potentiate the ingestion of certain bacteria, even at quite low concentrations.

Phagocytic ingestion of bacteria is potentiated by:

- Azlocillin
- Aztreonam
- Ceftriaxone
- Imipenem
- Spiramycin
- Ticarcillin.

Visual assays and radiometric methods have shown that tetracycline and doxycycline inhibit phagocytosis of *Escherichia coli* in vitro, even when the drug-treated PMNL were washed, implying that inhibition is irreversible. It has also been suggested that PMNL isolated from subjects taking oral tetracycline display reduced phagocytosis.

Postphagocytic events

Events which have been investigated as possible targets for antibiotics include activation of the hexose monophosphate shunt, release of lysosomal enzymes and induction of the respiratory burst. Again the methods used make it difficult to assess any clinical relevance. Observations include the inhibition by chloramphenicol of postphagocytic lysosomal fusion in cultured monocytes fed *Candida* cells and inhibition by polymyxin B of the release of lysosomal enzymes and the activation of the hexose monophosphate shunt in PMNL. It was unclear whether either or both of these activities had any effect on the ability of the phagocytic cells to kill bacteria.

Most investigations of postphagocytic events now use chemiluminescence to measure the phagocytic cell's respiratory burst (Table 8.1). However, the response varies with different particulate and soluble stimuli and with different light acceptor molecules. There is also much intersubject variability, as shown by differences in the level of activation found in fresh blood donations. Nevertheless, a number of drugs have been shown to enhance or depress the levels of chemiluminescence: tetracycline and amphotericin B may be inhibitory, whereas some cephalosporins such as cefotaxime and cefodizime may be

Table 8.1   *Direct effect of antibiotics on respiratory burst of PMNLs at therapeutic concentrations*

No effect	Increase respiratory burst	Decrease respiratory burst
Aminoglycosides	Cefotaxime	Amphotericin B
Most β-lactams	Cefpimizole	Erythromycin
Clindamycin		Rifampicin
Chloramphenicol		Roxithromycin
Fluconazole		Tetracycline
Fusidic acid		Trimethoprim
Metronidazole		
Quinolones		
Teicoplanin		
Vancomycin		

stimulatory. The enhanced activity induced by cefodizime is probably due to indirect binding of the drug to the cells, followed by release of activators. Amphotericin B appears to decrease the affinity of the cell receptor for the synthetic tripeptide f.met.leu.phe, while increasing the expression of the Fc receptor. Thus, the magnitude of the chemiluminescent response will be affected by the choice of a soluble or particulate stimulus. Tetracycline exerts its depressive effects on the oxidative burst through its ability to chelate Ca^{2+} and Mg^{2+}, cations well known to be involved in several cell functions.

Most β-lactam agents do not appear to affect the respiratory burst of PMNL directly, but cefotaxime and cefpimizole enhance the oxidative burst when PMNL are presented with opsonized particles (Labro 1993). No explanation has been proposed for such bioactivity. Certain macrolides, in particular erythromycin and roxithromycin, inhibit the oxidative burst, but only at concentrations in excess of 0.1 mg/l. However, josamycin (a macrolide with a 16-member ring) appears to have the opposite effect. The fact that each of these macrolides can be concentrated within the phagocytic cell may account for such immunomodulatory activity (Gemmell 1992a).

Two cephalosporins which are structurally related differ in the way in which they enhance the bactericidal activity of PMNL. Cefotaxime enhances the killing of *Staphylococcus aureus* by an effect on the cell's oxidative burst, but does not alter the efficacy of ingestion. In contrast, the enhancement of killing by cefodizime and cephalothin results from better phagocytosis of opsonized and non-opsonized bacteria (Labro et al 1987; Labro 1990). Cephalothin also stimulates non-oxygen dependent killing without affecting the oxidative response (Labro 1993).

In only a few instances has it been possible to show that the bioactivity displayed by these drugs in vitro also occurs in vivo. Unconfirmed reports suggest that cefpimizole enhances chemiluminescence and O_2^- production of PMNL in healthy elderly volunteers and cancer patients, and that cefodizime reverses reduced levels of chemiluminescence in

Table 8.2 *Effect of antibiotics on the cidal activity of phagocytic cells*

No effect	Increase cidal activity	Decrease cidal activity
Most β-lactams	Cefotaxime Ciprofloxacin Erythromycin Rifampicin	Teicoplanin

- Azithromycin
- Ciprofloxacin
- Clarithromycin
- Clindamycin
- Erythromycin
- Josamycin
- Lincomycin
- Ofloxacin
- Rifampicin
- Teicoplanin.

patients on chronic renal dialysis. Roxithromycin enhances oxidant production when given to volunteers, in contrast to its depressive action in vitro (Kita et al 1993). No explanation for these different effects has been proposed, but it is clear that the overall effect of any drug on the host's phagocytic cells in vivo must take into account the role of other immune modulators such as the cytokines.

Evaluation of the bioactivity of antibiotics on the terminal event of the phagocytic process, namely the killing of viable microorganisms, is difficult, because it is almost impossible to distinguish between the innate cidal activity of the phagocytes and the direct action of the antibiotics on the target bacterium.

Antimicrobial agents known to enhance the cidal activity of PMNL, monocytes and macrophages are shown in Table 8.2.

PENETRATION AND CONCENTRATION OF ANTIBIOTICS WITHIN PHAGOCYTIC CELLS

The discovery that certain antibiotics (e.g. penicillin) appear to enhance the intracellular killing of bacteria or are concentrated within the phagocytic cells (e.g. macrolides, rifampicin, the quinolones) has had a profound influence on the assessment of drug bioactivity. Intracellular penetration of antibiotics may be followed by a number of methods including high pressure liquid chromatography or fluorimetry, as well as radiologically and microbiologically. In some instances the drug quickly leaks out of the cell during the course of the experiment making it more difficult to assess whether long-term drug accumulation is possible in vivo (van der Auwera et al 1990).

Different types of phagocytic cell differ in their ability to concentrate antibiotics (Panteix et al 1993). For example, macrophages concentrate the aminoglycosides and several penicillins through pinocytosis, whereas a similar process is not found in PMNL. Intracellular drug accumulation can also be enhanced when the phagocytic cells are activated as in alveolar macrophages from cigarette smokers or PMNL engaged in active phagocytosis of particles. Antibiotics known to concentrate within phagocytic cells are:

Penetration of a drug is not a guarantee of intracellular bioactivity, since it may be bound or inactivated within the cell. The intracellular milieu may also influence adversely the action of an antibiotic. Phagocytosed bacteria are, for the most part, enclosed within the phagosome (*Legionella pneumophila* is an exception) which is normally at a neutral pH, but following phagosome–lysosome fusion the pH falls to that of the lysosomes themselves (pH 4.5–5.0). Many antibacterial agents (e.g. the aminoglycosides) operate poorly at such a pH and some (e.g. clindamycin) alkalinize the phagolysosomal contents. While improving the bioactivity of the drug, such a change undoubtedly affects the hydrolytic activity of the lysosomal enzymes. The low intraphagolysosomal pH is thought to explain the lack of activity of penicillins against intracellular bacteria. At pH values below 6.5, the growth of many bacteria is inhibited by these agents, but the normal autolytic process seen at higher pH fails to follow, probably because the autolytic enzymes are suppressed at a low pH.

The subcellular distribution of the antibacterial agent is important in determining its ultimate efficacy in eliminating intracellular pathogens. Some bacteria, such as *L. pneumophila* survive and multiply within phagocytic cells, especially alveolar macrophages. Erythromycin promotes intraphagocytic bactericidal activity against *L. pneumophila*, both in vitro and in vivo. *Staph. aureus*, which possesses a limited capacity for intracellular survival, can be eliminated by exposure to teicoplanin, ciprofloxacin or rifampicin, but not by vancomycin.

Modification or re-formulation of antibiotics may aid their intracellular penetration. One such approach, namely the incorporation of amphotericin B into liposomes or of aminoglycosides into nanoparticles, has already been successful.

EFFECT OF ANTIBIOTICS ON OTHER CELLS

In vitro measurement of T lymphocyte proliferation has in several instances shown that antibiotics may interfere with lymphocyte function. The quinolones potentiate radionucleotide uptake by phytohaemagglutin-stimulated lymphocytes when used at clinically attainable concentrations (Roche et al 1987, Rubinstein & Shalit 1993). In one report in patients given ofloxacin 300 mg twice daily for 5 days for either urinary tract or lower respiratory tract infection, some enhancement of lymphocyte proliferation was observed within 1 h of starting drug therapy and 5 days later. No information is available about any direct influence of antibiotics on B cells or their ability to synthesize immunoglobulin.

INDIRECT POTENTIATION OF PHAGOCYTIC CELL FUNCTION

Exposure of bacteria to low concentrations of antibiotics may enhance their susceptibility to phagocytic ingestion and killing as well as to their sensitivity to serum lysis (Gemmell 1992a). Although the cell wall of Gram-negative bacteria normally confers resistance to serum complement, growth of *Esch. coli* in ampicillin, ceftriaxone, netilmicin and some other drugs can alter its susceptibility to serum lysis. Antibiotics that render bacteria more susceptible to serum lysis are:

- Ampicillin
- Aztreonam
- Carumonam
- Ceftriaxone
- Cyclacillin
- Imipenem
- Netilmicin
- Rifampicin
- Streptomycin
- Tetracycline.

Drug-induced changes in bacterial susceptibility to phagocytosis may be due to changes in the ultrastructural topography of the bacteria, even at concentrations below the minimum inhibitory concentration (MIC). Some of these morphological changes (filamentation, thickened cell-walls, additional cross-walls) also occur in vivo following antibiotic therapy. Many in vitro studies have investigated the effect of such antibiotic-modified bacteria on opsonophagocytosis and killing (Milatovic 1982, van den Broek 1989, Gemmell 1992b). Expression of surface virulence factors is altered by exposure to various antibacterial agents such that both their opsonization and ingestion by PMNL is enhanced (Raponi et al 1989).

Table 8.3 lists those bacteria which are made more susceptible to phagocytosis in vitro on exposure to an antibiotic. In most instances the demonstration of increased susceptibility of bacterial cells to phagocytosis followed growth of the target bacteria for several hours in sub-MIC levels of the drug, and the presence or absence of a specific virulence factor was measured indirectly. Sometimes,

Table 8.3 *Modulation of virulence factors of bacteria by antibiotics rendering the pathogen more susceptible to phagocytosis*

Bacterium	Virulence factor	Antibiotic
Bacteroides fragilis	Capsule	Clindamycin, trospectinomycin
Escherichia coli	K antigen	Netilmicin, carumonam, ceftriaxone
Haemophilus influenzae	Capsule	ampicillin
Klebsiella pneumoniae	Capsule	Netilmicin
Pseudomonas aeruginosa	Outer membrane protein	Ceftazidime, ceftriaxone
Staphylococcus aureus	Protein A	Clindamycin, fusidic acid
Streptococcus pyogenes	M Protein	Clindamycin, erythromycin

inhibition of the expression of a cell-wall-associated virulence factor (M protein, capsule or protein A) was accompanied by inhibition of the biosynthesis of exotoxins (staphylococcal haemolysins, DNAase and coagulase or streptolysin O or S).

Most antibiotics that display this activity are inhibitors of protein biosynthesis (Gemmell 1992b), but the mechanism whereby the structural and soluble virulence factors are repressed has not been identified.

Subinhibitory concentrations of certain antibiotics alter surface structures of Gram-negative bacilli to such an extent that these structures no longer camouflage underlying epitopes. Sometimes, this type of change results in an opsonic recognition that did not occur (or occurred only to a minimal extent) without antibiotic treatment (Raponi et al 1993). Opsonic recognition of encapsulated *Esch. coli* after netilmicin or aztreonam treatment could be mediated either by complement or by polyclonal antibodies to rough mutants. Similar results have been obtained with some β-lactam antibiotics and quinolones.

Experiments in mice challenged with a virulent strain of *Esch. coli* revealed that mortality rates were lower in mice immunized with the bacteria exposed to ciprofloxacin than in mice immunized with untreated bacteria; aztreonam-treated *Esch. coli* did not protect mice in this way. These studies suggest that antibiotic-mediated effects on the bacteria may influence host defences against Gram-negative bacteria (Overbeek & Veringa 1991). This effect may be attributable to greater exposure of certain common antigens during antibiotic therapy.

Changes in the structural features of bacteria caused by exposure to sub-MIC concentrations of antibiotics may indirectly affect host immunological responsiveness. For example, ovoid cells of fosfomycin-treated *Salmonella* expressing higher levels of O-antigen in vitro consistently produced higher titres of specific antibody than did normal bacilli when injected into rabbits. T lymphocytes from the immunized animals also displayed a higher level of proliferation in response to stimulation with O-antigen. Also, vaccination of mice with penicillin treated *Esch. coli* and *Pseudomonas aeruginosa* resulted in increased numbers of plaque-forming splenic B cells producing antibody to lipopolysaccharide.

Postantibiotic leucocyte effect

Not long after the discovery of the clinical value of penicillin in the 1940s, it was recognized that satisfactory therapy of pneumococcal pneumonia could be achieved with regimens that produced concentrations of drug that were below the MIC for the pathogen for considerable periods of time. This postpenicillin stationary phase has since become known as the 'postantibiotic phase' and is found for a number of antibiotics and organisms (Pruul & McDonald 1988).

Postantibiotic suppression of growth is unlikely to be the complete explanation for the success achieved with discontinuous therapy. In vitro studies suggest that bacteria exposed to supra-MIC levels for a short period exhibit increased susceptibility to killing by PMNL. This phenomenon has been termed the 'postantibiotic leukocyte effect'. *Esch. coli* exposed to chloramphenicol or some quinolones becomes more susceptible to the bactericidal activity of PMNL than bacteria which have not been so exposed, as judged by a decrease in the numbers of viable intracellular bacteria.

Conclusion

It is becoming clear mainly from in vitro studies that certain antibiotics either directly or indirectly influence the body's immune system. Such agents might be classified as biological response modifiers in the same way as we already recognize some of the cytokines. For the future, adjunctive therapy with appropriate antibiotics and various cytokines or antagonists thereof might prove to be useful in changing the outcome of infection.

Although this chapter has concentrated upon the immunomodulatory activities of antibacterial agents either acting directly on the host's immune system or indirectly by rendering the bacterial pathogen more or less sensitive to attack, therapy might also be directed against the sequelae of bacterial infection and sepsis.

The development of septic shock follows the triggering of three main mechanisms: host cell activation, release of secondary mediators and development of multiple organ failure. There has been an explosion of research interest in the development of agents capable of providing selective inhibition of one or other target, e.g. anti-endotoxin or anti-cytokine therapies.

Many different cytokines are generated during bacterial sepsis as a direct result of activation of host cells. In particular, TNFα is one of the most potent pro-inflammatory agents and high serum levels of this cytokine correlate with poor clinical outcome. Antibody to this cytokine has been shown to be effective in animal models of Gram-negative bacteraemia and *Staph. aureus* shock and encouraging results in clinical trials have been repeated where early protection against mortality and shock has been recognized.

IL-1 is also an important secondary mediator whose biological activity might be the focus of attention in immunotherapy. However, in this case its receptor has been targetted as the most likely route to success.

An alternative strategy directed against the CD14 receptor found on neutrophils and macrophages which forms a complex with endotoxin and a serum binding protein (LBP) has been proposed but as yet few data are available to suggest clinical efficacy. The possible applications of these findings in clinical medicine are discussed in Chapter 41.

From the studies reported to date, it is unlikely that a single form of immunotherapy will prove effective in isolation (Lynn & Cohen 1995). It is more likely that, as in the use of antibiotic combinations to prevent the development of drug resistance in bacteria, it will be necessary to develop combination therapy comprising more than one agent together with an appropriate choice of antibiotics and the best supportive clinical care in order for real success in reducing the mortality rate from septic shock. In some cases, it might also be appropriate to consider selecting antibiotics which by their mode of action reduce the impact of the initial trigger, i.e. reduce the release of endotoxin from the bacterial cell.

References

Gemmell C G 1992a Antibiotics and neutrophil function – potential immunomodulating activities. *Journal of Antimicrobial Chemotherapy* 30B: 23–33

Gemmell C G 1992b Interaction between clindamycin and immune function. *Reviews in Contemporary Pharmacotherapy* 3: 321–327

Kita E, Sawaki M, Mikasa K 1993 Alteration of host response by long-term treatment of roxithromycin. *Journal of Antimicrobial Chemotherapy* 32: 285–294

Labro M T 1990 Cefodizime as a biological response modifier: a review of its in vivo, ex vivo and in vitro immunomodulatory properties. *Journal of Antimicrobial Chemotherapy* 26 (suppl C): 37–47

Labro M T 1993 Immunomodulation by antibacterial agents: is it clinically relevant? *Drugs* 45: 319–328

Labro M T, Amit N, Babin-Chevaye C, Hakim J 1987 Cefodizime (GR221) potentiation of human neutrophil oxygen-indpendent bactericidal activity. *Journal of Antimicrobial Chemotherapy* 19: 331–341

Lynn W A, Cohen J 1995 Adjunctive therapy for septic shock: a review of experimental approaches. *Clinics in Infectious Disease* 20: 143–158

Milatovic D 1982 Effect of subinhibitory antibiotic concentrations on the phagocytosis of *Staphylococcus aureus*. *European Journal of Clinical Microbiology* 1: 97–101

Overbeek B P, Veringa E M 1991 Role of antibodies and antibiotics in aerobic Gram-negative septicaemia: possible synergism between antimicrobial treatment and immunotherapy. *Reviews of Infectious Diseases* 13: 751–760

Panteix G, Guillaumond B, Harf R et al 1993 In vitro concentration of azithromycin in human phagocytic cells. *Journal of Antimicrobial Chemotherapy* 31 (suppl E): 1–4

Pruul H, McDonald P J 1988 Damage to bacteria by antibiotics in vitro and its relevance to antimicrobial chemotherapy: a historical perspective. *Journal of Antimicrobial Chemotherapy* 21: 695–700

Raponi G, Vreede R W, Rozenberg-Arska M, Hoepelman I M, Keller N, Verhoef J 1989 The influence of subminimal inhibitory concentrations of netilmicin and ceftriaxone on the interaction of *Escherichia coli* with host defences. *Journal of Antimicrobial Chemotherapy* 23: 565–576

Raponi G, Lun M T, Lorino G et al 1993 Reactivity and protective capacity of a polyclonal antiserum derived from mice immunised with antibiotic exposed *Escherichia coli*. *Journal of Antimicrobial Chemotherapy* 31: 117–128

Ritts R E 1990 Antibiotics as biological response modifiers. *Journal of Antimicrobial Chemotherapy* 26 (suppl C): 31–36

Roche Y, Gougerot-Pocidalo M A, Fay M, Etienne D, Forest N, Pocidalo J J 1987 Comparative effects of quinolones on human mononuclear leucocyte functions. *Journal of Antimicrobial Chemotherapy* 19: 781–790

Rubinstein E, Shalit I 1993 Effects of the quinolones on the immune system. In: Hooper D C, Wolfson J S (eds) Quinolone antimicrobial agents, 2nd edn., American Society of Microbiology, Washington, DC, p 519–526

van den Broek P J 1989 Antimicrobial drugs, microorganisms and phagocytes. *Review of Infectious Diseases* 11: 213–245

van der Auwera P, Bonnet M, Husson M, Jacobs F 1990 Antibiotics and phagocytic cell function: a critical review. In: Faist E, Meakins J L, Schildberg E (eds) Defence dysfunction in trauma shock and sepsis. Springer-Verlag, Heidelberg, p 167–173

Yourtree E L, Root R K 1982 Antibiotic–neutrophil interactions in microbial killing. In: Gallin J I, Fauci A S (eds) Advances in host defense mechanisms, vol 1. Raven Press, New York, p 187–209

General principles of chemotherapy

H. P. Lambert and F. O'Grady

Introduction

Antimicrobial drugs active in the laboratory against a large number of infectious agents are available, many of them of established value in the treatment of the diseases caused by these agents. But, as with most other drugs, their administration may be accompanied by unwanted effects. These naturally differ in their nature and severity from agent to agent, varying in their effects from trivial to life-threatening. However, in addition to the familiar problem of deciding the balance between benefit and risk (the therapeutic ratio) in the individual for whom any drug is prescribed, the administration of antimicrobial agents carries another problem, that of the selection and dissemination of resistant organisms. Drug resistance is discussed in detail in Chapter 3, but it is important here to note the cycle in which increasing use of a drug begets drug resistance and thus the requirement for new agents, only to be followed by resistance to the new agent in its turn. The problem of antibiotic resistance is far from theoretical, having led to the loss of many once-valuable agents: sulphonamides for meningococcal disease, sulphonamides and low-dose penicillin for gonorrhoea, ampicillin for Haemophilus influenzae *meningitis, can no longer be employed; many other examples are described in these pages. The constraints imposed by increasing drug resistance on antibiotic choice are most severe in the hospital environment, in which selection of resistant and virulent organisms takes place most easily.*

The optimal use of antimicrobial agents can best be considered first in the context of choice for the individual patient, and second in the context of policies for the control of antibiotic usage in general. These may be devised for a particular clinical problem or unit, or may form part of a control programme used in a hospital, or even nationally or internationally (see Ch. 12).

ANTIBIOTIC PRESCRIBING FOR THE INDIVIDUAL PATIENT

L. P. Garrod, the senior co-author of previous editions of this book, wrote that:

'successful chemotherapy must be rational, and rational treatment demands a diagnosis. This may only be provisional, and it may later be proved wrong, but the treatment chosen should be based on some explicit assumption as to the nature of the disease process. This may or may not carry with it an implication that the cause is a particular micro-organism'.

Many failures of therapy, sometimes with tragic consequences, result from neglecting to observe this basic precept. Thus, a patient may be treated for presumed postoperative septicaemia with agents appropriate only for Gram-negative aerobic bacteria when such a syndrome can as well be caused by Gram-positive cocci. The treatment must in fact be aimed at the microorganism and not at the disease as such. For a few diseases, the clinical diagnosis implies a specific microbial diagnosis with a known, or at least highly probable, drug susceptibility pattern. Thus diagnoses of erysipelas or scarlet fever imply causation by *Streptococcus pyogenes* and susceptibility to penicillin, meningococcal septicaemia with its almost pathognomonic rash implies causation by *Neisseria meningitidis* and, with occasional exceptions, susceptibility to penicillin, and severe chicken pox with primary pneumonia indicates causation by varicella-zoster virus and susceptibility to acyclovir.

In another group of infections, the causal organism is implicit in the clinical diagnosis but its antibiotic susceptibility cannot be inferred from the diagnosis. Examples such as typhoid fever caused by *Salmonella typhi*, or a carbuncle caused by *Staphylococcus aureus* can be cited. In these cases, when antibiotics need to be used before or without laboratory help, factors in drug choice must include previous local laboratory or epidemiological information which may indicate the likely susceptibility pattern.

Unfortunately, a large number of infections fit into neither of these categories. Syndromes such as pneumonia, meningitis or pyelonephritis can each be caused by diverse organisms, and clinical information is of limited value in deciding between them. Initial management, if early microbiological information is unavailable or has not contributed – indeed management throughout if laboratory facilities do not exist – must therefore be based on an explicit analysis of the likely or possible causal organisms and of their relative importance as pathogens. Clearly the decision pathway pursued by the clinician must vary considerably depending on the availability of laboratory services and on their degree of sophistication and skill. The role of microbiological diagnosis is crucial in the optimal management of infectious diseases and is discussed in Chapter 10.

Decision-making about antibiotic choice in the individual patient can be facilitated by the use of a simple check-list which may also be found of value in teaching students and junior staff good habits of antimicrobial drug use.

Beginning with the premise that the patient is presumed to have a microbial infection requiring treatment, the following aspects can be systematically considered.

- Which organism(s) is (are) the likely cause(s) of the syndrome and what is their relative importance?
- In the light of the presumed diagnosis what other steps should be taken to further diagnostic precision? Which specimens should be taken and how should they be handled? The answers obviously depend on the facilities available. Even when full laboratory facilities are available, many diagnostic failures are caused by poor handling of specimens, an aspect of diagnosis deserving more attention than it often receives.
- Which agents are available and active against the presumed cause or causes of the illness? Is their range of antimicrobial activity appropriate and what information is available about the likelihood of drug resistance?
- What are the unwanted effects of the agents under consideration, and how may they be balanced against the likely benefits of therapy with each agent? Special attention should be paid to the patient's renal function and possible deleterious effects on it.

These preliminary considerations are used to determine initial choice of therapy and should lead to a proper balance between appropriate and unnecessary use. Again, to quote Garrod:

'Prescribing habits are revealed in a brilliant and tragic light in reports of fatalities from the administration of antibiotics. An astonishing proportion of deaths from penicillin shock have followed an injection given for what seems an inadequate indication, including even a common cold, toothache and a sprained toe. Likewise, some deaths from marrow aplasia have been caused by chloramphenicol administered for minor catarrhal conditions: in some instances this has even been self-administration from a left-over bottle kept in the bathroom. These are extreme examples, but they can be supported by thousands of others in which more harm than good has been done, and by untold millions in which the drug has merely been wasted because the condition treated is by nature insusceptible to it.'

- Having decided the most appropriate agent, what is the correct dose and dose interval and what is the correct route of administration?

The object of systemic treatment is to attain a drug concentration in blood and tissue at least several-fold the minimal concentration necessary to inhibit or kill the infecting organism. Standard dose regimens, based as they are on antimicrobial susceptibility of the relevant organisms and on the pharmacological properties of the drugs concerned, are usually satisfactory, but it is essential also to consider dose in the individual patient. Thus, dosage often has to be reduced if the patient's renal function is impaired and the drug has a mainly renal route of excretion. On the other hand, dose may have to be increased when the site of infection is relatively inaccessible to the agent chosen, for example, in the treatment of meningitis by penicillins or cephalosporins (see Ch. 53).

Oral administration should be used if possible, but parenteral therapy is often necessary when speed of action is essential, when high serum concentrations need to be attained and when vomiting or bowel dysfunction make oral treatment potentially unreliable.

Local treatment at the site of infection is seldom necessary. Adequate antimicrobial drug concentrations can usually be achieved by high systemic dosage, even at relatively inaccessible sites such as cerebrospinal fluid (CSF) or joint cavities, and against the apparent advantage of local administration must be set the possibility of local tissue damage by the antibiotic solution used. If local treatment is thought necessary, careful attention to the correct preparation and dose is essential. The potential dangers of intrathecal administration are especially to be borne in mind, and many tragedies have resulted from miscalculation of the dose of penicillin appropriate for intrathecal use. Intrathecal agents, which are in any case rarely needed, should never be given except after careful discussion with informed authorities of the necessity of doing so, and most rigorous checking of preparation and dose.

- What is the correct duration of treatment? Antimicrobial drugs are often continued for an unnecessarily prolonged time or are discontinued too soon. Duration of therapy is discussed in relation to individual indications throughout this book, but frequent, at least daily, review of drug charts is a sound rule.

- Is the treatment working? Antimicrobial drug therapy cannot of course be considered in isolation and other aspects of therapy, many of them crucially important, must be taken into account in judging the effect of treatment. Even an 'appropriate' antibiotic may be ineffective if pus is not drained, bacterial shock treated and hypoxia and anaemia corrected. The main criteria of success are the normal clinical ones: well-being, resolution of fever, tachycardia and abnormal signs. In some infections, however, antibiotic assays are necessary to ensure that concentrations have reached effective but not toxic levels. The most common example in frequent use is the need for aminoglycoside assays (see p. 170).

- What is the cost of the drug? In publicly funded hospitals, this aspect is considered mainly in the formulation of hospital antibiotic policies rather than in individual treatment. In many countries and in private facilities, antibiotic cost is a major constraint on choice of agent.

Antibiotic combinations

Treatment with more than one agent is sometimes necessary, for a variety of reasons, classifiable in five groups:

1. To achieve adequate 'cover' of the range of possible pathogens before full diagnosis is reached
2. Mixed infections
3. Prevention of drug resistance
4. Reducing dosage of toxic agents
5. Antibacterial synergy.

1. The most frequent indication is found on the many occasions when treatment of a seriously ill patient has to be initiated before the microbial diagnosis is established, and when the organisms to be considered as possible pathogens cannot all be 'covered' by the use of one agent. The use is diminishing with the increasing variety of broad-spectrum agents. It is often then possible to switch to monotherapy when the responsible organism and its antimicrobial susceptibility are established.
2. In mixed infections, two agents are sometimes necessary to ensure activity against the pathogens concerned.
3. Combined treatment as a means of preventing the development of drug resistance is especially relevant to chronic infections and is of course firmly established as a cardinal feature in the treatment of tuberculosis and of leprosy (Ch. 59). This function of combined therapy is, however, sometimes important in acute infections such as those caused by *Pseudomonas aeruginosa*.
4. Occasionally, combined treatment can be used as a method of reducing dosage of a potentially toxic drug while achieving the same therapeutic end by its use in combination. The best authenticated example is the use

of reduced dosage of amphotericin in combination with flucytosine (itself unfortunately possessing substantial toxicity) in the treatment of cryptococcal meningitis (p. 870).

5. When antibiotics are combined in laboratory conditions, the combinations may prove additive, indifferent, synergic or antagonistic. Where the effect is additive, the agents together behave as though the concentration of either had been increased; where indifferent, the combined effect is no different from that of either alone; and where antagonistic, the effect of the combination is less than that of either agent alone. The word 'synergy' is used with slightly different connotations in the contexts of bacteristatic and bactericidal tests. In the former, synergy denotes a combined effect significantly greater than that of either drug acting alone. The best known example is that of sulphonamides and trimethoprim, acting as they do on different stages of bacterial folate synthesis. The clinical significance of this type of combined action is uncertain and is discussed on page 346.

Bactericidal synergy is used to describe the phenomenon in which two drugs are individually incompletely bactericidal but which acting together are able to kill the inoculum completely. An inhibitory concentration of one drug will be required, but complete killing may be produced by the addition of a subinhibitory concentration of the second.

This type of combined action is clinically important and is needed to achieve cure in certain cases of infective endocarditis, especially when the responsible organism is shown to be drug tolerant (p. 14), and in the treatment of septicaemia in the immune-suppressed.

These laboratory interactions and their clinical significance are discussed further in Part II.

THE ROLE OF THE LABORATORY IN DIAGNOSIS AND TREATMENT

Since it is often impossible to determine by clinical analysis the identity, let alone the drug susceptibility, of the causal agent, the importance of sound microbiological practice and of good liaison between ward or clinic and laboratory cannot be overemphasized. Nevertheless, even when laboratory service is not available, it is often possible, by employing the foregoing principles of antibiotics use, to make a logical and successful choice of agent. In many parts of the world sophisticated laboratory facilities and trained staff are absent, but simple laboratory methods are often available to the clinician, and the scope for diagnosis can be much enlarged by the ability reliably to perform a Gram-stain and a Ziehl–Neelsen stain on CSF or pus, to microscope urine and, if a somewhat higher level of laboratory work is available, to do blood, CSF and urine cultures.

When full laboratory facilities are available, it is essential that all appropriate specimens are taken before treatment is started (an occasional exception is the need sometimes to begin treatment in acute meningitis before lumbar puncture is done), and for the specimens to be handled properly and expeditiously. The responsibility for this stage in diagnosis, falling as it does between clinician and laboratory, is often badly executed and the cause of many missed opportunities for diagnosis. The laboratory receives dried saliva from a patient who may be coughing purulent sputum, or a dry swab with a slight discoloured tip from a patient just delivered of a litre of abdominal pus. The proper collection, handling and examination of specimens in the diagnosis and management of infection is most important.

In most regimens of antibiotic treatment it is assumed from data acquired before marketing that concentrations achieved at the site of infection are adequate and not excessive. The low toxicity of many antibiotic groups, notably of the β-lactam compounds, makes this a reasonable assumption in most circumstances. For compounds with a low therapeutic ratio, notably the aminoglycosides and vancomycin, assay of concentrations in blood and occasionally in other body fluids is essential, both to establish that adequate concentrations have been achieved and that concentrations are not excessive. This is especially important in patients with impaired renal function.

The stages of laboratory control of antibiotic therapy may thus be summarized as:

- Collection of appropriate specimens at the earliest possible moment and whenever possible before therapy has been started
- Efficient and rapid transport of specimens to the laboratory
- Microscopy, culture and identification
- Susceptibility testing of significant isolates
- When indicated, tests of combined antibiotic action
- When indicated, antibiotic assay in body fluids.

ANTIBIOTIC CONTROL POLICIES (see Ch. 12)

The search for rational and effective policies of antibiotic usage arise from increasing concern about the spread of resistant strains, the burden of unwanted effects from antimicrobial drugs and the mounting cost of the agents. Earlier studies on the use of antimicrobial drugs, mainly in hospitals, painted an alarming picture of widespread misuse, with a large proportion of prescriptions thought to be inappropriate, either because no antibiotic was indicated or because the agent and/or the dose chosen was incorrect. Later studies painted a less lurid picture, but it remains

clear that, whether used wisely or not, antibiotic prescription is extremely common. Whilst most therapeutic use appears reasonably judicious, some is undoubtedly inappropriate, with particular difficulty in prophylactic use (this is considered further here and in Chapter 42), which in a number of surveys has accounted for about one-third of antibiotic prescriptions. Antibiotic prescribing has also been studied in general practice. As might be supposed, variations in social and psychological history significantly affected the doctor's response and, despite a reasonably conservative prescribing pattern, there has been a trend towards an increase in antibiotic prescribing and a tendency to use a wider range of compounds. General practice formularies could do much to improve antibiotic prescribing practice.

In any type of practice, whether in hospital or in the community, the use of drugs is affected by a number of pressures: uncertainties of diagnosis, the wish to treat the patient successfully, the desire for treatment on the part of the patient and the cultural framework affecting expectations of drug treatment in the particular community. It is perhaps simpler for a research team to define the criteria for proper antimicrobial drugs usage than for the practising clinician to follow them. Moreover, even when social and psychological pressures are excluded, there is often substantial disagreement about what constitutes rational or irrational use of antimicrobial drugs, and in some of the studies the criteria might have been unreasonably rigorous. Nonetheless, for all these caveats, there is no doubt that antibiotic prescribing habits leave much room for improvement and much effort has been put into attempts to improve them.

There seems to be a strong case in favour of a positive policy for antibiotic prescribing which includes a prominent audit component enabling judgements to be made about the effect of the programme. While it is not unduly difficult to measure unwanted clinical effects of antibiotics and to monitor the consumption and cost of drugs, measurement of spread of the drug resistance, the third major disadvantage of antibiotic use, presents much greater difficulties. Many individual studies show that drug resistant organisms can be controlled by restrictive antibiotic policies, but the overall effects of even the most judicious prescribing policies are difficult to predict and require extensive study. These issues, and the measures which can be taken to develop antibiotic policies, are discussed fully in Chapter 12.

Three further general comments should be borne in mind in formulating antibiotic policies.

Many rational methods proposed for antibiotic control rely heavily on feedback from laboratory information (on isolation rates, antibiotic susceptibility patterns, etc.) and are thus inapplicable to antibiotic prescribing as it is practised in most parts of the world, including most general practice usage.

An important component of the problem is that of the

initial clinical assessment (does the patient have an infection, what might be the cause?). Thus, standards of undergraduate and postgraduate teaching in medicine and especially infectious diseases are likely to be as or more important than administrative policies in determining patterns of antibiotic usage.

Efforts to control antibiotic usage in order to limit the spread of resistant strains are likely to be unsuccessful unless they are combined with vigorous cross-infection control policies. Their success depends, too, on a combination of sound administrative policies with adequate staffing levels and high standards of professional practice.

WORLD HEALTH ORGANIZATION ESSENTIAL DRUG LIST

Control of antibiotic usage on a much larger canvas than that so far discussed is being attempted through the medium of the WHO Essential Drug List, a series of recommendations proposed by an international group of experts which, together with advice on other aspects of drug usage such as quality control, is published to act as a model for national policies. The list is updated from time to time and Table 9.1 gives the antibacterial agents included in current recommendations. It is important to note that some of the agents (as indicated in the table) are given as examples of a therapeutic group and that in these cases alternative agents may be preferred, depending on national factors such as cost and availability. The full list includes routes of administration, dosage forms, and strengths,

together with other information such as the need for dose adjustment in renal failure.

Table 9.1   *Antibacterial agents included in the WHO Essential Drug List*

Penicillins
Ampicillin
Benzathine penicillin
Benzylpenicillin
Cloxacillin
Phenoxymethylpenicillin
Piperacillin
Procaine benzylpenicillin
Other antibacterial drugs
Chloramphenicol
Erythromycin
Gentamicin
Metronidazole
Spectinomycin
Sulphadimidine
Sulfamethoxazole + trimethoprim
Tetracycline
(doxycycline, nitrofurantoin and trimethoprim are included in a complementary list)
Antileprosy drugs
Clofazimine
Dapsone
Rifampicin
Antituberculous drugs
Ethambutol
Isoniazid
Pyrazinamide
Rifampicin
Streptomycin
Thiacetazone + isoniazid

10

Laboratory control of antimicrobial therapy

D. C. Shanson

Introduction

Not all antimicrobial therapy requires laboratory help. Empirical therapy is perfectly adequate in many circumstances, for example, in the domiciliary treatment of urinary infection, especially if it is informed by knowledge of local resistance trends. In more serious infection the clinician cannot always afford to wait until laboratory results are available. Nonetheless, the laboratory often plays a vital part in the rational use of antimicrobial drugs by obtaining a microbiological diagnosis when infection is suspected. This initial step is most likely to succeed when there is close liaison between the clinical and laboratory staff, optimal collection and transport of appropriate samples – before the start of therapy whenever possible – and good microbiological practice (Shanson 1989, Stokes et al 1993). Once the causative organism is detected the antimicrobial drug susceptibilities can often be predicted, taking into account the results of national and local surveys of the susceptibility patterns of various pathogens to different antibiotics, and this may well assist the clinician to give more rational chemotherapy pending the results of susceptibility tests on the isolate or isolates. The determination of antibiotic susceptibility patterns of isolates from a given patient is of particular value when there is a serious infection and generally is of greater importance in hospital than in general practice as resistant strains are more often encountered in hospital. In hospital practice there is also an epidemiological reason for monitoring antibiotic susceptibility patterns of isolates. Surveillance of antibiotic-resistant organisms in different parts of the hospital is an important component of efforts to prevent and control the spread of resistant strains.

Limitations of susceptibility testing

CHOICE OF AGENT FOR TESTING

Plainly, the laboratory cannot carry out tests on all the antimicrobial agents that might be used in treatment. With some antibiotic groups, like the tetracyclines or sulphonamides, and in the special case of staphylococci that owe their resistance to β-lactam antibiotics to a change in a penicillin-binding protein, it is sufficient to test one representative of the whole family, since resistance to one normally extends to all the others. In other cases, including most β-lactam agents and aminoglycosides, where differences of activity and spectrum exist, the laboratory has to compromise by testing agents that are representative (sometimes incompletely) of a subclass; for example, cefotaxime to represent all extended spectrum cephalosporins and gentamicin to represent gentamicin, tobramycin and netilmicin. Within hospitals, the choice of agents to be tested by the laboratory should closely reflect the local policy of antibiotic use. The laboratory also needs to ensure that only clinically relevant antibiotics are reported for each significant isolate; for example, ampicillin, chloramphenicol and ciprofloxacin would be appropriate against *Salmonella typhi*, but gentamicin would not.

The results of some antibiotic susceptibility tests may be recorded in the laboratory, but not necessarily reported, as part of an agreed policy to restrict the use of selected 'reserve' antibiotics. This may also happen when the clinical significance of an isolate is uncertain, as for example when a coliform from a sputum sample is isolated from a patient in a general ward.

INTERPRETATION OF RESULTS

There are some potential pitfalls in the interpretation of antibiotic susceptibility tests. It is often difficult to distinguish between a clinically significant isolate and an organism that is merely colonizing a site sampled; if results are reported on a colonizing or contaminant organism, inappropriate therapy may be given as a consequence.

When the isolate is from a patient with serious infection and resistance to an antibiotic has been reported, a clinical response would generally not be obtained by giving that antibiotic, although the patient may improve for other reasons. Similarly, there are several factors that may limit the clinical correlation of response after giving an antibiotic to which an organism has been reported as susceptible. Thus, appropriate antimicrobial therapy may not achieve the desired result when there is a large collection of pus that needs surgical drainage; when there is chronic deep-seated infection; or when the host defences are greatly impaired, as with profound neutropenia following immunosuppression.

Antibiotic assays

Assays of antimicrobial drugs in serum or other body fluids may be helpful in providing optimal therapy for patients with serious infection who are receiving drugs with a narrow therapeutic margin such as aminoglycosides or glycopeptides. The results of assays may indicate whether concentrations obtained are high enough for effective therapy or whether there is an increased risk of adverse reactions associated with concentrations rising above those correlated with a toxicity risk. In these circumstances, appropriate changes to the dosing regimen can be suggested.

Definitions

ANTIBIOTIC SUSCEPTIBILITY

Antibiotic susceptibility (sensitive strain) is usually defined by inhibition of an organism at concentrations of antibiotic likely to be achieved in the blood after therapeutic doses. Ideally, the antibiotic concentration at the site of infection should exceed the minimum inhibitory concentration (defined below) by at least two- to four-fold in patients with serious infection. In practice, tissue concentrations are not precisely known and serum concentrations are used in the assessment of susceptibility.

MINIMUM INHIBITORY CONCENTRATION (MIC)

The MIC is defined as the lowest concentration of an antibiotic that produces no visible growth after overnight (16–20 h) incubation of a standard inoculum of the organism with a series of dilutions of the drug in broth or agar. Many antibiotics are subject to inoculum density effects that may profoundly affect the MIC. An inoculum of 10^5 colony-forming units/ml is commonly used in broth titrations, but the therapeutically 'correct' inoculum has not been defined.

MINIMUM BACTERICIDAL CONCENTRATION (MBC)

The MBC is usually defined as the minimum concentration of drug that reduces the colony count of viable organisms to less than 99.9% of its initial value after overnight incubation in broth; i.e. a 1000-fold reduction in the original inoculum. The MBC indicates the extent, but not the *rate* of killing, which may be more relevant to successful therapy in appropriate circumstances. Some antibiotics, notably β-lactam agents (in their action on Gram-positive cocci) and quinolones, exhibit an optimal dosage effect so that less killing is observed as the drug concentration is raised.

TOLERANCE

Organisms are said to be 'antibiotic tolerant' when the MBC exceeds the MIC by 16-fold or more. The term is usually used to describe staphylococci or streptococci that are less susceptible than usual to the bactericidal action of β-lactam antibiotics. The clinical significance of tolerance is usually uncertain, but it may have implications for the treatment of certain forms of infective endocarditis.

POSTANTIBIOTIC EFFECT

This term refers to the continued inhibition of an organism for a period of time (sometimes several hours) after the concentration of an antibiotic has ostensibly fallen to below the MIC. Demonstration of the phenomenon in vitro is prone to considerable variation depending on the conditions of the test, and the therapeutic significance is unclear.

BREAKPOINT

The breakpoint concentration of an antibiotic is the concentration used to judge whether an organism is considered 'sensitive' or 'resistant' in antimicrobial susceptibility tests. Sometimes two breakpoints are used to establish categories of *susceptible, resistant* and *reduced (intermediate) susceptibility.* The latter category implies that successful therapy may be possible if the drug is concentrated at the site of infection (e.g. excreted in high concentration in urine in urinary tract infection) or that high dosage might be appropriate.

Published breakpoints are generally estimated by consideration of serum concentrations achieved after standard dosage, sometimes modified according to known pharmacological properties of the drug, such as elimination half-life and extent of protein binding. Although breakpoints are arrived at by expert consensus, considerable differences often exist in recommendations made in different countries.

Breakpoint susceptibility testing refers to a method in which the susceptibility of organisms to an antibiotic is tested only at the agreed breakpoint or breakpoints for that antibiotic (see below).

Antibiotic susceptibility test methods

In general, routine susceptibility tests are applied only to the common aerobic bacteria. Particular problems relate to tests of fastidious and slow-growing organisms, including *Mycobacterium tuberculosis* (for which special methods are available) and many anaerobes. Susceptibility tests of fungi are beset by a number of technical problems and are not usually available on a routine basis.

Several methods of susceptibility testing are in common use for bacteria that are easy to grow; some form of agar diffusion method with discs or strips impregnated with standard amounts of antibiotic are generally most convenient. Many factors affect the reliability of each method. To minimize the risk of errors control organisms of known susceptibility or resistance to various antibiotics need to be tested alongside the organisms investigated from patients. To help ensure that high standards of antibiotic susceptibility test reports are issued consistently by a laboratory, regular participation in an external quality control scheme is recommended.

Rapid methods are generally preferred to help the prompt laboratory guidance of antibiotic therapy and, when practical, 'primary' (direct) susceptibility tests should be used rather than 'secondary' (indirect) tests alone. Primary tests are carried out by placing discs on an agar surface which has been inoculated directly with the patient's sample, and can usually be read within 16–24 h of receipt of the sample. Samples in which primary tests should be considered include urines from pyuric patients, turbid cerebrospinal fluid (CSF) samples, samples of pus and blood

cultures which look positive. The range of antibiotics tested in a primary method will largely depend on microscopy of a Gram-stained smear of the sample, although with urine samples a set of antibiotics appropriate to the common urinary pathogens is usually tested. Secondary antibiotic susceptibility tests are carried out with pure cultures of isolates, and have the advantage that the method used can be more carefully standardized. However, the results are not usually available until at least the second day after receipt of the sample.

For a discussion of detailed technical aspects of susceptibility testing, see Lorian (1991), Report (1991) and Reeves et al (1978).

ERICSSON'S DISC DIFFUSION TEST

With this standardized method a 'dense but not confluent' inoculum of the organism is flooded onto the surface of the agar plate and a high content disc of each antibiotic to be tested is applied. After incubation, the diameter of the inhibition zone is measured and compared to data in published charts based on regression lines plotted by comparing the log of the inhibition zone diameter of 100 organisms of varying sensitivity against the MICs of the organisms to that antibiotic. There are strict conditions required for the test, including the need to use the same agar medium which was used to prepare the regression data.

This test has been approved by an International Collaborative Survey Group (Ericsson & Sherris 1971) and is now mainly used in Scandinavia.

KIRBY–BAUER METHOD

Disc susceptibility testing in North America is frequently based on the Kirby–Bauer method (Bauer et al 1966). This method has been given official approval by the Food and Drug Administration in the USA and is the basis of the recommendations of the influential National Committee for Clinical Laboratory Standards (NCCLS) in that country. Only one type of medium is specified: Mueller–Hinton agar. The inoculum is prepared by using a swab immersed into a bacterial suspension of the same density as a barium sulphate standard to produce a standardized inoculum of just confluent growth. The other details of the test are similar to those of the Ericsson test.

The Kirby–Bauer test places great emphasis on standardization, with a view to achieving reproducibility between different laboratories carrying out susceptibility tests. It has no greater validity than other methods in terms of clinical correlates and suffers from the inherent weakness

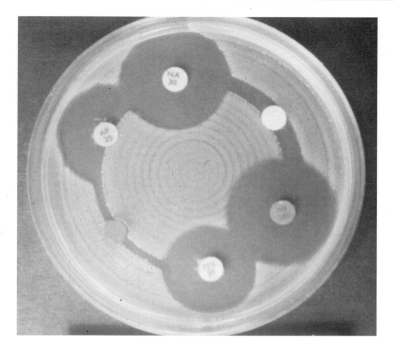

Fig. 10.1   *Stokes' comparative disc method of antibiotic susceptibility testing. The zones produced by the test strain in the centre of the plate are compared directly with those given by the control strain round the outer area plate.*

that batches of Mueller–Hinton medium may differ considerably in their performance.

STOKES' COMPARATIVE DISC METHOD

In Stokes' disc method (Stokes et al 1993) the inhibition zone obtained with the test organism is compared directly with that obtained with a fully sensitive control on the same agar plate (Fig. 10.1). The control organisms usually recommended include the Oxford strain of *Staphylococcus aureus* NCTC 6571 (for tests of Gram-positive cocci), *Escherichia coli* NCTC 10418 (for enteric Gram-negative bacilli), and *Pseudomonas aeruginosa* NCTC 10662 (for *Ps. aeruginosa* strains). Even though each disc is controlled there are many important details required to obtain satisfactory results as with any method. These include: appropriate choice of antibiotic; disc strength in relation to the site of infection; standardized inoculum (dense but not confluent); and an adequately nutritious sensitivity medium of suitable pH and ionic content, which is free of drug inhibitors (such as thymidine, which antagonizes trimethoprim and sulphonamides). The incubation conditions must be appropriate in respect of temperature, atmosphere and duration. Special methods are required for certain organisms such as methicillin resistant *Staph. aureus*

(MRSA), penicillin-resistant pneumococci and glycopeptide-resistant enterococci (Report 1991, Stokes et al 1993). Some of the variables affecting disc test results cannot be satisfactorily controlled by Stokes' comparative method. For example, with this method the genera of the bacterial strains tested are often different to those of the controls; this could be especially important when there is variation in the antibiotic content of the disc, and for interpretation of test inhibition zones which suggest 'intermediate sensitivity' (Brown 1990).

THE E TEST

The E test is a diffusion method that enables MIC values to be estimated directly. An extended series of two-fold dilutions of an initially high standard antibiotic concentration are distributed linearly along a special carrier strip. The strip is applied to a suitably inoculated plate and, after incubation overnight, the MIC is read where the inhibition ellipse intersects the calibrated scale (Fig. 10.2). Recommendations are provided by the manufacturers about standardization of the inoculum, type of medium to be used for different organisms and reading of the plates. The E test may especially help to detect pneumococci with resistance to penicillin and/or certain cephalosporins and enterococci

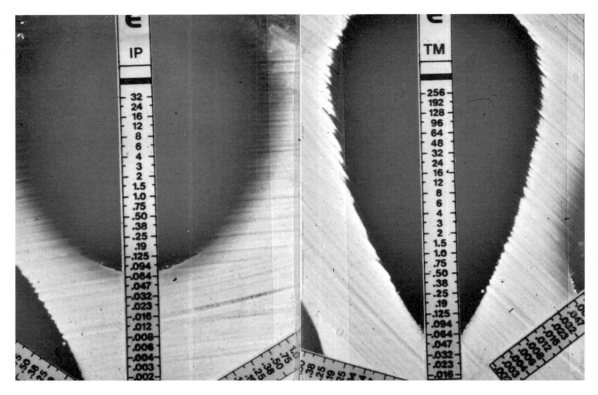

Fig. 10.2 *Estimation of minimum inhibitory concentrations by the E-test method.*

with resistance to aminoglycosides, ampicillin or vancomycin – examples of resistance which are sometimes not readily apparent with Stokes' comparative disc susceptibility method.

DILUTION TESTS

Dilution tests involving macro (tube) or micro (microtitration tray) broth, or agar methods have the advantage that known concentrations of drugs are tested, whereas with discs the antibiotic content may vary from 67% to 150% of the nominal value. Some of the factors that may influence the results of disc tests are less relevant to dilution methods, which may therefore give more reproducible results than disc tests. Other variables, such as inoculum density and constituents of the test medium, apply equally to both methods.

Broth or agar dilution methods are often used to provide 'gold standard' MIC data, but different factors govern the end-points of broth and agar dilution titrations and MIC values estimated in agar are commonly two- to four-fold lower than those found by broth methods. By use of a multi-

point inoculator with an agar dilution method, reproducible MIC results can be obtained on up to 36 different strains in each batch of tests. However, MIC tests are not usually necessary on large numbers of organisms except for survey or research purposes.

Broth dilution tests can be conveniently carried out in automated commercially available systems, sometimes together with semi-automated biochemical identification methods. There are pitfalls with the automated systems, including the possible undetected presence of mixed rather than pure cultures, and the unreliability of results obtained with some organisms, for example, methicillin-resistant staphylococci.

Dilution methods are more time consuming than diffusion methods and are more suitable for secondary susceptibility tests when a more accurate estimate of susceptibility than that provided by disc tests is needed. Occasionally, an MIC determination is desirable when the isolate is from a patient with septicaemia, meningitis or other life-threatening infections and when the disc test is giving unclear susceptibility results. MICs should always be determined for streptococci isolated from blood cultures of patients with endocarditis, as decisions about the choice of antibiotics and duration of treatment depend on the results. Broth rather than agar MIC tests should be considered, as further information about bacterial killing can readily be obtained by subculture and MBC values established. Combination tests of antibiotics on endocarditis isolates are best carried out in broth rather than agar (see antibiotic combinations, below).

BREAKPOINT ANTIBIOTIC SUSCEPTIBILITY TESTS

Some large laboratories have introduced breakpoint antibiotic susceptibility tests into the diagnostic laboratory to replace routine disc susceptibility tests. The test involves spot-inoculation of bacteria on plates containing antibiotic at one or two concentrations representing the agreed breakpoints for susceptibility or resistance. The method is suitable for laboratories with large workloads since economies of scale can be achieved by use of multipoint inoculation, with automatic scanning devices to read and record the results. Some laboratories use disc diffusion tests for most of the susceptibility tests but also include breakpoint tests for a few antibiotics, and for particular organisms, which are more difficult to test reliably with disc tests. These include: tests of susceptibility of gonococci to penicillin; tests of Gram-negative bacilli in which the disc test shows apparent intermediate susceptibility to aminoglycosides; and *Staph. aureus* with apparent intermediate susceptibility to methicillin.

With the breakpoint method, clear end-points to distinguish between susceptible, intermediately susceptible and resistant strains are obtained if appropriate antibiotic concentrations are used; as with all methods, other variables, such as medium and density of inoculum, must also be suitably controlled (Report 1991). For the method to work efficiently it is necessary to have a central antibiotic workstation in the laboratory so that work practices may need to be re-organized. The method is not as convenient as the disc test for primary sensitivities or for the recognition of mixed cultures, or strain variants, in the test inoculum which may have different susceptibilities to a given antibiotic.

Special susceptibility methods

KILLING CURVE TESTS

Time-kill tests, in which sequential viable counts are carried out on broth cultures of bacteria exposed to fixed concentrations of antibiotics, can give valuable data on the rate of killing of organisms, but are too labour intensive to be practical for most diagnostic laboratories. Tolerance to β-lactam antibiotics can be demonstrated by this method with some staphylococci and streptococci, in which an unusually slow rate of kill is demonstrated.

ANTIBIOTIC COMBINATIONS

Antibiotic combination tests are mainly required in routine practice for selecting suitable synergic therapy for patients with infective endocarditis or other serious infections in which synergic activity may be important to therapeutic success. Cross-diffusion tests may sometimes indicate synergy (or antagonism) but the most common method used is the *chessboard (checkerboard) combination test*. In this test two antibiotics are cross-titrated in either broth or agar so that a two-dimensional layout is produced in which each dilution of one antibiotic is combined with each dilution of the other. An MIC end-point is obtained for each antibiotic alone and in combination and the results used to plot a so-called *isobologram*, or to calculate the fractional inhibitory concentration (FIC). The FIC is the MIC in combination divided by the MIC of each antibiotic alone. The FIC index is the sum of the FICs (ΣFIC) and a value of ≤0.5 indicates synergy.

When the chessboard titration is carried out in broth, and the starting inoculum is known, the bactericidal effect of each antibiotic alone and in combination may be tested using a 99.9% reduction in colony count as the end-point for MBC and FBC (fractional bactericidal concentration) after incubation for a fixed time, usually 18 h. In this way a synergic bactericidal effect may be demonstrated between two antibiotics, and this may be helpful in the investigation of strains from patients with endocarditis. A simpler method for detecting bactericidal synergy between a β-lactam antibiotic, or glycopeptide, and an aminoglycoside, is to test a series of dilutions of the β-lactam antibiotic in broth containing a fixed concentration of aminoglycoside (e.g. gentamicin 1 mg/l) compared to parallel broths without the aminoglycoside.

When many different antibiotics need to be tested in combination with each other a 'half-chessboard' method may provide useful information. In this method each antibiotic is tested at a fixed concentration which relates to serum concentrations expected after therapeutic doses.

Chessboard titrations measure an overnight end-point, but do not indicate the rate of killing. For this purpose the killing curve method is more appropriate. Synergy may be demonstrated when the reduction in colony count achieved at a given time by a combination of antibiotics is 100-fold or more of that obtained with each antibiotic alone. Combination tests may similarly indicate antagonism (a reduction in bacterial killing), a simple additive effect, or indifference so that the activity of the more bactericidal drug prevails. These tests do not necessarily reflect the in vivo effects of the combination and share similar limitations to susceptibility tests in general.

TESTS FOR β-LACTAMASE

Coloured substrates, such as nitrocefin (a chromogenic cephalosporin), are useful for the rapid detection of β-lactamase produced by some penicillin-resistant strains of *Neisseria gonorrhoeae*, ampicillin-resistant *Haemophilus influenzae*, and β-lactamase-producing strains of enterococci, which are presently rare. Commercially available strips can be used for this purpose.

POSTANTIBIOTIC EFFECT

The continued effect of certain antibiotics, such as β-lactam antibiotics or aminoglycosides, after the concentration is reduced to below the MIC value, may be demonstrated in the time-kill test. Fresh broth is added after the desired period of antibiotic exposure to dilute the antibiotic sufficiently to reduce the concentration to below an inhibitory level. A postantibiotic effect is shown by a delay in recovery of growth. Aminoglycosides may have a postantibiotic effect lasting for several hours, and this has been suggested to contribute to the success of once-daily dosage regimens. Such a test is not practical in diagnostic laboratories, but can be used as a research tool.

MOLECULAR METHODS

Methods for the detection and characterization of plasmids conferring antibiotic resistance have been developed for many antibiotic-resistant strains of bacteria, but no test is commercially available for routine use.

Nucleic acid probes have been developed to detect the genes for various types of antibiotic resistance, including the Mec A gene present in MRSA, β-lactamases in some cephalosporin-resistant enterobacteria and glycopeptide resistance in vancomycin-resistant enterococci. At present, these are mainly used as research tools, but there is great future potential for the diagnostic use of such methods, provided the practical distinction between genotype and phenotype is recognized.

Antibiotic assay

Antibiotic assays are necessary to determine the concentrations of antibiotics achieved in serum and other body fluids, or tissues, to obtain a pharmacokinetic profile in healthy and diseased individuals, as part of the evaluation of any recently introduced antibiotic. However, the indications for antibiotic assay in clinical practice are relatively few and mainly involve drugs which have a narrow therapeutic margin, such as aminoglycosides and glycopeptides. Patients receiving aminoglycosides and vancomycin will need regular assays to check that rising toxic concentrations are not occurring and that concentrations likely to be effective are achieved after each dose. When patients have impairment of renal function, or are elderly, daily assays are usually necessary and rapid immunochemical methods are preferable to overnight microbiological assays.

The most meaningful assays are likely to be arranged when the wards and laboratory collaborate closely on the proper collection of samples that are clearly timed in relation to the last dose given, and when there is close liaison about interpretation of the results which may involve a change in antibiotic dosage. A pre-dose trough sample is usually collected during the 20 min before the dose, and a postdose peak sample is usually collected 1 h after the dose. If the trough gentamicin concentration is less than 1 mg/l and the peak concentration only 5 mg/l in, for example, a patient with klebsiella pneumonia and septicaemia, the dose should be increased so that the peak concentration is in the range 8–12 mg/l while keeping the trough level less than 2 mg/l – since peak levels greater than 8 mg/l are recommended for the most effective gentamicin treatment of Gram-negative pneumonia.

IMMUNOASSAY METHODS

Commercially available rapid immunoassay methods include enzyme immunoassay (EMIT, Syva) and fluorescence polarization assay (TDX or IMX, Abbott). Both are used for aminoglycoside assays and the latter can also be used for vancomycin assay. Regular participation in external quality-control schemes is recommended, as for all assay methods, to help ensure that an accurate and reproducible assay service is provided.

PLATE DIFFUSION METHODS

Most antibiotics can be assayed by a microbiological method and this is often useful when single antibiotics are used and time is not an important factor. However, there are many potential pitfalls in the technical performance of these assays, including factors such as the diluents and media used. Microbiological assay was formerly much used for gentamicin assays with klebsiella as the indicator organism. Adequate results may be obtained without the need for expensive equipment or reagents. Nonetheless, immunoassays are less liable to error, and give more rapid results, and are generally preferable to plate methods.

HIGH PRESSURE LIQUID CHROMATOGRAPHY (HPLC)

This technique depends on the test drugs, in a mobile phase, having differential retention times when passed under pressure down a special particle column. Metabolites of antimicrobial agents usually exhibit different retention times under suitable conditions and the method has the advantage of being able to resolve and quantify such compounds. HPLC is particularly useful for assays of drugs such as cephalosporins, but is more suitable for research than routine use.

SERUM BACTERICIDAL ASSAYS (BACK-TITRATIONS)

Back-titration of the patient's serum against the causative organism of infective endocarditis, or septicaemia in an immunosuppressed patient, has often been recommended to monitor therapy. Traditionally, a peak serum bactericidal titre of ≥ 1 in 8 in a sample taken about 1 h after the last dose of antibiotic has been regarded as evidence of satisfactory bactericidal activity, but there is a lack of consensus as to what might constitute a satisfactory trough bactericidal titre (Eykyn 1987). There are technical difficulties with this test, as there are also with the MBC tests, since the end-point may be difficult to read and there are many other variables. There are presently no internationally accepted guidelines to standardize the test. Surveys in the USA and the UK suggest that there is a general correlation between high peak bactericidal titres and bacteriological cure in patients with infective endocarditis (Eykyn 1987, Stratton 1987). However, the test is of limited value in an individual patient as the test is not reliable for predicting clinical outcome. For this reason many authorities no longer recommend the routine use of the back-titration test in patients treated for infected endocarditis. Nonetheless, for managing exceptional cases with particularly antibiotic-resistant causative organisms it may be helpful to compare titres obtained between different antibiotic combination regimens in the search for more effective therapy. Such a test should probably be done in a reference laboratory familiar with the many technical variables involved.

References

Bauer A W, Kirby W, Sherris J, Turck M 1966 Antibiotic susceptibility testing by a standardized single disk method. *American Journal of Clinical Pathology* 45: 493–496

Brown D F J 1990 The comparative methods of antimicrobial susceptibility testing – time for a change? *Journal of Antimicrobial Chemotherapy* 25: 307–310

Ericsson H M, Sherris J C 1971 Antibiotic sensitivity testing. Report of an international collaborative study. *Acta Pathologica et Microbiologica Scandinavica, Section B* (suppl 217): 1–90

Eykyn S J 1987 The role of the laboratory in assisting treatment – a review of current UK practices. *Journal of Antimicrobial Chemotherapy* 20 (suppl A): 51–70

Lorian V (ed) 1991 Antibiotics in laboratory medicine, 3rd edn. Williams & Wilkins, Baltimore

Reeves D S, Phillips I, Williams J D, Wise R 1978 Laboratory methods in antimicrobial chemotherapy. Churchill Livingstone, Edinburgh

Report 1991 A guide to sensitivity testing. *Journal of Antimicrobial Chemotherapy* 27 (suppl D): 1–50

Shanson D C 1989 Microbiology in clinical practice, 2nd edn. Wright, Oxford

Stokes E J, Ridgway G L, Wren M W 1993 Clinical microbiology, 7th edn. Edward Arnold, London

Stratton C W 1987 The role of the microbiology laboratory in the treatment of infective endocarditis. *Journal of Antimicrobial Chemotherapy* 20 (suppl A): 41–49

CHAPTER 11

Principles of chemoprophylaxis

H. P. Lambert

Introduction

In some circumstances antimicrobial agents can be used to prevent infection, or to prevent the progression of existing infection to manifest disease. The former method is sometimes described as primary prophylaxis and the latter as secondary prophylaxis. These methods may be especially useful when other methods of control such as vaccination are unavailable or cannot be employed in the prevailing conditions. Despite its evident attractions, however, chemoprophylaxis is not always successful and it is important to define the conditions in which it is most appropriately used.

Chemoprophylaxis is most readily applicable when directed at a single pathogen (or at least at a narrow range of pathogens) which is, and remains, fully susceptible to an easily available and non-toxic agent. A classical example is the prevention of recurrent infection by Streptococcus pyogenes in patients with rheumatic heart disease. By contrast, chemoprophylaxis has often failed when used in vulnerable patients in environments in which a variety of resistant organisms can emerge and cause the very types of infection it was intended to prevent. Examples of such failures are to be found in the former attempts at chemoprophylaxis in normal or premature infants, in unconscious or paralysed patients, or in patients with tracheostomies, and in the current uncertainties (see below and Ch. 44) on the role of selective decontamination. Nevertheless, advances in understanding of normal colonization and its disturbances has enabled some successes to be achieved, even in patients with immune suppression and in the hospital environment. Examples include the prevention of several infections to which patients with human immunodeficiency virus (HIV) infection are especially vulnerable (see Ch. 46) and the reduction of bacteraemic infection in neutropenia.

Chemoprophylaxis involves a diverse range of mechanisms, some of them still poorly understood. Antibiotics may be administered, as in contacts of meningococcal disease, in an attempt to prevent colonization, although it is often uncertain to what extent this is actually achieved and to what extent the process is one of early eradication of subclinical infection. Sometimes the agent is given following known or presumed infection, as in those exposed to infection with syphilis or gonorrhoea. In the chemoprophylaxis of tuberculosis isoniazid may be given to tuberculin-positive, and therefore already infected, subjects, with the aim of preventing progression to manifest disease or, in the case of neonatal contacts, in order to prevent primary infection. The duration of chemoprophylaxis varies greatly, from very short-term cover for dental procedures or surgery, to periods of many years, as in patients with rheumatic or congenital heart disease.

The success of proposed schemes of chemotherapy must be established, whenever possible, by clinical trials, since it cannot be assumed that an agent effective in established disease will necessarily be successful in prophylaxis. A notable example is that a number of agents, including penicillin, highly effective in the treatment of meningococcal septicaemia and meningitis, fail to eradicate naso-pharyngeal carriage of the organism. Another paradox is encountered in certain infections such as scrub typhus and leptospirosis, in which an agent of proven efficacy against the established disease may fail when used as a prophylactic agent, serving only to prolong the incubation period of the eventual illness.

Chemoprophylaxis is discussed throughout this book in the relevant chapters. Its medical applications are summarized here in Tables 11.1 and 11.2, in which we have thought it helpful to divide them according to the status of the host as either normal or with an underlying disease or other risk factor, while acknowledging that such a distinction is sometimes imprecise.

Table 11.1   *Applications of chemoprophylaxis in normal subjects*

Disease/pathogen	Prophylactic agent(s)	Comments	Refer to Chapter
Meningococcal disease	Rifampicin Ciprofloxacin Cefriaxone Sulphonamide	Effective individual protection. Not a major control measure	53
H. influenzae meningitis	Rifampicin	Effective individual protection. Not a major control measure	53
Traveller's diarrhoea	Doxycycline Co-trimoxazole Ciprofloxacin	Of some value. Often negated by drug resistance or unwanted effects	50
Cholera	Various	Modest value as a local control measure	50
Plague	Tetracycline		61
Leptospirosis	Doxycycline	Useful for short-term exposure	61
Scrub typhus	Doxycycline	Useful for short-term exposure	61
Syphilis	Penicillin	Contacts of cases	58
Gonorrhoea	Various	Major problems of antibiotic resistance in some areas	58
Pertussis	Erythromycin	Limited evidence of value. Use especially in institutional outbreaks	48
Tuberculosis	Isoniazid Rifampicin	Indicated in certain contact groups. See also in Table 11.2	59
Leprosy	Rifampicin	Contacts of lepromatous leprosy	59

Table 11.2   *Applications of chemoprophylaxis in groups with special susceptibility*

Patient group	Pathogen	Prophylactic agent(s)	Comment	Refer to Chapter
Rheumatic heart disease	*Str. pyogenes*	Penicillin	To reduce relapses of rheumatic fever and further cardiac damage	49
Rheumatic and congenital heart disease	*Str. viridans* Others	Ampicillin Clindamycin	To prevent endocarditis Best regimens disputed	49
Chronic bronchitis	Bacterial infections	Various antibiotics	Limited value. Usually given at the onset of exacerbation	48
Elderly: chronic chest and heart disease, diabetes, etc.	Influenza	Rimantidine Amantidine	Good evidence of value, but little used	48
Recurrent urinary tract infection	Various bacteria	Various schemes		56
HIV infection	*Pneumocystis* *Toxoplasmosis* *Candida* Herpes simplex Tuberculosis	Co-trimoxazole Pentamidine Various Fluconazole, etc. Acyclovir Antimycobacterial agents	Prevention of primary or recurrent infection with opportunistic pathogens of major importance in managing HIV	46

Table 11.2 *Cont'd*

Patient group	Pathogen	Prophylactic agent(s)	Comment	Refer to Chapter
Cancer/leukaemia	Bacteraemic infections	Various schemes	To diminish infections during neutropenic phases	43
Sickle cell disease/asplenia	*Str. pneumoniae*	Penicillin		page 147
Fetus	Syphilis	Penicillin	Indicated for positive serology in pregnancy	58
Fetus	*Toxoplasmosis*	Spiramycin, etc.	Efficacy in preventing fetal infection uncertain. Much variation in policies	63
Neonate	*Str. agalactiae*	Penicillin	Indications controversial	57
Neonate	Tuberculosis	Isoniazid	Mother found to have infectious tuberculosis in late pregnancy or puerperium	59
Neonate	HIV	Zidovudine	To reduce rate of transmission to infant	46

Principles of surgical prophylaxis

Important advances in the prevention of infection related to surgery have been achieved in recent decades. Detailed applications of surgical prophylaxis are taken up in Chapter 42, but the principles involved, of great importance for the formulation of hospital antibiotic policies, are discussed below, as is the special topic of infection in relation to splenectomy.

Postoperative infection may take the form of wound infections of widely varying severity, deep abscess formation or septicaemia sometimes accompanied by bacterial shock. At the least, postoperative infections cause distress, may prolong the patient's stay in hospital, and may add to the cost of management. At their worst, postoperative septicaemia and bacterial shock carry a high mortality. Infection rates vary greatly between different operations, surgeons and hospitals, and may also vary greatly from time to time within the same unit. Generally, however, rates are lowest with standard uncomplicated surgery at 'clean' sites, and highest when the integrity of a normally infected surface is breached, for example, after lower bowel and pelvic surgery.

Soon after their general introduction antimicrobial agents were used extensively, often for prolonged periods both before and after surgery, in attempts to prevent surgical infection. Such studies as were done often showed higher rates of infection in patients who had received regimens intended for prophylaxis and the infections which developed were often caused by antibiotic-resistant organisms which had become prevalent in the hospital environment. Experimental work providing a rational basis for successful

prophylaxis had its origin with the studies of Miles et al (1957). They established the important concept of a 'decisive period' in the development of a local infection, showing that beneficial influences such as an appropriate antibiotic, or detrimental ones such as local vasoconstriction, operate for a short period only, from just before to a few hours after the local infection is initiated. After this period has elapsed the ultimate size and severity of the local infection is uninfluenced by such interventions. Burke (1961) showed that this concept was equally applicable to experimental incisions and dermal lesions. These principles were tested in surgical practice by a few investigators, but progress was slow until the 1980s, when increasing concern about the prevalence of surgical infection and the cost of antibiotics led to improved trials and a consequent greater degree of precision in their prophylactic use.

There is now a substantial body of data enabling effective, operationally sensible and economic schemes of surgical prophylaxis to be established, based on the following principles:

- The best defence against infection is skilled surgery, in which tissue damage is minimized, suture lines are sound and accumulations of blood and tissue fluid are avoided. The likelihood of infection increases with duration of surgery.
- Prophylaxis is most clearly indicated in two main circumstances. First, in operations with known high rates of postoperative sepsis, in general those in which a heavily colonized surface is breached. Secondly, in operations following which infections, although rare, have disastrous consequences, for example, after heart

valve or joint replacement. Chemoprophylaxis is not usually given in normally 'clean' operations, but Platt et al (1990) showed that significant reduction in infection rates following herniorrhaphy and breast surgery could be achieved using single-dose preoperative prophylaxis. Whether the possible benefits of using perioperative chemoprophylaxis in a wider range of operations would outweigh the possible detriments in the form of increased antibiotic resistance and unwanted drug effects remains uncertain (Wenzel 1992).

- The likelihood of infection is closely related to the bacterial load in the wound at the time of surgery. The critical concentration seems to be about $10^5/g$ tissue. If this concentration is exceeded the infection rate rises steeply. Apart from excellence of technique, the microbial load at the operative site can be reduced by local or systemic use of antimicrobial agents, and in some circumstances by preoperative reduction of the bowel flora.

- Systemic prophylaxis should be given in such a way as to achieve adequate blood levels of the antibiotic just before surgery. An extensive analysis (Classen et al 1992) showed that prophylaxis was most effective if given in the 2 h before the incision. In practice, this generally means either intramuscular injection at the time of premedication, or intravenous administration at induction of anaesthesia. There is increasing evidence that for most operations a single injection of antibiotic reduces infection as much as do repeated injections, but if the duration of operation is longer than 2 h a second injection should be given.

The distinction between local methods, bowel decontamination and systemic treatment is often far from clear, because combinations of methods are sometimes used and because local methods often involve agents which are absorbed systemically.

- The agents chosen should be of low toxicity, should achieve tissue levels at the operative site and should have an antibacterial spectrum which covers the main organisms likely to cause infection after the particular operation. In the case of sites such as the lower bowel with a large anaerobic flora, the regimen should achieve both antianaerobic and antiaerobic activity.

Specific regimens are detailed in Chapter 42.

Colonization resistance and selective decontamination

Many infections affecting patients in hospital are preceded by progressive colonization of the gastrointestinal tract and oropharynx by Gram-negative aerobic bacteria. Because of the selective pressure of the hospital environment these organisms are often multiresistant and constitute an important source of nosocomial infection. A possible method of reducing these infections developed from the ideas of Van der Waaij and his colleagues on colonization resistance in the digestive tract. Working at first with gnotobiotic mice they showed that the normal anaerobic flora of the digestive tract, in association with other factors, acted as an important barrier to colonization by aerobic Gram-negative bacilli given by mouth, whereas germ-free animals could easily be colonized by low doses of the same organisms. The importance of anaerobes in maintaining colonization resistance in hospital patients and in those on antibiotics was also established (Van der Waaij & Berghuis de Vries 1974).

From this work arose the idea of selective decontamination – the use of agents to eliminate the Gram-negative bacillary and the fungal components of the bowel flora while preserving intact the protective anaerobes. This method of chemoprophylaxis has been applied most widely in neutropenic patients, as discussed in Chapter 43, and in intensive care units (see Ch. 44); it has also been applied in surgical prophylaxis (see Ch. 42). The method used varies between trials; a polymixin–aminoglycoside–amphotericin B mixture is usually administered by mouth, often combined with a local preparation to the oropharynx, and in many studies a cephalosporin is also given parenterally. The use of selective decontamination in intensive care units has been especially controversial, and units differ widely in their practice. A meta-analysis of 22 controlled trials (Selective Decontamination of the Digestive Tract Trialists' Collaborative Group 1993) concluded that selective decontamination significantly reduced respiratory tract infections in the intensive care unit. The effect on overall mortality was only moderate, reaching significant levels only in the subgroup of trials in which systemic and topical treatments were combined. Based on these more favourable trials, it was estimated that 6 (range 5–9) patients would need to be treated to prevent one respiratory infection, and 23 (13–139) to prevent one death.

Chemoprophylaxis in asplenia

Patients with absent or greatly reduced splenic function suffer an increased risk of infection by a number of different organisms. Although the increased rate of infection is small, estimated overall as 0.42% per year, the infections which do occur frequently have a fulminant course and carry a high mortality. This increased risk accompanies all forms of asplenia, but the degree of risk varies between different groups. Thus the risks are greater during the first 2 years after splenectomy, greater in children than in adults, and greater in those with haematological malignancy than after traumatic splenectomy. The risk is, however, life-long, and many reports record fatal infections years or even decades after splenectomy.

The most common cause of postsplenectomy infection is *Streptococcus pneumoniae* but *Haemophilus influenzae* and *Neisseria meningitidis* may be responsible. Other organisms of special importance in asplenic patients include malaria, babesiosis and *Capnocytophaga canimorsus* (DF2) following dog bites.

Attempts to prevent postsplenectomy infection rely on a combination of education, vaccination and chemoprophylaxis. The patient and their family should be fully informed of warning symptoms, and the patient should carry a suitable card or bracelet. Available vaccines against the capsulated bacteria should be given, but these are by no means a panacea since the serological response may be poor and severe pneumococcal infection has been caused both by strains represented in the vaccine and by non-vaccine strains.

The efficacy of chemoprophylaxis has been demonstrated in Jamaican children with homozygous sickle cell disease (John et al 1984), but there is much uncertainty about how best it should be employed in other at-risk groups. There is general agreement that it should be used in children up to the age of 16 years and in everyone during the first 2 years at least after splenectomy. Depending on the risk factors involved, chemoprophylaxis may then be stopped or continued, in some patients for life. If discontinued, patients should be given a supply of antibiotic to keep with them. The scientific and practical uncertainties in deciding the best policy for asplenic patients are revealed in a vigorous correspondence following an editorial on the topic (McMullin & Johnson 1993). The most common regimen is phenoxymethylpenicillin 500 mg twice daily (for adults) or amoxycillin 500 mg once daily. This policy will need to be kept under review should penicillin resistance in pneumococci become widespread. It is suggested that penicillin-allergic subjects are given erythromycin 250 mg twice daily (adult dose); in view of the ease with which erythromycin resistance emerges in streptococci, including pneumococci, it might be more advisable for such patients to be given a supply of erythromycin to take at the first sign of infection.

References

Burke J 1961 The effective period of preventive antibiotic action in experimental incisions and dermal lesions. *Surgery* 50: 161–168

Classen D C, Evans R S, Pestotnik S L, Horn S D, Menlove R L, Burke J P 1992 The timing of prophylactic administration of antibiotics and the risk of surgical wound infection. *New England Journal of Medicine* 326: 281–286

John A B, Ramlal A, Jackson H et al 1894 Prevention of pneumococcal infection in children with homozygous sickle cell disease. *British Medical Journal* 288: 1567–1570

McMullin M, Johnson G 1993 Long term management of patients after splenectomy. *British Medical Journal* 307: 1372–1373; 308: 131–133; 308: 598

Miles A A, Miles E M, Burke J 1957 The value and duration of defence reactions of the skin to the primary lodgement of bacteria. *British Journal of Experimental Pathology* 38: 79–96

Platt R, Zaleznik D F, Hopkins C C et al 1990 Perioperative antibiotic prophylaxis for herniorrhaphy and breast surgery. *New England Journal of Medicine* 322: 153–160

Selective Decontamination of the Digestive Tract Trialists' Collaborative Group 1993 Meta-analysis of randomised controlled trials of selective decontamination of the digestive tract. *British Medical Journal* 307: 525–532

Summerfield G 1994 Long term management after splenectomy. *British Medical Journal* 308: 598

Van der Waaij D, Berghuis de Vries J N 1974 Selective elimination of enterobacteriaceae from the digestive tract in mice and monkeys. *Journal of Hygiene (Cambridge)* 72: 205–211

Wenzel R P 1992 Preoperative antibiotic prophylaxis. *New England Journal of Medicine* 326: 337–339

CHAPTER 12

Antibiotic policies

P. G. Davey and D. Nathwani

Introduction

A recent survey found that 62% of 427 UK hospitals have a policy for antibiotic therapy and 75% have an antibiotic formulary (Working Party of the British Society of Antimicrobial Chemotherapy 1994). However, there was wide variation in the scope of policies and the methods that were used to implement them. For example, only half of the hospitals had a policy which included recommendations for surgical prophylaxis, 61% operated a formulary which included a restricted list of authorized antibiotics and 26% enforced automatic stop dates on antibiotic prescriptions. In this chapter we review the aims of antibiotic policies, the methods for policy implementation and, finally, the evidence that policies achieve their aims.

Stimuli for the introduction of antibiotic policies

Many of the stimuli for antibiotic policies are common to policies for other drug groups, but some are unique to antibiotics (Table 12.1). The general advantages of defining a core list of drugs which are used regularly have been

Table 12.1 General and specific advantages of an antibiotic policy

Category	Benefits
Knowledge	*General* Promotes awareness of benefits, risks and cost of prescribing. Facilitates educational and training programmes within the health care setting. Reduces the impact of aggressive marketing by the pharmaceutical industry. Encourages rational choice between drugs based on analysis of pharmacology, clinical effectiveness, safety and cost *Specific to antimicrobials* Provides education about local epidemiology of pathogens and their susceptibility to antimicrobials. Promotes awareness of the importance of infection control

Attitudes	*General*
	Acceptance by clinicians of the importance of setting standards of care and prescribing.
	Acceptance of peer review and audit of prescribing
	Specific to antimicrobials
	Recognition of the complex issues underlying antimicrobial chemotherapy.
	Recognition of the importance of the special expertise required for full evaluation of antimicrobial chemotherapy:
	    Diagnostic microbiology,
	    Epidemiology and infection control,
	    Clinical diagnosis and recognition of other diseases mimicking infection,
	    Pharmacokinetics and pharmacodynamics

Table 12.1 *Cont'd*

Category	Benefits
Behaviour	*General*
	Increased compliance with guidelines and treatment policies.
	Reduction of medical practice variation
	Specific to antimicrobials
	Improved liaison between clinicians, pharmacists, microbiologists and the infection control team
Outcome	*General*
	Improved efficiency of prescribing by increasing sensitivity (patients who can benefit receive treatment) and specificity (treatment is not prescribed to patients who will not benefit).
	Improved clinical outcome.
	Reduces medico-legal liability
	Specific to antimicrobials
	Limit emergence and spread of drug-resistant strains

recognized for many years by the World Health Organization (Hogerzeil 1995). The aim is to encourage rational prescribing, which is based on a knowledge of pharmacology, efficacy, safety and cost. Drug resistance amongst microbes is an unique stimulus to control of antibiotic prescribing (Cohen 1992, Neu 1992).

PRACTICAL ADVANTAGES OF LIMITING THE RANGE OF ANTIMICROBIALS PRESCRIBED

The prescription of an antimicrobial by a clinician has implications for nurses, pharmacists and microbiologists, all of whom will be involved in the preparation, administration and monitoring of the prescribed drug. Limiting the range of drugs used allows the team to become familiar with the necessary processes (Barber 1993). Many of the staff who take responsibility for these processes will rotate through several departments in the hospital or will provide cross-cover outside working hours. Having common policies within and between departments reduces the need for time-consuming re-training of staff as they move between clinical units. In the microbiology laboratory sensitivity testing of bacteria will clearly be facilitated by restricting the range of drugs prescribed, which has implications for the range of reagents which the laboratory must stock, the number of separate tests which must be carried out on each microbe and the range of procedures for which staff must be trained.

Providers of health care are increasingly being asked to provide evidence about quality assurance. Auditing practice is only possible if standards of care have been defined, and the narrower the range of drugs the easier it is to write and audit detailed standards of care. It is also likely that staff will find it easier to comply with policies which cover a limited range of drugs.

COST

Antibiotics account for 3–25% of all prescriptions, 2–21% of the total market value of drugs in a single country (Col & O'Connor 1987) and up to 50% of the drug budget in a hospital (Barriere 1985). New drugs are inevitably more expensive than old drugs, and new drugs will be heavily promoted by pharmaceutical companies. One of the aims of antibiotic policies is to encourage prescribers to continue to use older, more familiar drugs unless there are good reasons not to. Intravenous antibiotics are usually about 10-fold more expensive than equivalent oral formulations and intravenous administration requires additional consumables and staff time (Davey et al 1990). Policies which include specific recommendations about the route of administration may reduce costs considerably (Jewesson et al 1985, Quintiliani et al 1987, Smith 1988, Powers & Bingham 1990). Finally, limiting the range of drugs stocked allows the pharmacy to negotiate better prices for larger quantities of individual drugs and reduces the range of stock sitting on the pharmacy shelves.

QUALITY AND SAFETY OF PRESCRIBING

The importance of iatrogenic disease has been recognized and most countries now have national and local systems for monitoring drug safety. However, the major focus has been on drug safety and the identification of adverse drug reactions. Iatrogenic disease caused by avoidable prescribing errors is relatively difficult to study, but published data suggest that it is disturbingly common. For example, 47% of patients leaving a hospital emergency room in the USA had received a prescription for a new drug and 10% of these prescriptions introduced a potentially harmful drug interaction (Beers et al 1990). The risk of adverse

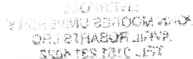

reactions is non-linearly related to the number of drugs prescribed; in other words, if the number of drugs which a patient is prescribed is increased from three to six, the risk of adverse effects is more than doubled (Smith et al 1966). Prescribing drugs which do not benefit the patients exposes them to unnecessary risk, and one study found that 26% of all adverse drug reactions in a hospital were caused by drugs which were prescribed unnecessarily (Ponge et al 1989). This is an alarming figure given that 8–10% of all admissions to a general medical ward are for adverse drug reactions and that 36% of inpatients will show some evidence of adverse drug reaction (Beers et al 1990). Unnecessary prescribing of antimicrobials carries additional risks for the patient (increased risk of superinfection with *Clostridium difficile*) and the environment (selection of drug resistant bacteria, e.g. *Enterococcus faecalis*). In general, administering drugs by the intravenous route is more hazardous than oral administration (Davey et al 1990, Parker & Davey 1992). Assessment of the quality of prescribing must therefore consider several elements, including the risks and benefits of introducing another drug and of intravenous versus oral administration.

In practice, it is very difficult to assess the appropriateness of an entire course of treatment, particularly in hospital. What is appropriate on one day may be inappropriate the next. This problem has been recognized in a practical system for reviewing each day of an antibiotic prescription and then computing the proportion of inappropriate days. The term 'inappropriate' covers a multitude of sins and encompasses both undertreatment and unnecessary overtreatment (Fig. 12.1). Inappropriate prescribing is associated with increased costs of care, although it is important to point out that prescribing errors may just be a marker for a generally poor quality of care (Dunagan et al 1989, 1991).

Monitoring of community prescribing is more difficult, especially where drugs are freely available over the counter (Kunin et al 1987, Obaseiki-Ebor et al 1987, Simon et al 1987, Thamlakitkul 1988, Lamikanra & Ndep 1989, Montefiore et al 1989, Urbina et al 1989). Unregulated availability of antibiotics from pharmacies in developing countries is a problem that has been discussed for several years. However, it is clear that both antibiotic prescribing and antibiotic resistance are growing in countries where antibiotics are only available by prescription from the doctor (Border 1994). Hogerzeil (1995) specifically identifies hospital antibiotic policies as a priority for education on rational prescribing in general, and recommends that more emphasis should be given to antibiotic policies in the training of undergraduates. There is no reason why the same policy of education should not be extended to prescribing in general practice (Wyatt et al 1990).

RESISTANCE

Other chapters in this book (see Chs. 3 and 9) describe the mechanisms and epidemiology of drug resistance. Control of antibiotic resistance has always been a primary stimulus to the development of antibiotic policies (Kunin et al 1973). The global escalation of antibiotic resistance might be seen as evidence that policies have failed – this question is addressed in more detail at the end of this chapter. At this stage we can conclude that the existence and increase in antibiotic resistance acts as a powerful stimulus to the development of antibiotic policies.

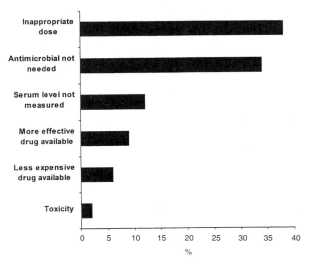

Fig. 12.1 *Reasons for classifying 1 day of antimicrobial chemotherapy in hospital as inappropriate. The data were obtained from 70 patients undergoing bone marrow transplantation who had a total of 749.5 days of treatment with an average of 1.824 antimicrobials per day, giving a product of 1367 antimicrobial days. Of these, 1188.5 (87%) were regarded as appropriate. The figure indicates the reasons for classifying the remaining days as inappropriate. (Figure drawn from data in Dunagan et al 1989.)*

Implementation of antibiotic policies

It is very easy to be too ambitious in setting aims for guidelines or policies. The first aim should be to change medical practice (Mant 1992), which may have a variety of secondary aims (e.g. reducing drug costs, improving quality of prescribing, limiting drug resistance). The success of a policy at achieving these secondary aims cannot be assessed unless it has achieved or maintained a specified standard of

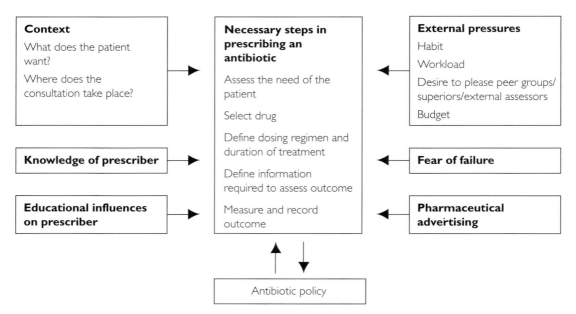

Fig. 12.2 *Influences on antibiotic prescribing. Ideally, antibiotic policies should inform all of the steps in prescribing and respond to information about the outcome of prescribing.*

practice. Ideally, antibiotic policies should recognize the complex process of prescribing an antibiotic (Fig. 12.2). Policies could address any or all of the steps in prescribing but, however comprehensive or limited the policy, it is essential that information flows both ways. The policy will only truly succeed if the results of implementation are audited and the policy is adapted in response to the information collected. This two-way exchange of information can also be represented in the form of an audit cycle (Fig. 12.3). Figures 12.2 and 12.3 are intended to represent an ideal; the fact that we are not there yet is no excuse for failing to try to improve practice. There is no harm in having a vision of an ultimate goal, provided that it is underpinned by a set of clear, measurable, achievable objectives.

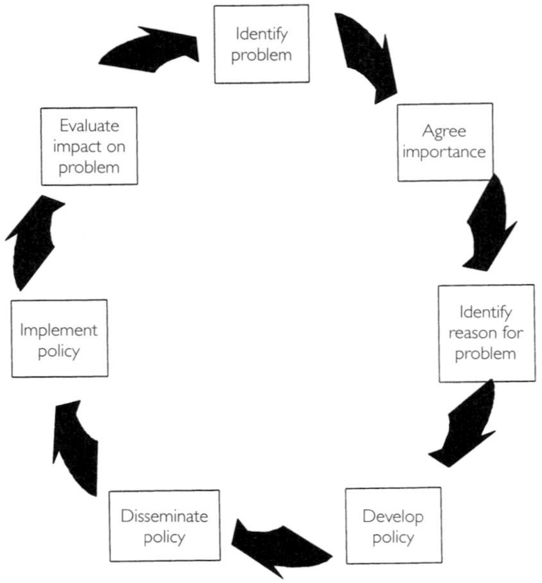

METHODS FOR IMPLEMENTATION OF ANTIBIOTIC POLICIES

These are summarized in Tables 12.2 and 12.3. Simply providing prescribers with educational information has been relatively unsuccessful (Table 12.2). Nonetheless, it is also relatively easy to perform. There have been very few comparative studies of different methods of implementation. Some papers describe a stepwise increase in effort to achieve a set goal (Feely et al 1990), but there have been few controlled trials (Avorn & Soumerai 1983, Schaffner et al 1983, Fowkes et al 1986, Cockburn et al 1992) and two papers cover other therapeutic areas (Fowkes et al 1986, Cockburn et al 1992). Nonetheless, it is worth looking beyond the antimicrobial literature to find alternative strategies which might be applied to implementation of antibiotic policies (Mugford et al 1991). The use of a

Fig. 12.3 *The audit cycle adapted to antimicrobial therapy.*

Table 12.2 *Examples of re-education and persuasive strategies used in controlling antibiotic usage. Educational strategies provide general advice, and persuasive strategies target specific topics, but both rely on mailed information rather than personal discussion, and neither strategy is restrictive*

Target	Strategy	Outcome	Reference
Re-education strategies			
Reduce use of specific drug	Mailed information	Transient effect, unsuccessful	Avorn & Soumerai 1983
Substitution of specific drugs	Drug bulletin	Successful	Fendler et al 1984
Compliance with formulary	Issuing formulary without feedback	Unsuccessful	Feely et al 1990
Persuasive strategies			
Reduction in costs of intravenous antibiotics	Feedback of costs to individual with peer comparison	Unsuccessful	Parrino 1989
Promote use of cheaper alternative agents	Educational advertising campaign using posters	Successful	Harvey et al 1986
Improve antibiotic dosing for parenteral antibiotics	Structured educational order form	Successful	Avorn & Soumerai 1983
Reduction in intravenous antibiotic costs	Information about cost added to microbiology form	Successful	Rubinstein et al 1988
Reduction in intravenous antibiotic costs	Guidelines for switching from intravenous to oral dosing	Successful	Quintiliani et al 1987

Table 12.3 *Facilitative and restrictive strategies used to control antibiotic usage. Facilitative strategies rely on regular feedback of information to prescribers about their own practice in comparison with peers, and usually involves personal communication as well as mailed information, but compliance with the policy remains voluntary. Power or restrictive strategies have a compulsory element*

Target	Strategy	Outcome	Reference
Facilitative strategies			
Substitution of specific drugs	Computerized feedback of potential cost savings	Successful	Evans et al 1986
Reduce use of specific drugs	Mailed information with feedback at interview	Successful	Avorn et al 1988
	Academic detailing	Successful	Avorn & Soumerai 1983
Compliance with formulary	Regular feedback to individual prescribers	Successful	Feely et al 1990
Reduce costs of surgical prophylaxis	Educational marketing	Successful	Landgren et al 1988
Identification of educational needs for 10 most commonly prescribed drugs	Individual tailored instruction packets	Successful	Manning et al 1986
Power or restrictive strategies			
Controlled use of expensive broad-spectrum parenteral drugs	Automatic stop orders for specific drugs	Successful	Marr et al 1988
	Prior approval of ID/microbiologist	Successful	Marr et al 1988
	Required ID consultation prior to prescription	Successful	Marr et al 1988
	Written justification by clinician	Transiently successful	McGowan & Findland 1974
Prescribing of injectable antibiotics	Guidelines posted to non-complying doctors and reimbursement denied for non-compliance	Successful	Brook & Williams 1976

personal approach directed at specific prescribers is generally the most effective strategy, a fact long known to the drug industry (Fowkes et al 1986, Cockburn et al 1992, Mant 1992). One of the most important steps in the audit cycle is to agree on the importance of the problem which is being audited. If this is achieved it becomes much easier to achieve a change in practice, otherwise audit may only change the practice of the auditors (Anderson et al 1988). Finally, as in most areas of medicine, it is not necessarily better to use the most complex and difficult strategy to achieve a change. Issuing educational information can work (Friis et al 1991, Kreling & Mott 1993).

WHO DEVELOPS THE POLICY?

The answer to this question is crucial to the success of the policy (Grimshaw & Russell 1994). Any set of guidelines can be developed by internal groups (composed entirely of the clinicians who will use them), intermediate groups (including some clinicians who will use them), or external groups (none of whom will use them) (Grimshaw & Russell 1993). Antibiotic policies should be developed by intermediate groups including senior clinicians who will use the policy as this will create an atmosphere of ownership of the policy, thereby facilitating compliance amongst all staff. For example, Putnam and Curry (1985) reported a greater increase in compliance when Canadian family physicians developed their own guidelines for five common conditions than when they received guidelines developed by others. The advocates of externally (national) developed guidelines indicate some evidence that they are being widely accepted (Gould 1990), especially in developing countries (Hogerzeil et al 1989). Nonetheless, comparative studies show the added advantage of involving representatives of the target audience in the design, implementation and review of policies (Fowkes et al 1986).

HOW IS THE POLICY PRESENTED?

The way in which an antibiotic policy is presented will determine how well it is accepted. It may be preferable to develop guidelines as opposed to 'policy' (from the Greek word for 'to police'), which may be seen as too dictatorial and inflexible. Algorithmic styles are often perceived by doctors to be too complex and lacking in flexibility (Institute of Medicine 1992). The need to be both practical and comprehensive can often be achieved by having a short summary of principal recommendations which can be consulted in clinical practice, underpinned by detailed documentation about the process of guideline development and the scientific basis (Grimshaw & Russell, 1994).

IS THE EFFECT OF THE POLICY SUSTAINED?

Feedback of information to prescribers appears to be particularly important for maintaining a change in practice. Feely et al (1990) examined the impact of the introduction of a hospital formulary with an intensive prescribing feedback programme over 1 year. Prescribing habits were monitored for a further year, but feedback was discontinued. In the year in which the intervention occurred generic prescribing rose by 50%: inappropriate prescribing and the overall use of third-generation cephalosporins fell and drug costs remained static against a projected increase for that year. During the next year, when no form of feedback intervention took place, previous gains were eroded and drug costs rose. The impact of different strategies on implementing and maintaining guidelines has not been widely subjected to scientific scrutiny. Probably the most rigorous was a multicentre trial of four strategies to reduce the use of routine, preoperative chest X-rays (Fowkes et al 1986). Establishing a utilization review group composed of radiologists and clinicians was the most successful strategy for changing practice. Moreover, this multidisciplinary review committee was the only strategy which maintained a change in practice for over a year, surviving a full change in junior medical staff.

HOW RESTRICTIVE SHOULD ANTIBIOTIC POLICIES BE?

Simple methods for controlling antibiotic prescribing include restricting access to the formulary and not allowing prescription outside the formulary list. These strategies are perceived as dictatorial or punitive and are likely to be less appealing to clinicians (Murray et al 1988). In health-care systems where there is reimbursement for medical costs, one such strategy has proved to be successful. Brook & Williams (1976) observed a dramatic reduction in the prescription of injectable antibiotics when payment was denied for claims not complying with guidelines. Whether these punitive methods should be used to implement policies is a moot point. Woolf (1993) recently acknowledged that practice guidelines achieve their greatest good by expanding medical knowledge, which may not be achieved by punitive measures. Nevertheless, he adds that there must be some rationale behind implementing guidelines of different qualities, and outlined a model for guideline enforcement. In essence, under this model, guidelines that define optimal care with certainty would be suitable for enforcement. Other guidelines, such as educational programmes that promote a change in behaviour, which have some scientific support but do not necessarily define all options would be suitable for less aggressive enforcement. As an example of this approach, we have been developing policies for surgical prophylaxis in Tayside, Scotland. Operations were divided into three categories: antibiotic prophylaxis mandatory, desirable and not indicated. The mandatory category included colorectal and joint-replacement surgery, for which several randomized controlled trials have shown that prophylaxis reduces mortality or long-term morbidity (Baum et al 1981, Kaiser 1994, Nichols 1994). In this category the evidence in favour of prophylaxis is so strong that it should be enforced and failure to administer prophylaxis correctly should be investigated. The remaining categories included operations such as biliary surgery, for which it may still be reasonable to restrict prophylaxis to defined high-risk groups (prophylaxis desirable), and operations such as hernia repair for which the majority of UK surgeons do not use prophylaxis (prophylaxis not indicated). In both these latter categories, individual clinicians are likely to have different views about the available evidence. The first aim is to get surgeons to define their own practice, this can then be compared, discussed or audited.

HOW SHOULD COMPLIANCE WITH POLICIES BE MONITORED?

Hospitals fortunate enough to have sophisticated information systems may be able to use these to monitor compliance with policies (Horn & Opal 1992). However, this is the exception rather than the rule. Less sophisticated information systems can still provide valuable information, but there is often no substitute for collection of data by hand (Cooke et al 1983, Fish et al 1992). This is not necessarily as daunting as it may seem – a 1-day prevalence survey of an entire hospital can be achieved in a few hours (Cooke et al 1983). In Tayside, we have involved a variety of staff in auditing policies, including trainee nurses, pharmacists, doctors and medical students. Audit is an educational activity, the process of data collection and analysis providing a valuable learning opportunity (Hogerzeil 1995). As with implementation, there are few studies comparing more than one method for monitoring compliance

with policies (Kreling & Mott 1993) and the published data do not allow conclusions to be drawn about the relative merits of different methods.

Including more than just drug choice in an antibiotic policy

Most antibiotic policies focus on which drug to prescribe, but there are several other important considerations (route of administration, dose, duration of treatment). Audits of the surgical prophylaxis policy at Ninewells Hospital, Dundee, Scotland, have shown good compliance with the recommended drug but not with other standards specified in the policy (Table 12.4). The policy recommends administration of a second dose of antibiotic in theatre if the operation lasts more than 2 h, but both audits showed that this was not happening at all. Clearly, surgeons need to be convinced about this aspect of the policy.

Perhaps the most important step in prescribing is the assessment of need for any antibiotic at all (see Fig. 12.2). In hospital, the decision to prescribe is often made by junior staff faced with a seriously ill patient and little or no results of investigation. It is unrealistic, and may well be undesirable, to try to prevent antibiotic prescribing under these circumstances. An alternative method for limiting unnecessary antimicrobial prescribing is to recommend that senior staff review the need for prescription 48–72 h after initiation. At this time laboratory information will be available, a non-infectious cause for the patient's symptoms may have been identified and the antibiotic can be stopped. This approach has led to a sustained reduction in antibiotic prescribing on one neonatal intensive care unit (Isaacs et al 1987). Outside intensive care units patient's with suspected infection will be less severely ill and the clinical evidence supporting prescription may be minimal (Moss et al 1981a–c). Under these circumstances it may be realistic to educate hospital doctors not to prescribe antibiotics at all. In the community, regular review of the patient's need for antibiotic is unrealistic. In this situation, development of decision rules may help to define the probability of bacterial infection and hence the risks and benefits of antibiotic prescription (Cebul

Table 12.4 *Results of audit of compliance with a policy for antibiotic prophylaxis of general surgery at Ninewells Hospital**

Audit criterion	1992 Audit (n = 108)	1993 Audit (n = 117)
Prophylaxis given	84 (78%)	92 (79%)
Correct drug	66/84 (79%)	66/92 (72%)
Correct timing (at induction of anaesthesia)	72/84 (86%)	91/92 (99%)
Prophylactic doses written in the once only section of the prescribing kardex	45/84 (54%)	86/92 (93%)
Additional doses given in theatre for operative procedures which lasted >2 h	0/58	0/31

* The audits were conducted by Gillian Malloch (pharmacist) and Ann Marie Skinner (medical student). *n*, Number of operations.

& Poses 1986, Pandey et al 1991). The number of prescriptions for antibiotics is rising steadily in the community and in hospital (Border 1994). We should all spend less time talking about which antibiotic to use and more time debating the need for any antibiotic at all. Bacteraemia provides a manageable focus for attention. Our own experience is very similar to previously published audits (Dunagan et al 1989, Gransden et al 1990, Wilkins et al 1991, Horn & Opal 1992). Review of patients with bacteraemia identifies patients who are being overtreated, including those with contaminated blood cultures. However, we regularly identify patients with significant bacteraemia who are receiving no antibiotic treatment at all.

Do antibiotic policies achieve their secondary aims?

EVIDENCE THAT ANTIBIOTIC POLICIES REDUCE HEALTH-CARE COSTS

Many published examples show that implementation of policies reduces antibiotic costs, in hospital (Dzierba et al 1986, Briceland et al 1988, Coleman et al 1991, Wilson et al 1991) or in the community (Friis et al 1989, Panton 1993). However, these studies suffer from two limitations: (1) they do not quantify the cost of designing, implementing and monitoring the policy, which may be considerable (Harvey et al 1986, Landgren et al 1988); and (2) monitoring the effects of the policy is generally restricted to antibiotic costs alone. Even inclusion of other drug costs may show that prescribing a cheaper, less-effective antibiotic can increase total drug costs due to increased prescription of drugs for symptomatic relief (Scott et al 1993). When treatment failure results in hospitalization, prescription of cheaper but less-effective drugs may dramatically increase health-care costs (Roach et al 1990). A recent review applied criteria for assessment of cost-effectiveness to published literature dealing with the reduction of prescribing cost (Kreling & Mott 1993). An adequate cost-effectiveness analysis was defined as one that compared more than one method for measuring the patterns of drug use, and/or efforts to alter drug use. Ideally, the outcomes of the interventions should be based on an analysis of the costs of the review or intervention methods employed, with a focus on efficiency (Kreling & Mott 1993). This review identified publications reporting 14 single studies and 34 continuing programmes for drug-utilization review. Of these, only three (21%) single studies and five (15%) programmes had systematically compared two or more methods for intervention or data collection. Even in these comparative

studies it was difficult to generalize the results because the programmes addressed different areas of prescribing and the end-point was usually the number of inappropriate prescriptions avoided. Clearly, the value of this outcome depends on the costs incurred by an inappropriate prescription. Probably the best method for comparing studies is to provide data on the financial cost of the review process (including implementation plus data collection) and estimates of the benefit resulting from a reduction of inappropriate prescribing (Table 12.5). These results generally show that the costs of drug-utilization review are offset by the savings achieved. However, the wide range of cost/benefit ratios should not be interpreted as showing that some methods are inherently superior to others, since the ratios are as much a function of the cost of inappropriate prescribing as of the effectiveness of methods for influencing prescribing. None of the studies considered the situation from the perspective of patients, which may well give different results, particularly if the primary aim of the programme is to reduce prescribing costs. The authors conclude that it is clear that the interventions described often do result in a change in prescribing behaviour, but it is unclear whether particular interventions are more cost-effective than others. Moreover, very few studies estimate the impact of interventions on total health-care costs, let alone on health outcomes (Kreling & Mott 1993). The implication is that, before embarking on a drug-utilization review it is important to estimate the costs of the programme and to compare these with the estimated benefits. Future research studies should provide a more comprehensive description of the costs and benefits of drug-utilization review.

DO ANTIBIOTIC POLICIES IMPROVE THE QUALITY OF PRESCRIBING?

Drugs with known dose-related side-effects may require therapeutic-drug monitoring to ensure that concentrations are within a therapeutic range, but standards of monitoring in clinical practice are liable to be well below those reported in clinical trials (Schiff et al 1991). Implementation of a policy and education programme has been shown to improve both the timing of serum sampling and the action taken in response to information about serum drug concentration (D'Angio et al 1990). Audit of aminoglycoside prescribing in our hospitals revealed major problems with gentamicin prescribing and monitoring. Of 255 patients in Dundee teaching hospitals prescribed gentamicin in 1990–1991, 82 (32%) did not have any measurement of serum concentration and 139 (80%) of the 173 remaining patients had been prescribed an inadequate dose, so that only 34 (13%) could be said to be receiving optimum treatment. These data were depressingly similar to other recent audits

Table 12.5 *Benefit/cost ratios for studies of drug utilization review which provide data about both elements. (Adapted from Kreling & Mott 1993.)*

Target for utilization review	Cost of intervention and monitoring to measure change in practice	Estimated savings achieved by the review programme	Benefit/cost ratio	Reference
Cephalexin, detropropoxyphene and vasodilators	$100 per physician per year	$19 740 decrease in prescribing costs in 1 year (average decrease $105 per physician per year)	1 : 1	Avorn & Soumerai 1983
Antibiotics for sore throat	$50 per month ($4200 for a total of 7 years)	$10 560 per case of acute rheumatic fever avoided	2.5 : 1	Barnett et al 1978
Antibiotics for sore throat	$1 per prescription audited	Approximate $1 reduction in average charges per patient	1 : 1	Grimm et al 1975
All drugs in a hospital-affiliated clinic	$924 over 9 months ($153 for set-up and $75 per month running cost)	Estimated savings in the final month of the programme $3259	44 : 1 in the final month (3259/75)	Hershey et al 1986
Prescription of H_2 antagonists and sucralfate for peptic ulcers	$3400 in the first year of the programme; $1040 per subsequent year	$14 600 saved on drug costs in the first year	4.3:1 in the first year	Mead & McGahn 1988
All drugs in a geriatric clinic	$2250 for 6 months	$6122 saved on drug costs in 6 months	2.7 : 1	Phillips & Carr-Lopez 1990
Non steroidal anti-inflammatory drugs	$1.30 per physician per year (total cost $10 775 in 6 months)	$0.45 reduction in drug costs per physician per year	0.35:1	Stergachis et al 1987

carried out in London (Shrimpton et al 1993) and in Sydney, Australia (Li et al 1989). Believing that the situation might be improved by once-daily dosing of aminoglycosides (Parker & Davey 1993) we established a multidisciplinary group to design and implement a policy based on experience at Hartford Hospital, Connecticut (Nicolau et al 1995). Launch of this policy in August 1994 was preceded by establishing a training programme for clinical pharmacists. In the 6 months since the launch of the new policy we have audited 66 patients, of whom 53 (80%) had correct dosing and monitoring, a marked improvement on the results of the previous audit.

Our audit of aminoglycoside prescribing also revealed examples of both overtreatment and undertreatment. For example, patients who were capable of taking oral medication and who were clinically stable continued to receive high-dose intravenous therapy unnecessarily, whereas patients with clinical signs of sepsis went untreated or received inappropriately low doses of oral drugs. There is published evidence that both these problems can be improved by design and implementation of policies (Huff et al 1988, Wilkins et al 1991, Allen et al 1992, Horn & Opal 1992) and we have used these as a basis for implementing local policies which are now being audited.

Other examples of the audit cycle applied to improve the quality of antimicrobial chemotherapy include a reduction in

the prescribing of tetracyclines to children (Kumana et al 1993) and training of junior medical staff in the safe administration of intravenous antibiotics (Cheng et al 1992). In all these cases the key to success has been the identification of a problem which prescribers agree to be important followed by identification of a practical method for improving practice.

DO ANTIBIOTIC POLICIES CONTROL RESISTANCE?

There is clearly a crude relationship between the overall use of antibiotics and the development of bacterial resistance (Levy et al 1988, Courcol et al 1989, Cohen 1992, Neu 1992), the question is whether or not antibiotic policies can limit the development of resistance. The literature contains many examples of the control of outbreaks of infection with drug-resistant bacteria which may be attributed to antibiotic-control measures (Table 12.6). However, it has been very difficult to eliminate confounding variables, such as other infection-control measures or a change in patient case mix (Table 12.6). The methodology of earlier studies was crude, in terms of both microbiology and epidemiology. More recent studies have used molecular techniques for precise definition of cross-

Table 12.6 *Evidence in support of a link between antimicrobial prescribing and the prevalence of drug-resistant strains of bacteria, with some of the potential confounding variables which could mean that it is wrong to interpret the association as simple cause and effect. (For more detailed analysis see McGowan (1983) and Richard et al (1994a, b).)*

Supporting evidence	Potential confounding variables
In the pre-antibiotic era pneumococci and other streptococci were common causes of nosocomial infection. In the antibiotic era they have been replaced by organisms such as *Pseudomonas aeruginosa*. In general, antimicrobial resistance is more prevalent in bacterial strains causing nosocomial infection than in organisms from community-acquired cases	There have been many other changes which may account for these observations (case mix, new medical technology)
Patients with resistant organisms are more likely to have received prior antibiotic therapy than are controls	Antibiotic use may just be a marker for patients who are more ill.
Concurrent variation between antimicrobial utilization and resistance has been noted for both increases and decreases in these two factors	Other reports document decreased prevalence of antimicrobial resistance without a corresponding decrease in antimicrobial use. It is difficult to separate control of antimicrobial prescribing from other infection-control measures which are used in the context of an outbreak of nosocomial infection with drug-resistant strains
There is a dose–response relationship between antimicrobial prescribing and the probability of infection with drug-resistant strains which operates at several different levels (individual patient, ward unit, hospital, country)	The association may be because of differences in underlying disease and/or aspects of management other than antimicrobial therapy
Interruption of transmission of resistant organisms (e.g. barrier isolation techniques) and control of antimicrobial prescribing are the only two measures which have been shown to be successful in limiting the prevalence of drug resistant bacteria.	It is virtually impossible to separate the effects of these two measures, which are almost always implemented concurrently

infection and more rigorous case control to minimize the impact of confounding variables (Richard et al 1994a, b). The association between prescribing and resistance is strengthened if the relationship can be demonstrated across a range of institutions. A study conducted in 18 centres in the USA identified a significant correlation between ceftazidime prescribing in intensive care units and the prevalence of ceftazidime-resistant *Enterobacter cloacae* (Ballow & Schentag 1992). Interestingly, one outbreak of ceftazidime-resistant *Pseudomonas aeruginosa* was successfully controlled by increasing the daily dose of ceftazidime in the intensive care unit treatment policy for pneumonia caused by this organism (Richard et al 1994b). Antibiotic control implies a reduction in antibiotic treatment, but this example shows that a thorough review of antibiotic treatment may well result in a recommendation for increased treatment.

The previous examples dealt with the difficulty of proving that antibiotic policies help to resolve a problem of resistance which has already emerged. It is even more difficult to prove that policies prevent the development of resistance. It is clear that antibiotic usage does increase the prevalence of drug-resistant bacteria in the normal human flora (Levy et al 1988, London et al 1994) and that this acts as a reservoir of resistant bacteria (Shanahan et al 1994). As we have already noted, most antibiotic policies are concerned with which antibiotic is prescribed (Bendall et al 1986) and it is more likely that development of

resistance will be contained by policies which also try to limit unnecessary prescribing of antibiotics. Although it is encouraging that hospitals which enforce policies also report low resistance rates (Sturm 1990), it is impossible to prove cause and effect. It is unrealistic to expect policies completely to prevent the development of drug resistance, because policies have a limited sphere of influence and reservoirs of resistant bacteria will inevitably arise elsewhere. For example, there is ample evidence of community reservoirs of resistance arising from prescribing of antibiotics in general medical or veterinary practice (Shanahan et al 1994) and, consequently, tight control of antibiotic prescribing in hospitals cannot eliminate the risk of introducing drug-resistant bacteria.

In summary, there is limited evidence to show that antibiotic policies prevent the spread of bacterial resistance, but this is mainly because of the virtual impossibility of controlling for all the other factors which influence the development of resistance. Advocates of antibiotic policies should certainly not allow this uncertainty to be used as an argument against the implementation of policies. We hope that the evidence reviewed here shows that antibiotic policies can definitely improve the quality of prescribing and may be used to limit prescribing costs. Limiting superinfection and antibiotic resistance should be viewed as additional potential benefits; they are probably not realistic primary aims for most policies.

References

Allen B, Naismith N W, Manser A J, Moulds R F W 1992 A campaign to improve the timing of conversion from intravenous to oral administration of antibiotics. *Australian Journal of Hospital Pharmacy* 22 (6): 434–439

Anderson C M, Chambers S, Clamp M et al 1988 Can audit improve patient care? Effects of studying use of digoxin in general practice. *British Medical Journal* 297: 113–114

Avorn J, Soumerai S B 1983 Improving drug-therapy decisions through educational outreach. A randomized controlled trial of academically based 'detailing'. *New England Journal of Medicine* 308: 1457–1463

Avorn J, Soumerai S B, Taylor W, Wessels M R, Janousek J, Weiner M 1988 Reduction of incorrect antibiotic dosing through a structured educational order form. *Archives of Internal Medicine* 148: 1720–1724.

Ballow C H, Schentag J J 1992 Trends in antibiotic utilization and bacterial resistance: report of the National Nosocomial Resistance Surveillance Group. *Diagnostic Microbiology and Infectious Disease* 15: 37S–42S

Barber N 1993 Improving quality of drug use through hospital directorates. *Quality in Health Care* 2: 3–4

Barnett G O, Winickoff R, Dorsey J L, Morgan M M, Lurie R S 1978 Quality assurance through automated monitoring and concurrent feedback using a computer based medical information system. *Medical Care* 16: 962–970

Barriere S L 1985 Cost containment of antimicrobial therapy. *Drug Intelligence and Clinical Pharmacy, The Annals of Pharmacotherapy* 19: 278–281

Baum M L, Anish D S, Chalmer T C, Sacks H S, Smith H, Fagerstrom R M 1981 A survey of clinical trials of antibiotic prophylaxis in colon surgery: evidence against further use of no-treatment controls. *New England Journal of Medicine* 305: 795–799

Beers M H, Storrie M, Lee G 1990 Potential adverse drug interactions in the emergency room. *Annals of Internal Medicine* 112: 61–64

Bendall M J, Ebrahim S, Finch R G, Slack R C, Towner K J 1986 The effect of an antibiotic policy on bacterial resistance in patients in geriatric medical wards. *Quarterly Journal of Medicine* 60: 849–854

Border P 1994 Diseases fighting back – the growing resistance of TB and other bacterial diseases to treatment. London, Parliamentary Office of Science and Technology, p 1–38

Briceland L L, Nightingale C H, Quintiliani R, Cooper B W 1988 Multidisciplinary cost-containment program promoting less frequent administration of injectable mezlocillin. *American Journal of Hospital Pharmacy* 45: 1082–1085

Brook R H, Williams K N 1976 Effect of medical care review on use of injections: a study of the New Mexico Experimental Care Review Organisation. *Annals of Internal Medicine* 85: 509–515

Cebul R D, Poses R M 1986 The comparative cost-effectiveness of statistical decision rules and experienced physicians in pharyngitis management. *Journal of the American Medical Association* 256: 3353–3357

Cheng E Y, Nimphius N, Hennen C R 1992 Training in antibiotic administration. *Anaesthesia and Analgesia* 74: 619–620

Cockburn J, Ruth D, Silagy C et al 1992 Randomised trial of three approaches for marketing smoking cessation programmes to Australian general practitioners. *British Medical Journal* 304: 691–695

Cohen M L 1992 Epidemiology of drug resistance: implications for a post-antimicrobial era. *Science* 257: 1050–1055

Col N F, O'Connor R W 1987 Estimating worldwide current antibiotic usage: report of Task Force 1. *Reviews of Infectious Diseases* 9 (suppl 3): S232–S243

Coleman R W, Rodoni L C, Kaubisch S, Granzella N B, O'Hanley P D 1991 Cost-effectiveness of prospective and continuous parenteral antibiotic control: experience at the Palo Alto Veterans Affairs Medical Center from 1987–1989. *American Journal of Medicine* 90: 439–444

Cooke D M, Salter A J, Phillips I 1983 The impact of antibiotic policy on prescribing in a London teaching hospital. A one-day prevalence survey as an indicator of antibiotic use. *Journal of Antimicrobial Chemotherapy* 11: 447–453

Courcol R J, Pinkas M, Martin G R 1989 A seven year survey of antibiotic susceptibility and its relationship with usage. *Journal of Antimicrobial Chemotherapy* 23: 441–451

D'Angio R G, Stevenson J G, Lively B T, Morgan J E 1990 Therapeutic drug monitoring: improved performance through educational intervention. *Drug Monitoring* 12: 173–181

Davey P, Dodd T, Kerr S, Malek M 1990 Audit of iv antibiotic administration. *Pharmaceutical Journal* June 30: 793–796

Dunagan W C, Woodward R S, Medoff G et al 1989 Antimicrobial misuse in patients with positive blood cultures. *American Journal of Medicine* 87: 253–259

Dunagan W C, Woodward R S, Medoff G et al 1991 Antibiotic misuse in two clinical situations: Positive blood culture and administration of aminoglycosides. *Reviews of Infectious Diseases* 13: 405–412

Dzierba S H, Reilly R T, Caselnova D A 1986 Cost savings achieved through cephalosporin use review and restriction. *American Journal of Hospital Pharmacy* 43: 2194–2197

Evans R S, Larsen R A, Burke J P et al 1986 Computer surveillance of hospital acquired infections and antibiotic use. *Journal of the American Medical Association* 256: 1007–1011

Feely J, Chan R, Cocoman L, Mulpeter K, O'Commor P 1990 Hospital formularies: need for continuous intervention. *British Medical Journal* 300: 28–30

Fendler K J, Gumbhir A K, Sall K 1984 The impact of drug bulletins on physician prescribing habits in a health maintenance organisation. *Drug Intelligence and Clinical Pharmacy* 300: 28–30

Fish C A, Kirking D M, Martin J M 1992 Information systems for evaluating the quality of prescribing. *Annals of Pharmacotherapy* 26: 392–398

Fowkes F G R, Evans K T, Hartley G et al 1986 Multicentre trial of four strategies to reduce use of a radiological test. *The Lancet* i: 367–369

Friis H, Bro F, Mabeck C E, Vejlsgaard R 1991 Changes in prescription of antibiotics in general practice in relation to different strategies for drug information. *Danish Medical Bulletin* 38 (4): 380–382

Gould I M 1990 Current prophylaxis and prevention of infective endocarditis. *British Dental Journal* 168: 409–410

Gransden W R, Eykyn S J, Phillips I, Rowe B 1990 Bacteraemia due to *Escherichia coli*: a study of 861 episodes. *Reviews of Infectious Diseases* 12: 1008–1018

Grimm R H, Shimoni K, Harlan W R, Estes E H 1975 Evaluation of patient care protocol use by various providers. *New England Journal of Medicine* 292: 507–511

Grimshaw J M, Russell I T 1993 Achieving health gain through clinical guidelines. I: Developing scientifically valid guidelines. *Quality in Health Care* 2: 243–248

Grimshaw J M, Russell I T 1994 Achieving health gain through clinical guidelines. II: Ensuring guidelines change medical practice. *Quality in Health Care* 3 (1): 45–52

Harvey K J, Stewart R, Hemming M, Naismith N, Moulds R F W 1986 Educational antibiotic advertising. *The Medical Journal of Australia* 145: 28–32

Hershey C O, Porter D K, Breslau D, Cohen D I 1986 Influence of simple computerized feedback on prescription charges in an ambulatory clinic: a randomized clinical trial. *Medical Care* 24: 472–481

Hogerzeil H V 1995 Promoting rational prescribing: an international perspective. *British Journal of Clinical Pharmacology* 39: 1–6

Hogerzeil H V, Sallami A O, Walker G J A, Fernando G 1989 Impact of an essential drugs programme on availability and rational use of drugs. *The Lancet* i: 141–142

Horn D L, Opal S M 1992 Computerized clinical practice guidelines for review of antibiotic therapy for bacteremia. *Infectious Diseases in Clinical Practice* 1: 169–173

Huff J C, Bean B, Balfour H H et al 1988 Therapy of herpes zoster with oral acyclovir. *The American Journal of Medicine* 85 (suppl 2A): 84–89

Institute of Medicine 1992 In: Anon (ed) Guidelines for clinical practice: from development to use. National Academy Press, Washington, DC, p 248

Isaacs D, Wilkinson A R, Moxon E R 1987 Duration of antibiotic courses for neonates. *Archives of Disease in Childhood* 62: 727–728

Jewesson P J, Bachand R L, Bell G A, Ensom R J, Chow A W 1985 Quality of use of parenteral metronidazole therapy in a teaching hospital. *Canadian Medical Association Journal* 132: 785–789

Kaiser A B 1994 Antimicrobial prophylaxis in surgery. *New England Journal of Medicine* 315: 1129–1137

Kreling D H, Mott D A 1993 The cost effectiveness of drug utilisation review in an outpatient setting. *PharmacoEconomics* 4: 414–436

Kumana C R, Kou M, Wong B C Y, Lee P W, Li K Y 1993 Drug audit in Hong Kong with special reference to antibiotics. *Journal of the Hong Kong Medical Association* 45: 177–180

Kunin C M, Tupasi T, Craig W A 1973 Use of antibiotics: a brief exposition of the problem and some tentative solutions. *Annals of Internal Medicine* 79: 555–560

Kunin C M, Lipton H L, Tupasi T et al 1987 Social, behavioral, and practical factors affecting antibiotic use worldwide: report of Task Force 4. *Reviews of Infectious Diseases* 9 (suppl 3): S270–S285

Lamikanra A, Ndep R B 1989 Trimethoprim resistance in urinary tract pathogens in two Nigerian hospitals. *Journal of Antimicrobial Chemotherapy* 23: 151–154

Landgren F T, Harvey K J, Mashford M L, Moulds R F W, Guthrie B, Hemming M 1988 Changing antibiotic prescribing by educational marketing. *The Medical Journal of Australia* 149: 595–599

Levy S B, Marshall B, Schluederberg S, Rowse D, Davis J 1988 High frequency of antimicrobial resistance in human fecal flora. *Antimicrobial Agents and Chemotherapy* 32: 1801–1806

Li S C, Ioannides-Demos W, Spicer W J et al 1989 Prospective audit of aminoglycoside usage in a general hospital with assessments of clinical processes and adverse clinical outcomes. *The Medical Journal of Australia* 151: 224–232

London N, Nijsten R, Mertens P, Bogaard A v d, Stobberingh E 1994 Effect of antibiotic therapy on the antibiotic resistance of faecal *Escherichia coli* in patients attending general practitioners. *Journal of Antimicrobial Chemotherapy* 34: 239–246

McGowan J E, Findland M 1974 Usage of antibiotics in a general hospital: effect of requiring justification. *Journal of Infectious Diseases* 130: 165

McGowan J E J 1983 Antimicrobial resistance in Hospital Organisms and its relation to antibiotic use. *Reviews in Infectious Diseases* 5: 1033–1048

Manning P R, Lee P V, Clintworth W A, Denson T A, Oppenheimer P R, Gilman N J 1986 Changing prescribing practices through individual continuing education. *Journal of the American Medical Association* 256: 230–232

Mant D 1992 Facilitating prevention in primary care. *British Medical Journal* 304: 652–653

Marr J J, Moffet H L, Kunic C M 1988 Guidelines for improving the use of antimicrobial agents in hospitals: a statement by the Infectious Diseases Society of America. *Journal of Infectious Diseases* 157: 869–876

Mead R A, McGahn W F 1988 Use of histamine-2-receptor blocking agents and sucralfate in a health maintenance organization following continued clinical pharmacist intervention. *Drug Intelligence and Clinical Pharmacy, The Annals of Pharmacotherapy* 22: 466–469

Montefiore D, Rotimi V O, Adeyemi-Doro F A B 1989 The problem of bacterial resistance to antibiotics among strains isolated from hospital patients in Lagos and Ibadan, Nigeria. *Journal of Antimicrobial Chemotherapy* 23: 641–651

Moss F, McNicol M W, McSwiggan D A, Miller D L 1981a Survey of antibiotic prescribing in a district general hospital. I. Pattern of use. *The Lancet* ii: 349–352

Moss F, McNicol M W, McSwiggan D A, Miller D L 1981b Survey of antibiotic prescribing in a district general hospital. III. Urinary tract infection. *The Lancet* ii: 461–462

Moss F, McNicol M W, McSwiggan D A, Miller D L 1981c Survey of antibiotic prescribing in a district general hospital. II. Lower respiratory tract infection. *The Lancet* ii: 407–409

Mugford M, Banfield P, O'Hanlon M 1991 Effects of feedback of information on clinical practice: a review. *British Medical Journal* 303: 398–402

Murray M D, Kohler R B, McCarthy M C, Main J W 1988 Attitudes of those physicians concerning various antibiotic use control programs. *American Journal of Hospital Pharmacy* 45: 584–588

Neu H C 1992 The crisis in antibiotic resistance. *Science* 257: 1064–1073

Nichols R L 1994 Antibiotic prophylaxis in surgery. *Current Opinion in Infectious Diseases* 7: 647–652

Nicolau D P, Freeman C D, Bellivieau P P, Nightingale C H, Ross J W, Quintiliani R 1995 Experience with a once-daily aminoglycoside program administered to 2,184 adult patients. *Antimicrobial Agents and Chemotherapy* 39 (3): 650–655

Obaseiki-Ebor E E, Akerele J O, Ebea P O 1987 A survey of antibiotic outpatient prescribing and antibiotic self-medication. *Journal of Antimicrobial Chemotherapy* 20: 759–763

Pandey R M, Daulaire N M, Starbuck E S, Houston R M, McPherson K 1991 Reduction in total under-five mortality in western Nepal through community-based antimicrobial treatment of pneumonia. *The Lancet* 338: 993–997

Panton R 1993 FHSAs and prescribing. *British Medical Journal* 306: 310–314

Parker S E, Davey P G 1992 Pharmacoeconomics of intravenous drug administration. *PharmacoEconomics* 1: 103–115

Parker S E, Davey P G 1993 Practicalities of once-daily aminoglycoside dosing. *Journal of Antimicrobial Chemotherapy* 31: 4–8

Parrino T A 1989 The nonvalue of retrospective peer comparison feedback in containing hospital antibiotic costs. *American Journal of Medicine* 86: 442–448

Phillips S L, Carr-Lopez S M 1990 Impact of a pharmacist on medication discontinuation in a hospital-based geriatric clinic. *American Journal of Hospital Pharmacy* 47: 1075–1079

Ponge T, Cottin S, Fruneau P, Ponge A, Van Wassenhove L, Larousse C 1989 Iatrogenic disease. Prospective study, relation to drug consumption. *Therapie* 44 (1): 63–66

Powers T, Bingham D H 1990 Clinical and economic effect of ciprofloxacin as an alternative to injectable antimicrobial therapy. *American Journal of Public Health* 47: 1781–1784

Putnam R W, Curry L 1985 Impact of patient care appraisal on physician behaviour in the office setting. *Canadian Medical Association Journal* 132: 1025–1029

Quintiliani R, Cooper B W, Briceland L L, Nightingale C H 1987 Economic impact of streamlining antibiotic administration. *American Journal of Medicine* 82 (suppl 4A): 391–394

Richard P, Delangle M, Merrien D et al 1994a Fluoroquinolone use and fluoroquinolone resistance: is there an association? *Clinical Infectious Diseases* 19: 54–59

Richard P, Le Floch R, Chamoux C, Pannier M, Espaze E, Richet H 1994b *Pseudomonas aeruginosa* outbreak in a burn unit: role of antimicrobials in the emergence of multiply resistant strains. *Journal of Infectious Diseases* 170: 377–383

Roach A C, Kernodle D S, Kaiser A B 1990 Selecting cost-effective antimicrobial prophylaxis in surgery: are we getting what we pay for? *Drug Intelligence and Clinical Pharmacy, The Annals of Pharmacotherapy* 24: 183–185

Rubinstein E, Barzilai A, Segev S et al 1988 Antibiotic cost reduction by providing cost information. *European Journal of Clinical Pharmacology* 35: 269–272

Schaffner W, Ray W A, Federspiel C, Miller W O 1983 Improving antibiotic prescribing in office practice: a controlled trial of three educational methods. *Journal of the American Medical Association* 250: 1728–1732

Schiff G D, Hedge H K, LaCloche L, Hryhorczuk D O 1991 Inpatient theophylline toxicity: preventable factors. *Annals of Internal Medicine* 114: 748–753

Scott W G, Tilyard M W, Dovey S M, Cooper B, Scott H M 1993 Roxithromycin versus cefaclor in lower respiratory tract infection: a general practice pharmacoeconomic study. *PharmacoEconomics* 4: 122–130

Shanahan P M A, Thomson C J, Amyes S G B 1994 The global impact of antibiotic-resistant bacteria: their sources and reservoirs. *Reviews in Medical Microbiology* 5 (3): 174–182

Shrimpton S B, Milmoe M, Wilson A P R et al 1993 Audit of prescription and assay of aminoglycosides in a UK teaching hospital. *Journal of Antimicrobial Chemotherapy* 31: 599–606

Simon H J, Folb P I, Rocha H 1987 Policies, laws and regulations pertaining to antibiotics: report of Task Force 3. *Reviews of Infectious Diseases* 9 (suppl 3): S261–S269

Smith A L 1988 Oral antibiotic therapy for serious infections. *Annual Review of Medicine* 39: 171–184

Smith J W, Seidl L G, Cluff L E 1966 Studies on the epidemiology of adverse drug reactions V. Clinical factors influencing susceptibility. *Annals of Internal Medicine* 65: 629–640

Stergachis A, Fors M, Wagner E H, Sims D D, Penna P 1987 Effect of a clinical pharmacist on drug prescribing in a primary care clinic. *American Journal of Hospital Pharmacy* 77: 1518–1523

Sturm A W 1990 Effects of a restrictive antibiotic policy on clinical efficacy of antibiotics and susceptibility patterns of organisms. *European Journal of Clinical Microbiology and Infectious Diseases* 9: 381–389

Thamlakitkul V 1988 Antibiotic dispensing by drug store personnel in Bangkok, Thailand. *Journal of Antimicrobial Chemotherapy* 21: 125–131

Urbina R, Prado V, Canelo E 1989 Trimethoprim resistance in enterobacteria in Chile. *Journal of Antimicrobial Chemotherapy* 23: 143–149

Wilkins E G L, Hickey M M, Khoo S 1991 Northwick Park Infection Consultation Service. Part II. Contribution of the service to patient management: an analysis of results between September 1987 and July 1990. *Journal of Infection* 23: 57–63

Wilson J, Gordon A, French S, Aslam M 1991 The effectiveness of prescribers newsletters in influencing hospital drug expenditure. *Hospital Pharmacy Practice* May: 33–38

Woolf S H 1993 Practice guidelines: A new reality in medicine. *Archives Internal Medicine* 153: 2646–2655

Working Party of the British Society of Antimicrobial Chemotherapy 1994 Working Party report – hospital antibiotic control measures in the UK. *Journal of Antimicrobial Chemotherapy* 34: 21–42

Wyatt T D, Passmore C M, Morrow N C, Reilly P M 1990 Antibiotic prescribing: the need for a policy in general practice. *British Medical Journal* 300: 441–444

Aminoglycosides and aminocyclitols

I. Phillips and K. P. Shannon

Introduction

This large group of naturally occurring or semi-synthetic polycationic compounds includes a number of therapeutic importance. They are nearly all potent bactericidal agents that share the same general range of antibacterial activity, pharmacokinetic behaviour, a tendency to damage one or other branch of the eighth nerve and some tendency to cause renal damage, or at least to impair further the function of an already damaged kidney. The degree of toxicity varies; for some it is so great as to preclude systemic use.

The therapeutically important members of the group have aminosugars glycosidically linked to aminocyclitols. Consequently, they should properly be described as 'aminoglycosidic aminocyclitols', but the name 'aminoglycosides', which was used before the detailed structures of the compounds was known, is now too well established to be easily displaced by a more cumbersome title. At the extremes of the group are kasugamycin, which contains an aminoglycoside but no aminocyclitol and is hence a 'pure aminoglycoside', and spectinomycin, which contains an aminocyclitol but no aminoglycoside and is hence a 'pure aminocyclitol'.

The main agents fall into two major groups depending upon the aminocyclitol they contain. The first, small group, in which the aminocyclitol is streptidine, consists of streptomycin and its close relatives dihydrostreptomycin and bluensomycin, neither of which is used clinically. The second, larger group, in which the aminocyclitol is 2-deoxystreptamine, is subdivided into the neomycin group (in which there are substitutions at positions 4 and 5 of 2-deoxystreptamine) which includes neomycin and paromomycin, and the 4,6-substituted group which is itself subdivided into the kanamycin and gentamicin subgroups. The nomenclature of the aminoglycoside structure is illustrated by that of kanamycin B:

The carbon atoms in the 2-deoxystreptamine ring are labelled 1 to 6; those in the amino sugar substituted at position 4 are labelled 1' to 6' and those in the 6-position amino sugar 1" to 6". The kanamycin subgroup includes kanamycins, tobramycin and their semi-synthetic derivatives amikacin and dibekacin. The gentamicin group includes gentamicins, sissomicin and its semisynthetic derivative netilmicin.

Several of the natural agents consist of mixtures of closely related compounds. For example, there are numerous gentamicins, three kanamycins and two neomycins. Moreover, there are close relationships between some of the differently named compounds. For example, tobramycin is 3'-deoxykanamycin B and the substitution of an amino for a hydroxyl group in paromomycin I gives neomycin B. The chemical differences are particularly important in determining sensitivity of the compounds to inactivation by bacterial enzymes.

Antimicrobial activity

The activity of the more important aminoglycosides against

common pathogens is summarized in Table 13.1. To different degrees the aminoglycosides are active against *Staphylococcus aureus*, coagulase-negative staphylococci and *Corynebacterium* spp., but the activity against many other Gram-positive bacteria, including streptococci, is limited. As a group, they are widely active against the Enterobacteriaceae and other aerobic Gram-negative bacilli including, for some compounds, *Pseudomonas aeruginosa*. Several are active against *Mycobacterium tuberculosis* and some other mycobacteria. However, the number of investigations is small and there are some conflicting reports; for example, early studies suggested that gentamicin was active against *M. tuberculosis* in vitro, although not in vivo, but a later study found gentamicin, sissomicin and tobramycin to have very little activity against this organism. Aminoglycosides are not active against anaerobic bacteria.

Diffusion of such highly polar cationic compounds across the cell membrane is very limited and intracellular accumulation of the drugs is brought about by active transport, which occurs in three phases. There is an initial energy-independent binding of the compounds to the exterior of the cell, which is inhibited by Ca^{2+} and Mg^{2+} ions. This is followed by energy-dependent phase I (so called because it is abolished by treatments that inhibit energy metabolism) in which aminoglycosides associate with membrane transporters on the basis of their positive electrical charge and are driven across the cytoplasmic membrane by the electrical potential difference which is negative on the interior of the membrane. A faster rate of aminoglycoside uptake, energy-dependent phase II, starts after aminoglycosides have bound to ribosomes and seems to be an effect, rather than a cause, of their action on the cell. Aminoglycoside uptake is adversely affected by low pH and

Table 13.1 MICs (mg/l) of aminoglycosides for common pathogenic bacteria*

	Gentamicin	Netilmicin	Tobramycin	Amikacin	Kanamycin	Neomycin	Streptomycin	Spectinomycin
Staphylococcus aureus	0.25	0.25	0.25	1	1	0.5	4	64
Coagulase-negative staphylococci	0.03	0.03	0.03	0.25	0.5	0.06	2	32
Streptococcus pyogenes	4	4	16	32	32	16	8	32
Streptococcus pneumoniae	4	8	16	64	64	128	32	8
Enterococcus faecalis	16	8	16	128	64	32	128	64
Clostridium perfringens	R	R	R	R	R	R	R	R
Mycobacterium tuberculosis	>64		>64	1	8	0.5	0.5	
Mycobacterium avium/intracellulare	4			8	4		2	
Neisseria meningitidis	16	16	16	32	32	4		8
Neisseria gonorrhoeae	4	4	4	16	16	16	8	16
Haemophilus influenzae	0.5	0.5	1	1	1	2	2	4
Escherichia coli	0.5	0.5	1	2	4	1	8	8
Klebsiella spp.	0.5	0.5	0.5	2	2	1	4	16
Enterobacter spp.	0.5	0.5	0.5	2	2	1	4	16
Proteus mirabilis	1	1	1	4	4	4	16	32
Proteus vulgaris/Morganella morganii	0.5	0.5	0.5	2	1	1	4	32
Providencia stuartii	8	8	8	2	2	32	128	>128
Salmonella spp.	0.25	0.25	0.5	1	2	2	4	4
Shigella spp.	1	1	0.5	2	4	8	2	4
Serratia marcescens	0.25	0.5	1	1	1	1	2	8
Pseudomonas aeruginosa	2	4	0.5	4	64	8	32	>128
Stenotrophomonas maltophilia	1	8	2	8	>128	32	32	>128
Bacteroides spp.	R	R	R	R	R	R	R	R

*The values shown are median MICs (MIC_{50}). Resistance to each agent occurs in at least some strains of most organisms, so knowledge of the local prevalence of resistance is necessary. R indicates that all strains are resistant.

reduced oxygen tension. Consequently, activity of the drugs in vitro is reduced in acid media or anaerobic conditions and by the presence of divalent cations; the susceptibility of *Ps. aeruginosa* is particularly sensitive to the cation concentration. Because of the effects of pH on activity, it is hard to be sure that the relatively high minimum inhibitory concentrations (MICs) seen for organisms that require carbon dioxide truly reflects their degree of resistance.

Aminoglycosides are generally bactericidal in concentrations close to the MIC and the rate of killing increases directly with the concentration. They show bactericidal synergy with β-lactams and some other agents that act on the cell envelope, notably against organisms that owe their limited susceptibility to aminoglycosides to relatively poor uptake of the compounds.

Acquired resistance

Resistance in many organisms originally susceptible to the older compounds is now widespread, and resistance to the more recently introduced agents has increased. The geographical distribution of resistant strains is diverse, as confirmed by surveys that have shown resistance to be more prevalent in southern than in central or northern Europe. Marked changes have also occurred over the years. For example, resistance to streptomycin or kanamycin was fairly common by the mid-1970s in the UK, but resistance to gentamicin, tobramycin or amikacin was very rare. Since then the incidence of gentamicin resistance among Gram-negative bacilli increased until the mid-1980s; thereafter it generally declined. Many strains with plasmid-encoded extended-spectrum β-lactamases are also aminoglycoside resistant, so large outbreaks of infection with such strains may result in an increase in aminoglycoside resistance rates.

There are three mechanisms of resistance to aminoglycosides: alteration in the ribosomal binding of the drug; reduced uptake; and inactivation by specific aminoglycoside-modifying enzymes. Single step mutation, usually in the *rpsL* gene, to high resistance resulting from alteration of a single ribosomal protein occurs only to streptomycin in clinical isolates. Of the three mechanisms, that mediated by aminoglycoside-modifying enzymes is the most important because it is the most common and generally confers a higher degree of resistance than reduced uptake. The enzymes are usually, though not always, plasmid encoded and the resistances conferred are frequently transferable. This mechanism of resistance shares many features with β-lactamase production by organisms resistant to penicillins or cephalosporins in that the cells owe their survival to the inactivation of the agent to which they remain intrinsically susceptible and in that a considerable, and growing, number of enzymes have been identified from different bacterial species and strains.

Aminoglycoside-modifying enzymes

There are three classes of aminoglycoside-modifying enzyme, which differ in the nature of the sites modified: *N*-acetyltransferases (AAC) modify amino groups whereas *O*-phosphotransferases (APH) and *O*-nucleotidyltransferases (ANT) modify hydroxyl groups. *O*-Nucleotidyltransferases are also known as *O*-adenyltransferases, but this name is less appropriate since, although adenylated aminoglycoside is the major product, guanylate and inosinate can also be found. The sites of attack of these enzymes on gentamicin are as shown:

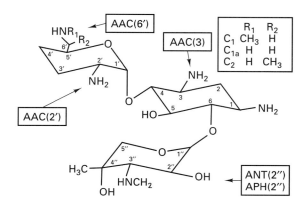

The position of the group attacked and the ring that carries it is indicated by the number of the enzyme: thus AAC(3) is the acetyltransferase that modifies the amino group in the 3-position on the central aminocyclitol ring; AAC(2') is the acetyltransferase that modifies the amino group in the 2-position on the 4-substituent ring; and ANT(2") and APH(2") modify the hydroxyl group at the 2-position on the 6-substituent ring.

Where two enzymes act at the same position, but differ in the aminoglycosides modified, they are distinguished by roman numerals. The most important differences occur with AAC(3) and AAC(6'). For example, all types of AAC(3) modify gentamicin; AAC(3)I modifies tobramycin so poorly that it does not confer resistance to it; AAC(3)II confers resistance to tobramycin and netilmicin as well as to gentamicin; AAC(3)III adds kanamycin and neomycin but loses netilmicin, and AAC(3)IV is one of the few enzymes to modify apramycin. Other AAC(3) enzymes have also been described. The widespread AAC(3)V has subsequently been recognized to be the same as AAC(3)II. The resistance of important 2-deoxystreptamine-containing aminoglycosides to the principle enzymes so far characterized is shown in Table 13.2. Various phosphotransferases and nucleotidyl-transferases modify streptomycin and its relatives (and sometimes also spectinomycin), but there is no crossover between the streptomycin and 2-deoxystreptamine groups in terms of sensitivity to aminoglycoside-modifying enzymes.

Table 13.2 *Range of activity of enzymes that modify 2-deoxystreptamine-containing aminoglycosides*

Enzyme	Modification of						
	Kanamycin A	Neomycin	Amikacin	Tobramycin	Gentamicin, sissomicin	Netilmicin	Apramycin
APH(3')I & II	+	+	–	0	0	0	0
APH(3')III & VI	+	+	+	0	0	0	0
APH(2")	+	0	–	+	+	–	0
ANT(4')(4")	+	+	+	+	0	0	0
ANT(2")	+	0	–	+	+	–	0
AAC(3)I	–	–	–	–	+	–	–
AAC(3)II	±	–	–	+	+	+	–
AAC(3)III	+	+	–	+	+	–	–
AAC(3)IV	±	+	–	+	+	+	+
AAC(2')	0	+	0	+	+	+	0
AAC(6')I	+	+	+	+	Variable*	+	0
AAC(6')II	+	–	–	+	+	+	0

+, Modified; ±, poorly modified; –, not modified; 0, substituent necessary for modification absent.
* gentamicin C_{1a}, C_2 and sissomicin +, gentamicin C_1 ±/–.

Many aminoglycoside-modifying enzymes that are apparently identical in terms of resistance profile have been shown to have different amino acid sequences. Lower case letters are used to designate the different subgroups: thus, AAC(6')Ia and AAC(6')Ib are two unique proteins conferring identical resistance profiles. It is often found that one particular subgroup is responsible for the majority of instances of the resistance profile. For example, the *aac(3)IIa* gene was found in 85% of isolates with the AAC(3)II phenotype while *aac(3)IIb* was found in 6%. The *aac(3)IIb* gene was 72% identical to *aac(3)IIa*. A third gene, *aac(3)IIc*, was 97% identical to *aac(3)IIa* with changes in only 26 bases resulting in 12 amino acid changes; it is likely that strains possessing this gene would hybridize with a DNA probe for the *aac(3)IIa* gene. Consequently, the subgroups of enzymes should perhaps be regarded as related families of enzymes, analogous to the TEM and SHV groups of plasmid-determined β-lactamases, rather than as particular amino acid sequences. As with β-lactamases, single amino acid changes can have significant effects on substrate profiles; for example, changing the leucine at position 130 of AAC(6')Ib to serine results in an enzyme with the AAC(6')II phenotype.

Resistance to aminoglycosides results from the interplay between the rate of drug inactivation by the modifying enzyme and the rate of drug transport. Thus the resistance phenotype of a particular microorganism depends on the concentration of enzyme, its V_{max}, the K_m for a given substrate and the rate of drug uptake. Resistance caused by modifying enzymes is sometimes expressed not as the usual decrease in bacteriostatic activity but rather as a reduced bactericidal activity or abolition of bactericidal synergy with other antibiotics.

Reduced permeability

Another variety of resistance to aminoglycosides which is not caused by antibiotic inactivation by specific modifying enzymes may also be clinically significant. This resistance is the result of impaired uptake of the drugs, as a result of changes in energy metabolism or outer membrane structure, and is conveniently, though probably inaccurately, termed 'reduced permeability'. It is often the result of selection of mutants as a result of exposure to the drug (notably topically). Its clinical significance is that newer aminoglycosides that are active against strains resistant to older members of the group by virtue of their resistance to aminoglycoside-modifying enzymes may show no advantage against relatively impermeable strains – in fact the reverse may be true.

Prevalence of resistance mechanisms

Most of the aminoglycoside-modifying enzymes are plasmid- or transposon-encoded; however, a few are believed to be chromosomally-determined with the presence of the gene, if not its expression in terms of resistance profile, characteristic of the species. The most notable examples are *aac(2')Ia*, which is characteristic of *Providencia stuartii*, and *aac(6')Ic*, which is characteristic of *Serratia marcescens*. The expression of these two genes appears to be tightly regulated. Although the chromosomal *aac(6')Ic* gene is found in all *Ser. marcescens* strains, most are aminoglycoside-susceptible with little or no *aac(6')Ic* mRNA detectable. Mutation to aminoglycoside resistance is accompanied by abundant mRNA production. It is not known if the *aac(6')Ic* gene has a role, other than conferring aminoglycoside resistance when derepressed. *Enterococcus faecium* synthesizes a chromosomally-encoded AAC(6'), although, not surprisingly, it is distinct from the *Ser. marcescens* enzyme, being encoded by *aac(6')Ii*.

Expression of the plasmid- or transposon-encoded aminoglycoside-modifying enzymes does not appear to be regulated. Transcription of these genes is constitutive, which although costly in terms of cellular energy provides constant protection against the presence of aminoglycosides.

Differences occur between organisms, both in location and with time in the aminoglycoside-modifying enzymes detected. Apart from the chromosomally-determined enzymes mentioned above, Enterobacteriaceae tend to produce AAC(3)I, II or IV, AAC(6')I, ANT(2") and APH(3'); *Ps. aeruginosa* tends to produce AAC(3)I, AAC(3)III, AAC(6')I or II, ANT(2") and APH(3'); staphylococci and *Ent. faecalis* tend to produce ANT(4')(4") or the protein with bifunctional AAC(6') + APH(2") activity. In the most recently published European survey, resistance in Enterobacteriaceae was usually associated with ANT(2"), AAC(3)II or AAC(6')I. In an earlier study of geographical differences of resistance patterns, a similar pattern of ANT(2"), AAC(3) and AAC(6') prevalence was found in the USA, whereas AAC(3)II predominated in South America and AAC(6') in the Far East. At St Thomas' Hospital, London, resistance in enterobacteria (other than *Providencia* spp.) was predominantly associated with AAC(3)I in the mid-1970s, but by the 1980s AAC(3)II and ANT(2") had become the most common enzymes; these were joined by AAC(3)IV in the 1990s, but the latter enzyme was found mostly in *Escherichia coli* and not in *Klebsiella* spp.

Although some strains produce a single aminoglycoside-modifying enzyme, others produce several. Strains with resistance to gentamicin or tobramycin often also produce APH(3')I or II and a phosphotransferase or nucleotidyl-transferase that confers resistance to streptomycin. An increasing number of strains appear to produce two or more enzymes active against gentamicin group aminoglycosides.

Formal demonstration of the presence of these enzymes, by use of the cellulose phosphate paper binding method or by identification of their products by chromatography, is beyond the capability of most diagnostic microbiology laboratories. However, by a judicious choice of test agents their presence can be deduced with varying degrees of confidence from the resistance patterns of the organisms. Compounds not readily available, such as fortimicin and the 2' and 6'-*N*-ethyl derivatives of netilmicin can be particularly helpful in the determination of aminoglycoside resistance mechanisms. Table 13.3 shows the deductions that can be made for most Gram-negative organisms (but not always *Acinetobacter* spp., *Flavobacterium* spp. or *Stenotrophomonas maltophilia*) and staphylococci. The presence of multiple enzymes complicates the deductions, but it is usually possible to infer the presence of APH(3') plus an enzyme that confers resistance to gentamicin.

Since the prevalence of these enzymes differs from place to place and time to time, presumably as a result of local differences in the availability of organisms receptive to the plasmids that encode them, in antibiotic prescribing habits and in the opportunities for resistant organisms to spread, it is imperative that the local prevalence of resistance to individual agents be established when choosing between aminoglycosides. This is particularly important for the treatment of severe sepsis of undetermined origin.

Pharmacokinetics

Being highly polar polycations, the aminoglycosides are very poorly absorbed from the gut, less than 1% of the oral dose reaching the plasma. Some absorption may occur on prolonged administration or in the presence of inflammatory bowel disease. All are rapidly absorbed after intramuscular injection or instillation into serous cavities. Their binding to plasma protein is low and they are distributed in the extracellular water. There is little penetration into cells, tissues or secretions, including the aqueous humour and cerebrospinal fluid (CSF), although this may unpredictably increase in the presence of inflammation. It has been suggested that dosage would be more appropriately based on the lean body mass, of which the body water is consistently 70%. There is widespread binding to tissue sites, and saturation of these is responsible for incomplete excretion of the drugs over the first few days of administration and their relatively prolonged excretion after cessation of treatment.

β-Lactam degradation

β-Lactam antibiotics, particularly penicillins and cephalosporins, are commonly prescribed in combination with aminoglycosides to secure bactericidal synergy, or breadth of spectrum, and it is unfortunate that the agents frequently inactivate one another if mixed together in infusion fluids. Depending on the identity and concentration of the agents, and amongst other factors, the composition, pH and temperature of the fluid, the β-lactam or the aminoglycoside may be the more severely affected. When carbenicillin and gentamicin are mixed in an intravenous fluid and the concentration of carbenicillin is significantly higher, the gentamicin is progressively inactivated, while in a mixture of methicillin and kanamycin it is the penicillin and not the aminoglycoside that suffers. Amikacin has been claimed to be stable in the presence of carbenicillin and piperacillin, while gentamicin and tobramycin showed considerable loss of activity over 8 h at 25°C or 4°C. Cefotaxime and latamoxef (moxalactam) were without effect. The process, which is due in the case of gentamicin to the opening of the β-lactam ring with inactivation of the penicillin and reaction with the methylamino group of the aminoglycoside to form an inactive amine, takes several

Table 13.3 *Aminoglycoside resistance mechanisms inferred from resistance patterns*

Aminoglycoside						Mechanism	Comments
Gentamicin	Netilmicin	Tobramycin	Amikacin	Kanamycin	Neomycin		
Gram-negative organisms							
R	S	S	S	S	S	AAC(3)I	Resistant to fortimicin
R	R	R	S	r	S	AAC(3)II	Higher level resistance to gentamicin than to tobramycin or netilmicin
R	S	R	S	R	R	AAC(3)III	Reduced susceptibility to 5-epi-sissomicin
R	R	R	S	r	R	AAC(3)IV	Resistant to apramycin
R	R	R	S	S	R	AAC(2')	Susceptible to 2'-N-ethyl netilmicin, resistant to 6'-N-ethyl netilmicin
S/r	R	R	R/S	R	R	AAC(6')I	Susceptible to 6'-N-ethyl netilmicin, resistant to 2'-N-ethyl netilmicin
R	R	R	S	R	S	AAC(6')II	Susceptible to 6'-N-ethyl netilmicin, resistant to 2'-N-ethyl netilmicin found in *Ps. aeruginosa*
R	S	R	S	R	S	ANT(2")	Equal resistance to gentamicin and tobramycin. Susceptible to 5-epi-sissomicin, in contrast to AAC(3)III producers
S	S	R	R	R	S	ANT(4')II	Differs from the staphylococcal enzyme, ANT(4')(4")I, which also confers reduced susceptibility to dibekacin
S	S	S	S	R	R	APH (3')I & II	Usually higher level resistance to kanamycin than to neomycin. APH(3')I and APH(3')II can be distinguished by butirosin and lividomycin resistance
S	S	S	R	R	R	APH(3')VI	APH(3')VI has been sequenced from *Acinetobacter*; this resistance pattern in other Gram-negative bacteria may be caused by a related but different gene product. The mechanism should be confirmed by molecular or enzymological methods
R	R	R	R	R	R	Reduced permeability	Changes in susceptibility should be of a similar magnitude for all compounds so that the relative activities are the same as normal strains. Usually low level but high level resistance can occur in *Pseudomonas* spp.
Staphylococci							
S	S	R	R	R	S	ANT(4')(4")I	Reduced susceptibility to dibekacin but MICs much lower than those of tobramycin
R	r	R	r	R	r	APH(2") + AAC(6')	Gentamicin MICs ≥ tobramycin MICs. If tobramycin MIC > gentamicin MIC suspect APH(2") + AAC(6') + ANT(4')4")I (dibekacin MIC should be lower than tobramycin MIC, but the mechanism should be confirmed by molecular or enzymological methods)
S	S	S	S	R	R	APH(3')	
S	S	S	R	R	R	APH(3')III	

S, Susceptible; r, reduced susceptibility; R, resistant.

hours and is seen in clinical practice only if the agents are mixed in a bottle for slow parenteral infusion and in severe renal failure where the agents persist for long periods in the plasma.

Excretion
Excretion of aminoglycosides is almost entirely by glomerular filtration, and high concentrations of unchanged agent are found in the kidney substance and the urine. Consequently, they are retained in relation to the degree of reduction of renal function, and dosage must be appropriately monitored and adjusted in renal failure in order to ensure plasma concentrations that are therapeutically adequate, but below toxic concentrations.

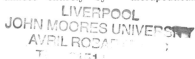

Clearance depends in part on accumulation in the deep compartment, which can be saturated, especially the kidneys, where the concentration of some agents in the cortex reaches 1 mg/g. Aminoglycosides are removed reasonably effectively by haemodialysis but not by peritoneal dialysis.

Blood concentrations and dosage adjustment

Because aminoglycosides can produce concentration-related ototoxicity and nephrotoxicity, it is important to ensure that plasma concentrations do not exceed toxic concentrations. It is equally important to ensure that fear of toxicity does not result in therapeutically inadequate dosage. Plasma concentrations in patients receiving aminoglycosides must therefore be monitored, and dosage adjusted appropriately. Means of achieving this in patients with renal impairment are described in Chapter 5, but retention of the drugs because of relatively inefficient renal excretion must also be anticipated and the dosage appropriately adjusted in infants and the elderly. Repeated courses of aminoglycoside therapy, which patients with cystic fibrosis are likely to have received, may also lead to toxic effects, at least subclinically. The need for individualized as against standard dosage and the benefits of less frequent dosage have been repeatedly emphasized, but – no doubt in part as a result of the heterogeneity of patient groups – unequivocal benefit in terms of efficacy or toxicity is difficult to establish. Nevertheless, once-daily aminoglycoside therapy, which tends to produce higher peak plasma concentrations but lower trough levels, is believed to be at least as efficacious and safe as conventional dosing regimens for non-neutropenic patients.

There are several special situations that alter the pharmacokinetics of aminoglycosides. Since the compounds do not penetrate adipose tissue well, excessively high serum concentrations will be achieved in obese patients if the dose is based on total body weight; it has been suggested that addition of 40% of the adipose mass to the lean body mass be used to calculate the dose for patients who are less than 80% overweight with 60% added for patients more than 80% overweight. Higher doses and perhaps more frequent doses may be necessary in patients with cystic fibrosis. Higher and more frequent doses may also be necessary for burns patients.

Various methods have been developed to monitor aminoglycoside concentrations during therapy, and because of the need for rapidity and specificity, immunological methods (e.g. EMIT and TDX) that can give answers in a few minutes are now generally used.

Both manual and computerized nomograms have been used to determine appropriate aminoglycoside doses. However, a comparison of a newly developed set of guidelines with five other previously published nomograms (Mawer, Chan, Hull–Sarubbi, rule-of-eight, and Dettli) found that the new guidelines, the Dettli nomogram, and the Hull–Sarubbi table achieved similar percentages (52–57%) of patients within the target ranges (5–10 mg/l for peak and less than 2 mg/l for trough), although 28% of patients had predicted peak concentrations below 5 mg/l with the new method compared to 15% with the other two. Only 38% of patients were within both ranges when the Mawer nomogram and the rule-of-eight methods were used. Consequently, since a large percentage of patients would have achieved concentrations outside of the target ranges no matter which nomogram was used, it was concluded that serum concentration monitoring is still recommended to confirm dose requirements.

A multistage protocol, involving physicians, nurses and pharmacists, has been developed to ensure that surgical patients prescribed aminoglycosides were quickly and consistently put on a safe and effective course of therapy. The medical practitioner selects an aminoglycoside and calculates a loading dose and initial maintenance dosage by using a nomogram printed on an antimicrobial order form; nurses are trained to administer and document aminoglycoside doses accurately and to draw blood samples at the correct times; pharmacists order serum aminoglycoside concentration assays, analyse the results, and recommend changes in dosage when necessary. An evaluation of the effectiveness of the dosing protocol found that, compared with the control group, a higher percentage of patients treated under the protocol were receiving therapeutic, nontoxic dosages of aminoglycosides within 48 h of the start of therapy. In addition, fewer serum drug concentration tests were ordered per patient under the protocol, and the percentage of concentration determinations useful for analysis was higher. The mean duration of aminoglycoside therapy was identical before and after the protocol was instituted, and nephrotoxic reactions tended to be less common among the protocol patients.

Liposomal aminoglycosides

Liposomal aminoglycosides are microscopic vesicles with the aminoglycosides bound by one or more phospholipid bilayers and may represent an advance in the therapeutic use of aminoglycosides. When administered intravenously, they are rapidly cleared from the blood by phagocytes, especially those of the liver and spleen. The drug is then slowly released from the phagocytes so the serum half-life is significantly prolonged and there is a greater AUC than after administration of the free drug. The use of liposomal preparations also reduces the volume of distribution and the peak serum concentration and increases the maximum tolerated dose. It may reduce renal toxicity by shifting drug accumulation from the kidney to phagocyte-rich organs such as the liver and spleen. The effect of liposomal aminoglycosides on the inner ear is unknown. Animal experiments have confirmed the efficacy of liposomal aminoglycosides in enhancing the killing of various bacteria, especially intracellular pathogens such as mycobacteria and brucellae. There is, as yet, little information on their effects in humans but liposome-encapsulated gentamicin has been used successfully to reduce the numbers of organisms in the blood of acquired immune deficiency syndrome (AIDS) patients with *Mycobacterium avium/Mycobacterium intracellulare* bacteraemia.

Toxicity and side-effects

Adverse effects include pain and irritation at the site of infection, hypersensitivity, eosinophilia with, or without, other allergic manifestations, circumoral paraesthesiae and other peripheral and central nervous effects, mild haematological disturbances and abnormal liver function tests. However, by far the most important toxic effects are those exerted on the eighth nerve and kidney. There are considerable differences amongst the agents in their relative toxicities, which are summarized for some of the older compounds in Table 13.4. Netilmicin shows lower toxicity than gentamicin, particularly when much higher doses than would be used therapeutically are tested; however, the nephrotoxicity dose–response curves of netilmicin compared to other aminoglycosides are not parallel so its advantages are less unambiguous when doses equivalent to those used therapeutically are used. Nevertheless, a comparison of clinical trials suggested that netilmicin was less ototoxic and nephrotoxic than gentamicin, tobramycin or amikacin, when conventional two or three times daily doses were given. However, for reasons that are not understood, the frequency of adverse reactions to gentamicin is greater in trials in which the drug is compared with tobramycin than in those in which it is compared with netilmicin; no major differences in adverse reactions were noticed in the comparative trials of gentamicin and netilmicin. When once-daily gentamicin and netilmicin were compared, no significant differences were found between the regimens with regard to hearing loss, prodromal signs of ototoxicity or nephrotoxicity.

Table 13.4 *Relative toxicity index* of aminoglycosides*

	Vestibular	Auditory	Renal
Streptomycin	4	1	<1
Neomycin	1	4	4
Kanamycin	1	2	1
Gentamicin	3	2	2
Tobramycin	2	2	2

*1–4: least to most toxic. Based on Price K E, Godfrey J C, Kawaguchi H 1974 *Advances in Applied Microbiology* 18: 191–307

Ototoxicity

The aminoglycosides are potentially toxic to varying degrees to the vestibular and cochlear branches of the eighth nerve. Ototoxicity results from accumulation of the drugs in the perilymph of the inner ear. Penetration is facilitated by high plasma concentrations and persistence by elevated trough concentrations, which impair back diffusion of the agents into the plasma. It follows that the danger of ototoxicity is likely to be markedly increased in the presence of impaired renal function. Toxicity is due to injury to the sensory cells of the inner ear which may progress to destructive changes with consequent permanent functional impairment. Ataxia and oscillopsy may be less well recognized (and more distressing) manifestations of toxicity than vertigo.

Vestibular toxicity develops before the cochlear effects, and both may be prevented by stopping the drug when caloric irrigation indicates vestibular impairment; but formal testing of auditory or vestibular function commonly reveals evidence of subclinical injury in a relatively high proportion of patients.

Simultaneous or sequential administration of other potentially ototoxic agents, including repeated treatment with the same or other aminoglycosides, potent diuretics such as ethacrynic acid or frusemide or certain cephalosporins, may potentiate the adverse effects of aminoglycosides, which are likely to be greater in the elderly and those with pre-existing hearing impairment. The predictive value of such factors has been disputed and auditory toxicity has also been correlated with longer treatment, bacteraemia, higher temperature, liver dysfunction, urea/serum creatinine ratio and low haematocrit.

Nephrotoxicity

Renal damage is produced to very different degrees by the various agents and is related to the accumulation of high concentrations of the drugs in the renal cortex. Views about the frequency of nephrotoxicity from the systematically administered agents differ markedly from around 2% to 60% depending on the patient population, dosage and criteria of renal damage. In volunteers, the percentage of drug excreted was highest for netilmicin (99%) and lowest for gentamicin (80%), which showed the highest degree of net reabsorption and is generally regarded as the more nephrotoxic. The abnormal persistence of aminoglycosides in the plasma between doses may be the earliest and most sensitive indication of the onset of renal impairment.

If acute tubular necrosis develops it usually does so towards the end of the first week of administration, during which time the drugs are accumulated at tissue binding sites. Regeneration of damaged tubular epithelium with the restoration of function usually occurs if the drug is discontinued. The precise value of measurements of renal enzymes or β_2 microglobulin excretion as early indicators of renal damage has been debated; but the appearance of brush border membrane fragments in the urine or new cylindruria are strongly correlated with decline of renal function.

Many putative risk factors including dosage and duration of therapy, plasma concentrations and renal function have proved to be related to age which has emerged in some studies as the dominant or even sole independent determinant of toxicity risk.

As in the case of ototoxicity, it is generally held that renal damage is more likely, and probably more severe, with simultaneous use of other agents that act on the kidney. This applies particularly to some potent diuretics, cisdiamine dichlorplatinum and cephalosporins, especially cephaloridine, which may act by preventing escape of the aminoglycoside from the proximal tubular cells. However, the situation is not clear-cut. In a number of clinical studies, the effect of alleged risk factors has not reached statistical significance and, in experimental animals, cephalosporins increase nephrotoxicity if given before gentamicin but decrease it if given simultaneously or later.

Neuromuscular blockade

Aminoglycosides can produce neuromuscular blockade, probably by functioning as membrane stabilizers in the same way as curare. If D-tubocurarine is assigned a blocking value of 1000, neomycin has a value of 2.5, streptomycin 0.7 and kanamycin 0.5. Their effect is therefore relatively feeble, and it is rare for them to produce any effect in those whose neuromuscular function is normal. However, antibiotics are customarily given in much larger amounts than curare, and patients who are also receiving muscle relaxants or anaesthetics or who are suffering from myasthenia gravis are at special risk. Analogous effects which can be reversed by calcium have been described on the gut and uterus.

Clinical use

Aminoglycosides are the mainstay of the treatment of severe sepsis caused by enterobacteria and some other Gram-negative aerobic bacilli. For the treatment of severe sepsis of undetermined cause (pp. 589, 618) they are frequently administered in combination with agents active against Gram-positive or anaerobic bacteria as appropriate. Some are also used for a number of specialized infections described under the individual agents, including endocarditis (p. 700), and respiratory (Ch. 48) infections and tuberculosis (Ch. 59).

Streptomycin has a few specific clinical uses in addition to its now very limited place in the treatment of tuberculosis; it is used in the treatment of plague and tularaemia and may also possibly be used (together with a tetracycline) in brucellosis. Neomycin, orally, is used for reducing the gut flora prior to surgery and in the management of hepatic failure.

For general clinical use, one has a choice of gentamicin, netilmicin, tobramycin and amikacin. There is no clear choice on the grounds of toxicity since differences between the various members of the groups are of no proven clinical relevance, although the indication that netilmicin may be the least toxic should be considered. Differences in in vitro activity depend largely on the local prevalence of particular resistance mechanisms; in some locations most gentamicin-resistant strains are susceptible to netilmicin or tobramycin. However, in general, amikacin has the greatest activity against gentamicin-resistant strains. The necessity for assay procedures to be available must also be borne in mind when considering a policy for the use of aminoglycosides. A recent review considers that gentamicin is the all purpose, first choice agent for patients without renal functional deficit; that tobramycin should be considered for *Ps. aeruginosa* infections; that amikacin is preferred if there is resistance to another aminoglycoside; and that netilmicin is preferred in patients with auditory or vestibular deficits or with established or impending renal insufficiency including the elderly. The British National Formulary suggests that netilmicin may cause less ototoxicity in patients needing treatment for longer than 10 days.

We believe that it is sensible to restrict the use largely to just two agents and that gentamicin should remain the aminoglycoside of first choice for the treatment of suspected or confirmed infections caused by Gram-negative bacilli unless resistance is a major problem. Gentamicin, in combination with amoxycillin and metronidazole as appropriate, can also be used for the treatment of microbiologically undiagnosed severe infection, unless microbiological or epidemiological evidence indicates a high probability of resistance in any individual case. Netilmicin can replace gentamicin when this is desirable for toxicological reasons. Amikacin would be reserved for the treatment of infections proven or strongly suspected to be caused by gentamicin-resistant amikacin-susceptible organisms.

Further information

Aminoglycoside Resistance Study Groups 1994 Resistance to aminoglycosides in *Pseudomonas. Trends in Microbiology* 2: 347–353

British National Formulary 1993 Aminoglycosides – in the British National Formulary 26, p 214–216. British Medical Association and the Royal Pharmaceutical Society, London

Bryan L E 1988 General mechanisms of resistance to antibiotics. *Journal of Antimicrobial Chemotherapy* 22 (suppl A): 1–15

D'Amico D J, Caspers-Velu L, Libert J et al 1985 Comparative toxicity of intravitreal aminoglycoside antibiotics. *American Journal of Ophthalmology* 1000: 264–275

Davey P G, Finch R G, Wood M J (eds) 1991 Once daily amikacin. *Journal of Antimicrobial Chemotherapy* 27 (suppl C): 1–152

Dornbusch K, Miller G H, Hare R S, Shaw K J, ESGAR Study Group 1990 Resistance to aminoglycoside antibiotics in Gram-negative bacilli and staphylococci isolated from blood. Report from a European collaborative study. *Journal of Antimicrobial Chemotherapy* 26: 131–144

Flournoy D J 1985 Influence of aminoglycoside usage on susceptibilities. *Chemotherapy* 31: 178–180

Franson T R, Quebbeman E J, Whipple J et al 1988 Prospective comparison of traditional and pharmakokinetic aminoglycoside dosing methods. *Critical Care Medicine* 16: 840–843

Gilbert D N 1991 Once-daily aminoglycoside therapy. *Antimicrobial Agents and Chemotherapy* 35: 399–405

Jedeikin R, Dolgunski E, Kaplan R, Hoffman S 1987 Prolongation of neuromuscular blocking effect of vecuronium by antibiotics. *Anaesthesia* 42: 858–860

Klastersky J, Phillips I (eds) 1986 Aminoglycosides in combination in severe infections. *Journal of Antimicrobial Chemotherapy* 17 (suppl A): 1–66

Kumana C R, Yuen K Y 1994 Parenteral aminoglycoside therapy: selection, administration and monitoring. *Drugs* 47: 902–913

Lynch T J, Possidente C J, Cioffi W G, Hebert J C 1992 Multidisciplinary protocol for determining aminoglycoside dosage. *American Journal of Hospital Pharmacy* 49: 109–115

Mattie H, Craig W A, Pechère J C 1989 Determinants of efficacy and toxicity of aminoglycosides. *Journal of Antimicrobial Chemotherapy* 24: 281–293

Mendelman P M, Smith A L, Levy J, Weber A, Ramsey B, Davis R L 1985 Aminoglycoside penetration, inactivation and efficacy in cystic fibrosis sputum. *American Review of Respiratory Diseases* 131: 761–765

Nightingale S D, Saletan S L, Swenson C E et al 1993 Liposome-encapsulated gentamicin treatment of *Mycobacterium avium–Mycobacterium intracellulare* complex bacteremia in AIDS patients. *Antimicrobial Agents and Chemotherapy* 37: 1869–1872

Nordström L, Ringberg H, Cronberg S, Tjernström O, Walder M 1990 Does administration of an aminoglycoside in a single daily dose affect its efficacy and toxicity? *Journal of Antimicrobial Chemotherapy* 25: 159–173

Palla R, Marchitiello M, Tuoni M 1985 Enzymuria in aminoglycoside-induced kidney damage. Comparative study

of gentamicin, amikacin, sisomicin and netilmicin. *International Journal of Clinical Pharmacology Research (Geneva)* 5: 351–355

Phillips I, King A, Shannon K 1986 Prevalence and mechanisms of aminoglycoside resistance. A ten year study. *American Journal of Medicine* 80 (suppl 6B): 48–55

Phillips I, King A, Gransden W R, Eykyn S J 1990 The antibiotic sensitivity of bacteria isolated from the blood of patients in St Thomas' Hospital, 1969–1988. *Journal of Antimicrobial Chemotherapy* 25 (suppl C): 59–80

Prins J M, Büller H R, Kuijper E J, Tange R A, Speelman P 1994 Once-daily gentamicin versus once-daily netilmicin in patients with serious infections – a randomized clinical trial. *Journal of Antimicrobial Chemotherapy* 33: 823–835

Shaw K J, Rather P N, Hare R S, Miller G H 1993 Molecular genetics of aminoglycoside resistance genes and familial relationships of the aminoglycoside-modifying enzymes. *Microbiological Reviews* 57: 138–163

Silva V L, Gil F Z, Nascimento G, Cavanal M F 1988 Aminoglycosides and nephrotoxicity. *Renal Physiology* 10: 327–337

Thomson A H, Campbell K C, Kelman A W 1990 Evaluation of six gentamicin nomograms using a bayesian parameter estimation program. *Therapeutic Drug Monitoring* 12: 258–263

Wallace S M, Chan L Y 1985 In vitro interaction of aminoglycosides with beta-lactam penicillins. *Antimicrobial Agents and Chemotherapy* 28: 274–281

Watanakunacorn C 1989 The prevalence of high level aminoglycoside resistance among enterococci isolates from blood culture during 1980–1988. *Journal of Antimicrobial Chemotherapy* 24: 63–68

Young E J, Sewell C M, Koza M A, Clarridge J E 1985 Antibiotic resistance patterns during aminoglycoside restriction. *American Journal of the Medical Sciences* 290: 223–227

Zetany R G, El Saghir N S, Santosh-Kumar C R, Sigmon M A 1990 Increased aminoglycoside requirements in haematological malignancy. *Antimicrobial Agents and Chemotherapy* 34: 702–708

Gentamicin group

In this group we include gentamicin, isepamicin (HAPA gentamicin B), sisomicin (a dehydro derivative of gentamicin C_{1a}) – and its derivatives 5-epi-sisomicin and netilmicin (1-N-ethylsissomicin) – and verdamicin (dehydro gentamicin C_2).

GENTAMICIN

A mixture of fermentation products of *Micromonospora purpurea*. The gentamicin used clinically is a mixture of gentamicins C; components C_1, C_{1a} and C_2 are required to be present in the commercial product in certain proportions. Minute amounts of gentamicin C_{2b} (also known as sagamicin) are also present. Supplied as the sulphate. Usually sterilized by filtration but aqueous solutions to which sodium metabisulphate (80 mg/l) is added can be autoclaved without discoloration or loss of activity.

Gentamicin	R_1	R_2	R_3	R_4	R_5	R_6
A	NH_2	OH	OH	H	OH	H
B	OH	OH	OH	H	NH_2	CH_3
B_1	OH	OH	OH	CH_3	NH_2	CH_3
C_1	NH_2	H	H	CH_3	$NHCH_3$	CH_3
C_{1a}	NH_2	H	H	H	NH_2	CH_3
C_2	NH_2	H	H	CH_3	NH_2	CH_3
C_{2b}	NH_2	H	H	H	$NHCH_3$	CH_3
X	NH_2	OH	OH	H	OH	CH_3

Antimicrobial activity

The activity of gentamicin against common pathogenic bacteria is shown in Table 13.1. It is active against *Staph. aureus* and coagulase-negative staphylococci, but streptococci and pneumococci are at least moderately resistant. Gram-positive bacilli, including *Actinomyces* and *Listeria* spp. are moderately susceptible, but clostridia and other obligate anaerobes are resistant. There is no useful activity at clinically attainable concentrations against mycobacteria. Gentamicin is active against most enterobacteria, including *Esch. coli, Klebsiella, Citrobacter, Enterobacter, Proteus, Serratia* and *Yersinia* spp., and also against some other aerobic Gram-negative bacilli including *Acinetobacter, Brucella, Francisella* and *Legionella* spp., though its in vitro activity against intracellular parasites such as *Brucella* spp. is of doubtful usefulness. It is active

against *Ps. aeruginosa* and other members of the fluorescens group, but other pseudomonads are often resistant and *Flavobacterium* spp. are always resistant.

As with other aminoglycosides, activity is increased by low Mg^{2+} and Ca^{2+} concentrations and diminished under anaerobic or hypercapnic conditions. The . MIC for susceptible strains of *Ps. aeruginosa* can vary more than 300-fold with the Mg^{2+} content of the medium.

The effect of pH on activity is demonstrated by the finding that at pH 7.4 the mean MIC for *Ps. aeruginosa* was 0.9 and the mean MBC (minimum bactericidal concentration) 2.1 mg/l, with no inoculum effect. At pH 7.0, the MIC for a third of the strains was 16 mg/l and no MICs were <8 mg/l; in addition, there was a two-fold or greater increase in MIC with a 100-fold increase in inoculum. In urine, MICs were 4–32 times those in broth, but reduced osmolality increased the susceptibility of *Ps. aeruginosa*. The reduction in susceptibility as pH fell was counterbalanced by the osmolality effect due to reduction in Mg^{2+} and Ca^{2+}. Activity against *Ps. aeruginosa* has also been found to be significantly less in serum or sputum compared with ion-depleted broth, as a result both of binding (more in sputum than in serum) and antagonism by ions.

The action of gentamicin is bactericidal and increases with pH, but to different degrees against different bacterial species. Marked bactericidal synergy is commonly demonstrable with β-lactams, notably with ampicillin or benzylpenicillin against *Ent. faecalis*, and with vancomycin against streptococci and staphylococci. Bactericidal synergy with a wide variety of β-lactam antibiotics can also be demonstrated in vitro against many Gram-negative rods, including *Ps. aeruginosa*. Antagonism has been demonstrated in vitro with chloramphenicol, but the clinical significance of this is doubtful.

Acquired resistance

Acquired resistance to gentamicin was extremely rare in the UK before the mid-1970s. However, gentamicin-resistant strains of staphylococci, enterobacteria, *Pseudomonas* and *Acinetobacter* spp. have now been reported from many centres, often from burns and intensive care units where the agent has been used extensively. At St Thomas' Hospital, resistance in enterobacteria increased during the second half-of the 1970s, so that by the early 1980s approximately 10% of isolates of *Klebsiella* spp. were resistant. Subsequently, there was a fall in the prevalence of resistance and by 1992 only about 1% of isolates were resistant. Resistance was much less common in *Esch. coli*, never exceeding 1%. The findings at this one hospital agree with those of a multicentre UK study conducted in 1986 that found 6% of urinary isolates of *K. pneumoniae*, 13% of *K. oxytoca* but only 0.6% of *Esch. coli* to be gentamicin resistant.

Klebsiella spp. form an important source of multiple resistance for other, more pathogenic, species, since the great majority of multiply-resistant klebsiellae can transfer resistances to *Esch. coli*, usually via a single plasmid: amongst more than 100 epidemiologically distinct klebsiellae from six countries, a few types (K2, K17 and K21) accounted for a third of the strains and almost all were resistant to at least 10 other antibiotics and almost a third to at least 15. All were resistant to ampicillin and carbenicillin (which is characteristic of the organism), more than 70% to assorted aminoglycosides, cephalosporins, sulphonamides, tetracycline and chloramphenicol and 40% to trimethoprim.

There are considerable geographical differences in the prevalence of gentamicin resistance, with a figure of about 3% for Gram-negative organisms from Scandinavia and Great Britain in a study conducted in 1987–88, 9–14% for Belgium, Germany, Austria, France and Spain, 21% for Italy, 31% for Portugal and 41% for Greece. Findings in the USA tend to be similar to those in Northern Europe, but many developing countries, where control of the prescription of antibiotics may be lax, have very high rates, for example 38% in Brazil and 47% in Thailand for *Klebsiella* spp. However, resistance was less common in Riyadh, Saudi Arabia, where antibiotics were freely available until 1982, with a rate of 1.6% for *Esch. coli* and 9% for *Klebsiella* spp. for organisms collected in 1983–84.

Acquired resistance in Gram-negative organisms is usually, but not exclusively, caused by aminoglycoside-modifying enzymes. There is some geographical variation in the prevalence of the different enzymes. ANT(2") is the most common in the USA, but in Europe various forms of AAC(3), particularly AAC(3)II, are more or less as common as ANT(2"). ANT(2") is also common in the Far East, usually accompanied by AAC(6'), but is rare in Chile. The importance of geographical differences in distribution of strains with particular enzymes is illustrated by experience in Belgium where 90% of gentamicin-resistant Gram-negative rods were susceptible to amikacin but only 13–14% to netilmicin and tobramycin due to the local predominance of AAC(3)II. In contrast, in the USA where ANT(2") predominates, most gentamicin-resistant isolates would be expected to be susceptible to amikacin and netilmicin, but resistant to tobramycin.

Urine from patients receiving gentamicin or treated topically has proved to be an important source of strains that owe their resistance not to the enzymatic degradation of the agent, but to a non-specific decrease in uptake of aminoglycosides (p. 167). Such strains, which have been involved in outbreaks of hospital-acquired infection, are cross-resistant to all aminoglycosides.

Gentamicin resistance in staphylococci and high level resistance in enterococci is usually caused by the bifunctional APH(2")/AAC(6') enzyme. Other aminoglycoside-modifying enzymes, e.g. ANT(4')(4") and APH(3'), may also occur in these organisms but do not contribute to gentamicin resistance. Gentamicin-resistant staphylococci began to emerge in the mid-1970s, and by 1986 when a multicentre study was conducted in the UK about 3% of *Staph. aureus* and 25% of coagulase-negative staphylococci were gentamicin-resistant. As with Gram-negative organisms, higher rates of resistance are found for staphylococci in central and southern than in northern Europe. Epidemic multiply-resistant *Staph. aureus* (MRSA) strains are gentamicin resistant.

Since first being described in 1979, high-level resistance to gentamicin (MIC > 2000 mg/l) in enterococci has spread world-wide and has been responsible for serious infections; penicillin–gentamicin combinations do not exert synergistic bactericidal activity against such strains. In UK studies, high level gentamicin resistance was found in 7% and 8.2% of *Ent. faecalis* isolates in London and Newcastle, respectively, and in 6.7% and 13% of all enterococci in Cambridge and Nottingham respectively. At a USA hospital, the first blood culture isolate of *Ent. faecalis* with high-level gentamicin resistance was seen in 1985, and the prevalence of high-level gentamicin resistance among enterococci isolated from blood cultures during 1985–88 was 9% but increased to 35% during the period 1989–91. Similarly, in London, high level resistance appeared in the mid 1980s and was found in about one-third of blood culture isolates from 1986 to 1990. High level gentamicin resistance is much less common in *Ent. faecium*, but has been reported in the UK, the USA and Asia.

Pharmacokinetics

Gentamicin is almost unabsorbed from the alimentary tract. In normal subjects there are wide variations between individuals in the peak plasma concentrations and half-lives of the drug observed after similar doses, but individual patients tend to behave consistently. Some patients with normal renal function develop unexpectedly high and some develop unexpectedly low peak values on conventional doses of gentamicin. Fever appears to be a significant factor in reducing the peak concentration, and anaemia has been found by some workers to be a significant factor in raising it. The mechanisms involved in these effects have not been elucidated, but it is suggested that haemodynamic changes associated with fever and anaemia might facilitate mobilization of the drug from intramuscular injection sites to raise the peak concentration or to modify drug distribution and renal handling in such a way as to lower it.

Following a dose of 80 mg i.m. in the adult, peak plasma concentrations of 4–12 mg/l are obtained at 0.5–2 h. Similar results are achieved by i.v. infusion over 20–30 min. In a comparison in volunteers of bolus injection versus infusion over 15 min, plasma concentrations at the end of administration were around 18 and 8 mg/kg, respectively. At 1 h, the concentrations were not significantly different (around 4 mg/kg) with half-lives around 2.3 h. The peak plasma concentration increases proportionally with dose. Mean initial serum peak concentrations were 10.2 mg/l in patients given 4 mg/kg once daily compared to 5.2 mg/l in patients given 1.33 mg/kg three times daily. Binding to plasma protein is 20–30%. Despite the very high bronchial concentrations achieved, aerosol administration does not give rise to detectable plasma concentrations.

Absorption of half the dose was achieved when 100 mg was added to 2 l of dialysate in patients on CAPD. On a 6 h cycle, clearance by dialysis was 2.9 ml/min.

There is a marked effect of age: in children up to 5 years the peak plasma concentration is about half and for children between 5 and 10 years about two-thirds of the concentration produced by the same dose per kilogram in adults. This difference can be eliminated to a large extent by calculating dosage not on the basis of weight but on surface area, which is more closely related to the volume of the extracellular fluid in which gentamicin is distributed.

The initial plasma half-life is about 2 h, but a significant proportion is eliminated much more slowly, the terminal half-life being of the order of 12 days. There is again much individual variation. In a study of more than 1600 patients treated for infection with Gram-negative bacteria, the elimination half-life of the drug ranged from 0.4 to 32.7 h in those with normal serum creatinine concentrations and from 0.4 to 7.6 h in those with normal creatinine clearances. Factors influencing the results, in addition to creatinine clearance, were age, the volume of distribution, sex and haematocrit. As a result of these variations, the daily dose needed to achieve a therapeutic concentration in the serum ranged from 0.5 to 25.8 mg/kg.

Young narcotic abusers treated for severe infections were found to eliminate the drug rapidly and this was associated, by comparison with older subjects, with a larger volume of distribution, lower serum creatinine concentration and enhanced creatinine clearance, although none of these factors could be used as a reliable predictor of appropriate dosage regimens.

Some febrile neutropenic patients do not differ from normal subjects in their pharmacokinetics, but in others, as in patients with cystic fibrosis, gentamicin clearance is enhanced and dosage adjustment is necessary.

β-Lactam degradation. Like other aminoglycosides, gentamicin is degraded in the presence of high concentrations of some β-lactams. The serum concentration of gentamicin in patients given 80 mg of the drug plus 5 g ticarcillin by i.v. infusion over 30 min was consistently lowered, while that of ticarcillin was unaffected. The ureidopenicillins mezlocillin and piperacillin were without effect. Others found that in patients in end-stage renal failure off dialysis, the elimination half-life of gentamicin fell from around 60 h when administered alone to 19 h when administered with carbenicillin and 38 h when administered with piperacillin.

Distribution

Gentamicin does not enter cells so intracellular organisms, for example *Salmonella typhi*, are protected from its action. Fat contains less extracellular fluid than other tissues and pharmacokinetic comparisons indicate that the volume of distribution in obese patients approximates to the lean body mass plus 40% of the adipose mass.

Sputum. Access to the lower respiratory tract is limited, and it appears that rapid intravenous infusion produces the highest but shortest-lived intrabronchial concentrations, while i.m. injection produces lower but more sustained concentrations.

CSF. Gentamicin does not reach the CSF in useful concentrations after systemic administration. In patients receiving 3.5 mg/kg per day plus 4 mg intrathecally, CSF concentrations of 20–25 mg/l have been found.

Serous fluids and exudates. Concentrations in pleural, pericardial and synovial fluids are less than half the simultaneous plasma concentrations but may rise in the presence of inflammation. In cirrhotic patients with bacterial peritonitis treated with 3–5 mg/kg per day, concentrations of 4.2 mg/kg were found in the peritoneal fluid with a fluid to serum ratio of 0.68. The maximum concentration in inflammatory exudate is less than that in the plasma, partly because it is reversibly bound (it is thought by chromatin released from lysed neutrophils) in purulent exudates, but it persists much longer.

Skin and muscle. Concentrations in skin and muscle, as judged from assay of decubitus ulcers excised 150 min after patients had received 80 mg i.m., were 5.8 and 6.5 mg/kg, respectively, the serum concentrations at that time being 5.1 and 5.4 mg/l.

Fetus. Gentamicin traverses the placenta, producing a concentration in the fetal blood about one-third of that in the maternal blood.

Excretion

Gentamicin accumulates in the renal cortical cells, and over the first day or two of treatment only about 40% of the dose is recovered. The renal clearance is around 60 ml/min. Subsequently, it is excreted almost quantitatively unchanged in the urine, principally by glomerular filtration, but there is probably an element of tubular secretion. In severely oliguric patients some extra renal elimination by unidentified routes evidently occurs. Urinary concentrations of 16–125 mg/l are found in patients with normal renal function receiving 1.5 mg/kg per day. In the presence of severe renal impairment with persistence of the drug in the circulation, urinary concentrations as high as 1000 mg/l may be found.

The clearance of the drug is linearly related to that of creatinine, and this relationship is used as the basis of the modified dosage schedules which are required in patients with impaired renal function in order to avoid accumulation of the drug (p. 77).

Haemodialysis can remove the drug at about 60% of the rate at which creatinine is cleared, but the efficiency of different dialysers varies markedly. Peritoneal dialysis removes only about 20% of the administered dose over 36 h – a rate that does not add materially to normal elimination.

Little gentamicin enters the bile, concentrations being less than half the simultaneously measured plasma concentrations.

Toxicity and side-effects

Ototoxicity

Vestibular function is usually affected, but labyrinthine damage has been reported in about 2% of patients, usually in those with peak plasma concentrations in excess of 8 mg/l. Symptoms range from acute Menière's disease to tinnitus and are usually permanent. Deafness is unusual but may occur in patients treated with other potentially ototoxic agents. Onset of ototoxicity after the cessation of treatment is very rare. In an extensive study, the overall incidence of ototoxicity was 2%. Vestibular damage accounted for two-thirds of this and impaired renal function was the main determinant.

Nephrotoxicity

Some degree of renal toxicity has been observed in 5–10% of patients. Among 97 patients receiving 102 courses of the drug in dosages adjusted in relation to renal function, nephrotoxicity was described as definite in 9.8% and possible in 7.8%. In patients treated for 39–48 days, serum creatinine has been reported to increase initially with retention of gentamicin, but renal function recovered after 3–4 weeks despite continuing treatment. However, many patients are treated for severe sepsis associated with shock or disseminated intravascular coagulopathy, or from other disorders that are themselves associated with renal failure. In critically ill patients with severe sepsis, treatment has been complicated by nephrotoxicity in 23–37%.

Mechanism. Selective accumulation of the drug by the proximal renal tubules may lead to cloudy swelling and progress to tubular necrosis. Autoradiographic localization indicates that gentamicin is very selectively localized in the proximal convoluted tubules, and a specific effect on potassium excretion may both indicate the site of toxicity and provide an early indication of renal damage. Accumulation of the drug and excretion of proximal tubular enzymes may precede any rise in the serum creatinine.

Detection. Alanine aminopeptidase excretion has been found to be very variable in normal subjects and an unreliable predictor of renal damage. β_2-Microglobulin excretion has been found by some observers to show decreased tubular function both before and during treatment of patients with urinary tract infection which improved with successful therapy. Excretion of the protein has also been shown to parallel increases in elimination half-life in patients on well-controlled therapy in whom reduction of creatinine clearance occurred, although the serum creatinine concentration remained within normal limits. When more severe and less readily reversible nephrotoxicity occurs, it is almost invariably seen in patients with pre-existing renal disorders. Nephrotoxicity is presumably related to the high concentrations of gentamicin that develop in the kidney.

Drug combinations. Nephrotoxicity in patients treated with combinations of gentamicin and cephalosporins, notably cephaloridine, has been regarded as an example of 'synergic toxicity' where each of the agents exerts a detrimental effect on the same organ which is generally clinically insignificant when the agents are given alone but notable when they are given together. However, the interaction is complex and whether the combination proves to be more or less toxic depends on the relative doses and order in which the agents are given.

Other effects

Neuromuscular blockade is possible but unlikely in view of the small amounts of the drug administered. Intrathecal injection may result in radiculitis, fever and persistent pleocytosis. Significant hypomagnesaemia may occur, particularly in patients also receiving cytotoxic agents.

Clinical use

Gentamicin treatment is principally used for serious Gram-negative bacillary infection. In the urinary tract, it may be indicated for infection with *Ps. aeruginosa* or organisms resistant to other agents. The urine should be alkalinized. Dosage must be determined in relation to the patient's age, weight and renal function and monitored as described on page 79 in order to ensure adequate therapeutic but non-toxic plasma concentrations. In Gram-negative septicaemia many regard gentamicin as the antibiotic of choice, though newer cephalosporins or quinolones are now often preferred. In severe sepsis of unknown origin, it is usually combined with an agent active against Gram-positive organisms, and where they are thought likely to be implicated, an agent active against anaerobes. *Ps. aeruginosa* meningitis and Gram-negative pneumonia have been successfully treated in adults, although mortality remains high. In systemic *Ps. aeruginosa* infections it is advisable to combine gentamicin with an antipseudomonal penicillin or cephalosporin. Gentamicin has been combined with a cephalosporin for *Klebsiella* infections, particularly pneumonia, with ampicillin for *Esch. coli* and *Proteus mirabilis* infections and with β-lactams for streptococcal endocarditis. It should be noted that sustained concentrations of β-lactams in patients with renal failure may degrade gentamicin (p. 168).

Gentamicin has been used to treat severe infection in neonates, including septicaemia and meningitis, for which intrathecal or intraventricular injections may be necessary. Its efficacy is discussed on p. 751.

Gentamicin was used for the treatment of severe infections due to *Staph. aureus* infected burns, bed sores, various superficial skin disorders and nasal carriage sites. Such applications have in many cases been complicated by the emergence of gentamicin-resistant strains.

Gentamicin eye drops are effective for the treatment of conjunctival infections with susceptible organisms. Gentamicin drops, often in combination with hydrocortisone, are also used for infections of the external ear, though malignant otitis externa caused by *Ps. aeruginosa* requires systemic therapy, possibly with a quinolone.

Oral administration of 50 mg gentamicin has been used for preoperative suppression of the bowel flora and in combination with clindamycin or metronidazole for prophylaxis of large bowel surgery (p. 603) and in combination with nystatin and vancomycin in the suppression of bowel flora in neutropenic patients. Reference is also made to its use in brucellosis (p. 883), tularaemia (p. 884) and listeriosis (p. 809).

Preparations and dosage

Proprietary names: Genticin, Cidomycin.

Preparations: Injection, various topical.

Dosages: Adult, i.m., i.v., i.v. infusion 2–5 mg/kg per day in divided doses every 8 hours.

Children aged up to 2 weeks, 3 mg/kg every 12 h; aged 2 weeks to 12 years, 2 mg/kg every 8 h. In the elderly and those with renal impairment the dose must be suitably modified.

Further information

Backus R M, DeGroot J C, Tange R A, Huizing E H 1987 Pathological findings in the human auditory system following long-standing gentamicin ototoxicity. *Archives of Otolaryngology* 244: 69–73

Bianco T M, Dwyer P N, Bertino J S Jr 1989 Gentamicin pharmacokinetics, nephrotoxicity and prediction of mortality in febrile neutropenic patients. *Antimicrobial Agents and Chemotherapy* 33: 1890–1895

Davey P, Gozzard D, Goodall M, Leyland M J 1985 Hypomagnesaemia: an under-diagnosed interaction between gentamicin and cytotoxic chemotherapy for non-lymphoblastic leukaemia. *Journal of Antimicrobial Chemotherapy* 15: 623–628

Fisher G M, Kelsey M C, Cooke E M 1986 An investigation of the spread of gentamicin resistance in a district general hospital. *Journal of Medical Microbiology* 22: 69–77

Glasser D B, Gardner S, Ellis J G, Pettit T H 1985 Loading doses and extended dosing intervals in topical gentamicin therapy. *American Journal of Ophthalmology* 99: 329–332

Gray J W, Pedler S J 1992 Antibiotic-resistant enterococci. *Journal of Hospital Infection* 21: 1–14

Kasik J W, Jenkins S, Leuschen M P, Bolam D L, Nelson R M 1985 Postconceptional age and gentamicin elimination half-life. *Journal of Paediatrics* 106: 502–505

Lowite J S, Gorvoy J D, Smaldone G C 1987 Quantitative deposition of aerosolised gentamicin in cystic fibrosis. *American Review of Respiratory Disease* 136: 1445–1449

MacArthur R D, Lehman M H, Currie-McCumber C A, Shlaes D M 1988 The epidemiology of gentamicin-resistant *Pseudomonas aeruginosa* in an intermediate care unit. *American Journal of Epidemiology* 128: 821–827

Maes P 1987 Evaluation of resistance mechanisms of gentamicin-resistant Gram-negative bacilli and their susceptibility to tobramycin, netilmicin and amikacin. *Journal of Antimicrobial Chemotherapy* 15: 283–289

Matzke G R, Jameson J J, Halstenson C E 1987 Gentamicin deposition in young and elderly patients with various degrees of renal function. *Journal of Clinical Pharmacology* 27: 216–220

Melby M J, Heissler J F, Grochowski E C, Stockmar R A 1985 Predicting serum gentamicin concentration in patients undergoing haemodialysis. *Clinical Pharmacy* 3: 509–516

Meunier F, Van der Auwera P, Schmitt H, de Maertelaer V, Klastersky J 1987 Pharmacokinetics of gentamicin after i.v. infusion or i.v. bolus. *Journal of Antimicrobial Chemotherapy* 19: 225–231

Phillips I, King A, Gransden W R, Eykyn S J 1990 The antibiotic sensitivity of bacteria isolated from the blood of patients in St Thomas' Hospital, 1969–1988. *Journal of Antimicrobial Chemotherapy* 25 (suppl C): 59–80

Pons G, d'Athis P, Rey E et al 1988 Gentamicin monitoring in neonates. *Therapeutic Drug Monitoring* 10: 421–427

Prins J M, Buller H R, Kuijper E J, Tange R A, Speelman P 1993 Once versus thrice daily gentamicin in patients with serious infections. *Lancet* 341: 335–339

Regec A L, Trifillis A L, Trump B F 1986 The effect of gentamicin on human renal proximal tubular cells. *Toxicologic Pathology* 14: 238–241

Smyth E G, Stevens P J, Holliman R E 1989 Prevalence and susceptibility of highly gentamicin resistant *Enterococcus faecalis* in a South London teaching hospital. *Journal of Antimicrobial Chemotherapy* 23: 633–639

Takahashi S, Nagano Y 1985 Dissemination of gentamicin-resistant plasmids among strains of Enterobacteriaceae. *Journal of Hospital Infection* 6: 46–59

Viollier A F, Standiford H C, Drusano G L, Tatem B A, Moody M R, Schimpff S C 1985 Comparative pharmacokinetics and serum bactericidal activity of mezlocillin, ticarcillin and piperacillin with and without gentamicin. *Journal of Antimicrobial Chemotherapy* 15: 597–606

Winstanley T G, Hastings J G M 1990 Synergy between penicillin and gentamicin against enterococci. *Journal of Antimicrobial Chemotherapy* 25: 551–560

Zervos M J, Kaufmann C A, Therasse P M, Bergman A E, Mikesell T S, Schaberg D R 1987 Nosocomial infection by gentamicin-resistant *Streptococcus faecalis*. An epidemiological study. *Annals of Internal Medicine* 106: 687–691

ISEPAMICIN
Hapa-gentamicin B

There has naturally been considerable interest in the possibility of modifying gentamicin in such a way as to preserve its activity but render it resistant to microbial inactivation. One such compound, hapa-gentamicin B, is structurally related to both the gentamicin C group and kanamycin. It is slightly more active than amikacin and,

because of its resistance to most aminoglycoside-modifying enzymes, retains activity against some strains resistant to a variety of other aminoglycosides. However, like amikacin, it is inactivated by AAC(3)III and AAD(4')(4") (mostly from Gram-positive organisms) and AAC(3)-VI (mostly from *Acinetobacter*). Its main difference from amikacin in terms of sensitivity to aminoglycoside-modifying enzymes is its resistance to AAC(6').

Isepamicin is also active in vitro against *M. avium/M. intracellulare* (*M. avium* complex) and *Nocardia asteroides*. The degree of inactivation of isepamicin by β-lactams was significantly less than that of amikacin or gentamicin. As is typical of aminoglycosides, excretion of isepamicin is reduced in patients with renal impairment. Like other aminoglycosides isepamicin is ototoxic; however, the degree of ototoxicity is less than that of amikacin.

Further information

Barrett M S, Jones R N, Erwin M E, Koontz F P 1992 CI-960 (PD127391 or AM-1091), sparfloxacin, WIN 57273, and isepamicin activity against clinical isolates of *Mycobacterium avium–intracellularae* complex, *M. chelonae*, and *M. fortuitum*. *Diagnostic Microbiology and Infectious Disease* 15: 169–171

Halstenson C E, Kelloway J S, Affrime M B, Lin C C, Teal M A, Shapiro B E, Awni W M 1991 Isepamicin disposition in subjects with various degrees of renal function. *Antimicrobial Agents and Chemotherapy* 35: 2382–2387

Khardori N, Shawar R, Gupta R, Rosenbaum B, Rolston K 1993 In vitro antimicrobial susceptibilities of *Nocardia* species. *Antimicrobial Agents and Chemotherapy* 37: 882–884

Mainardi J L, Zhou X Y, Goldstein F et al 1994 Activity of isepamicin and selection of permeability mutants to beta-lactams during aminoglycoside therapy of experimental endocarditis due to *Klebsiella pneumoniae* CF104 producing an aminoglycoside acetyltransferase 6' modifying enzyme and a TEM-3 β-lactamase. *Journal of Infectious Diseases* 169: 1318–1324

Takumida M, Nishida I, Nikaido M, Hirakawa K, Harada Y, Bagger-Sjoback D 1990 Effect of dosing schedule on aminoglycoside ototoxicity: comparative cochlear ototoxicity of amikacin and isepamicin. *ORL Journal of Otorhinolaryngology and its Related Specialities* 52: 341–349

Walterspiel J N, Feldman S, Van R, Ravis W R 1991 Comparative inactivation of isepamicin, amikacin, and gentamicin by nine β-lactams and two β-lactamase inhibitors, cilastatin and heparin. *Antimicrobial Agents and Chemotherapy* 35: 1875–1878

SISSOMICIN
Sisomicin, Rickamicin

A fermentation product of *Micromonospora inyoensis* supplied as the sulphate. Chemically, sissomicin is a dehydro derivative of gentamicin C_{1a}.

	R_1	R_2
sissomicin	OH	H
5-epi-sissomicin	H	OH

Antimicrobial activity

It is active against *Staph. aureus* and widely active against enterobacteria and *Ps. aeruginosa*. As with other amino-glycosides (p. 168), its action against *Pseudomonas* is depressed in the presence of Mg^{2+} and Ca^{2+}. Streptococci and anaerobes are resistant. The combination with mezlocillin is said to be active against most carbenicillin-resistant strains of *Ps. aeruginosa*. Its bactericidal activity, exerted at concentrations close to the MIC, increases with pH. Typical aminoglycoside synergy with appropriate β-lactams can be demonstrated against *Staph. aureus*, streptococci, enterobacteria and *Ps. aeruginosa*.

Acquired resistance

Cross-resistance with gentamicin is due to almost identical sensitivity of the two drugs to aminoglycoside-modifying enzymes (Table 13.2). Sissomicin, being a derivative of gentamicin C_{1a}, is sensitive to AAC(6'), to some types of which gentamicin is relatively resistant.

Pharmacokinetics

Sissomicin appears to be virtually identical with gentamicin in pharmacokinetic behaviour. Following i.m. doses of 1–1.5 mg/kg, mean peak plasma concentrations of 1.5–9.0 mg/l have been found at 0.5–1 h. It is widely distributed in the body water, but concentrations in CSF are low, even in the presence of inflammation.

It is eliminated unchanged almost completely over 24 h in the glomerular filtrate. Excretion decreases proportionately with renal impairment and because of the virtual identity of the behaviour of the two compounds, a gentamicin nomogram can be used to adjust dosage. About 40% of the dose is eliminated during a 6 h dialysis period, during which the elimination half-life falls to about 8 h.

Toxicity and side-effects

Mild and reversible impairment of renal function, as evidenced by a 50% rise in serum creatinine concentration, occurs in about 5% of patients. Nephrotoxicity is more likely to be seen in those with pre-existing renal disease or treated concurrently with other potentially nephrotoxic drugs.

Ototoxicity mainly affecting vestibular function has been found in about 1% of patients. Neuromuscular blockade and other effects common to aminoglycosides including rashes, paraesthesiae, eosinophilia and abnormal liver function tests have been described.

Clinical use

Its uses are identical with those of gentamicin which it closely resembles.

Preparations and dosage

Proprietary names: Baymicine, Sissoline (France), Extramycin (Germany), Mensiso, Sisobiotic, Sisomin (Italy), Sisomina (Spain).

Preparation: Injection.

Dosages: Adult i.m., i.v. 3 mg/kg per day in three divided doses. The dose should be reduced in renal impairment. Limited availability, not UK or USA.

5-EPI-SISSOMICIN

This semi-synthetic derivative, in which the hydroxyl group at position 5 of the deoxysteptamine ring is reorientated, is more resistant to aminoglycoside-modifying enzymes including AAD(2"), APH(2"), AAC(3)I, AAC(3)II and AAC(2'). It is widely active against enterobacteria, including gentamicin- and sissomicin-resistant strains elaborating those enzymes. It is also said to be more potent against strains of *Ps. aeruginosa* which owe their resistance to reduced aminoglycoside uptake.

In volunteers receiving 1 mg/kg i.m. mean peak plasma concentrations of 3.0–4.8 mg/l have been found at 0.5–0.75 h. The elimination half-life has been reported to be 2.3–3.9 h. Excretion is predominantly renal, 75–85% of the dose appearing in the urine within 24 h.

Further information

Amirak I D, Williams R J, Chung M, Noone P 1985 The single dose pharmacokinetics of 5-epi-sisomicin (Sch 22591) in human volunteers. *Journal of Antimicrobial Chemotherapy* 15: 607–611

Symposium 1979 New aspects in aminoglycoside therapy: sisomicin. *Infection* 7 (suppl 3): S240–S304

Tamura K, Iwakiri R, Amamoto T, Seith M 1985 Serum concentration of sisomicin by intravenous infusion and its clinical response as a single agent. *Japanese Journal of Antibiotics* 38: 1552–1556

NETILMICIN

Semi-synthetic 1-*N*-ethyl sissomicin. Supplied as the sulphate.

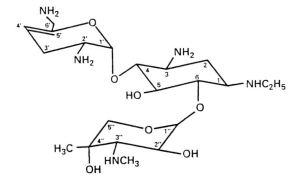

Antimicrobial activity

Netilmicin is active against staphylococci, including β-lactamase-producing, methicillin-resistant and coagulase-negative strains. Streptococci are resistant. Nocardia are inhibited by 0.04–1 mg/l. It is active against a wide range of enterobacteria, *Acinetobacter* and *Pseudomonas*, but *Providencia* are generally resistant. Most anaerobic bacteria are resistant. The susceptibility of common pathogenic bacteria is shown in Table 13.1.

It is active against some gentamicin-resistant strains, particularly those that synthesize AAD(2″) or AAC(3)I. It exhibits such typical aminoglycoside properties as bactericidal activity at or close to the MIC, greater activity at alkaline pH, depression of activity against *Pseudomonas* by divalent cations and synergy with β-lactam antibiotics. Bactericidal synergy can be demonstrated regularly with benzyl penicillin against viridans streptococci and *Ent.*

faecalis, including penicillin-tolerant strains, but seldom against *Ent. faecium*, which characteristically synthesizes AAC(6′) to which netilmicin is sensitive.

Acquired resistance

Although it is related to gentamicin, netilmicin differs in its sensitivity to aminoglycoside modifying enzymes, being resistant to AAD(2″), AAC(3)I and AAC(3)III to which gentamicin is sensitive, but being sensitive to AAC(6′) to some forms of which gentamicin is resistant. AAC(3)II confers resistance to netilmicin but generally to a smaller degree than to gentamicin.

Netilmicin resistance rates of 5% or less were found for Gram-negative organisms in the UK, the Netherlands, Switzerland, Denmark and Sweden in a European collaborative study; rates of 6–10% were found for Germany, Austria and Finland, 11–20% for Belgium, France and Spain, and over 20% for Italy, Portugal and Greece. Resistance rates for netilmicin were generally about the same as, or a little lower than, those for gentamicin.

Pharmacokinetics

Intramuscular injection of 1 mg/kg in the adult produces peak plasma concentrations of 3–5 mg, 30–40 min after the dose. Doubling the dose approximately doubles the peak plasma concentration. Administration of 2 or 3 mg/kg by i.v. infusion over 30 min produces terminal concentrations around 12 and 16 mg/l. In patients receiving 200 mg (2.2–3.6 mg/kg) i.m. 8-hourly for 10 days a mean peak plasma concentration of around 14 mg/l was found. When once-daily doses of about 6 mg/kg were used in febrile neutropenic patients, the peak plasma concentrations were about 15 mg/l. Peak concentrations of about 10 mg/l were found in children with pyelonephritis treated with 5 mg/kg once daily compared to peaks of about 5 mg/l in children given 2 mg/kg three times per day. Binding to plasma protein is very low. The serum half-life is 2–2.5 h in normal adults and linearly inversely related to creatinine clearance.

In the newborn, i.m. injection of 2.5 mg/kg produces peak plasma concentrations of 1–5 mg/l 1 h after the dose, with a plasma half-life of 4 h. In children with cystic fibrosis, a terminal half-life of 2.3 versus 1.4 h in unaffected children has been found.

Distribution

Netilmicin is distributed in the extracellular water. In patients with cystic fibrosis the apparent volume of distribution is increased and the total body clearance prolonged.

Very little reaches the CSF even in the presence of inflammation. In patients with uninflamed meninges who received 150 mg i.m. or i.v., none could be detected in the CSF after the first dose, although up to 0.18 mg/l could be found in some patients after later doses. Concentrations of 0.13–0.45 mg/l were found in the CSF of patients without meningeal inflammation following an intravenous dose of 400 mg. In patients with meningitis, the drug was still undetectable in some, although concentrations of 0.2–5 mg/l could be found later in the course of treatment in others.

Excretion

Netilmicin is incompletely excreted unchanged in the urine over 24 h in the glomerular filtrate, with some tubular reabsorption. Over the first 6 h, about 50% and by 24 h about 80% of the dose appears. The remainder is metabolized or disposed of by unidentified mechanisms. Clearance on haemodialysis is similar to that reported for gentamicin.

Toxicity and side-effects

Netilmicin appears to be distinctly less nephrotoxic than gentamicin, a difference not easily explained since the renal clearance and renal and medullary concentrations of the drugs appear to be similar. Both vestibular and cochlear toxicity appear to be low and vestibular toxicity without audiometric abnormality is rare. In some patients, plasma concentrations up to 30 mg/l over periods exceeding 1 week have not resulted in ototoxicity. Evidence of some renal toxicity in the excretion of granular casts has occurred fairly frequently in patients receiving 7.5 mg/kg per day, and is more likely to occur in the elderly and in those receiving higher doses or longer courses. In patients treated for an average of 35 days with 2.4–6.9 mg/kg per day, there was no effect on initially normal renal function, even in the elderly. Long-term treatment led to an increase in elimination half-life from 1.5 to 1.9 h. Nephrotoxicity has been observed in some diabetic patients. Overall estimates of the frequency of nephrotoxicity have ranged from 1% to 18%. Increases in SGOT and serum alkaline phosphatase concentrations have been seen in some patients without other evidence of hepatic impairment.

Once-daily dosing of netilmicin is thought to be, if anything, safer than twice or three times daily dosing.

Clinical use

Netilmicin has been used to treat severe Gram-negative bacillary infection, complicated urinary infections and, in combination, severe undiagnosed sepsis. It is particularly indicated in infections that would otherwise be treated with gentamicin when the infecting organism is resistant to that agent.

Preparations and dosage

Proprietary name: Netillin.

Preparation: Injection.

Dosage: Adults, i.m., i.v, i.v. infusion 4–6 mg /kg per day in a single dose or divided doses every 8–12 h. In severe infections up to 7.5 mg/kg per day in divided doses every 8 h, reduced as soon as is clinically indicated, usually within 48 h. Widely available.

Further information

Craig W A, Gudmundsson S, Reich R M 1983 Netilmicin sulfate: a comparative evaluation of antimicrobial activity, pharmacokinetics, adverse reaction and clinical efficacy. *Pharmacotherapy* 3: 305–315

Dahlager J I 1980 The effect of netilmicin and other aminoglycosides on renal function. A survey of the literature on the nephrotoxicity of netilmicin. *Scandinavian Journal of Infectious Diseases* 23 (suppl): 96–102

Dornbusch K, Miller G H, Hare R S, Shaw K J, ESGAR Study Group 1990 Resistance to aminoglycoside antibiotics in Gram-negative bacilli and staphylococci isolated from blood. Report from a European collaborative study. *Journal of Antimicrobial Chemotherapy* 26: 131–144

Guay D R 1983 Netilmicin (Netromycin, Schering-Plough). *Drug Intelligence and Clinical Pharmacy* 17: 83–91

Kahlmeter G 1980 Netilmicin: clinical pharmacokinetics and aspects of dosage schedules. An overview. *Scandinavian Journal of Infectious Diseases* 23 (suppl): 74–81

Kuhn R J, Nahata M C, Powell D A, Bickers R G 1986 Pharmacokinetics of netilmicin in premature infants. *European Journal of Clinical Pharmacology* 29: 635–637

Nau R, Scholz P, Sharifi S, Rohde S, Kolenda H, Prange H W 1993 Netilmicin cerebrospinal fluid concentrations after an intravenous infusion of 400 mg in patients without meningeal inflammation. *Journal of Antimicrobial Chemotherapy* 32: 893–896

Noone P 1984 Sisomycin, netilmicin and dibekacin. A review of their antibacterial activity and therapeutic use. *Drugs* 27: 548–578

Nordstrom L, Ringberg H, Cronberg S, Tjernstrom O, Walder M 1990 Does administration of an aminoglycoside in a single daily dose affect its efficacy and toxicity? *Journal of Antimicrobial Chemotherapy* 25: 159–173

Rahal J J, Simberkoff M S 1986 Comparative bactericidal activity of penicillin–netilmicin and penicillin–gentamicin against enterococci. *Journal of Antimicrobial Chemotherapy* 17: 585–591

Rozdzinski E, Kern W V, Reichle A et al 1993 Once-daily versus thrice-daily dosing of netilmicin in combination with β-lactam antibiotics as empirical therapy for febrile neutropenic patients. *Journal of Antimicrobial Chemotherapy* 31: 585–598

Shawson D C, Tadayon M, Bakhtiar M 1986 Bactericidal activity of netilmicin, compared with gentamicin and streptomycin, alone and in combination with penicillin against penicillin tolerant viridans streptococci and enterococci. *Journal of Antimicrobial Chemotherapy* 18: 479–490

Solberg C O, Reeves D, Phillips I (eds) 1984 Netilmicin. *Journal of Antimicrobial Chemotherapy* 13 (suppl A): 1–81

Tulkens P M 1991 Pharmacokinetic and toxicological evaluation of a once-daily regimen versus conventional schedules of netilmicin and amikacin. *Journal of Antimicrobial Chemotherapy* 27 (suppl C): 49–61

Vigano A, Principi N, Brivio L, Tommasi P, Stasi P, Villa A D 1992 Comparison of 5 milligrams of netilmicin per kilogram of body weight once daily versus 2 milligrams per kilogram thrice daily for treatment of Gram-negative pyelonephritis in children. *Antimicrobial Agents and Chemotherapy* 36: 1499–1503

SAGAMICIN
Gentamicin C$_{2b}$

Sagamicin is produced in substantial amounts, together with its precursor, gentamicin C$_{1a}$, by a mutant of *Micromonospora purpurea* and by *Micromonospora sagamiensis* var. *nonreducans*. It closely resembles gentamicin in antibiotic activity and spectrum, but is more resistant to AAC(6').

VERDAMICIN

This is the dehydro derivative of gentamicin C$_2$. Its in vitro activity resembles that of gentamicin and sissomicin.

Kanamycin group

In this group we include kanamycin A and its derivatives amikacin and butikacin, and the derivatives of kanamycin B, *dibekacin (dideoxy kanamycin B) – and its derivative, habekacin – and tobramycin (3'-deoxy kanamycin B).*

KANAMYCIN

Fermentation product of *Streptomyces kanamyceticus*. There are three kanamycins, A, B and C. Kanamycin B has twice the activity and twice the acute toxicity of kanamycin A. Kanamycin C is significantly less active and more toxic than kanamycin A. The content of kanamycin B in commercial preparations is required to be less than 3% (BP) or less than 5% (USP). Kanamycin A is very stable, losing less than 10% of its activity on autoclaving at 120°C for 1 h.

	R$_1$	R$_2$
kanamycin A	OH	NH$_2$
B	NH$_2$	NH$_2$
C	NH$_2$	OH

Antimicrobial activity

Kanamycin is active against *Staph. aureus*, including β-lactamase-producing and methicillin-resistant strains, and against *Staph. epidermidis*, including methicillin-resistant strains. Other aerobic and anaerobic Gram-positive cocci and the majority of Gram-positive rods are resistant. *M. tuberculosis* is susceptible. It is active against Neisseria including penicillin-resistant *N. gonorrhoeae*. It is widely active against enterobacteria; *Acinetobacter, Alkaligenes, Campylobacter, Legionella* and *Pasteurella* spp. are also susceptible *in vitro*, but *P. cepacia* and *Sten. maltophilia* are resistant. *Flavobacterium* spp. and *Bacteroides melaninogenicus* are moderately susceptible, but the majority of other *Bacteroides* spp. are resistant. *Treponema pallidum, Leptospira* and *Mycoplasma* spp. are all resistant. The susceptibility of common pathogenic bacteria is shown in Table 13.1. It is more active at alkaline pH and exerts a rapid bactericidal effect at concentrations a little above the MIC. Bactericidal synergy is generally demonstrable with penicillins against *Ent. faecalis*.

Acquired resistance

Resistance in *Staph. aureus* and many enterobacteria at one time became common, but is believed to have declined in many places with decreased use of the agent. However, since susceptibility to kanamycin is no longer tested routinely, it is not possible to be certain about the current situation. Clinically significant resistance is usually multiple, plasmid-borne and due to enzymatic inactivation of the drug. Kanamycin A is sensitive to many of the aminoglycoside-modifying enzymes that inactivate gentamicin or tobramycin and in addition is sensitive to APH(3'); however, it is resistant to AAC(2') so *Prov. stuartii* is usually susceptible to kanamycin (see Table 13.2). Resistance due to reduced permeability has also been encountered, as in an outbreak due to resistant *Klebsiella* spp. in a neonatal intensive care unit where gentamicin had been extensively used and the strains were resistant to a broad range of aminoglycosides. Relative resistance has been encountered in *N. gonorrhoeae* where kanamycin has been commonly used.

Pharmacokinetics

Very little is absorbed from the intestinal tract. After an oral dose of 6 g, the concentration in faeces was found to be 25 mg/g while that in urine was 12 mg/ml. Kanamycin is normally administered by i.m. injection when a dose of 500 mg produces peak plasma concentrations after 1 h of about 15–20 mg/l and doses of 1 g about 20–35 mg/l. The proportion bound to plasma protein is very low. The plasma half-life is around 2.5 h. The peak plasma concentration in the neonate is dose related: concentrations of 8–30 mg/l (mean 18 mg/l) have been found 1 h after a 10 mg/kg dose.

The volume of distribution indicates that the drug is confined to the extracellular fluid. The concentration in serous fluids is said to equal that in the plasma, but it does not enter the CSF in therapeutically useful concentrations even in the presence of meningeal inflammation.

Excretion

Kanamycin is excreted almost entirely by the kidneys and almost exclusively in the glomerular filtrate, so that probenecid has no effect on its plasma concentration. Renal clearance is about 80 ml/min, indicating some tubular reabsorption. Up to 80% of the dose appears unchanged in the urine over the first 24 h, producing concentrations around 100–500 mg/l. It is retained in proportion to reduction in renal function. Less than 1% of the dose appears in the bile. In patients receiving 500 mg i.m. preoperatively, concentrations of 2–23 mg/l have been found in bile and 8–14 mg/g in gallbladder wall, through which some entry evidently occurs since the drug can still be detected when the cystic duct is obstructed. The fate of the remaining 20% or so has not been established.

Toxicity and side-effects

Intramuscular injections are moderately painful, and minor side-effects similar to those encountered with streptomycin (p. 196) have been described. Eosinophilia in the absence of other manifestations of allergy, occurs in up to 10% of patients. Other manifestations of hypersensitivity are rare. As with other aminoglycosides, the most important toxic effects are on the eighth nerve and much less frequently, but more importantly, on the kidney.

Nephrotoxicity

Renal damage is seen principally in patients with preexisting renal disease or treated concurrently or sequentially with other potentially nephrotoxic agents. The drug accumulates in the renal cortex, producing cloudy swelling, which may progress to acute necrosis of proximal tubular cells with oliguric renal failure. The resulting renal impairment usually resolves on stopping the drug, but may take months to do so. The appearance of protein, red cells and casts in the urine of treated patients is relatively common. Less dramatic deterioration of renal function, particularly exaggeration of the potential nephrotoxicity of other drugs or of existing renal disease, is principally important because it increases the likelihood of ototoxicity.

Ototoxicity

Vestibular damage is uncommon but may be severe and prolonged. Hearing damage is usually bilateral, and fortunately typically affects frequencies above the conversational range. Acute toxicity is most likely in patients in whom the plasma concentration exceeds 30 mg/l, but chronic toxicity may be seen in patients treated with the drug over long periods. Toxicity has been seen in up to 40% of patients treated for tuberculosis but in less than 2% of patients treated for acute conditions. Auditory toxicity may be potentiated by concurrent treatment with potent diuretics like ethacrynic acid. If tinnitus – which usually heralds the onset of auditory injury – develops, the drug should be withdrawn.

Neuromuscular blockade

This is seen particularly in patients receiving other muscle relaxants or suffering from myasthenia gravis and may be reversed by neostigmine. Prolonged oral use may be associated with malabsorption or, rarely, complicated by superinfection with resistant *Staph. aureus* leading to severe enteritis.

Clinical use

Kanamycin has been used topically and orally for much the same purposes as neomycin (p. 193). Prolonged oral administration may lead to systemic toxicity, but this and malabsorption are said to be less likely than with neomycin. In combination with a cephalosporin, it has been commended for the treatment of *Klebsiella* pneumonia and of infection due to methicillin-resistant staphylococci. It has been used for the treatment of intractable *Proteus* urinary infections, where the alkalinity of the urine favours its action. It may prove on laboratory testing to be the aminoglycoside of choice for combination with a β-lactam in the therapy of bacterial endocarditis, including that due to *Staph. aureus*. It has been used in the treatment of gonorrhoea due to penicillin-resistant strains.

Preparations and dosage

Proprietary name: Kannasyn.

Preparations: Injection, ophthalmic.

Dosage: Adults, i.m. injection 250 mg every 6 h, or 500 mg every 12 h. Adults and children, i.v. infusion, 15–30 mg/kg per day in divided doses every 8–12 h.

Widely available.

Further information

Davis R R, Brummett R E, Bendrick T W, Himes D L 1984 Dissociation of maximum concentration of Kanamycin in plasma and perilymph from ototoxic effect. *Journal of Antimicrobial Chemotherapy* 14: 291–302

Garrod L P, Lambert H P, O'Grady F 1981 Antibiotic and chemotherapy, 5th edn. Churchill Livingstone, Edinburgh

Shannon K P, Phillips I, King B A 1978 Aminoglycoside resistance among *Enterobacteriaceae* and *Acinetobacter* species. *Journal of Antimicrobial Chemotherapy* 4: 131–142

AMIKACIN
BBK8

A semi-synthetic derivative of kanamycin A in which the 1-amino group of the deoxystreptamine moiety is replaced by the HABA (hydroxyaminobutyric acid) group (NH–COCH(OH)CH$_2$NH$_2$) found in the natural aminoglycoside, butirosin. Supplied as the sulphate.

Antimicrobial activity

Amikacin is active against a wide range of enterobacteria, and *Ps. aeruginosa*, also *Staph. aureus* and *Staph. epidermidis* including methicillin-resistant strains, but other Gram-positive cocci, including streptococci, pneumococci and the majority of Gram-positive rods are resistant. *Myc. tuberculosis*, including most streptomycin-resistant strains, is susceptible. Like other aminoglycosides, it is inactive against anaerobic bacteria. Its activity against common pathogenic bacteria is shown in Table 13.1.

Amongst other organisms, *Acinetobacter, Alkaligenes, Arizona, Campylobacter, Citrobacter, Hafnia, Legionella, Pasteurella, Providencia, Serratia* and *Yersinia* spp. are usually susceptible in vitro. *Sten. maltophilia*, many non-aeruginosa pseudomonads and *Flavobacterium* spp. are resistant. *M. tuberculosis* and some other mycobacteria including *M. fortuitum* (MIC 4 mg/l) are susceptible; most other mycobacteria, including *M. kansasii* and *M. avium/M. intracellulare* (*M. avium* complex), are resistant. *Nocardia asteroides* is susceptible.

Amikacin exhibits typical aminoglycoside characteristics, including an effect of divalent cations on its activity against *Ps. aeruginosa* analogous to that seen with gentamicin (p. 174) and synergistic activity with β-lactams. The degree of synergy differs with the degree of β-lactam activity, but may be demonstrable against organisms 'resistant' in conventional terms. Synergy has been demonstrated with imipenem against about a third of *Staph. aureus* and gentamicin-resistant enterobacteria, but rarely against *Ps. aeruginosa*.

Its particular interest is that like butirosin from which its side-chain is derived, it is little or not affected by the majority of enzymes that inactivate gentamicin and tobramycin (Table 13.2) and is consequently active against staphylococci, enterobacteria and pseudomonas that owe their resistance to the elaboration of those enzymes. However, AAC(6'), AAD(4')(4") and some forms of APH(3') can confer amikacin resistance; since these enzymes generally do not confer gentamicin resistance, amikacin resistant strains can be missed in routine susceptibility tests when gentamicin is used as the representative aminoglycoside.

Acquired resistance

Resistant strains of *Ps. aeruginosa* and other pseudomonads, *Acinetobacter, Serratia* spp. and a number of other enterobacteria have already been described. There have been reports of amikacin resistance arising during treatment of infections due to *Serratia* spp. and *Ps. aeruginosa.* Outbreaks of infection due to multi-resistant strains of enterobacteria and *Ps. aeruginosa* have occurred where amikacin has been used extensively, particularly in burns units. Strains of *Staph. aureus* and coagulase-negative staphylococci that owe their resistance to the synthesis of AAD(4')(4") have been described; this enzyme has recently been found in *Esch. coli, Klebsiella* spp. and *Ps. aeruginosa.* In *Ent. faecalis,* resistance to penicillin–aminoglycoside synergy has been associated with plasmid-mediated APH(3'); A derivative of amikacin that lacks the 4'-OH group (BB-K311) is a very poor substrate for the enzyme and is active against strains that produce it.

Gentamicin- or multiply-resistant enterobacteria strains are generally susceptible. Resistance in Gram-negative organisms is usually caused by reduced uptake of the drug or by the aminoglycoside-modifying enzymes AAC(6') or AAC(3)VI. The latter enzyme is usually found in *Acinetobacter* spp., but has also been found, encoded by a transposon, in *Prov. stuartii.* One type of AAC(6) is chromosomally encoded by *S. marcescens,* though not usually expressed.

The prevalence of resistance can change rapidly with increased usage of the drug. In New York, resistant strains rose from 2% to almost 8% in 18 months during which there had been a three-fold increase in usage; most resistance, associated with AAC(6'), was seen in *Klebsiella, Serratia* and *Pseudomonas* spp. The spread of extended-spectrum β-lactamases belonging to the TEM and SHV families may result in an increase in amikacin resistance, since most strains that produce such enzymes also produce AAC(6').

Pharmacokinetics

The pharmacokinetic behaviour of amikacin is virtually identical with that of its parent, kanamycin. Particular stability has been claimed for amikacin in the presence of penicillins and in patients on chronic haemodialysis, the serum concentrations and clearance were unaffected by simultaneous administration of carbenicillin. Binding to plasma protein is 3–4%.

Mean peak plasma concentrations around 20 and 30 mg/l have been found 1 h after i.m. doses of 0.5 g and 7.5 mg/kg,

respectively. Rapid i.v. injection of 7.5 mg/kg produced concentrations in excess of 60 mg/l shortly after injection. Following i.v. infusion of 0.5 g over 30 min, concentrations of 35–50 mg/l have been found. In volunteers, intravenous infusion of 3.33 mg/kg for 6 h followed by 1 mg/kg produced a steady state concentration around 12 mg/l. The half-life is 2–2.3 h by the i.v. route and 2.8 h by the i.m. route. Most pharmacokinetic parameters follow an almost linear correlation when the high once daily doses (~15 mg/kg) are compared with the traditional 7.5 mg/kg twice daily.

In patients on CAPD, there was no difference in mean peak plasma concentration or volume of distribution whether the drug was given intravenously or intraperitoneally.

Infants

In infants receiving 7.5 mg/kg by i.v. injection, peak plasma concentrations were 17–20 mg/l. No accumulation occurred on 12 mg/kg per day for 5–7 days, but infusion over 20 min produced very low concentrations. There was little change in the plasma concentration or the half-life (1.7 and 1.9 h) on the third and seventh days of a period over which 150 mg/m² was infused over 30 min every 6 hours. When the dose was raised to 200 mg/m² the concentration never fell below 8 mg/l. The plasma half-life was longer in babies of lower birthweight and was still 5–5.5 h in babies aged 1 week or older. The importance of dosage control in the neonate is emphasized by the findings that there is an inverse linear relationship between postconception age and plasma elimination half-life – leading to potential underdosing on standard regimens – with the complication that toxicity in the neonate is not clearly related to plasma concentration.

Distribution

The apparent volume of distribution (23–38%) indicates distribution throughout the extracellular water. In blister fluid following an iv. bolus of 0.5 g, peak concentrations were around 12 mg/l with a mean elimination half-life of 2.3 h. In patients with impaired renal function, penetrance and peak concentration increased linearly with decrease in creatinine clearance.

In patients with purulent sputum, a loading dose of 4 mg/kg i.v. plus 8 h infusions of 7–12 mg/kg produced concentrations around 2 mg/l with a mean sputum/serum ratio of 0.15. With brief infusions over 10 min for 7 days, sputum concentrations of around 9% of the simultaneous serum values have been found.

Concentrations of amikacin in the CSF of adult volunteers receiving 7.5 mg/kg i.m. were less than 0.5 mg/l and virtually the same in patients with meningitis. Rather higher but variable concentrations up to 3.8 mg/l have been found in neonatal meningitis.

Amikacin crosses the placenta, and concentrations of 0.5–

6 mg/l have been found in the cord blood of women receiving 7.5 mg/kg in labour.

Excretion

Up to 95% of the unchanged drug is eliminated in the urine over 24 h, producing urinary concentrations between 150 and 3000 mg/l. Renal clearance is 70–84 ml/min, and this, with the ratio of amikacin to creatinine clearance (around 0.7), indicates that it is filtered and tubular reabsorption is insignificant. It accumulates in proportion to reduction in renal function, although there may be some extrarenal elimination in anephric patients. The mean plasma half-life in patients on, or recently off, haemodialysis was around 4 h, while that on peritoneal dialysis was 28 h.

In patients receiving 500 mg/kg preoperatively, concentrations in gallbladder wall reached 34 mg/l and in bile 7.5 mg/l in some patients. In patients given 500 mg i.v. 12 h before surgery and 12 hourly for four doses thereafter, the mean bile/serum ratio 1 h after the dose was around 0.4.

Toxicity and side-effects

Ototoxicity

Neurosensory hearing loss (mainly high-tone deafness) has been detected by audiometry and labyrinthine injury by coloric testing, but have seldom been severe. High-frequency hearing loss and vestibular impairment have been described in about 5% of patients and conversational loss in about 0.5%; more in patients monitored audiometrically (29%) and by caloric testing (19%). Toxicity was found to be significantly more common in males. Cochlear damage has appeared after cessation of treatment.

Hearing loss appears to be reversible when the drug is discontinued. Patients with high-tone hearing loss have generally received more drug for longer than patients without. Over half the patients with peak serum concentrations exceeding 30 mg/l or trough concentrations exceeding 10 mg/l developed cochlear damage. The main contributory factor was previous treatment with other aminoglycosides.

Nephrotoxicity

Impairment of renal function, usually mild or transient, has been observed in 3–13% of patients, notably in the elderly or those with preexisting renal disorders or treated concurrently or previously with other potentially nephrotoxic agents.

Other reactions

Adverse effects common to aminoglycosides occur, including hypersensitivity, gastro-intestinal disturbances, headache, drug fever, peripheral nervous manifestations, eosinophilia, mild haematological abnormalities and disturbed liver function tests without other evidence of hepatic derangement.

Clinical use

Amikacin is principally used for the treatment of infections due to organisms resistant to other aminoglycosides because of their ability to degrade them. It may be valuable in hospitals where gentamicin-resistant strains are known to be common, or in the control of hospital outbreaks. It may show no advantage against strains which owe their resistance to reduced permeability (p. 167) and is unlikely to be effective in outbreaks with producers of extended-spectrum β-lactamases. It has also been used in the treatment of febrile episodes in neutropenic patients or in sepsis of unknown origin (when it should be combined with a β-lactam or agent active against anaerobic organisms as appropriate) and in staphylococcal septicaemia, neonatal meningitis and urinary tract infection. Dosage must be monitored and adjusted in patients with renal impairment as described on p. 176. It has been suggested that peak concentrations should not exceed 30 mg/l and that a trough concentration of 10 mg/l should be maintained to achieve therapeutic effects. However, high peak concentrations would be expected if the once-daily regimen with 15 mg/kg were used.

Preparations and dosage

Proprietary name: Amikin.

Preparation: Injection.

Dosage: Adults and children, i.m., i.v., 15 mg/kg per day in two divided doses. Neonates and premature infants, an initial loading dose of 10 mg/kg followed by 15 mg/kg per day in two equally divided doses. The dose must be reduced if renal function is impaired, and in the elderly.

Widely available.

Further information

Adelman R D, Wirth F, Rubio T 1987 A controlled study of the nephrotoxicity of mezlocillin and amikacin in the neonate. *American Journal of Diseases in Children* 141: 1175–1178

Autret E, Marchand S, Breteau M, Grenier B 1986 Pharmacokinetics of amikacin in cystic fibrosis: a study of bronchial diffusion. *European Journal of Clinical Pharmacology* 31: 79–83

Beaubien A R, Destardins S, Ormsby E et al 1989 Incidence of amikacin ototoxicity: a sigmoid function of total drug exposure independent of plasma levels. *American Journal of Otolaryngology* 10: 234–243

Davey P G, Finch R G, Wood M J (eds) 1991 Once daily amikacin. *Journal of Antimicrobial Chemotherapy* 27 (suppl C): 1–152

Dillon K R, Dougherty S H, Casner P, Polly S 1989 Individualised pharmacokinetics versus standard dosing of amikacin: a comparison of therapeutic outcomes. *Journal of Antimicrobial Chemotherapy* 24: 581–589

Gerding D N, Larson T A, Hughes R A, Weiler M, Shanholtzer C, Peterson L R 1991 Aminoglycoside resistance and aminoglycoside usage: ten years of experience in one hospital. *Antimicrobial Agents and Chemotherapy* 35: 1284–1290

Jacoby G A, Blaser M J, Santanam P et al 1990 Appearance of amikacin and tobramycin resistance due to 4'-amino-glycoside nucleotidyltransferase [ANT(4')-II] in Gram-negative pathogens. *Antimicrobial Agents and Chemotherapy* 34: 2381–2386

Kenyon C F, Knoppert D C, Lee S K, Vandenberghe H M, Chance G W 1990 Amikacin pharmacokinetics and suggested dosage modifications for the preterm infant. *Antimicrobial Agents and Chemotherapy* 34: 265–268

Lambert T, Gerbaud G, Bouvet P, Vieu J F, Courvalin P 1990 Dissemination of amikacin resistance gene *aphA6* in *Acinetobacter* spp. *Antimicrobial Agents and Chemotherapy* 34: 1244–1248

Lambert T, Gerbaud G, Courvalin P 1994 Characterization of transposon Tn1528, which confers amikacin resistance by synthesis of aminoglycoside 3'-O-phosphotransferase type VI. *Antimicrobial Agents and Chemotherapy* 38: 702–706

Maes P, Vanhoof R 1992 A 56-month prospective surveillance study on the epidemiology of aminoglycoside resistance in a Belgian general hospital. *Scandinavian Journal of Infectious Diseases* 24: 495–501

Maller R, Isaksson B, Nilsson L, Soren L 1988 A study of amikacin given once versus twice daily in serious infections. *Journal of Antimicrobial Chemotherapy* 22: 75–79

Ristuccia A M, Cunha B A 1985 An overview of amikacin. *Therapeutic Drug Monitoring* 7: 12–29

Schiff T A, McNeil M M, Brown J M 1993 Cutaneous *Nocardia farcinica* infection in a nonimmunocompromised patient: case report and review. *Clinical Infectious Disease* 16: 756–760

Smelzer B D, Schwartzman M S, Bertino J S Jr 1988 Amikacin pharmacokinetics during continuous ambulatory peritoneal dialysis. *Antimicrobial Agents and Chemotherapy* 32: 236–240

Tran Van Nhieu G, Bordon F, Collatz E 1992 Incidence of an aminoglycoside 6'-N-acetyltransferase, ACC(6')-1b, in amikacin-resistant clinical isolates of Gram-negative bacilli, as determined by DNA-DNA hybridisation and immunoblotting. *Journal of Medical Microbiology* 36: 83–88

Williams P J, Hull J H, Sarubbi F A, Rogers J F, Wargin W A 1986 Factors associated with nephrotoxicity and clinical outcome in patients receiving amikacin. *Journal of Clinical Pharmacology* 26: 79–86

BUTIKACIN
UK-18,892

Butikacin, the 1-*N*-(4-amino-2-hydroxybutyl) derivative of kanamycin A, is closely related chemically to amikacin, which it resembles in activity, resistance to aminoglycoside-modifying enzymes and pharmacokinetics.

Further information

Andrews R J, Brammer K W, Cheeseman H E, Jevons S 1978 UK-18,892: resistance to modification by aminoglycoside-inactivating enzymes. *Antimicrobial Agents and Chemotherapy* 14: 846–850

Jevons S, Cheeseman H E, Brammer K W 1978 In vitro studies with UK-18,892, a new aminoglycoside antibiotic. *Antimicrobial Agents and Chemotherapy* 14: 277–280

Kendall M J, Wise R, Andrews J M, Bedford K A 1978 A pharmacological study of UK-18,892 and amikacin. *Journal of Antimicrobial Chemotherapy* 4: 459–463

DIBEKACIN
DKB

Semisynthetic 3',4'-dideoxy kanamycin B. Supplied as the sulphate. Closely related to the natural compound tobramycin, which chemically is 3'-deoxy kanamycin B.

Antimicrobial activity

Dibekacin is active against staphylococci including methicillin-resistant strains, a wide range of enterobacteria, *Acinetobacter* and *Pseudomonas* spp. It is also active against *M. tuberculosis* and *M. avium/M. intracellulare* (*M. avium* complex: MICs 4–16 mg/l). It exhibits the usual aminoglycoside properties of bactericidal activity at concentrations close to the MIC and bactericidal synergy with selected β-lactams. Absence of hydroxyl groups present in the parent kanamycin B renders it resistant to phosphorylation by APH(3'). It is also resistant to some forms of AAD(4'). However, the type of this enzyme, AAD(4')(4"), found in some Gram-positive organisms modifies dibekacin at the 2"-hydroxyl group; nevertheless dibekacin has much greater activity than tobramycin against organisms that produce the enzyme.

Pharmacokinetics

In volunteers, a dose of 1 mg/kg by i.v. bolus produced peak plasma concentrations around 5 mg/l with a mean elimination half-life of 2.3 h. In another study, following 1.5 mg/kg by i.v. bolus the mean peak plasma concentration in young subjects was around 14 mg/kg with a half-life of 1 h. In elderly subjects the half-life was around 3.4 h. Following i.m. injection in volunteers, 1 mg/l has produced mean peak plasma concentrations of 4.4 mg/kg with a half-life of around 2 h, while a dose of 100 mg produced a mean peak plasma concentration of around 10 mg/l with an elimination half-life of around 2.2 h. As with other aminoglycosides, dibekacin is inactivated in the presence of high concentrations of certain β-lactams and at a dibekacin/β-lactam ratio of 1/100, the loss of activity over 48 h in the presence of different penicillins was: ticarcillin, 99%; carbenicillin, 90% and ampicillin 65%.

Dibekacin is eliminated principally by the renal route, 75–80% of the dose appearing in the urine in the first 24 h. Elimination is inversely related to renal function, and in patients maintained on chronic haemodialysis, the half-life has been found to rise to 54 h between dialyses and fall to 6–7 h on dialysis.

Toxicity and side-effects

Toxic effects are those typical of aminoglycosides (p. 171) and it has been found to exhibit toxicity similar to or less than that of gentamicin. In volunteers given 3 mg/kg per day as two i.m. doses over 10 days, peak N-acetyl-β-glucosaminidase excretion was significantly less than that in volunteers receiving a similar regimen of gentamicin, but the significance of this index of renal toxicity has been questioned. In a study in guinea-pigs dibekacin was found to have greater auditory toxicity than tobramycin but lower vestibular toxicity.

Clinical use

Dibekacin may be used in the treatment of infections due to organisms resistant to established aminoglycosides.

Preparations and dosage

Preparation: Injection.

Dosage: Adults, i.m., i.v., 1–3 mg/kg per day in divided doses.

Available in continental Europe, not the UK or USA.

Further information

Arancibia A, Chavez J, Ibarra R, Ruiz I, Icarte A, Thambo S, Chavez H 1987 Disposition kinetics of dibekacin in normal subjects and in patients with renal failure. *International Journal of Cinical Pharmacology, Therapy and Toxicology* 25: 38–43

Courcol R J, Loeuille G A, Delnatte J, Martin G R 1985 Pharmacokinetics of dibekacin in children with cystic fibrosis. *International Journal of Clinical Pharmacology Research* 5: 87–91

Jacoby G A, Blaser M J, Santanam P et al 1990 Appearance of amikacin and tobramycin resistance due to 4'-aminoglycoside nucleotidyltransferase [ANT(4')-II] in Gram-negative pathogens. *Antimicrobial Agents and Chemotherapy* 34: 2381–2386

Kitsato I, Yokota M, Inouye S, Igarishi M 1990 Comparative ototoxicity of ribostamycin, dactimicin, dibekacin, kanamycin, amikacin, tobramycin, gentamicin, sisomicin and netilmicin in the inner ear of guinea pigs. *Chemotherapy* 36: 155–168

Navarro A S, Lanao J M, Dominguez-Gil Huale A 1986 In-vitro interaction between dibekacin and penicillin. *Journal of Antimicrobial Chemotherapy* 17: 83–89

HABEKACIN
Arbekacin

The 1-*N*-(4-amino-2-hydroxybutyryl) derivative of dibekacin – to which it bears the same relation as amikacin bears to kanamycin A. Its activity is comparable with that of amikacin against susceptible and a number of gentamicin- and tobramycin-resistant strains. In volunteers given 3 mg/kg i.v., mean peak plasma concentrations around 8 mg/l were reached in less than 1 h. The plasma elimination half-life is around 2 h. Habekacin is retained in renal failure, but moderately well removed by haemodialysis.

Further information

Fillastre J P, Leroy A, Humbert G, Moulin B, Bernadet P, Josse S 1987 Pharmacokinetics of habekacin in patients with renal insufficiency. *Antimicrobial Agents and Chemotherapy* 31:575–577

TOBRAMYCIN

Nebramycin factor 6; 3'-deoxy kanamycin B

A fermentation product of *Streptomyces tenebraeus* supplied as the sulphate.

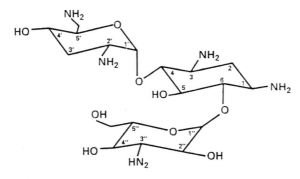

Antimicrobial activity

Tobramycin is active against staphylococci, including β-lactamase-producing, methicillin-resistant and coagulase-negative strains, a wide variety of enterobacteria and *Ps. aeruginosa*, including some strains with acquired resistance to gentamicin. In general it has somewhat greater in vitro activity than gentamicin against *Ps. aeruginosa*, but against other organisms its activity is generally the same as, or a little lower than, that of gentamicin. Other *Pseudomonas* species are generally resistant, as are streptococci and most anaerobic bacteria. The susceptibility of common pathogenic organisms is shown in Table 13.1. Other organisms usually susceptible in vitro include *Acinetobacter*, *Legionella* and *Yersinia* spp. Alkaligenes, Flavobacterium spp. and Mycobacterium spp. are resistant. Tobramycin exhibits bactericidal activity at concentrations close to the MIC and bactericidal synergy typical of aminoglycosides in combination with penicillins or cephalosporins.

Acquired resistance

Many aminoglycoside-modifying enzymes that attack gentamicin also attack tobramycin. However, AAC(3)I does not confer tobramycin resistance and AAC(3)II confers a lower degree of tobramycin resistance than of gentamicin resistance. Conversely, AAD(4')(4") confers tobramycin but not gentamicin resistance, as do some types of AAC(6').

Overproduction of APH(3') has been reported to confer a low degree of tobramycin resistance (MIC 8 mg/l), but not gentamicin resistance (MIC 2 mg/l); the resistance was ascribed to 'trapping' rather than phosphorylation.

Tobramycin resistance rates of 5% or less were found for Gram-negative organisms in the UK, the Netherlands, Switzerland, Denmark, Sweden and Finland in a European collaborative study; rates of 6–10% were found for Belgium, Germany and Austria, 11–20% for France, Spain and Italy, and over 20% for Portugal and Greece. These rates were generally about the same as those of gentamicin, except for Finland and Austria for which they were about half those for gentamicin.

Pharmacokinetics

Tobramycin is effectively not absorbed from the gut and its pharmacokinetic behaviour after systemic administration closely resembles that of gentamicin. Mean peak plasma concentrations of 3–4 mg/l have been found 30 min after intramuscular injection of 80 mg and 6–7 mg/l have been found 30 min after i.v. injection of 1 mg/kg. In patients treated for prolonged periods with 2.5 mg/kg i.v. 12 hourly, average peak steady-state values were 6.5 mg/l after 30 weeks and 7.1 mg/l after 40 weeks. Continuous i.v. infusion of 6.6 mg/h and 30 mg/h produced steady-state concentrations of 1 and 3.5–4.5 mg/l, respectively. Higher concentrations (10–12 mg/l) have been obtained by bolus injection over about 3 min. Peak concentrations of around 50 mg/l have been reported in cystic fibrosis patients given 9 mg/kg once daily. Binding to plasma protein is said to be up to 30%. The plasma half-life following rapid i.v. injection has been variously reported to lie between 1.5 and 3 h. In patients dosed repeatedly or continuously for some weeks, the elimination half-life declined from 9.3–11.3 h initially to 5.6 h. Accumulation occurs over the first few days of treatment, due probably to tissue binding, and excretion continues for up to 3 weeks after cessation of treatment.

As with a number of other agents, clearance is more rapid in patients with cystic fibrosis. In the neonate, peak plasma concentrations of 4–6 mg/l have been found 0.5–1 h after doses of 2 mg/kg. Mean plasma elimination half-lives of 4.6–8.7 h were inversely proportional to the birthweight and creatinine clearance. The half-life was found to be initially extremely variable (3–17 h) in infants weighing 2.5 kg at birth, but considerably more stable (4–8 h) at the end of therapy 6–9 days later.

β-Lactam inactivation

In common with other aminoglycosides, tobramycin interacts with certain β-lactams, but is said to be stable in the presence of ceftazidime, imipenem and aztreonam. In mixtures containing 80 mg tobramycin and 4–5 mg carbenicillin or ticarcillin per litre, 30–40% of tobramycin activity was lost over 1 h. Of the penicillins tested, piperacillin caused least inactivation in vitro.

Distribution

The volume of distribution (17 l) slightly exceeds the extracellular water volume. In tracheostomized or intubated patients given a loading dose of 1 mg/kg and then 8 hourly i.v. infusions of 2–3.5 mg/kg, average concentrations in the bronchial secretions were 0.7 mg/l with a mean serum/secretion ratio of 0.18.

In patients with cystic fibrosis, receiving 10 mg/kg of the drug per day, the bronchial secretions may contain 2 mg/l or more. Concentrations are low in peritoneal fluid but can rise to 60% of the plasma concentration in peritonitis and in synovial fluid.

Tobramycin crosses the placenta, and concentrations of 0.5 mg/l have been found in the fetal serum when the mother was receiving a dose of 2 mg/kg.

Access to the CSF resembles that of gentamicin (p. 176).

Excretion

Tobramycin is eliminated in the glomerular filtrate and is unaffected by probenecid. Renal clearance is 90 ml/min. About 60% of the administered dose is recovered from the urine over the first 10 h, producing urinary concentrations after a dose of 80 mg of 90–500 mg/l over the first 3 h. The nature of the extrarenal disposal of the remaining 40% of the drug has not been established. In the neonate, urinary concentrations after doses of 2 mg/kg ranged around 10–100 mg/l over the first 8 h, but the total urinary recovery has varied widely. In patients with impaired renal function, urinary concentrations of the drug are depressed and the plasma half-life prolonged in proportion to the rise in serum creatinine, reaching 6–8 h, at a creatinine concentration of 350 μmol/l. In view of the virtually identical behaviour of the two drugs, modification of tobramycin dosage in patients with impaired renal function may be based on the procedures used for gentamicin (p. 176). About 70% of the drug is removed by haemodialysis over 12 h, but the efficiency of different dialysers varies markedly.

Toxicity and side-effects

Ototoxicity

The effect of tobramycin is predominantly on the auditory branch of the eighth nerve; vestibular function is seldom affected. Experimental evidence suggests that comparable effects on cochlear electrophysiology and histology require doses of tobramycin about twice those of gentamicin. In patients, electrocochleography has shown an immediate dramatic reduction of cochlear activity when the serum tobramycin concentration exceeded 8–10 mg/l, but there were no associated symptoms and function recovered fully as the drug was eliminated. Clinical ototoxicity is rare and most likely to be seen in patients with renal impairment or treated concurrently or sequentially with other potentially ototoxic agents.

Nephrotoxicity

Renal impairment with proteinuria, excretion of granular casts, oliguria and rise of serum creatinine has been noted in 1–2% of patients. Some evidence of nephrotoxicity has been found in about 10% of patients, depending on the sensitivity of the tests employed. In patients treated for urinary tract infection, β_2-microglobulin excretion indicated reduced renal tubular function before and during treatment which improved as infection was eliminated. In patients treated with 120 mg loading dose and 80 mg 8 hourly, renal enzyme excretion increased and there was a small but significant reduction in chrome-EDTA clearance even when the clinical condition improved. It has been suggested that intermittent dosage with large but infrequent plasma peaks may be less toxic than, and as efficacious as, continuous dosing. It is generally held that the likelihood of toxicity increases with pre-existing renal impairment and higher or more prolonged dosage, but in a comparison of patients treated with 8 mg/kg per day for *Pseudomonas* endocarditis with those treated with 3 mg/kg per day for Gram-negative sepsis, there was no evidence of renal impairment in either group. Although there was audiological evidence of high frequency loss in some patients receiving the high dosage, there was no sustained loss of conversational hearing. Nor does there seem to be a significant effect of age: in patients aged 20–39 years, the mean elimination half-life of the drug at the end of treatment was 2.3 h while in those aged 60–79 years it was 2.4 h. In severely ill patients, evidence of renal toxicity may be found in 20%.

Other reactions

Other toxic manifestations are rare. Local reactions sometimes occur at the site of injection. Rashes and eosinophilia in the absence of other allergic manifestations are seen. Increased SGOT values may occur in the absence of other evidence of hepatic derangement.

Clinical use

Therapeutic use is for practical purposes identical to that of gentamicin, except possibly for *Pseudomonas* infection, where it has somewhat greater activity against gentamicin-susceptible and some gentamicin-resistant strains. Its use as a possible substitute for gentamicin in the speculative treatment of severe undiagnosed infection is offset by its lower activity against other possibly implicated organisms. It has been successfully used for the treatment of

Pseudomonas septicaemia and pneumonia and infection in cystic fibrosis (p. 691) where, despite the increased dosage required to offset enhanced elimination, toxicity has generally not been a problem. Large doses are required to ensure adequate tissue concentrations and combination with an anti-pseudomonal penicillin is recommended. Used alone, it has been successful in pseudomonal infections of the urinary tract, meninges and soft tissues. It has been used in combination with cephalosporins or clindamycin in the control of febrile episodes in neutropenic patients and in the prophylaxis of abdominal surgery.

Preparations and dosage

Proprietary names: Nebcin, Trobalex, Brulamycin, Tobrasix, Tobrex (Austria), Obracin (Belgium), Nebcine (France), Gernebcin, Tobramaxin (Germany), Nebicina, Tobral (Italy), Nebcina (Norway) Mytobrin (South Africa), Tobradistin (Sweden).

Preparations: Injections, eye drops.

Dosage: Adults i.m., i.v., 3 mg/kg per day in three equal doses every 8 h; 5 mg/kg per day in three to four equal doses may be used for life-threatening infections. The higher dose should be reduced as soon as clinically indicated. Children 6–7.5 mg/kg per day in three to four equally divided doses. Premature or full term neonates up to 4 mg/kg per day in two equal doses every 12 h.

Further information

Burkle W S 1986 Is tobramycin less nephrotoxic than gentamicin? *Clinical Pharmacy* 5: 514–516

Horrevorts A M, Degener J E, Dzoljic-Danilovic G et al 1985 Pharmacokinetics of tobramycin in patients with cystic fibrosis. Implications for the dosing interval. *Chest* 88: 260–264

Horrevorts A M, de Witte T, Degener J E et al 1987 Tobramycin in patients with cystic fibrosis. Adjustments in dosing interval for effective treatment. *Chest* 22: 844–448

Jacoby G A, Blaser M J, Santanam P et al 1990 Appearance of amikacin and tobramycin resistance due to 4'-aminoglycoside nucleotidyltransferase [ANT(4')-II] in Gram-negative pathogens. *Antimicrobial Agents and Chemotherapy* 34: 2381–2386

Mayer P R, Brown C H, Carter R A, Welty T E, Millican M D, Eberhard N K 1986 Pharmacokinetics in geriatric patients. *Drug Intelligence and Clinical Pharmacy* 20: 611–615

Menard R, Molinas C, Arthur M, Duval J, Courvalin P, Leclercq R 1993 Overproduction of 3'-aminoglycoside phospho-transferase type I confers resistance to tobramycin in *Escherichia coli. Antimicrobial Agents and Chemotherapy* 37: 78–83

Murray K M, Bauer L A, Koup J R 1986 Predictive performance of computer dosing methods for tobramycin using two pharmacokinetic models and two weighting algorithms. *Clinical Pharmacy* 5: 411–414

Pasturek J G 2nd, Ragan F A Jr, Phelan M 1987 Tobramycin dosing in the puerperal patient. *Journal of Reproductive Medicine* 32: 343–346

Pedersen S S, Jensen T, Osterhammel D, Osterhammel P 1987 Cumulative and acute toxicity of repeated high-dose tobramycin treatment in cystic fibrosis. *Antimicrobial Agents and Chemotherapy* 31: 594–599

Spruill W J, McCall C Y, Francisco G E 1985 In vitro inactivation of tobramycin by cephalosporins. *American Journal of Hospital Pharmacy* 42: 2506–2509

Walshe J J, Morse G D, Janicke D M, Apicella M A 1986 Cross-over pharmacokinetic analyses comparing intravenous and intraperitoneal administration of tobramycin. *Journal of Infectious Diseases* 153: 796–799

Williams J D (ed) 1978 Tobramycin – comparative toxicity of aminoglycoside antibiotics. *Journal of Antimicrobial Chemotherapy* 4 (suppl A): 1–101

Winslade N E, Adelman M H, Evans E J, Schentag J J 1987 Single-dose accumulation pharmacokinetics of tobramycin and netilmicin in normal volunteers. *Antimicrobial Agents and Chemotherapy* 31: 605–609

Neomycin group

In contrast to the gentamicin and kanamycin groups, the neomycin group is based on 4,5-disubstituted 2-deoxy-streptamine. It includes neomycin, framycetin and paromomycin.

NEOMYCIN

Neomycins A, B and C are fermentation products of *Streptomyces fradii*. The product marketed as 'neomycin' is an isomeric mixture of neomycins B and C supplied as the sulphates. Solutions are stable at room temperature. Framycetin (see p. 194) is essentially neomycin B. Paromomycins I and II (see p. 194) are closely related to neomycin.

	R_1	R_2	R_3
neomycin B	NH_2	H	CH_2NH_2
C	NH_2	CH_2NH_2	H
paromomycin I	OH	H	CH_2NH_2
II	OH	CH_2NH_2	H

Antimicrobial activity

Neomycin is active against staphylococci and a wide range of enterobacteria, but Streptococci, Gram-positive rods and the majority of anaerobic bacteria are resistant. Amongst other organisms susceptible in vitro (MIC 4–8 mg/l) are *Pasteurella*, *Vibrio*, *Borellia* and *Leptospira* spp. It is active against *M. tuberculosis*, including streptomycin-resistant strains. The susceptibility of common pathogenic bacteria is shown in Table 13.1.

Neomycin exerts a rapid bactericidal effect which is enhanced at alkaline pH; when the pH is raised from 5.5 to 8.5, activity is increased 64-fold.

Acquired resistance

Resistance is acquired in a step-wise fashion and, particularly as a result of long continued topical use, in some hospitals resistance in staphylococci became common. The use of neomycin–bacitracin–polymyxin mixtures may have contributed to this, as many strains resistant to neomycin are also resistant to bacitracin. Amongst enterobacteria, *Salmonella* and *Shigella* spp. and strains of *Esch. coli* from infants are commonly resistant. Resistant enterobacteria may appear in the faeces of patients treated orally and in those treated for prolonged periods, most have been found to possess multiple transferable antibiotic resistance. Cross-resistance with kanamycin is often due to the synthesis of APH(3'), though AAC(6'), some forms of AAC(3) and AAD(4')(4") also modify both neomycin and kanamycin. Resistant strains of *Staph. aureus* are usually more resistant to kanamycin than to neomycin. The rare enzyme AAC(1) confers resistance to neomycin, paromomycin and apramycin, but not to other aminoglycosides.

Pharmacokinetics

Very little is absorbed after oral administration and more than 95% is eliminated unchanged in the faeces. Peak plasma concentrations of less than 4 mg/l have been found after an oral dose of 3 g. After i.m. injection of 0.5 g the peak plasma concentration is around 20 mg/l at 1 h. Distribution and excretion resemble that of streptomycin, but the toxicity of neomycin precludes systemic administration except in the most extreme cases.

Toxicity and side-effects

Neomycin is the most liable of all the aminoglycosides to damage the kidneys and the auditory branch of the 8th nerve (Table 13.4). This has almost entirely restricted it to topical and oral use.

Irreversible deafness may develop even if the drug is stopped at the first sign of damage. Loss of hearing may occur as a result of topical applications to wounds or other denuded areas, particularly if renal excretion is impaired. Instillation of ear drops containing neomycin can result in deafness. This generally develops in the second week of treatment and is usually reversible.

Rashes have been described in 6–8% of patients treated topically and these patients may be rendered allergic to other aminoglycosides. Nausea and protracted diarrhoea may follow oral administration. Sufficient drug may be absorbed from the gut on prolonged oral administration to produce deafness but not renal damage. Intestinal malabsorption and superinfection have been seen in patients receiving 4–9 g/day and may develop in patients receiving as little as 3 g/day of the drug. Precipitation of bile salts by the drug may impair the hydrolysis of long-chain triglycerides. Large doses instilled into the peritoneal cavity at operation may be absorbed, with resultant systemic toxicity, and patients concurrently exposed to anaesthetics and muscle relaxants, are liable to suffer neuromuscular blockade, which is reversible by neostigmine.

Neomycin is a useful reagent in the investigation of phospholipase activity as, for example, in arachidonic acid release.

Clinical use

Neomycin has been used extensively for the local treatment of superficial infections with staphylococci and Gram-negative bacilli, either alone or in combination with bacitracin, chlorhexidine or polymyxin. In combination with chlorhexidine or bacitracin, it has also been used in the treatment of staphylococcal nasal carriers, but the appearance of neomycin-resistant strains has reduced its value for this purpose. Prolonged application to the skin may cause sensitization and has proved a fruitful means of facilitating the emergence of resistance. Solutions have been instilled in the urinary bladder for prophylaxis after instrumentation and in the test to distinguish infection of the upper and the lower urinary tract. It has been introduced into the peritoneal cavity at operation for the prevention or treatment of peritonitis and by subconjunctival injection for the treatment of ocular infections, but it is readily absorbed from these sites, with the danger of systemic toxicity or neuromuscular blockade.

Neomycin has been used orally often in combination with other agents, in patients prior to abdominal surgery, or in those at special risk from opportunistic infections with gut bacteria. Oral doses of 4–8 g/day are used to reduce the colonic population of bacteria that generate ammonia or other aminotoxins believed to be responsible for hepatic encephalopathy. Such large doses administered for long periods may result in atrophic changes in the intestinal mucosa with malabsorption of fats, carbohydrates and some drugs, and sufficient may be absorbed to cause deafness. Oral treatment has been used in travellers' diarrhoea and salmonellosis. It exerts a hypocholesterolaemic effect by a mechanism which resembles that of bile acid sequestrants, but its prolonged administration for this purpose may lead to the development of resistance in the bowel flora.

Naka S H, Ima S, Tohmatsu T, Shirato L, Takenaka A, Nozawa Y 1987 Neomycin as a potent agent for arachidonic acid release in human platelets. *Biochemical and Biophysical Research Communications* 146: 820–826

Rappoport B Z 1986 A prospective study of high-frequency auditory function in patients receiving oral neomycin. *Scandinavian Audiology* 15: 67–71

Witebsky F G 1986 Effect of oral neomycin treatment of hyperlipoproteinaemia on antibiotic susceptibilities of stool enteric flora. *American Journal of Cardiology* 58: 375–376

FRAMYCETIN
Neomycin B

A fermentation product of *Streptomyces fradii* and *Streptomyces lavendulae*. Supplied as the sulphate. Buffered aqueous solutions (pH 7) are stable at room temperature. It is required to contain not more than 3% neomycin C and not more than 1% neomycin A.

It is now available only in preparations for oral or topical use. Its properties are those of neomycin (p. 192) which is an isomeric mixture of neomycins B and C.

Preparations and dosage

Proprietary names: Mycifradin, Nivemycin.

Preparations: Tablets, elixir, topical.

Dosage: Adults, oral, 1 g every 4 h for a maximum of 72 h.

Widely available.

Preparations and dosage

Proprietary name: Soframycin.

Preparations: Tablets, topical ophthalmic, aural.

Dosage: Adult, oral, 2–4 g/day in divided doses.

Widely available. Oral preparations not available in the UK.

Further information

DiPitro J T 1985 Oral neomycin sulfate and erythromycin base before colon surgery: a comparison of serum and tissue concentrations. *Pharmacotherapy* 5: 91–94

Jagelman D G 1985 A prospective, randomised, double-blind study of 10% mannitol mechanical bowel preparation combined with oral neomycin and short-term perioperative intravenous Flagyl as prophylaxis in elective colorectal resections. *Surgery* 98: 861–865

Lovering A M, White L O, Reeves D S 1987 AAC(1): a new aminoglycoside-acetylating enzyme modifying the C_1 amino group of apramycin. *Journal of Antimicrobial Chemotherapy* 20: 803–813

Further information

Garrod L P, Lambert H P, O'Grady F 1981 Antibiotic and chemotherapy, 5th edn. Churchill Livingstone, Edinburgh

PAROMOMYCIN
Aminosidin, catenulin, crestomycin, hydroxymycin, estomycin, monomycin A, neomycin E, paucimycin

A fermentation product of *Streptomyces* sp. supplied as the sulphate. The commercial product is a mixture of the two isomeric paromomycins I and II; the chemical structure is shown on p. 193.

Its antibacterial activity is almost identical with that of neomycin; since the structures of its components differ from those of neomycin in having a hydroxyl rather than an amino group at the 6'-position it is not sensitive to AAC(6'). It is active against *M. tuberculosis*, including multidrug-resistant strains, and the *M. avium* complex. Paromomycin differs from other aminoglycosides in being active against *Entamoeba histolytica* and also some helminths. In its pharmacokinetic behaviour and liability to produce deafness and intestinal malabsorption it closely resembles neomycin. As an antibacterial agent, its uses have been similar to those of neomycin, but it has also been successfully used in the treatment of amoebic dysentery and as a single oral dose to eliminate *Taenia saginata*, *Taenia solium*, and *Diphyllobothrium latum*. Repeated doses are necessary to eliminate *Hymenolepsis nana*. It has been used for the treatment of leishmaniasis and has also been used to treat cryptosporidiosis in patients with AIDS.

Preparations and dosage

Proprietary names: Grabbomycin, Humagel, Humatin, Gabbroral (Belgium), Sinosid (Italy).

Preparations: Capsules or syrup.

Dosage: Adult oral dose 25–35 mg/kg per day in three divided doses for 5–10 days.

Limited availability including USA, not UK.

Further information

Armitage K, Flanigan T, Carey J et al 1992 Treatment of cryptosporidiosis with paromomycin. A report of five cases. *Archives of Internal Medicine* 152: 2497–2499

Kayok T P, Reddy M V, Chinnaswamy J, Danziger L H, Gangadharam P R 1994 Activity of aminosidine (paromomycin) for *Mycobacterium tuberculosis* and *Mycobacterium avium*. *Journal of Antimicrobial Chemotherapy* 33: 323–327

Scott J A, Davidson R N, Moody A H et al 1992 Aminosidine (paromomycin) in the treatment of leishmaniasis imported into the United Kingdom. *Transactions of the Royal Society of Tropical Medicine and Hygiene* 86: 617–619

Streptomycin group

Streptomycin itself is the only important member of this group, which also includes dihydrostreptomycin.

STREPTOMYCIN
Estreptomicina

A fermentation product of *Streptomyces griseus*. Available in some countries as the calcium chloride or as the hydrochloride, but usually supplied as the sulphate. Solutions are stable for long periods in the cold.

Antimicrobial activity

Streptomycin is particularly active against Mycobacteria, enterobacteria and some strains of staphylococci. Streptococci and pneumococci are relatively, and anaerobic bacilli and fungi almost completely, resistant (Table 13.1). *M. kansasii* and most strains of *M. ulcerans* are susceptible, as are *Brucella* (MIC 0.5 mg/l), *Francisella*, *Pasteurella* spp. and *Yersinia pestis*.

The antibacterial activity is greatest in a slightly alkaline medium (pH 7.8) and is considerably reduced in media with a pH of 6.0 or less. It is so sensitive to the effect of pH that the natural acidity of a solution of streptomycin sulphate may be sufficient to depress its antibacterial activity: pneumococci inhibited by 20 mg streptomycin sulphate/l (pH 7.1), were not inhibited by 50 mg/l (pH 6.8).

It is actively bactericidal, the velocity of killing increasing progressively with concentration.

Acquired resistance

In contrast to the situation with most other aminoglycosides, high level resistance can result from a single-step mutation (at least for *Esch. coli*) in the *rpsL* gene which encodes ribosomal protein S12 which alters the protein so that binding of streptomycin is reduced. Streptomycin resistance in some clinical isolates of *M. tuberculosis* is associated either with missense mutations in the *rpsL* gene, or with base substitutions at position 904 in the 16S rRNA.

Resistance can also be caused by aminoglycoside-modifying enzymes. Phosphotransferases that modify the 3"-hydroxyl group have been found in both Gram-negative and Gram-positive organisms, a phosphotransferase that modifies the 6-hydroxyl group in *Pseudomonas* spp. and a nucleotidyltransferase that modifies the 3"-hydroxyl group (plus the 9-hydroxyl of spectinomycin) in Gram-negative organisms.

Increase in resistance to streptomycin often occurs within a few days (for *M. tuberculosis* a few weeks) of the beginning of streptomycin treatment, and resistance of many species is now common. Primary streptomycin resistance in *M. tuberculosis* had become uncommon in the UK and USA, though found in more than a third of cases in the Far East. However, since 1990 several clusters of multidrug-resistant tuberculosis have been identified among hospitalized patients with AIDS in the USA.

Low level resistance is due to decreased uptake of the antibiotic. An important therapeutic consequence of this is seen in enterococci, wild strains of which show two distinct levels of resistance. Moderate resistance (MIC 62–500 mg/l) is due to impermeability of the bacterial cell which prevents the drug reaching the ribosome. This impermeability can be overcome by simultaneous exposure to agents such as penicillin, which interfere with synthesis of the bacterial cell wall (p. 11) where the permeability barrier is presumably located. As a result, strains showing moderate resistance to streptomycin exhibit synergy with penicillin, but strains showing high levels of resistance (MIC 1000 mg/l) have ribosomes which are resistant to streptomycin and hence simultaneous treatment with penicillin is without effect.

Ps. aeruginosa can have high level resistance due to ribosomal change or streptomycin-modifying enzymes and low level resistance (up to 200 mg/l) due to decreased uptake of the drug. More than one mechanism of streptomycin resistance also exists in *Staph. aureus*, in some strains of which resistance is plasmid borne, while in others it is probably due to ribosomal modification resulting from mutation at a single chromosomal locus.

No streptomycin resistance was found in the isolates of *Yersinia pestis* from the 1991 outbreak of plague in Tanzania.

It is not infrequent to find strains of meningococci, *Staph. aureus*, *Esch. coli*, *Ps. aeruginosa*, *Proteus* and *M. tuberculosis* which are actually favoured by the presence of the antibiotic or completely dependent on it. Isolated ribosomes from streptomycin-dependent *Esch. coli* show a change in the same single ribosomal protein that determines resistance and synthesize peptides only in the presence of the drug.

Cross-resistance between streptomycin and neomycin and kanamycin is usually one way: strains resistant to neomycin and kanamycin are nearly always resistant to streptomycin, while streptomycin-resistant bacteria are frequently still sensitive to neomycin and kanamycin. However, there is no enzymatic basis for this cross-resistance, which is not universal. Enterococci with high level resistance to gentamicin, and consequent resistance to gentamicin–β-lactam synergy, may show synergy between the β-lactam and streptomycin.

Pharmacokinetics

Streptomycin is not absorbed in any quantity from the intestinal tract. In adults receiving 0.5 or 1 g i.m., peak plasma concentrations of 25–50 and 26–58 mg/l, respectively, are obtained at 0.5–1.5 h. The plasma elimination half-life is 2.4–2.7 h. In patients treated for tuberculosis, considerable variation has been encountered on repeat dosing, the peak concentrations following a dose of 0.75 g, sometimes differing by as much as 50 mg/l. Binding to plasma protein is 35%.

In premature infants, 10 mg/kg produced peak plasma concentrations of 17–42 mg/l at about 2 h with a half-life of 7 h. In patients over the age of 40 years, excretion is delayed and in older subjects commonly incomplete at 24 h. In such patients, a dose of 0.75 g i.m. produces peak plasma concentrations around 25–60 mg/l with a half-life up to 9 h.

Distribution

Streptomycin diffuses fairly rapidly into most body tissues, but is distributed only in the extracellular fluid. It appears in the peritoneal fluid in concentrations of about one-quarter to one-half those present in the blood, and in pleural fluid the concentrations may equal those in the blood. It does not penetrate into the CSF or thick-walled abscesses, but significant amounts are usually present in tuberculous cavities. Concentrations in cord blood are similar to those in maternal blood.

Excretion

Streptomycin is rapidly excreted by glomerular filtration and is unaffected by agents which block tubular secretion. The renal clearance is 30–70 ml/min and 30%–90% of the dose is usually excreted in the first 24 h. Concentrations in the urine often reach 400 mg/l after doses of 0.5 g and 1000 mg/l or more after doses of 1 g. In oliguria, the plasma half-life is prolonged and dosage must be reduced if toxic concentrations are to be avoided. Less than 1% appears in the bile, where concentrations of 3–12.5 mg/l have been recorded.

Toxicity and side-effects

Pain and irritation at the site of injection are common, and sterile inflammatory reactions or peripheral neuritis from direct involvement of a nerve sometimes occur. Many patients experience paraesthesiae in and around the mouth, vertigo and ataxia, headaches, lassitude and 'muzziness in the head'.

Renal dysfunction is rare but has been described in patients receiving 3–4 g/day.

Ototoxicity

The most common serious toxic effect is vestibular disturbance, which is related to total dosage and excessive blood concentrations, and hence to the age of the patient and the state of renal function. In older patients the risk of damage is higher and compensation is less than in young patients. Active secretion into the endolymph or persistence of the drug in the perilymph after the plasma concentration has fallen may play an important part in such ototoxicity. There is no significant relation between incidence of dizziness and peak streptomycin concentration, but a highly significant relation to plasma concentrations exceeding 3 mg/l at 24 h. The risk to hearing is much less, but damage sometimes occurs after only a few doses. Congenital hearing loss or abnormalities in the caloric test or audiogram have several times been described in children born to women treated with streptomycin in pregnancy. There is considerable individual variation in susceptibility to its toxic effects which may be partly genetically determined.

Allergy

In addition to eosinophilia unassociated with other allergic manifestations, rashes and drug fever occur in about 5% of treated patients. These are usually trivial and respond to antihistamine treatment, so that in most cases therapy can be continued, although this should be done with caution, since occasionally severe and even fatal exfoliative dermatitis may develop. Skin sensitization is also common in nurses and dispensers who handle streptomycin and may lead to severe dermatitis, sometimes associated with periorbital swelling and conjunctivitis. Reactions most frequently develop between 4 and 6 weeks, but may appear after the first dose or after 6 months' treatment. Patients who develop hypersensitivity during prolonged therapy can generally be desensitized by giving 20 mg prednisolone daily plus 10 daily increments from 0.1 to 1.0 g when normal dosage will usually be tolerated, or by giving increased doses of streptomycin every 6 h.

Neuromuscular blockade

It is rare for neuromuscular blockade to develop in those whose neuromuscular mechanisms are normal, but patients who are also receiving muscle relaxants or anaesthetics or are suffering from myasthenia gravis are at special risk.

Other effects

Rare neurological manifestations include peripheral neuritis and optic neuritis with scotoma. Other rare effects have been aplastic anaemia, agranulocytosis, haemolytic anaemia, thrombocytopenia, hypocalcaemia and severe bleeding associated with a circulating factor V antagonist.

Clinical use

The most important use of streptomycin is in the treatment of tuberculosis (Ch. 59). It has also been used in the treatment of infection due to *M. kansasii*.

Apart from this, streptomycin is the most effective antibiotic for the treatment of plague (p. 885) and tularaemia (p. 884). It has been frequently used in combination with penicillin, in the treatment of bacterial endocarditis and in combination with a tetracycline has been considered to be an effective treatment for brucellosis (p. 883). It has been used in combination with sulphonamides or rifampicin in the treatment of the variety of mycetoma due to *Actinomyces* spp. Oral streptomycin is of no value in the treatment of enteric infections. Reference is also made to its use in bartonellosis (p. 886) and Whipple's disease (p. 714).

The vestibular end organs are essential to the development of motion sickness, and depression of the vestibular function by streptomycin has been used in the treatment of patients suffering from Meniere's disease.

Preparations and dosage

Proprietary names: Streptomycin sulphate, Strepto-Fatol (Germany), Streptocol (Italy), Novostrep, Solustrep (South Africa), Cidan Est (Spain).

Preparation: Injection.

Dosage: Tuberculosis: Adults i.m. 1 g daily (750 mg daily for adults over 40 years of age). Children i.m. 20 mg/kg per day.

Widely available.

Further information

Edlin B R, Tokars J I, Grieco M H et al 1992 An outbreak of multidrug-resistant tuberculosis among hospitalized patients with the acquired immunodeficiency syndrome. *New England Journal of Medicine* 326: 1514–1521

Honore N, Cole S T 1994 Streptomycin resistance in mycobacteria. *Antimicrobial Agents and Chemotherapy* 38: 238–242

Lyamuya E F, Nyanda P, Mohammedali H, Mhalu F S 1992 Laboratory studies on *Yersinia pestis* during the 1991 outbreak of plague in Lushoto, Tanzania. *Journal of Tropical Medicine and Hygiene* 95: 335–338

Moretz W H Jr, Shea J J Jr, Orchik D J, Emmett J R, Shea J J 3rd 1987 Streptomycin treatment in Meniere's disease. *Otolaryngology – Head and Neck Surgery* 96: 256–259

Nachamkin I, Axelrod P, Talbot G H et al 1988 Multiply high-level-aminoglycoside-resistant enterococci isolated from patients in a University Hospital. *Journal of Clinical Microbiology* 26: 1287–1291

Nicholls W W 1989 The enigma of streptomycin transport. *Journal of Antimicrobial Chemotherapy* 23: 673–676

Yee Y, Farber B, Mates S 1986 Mechanism of penicillin-streptomycin synergy for clinical isolates of viridans streptococci. *Journal of Infectious Disease* 154: 531–534

Zenilman J M, Miller M H, Mandel L J 1986 In vitro studies simultaneously examining effect of oxacillin on uptake of radio-labeled streptomycin and on associated bacterial lethality in *Staphylococcus aureus*. *Journal of Antimicrobial Chemotherapy* 10: 877–882

DIHYDROSTREPTOMYCIN

Obtained by catalytic reduction of streptomycin. Also produced naturally by *Streptomyces humidis*. Supplied as the sulphate.

Dihydrostreptomycin closely resembles streptomycin in its properties, but it is much more liable to produce deafness which is often complete, permanent and may not become evident until after treatment is completed. There is no indication for its use in man.

Further information

Garrod L P, O'Grady F 1971 Antibiotic and chemotherapy, 3rd edn. E & S Livingstone, Edinburgh, p 112–113

Miscellaneous compounds

This group contains a number of compounds that do not fit into the other groups. We include the 'pure aminocyclitol' (see p. 164) spectinomycin and its derivative trospectomycin, apramycin, fortimicin and the 'pure aminoglycoside' (see p. 164) kasugamycin.

SPECTINOMYCIN
Aminospectacin, actinospectacin

A fermentation product of *Streptomyces spectabilis* and *Streptomyces flavopersicus*. Supplied as the dihydrochloride and the sulphate.

	R
spectinomycin	CH_3
trospectomycin	$CH_2CH_2CH_2CH_3$

Antimicrobial activity

Its activity is modest (Table 13.1) and markedly affected by medium composition and pH. It exerts only moderate activity against Gram-positive organisms. It is widely active against enterobacteria but *Providencia* spp. are resistant. Anaerobic bacteria are resistant.

Of particular interest is its activity against *N. gonorrhoeae*, including β-lactamase-producing strains. Amongst other sexually-acquired organisms, *Ureaplasma urealyticum* is susceptible and *Chlamydia trachomatis* and *T. pallidum* resistant.

For most organisms, the MBC is at least four times the MIC and it is regarded as essentially bacteriostatic. In contrast, it is bactericidal for gonococci in concentrations close to the MIC, which is of the order of 2–16 mg/l for both penicillin-susceptible and resistant strains.

Acquired resistance

N. gonorrhoeae resistant to spectinomycin have emerged in South-East Asia, the USA and the UK; the resistance of UK isolates was not attributable to aminoglycoside-modifying enzymes. Spectinomycin was first used as the primary drug of choice against gonorrhoea in the Philippines and Korea in 1981, and in Thailand in 1983; spectinomycin resistance reached 22% in the Philippines by 1988 and 9% in Thailand by 1990.

Acquired resistance in enterobacteria, enterococci and staphylococci can be caused by nucleotidyltransferases that modify the drug at position 9. The enzyme from Gram-negative organisms [ANT(3")(9)] also modifies streptomycin at position 3", thus conferring cross-resistance to the two drugs. There is no enzymatic cross-resistance with 2-deoxystreptamine-containing aminoglycosides.

Pharmacokinetics

Spectinomycin is poorly absorbed on oral administration. Binding to plasma protein is very low. Plasma concentrations produced by intramuscular doses are around 60–80 mg/l,

1 h after 25 mg/kg and 40–160 mg/l 1 h after a dose of 3 g. The plasma half-life is of the order of 2–3 h. It is almost completely excreted unchanged in the urine over 24 h, concentrations on conventional dosage reaching 1 g/l. Excretion is unaffected by probenecid.

Toxicity and side-effects

Toxicity is low. Transient headache, dizziness, pain at the site of injection and occasional fever have been described. No evidence of ototoxicity or renal toxicity has been found in volunteers receiving doses of 2 g 6-hourly for 3 weeks, amounts much in excess of those used therapeutically.

Clinical use

The use of spectinomycin is restricted to the single-dose treatment of gonorrhoea in penicillin-allergic patients or due to penicillin-resistant strains.

Preparations and dosage

Proprietary name: Trobicin, Trobicine, Stanilo, Kempi (Sweden).

Preparation: Injection.

Dosage: Deep i.m. injection adults, 2 g as a single dose of 4 g in two separate i.m. sites in those difficult to treat and areas of assistance.

Widely available.

Further information

Boslego J W, Tramont E C, Takafuji E T et al 1987 Effect of spectinomycin use on the prevalence of spectinomycin-resistant and of penicillinase-producing *Neisseria gonorrhoeae*. *New England Journal of Medicine* 317: 272–278

Clendennen T E, Echeverria P, Saengeur S, Kees E S, Boslego J W, Wignall F S 1992 Antibiotic susceptibility survey of *Neisseria gonorrhoeae* in Thailand. *Antimicrobial Agents and Chemotherapy* 36: 1682–1687

Zenilman J M, Nims L J, Menegus M A, Nolte F, Knapp J S 1987 Spectinomycin-resistant gonococcal infections in the United States 1985–1986 *Journal of Infectious Diseases* 156: 1002–1004

TROSPECTOMYCIN
U-63366F

A propyl derivative of spectinomycin. It is 4–32 times more active than spectinomycin against Gram-positive organisms, *Neisseria* spp., *H. influenzae* and *C. trachomatis*. It is active against anaerobes with 88% of *Bacteroides fragilis* group

isolates, and larger proportions of other anaerobes, inhibited by 32 mg/l. Against most enterobacteria its activity resembles that of the parent compound with which there is complete cross-resistance and identity of sensitivity to aminoglycoside-modifying enzymes. It inhibits aminoglycoside-resistant strains of *Ent. faecalis* at 4 mg/l and *Ent. faecium* at 8 mg/l, but it is not bactericidal even in the presence of ampicillin.

In volunteers given 1 g i.m., mean peak plasma concentrations around 28 mg/l were obtained at about 1 h. The plasma elimination half-life was around 1.9 h. It was generally well tolerated apart from mild and transient pain at the site of injection and mild neurological symptoms and disturbance of liver function tests common to aminoglycosides.

Further information

Appelbaum P C, Spangler S K, Jacobs M R 1991 Susceptibilities of 394 *Bacteroides fragilis*, non-*B. fragilis* group *Bacteroides* species, and *Fusobacterium* species to newer antimicrobial agents. *Antimicrobial Agents and Chemotherapy* 35: 1214–1218

Khardori N, Gandhi M, Adame J, Kalvakuntla L, Rosenbaum B, Bodey G P 1990 The activity in-vitro of trospectinomycin sulphate (U-63366F) against aminoglycoside-resistant enterococci. *Journal of Antimicrobial Chemotherapy* 25: 777–785

Novak E, Paxton L M, Bye A, Patel R, Zurenko G E, Francom S F 1990 Human safety and pharmacokinetics of a single intramuscular dose of a novel spectinomycin analog, trospectomycin (U-63366F). *Antimicrobial Agents and Chemotherapy* 34: 2342–2347

Zurenko G E, Yagi B H, Vavra J J, Wentworth B B 1988 In vitro antibacterial activity of trospectomycin (U-63366F) a novel spectinomycin analog. *Antimicrobial Agents and Chemotherapy* 32: 216–223

APRAMYCIN

Apramycin (nebramycin factor 2) is one of a group of antibiotics produced by a strain of *Streptomyces tenebrarius*. It is a 4-substituted deoxystreptamine with a unique octadiose in bicyclic form together with the rare 4-aminoglucose. It has relatively low intrinsic activity for an aminoglycoside and is used in veterinary medicine for the treatment of intestinal bacterial infections in animals. It is resistant to all known aminoglycoside-modifying enzymes apart from AAC(3)IV and the rare AAC(1). AAC(3)IV was initially found in bacteria from animals, but subsequently has appeared in strains from humans.

Further information

Chaslus-Dancla E, Glupcznski Y, Gerbaud G, Lagorce M, Lafont J P, Courvalin P 1989 Detection of apramycin resistant *Enterobacteriaceae* in hospital isolates. *FEMS Microbiology Letters* 52: 261–265

Hunter J E, Hart C A, Shelley J C, Walton J R, Bennett M 1993 Human isolates of apramycin-resistant *Escherichia coli* which contain the genes for the AAC(3)IV enzyme. *Epidemiology and Infection* 110: 253–259

Johnson A P, Burns L, Woodford N et al 1994 Gentamicin resistance in clinical isolates of *Escherichia coli* encoded by genes of veterinary origin. *Journal of Medical Microbiology* 40: 221–226

Lovering A M, White L O, Reeves D S 1987 AAC(1): a new aminoglycoside-acetylating enzyme modifying the C1 aminogroup of apramycin. *Journal of Antimicrobial Chemotherapy* 20: 803–813

Wray C, Hedges R W, Shannon K P, Bradley D E 1986 Apramycin and gentamicin resistance in *Escherichia coli* and salmonellas isolated from farm animals. *Journal of Hygiene (London)* 97: 445–456

FORTIMICIN
Astromicin

Fortimicin A (astromicin, KW-1070) is a pseudodisaccharide aminoglycoside produced by *Micromonospora olivoastero-spora*. Two derivatives, 3-*O*-demethyl fortimicin A and dactimicin, originally isolated from *Dactylosporangium matsuzakienzae* and which chemically is the formimidoyl derivative of fortimicin A, have also been investigated. Fortimicin A has the spectrum of activity expected for aminoglycosides with intrinsic activity similar to that of amikacin for most groups of organisms but shows relatively poor activity against *Ps. aeruginosa*. 3-*O*-Demethyl fortimicin A tends to have slightly higher activity; its activity against *Ps. aeruginosa* is approximately three-fold higher than that of fortimicin A. Dactimicin is similar to astromicin in in vitro activity. The three compounds are active against many strains that produce aminoglycoside-modifying enzymes. Fortimicin A and 3-*O*-demethyl fortimicin A are sensitive to AAC(3) and the APH(2")/AAC(6') bifunctional enzyme, but dactimicin is more resistant than astromicin to AAC(3)I, probably owing to the protective action of the formimidoyl group.

	R_1	R_2
Fortimicin A	CH_3	H
O-Demethyl fortimicin A	H	H
Dactimicin	CH_3	CH=NH

Peak concentrations of 10–12 mg/l fortimicin A were found in the blood following 200 mg i.v. or i.m. administration to volunteers; over 85% of the drug was recovered in urine during the 8 hours following administration.

Preparations and dosage

Preparation: Injection.

Dosage: Adults, 400 mg daily in 2 divided doses.

Limited availability. Not available in the UK.

Further information

Felmingham D, Jones K 1989 In vitro activity of dactimicin and other aminoglycosides against bacteria producing aminoglycoside-modifying enzymes. *Drugs under Experimental and Clinical Research* 15: 133–136

Matsuhashi Y, Yoshida T, Hara T, Kazuno Y, Inouye S 1985 In vitro and in vivo antibacterial activities of dactimicin, a novel pseudodisaccharide aminoglycoside, compared with those of other aminoglycoside antibiotics. *Antimicrobial Agents and Chemotherapy* 27: 589–594

Nakashima M, Takiguchi Y, Inoue A, Kobayashi S 1986 A phase I study on intravenous drip infusion of astromicin. *Japanese Journal of Antibiotics* 39: 1453–1472

Omoto S, Yoshida T, Kurebe M, Inouye S 1987 Dactimicin, a new, less toxic aminoglycoside antibiotic active against resistant bacteria. *Drugs under Experimental and Clinical Research* 13: 719–725

KASUGAMYCIN

A fermentation product of *Streptomyces kasugaensis*. Its antibacterial activity is generally weak, but attention has been paid to its activity against mycobacteria, *Pseudomonas* (MIC 16–32 mg/l) and *Leptospira*. The most striking contrast with major aminoglycosides is that up to 40% can be recovered from the urine after oral administration. After a dose of 1 g i.v., peak plasma concentrations are around 100 mg/l and after the same dose i.m. between 20 and 25 mg/l at 1–2 h. The plasma elimination half-life is around 3 h and peak concentrations in the urine exceed 1000 mg/l. The drug has been used to some effect in the treatment of Pseudomonas urinary infection, but anorexia, which is often severe, is relatively common and this, combined with indications of nephrotoxicity, has deprived it of much therapeutic interest.

Further information

Garrod L P, Lambert H P, O'Grady F 1981 Antibiotic and chemotherapy, 4th edn. Churchill Livingstone, Edinburgh, p 117

β-Lactams: cephalosporins

R. Wise

Introduction

The compounds are based on cephalosporin C, which together with other antibiotics was found among the fermentation products of *Cephalosporium acremonium* cultivated from a Sardinian sewage outfall by Professor Giuseppe Brotzu in 1948. Since then the number of semi-synthetic cephalosporins developed has exceeded 100, all with similar names and often similar properties. It should be remembered that the properties shared by this group of compounds are more numerous and important than the differences between them, which tend to be magnified by commercial pressures. This is not to say that the more recently available agents are not significantly different from those of 20–30 years ago.

The cephalosporins and related cephamycins all have a 6-membered dihydrothiazine ring (as against penicillins which have a 5-membered thiazolidine ring) fused to the β-lactam ring (see Ch. 16). They are derivatives of 7-aminocephalosporanic acid (7-ACA) which can be modified at a number of positions: alterations at the C-3 position

tend to affect the pharmacokinetic and metabolic properties; introduction of an oxymethyl group at C-7 yields a cepha-mycin with enhanced β-lactamase stability, especially for the cephalosporinases of certain *Bacteroides* spp.; other changes at the C-7 or C-12 positions alter, in general, the antibacterial and/or β-lactamase stability – for example, an aminothiazolyl group confers high activity against Gram-negative bacilli.

Other compounds conveniently considered alongside the cephalosporins include the oxacephems, in which the sulphur of the dihydrothiazine ring is replaced by oxygen, and the carbacephems in which the replacement is carbon.

Classification

Attempts to classify the cephalosporins are either too simplistic, such as those describing the agents as 'first', 'second', 'third' and, possibly, 'fourth' generation cephalosporins based upon increasing activity (usually against Gram-negative bacilli) and enhanced β-lactamase stability, or are overcumbersome. The following grouping is adopted here:

Box 14.1

Group 1	Group 2	Group 3	Group 4	Group 5	Group 6	Group 7
Cefazaflur	Cefaclor	Cefbuperazone*	Cefmenoxime	Cefdinir	Cefoperazone	Cefepime
Ceforanide	Cefadroxil	Cefmetazole*	Cefodizime	Cefetamet	Cefpimizole	Cefpirome
Ceftezole	Cefatrizine	Cefminox*	Cefotaxime	Cefixime	Cefpiramide	
Cephacetrile	Cefroxadine	Cefonicid	Ceftizoxime	Cefpodoxime	Cefsulodin	
Cephaloridine	Cephalexin	Cefotetan*	Ceftriaxone	Cefprozil	Ceftazidime	
Cephalothin	Cephradine	Cefotiam	Latamoxef†	Ceftibuten		
Cephapirin	Loracarbef‡	Cefoxitin*				
Cephazolin		Cefuroxime				
		Cephamandole				

*7-Methoxycephalosporin (cephamycin).
†7-Methoxyoxacephem.
‡1-Carbacephem.

Group 1: parenteral compounds of moderate antimicrobial activity and resistance to staphylococcal β-lactamase, hydrolysed by a wide variety of enterobacterial β-lactamases.

Group 2: oral compounds of moderate antimicrobial activity resistant to staphylococcal β-lactamase and moderately resistant to some enterobacterial β-lactamases.

Group 3: parenteral compounds of moderate antimicrobial activity resistant to a wide range of β-lactamases.

Group 4: parenteral compounds with potent antimicrobial activity and resistance to a wide range of β-lactamases.

Group 5: oral compounds with potent antimicrobial activity and resistance to a wide range of β-lactamases.

Group 6: parenteral compounds with activity against *Pseudomonas aeruginosa* and resistance to a wide range of β-lactamases.

Group 7: parenteral compounds with potent activity against enterobacteria, modest activity against *Ps. aeruginosa*, enhanced β-lactamase stability and enhanced anti-staphylococcal activity.

Groups 1 and 2 belong to the 'first' generation compounds; group 3 to the 'second'; groups 4–6 to the 'third'; and group 7 to the possible 'fourth' (see Box 14.1).

Antimicrobial activity

Cephalosporins are generally active against *Staphylococcus aureus* and coagulase-negative staphylococci, including β-lactamase-producing strains, although the degree of activity varies among different members of the group. Methicillin-resistant staphylococci are usually resistant. Streptococci, including pneumococci, are susceptible but *Enterococcus faecalis* and *Enterococcus faecium*, despite their susceptibility to ampicillin and benzylpenicillin, are virtually completely resistant. *Streptococcus pneumoniae* with altered penicillin-binding proteins (PBPs) rendering them less susceptible to penicillin, are also less susceptible to the cephalosporins (overuse of which may have led to resistance in the first place); however, different cephalosporins vary in their affinity for these target sites. Cephalosporins of groups 4–6 are often more active than others against these strains, but susceptibility should be confirmed (by minimum inhibitory concentration (MIC) titration) in each case. Many Gram-negative species including neisseriae, *Haemophilus influenzae*, *Escherichia coli*, salmonellae, some klebsiellae and *Proteus mirabilis* are sensitive to varying degrees. Inoculum-related effects are common, particularly when compounds of groups 1 and 2 are tested against Gram-negative bacilli. *Ps. aeruginosa* is sensitive only to group 6 compounds. Bactericidal synergy is commonly demonstrable with aminoglycosides and a number of other agents, and cephalosporins figure largely in combinations intended to provide very broad-spectrum cover, particularly in immunocompromised patients. Mycobacteria, mycoplasmas and fungi are generally resistant.

Cephalosporins act at the same sites in the bacterial cell as the penicillins, inducing the same spectrum of concentration-dependent morphological changes and exhibiting similar variation in their affinities for the various PBPs. Group 2 compounds, pre-eminently cephalexin and cephradine, do not prevent elongation of susceptible enterobacteria, which continue to grow into filaments. For this reason they are much more slowly bactericidal than group 1 compounds, which induce spheroplast formation and prompt lysis of the cells.

Acquired resistance

The most important form of resistance is that due to the elaboration of β-lactamases (p. 319). The degree of stability to staphylococcal β-lactamase differs and some agents, notably cephazolin and cephaloridine, are hydrolysed quite rapidly. Three categories of stability to *Staph. aureus* β-lactamase are distinguished according to the rate of hydrolysis relative to that of benzylpenicillin (100): high (>10) – cephaloridine and cephazolin; moderate (1–10) – cephalexin and cephradine; and low (<1) – cefatrizine and cefaclor.

The chromosomal β-lactamase of *Esch. coli*, which has virtually no hydrolytic activity against ampicillin, slowly degrades some of the earlier cephalosporins, including cephalothin, cephaloridine and cephazolin, and is responsible for the inoculum effect observed with *Esch. coli*. The *Bacteroides fragilis* group also possess chromosomal β-lactamases that are more active against cephalosporins than against penicillins. These enzymes are able to inactivate most cephalosporins, including cefuroxime, cefotaxime and ceftizoxime. Cephamycins and latamoxef are not hydrolysed.

Genera, including *Citrobacter*, *Enterobacter* and *Serratia*, with an inducible, or derepressible chromosomal β-lactamase (p. 319) exhibit decreased susceptibility to a wide variety of β-lactam agents, including group 4 cephalosporins. Cephalosporins vary in their efficiency as inducers. Cefoxitin and cefmetazole are more potent inducers than are cephazolin and cefotiam of the *Enterobacter cloacae* and *Citrobacter* enzymes and cephazolin and cefuroxime are more potent inducers of those of *Serratia* and *Morganella*. Cefmenoxime, cefotaxime, ceftizoxime, ceftriaxone and cefuroxime are poor inducers.

In addition to chromosomal β-lactamases, Gram-negative bacilli may possess plasmid-mediated enzymes (p. 319) against which different cephalosporins exhibit considerable variation in stability. Transmissible resistance to cefotaxime and cefuroxime has been demonstrated in *Klebsiella pneumoniae* and to cefotaxime, ceftriaxone and ceftazidime in *Esch. coli*. Variants of the TEM-1, TEM-2 and SHV series of β-lactamases can hydrolyse all cephalosporins to varying extents. For example, the TEM-5 enzyme will hydrolyse ceftazidime more efficiently than cefotaxime, yet this is reversed with TEM-9. Generally, the group 5 oral agents are more resistant to plasmid-mediated β-lactamase hydrolysis than are the group 2 agents. The common TEM and PSE enzymes are predominantly responsible for the resistance of *Ps. aeruginosa* to cefoperazone and cefsulodin; but other mechanisms are involved in resistance to other antipseudomonal cephalosporins.

The resistance of Gram-negative bacilli does not depend solely on β-lactamase formation. It varies also with the extent to which the antibiotic can penetrate the outer cell membrane and reach the site of enzyme formation. This property, known as crypticity, can be measured by comparing the enzyme activity of intact and disrupted cells. Resistance may also be intrinsic resulting from a change in the biochemical target of the antibiotic; that is the PBPs.

Pharmacokinetics

The oral agents in group 2 are generally well absorbed with the bioavailability of cefadroxil, cefazaflur, cefroxadine, cephalexin and cephradine in excess of 85%. The bioavailability of some of the agents in other groups is enhanced by prodrug formulation, for example cefetamet pivoxyl, cefuroxime axetil and cefpodoxime proxetil. These latter agents tend to have improved absorption following food, whereas food has little or a deleterious effect on the absorption of group 2 compounds. Cefaclor is relatively unstable in the body.

Cephalosporins carrying an acetoxymethyl group at C-3, which include cephalothin, cephaloglycin, cephapirin, cephacetrile and cefotaxime, are susceptible to mammalian esterases which remove the acetyl group to form the corresponding hydroxymethyl compound. Such desacetyl-cephalosporins generally exhibit poorer antibacterial activity than the parent compounds, and spontaneous cyclization of the hydroxyl group with the carboxyl at C-4 may occur. The relevance (if any) of deacetylation to therapy has not been established. Most cephalosporins are rapidly eliminated with plasma half-lives of 1–2 h, but some are more persistent with half-lives of 3.5 h (cefotetan), 4.5 h (cefonicid), 5 h (cefpiramide) and 8.5 h (ceftriaxone).

Cephalosporins are well distributed, achieving high concentrations in the tissues and serous cavities, but penetration into the eye and the cerebrospinal fluid (CSF) is poor. They cross the placenta. They are generally excreted in high concentrations in the urine by both glomerular filtration and tubular secretion and their elimination is depressed by probenecid and renal failure. Cephaloridine is exclusively excreted in the glomerular filtrate, but concentrated by the proximal tubular cells – a property which it shares with aminoglycosides – and which is responsible for its effect on renal function (p. 75). The less active metabolites resulting from removal of acetoxymethyl groups at

C-3 are also excreted in the urine. Some excretion is via the bile, and notably high concentrations of cephazolin, cephamandole, cefbuperazone, cefmenoxime, cefoperazone, ceftriaxone and latamoxef may be achieved. In the case of ceftriaxone transient biliary 'sludge' of calcium ceftriaxone may occur.

The clearance of a number of compounds (cephalothin, cephapirin, cefotaxime) depends to a significant degree on hepatic metabolism. Hepatic uptake and transport tend to be a feature of drugs that are highly protein bound, and are apparently related to ability to bind to a liver protein and also to molecular weight (MW) >500 (ceftriaxone, cefotaxime, cefoperazone). Cefoperazone, which has the highest molecular weight (667) of current congeners, is 60–80% excreted in bile, in contrast, for example, to 10% for ampicillin (MW 371) or carbenicillin (MW 422).

Hepatic clearance tends to be lower in biliary obstruction than in cirrhosis but the correlation with type of disease is poor, partly because compensatory changes in drug distribution and renal excretion may be extensive. Where compounds are deacetylated to inactive metabolites which are excreted predominantly by the kidney, hepatic failure has little effect on the plasma half-life, in part because deacetylating enzymes are widely distributed. The presence of ascites and oedema in liver failure increases the volume of distribution, reducing the plasma concentration and increasing the elimination half-life, and reduction of serum albumen and accumulation of inhibitors of protein binding such as bilirubin can increase the unbound fraction of highly bound compounds, facilitating their elimination in the glomerular filtrate. The compensatory role of the kidney is well exemplified, for example, by cefoperazone, of which the renal excretion rises from around 20% in normal subjects to around 90% in patients in hepatic failure.

Toxicity and side-effects

Severe local pain (requiring the addition of lidocaine) and thrombophlebitis are most common with cefoxitin and cephalothin. Hypersensitivity occurs in 0.5–10% of patients, mostly in the form of rashes, eosinophilia, drug fever and serum sickness. In addition to immediate reactions, a maculopapular rash with or without fever, lymphadenopathy and eosinophilia may appear after several days' treatment. Severe reactions are very rare. As with penicillins, allergy to cephalosporins is based on major (cephaloyl) and minor antigenic determinants. These cross-react with antibodies to penicillins, but clinical reactions to cephalosporins in penicillin-allergic patients are rare. About 10% of such reactions are said to occur, generally in patients who react to a variety of drugs. Nonetheless, the generally accepted advice is that cephalosporins should not be given to patients who have previously suffered a well-documented severe reaction to penicillins. Specific allergy to cephalosporins also occurs, but there is no evidence that the compounds differ markedly in allergenicity. A number of cephalosporins interfere with: alkaline copper reduction tests for glucose, but not enzyme-based tests; the Porter–Silber reaction for 17-hydroxycorticosteroids; and the alkaline picrate assay of creatinine giving falsely elevated values.

Group 1

These compounds are generally well tolerated. A positive direct Coombs' test has been found in up to 5% of patients receiving cephalothin which is due to non-specific red cell adhesion caused by cephalothin protein complexes, generally without clinical consequences. Specific anticephalosporin antibodies rarely develop, but can lead to haemolytic anaemia. Reversible abnormalities of platelet function and coagulation resulting from several different mechanisms have been described. Unlike those encountered with some group 4 agents, these are of little clinical significance, but the possibility of potentiation of coumarin anticoagulants has been raised. Thrombocytopenia and neutropenia are occasionally seen. Transient abnormalities of liver function tests without other evidence of hepatotoxicity and gastro-intestinal disturbances have also occurred. In patients receiving excessive doses, especially in the presence of renal failure, central nervous system (CNS) disturbances may occur.

The most important toxic manifestation produced by a group 1 agent is the drug-related renal toxicity of cephalo-ridine. This risk, which is increased by pre-existing renal disease, or administration of potent diuretics such as frusemide, is related to the special transport characteristics of cephaloridine and is much less likely to occur with other agents of the group. Cephazolin renal toxicity can be inhibited by probenecid and appears to depend on the same mechanism, but weight for weight cephazolin is 3 or 4 times less toxic than cephaloridine. Rare disturbances of renal function attributed to other agents in this group appear to have the direct toxic or allergic origins described for penicillins. Claims that the nephrotoxicity of cephalosporins is potentiated by aminoglycosides have been disputed.

Group 2

These agents are generally well tolerated and show side-effects essentially similar to those seen with those of group 1 agents. Gastro-intestinal disturbances and hyper-sensitivity reactions may occur. Candida overgrowth with vaginitis has been a feature of some studies. There is no evidence of significant renal toxicity. Rare reversible haematological abnormalities have been described. As with other β-lactam antibiotics, if very high concentrations are achieved, there may be CNS disturbances and, if they are given in excessive doses, particularly to patients with renal failure, there may be convulsions. Serum sickness has been seen with cefaclor.

Groups 3 and 4

On the whole, these are well tolerated and reactions to them have generally been those encountered with earlier cephalosporins. Pain at the site of intramuscular injection and phlebitis at the site of intravenous administration have been fairly common. Hypersensitivity, principally in the form of rashes, has been seen, but severe reactions have been very rare and the degree of cross-allergenicity with penicillin does not appear to differ from the earlier agents. Diarrhoea has been encountered in about 5% of patients and pseudo-membranous colitis has been described.

Among the agents with a methylthiotetrazole (MTT) side-chain (cefbuperazone, cefmenoxime, cefmetazole, cefminox, cefoperazone, cefotetan, cephamandole, latamoxef), a disulfuram-like reaction, evidently due to inhibition of aldehyde dehydrogenase, has occurred relatively fre-quently. The MTT group leaves the molecule when the β-lactam ring is opened, on binding to protein and in solution. It is released and reabsorbed after biliary excretion of the parent cephalosporin. Free MTT is demonstrable in the blood of patients and in solutions prepared for intravenous (i.v.) infusion. MTT does not itself inhibit aldehyde dehydrogenase and the disulfuram-like effect appears to be due to the disulphide dimer. Despite the presence of the MTT group, there is some evidence that the mechanism of ethanol metabolism inhibition by latamoxef is different and the major problems have been associated with this compound. Patients should be advised to avoid alcohol during and 3 days after treatment with these agents. The MTT side-chain is also associated with hypoprothrombin-aemia (see below).

Platelet abnormalities. Abnormalities of coagulation have been associated with β-lactams since platelet dysfunction was first attributed to benzylpenicillin. It is particularly noted in patients receiving carbenicillin and ticarcillin in high dosage and results in gross prolongation of the template bleeding time to >20 min. Patients with severe renal impair-ment are most at risk from the combination of high β-lactam plasma concentrations and uraemic platelet dysfunction. The effect results from interference with platelet–receptor inter-action and is common to all β-lactams, but is much less frequently seen with cephalosporins, with the exception of latamoxef which shares an α-carboxy substituent with the carboxypenicillins.

High concentrations (2–3 g/l) of most β-lactams will depress in vitro the aggregation response of platelets to adenosine diphosphate and other aggregatory agonists, but these concentrations are well above those achieved thera-peutically and potency in such tests is poorly correlated with bleeding tendency and prolonged template bleeding time. In volunteers, therapeutic doses of benzylpenicillin, a number of other penicillins and latamoxef all increase the bleeding time in a time and concentration dependent manner.

Hypoprothrombinaemia. Although penicillins have long been associated with clotting abnormalities, it was cephalosporins that brought bleeding associated with β-lactams into prominence when cephamandole, cefoperazone, latamoxef and other compounds with a C-3 MTT side-chain (see above), were found to induce severe hypoprothrombinaemia, especially in patients who were malnourished, had renal failure or were treated for prolonged periods. The deficiency is readily reversed by vitamin K_1.

Changes in bowel flora, sometimes accompanied by emergence of resistant organisms, including *Clostridium difficile*, are particularly likely with those potent agents which are extensively excreted in the bile and because of their non-absorption achieve substantial faecal concentrations. Particular concern has naturally been expressed that such changes could be a feature of group 5 agents. The more recent agents do not appear to exert significant renal, hepatic or CNS toxicity.

Clinical use

Group 1

Cephaloridine and cephazolin are relatively unstable to staphylococcal β-lactamase and should not be used to treat patients suffering from such infections. Cephalothin (which cephacetrile and cephapirin resemble) is similar in efficacy to β-lactamase-stable penicillins in the treatment of severe staphylococcal disease and has been substituted in penicillin-allergic patients. Strains resistant to methicillin are also resistant to these cephalosporins. By contrast, they may be active against some otherwise resistant strains of *Staphylococcus epidermidis* and have been used for the treatment of such infections.

They have been successful in the treatment of Gram-negative infections of the urinary tract. For the treatment of severe respiratory tract or generalized infection with enterobacteria they are not reliable when used alone, and the addition of an aminoglycoside to improve bactericidal activity is necessary. They should be avoided in the treatment of diseases where *H. influenzae* or enterococci may be implicated. They are not reliable agents for use alone in the treatment of severe undiagnosed sepsis. They have been used in gonorrhoea and syphilis, especially in penicillin-allergic patients. They have been used extensively and with some good reported results, for the chemoprophylaxis of large bowel surgery, total hip replacement and cardiac surgery, but it should be noted that unnecessary prophylaxis with cephalosporins has been identified in a number of series as the major single cause of antibiotic misuse.

Because of its higher biliary concentration, cephazolin has been used in the prophylaxis and treatment of biliary infection. Among agents of this group, cephazolin is preferred by some prescribers because of its longer half-life. Unreliable access to the CSF casts doubt on the wisdom of their use in meningitis, although they have been used successfully.

Group 2

These agents have had widespread use for the treatment of upper respiratory, urinary, soft tissue and a variety of other infections. They are possible alternatives to benzylpenicillin in allergic patients for the treatment of streptococcal, pneumococcal and staphylococcal infections. Because of the prevalence of resistant strains, they should not be used as penicillin substitutes in the prophylaxis or treatment of clostridial infections.

They are less effective than established agents as single dose therapy for uncomplicated urinary infection, but may be useful for the long term treatment of selected patients with persistent or recurrent infection due to sensitive organisms. They are inactive against enterococci which may emerge in the course of treatment. They have been used in gonorrhoea and also for the prophylaxis and treatment of bone and joint infections. With the exception of cefaclor they should not be used for the treatment of infections in which *H. influenzae* is known, or likely, to be implicated.

Groups 3 and 4

These agents have been used successfully to treat a variety of Gram-negative bacterial infections, but their principal place is in the management of infection due to organisms resistant to older agents. They have been successfully used in hospital-acquired pneumonia, particularly that due to enterobacteria. They are inactive against *Legionella pneumophila*, *Mycoplasma pneumoniae* and *Coxiella burnetii*. Their in vitro properties strongly commend them for the treatment of severe sepsis of unknown or possibly mixed bacterial origin. It is not established that the superior activity in vitro of group 4 over group 3 compounds is reflected in greater clinical efficacy. Despite the difference in potency, it is customary to give similar doses of compounds in both groups, partly because the very high activity seen against enterobacteria is not exhibited against Gram-positive organisms.

Where pseudomonas infection is unlikely and infection does not arise from sites in which enterococci or bacteroides are likely to be involved, cefuroxime and cefotaxime have been used successfully for the treatment of severe undiagnosed infection, either alone or in conjunction with other agents. Superinfection with enterococci may complicate treatment and relatively frequently resistance has developed during treatment of infections due to *Ps. aeruginosa* or *Enterobacter* spp.

Group 4 agents now have an established place in the treatment of meningitis due to many enterobacteria and β-lactamase-producing *H. influenzae*. They are not effective in the treatment of meningitis due to *Listeria monocytogenes*, *Enterobacter*, *Ps. aeruginosa* or *Serratia* spp. Despite their in vitro potency, they do not appear to offer any advantage over established therapy in the treatment of meningitis due to *H. influenzae* or *Neisseria meningitidis*. Their activity and resistance to β-lactamases has led to their successful use for the treatment of infection due to β-lactamase-producing gonococci.

Group 5

Those oral compounds may well replace the group 2 agents if resistance to the earlier compounds becomes significant. The relatively lower activity of cefixime and ceftibuten against Gram-positive cocci suggests they should be used with caution in infections with these organisms. The incidence of side-effects is generally low, but gastro-intestinal problems may be higher with these more active compounds than with those in group 2.

Group 6

Ceftazidime has achieved success in infection due to *Ps. aeruginosa*, particularly in patients with cystic fibrosis, and as a single agent in the management of such problems as sepsis of unidentified origin in immunocompromised patients. Cefsulodin and cefoperazone are indicated only in proven or highly suspected pseudomonas infection and have often been given in combination with an appropriate aminoglycoside.

Group 7

Cefpirome and cefepime are relative newcomers to the field. Their major properties are similar to those of group 4 agents. They will probably be reserved for use in patients with severe infections caused by bacteria with plasmid and chromosomally mediated β-lactamases, and as such will generally be used in hospital-acquired infections or in serious problems in the neutropenic patient.

Further information

Anonymous 1993 Antimicrobial prophylaxis in surgery. *Medical Letter* 35: 91–94

Bignall C 1994 The eradication of gonorrhoea. *British Medical Journal* 309: 1103–1104

Blanca M, Fernandez J, Miranda A et al 1989 Cross-reactivity between penicillins and cephalosporins: clinical and immunologic studies. *Journal of Allergy and Clinical Immunology* 83: 381–385

Cherubin C E, Eng R H, Norrby R, Modal J, Humbert G, Overturf G 1989 Penetration of newer cephalosporins into cerebrospinal fluid. *Reviews of Infectious Diseases* 11: 526–548

Cojocel C, Gottsch U, Tolle K L, Baumann K 1988 Nephrotoxic potential of first-, second-, and third-generation cephalosporins. *Archives of Toxicology* 62: 458–464

Cunha B A, Gossling H R, Pasternak H S, Nightingale C H, Quintilliani R 1984 Penetration of cephalosporins into bone. *Infection* 12: 80–84

de Lalla F, Privitera G, Ortisi G et al 1989 Third generation cephalosporins as a risk factor for *Clostridium difficile* associated disease: a four year survey in a general hospital. *Journal of Antimicrobial Chemotherapy* 23: 623–631

Eichenwald H F, Schmitt H J 1986 The cephalosporin antibiotics in pediatric practice. *European Journal of Pediatrics* 144: 532–538

Fassbender M, Lode H, Schaberg T, Borner K, Koeppe P 1993 Pharmacokinetics of new oral cephalosporins, including a new carbacephem. *Clinical Infectious Diseases* 16: 646–653

Follath F, Costa E, Thommen A, Frei R, Burdeska A, Meyer J 1987 Clinical consequences of development of resistance to third generation cephalosporins. *European Journal of Clinical Microbiology* 6: 446–450

Fry D E 1986 Third generation cephalosporins in surgical practice. *American Journal of Surgery* 15: 306–313

Goldstein R S, Smith P F, Tarloffj B, Contardi L, Rush G F, Hook J B 1988 Biochemical mechanisms of cephaloridine nephrotoxicity. *Life Sciences* 42: 1809–1816

Gustafero C A, Steckelberg J M 1991 Cephalosporin antimicrobial agents and related compounds. *Mayo Clinic Proceedings* 66: 1064–1073

Harding S M 1985 Pharmacokinetics of the third-generation cephalosporins. *American Journal of Medicine* 79 (2A): 21–24

Ives T J, Frey J J, Furr S J, Bentz E J 1987 Effect of an educational intervention on oral cephalosporin use in primary care. *Archives of Internal Medicine* 147: 44–47

Izhar M 1994 Cephalosporins: a guide to use in general practice. *Prescriber* 5: 55–74

Jones R N 1989 A review of cephalosporin metabolism: a lesson to be learned for future chemotherapy. *Diagnostic Microbiology and Infectious Disease* 12: 25–31

Kitson T M 1987 The effect of cephalosporin antibiotics on alcohol metabolism: a review. *Alcohol* 4: 143–148

Meyers B R 1985 Comparative toxicities of third generation cephalosporins. *American Journal of Medicine* 79: 96–103

Murphy M F, Metcalf P, Grint P C et al 1985 Cephalosporin-induced immune neutropenia. *British Journal of Haematology* 59: 9–14

Nanji A A, Poon R, Hinberg I 1987 Interference by cephalosporins with creatinine measurement by desk-top analysers. *European Journal of Clinical Pharmacology* 33: 427–429

Nichols R L, Wikler M A, McDevitt J T, Lentek A L, Hosutt J A 1987 Coagulopathy associated with extended-spectrum cephalosporins in patients with serious infections. *Antimicrobial Agents and Chemotherapy* 31: 281–285

Nicolle L E 1988 Prior antimicrobial therapy and resistance of *Enterobacter, Citrobacter* and *Serratia* to third generation cephalosporins. *Journal of Hospital Infection* 11: 321–327

Norrby S R 1986 Adverse reactions and interactions with newer cephalosporin and cephamycin antibiotics. *Medical Toxicology* 1: 32–46

Quin J D 1989 The nephrotoxicity of cephalosporins. *Adverse Drug Reactions and Acute Poisoning Reviews* 8: 63–72

Sabath L D 1989 Reappraisal of the antistaphylococcal activities of first generation (narrow-spectrum) and second-generation (expanded spectrum) cephalosporins. *Antimicrobial Agents and Chemotherapy* 33: 407–411

Sanders W E, Sanders C C 1988 Inducible beta-lactamases: clinical and epidemiologic implications for use of newer cephalosporins. *Reviews of Infectious Diseases* 10: 830–838

Sattler F R, Weitekamp M R, Ballard J O 1986 Potential for bleeding with the new beta-lactam antibiotics. *Annals of Internal Medicine* 105: 924–931

Schentag J J, Welage L S, Williams J S et al 1988 Kinetics and action of N-methyl-thiotetrazole in volunteers and patients. Population-based clinical comparisons of antibiotics with and without this moiety. *American Journal of Surgery* 155 (5A): 40–44

Seminar-in-print 1987 The cephalosporin antibiotics. *Drugs* 34 (suppl 2): 1–258

Shearer M J, Bechtold H, Andrassy K et al 1988 Mechanism of cephalosporin-induced hypoprothrombinaemia: relation to cephalosporin side chain vitamin K metabolism and vitamin K status. *Journal of Clinical Pharmacology* 28: 88–95

Stork C, Etzel J V, Brocavich J M, Forlenza S 1994 Cephalosporin-associated hypoprothrombinemia: Case and review of the literature. *Journal of Pharmacy Technology* 10: 5–13

Tan J S, Salstrom S J 1984 Diffusibility of the newer cephalosporins into human interstitial fluids. *American Journal of Medicine* 77 (4C): 33–36

Thompson J W, Jacobs R F 1993 Adverse effects of newer cephalosporins – an update. *Drug Safety* 9: 132–142

Thornberry C 1985 Review of the in vitro activity of third-generation cephalosporins and other newer beta-lactam antibiotics against clinically important bacteria. *American Journal of Medicine* 79 (2A): 14–20

Van der Auwera P 1990 In-vitro tests of the function of phagocytic cells and their interaction with antimicrobial agents: a critical review. *Journal of Antimicrobial Chemotherapy* 26: 168–173

Williams J D 1987 The cephalosporin antibiotics. *Drugs* 34 (suppl 2): 1–258

Wise R 1990 The pharmacokinetics of the oral cephalosporins – a review. *Journal of Antimicrobial Chemotherapy* 26 (suppl E): 13–20

Wise R 1994 Antibacterial agents: oral cephalosporins. *Prescribers Journal* 34: 110–115

Wright D N, Marble D A, Saxon B, Johnson C C, Bosso J A, Matsen J M 1988 In vitro inactivation of aminoglycosides by cephalosporin antibiotics. *Archives of Pathology and Laboratory Medicine* 112: 526–528

Yogev R 1986 A strategy for evaluating which of the new cephalosporins to use. *Pediatric Annals* 15: 470–471, 474–477

Group 1

Parenteral cephalosporins with broad-spectrum moderate antimicrobial activity and resistance to staphylococcal β-lactamase, but hydrolysed by various enterobacterial β-lactamases. In general, cephazolin and cefazaflur are the most, and ceforanide the least active (Table 14.1).

CEFAZAFLUR

Its activity against common pathogenic bacteria is shown in Table 14.1. Following intramuscular (i.m.) injection of 1 g, mean peak plasma levels around 25 mg/l are achieved at about 0.5 h. The mean plasma half-life is about 50 min; 90% of the dose is eliminated in the urine in the first 6 h.

Further information

Aswapokee N, Neu H C 1979 In vitro activity and β-lactamase stability of cefazaflur compared with those of β-lactamase-stable cephalosporins. *Antimicrobial Agents and Chemotherapy* 15: 444–446

Table 14.1   *Activity of group 1 cephalosporins against common pathogenic bacteria: MIC (mg/l)*

	Cefazaflur	Ceforanide	Ceftezole	Cephacetrile	Cephaloridine	Cephalothin	Cephapirin	Cephazolin
Staph. aureus	0.5	1–4	1	0.5–1	0.1–0.25	0.25–0.5	0.25	0.25–0.5
Str. pyogenes	0.1	0.1–0.5	0.25	0.1–0.25	0.01–0.03	0.1	0.1	0.1–0.25
Str. pneumoniae	0.1	0.1–0.5	0.25	0.25	0.03–0.06	0.06–0.1	0.1	0.1
Ent. faecalis	R	R	32	16	16–32	32	32	R
N. gonorrhoeae	2	1–2	0.5	4	0.25–2	0.25–2	4	0.1–0.5
N. meningitidis		0.1			0.5	0.5		
H. influenzae	0.25	4–8	4	2	4–8	4–8	2–4	2–8
Esch. coli	0.25	1–4	8	4–8	2–4	4–8	4	0.5–4
Klebsiella spp.	0.5	1–8	8	4–8	4	4	4	1–4
Enterobacter spp.	R	16–32	R	R	R	R	32–R	32–R
Pr. mirabilis	1	1	16	8	4	2–4	1–4	4
Pr. vulgaris	R	R	R	R	R	R	R	R
Morganella/Providencia	R	R	R	R	R	R	R	R
Salmonella spp.		0.5		4–8	2	2	1	1–2
Shigella spp.		0.5			2	2	1	
Ser. marcescens	R	R	R	R	R	R	R	R
Citrobacter spp.		32			R	64		2–R
Ps. aeruginosa	R	R	R	R	R	R	R	R
B. fragilis		R			32–64	32–64		16–32

CEFORANIDE

A semi-synthetic cephalosporin of group 1.

Antimicrobial activity

It is broadly active against Gram-positive and Gram-negative organisms (Table 14.1) but its activity in vitro is significantly reduced in the presence of serum. Some strains of *Mycobacterium tuberculosis* are inhibited by as little as 4 mg/l.

Pharmacokinetics

In patients receiving 2 g i.v. over 30 min, concentrations around 250 mg/l have been found with a plasma half-life of 2.5 h. In patients similarly receiving 0.25, 0.5 and 1 g the response is essentially linear, with mean end-infusion concentrations of around 40, 70 and 135 mg/l, respectively. Similar i.m. doses produced mean peak values of around 20, 40 and 70 mg/l. Administration of 2 g probenicid orally had no effect on the plasma, urinary or salivary levels. Binding to plasma protein is 81–88%. The plasma half-life is said to be shorter in 1- to 2-year-olds than in younger or older children.

Excretion

It is almost entirely eliminated in the urine, 80–95% being recovered in the first 12 h. As a result, the half-life is inversely related to renal function, rising to around 20 h when the creatinine clearance falls below 5 ml/min. Haemodialysis over 6 h removed 50%, reducing the plasma half-life to around 5 h.

Bile. In patients with normal biliary tracts given 1 g i.v. over 10 min preoperatively, mean concentrations rising to around 180 mg/l at 4 h have been found. When the duct was occluded, values were much lower, but concentrations in common duct bile were similar.

Toxicity and side-effects

It is generally well tolerated; phlebitis and pain at the site of injection are reported in some patients with occasional transient neutropenia and increased transaminase levels.

Pseudomembranous colitis has been described.

Clinical use

It has been principally used for the treatment of infections due to Gram-positive cocci, including staphylococcal and streptococcal soft tissue infections and for staphylococcal and non-enterococcal streptococcal endocarditis. It has been used for the treatment of chest infection, where it has been effective in eliminating *Str. pneumoniae* but not *H. influenzae*.

Preparations and dosage

Proprietary name: Precef.

Preparation: Injection

Dosage: Adults, i.m., i.v., i.v. infusion, 0.5–1 g every 12 h.

Available in the USA.

Further information

Campoli-Richards D M, Lackner T E, Monk J P 1987 Ceforanide. A review of its antibacterial activity, pharmacokinetic properties and clinical efficacy. *Drugs* 34: 411–437

Lefrock J L, Holloway W, Carr B B, Schell R F 1984 in vitro and clinical evaluation of ceforanide. *American Journal of Medical Science* 287: 21–25

Souney P F, Fisher S, Tuomala R E, Polk B F, Simpson C 1988 Plasma and tissue concentrations of ceforanide and cefazolin in women undergoing hysterectomy. *Chemotherapy* 34: 185–190

CEFTEZOLE

A semi-synthetic cephalosporin of group 1. Its activity against common pathogenic bacteria is shown in Table 14.1.

Preparations

Proprietary name: Celoslin.

Available in Italy and Japan.

Further information

Fraschini F, Scaglione F, DePascale A, Del Mastro S 1986 Pharmacokinetic studies on ceftezole. *Chemioterapia* 5: 388–390

Nishida M, Murakawa T, Kamimura T et al 1976 in vitro and in vivo evaluation of ceftezole, a new cephalosporin derivative. *Antimicrobial Agents and Chemotherapy* 10: 1–13

CEPHACETRILE

A semi-synthetic cephalosporin of group 1 supplied as the sodium salt.

Antimicrobial activity

Its spectrum resembles that of cephalothin (Table 14.1). It is active against aerobic and anaerobic Gram-positive rods and cocci, except *Ent. faecalis*. Neisseria, but not β-lactamase-producing *N. gonorrhoeae*, are susceptible, as are *Bordetella* spp. *Enterobacter*, *Providentia*, *Serratia* spp. and *Pr. vulgaris* are all resistant. Many *Bacteroides* species, fusobacteria and veillonella are susceptible, but *B. fragilis* is resistant.

Pharmacokinetics

Following i.m. doses of 0.5 and 1 g, peak plasma concentrations around 10 and 15 mg/l, respectively, are achieved at 1 h. A few minutes after i.v. injection of 1 g the plasma level is around 100 mg/l. About 25% is bound to plasma protein and the apparent volume of distribution is 19–23 mg/l. Some of the drug is desacetylated.

Penetration into the CSF is limited, concentrations of 0.5 mg/l being found 1 h after a 2 g dose but up to 15 mg/l 30 min after three 3 g i.v. doses, with concentrations of 2–4 mg/l persisting after 5 days. It crosses the placenta, and in cord blood concentrations of 10 mg/l have been found 2–4 h after a dose of 500 mg/h i.v.

The bulk of the drug is excreted in the urine, 80% being recovered in the first 6 h, producing concentrations in excess of 1 g/l, 25% of which is in the desacetylated form. Renal clearance is 313 ml/min following a dose of 1 g i.v. and involvement of tubular secretion is shown by depression of clearance by probenecid. Renal excretion is depressed in renal failure. Little is excreted in the bile, concentrations of 1.9 mg/l being found 4 h after a 1 g dose in T-tube bile.

Toxicity and side-effects

Eosinophilia in the absence of other manifestations of hypersensitivity and in patients not known to be allergic to β-lactams is common and fever occurs. Minor biochemical abnormalities common to cephalosporins also occur.

Clinical use

As for group 1 cephalosporins (p. 206).

Further information

Dettli L, Spring P, Lomar A V 1977 Pharmacokinetics of cephalosporins in the cerebrospinal fluid. In: Gladtke E, Marget W, Muller A A (eds) Cephacetrile – a review of progress to date. CIBA, p 61–75

Hierholzer G, Hierholzer S 1977 Cephalosporins in traumatology. In: Gladtke E, Marget W, Muller A A (eds) Cephacetrile – a review of progress to date. CIBA, p 76–85

CEPHALORIDINE

A semi-synthetic cephalosporin of group 1.

Antimicrobial activity

Its activity and spectrum are similar to those of cephalothin (Table 14.1). It is much less resistant to staphylococcal β-lactamase than was at first believed and its activity against β-lactamase-producing *Staph. aureus* declines rapidly as the inoculum size is increased.

Pharmacokinetics

Doses of 0.5 and 1 g produce peak plasma levels at 1 h of 18–20 and 20–40 mg/l, respectively. A 1 g dose given by rapid i.v. injection produces levels a few minutes after administration of 80–100 mg/l. The plasma half-life is 1.5 h. It is not significantly metabolized. It is about 20% bound to plasma protein.

Distribution

Concentrations in serous fluids and sputum have been found to be 30–50% of the simultaneous plasma levels. Entry into the CSF across normal meninges is poor but in the presence of inflammation concentrations of around 25% of those simultaneously present in the plasma have been obtained.

Excretion

It is excreted unchanged in the urine, mainly in the glomerular filtrate, 55–60% being recovered in the first 6 h. In patients on chronic renal dialysis the plasma half-life progressively declines, presumably due to the recruitment of extrarenal mechanisms of disposal. In T-tube bile, concentrations around 20 mg/l have been found after a dose of 1 g but this route of excretion accounts for less than 0.1% of the total drug administered.

Toxicity and side-effects

Moderate doses produce many hyaline casts in the urine and larger doses (6 g/day or more) have sometimes caused proximal tubular necrosis with increasing proteinuria and raised blood urea, going on in some cases to oliguria and renal failure. The renal toxicity of cephaloridine is enhanced by frusemide and ethacrynic acid. Claims that it is also enhanced by aminoglycosides have been disputed. Like other β-lactam antibiotics, cephaloridine is taken into the proximal tubular cells by a transport pump common to organic anions but, unlike other agents, fails to diffuse sufficiently rapidly across the luminal membrane of the cell to prevent intracellular accumulation and, if the dosage is sufficiently high, cellular damage. It is otherwise generally well tolerated, but hypersensitivity reactions and effects on biochemical, Coombs' and prothrombin tests common to cephalosporins have been described.

Clinical use

As for group 1 cephalosporins (p. 206). Its susceptibility to staphylococcal β-lactamase makes it a suspect choice for the treatment of such infections, but is has nonetheless been used successfully. With the accumulation of substitute agents, its nephrotoxicity has led to its withdrawal in a number of countries.

Further information

Mandell G L 1973 Cephaloridine. *Annals of Internal Medicine* 79: 561–565

Norby R, Stenqvist K, Elgefors B 1976 Interaction between cephaloridine and furosamide in man. *Scandinavian Journal of Infectious Diseases* 8: 209–212

Tune B M 1975 Relationship between the transport and toxicity of cephalosporins in the kidney. *Journal of Infectious Diseases* 132: 189–194

CEPHALOTHIN

A semi-synthetic cephalosporin supplied as the sodium salt.

Antimicrobial activity

Its activity against common pathogenic bacteria is shown in Table 14.1. It is stable to staphylococcal β-lactamase and hence active against β-lactamase-producing *Staph. aureus*. Streptococci, including penicillin-sensitive pneumococci, but not enterococci, are highly susceptible. Anaerobic Gram-positive bacilli are generally susceptible, although *Listeria* spp. are resistant. It is active against a range of enterobacteria, *Pasteurella* and *Vibrio* spp. *H. influenzae*, *Bordetella* and *Brucella* spp. are moderately resistant. *Campylobacter, Citrobacter, Enterobacter* and *Pseudomonas* spp. are resistant. Most species of *Bacteroides*, with the exception of *B. fragilis*, fusobacteria and veillonella are susceptible. *Treponema pallidum* and *Leptospira* spp. are susceptible, but mycobacteria and mycoplasma are resistant. It is hydrolysed by many enterobacterial β-lactamases (p. 316).

Pharmacokinetics

Intramuscular administration, which is commonly painful, produces peak plasma levels 30 min to 1 h after doses of 0.5 or 1 g of 6–8 and 15–20 mg/l, respectively. The normal route of administration is intravenous; 15 min after i.v. injection of 1 g the plasma level is about 30 mg/l, falling to 3–12 mg/l at 1 h. Continuous infusion of 12 g/day produced steady-state levels of 10–30 mg/l. It is 60–70% bound to plasma protein. It is metabolized by hepatic esterases to the microbiologically less active desacetyl compound, which accounts for 20–30% of the concentrations in serum and urine. As a result, it has a short plasma half-life of 0.6 h. Degradation causes the concentration to fall when the drug is incubated in serum in vitro. The desacetyl compound has about 20% of the activity of the parent compound against a number of species. Trivial amounts of other products which are microbiologically inactive can also be detected.

Distribution

Concentrations up to 70 mg/l have been achieved in pleural fluid 1 h after 1 g i.v. and 30–60 mg/l in serous fluid follow-ing 2 g i.v. of the drug. Lower concentrations have been found in ascitic fluid, of the order of 3 mg/l following 1 g i.v. Penetration into the CSF is very poor, rising in the presence of inflammation to less than 2 mg/l following 2 g i.v. Concentrations in sputum are 10–25% of the corresponding serum levels. The sputum content has been said to improve markedly from a maximum of around 3 mg/l to around 13 mg/l when serum concentrations in excess of 20 mg/l are achieved. Concentrations in bone around 4 mg/g have been described following an intravenous dose of 1 g. Concentrations of 2–6 mg/l in amniotic fluid and around 3 mg/l in cord blood have been found after 1 g i.m. Concentrations about 25% of the simultaneous plasma levels have been found in prostatic fluid.

Excretion

Most of the dose is recovered in the urine, 70% following intravenous administration and 50% following intramuscular administration, producing urinary concentrations of 500–2000 mg/l during the first 6 h after a 1 g dose. Urinary excretion is depressed by probenecid indicating significant tubular secretion and by renal failure, although, because of metabolism, the plasma half-life of the drug is only moderately prolonged to about 3 h, while that of the principal metabolite rises to 12 h or more. Impaired tubular secretion is responsible for the elevated levels of the drug found in newborn and premature infants. Biliary excretion is trivial, producing levels of 1–17 mg/l after 1 g i.v. and liver disease has little effect on its half-life or plasma protein binding.

Toxicity and side-effects

Hypersensitivity reactions, occasionally severe, and disturbances of laboratory tests common to cephalosporins occur. In volunteers receiving very large doses (8 g daily for 2–4 weeks) a serum-sickness-like illness developed. Positive Coombs' reactions associated with red cell agglutination, but very seldom with haemolysis, are common. Thrombocytopenia and leucopenia possibly mediated by analogous mechanisms have been described. A coagulopathy with prolonged prothrombin time has been encountered in patients with renal failure or very high plasma levels resulting from excessive dosage. Evidence has been cited of exaggeration of pre-existing renal disease or renal damage, perhaps enhanced by simultaneous administration of aminoglycosides or frusemide, in which direct tubular injury or allergic nephritis may have been involved.

Clinical use

As for group 1 cephalosporins (p. 206).

Further information

Durham D S, Ibels L S 1981 Cephalothin-induced acute allergic interstitial nephritis. *Australian and New Zealand Journal of Medicine* 11: 266–267

Klein J O, Eickhoff T C, Tilles J G, Finland M 1964 Cephalothin: activity, in vitro absorption and excretion in normal subjects and clinical observations in 40 patients. *American Journal of Medical Science* 248: 640–656

Munch R, Steurer J, Luthy R, Seigenthaler W, Kuhlmann U 1983 Serum and dialysate concentrations of intraperitoneal cephalothin in patients undergoing continuous ambulatory peritoneal dialysis. *Clinical Nephrology* 20: 40–43

Nilsson-Ehle I, Nilsson-Ehle P 1979 Pharmacokinetics of cephalothin: accumulation of its deacetylated metabolite in uremic patients. *Journal of Infectious Diseases* 139: 712–716

CEPHAPIRIN

A semi-synthetic cephalosporin of group 1.

Antimicrobial activity

Its antibacterial spectrum is almost identical with that of cephalothin (Table 14.1), but it is more labile to staphylococcal β-lactamase.

Pharmacokinetics

Intramuscular injections can be painful, but the inflammation resulting from i.v. infusion is said to be less than that produced by cephalothin. A peak plasma concentration of 15–25 mg/l is obtained 0.5 h after intramuscular injection of 1 g. A few minutes after intravenous administration of the same dose, the plasma concentration is 100–130 mg/l. The plasma half-life is 0.4–0.8 h. It is 45–55% bound to plasma protein and metabolized to the desacetyl form; only 5–10%

of the metabolite appears in the plasma, but it accounts for almost half the drug in the urine.

Excretion

Following an i.v. dose of 1 g, 55–70% is recovered in the urine over the first 8 h and 55–65% following an i.m. dose producing levels of 300–2500 mg/l. Renal clearance is around 340 ml/min and declines in renal failure, although the plasma half-life, because of metabolism of the drug, rises only modestly to around 1.5 h. Less than 1% of the dose appears in the bile.

Toxicity and side-effects

Mild hypersensitivity reactions, interference with laboratory tests common to cephalosporins on infusion of large doses, and a serum-sickness-like illness analogous to that seen with cephalothin have been observed.

Clinical use

As for group 1 cephalosporins (p. 206).

Further information

Axelrod J, Meyers B R, Hirschman S Z 1972 Cephapirin: pharmacology in normal human volunteers. *Journal of Clinical Pharmacology* 12: 84–88

Creatsas G, Pavlatos M, Lolis D, Kaskarelis D 1980 A study of the kinetics of cephapirin and cephalexin in pregnancy. *Current Medical Research and Opinion* 7: 43–46

CEPHAZOLIN

A semi-synthetic cephalosporin of group 1 supplied as the sodium salt.

Antimicrobial activity

It is active against *Staph. aureus*, but it is more susceptible to staphylococcal β-lactamases than is cephalothin and more resistant than cephaloridine. Aerobic and anaerobic Gram-positive cocci (except enterococci) and bacilli are susceptible. Neisseria including penicillin-resistant, but not β-lactamase-producing *N. gonorrhoeae* are also susceptible. *Enterobacter, Klebsiella, Providencia, Serratia* spp. and *Pr. vulgaris* are all resistant. *B. fragilis* is resistant, but other

Bacteroides spp., fusobacteria and *Veillonella* spp. are susceptible. Its activity against common pathogenic bacteria is shown in Table 14.1.

Acquired resistance

Generally there is complete cross-resistance with other group 1 cephalosporins.

Pharmacokinetics

Intramuscular injections of 0.5 and 1 g produce peak plasma levels at 1 h of 35 and 65–70 mg/l, respectively. A few minutes after rapid i.v. injection of 1 g the plasma concentration is 180–200 mg/l. The plasma half-life is 1.5–2.0 h. Continuous infusion of 6 g/day produced steady-state levels around 50 mg/l. It is not metabolized. It is 75–85% bound to plasma protein and the volume of distribution is about 10 l (the smallest of the cephalosporins in group 1). High plasma levels may therefore be an indication of relative confinement to the plasma space. In hepatic cirrhosis lowered serum albumen is associated with reduced binding to plasma protein and reduction in plasma half-life, probably due to enhanced renal clearance.

Distribution

It crosses inflamed synovial membranes, but the levels achieved are well below those of the simultaneous serum levels and entry to the CSF is poor. In patients receiving 10 mg/kg by i.v. bolus mean concentrations in cancellous bone were 3.0 mg/l when the mean serum concentration was 33 mg/l, giving a bone/serum ratio of 0.06. Some crosses the placenta, but the concentrations found in the fetus and membranes are low.

Excretion

It is almost completely recovered unchanged in the urine (60% of the dose within the first 6 h), producing concentrations in excess of 1 g/l. The involvement of tubular secretion is shown by the depression of excretion by probenecid. The renal clearance is around 65 ml/min and declines in renal failure, when the half-life may rise to 40 h, although levels in the urine sufficient to inhibit most urinary pathogens are still found. It is moderately well removed by haemodialysis and less well by peritoneal dialysis.

Bile. Levels sufficient to inhibit a number of enteric organisms likely to infect the biliary tract are found in T-tube bile (17–31 mg/l following a 1 g i.v. dose), but this is principally due to the high serum levels of the drug and the total amounts excreted via the bile are small.

Toxicity and side-effects

Eosinophilia is common and fever occurs. Nephrotoxicity is low, with no evidence of renal damage resulting from the administration of 12 g per day, although very high doses are nephrotoxic in animals. Other side-effects are those common to group 1 cephalosporins (p. 205), including rare bleeding disorders and encephalopathy in patients in whom impaired excretion, or direct instillation leads to very high CSF levels. Neutropenia has been described and hypoprothrombinaemic bleeding has been attributed to the side-chain which is said to be a more potent inhibitor of carboxylation of glutamic acid than is cephazolin itself.

Clinical use

As for group 1 cephalosporins (p. 206). It has been commended for biliary infection because of the moderately high concentrations achieved in bile. It is commonly used in the prophylaxis of abdominal surgery.

Preparations and dosage

Proprietary name: Kefzol.

Preparation: Injection.

Dosage: i.m., i.v., i.v. infusion. Adults 0.5–1 g every 6–12 h; children, 25 mg/kg daily in divided doses, increasing to 100 mg/kg daily in severe infection.

Widely available.

Further information

Bunke C M, Aronoff G R, Brier M E, Sloan R S, Luft F C 1983 Cefazolin and cephalexin kinetics in continuous ambulatory peritoneal dialysis. *Clinical Pharmacology and Therapeutics* 33: 66–72

Cunha B A, Ristuccia A M, Honas M, Ristuccia P A, Jannelli D E 1982 Tissue penetration characteristics of ceftizoxime and cefazolin in human bile and gall bladder wall. *Journal of Antimicrobial Chemotherapy* 10 (suppl C): 117–120

Decroix M O, Zini R, Chaumeil J C, Tillementi P 1988 Cefazolin serum protein binding and its inhibition by bilirubin, fatty acids and other drugs. *Biochemical Pharmacology* 37: 2807–2814

Deguchi Y, Koshida R, Nakashima E et al 1988 Interindividual changes in volume of distribution of cefazolin in newborn infants and its prediction based on physiological pharmacokinetic concepts. *Journal of Pharmaceutical Sciences* 77: 674–678

Dekel A, Elian I, Gibory Y, Goldman J A 1980 Transplacental passage of cefazolin in the first trimester of pregnancy. *European Journal of Obstetrics, Gynaecology and Reproductive Biology* 10: 303–307

Frame P T, Watanakunakorn C, McLaurin R L, Khodadad G 1983 Penetration of nafcillin, methicillin and cefazolin into human brain tissue. *Neurosurgery* 12: 142–147

Herd A M, Ross C A, Bhattacharja J K 1989 Acute confusional state with postoperative intravenous cefazolin. *British Medical Journal* 299: 393–394

Manzella J P, Paul R L, Butler I L 1988 CNS toxicity associated with intraventricular injection of cefazolin. Report of three cases. *Journal of Neurosurgery* 68: 970–971

Ortiz A, Martin-Llonch N, Garron M P et al 1991 Cefazolin-induced encephalopathy in uremic patients. *Reviews of Infectious Diseases* 13: 772–774

Periti P, Mazzei T, Orlandini F et al 1988 Comparison of the antimicrobial prophylactic efficacy of cefotaxime and cephazolin in obstetric and gynaecological surgery: a randomised multicentre study. *Drugs* 35: 133–138

Philipson A, Stiernstedt G, Ehrnebo M 1987 Comparison of the pharmacokinetics of cephradine and cefazolin in pregnant and nonpregnant women. *Clinical Pharmacokinetics* 12: 136–144

Thompson J R, Garber R, Ayers J, Oki J 1987 Cefazolin-associated neutropenia. *Clinical Pharmacy* 6: 811–814

Townsend T R, Reitz B A, Bilker W B, Bartlett J G 1993 Clinical trial of cefamandole, cefazolin, and cefuroxime for antibiotic prophylaxis in cardiac operations. *Journal of Thoracic and Cardiovascular Surgery* 106: 664–670

Walker P C, Kaufmann R E, Massoud N 1986 Compatibility of cefazolin and gentamicin in peritoneal dialysis solutions. *Drug Intelligence and Clinical Pharmacy* 20: 697–700

Group 2

Oral cephalosporins with broad-spectrum moderate antimicrobial activity, resistant to staphylococcal β-lactamase and moderately resistant to some enterobacterial β-lactamases (Table 14.2).

CEFACLOR

A semi-synthetic cephalosporin of group 2 differing from cephalexin by the substitution of Cl for CH_3 at C-3. Aqueous solutions are stable at room temperature and 4°C for 72 h at pH 2.5 but rapidly lose activity at pH 7.

Table 14.2 *Activity of group 2 cephalosporins against common pathogenic bacteria: MIC (mg/l)*

	Cefaclor	Cefadroxil	Cefatrizine	Cefroxadine	Cephalexin	Cephradine	Loracarbef
Staph. aureus	2–4	2–4	0.5–1	2	2–4	2–4	1–8
Str. pyogenes	0.25	0.1–0.5	0.03–0.1	0.5	0.5–2	0.5–2	0.12–1
Str. pneumoniae	0.5–1	1	0.25–0.5	2	2	2–4	0.5–2
Ent. faecalis	R	R	R	R	R	R	R
N. gonorrhoeae	0.1–0.5	4	0.25–0.5	0.5	0.5–4	0.5–4	0.12–0.25
H. influenzae	1–2	16–32	2–8	8	8–32	8–32	0.5–2
Esch. coli	2–8	8–16	2–8	16	8	16	1–2
Klebsiella spp.	4–8	8–16	8	16	8	16	1–8
Enterobacter spp.	R	R	R	R	R	R	R
Pr. mirabilis	2–16	8–16	4–8	16	8–16	16	1–8
Pr. vulgaris	R	R	16–R	R	R	R	R
Morganella/Providencia	R	R		R	R	R	R
Salmonella spp.	2	8	8		2	8	1–2
Ser. marcescens	R	R	R		R	R	R
Ps. aeruginosa	R	R	R	R	R	R	R
B. fragilis	R		R	32	R		R

Antimicrobial activity

It is active against *Esch. coli*, *Pr. mirabilis* and *K. pneumoniae*, and notably against *N. gonorrhoeae* and *H. influenzae* including β-lactamase-positive strains. There is a marked inoculum effect against *H. influenzae*, the MIC of 1–2 mg/l at 10^4–10^5 cfu rising to >256 mg/l at 10^8 cfu. Its activity is less against streptococci and staphylococci and it is relatively susceptible to staphylococcal β-lactamase. *P. vulgaris* and *Providencia*, *Acinetobacter* and *Serratia* spp. are resistant. Anaerobic Gram-positive cocci are sensitive but clostridia resistant. *B. fragilis* is resistant but other *Bacteroides* spp. are commonly susceptible. Its activity against common pathogenic bacteria is shown in Table 14.2.

Pharmacokinetics

It is rapidly absorbed when given by mouth, the mean peak plasma levels after a 250 mg dose being 6–7 mg/l at about 50 min. There is no accumulation of the drug during repeated administration. In patients receiving 500 mg 8-hourly for 10 days, mean peak serum levels were 8.9 mg/l on day 1 and 7.1 mg/l on day 7. In volunteers receiving 1 g 8-hourly for 8 days, mean peak serum levels of around 29 mg/l were found on day 1 and on day 8; in each case the peak occurred around 1.3 h.

The plasma half-life is 0.5–1 h. Food intake increases the time taken to reach peak plasma levels and reduces the peak by 25–50%. The actual amount absorbed is unaffected. In children receiving 15 mg/kg per day (maximum daily dose 1 g) the mean peak serum level was 16.8 mg/l at 0.5–1 h. A 'long-acting' formulation is available; the half-life is increased to about 1.5 h.

Distribution

In patients receiving 500 mg 8-hourly for 10 days, concentrations in mucoid sputum have been found to be 0–1.7 (mean 0.5) mg/l and 0–2.8 (mean 1.0) mg/l in purulent sputum. In children with chronic serous otitis media, receiving 15 mg/kg daily, the mean peak concentration in middle ear secretion was 3.8 mg/l within 30 min of the dose when the mean simultaneous serum concentration was 12.8 mg/l.

Excretion

About half of the dose is recovered from the urine in the first 6 h and 70% in 24 h. Probenecid prolongs the plasma levels but in renal insufficiency the plasma half-life is only moderately increased, suggesting non-renal mechanisms of elimination, although no metabolites have been identified. The drug probably chemically degrades in serum. In patients with creatinine clearance values of 5–15 ml/min the mean plasma elimination half-life rose to 2.3 h and the 24 h urinary excretion fell to less than 10%. In patients requiring intermittent haemodialysis and receiving 500 mg 8-hourly for 10 days, the half-life rose to 2.9 h between and 1.5 h on

dialysis. Dialysis was calculated to remove 34% of the dose. The corrected creatinine clearance proved to be the best indicator of plasma half-life.

Toxicity and side-effects

Apart from mild gastro-intestinal disturbance, the drug is well tolerated. In one series, 6% of patients developed transiently increased transaminase levels and 12% symptomatic vaginal candidiosis. Serum sickness has been noted.

Clinical use

As for group 2 cephalosporins (p. 206). It has been particularly commended for respiratory infections because of its activity against *H. influenzae* (p. 691).

Preparations and dosage

Proprietary name: Distaclor.

Preparations: Tablets, modified-release suspension, capsules.

Dosage: Adults, oral, 250–500 mg every 8 h, depending on severity of infection. Children, 20 mg/kg per day in divided doses every 8 h. In more severe infections, 40 mg/kg per day in divided doses, up to a daily maximum of 1 g.

Widely available.

Further information

Blumer J L, McLinn S E, DeAbate C A et al 1995 Multinational multicenter controlled trial comparing ceftibuten with cefaclor for the treatment of acute otitis media. *Pediatric Infectious Disease Journal* 14: S115–S120

Brady M T, Barson W J, Cannon H J Jr, Grossman L K 1987 Onset of *Haemophilus influenzae* type-b meningitis during cefaclor therapy for preseptal cellulitis. *Clinical Pediatrics (Philadelphia)* 26: 132–134

Hyslop D L 1988 Cefaclor safety profile: a ten-year review. *Clinical Therapeutics* 11 (suppl A): 83–94

Kearns G L, Wheeler J G, Childress S H, Letzig L G 1994 Serum sickness-like reactions to cefaclor: role of hepatic metabolism and individual susceptibility. *Journal of Pediatrics* 125: 805–811

Levine L R 1985 Quantitative comparison of adverse reactions to cefaclor vs. amoxycillin in a surveillance study. *Pediatric Infectious Diseases* 4: 358–361

Neu H C, Fu K P 1978 Cefaclor: in vitro spectrum of activity and beta-lactamase stability. *Antimicrobial Agents and Chemotherapy* 13: 584–588

Verhoef J 1988 Cefaclor in the treatment of skin, soft tissue and urinary tract infections: a review. *Clinical Therapeutics* 11 (suppl A): 71–82

Vial T, Pont J, Pham E, Rabilloud M, Descotes J 1992 Cefaclor-associated serum sickness-like disease: eight cases and review of the literature. *Annals of Pharmacotherapy* 26: 910–914

CEFADROXIL

p-Hydroxycephalexin; a semi-synthetic cephalosporin of group 2. It is available as the mono- and trihydrate.

Antimicrobial activity

Resembles closely that of cephalexin (Table 14.2).

Pharmacokinetics

Following an oral dose of 0.25, 0.5 or 1 g in adult volunteers, mean peak plasma levels of 9.0, 17.9 and 35.2 mg/l have been found after 1.2, 1.2 and 1.6 h, respectively. Accumulation occurred when volunteers were given 1 g 8 hourly for 8 days. On day 1 the mean peak plasma concentration was 27.5 mg/l at 2.5 h and on day 8 it was 35.5 mg/l at 1.5 h after the dose. Doubling the dose up to 500 mg approximately doubles the plasma level. The plasma half-life is 1.2 h. Protein binding is 20%. Absorption is little affected by administration with food. Distribution is similar to that of cephalexin.

It is eliminated by both glomerular filtration and tubular secretion, and 90% of the dose appears in the urine over 24 h, most in the first 6 h, producing concentrations around 500–2500 mg/l. Loss of linearity in the relation between peak plasma concentration and dose above 500 mg may be due to saturation of renal tubular clearance.

Toxicity and side-effects

It is generally well tolerated. Such side-effects as have been described are those common to group 2 cephalosporins.

Clinical use

As for group 2 cephalosporins (p. 206). It has been successfully used for the treatment of upper respiratory tract infection and community-acquired pneumonia.

Preparations and dosage

Proprietary name: Baxan.

Preparations: Capsules, suspension.

Dosage: Adults, oral, 40 kg and over, 0.5–1 g twice a day. Children under 1 year, 25 mg/kg daily in divided doses; children 1–6 years, 250 mg twice daily; children over 6 years, 500 mg twice daily.

Widely available.

Further information

Akimoto Y, Komiya M, Kaneko K, Fujii A, Peterson L J 1994 Cefadroxil concentrations in human serum, gingiva, and mandibular bone following a single oral administration. *Journal of Oral and Maxillofacial Surgery* 52: 397–401

Casewell M W, Bragman S G 1987 The in-vitro activity of cefadroxil and the interpretation of disc-susceptibility testing. *Journal of Antimicrobial Chemotherapy* 19: 597–603

Hampel B, Lode H, Wagner J, Koeppe P 1982 Pharmacokinetics of cefadroxil and cefaclor during an 8-day dosage period. *Antimicrobial Agents and Chemotherapy* 22: 1061–1063

Hebert A A, Still J G, Reuman P D 1993 Comparative safety and efficacy of clarithromycin and cefadroxil suspensions in the treatment of mild to moderate skin and skin structure infections in children. *Pediatric Infectious Disease Journal* 12 (suppl): S112–S117

Miller L M, Mooney C J, Hansbrough J F 1989 Comparative evaluation of cefaclor versus cefadroxil in the treatment of skin and skin structure infections. *Current Therapeutic Research* 46: 405–410

Seminar-in-print 1986 Cefadroxil and respiratory tract infections. *Drugs* 32 (suppl 3): 1–56

Stromberg A, Friberg U, Cars O 1987 Concentrations of phenoxymethyl-penicillin and cefadroxil in tonsillar tissue and tonsillar surface fluid. *European Journal of Clinical Microbiology* 6: 525–529

CEFATRIZINE

A semi-synthetic cephalosporin of group 2.

Antimicrobial activity

Its spectrum is similar to that of cephalexin but it is more active against *H. influenzae*. It is active against *Esch. coli*, *Enterobacter*, *Klebsiella* and *Proteus* spp. (Table 14.2). Wide strain variations in susceptibility have been reported. Activity is much affected by medium composition and inoculum size.

Pharmacokinetics

It is only partially absorbed when given by mouth. The peak blood level attained after an oral dose of 500 mg is around 6 mg/l 1–2 h after the dose, with a half-life of 2.5 h. Intramuscular administration of a similar dose produces an average peak plasma level of around 12 mg/l at 30 min after injection, with a half-life of 1.5 h. There is some accumulation after repeated doses. The half-life is extended to 5.5 h in end-stage renal failure. It is 40–60% bound to plasma protein. Distribution resembles that of cephalexin. It crosses the placenta readily.

Urinary recovery in 6 h is 35% of an oral dose and 45% of an i.m. dose, producing urinary levels of 50–400 and 50–1600, respectively. It is presumed that the remainder is metabolized, but no metabolites have been identified.

Toxicity and side-effects

Apart from some mild diarrhoea, it appears to be well tolerated.

Clinical use

As for group 2 cephalosporins (p. 206).

Preparations and dosage
Dosage: Adults, oral, 500 mg twice daily.
Very limited availability.

Further information

Carlone N A, Cuffini A M, Forno P, Izzoglio M, Cavallo G 1985 Susceptibility of clinical isolates of Gram-positive and Gram-negative organisms to cefatrizine. *Drugs Under Experimental and Clinical Research* 11: 447–451

Pfeffer M, Gaver R C, Ximinez J 1983 Human intravenous pharmacokinetics and absolute oral bioavailability of cefatrizine. *Antimicrobial Agents and Chemotherapy* 24: 915–920

CEFROXADINE

A semi-synthetic cephalosporin of group 2.

The antimicrobial spectrum is identical with that of cephalexin (Table 14.2), but it is said to be more actively bactericidal. A dose of 1 g as film-coated tablets produced mean peak plasma levels of 25 mg/l at 1 h. Absorption was depressed and delayed by administration with food. The plasma elimination half-life was 0.8 h, rising to 40 h in end-stage renal failure and falling to 3.4 h during haemodialysis. Urinary recovery was 85%. Its clinical uses are those of group 2 cephalosporins.

Preparations and dosage
Proprietary name: Oraspor.
Dosage: Adults, oral, 0.5–2 g/day in divided doses.
Very limited availability.

Further information

Gerardin A, Lecaillon J B, Schoeller J P, Humbert G, Guibert J 1982 Pharmacokinetics of cefroxadine (CGP 9000) in man. *Journal of Pharmacokinetics and Biopharmacy* 10: 15–26

Lecaillon J B, Hirtz J L, Schoeller J P, Humbert G, Vischer W 1980 Pharmacokinetic comparison of cefroxadine (CGP 9000) and cephalexin by simultaneous administration to humans. *Antimicrobial Agents and Chemotherapy* 18: 656–660

Nieto M J, Lanao J M, Dominiguez-Gil A, Tabernero J M, Macias J F 1983 Elimination of cefroxadine from patients undergoing dialysis. *European Journal of Clinical Pharmacology* 24: 109–112

Yasuda K, Kurashige S, Mitsuhashi S 1980 Cefroxadine (CGP 9000), an orally active cephalosporin. *Antimicrobial Agents and Chemotherapy* 18: 105–110

CEPHALEXIN

A semi-synthetic cephalosporin of group 2 supplied as the monohydrate.

Antimicrobial activity

Its antibacterial spectrum is similar to that of group 1 cephalosporins, but with a somewhat lower degree of activity against most species, particularly Gram-positive cocci (Table 14.2). It is relatively resistant to staphylococcal β-lactamase, but has no useful activity against methicillin-resistant strains. It is active otherwise against both aerobic and anaerobic Gram-positive cocci, with the exception of enterococci, but Gram-positive rods are relatively resistant. Neisseria, including β-lactamase-producing *N. gonorrhoeae*, are moderately susceptible, while *Bordetella* spp. and *H. influenzae* are moderately resistant. It is active against a range of enterobacteria, but it is degraded by many entero-bacterial β-lactamases. *Citrobacter, Edwardsiella, Entero-bacter, Hafnia, Providencia* and *Serratia* spp. are all resistant. *Bacteroides* spp. (with the exception of *B. fragilis*), fusobacteria and veillonella are susceptible. Because of its mode of action it is only slowly bactericidal to Gram-negative bacilli.

Pharmacokinetics

It is stable to gastric acid and almost completely absorbed when given by mouth, the peak concentration being depressed or delayed by food. Mean peak plasma concentrations of 9 and 18 mg/l are obtained after 0.5 and 1 g orally, respectively. The half-life is about 0.8 h. There is accumulation after 1 g, but not 0.5 g, 6-hourly. Intravenous injection of 1 g over 5 min produces levels of 60–70 mg/l shortly after injection. The plasma half-life by this route is about 1.1 h. Intramuscular injection is painful and produces delayed peak plasma concentrations considerably less than those obtained by oral administration: 10 mg/l 2 h after a dose of 1 g. Preparations for parenteral administration are not generally available. There is no biodegradation or transformation. It is 10–15% bound to plasma protein.

Distribution
In synovial fluid, levels of 6–38 mg/l have been described after a 4 g oral dose, but penetration into the CSF is poor: 1.3 mg/l 3–4 h after an oral dose of 0.75 g. Useful levels are achieved in bone (1.3 mg/l at 3 h after 0.5, and 9–44 mg/l after 1 g orally) and in purulent sputum. Concentrations of 10–20 mg/l have been found in breast milk. Concentrations in cord blood following a maternal oral dose of 0.25 g were minimal.

Excretion
Almost 100% of the dose is recoverable from the urine within the first 6 h, producing urinary concentrations exceeding 1 g/l. The involvement of tubular secretion is indicated by the increased plasma peak concentration and reduced urinary excretion produced by probenecid. Renal clearance is around 200 ml/min and is depressed in renal failure, although therapeutic concentrations are still obtained in the urine. It is removed by both peritoneal and haemodialysis. Some is excreted in the bile, in which therapeutic concentrations may be achieved.

Toxicity and side-effects

Diarrhoea, vomiting and abdominal discomfort are relatively common. Pseudomembranous colitis has been described and overgrowth of *Candida* with vaginitis may be troublesome. Otherwise, mild hypersensitivity reactions and biochemical changes common to cephalosporins occur. There is no evidence that pre-existing renal disease is aggravated. Very rare neurological disturbances have been described, particularly in patients in whom very high plasma levels have been achieved. There are also rare reports of Stevens–Johnson syndrome and toxic epidermal necrolysis.

Clinical use

As for group 2 cephalosporins (p. 206). It should not be used in infections in which *H. influenzae* is, or is likely to be, implicated. It should not be used as an alternative to penicillin in syphilis.

Preparations and dosage
Proprietary names: Keflex, Ceporex.
Preparations: Capsules, tablets, suspension.
Dosage: Adults, oral, 1–2 g/day in divided doses; for severe infections, increase dose to 1 g three times daily or 3 g twice daily. Children, 25–60 mg/kg per day; for severe infection increase dose to 100 mg/kg per day, with a maximum of 4 g/day.
Widely available.

Further information

Dave J, Heathcock R, Fenelon L, Bihari D J, Simmons N A 1991 Cephalexin induced toxic epidermal necrolysis. *Journal of Antimicrobial Chemotherapy* 28: 477–488

Davis G M, Forland S C, Cutler R E 1985 Serum and dialysate concentrations of cephalexin following repeated dosing in CAPD patients. *American Journal of Kidney Diseases* 6: 177–180

Hori R, Okumura K, Nihira H, Nakano H, Akagi K, Kamiya A 1985 A new dosing regimen in renal insufficiency: application to cephalexin. *Clinical Pharmacology and Therapeutics* 38: 290–295

Jackson H, Vion B, Levy P M 1988 Generalised eruptive pustular drug rash due to cephalexin. *Dermatologica* 177: 292–294

Martine F C, Kindrachuk R W, Thomas E, Stamey T A 1985 Effect of prophylactic, low dose cephalexin on fecal and vaginal flora. *Journal of Urology* 133: 994–996

Speight T M, Brogden R N, Avery G S 1972 Cephalexin: a review of its antibacterial, pharmacological and therapeutic properties. *Drugs* 3: 9–76

CEPHRADINE

A semi-synthetic cephalosporin of group 2 available in both oral and injectable forms.

Antimicrobial activity

Its antibacterial spectrum is almost identical to that of cephalexin (Table 14.2). It is active against aerobic and anaerobic Gram-positive cocci (with the exception of enterococci) and bacilli. Neisseria, including β-lactamase positive strains, are moderately susceptible. *H. influenzae* is resistant. It is active against a variety of enterobacteria but susceptible to many enterobacterial β-lactamases.

Pharmacokinetics

It is practically completely absorbed when given by mouth. The peak is delayed and reduced by food, but the half-life and the area under the curve (AUC) are not altered. Absorption is depressed by some intestinal disorders. After an oral dose of 0.5 g, a peak plasma level of 18–20 mg/l is obtained at about 1 h. The peak rises to 20–34 mg/l 1–2 h after a dose of 1 g. A 1 g dose of the parenteral preparation produces a peak plasma concentration at 1–2 h of 10–12 mg/l and the same dose intravenously produces levels a few minutes after injection of 50–90 mg/l. The plasma half-life is 0.8–1 h. It is 8–12% bound to plasma protein.

Distribution

Concentrations of up to 40% of those simultaneously found in the serum have been demonstrated in lung tissue. Penetration into the CSF is poor, concentrations of 1.4–4.5 mg/l being found after doses of 150–300 mg/kg in children. Levels in sputum were about 20% of those simultaneously present in the plasma following a 1 g oral dose and similar levels have been found in bone – around 10 mg/g 20 min after 1 g i.v. Breast milk concentrations approaching 1 mg/l have been found following 500 mg orally 6-hourly and similar concentrations have been found in amniotic fluid. Cord blood concentration is said to be similar to that in the maternal blood.

Excretion

It is excreted unchanged in the urine, 90–100% being recovered in the first 6 h, the excretion being more rapid after oral than i.m. administration. Probenecid produces a marked delay in the peak and a 40–70% increase in the plasma concentration. The AUC is correspondingly increased but concentrations exceeding 1 g/l are still found in the urine. There is some biliary excretion, concentrations of 2–40 mg/l being found up to 8 h following an oral dose of 500 mg.

Toxicity and side-effects

The parenteral forms may give rise to local pain or thrombophlebitis. Hypersensitivity manifestations and interference with laboratory tests common to cephalosporins have been described. In some patients *Candida* vaginitis has been troublesome. Increase of blood urea has been reported in some patients but there is no unequivocal evidence of renal toxicity. Joint pain is reported in some patients. Very rarely, diffuse interstitial infiltrates occur.

Clinical use

As for group 2 cephalosporins (p. 206). It has been favoured by some for the prophylaxis and treatment of bone infection.

Preparations and dosage
Proprietary name: Velosef.
Preparations: Capsules, syrup, injection.
Dosage: Adults, oral, 250–500 mg every 6 h, or 0.5–1 g every 12 h. Children, 25–100 mg/kg per day in 2 or 4 equally divided doses. Adults, i.m., i.v, 2–8 g/day in divided doses depending on severity of infection. Children, 50–100 mg/kg per day in 4 divided doses; more serious illnesses may require 200–300 mg/kg per day.
Widely available.

Further information

Adam D, Hofstetter A G, Jacoby W, Reichart B 1976 Studies on the diffusion of cephradine and cephalothin into human tissue. *Infection* 4 (suppl 2): S105–S107

Klastersky J, Daneau D, Weerts D 1973 Cephradine. Antibacterial activity and clinical effectiveness. *Chemotherapy* 18: 191–204

Leigh D A 1989 Determination of serum and bone concentrations of cephradine and cefuroxime by HPLC in patients undergoing hip and knee replacement surgery. *Journal of Antimicrobial Chemotherapy* 23: 877–883

Middlehurst R J, Pedlar J, Barker G R, Rood J P 1989 Cephradine penetration of mandibular bone. *Journal of Oral and Maxillofacial Surgery* 47: 672–673

Philipson A 1987 Comparison of the pharmacokinetics of cephradine and cefazolin in pregnant and non-pregnant women. *Clinical Pharmacokinetics* 12: 136–144

Zaki A, Schreiber E C, Weliky I, Knill J R, Hubsher J A 1974 Clinical pharmacology of oral cephradine. *Journal of Clinical Pharmacology* 14: 118–126

LORACARBEF

An oral carbacephem, closely related to cefaclor, but with carbon replacing sulphur in the fused ring structure, and consequently improved chemical stability.

Its activity corresponds closely to that of cefaclor, with moderate activity against staphylococci (but not methicillin-resistant strains), streptococci and some enterobacteria. Enterococci, *Ps. aeruginosa* and *B. fragilis* are resistant (Table 14.2). Like cefaclor, it is hydrolysed by many enterobacterial β-lactamases, including the common TEM and OXA enzymes (p. 316).

Oral administration of a single 500 mg dose to healthy adult volunteers yielded a mean peak plasma concentration of 16 mg/l after 1.3 h. Food delays absorption. The apparent volume of distribution is 20–28 l. In a study of children with upper respiratory tract infection, concentrations of 12.6 mg/l and 18.7 mg/l were achieved 45 min after doses of 7.5 and 15 mg/kg, respectively, given as an oral suspension. Similar doses administered to children with acute otitis media achieved concentrations of 2 and 4 mg/l (48% and 42% of the corresponding plasma level) in middle ear fluid after 2 h.

Most of the dose is excreted into urine unchanged, 60% within 12 h. The elimination half-life is about 1 h, with corresponding increases in patients with impaired renal function. Probenecid delays excretion.

It is well tolerated. Diarrhoea is the most prominent side-effect, occurring in about 4% of patients. Other gastro-intestinal upsets are also reported.

It is used for the oral treatment of upper respiratory tract infection, particularly acute otitis media in children, in skin and soft-tissue infections, and in uncomplicated urinary tract infection caused by sensitive organisms.

Further information

Brogden R N, McTavish D 1993 Loracarbef: a review of its antimicrobial activity, pharmacokinetic properties and therapeutic efficacy. *Drugs* 45: 716–736

Doern G V, Vautour R, Parker D, Tubert T, Torres B 1991 In vitro activity of loracarbef (LY163892), a new oral carbacephem antimicrobial agent, against respiratory isolates of *Haemophilus influenzae* and *Moraxella catarrhalis*. *Antimicrobial Agents and Chemotherapy* 35: 1504–1507

Force R W, Nahata M C, Perez A, Demers D 1993 Loracarbef: a new orally administered carbacephem antibiotic. *Annals of Pharmacotherapy* 27: 321–329

Gan V N, Kusmiesz H, Shelton S, Nelson J D 1991 Comparative evaluation of loracarbef and amoxicillin-clavulanate for acute otitis media. *Antimicrobial Agents and Chemotherapy* 35: 967–971

Hamilton-Miller J M T, Brumfitt W 1991 Comparative in vitro activity of cefixime, cefaclor and loracarbef against urinary pathogens. *Drugs under Experimental and Clinical Research* 17: 517–519

Jones R N, Barry A L 1988 Antimicrobial activity of LY163892, an orally administered 1-carbacephem. *Antimicrobial Agents and Chemotherapy* 22: 315–320

Kusmiesz H, Shelton S, Brown O, Manning S, Nelson J D 1990 Loracarbef concentrations in middle ear fluid. *Antimicrobial Agents and Chemotherapy* 34: 2030–2031

Nahata M C, Koranyi K I 1992 Pharmacokinetics of loracarbef in pediatric patients. *European Journal of Drug Metabolism and Pharmacokinetics* 17: 201–204

Sitar D S, Hoban D J, Aoki F Y 1994 Pharmacokinetic disposition of loracarbef in healthy young men and women at steady state. *Journal of Clinical Pharmacology* 34: 924–929

Group 3

Parenteral cephalosporins with broad-spectrum antimicrobial activity, resistant to a wide range of β-lactamases. They exhibit modest activity against Gram-positive organisms and their effect on enterobacteria depends more on their stability to β-lactamases than on their intrinsic activity. Cefotiam and cephamandole display the best overall activity although their β-lactamase stability is inferior to that of cefoxitin and cefuroxime which are intrinsically less active (Table 14.3).

CEFBUPERAZONE

A semi-synthetic cephamycin of group 3.

It has been particularly noted for its activity against anaerobes. Most *B. fragilis* strains are inhibited by 32 mg/l and it is active against *B. vulgatus* among other species, but not against *B. distasonis* or *B. thetaiotaomicron*. Fuso-

Table 14.3 *Activity of group 3 cephalosporins against common pathogenic bacteria: MIC (mg/l)*

	Cefbuperazone	Cefmetazole	Cefminox	Cefonicid	Cefotetan	Cefotiam	Cefoxitin	Cefuroxime	Cephamandole
Staph. aureus	8	1	8–16	1–4	8–16	1	2–8	1–4	0.5–1
Str. pyogenes	2–8	0.5	4–8	0.5–2	1	0.03	0.25–1	0.03–0.1	0.06–1
Str. pneumoniae	2–4	0.5	0.5–2	1–2	2	0.25	1–2	0.03–0.1	0.06–25
Ent. faecalis	R	R	R	R	R	R	R	R	32–R
N. gonorrhoeae		0.5	0.5–1	1	0.5–1	0.1	0.1–0.5	0.06–0.1	0.06
N. meningitidis		0.25		0.25	0.1	0.06	0.25	0.06	0.1–0.5
H. influenzae	1	4–8	0.25–2	0.5–1	1–4	0.5	2–4	0.5	0.25–2
Esch. coli	0.25	1–2	0.25–2	1	0.1–0.5	0.1	2–8	1–4	0.5–4
Klebsiella spp.	0.5	1–2	0.5–1	4–8	0.1–0.5	0.5	2–8	2–4	0.5–2
Pr. mirabilis	2	1–4	0.25–0.5	0.5	0.1–0.5	0.5	2–8	0.5–4	0.5–2
Pr. vulgaris	4	4–8	0.1–0.5	8–R	0.5–2	0.25–R	2–8	4–R	8–R
Morganella/Providencia	1–8		0.2–16		4–32	R	R	R	R
Enterobacter spp.	1	R	32–R	32–R	8–64	0.5–R	R	16–32	32–R
Salmonella spp.	0.5–4	0.5	0.25–0.5		0.25–1	0.25	1–8	1–4	0.1–0.5
Shigella spp.						0.5	32	2	0.5
Ser. marcescens	8	R	8–R	64–R	0.1–1	4–R	16–32	8–64	R
Citrobacter spp.	8	R	4–R		0.5–R		16–R	8	8
Ps. aeruginosa	R	R	R	R	R	R	R	R	R
B. fragilis	2	4–R	0.5–4	R	4–32	R	4–32	4–64	64–R

bacteria, propionibacteria and some clostridia are also susceptible. It is not hydrolysed by common β-lactamases and as a result its activity is not affected by inoculum size. Its activity against common pathogenic bacteria is shown in Table 14.3. It is not active against cefoxitin-resistant strains.

Preparations

Proprietary names: Keiperazon, Tomiproan.
Available in Japan.

Further information

Del Bene V E, Carek P J, Twitty J A, Burkey L J 1985 In vitro activity of cefbuperazone compared with that of other new β-lactam agents against anaerobic Gram-negative bacilli and contribution of β-lactamase to resistance. *Antimicrobial Agents and Chemotherapy* 27: 817–820

Karger L 1986 Impact of cefbuperazone on the colonic microflora in patients undergoing colorectal surgery. *Drugs under Experimental and Clinical Research* 12: 983–986

Tanaka H, Nishino H, Sawada T et al 1987 Biliary penetration of cefbuperazone in the presence and absence of obstructive jaundice. *Journal of Antimicrobial Chemotherapy* 20: 417–420

CEFMETAZOLE

A semi-synthetic cephamycin of group 3.

It is active against *Staph. aureus*, *Staph. epidermidis*, *Esch. coli*, *K. pneumoniae*, *Pr. mirabilis*, *Pr. vulgaris*, *Morganella morganii*, *Yersinia* spp. and *B. fragilis* (MIC 2–32 mg/l); clostridia are inhibited by 0.25–32 mg/l and anaerobic Gram-positive cocci by 0.25–8 mg/l. *Ser. marcescens* is moderately susceptible, but *Ps. aeruginosa* and *Ent. faecalis* are resistant. It is active against *Mycobacterium fortuitum* and some strains of *Mycobacterium chelonei*. Its activity against common pathogenic bacteria is shown in Table 14.3. It is resistant to a wide range of β-lactamases.

In volunteers given 30 mg/kg by i.v. bolus, the mean plasma concentrations after 15 min were around 215 mg/l; 1 g by i.v. infusion over 1 h produced mean concentrations of 77 mg/l with half-life of 0.8 h. By i.m. injection, a dose of 30 mg/kg produced mean peak serum levels of 78 mg/l at

0.75 h. The mean plasma half-life was 1.3 h. It is 68% bound to plasma proteins and its apparent volume of distribution is 17.5 l.

The principal route of excretion is the urine, where 70% is recovered over the first 6 h, falling to less than 10% in patients whose creatinine clearance is less than 10 ml/min, in whom plasma levels are elevated and plasma half-life increased to around 15 h.

Toxicity, side-effects and use are those common to group 3 cephalosporins.

Preparations and dosage

Preparation: Injection.

Dosage: Adults, i.v., 2 g every 6–12 h.

Available in Spain and Japan.

Further information

Borin M T, Peters G R, Smith T C 1990 Pharmacokinetics and dose proportionality of cefmetazole in healthy young and elderly volunteers. *Antimicrobial Agents and Chemotherapy* 34: 1944–1948

Cornick N A, Jacobus N V, Gorbach S L 1987 Activity of cefmetazole against anaerobic bacteria. *Antimicrobial Agents and Chemotherapy* 31: 2010–2012

Finch R, Moellering R C, Speller D 1988 Cefmetazole: a clinical appraisal. *Journal of Antimicrobial Chemotherapy* 23 (suppl D): 1–139

Halstenson C E, Guay D R P, Opsahl J A et al 1990 Disposition of cefmetazole in healthy volunteers and patients with impaired renal function. *Antimicrobial Agents and Chemotherapy* 34: 519–523

Ito M K, Gill M A, Chenella F C et al 1988 Intraoperative serum, bile and gallbladder-wall concentrations of cefmetazole in patients undergoing cholecystectomy. *Clinical Pharmacy* 7: 467–468

Jones R N, Barry A L, Fuchs P C, Thornsberry C 1986 Antimicrobial activity of cefmetazole (CS-1170) and recommendations for susceptibility testing by disk diffusion, dilution and anaerobic methods. *Journal of Clinical Microbiology* 24: 1055–1059

Schentag J J 1991 Cefmetazole sodium: pharmacology, pharmacokinetics, and clinical trials. *Pharmacotherapy* 11: 2–19

Stanfield J A, DiPiro J T 1988 Interference of cefmetazole sodium and cefotetan disodium with urine-glucose testing systems. *American Journal of Hospital Pharmacy* 45: 625–626

Uchihara T, Tsukagoshi H 1988 Myoclonic activity associated with cefmetazole, with a review of neurotoxicity of cephalosporins. *Clinical Neurology and Neurosurgery* 90: 369–371

CEFMINOX

A semi-synthetic cephamycin of group 3.

Its activity is similar to that of cefoxitin and cefotetan, but the activity against enterobacteria and *B. fragilis* is somewhat better (Table 14.3). *Cl. difficile* is inhibited by 4–16 mg/l. It is stable to the common β-lactamases of enterobacteria and *Bacteroides* spp., but some enzymes from *B. fragilis*, notably zinc-dependent metallo-enzymes (p. 319) hydrolyse cefminox and other cephamycins. The effect is bactericidal at concentrations close to the MIC and there is little inoculum effect. Immunomodulatory activity has been shown in the serum of volunteers receiving 2 g cefminox i.v.: attachment of *Candida albicans* to polymorphonuclear neutrophils was increased, but the number of yeasts ingested or killed was reduced.

Doses of 1 or 2 g administered by i.v. infusion over 15 min to healthy volunteers achieved plasma concentrations of about 30 and 52 mg/l after 1 h. The elimination half-life was about 2 h. Plasma protein binding is 68%.

Postmarketing surveillance in Japan over a 4-year period revealed no unusual side-effects in groups that included the elderly and pregnant women. Its uses are similar to those of other cephamycins.

Preparations

Proprietary name: Meicelin.

Available in Japan.

Further information

Aguilar L, Esteban C, Frias J, Pérez-Balcabao I, Carcas A J, Dal-Ré R 1994 Cefminox: correlation between in-vitro susceptibility and pharmacokinetics and serum bactericidal activity in healthy volunteers. *Journal of Antimicrobial Chemotherapy* 33: 91–101

Corrales I, Aguilar L, Mato R, Frias J, Prieto J 1994 Immunomodulatory effect of cefminox. *Journal of Antimicrobial Chemotherapy* 33: 372–374

Inouye S, Goi H, Watanabe T et al 1984 In vitro and in vivo antibacterial activities of MT-141, a new semisynthetic cephamycin, compared with those of five cephalosporins. *Antimicrobial Agents and Chemotherapy* 26: 722–729

Mayama T, Koyama Y, Sebata K, Tanaka Y, Shirai S, Sakai H 1995 Postmarketing surveillance on side-effects of cefminox sodium (Meicelin). *International Journal of Clinical Pharmacology and Therapeutics* 33: 149–155

Soriano F, Edwards R, Greenwood D 1991 Comparative susceptibility of cefminox and cefoxitin to β-lactamases of *Bacteroides* spp. *Journal of Antimicrobial Chemotherapy* 28: 55–60

Soriano F, Edwards R, Greenwood D 1992 Effect of inoculum size on bacteriolytic activity of cefminox and four other β-lactam antibiotics against *Escherichia coli*. *Antimicrobial Agents and Chemotherapy* 36: 223–226

Watanabe S, Omoto S 1990 Pharmacology of cefminox, a new bactericidal cephamycin. *Drugs under Experimental and Clinical Research* 16: 461–467

CEFONICID

A semi-synthetic cephalosporin of group 3.

It is widely active against Gram-positive and Gram-negative organisms (Table 14.3) but its bacteriostatic and bactericidal activity in vitro is depressed by the presence of 50% serum.

It is highly bound to plasma protein (98%), the free fraction in volunteers receiving 30 mg/kg i.v. over 5 min immediately falling to 2%. Following 1 g i.m. a mean peak plasma concentration of 83 mg/l has been found. Following a dose of 1 g by i.v. bolus mean peak plasma concentrations of 130–300 mg/l have been reported with a half-life of 5 h. In volunteers, doses of 7.5 mg/kg i.v. over 5 min produced peak plasma concentrations of 95–156 mg/l with a half-life of 4.4 h. In patients treated for community-acquired pneumonia, concentrations of 2–4 mg/l have been found in sputum. Disposition is not altered in patients with severe skin or soft-tissue infections.

It is predominantly excreted by renal secretion, 83–89% being recovered unchanged in the urine over 24 h. Plasma half-life is linearly related to creatinine clearance. As a result of its high protein binding it is not removed by haemodialysis.

It is generally well tolerated; pain on i.m. injection, rash and positive Coombs' test are reported in some patients. It has been used to treat respiratory, soft tissue and urinary infections, its long half-life being claimed to be an advantage.

Preparations and dosage

Preparation: Injection.

Dosage: Adults, 500 mg to 2 g once daily depending on severity of infection.

Available in Italy.

Further information

Cazzola M, Polverino M, Guidetti E et al 1990 Penetration of cefonicid into human lung tissue and lymph nodes. *Chemotherapy* 36: 325–331

Fillastre J-P, Fourtillan J-B, Leroy A et al 1986 Pharmacokinetics of cefonicid in uraemic patients. *Journal of Antimicrobial Chemotherapy* 18: 203–211

Furlan G, Besa G, Broccali G, Gusmitta A 1989 Pharmacokinetics of cefonicid in serum and its penetration into lung tissue, bronchial mucosa and plasma. *International Journal of Clinical Pharmacology Research* 9: 49–53

Furlanut M, D'Elia R, Riva E, Pasinelli F 1989 Pharmacokinetics of cefonicid in children. *European Journal of Clinical Pharmacology* 36: 79–82

Heim-Duthoy K L 1988 Pharmacokinetics of cefonicid in patients with skin and skin structure infection. *Antimicrobial Agents and Chemotherapy* 32: 485–487

Liebergall M, Mosheiff R, Rand N et al 1995 A double-blinded, randomized, controlled clinical trial to compare cefazolin and cefonicid for antimicrobial prophylaxis in clean orthopedic surgery. *Israel Journal of Medical Sciences* 31: 62–64

Saltier E, Brogden R N 1986 Cefonicid. A review of its antibacterial activity pharmacological properties and therapeutic use. *Drugs* 32: 222–259

Tanos V, Rajansky N, Anteby S O 1994 Comparison of cefonicid and cefazolin prophylaxis in abdominal hysterectomy. *Gynecologic and Obstetric Investigation* 37: 115–117

Trang J M, Monson T P, Ackermann B H, Underwood F L, Manning J T, Kearns G L 1989 Effect of age and renal function on cefonicid pharmacokinetics. *Antimicrobial Agents and Chemotherapy* 33: 142–146

CEFOTETAN

A semi-synthetic cephamycin of group 3.

Antimicrobial activity

It exhibits potent activity against enterobacteria, most of which are inhibited by <1 mg/l, and modest activity against *Staph aureus* and *Bacteroides* spp.; enterococci are resistant (Table 14.3).

Pharmacokinetics

A few minutes after rapid i.v. doses of 0.5 and 1.0 g, plasma concentrations of 80–120 and 140–180 mg/l are found. There is no evidence of accumulation on a dosage of 1 g 12-hourly. It is 88% bound to plasma proteins and its apparent volume of distribution is 10.3 l. It is partially converted to a tautomer which can occasionally be detected in the plasma. The plasma half-life is 3–3.5 h.

Distribution

Tissue fluid concentrations were about 30% of the simultaneous serum level. In patients given 1 g by i.v. bolus preoperatively, concentrations were detectable within minutes in the peritoneal fluid, reaching 44% of the simultaneous serum level at 0.5 h and 115% at 3 h.

Excretion

About 85% of the drug is eliminated in the urine over 24 h. Accumulation in renal failure is inversely linearly related to the creatinine clearance, the plasma half-life, rising to 20 h in patients requiring haemodialysis. During haemodialysis the half-life falls to around 7.5 h and on continuous ambulatory peritoneal dialysis (CAPD) it falls to 15.5 h, 5–10% of the dose being recovered in the dialysate over 24 h. Excretion of the tautomer is not affected by the degree of renal failure.

Toxicity and side-effects

Reactions are generally those typical of the group. Anaphylaxis has been described and there is some risk of disulphiram-like reactions. It inhibits vitamin K 2,3-epoxide reductase and hypoprothrombinaemia can occur. Immunologically determined thrombocytopenia has been seen. In volunteers receiving the drug intravenously, there was a marked reduction in faecal *Esch. coli* and *B. fragilis*, with appearance of *Cl. difficile* in a few subjects.

Clinical uses

Those of group 3 cephalosporins (p. 206).

Preparations and dosage

Preparation: Injection.

Dosage: Adults, i.m., i.v., 1–3 g every 12 h depending on severity of infection.

Available in Italy, France, USA.

Further information

Bloomberg R J 1988 Cefotetan-induced anaphylaxis. *American Journal of Obstetrics and Gynecology* 159: 125–126

Browning M J, Holt H A, White L O et al 1986 Pharmacokinetics of cefotetan in patients with end-stage renal failure on maintenance dialysis. *Journal of Antimicrobial Chemotherapy* 18: 103–106

Christie D J, Lennon S S, Drew R L, Swinehart C D 1988 Cefotetan-induced immunologic thrombocytopenia. *British Journal of Haematology* 70: 423–426

Eckrich R J, Fox S, Mallory D 1994 Cefotetan-induced immune hemolytic anemia due to the drug-adsorption mechanism. *Immunohematology* 10: 51–54

Jones R N 1988 Cefotetan: a review of the microbiologic properties and antimicrobial spectrum. *American Journal of Surgery* 155: 16–23

Kline S S, Mauro V F, Forney R B, Freimer E H, Somani P 1987 Cefotetan-induced disulfiram-type reactions and hypoprothrombinemia. *Antimicrobial Agents and Chemotherapy* 31: 1328–1331

Martin C, Thomachet L, Albanese J 1994 Clinical pharmacokinetics of cefotetan. *Clinical Pharmacokinetics* 26: 248–258

Quintiliani R, Nightingale C H, Stevens R C, Outman W R, Deckers P J, Martens M G 1988 Comparative pharmacokinetics of cefotetan and cefoxitin in patients undergoing hysterectomies and colorectal operations. *American Journal of Surgery* 155: 67–70

Ripa S, Mignini F, Prenna M 1987 Pharmacokinetics of cefotetan in elderly subjects after intramuscular administration. *Chemioterapia* 6: 359–363

Shwed J A, Danziger L H, Wojtynek J, Rodvold K A 1991 A comparative evaluation of the safety and efficacy of cefotetan and cefoxitin in surgical prophylaxis. *Drug Intelligence and Clinical Pharmacy, Annals of Pharmacotherapy* 25: 10–13

Triger D R, Malia R D, Preston F E 1988 Platelet function and coagulation in patients with hepatobiliary disorders receiving cefotetan prophylaxis. *Infection* 16: 105–108

Wagner B K J, Heaton A H, Flink J R 1992 Cefotetan disodium-induced hemolytic anemia. *Annals of Pharmacotherapy* 20: 199–200

Ward A, Richards D M 1985 Cefotetan. A review of its antibacterial activity, pharmacokinetic properties and therapeutic use. *Drugs* 30: 382–426

CEFOTIAM

A semi-synthetic cephalosporin of group 3.

Antimicrobial activity

It is active against *Staph. aureus*, including β-lactamase producing strains; *Str. pyogenes* and *Str. pneumoniae* are very susceptible but *Ent. faecalis* is resistant. Neisseriae, including β-lactamase-positive strains, are very susceptible. It is active against *H. influenzae* and a wide range of enterobacteria, but not *B. fragilis* (Table 14.3). There is little effect of 75% serum on inhibitory activity.

Pharmacokinetics

A few minutes after i.v. bolus administration, plasma concentrations around 100 and 200 mg/l are obtained following doses of 0.5 and 1.0 g, respectively. In volunteers given 1 or 2 g i.v. over 30 min, the concentrations 15 min after the end of infusion were around 35 and 80 mg/l, respectively. Intramuscular injections of 0.5 and 1 g produced mean peak plasma levels around 8 and 17 mg/l, respectively. The plasma half-life is 0.6–1.1 h. Administration with lidocaine produced no change in pharmacokinetics in volunteers. There is no evidence of accumulation on repeated dosage. Plasma protein binding is 40% and the apparent volume of distribution is 35 l.

Distribution
In parturient patients given 1 g i.v., peak concentration at 15–30 min in umbilical cord blood was 13–24 mg/l and in amniotic fluid was 19.6–23.5 mg/l at around 2.5 h.

Excretion
Urinary excretion is almost complete 4 h after the end of i.v. infusion, but only 50–67% is recovered unchanged; there is substantial non-renal elimination and some evidence of saturation of renal tubular excretion at doses above 2 g. In anuria the plasma elimination half-life rises to 13 h and plasma and renal clearances parallel creatinine clearance. Biliary excretion accounts for 0.2% of the dose. In patients with cholelithiasis given 0.5 or 1 g i.v., mean concentrations in gallbladder bile and gallbladder wall 30 min after the dose were around 17 and 32 mg/l, respectively. In patients with normal liver function hepatic bile concentrations can exceed 1 g/l.

Cefotiam hexetil
The pro-drug ester of cefotiam allowing oral administration. Bioavailability is around 65% and food delays absorption. In patients with chronic maxillary sinusitis given two 200 mg doses of the pro-drug 12 h apart, plasma concentrations 1 h after the second dose were about 1 mg/l with similar concentrations in sinus fluid.

Toxicity and side-effects

It is generally well tolerated, apart from superficial phlebitis in some patients. Failure of therapy has been associated with superinfection, and colonization with resistant Gram-negative organisms has also been observed.

Clinical use

It has been successfully used to treat lower respiratory infections due to *Str. pneumoniae*, *K. pneumoniae* and *H. influenzae* and to treat skin and soft-tissue infection.

Preparations and dosage
Preparation: Injection.
Dosage: Adults, i.m., i.v., up to 6 g/day in divided doses.
Limited availability in continental Europe.

Further information

Brogard J M, Jehl F, Willemin B, Lamalle A M, Blickle J F, Monteil H 1989 Clinical pharmacokinetics of cefotiam. *Clinical Pharmacokinetics* 17: 163–174

Brouard R, Tozer T N, Merdjan H, Guillemin A, Baumelou A 1988 Transperitoneal movement and pharmacokinetics of cefotiam and cefsulodin in patients on continuous ambulatory peritoneal dialysis. *Clinical Nephrology* 30: 197–206

Carbon C, Chatelin, Bingen E et al 1995 A double-blind randomized trial comparing the efficacy and safety of a 5-day course of cefotiam hexetil with that of a 10-day course of penicillin V in adult patients with pharyngitis caused by group A β-haemolytic streptococci. *Journal of Antimicrobial Chemotherapy* 35: 843–854

Cherrier P, Tod M, Le-Gros V, Petitjean O, Brion N, Chatelin A 1992 Cefotiam concentrations in the sinus fluid of patients with chronic sinusitis after administration of cefotiam hexetil. *European Journal of Clinical Microbiology and Infectious Diseases* 12: 211–215

Imada A, Hirai S 1995 Cefotiam hexetil. *International Journal of Antimicrobial Agents* 5: 85–99

Maier H, Attalan M, Weidauer H 1992 Efficacy and safety on cefotiam hexetil in the treatment of ear, nose and throat infections. *Arzneimittelforschung* 42: 980–982

Rouan M C, Binswanger U, Bammatter F, Theobald W, Schoeller J P, Guibert J 1984 Pharmacokinetics and dosage adjustment of cefotiam in renal impaired patients. *Journal of Antimicrobial Chemotherapy* 13: 611–618

Satake K, Cho K, Taniura M, Oka I, Koo I 1982 Cefotiam concentrations in bile and in the wall of the gallbladder in patients with biliary disease. *Journal of Antimicrobial Chemotherapy* 10: 141–145

CEFOXITIN

A semi-synthetic cephamycin of group 3.

Antimicrobial activity

It is moderately active against *Staph. aureus* and other Gram-positive cocci, but enterococci and *L. monocytogenes* are resistant. Anaerobic Gram-positive cocci and Gram-positive bacilli, including clostridia and actinomyces, are susceptible. About half the strains of *M. fortuitum* and 10% of *M. chelonei* tested were inhibited by 16 mg/l. It exhibits a high degree of activity against various Gram-negative bacilli, including *Citrobacter, Legionella, Providencia, Serratia* and some *Acinetobacter* spp. *Enterobacter* spp. are resistant. It is moderately active against *Bacteroides* spp., but the MIC_{90} for *B. fragilis* is 16–32 mg/l and considerable strain variation in susceptibility occurs. Its activity against common pathogenic bacteria is shown in Table 14.3. It is rapidly bactericidal to enterobacteria at concentrations close to the MIC. It is resistant to many Gram-negative β-lactamases and is active against organisms elaborating them.

Acquired resistance

Resistant strains of *Bacteroides* (which may be cross-resistant to imipenem) have been described. Resistance may be transferable to other *Bacteroides* spp. In some, but not all, strains resistance is associated with a β-lactamase which slowly hydrolyses cefoxitin. It is a potent inducer of chromosomal cephalosporinases of certain Gram-negative bacilli and can antagonize the effect of cefotaxime and other β-lactam agents.

Pharmacokinetics

Cefoxitin is not absorbed by oral administration, but is very rapidly absorbed from intramuscular sites, doses of 0.5 and 1 g producing peak plasma concentrations 20 min after injection of 11 and 23 mg/l, respectively. A few minutes after rapid i.v. administration of 1 g the plasma concentration is around 150 mg/l and after 2 g, 220 mg/l. Doubling the dose approximately doubles the plasma level. It is absorbed from suppositories to varying degrees depending on the adjuvants: peak serum levels around 9.8 mg/l have been obtained after a dose of 1 g, giving a bioavailability of around 20%. It is 65–80% bound to plasma protein and its apparent volume of distribution is 7 l. Less than 5% of the drug is desacetylated and in a few subjects deacylation of 1 or 2% of the dose to the antibacterially inactive descarbamyl form also occurs. The plasma half-life is 45 min. In infants and children treated with 150 mg/kg daily, mean serum concentrations 15 min after i.v. and i.m. administration were 81.9 and 68.5 mg/l, with elimination half-lives of 0.70 and 0.67 h, respectively.

Distribution

About 20% of the corresponding serum levels are found in sputum following 2 g i.v. of the drug. In patients given 1 g by i.v. bolus preoperatively concentrations in lung tissue at 1 h were around 13 mg/g.

Penetration into normal CSF is very poor; in most patients with aseptic meningitis receiving 2 g i.v. none could be detected in the CSF. In patients with purulent meningitis treated with three 6-hourly i.v. bolus doses of 2 g, CSF concentrations peaked between 2 and 6 h at 1–22 mg/l, concentrations in most patients not exceeding 6 mg/l. In patients with bacterial meningitis treated with 2 g i.v. 4-hourly for 10 days, mean CSF concentrations of 3.3, 4.7 and 2.9 on days 1, 3 and 10 were raised to 8.6, 12.3 and 4.3 mg/l when 0.5 g probenecid was given 6–8 hourly. In children with meningitis receiving 75 mg/kg 6-hourly, peak concentrations of 5–6 mg/l were found around 1 h after the dose. In patients receiving 2 g i.v. before surgery, the mean penetrance into peritoneal fluid was 86%. Concentrations fell in parallel with those in serum, giving an elimination half-life around 0.72 h. In patients receiving 2 g i.m. before hysterectomy, mean concentrations in pelvic tissue were 7.8 mg/g. Breast milk has been found to contain 5–6 mg/l after 1 g i.v.

Excretion

It is almost entirely excreted in the urine by both glomerular filtration and tubular secretion, about 90% being found in the first 12 h following an i.m. dose and 80% following an i.v. dose, producing concentrations in excess of 1 g/l. Frusemide in doses of 40–160 mg had no effect on the elimination half-life of doses of 1 or 2 g. Probenecid delays the plasma peak and decreases the renal clearance and urine concentration. The plasma half-life and volume of distribution have been variously said to be decreased or unaffected. The renal clearance has been calculated variously to lie between 225 and 330 ml/min. The plasma half-life increases inversely with creatinine clearance to reach 24 h in oliguric patients, with corresponding reduction in total body clearance. In patients on CAPD, peritoneal clearance accounted for only 7.5% of mean plasma clearance and the mean plasma half-life during 6 h dialysis was 7.8 h.

Bile. Concentrations up to 230 mg/l have been found in bile after 2 g i.v., with bile:serum ratios at various times after the dose up to 16.7.

Toxicity and side-effects

Reactions have been those common to cephalosporins. Transient neutropenia, eosinophilia and increased transaminase levels have occurred. Evidence of renal damage, including proteinuria with or without increase of blood urea, has been described in patients with pre-existing renal disease or other aggravating factors. Pain on intramuscular, and thrombophlebitis on intravenous injection occur. Substantial changes can occur in the faecal flora, with virtual eradication of susceptible enterobacteria and non-*fragilis Bacteroides* and appearance of, or increase in, enterococci, staphylococci, resistant enterobacteria, *Ps. aeruginosa, B. fragilis* and, in some cases, *Cl. difficile.* Development of meningitis due to *H. influenzae* and *Str. pneumoniae* in patients treated for other infections has been observed. It may interfere with the Jaffe reaction for creatinine.

Clinical use

As for group 3 cephalosporins, with particular emphasis on mixed infections including anaerobes, notably abdominal and pelvic sepsis (Ch. 42). In considering its use, its low activity against aerobic Gram-positive cocci should be noted. Reference is made to its use in endocarditis (Ch. 49) and septicaemia (Ch. 41).

Preparations and dosage

Proprietary name: Mefoxin.

Preparation: Injection.

Dosage: Adults, i.m., i.v., 1–2 g every 6–8 h with a maximum of 12 g/day. Children, <1 week, 20–40 mg/kg every 12 h; children 1–4 weeks, 20–40 mg/kg every 8 h; children >1 month, 20–40 mg/kg every 6–8 h.

Widely available.

Further information

Alexander D P, Becker J M 1988 Cefoxitin disposition in colorectal surgery. Implications for the effective use of prophylactic antibiotics. *Annals of Surgery* 208: 162–168

Berne T V, Yellin A E, Appleman M D, Gill M A, Chenella F C, Heseltine P N R 1990 Controlled comparison of cefmetazole with cefoxitin for prophylaxis in elective cholecystectomy. *Surgery, Gynecology and Obstetrics* 170: 137–140

Brogden R N, Heel R C, Speight T M, Avery G S 1979 Cefoxitin: a review of its antibacterial activity, pharmacological properties and therapeutic use. *Drugs* 17: 1–37

Brown R B, Klar J, Lemeshow S, Teres D, Pastides H, Sands M 1986 Enhanced bleeding with cefoxitin or moxalactam. Statistical analysis within a defined population of 1493 patients. *Archives of Internal Medicine* 146: 2159–2164

Carver P L, Nightingale C H, Quintiliani R 1989 Pharmacokinetics and pharmacodynamics of total and unbound cefoxitin and cefotetan in healthy volunteers. *Journal of Antimicrobial Chemotherapy* 23: 99–106

Feldman W E, Moffitt S, Manning N S 1982 Penetration of cefoxitin into cerebrospinal fluid of infants and children with bacterial meningitis. *Antimicrobial Agents and Chemotherapy* 21: 468–471

Garcia M J, Dominiguez-Gil A, Tabernero J M, Diaz Molina M 1983 Pharmacokinetics of cefoxitin during haemofiltration. *European Journal of Clinical Pharmacology* 25: 395–398

Gonik B, Cotton D, Feldman S, Cleary T G, Pickering K 1984 Comparative pharmacokinetics of cefoxitin in postpartum normotensive and pregnancy-induced hypertensive patients. *American Journal of Obstetrics and Gynecology* 148: 1088–1091

Roex A J, van Loenen A C, Puyenbroek J I, Arts N F 1987 Secretion of cefoxitin in breast milk following short-term prophylactic administration in caesarian section. *European Journal of Obstetrics, Gynecology and Reproductive Biology* 25: 299–302

Shwed J A, Danziger L H, Wojtynek J, Rodvold K A 1991 A comparative evaluation of the safety and efficacy of cefotetan and cefoxitin in surgical prophylaxis. *Drug Intelligence and Clinical Pharmacy, Annals of Pharmacotherapy* 25: 10–13

Sieradzan R R, Bottner W A, Fasco M J, Bertoni J S Jr 1988 Comparative effects of cefoxitin and cefotetan on vitamin K metabolism. *Antimicrobial Agents and Chemotherapy* 32: 1446–1449

Stark C, Edlund C, Hedberg M, Nord C E 1995 Induction of β-lactamase production in the anaerobic microflora by cefoxitin. *Clinical Infectious Diseases* 20 (suppl 2): S350–S351

Van Hoogdalem E J, Wackwitz A T, DeBoer A G, Cohen A F, Breimer D D 1989 Rate-controlled rectal absorption enhancement of cefoxitin by coadministration of sodium salicylate or sodium octanoate in healthy volunteers. *British Journal of Clinical Pharmacology* 27: 75–81

CEFUROXIME

A semi-synthetic cephalosporin of group 3 supplied as the sodium salt, or as the acetoxyethyl ester.

Antimicrobial activity

It is active against *Staph. aureus* and most streptococci but not against penicillin-resistant *Str. pneumoniae*. It is active against most enterobacteria, including the great majority of multiply-resistant strains. *Acinetobacter* spp., *Ser. marcescens* and *Ps. aeruginosa* are resistant, although some other pseudomonads, including *Burkholderia* (*Ps.*) *cepacia*, are susceptible. Some anaerobic Gram-negative rods are susceptible, but *B. fragilis* is resistant. The minimum immobilizing concentration for the Nichol's strain of *T. pallidum* is 0.01 mg/l. Its activity against common pathogenic bacteria is shown in Table 14.3.

For most susceptible species, it is bactericidal at concentrations close to the MIC. Synergy with aminoglycosides is demonstrable against a number of species. It is completely stable to some Gram-negative β-lactamases and hydrolysed only slowly by most others.

Pharmacokinetics

It is highly ionized at physiological pH and poorly lipid soluble, so that very little is absorbed by mouth: after oral administration of the sodium salt only about 1% of the drug is recovered in the urine. A peak plasma level around 18–25 mg/l is obtained 0.5 h after an i.m. dose of 0.5 g and 26–40 mg/l 1 h after a dose of 1 g. A few minutes after rapid i.v. administration of 0.75, 1 or 1.5 g, the mean plasma concentrations were around 75, 110 and 200 mg/l, respectively. It is 30% bound to plasma protein and the apparent volume of distribution is 11–15 l. There is very little biotransformation. The mean plasma elimination half-life (1.1–1.4 h) is prolonged in the elderly up to 2.35 h.

In children given 50 or 75 mg/kg i.v. over 15 min mean peak serum concentrations were around 105 and 150 mg/l, respectively. There was little accumulation in those treated with 50 mg/kg 6-hourly. At the end of a 30-min i.v. infusion of 0.5 g the plasma level was around 85 mg/l. The mean plasma half-life is 1.5 h.

Distribution
In patients with severe meningeal inflammation, the mean

CSF concentration after 1.5 g i.v. has been in the range 1.5–3.7 mg/l in the presence of mild to moderate inflammation, and in viral meningitis 0.1–2 mg/l. In about a third of patients with normal CSF, no drug could be detected and in the remainder concentrations ranged from 0.2 to 1 mg/l. In children treated for meningitis with 50 or 75 mg/kg, the CSF:serum ratio was 0.07 and 0.10, respectively. Concentrations in pleural drain fluid after thoracic surgery approximated to serum levels at 2 h after doses of 1 or 1.5 g and exceeded serum levels at 4 h when they were still around 10 mg/l. Levels in pericardial fluid were similar, with fluid: serum ratios between 0.5 and 2 h of 0.44. In patients receiving 1.5 g by i.v. bolus preoperatively, concentrations around 22 mg/g were found in subcutaneous tissue at about 5 h with an elimination half-life of about 1.5 h.

Mean concentrations in the femoral head after 750 mg i.m. given with premedication or 1.5 g by i.v. bolus at the time of induction, gave bone:serum ratios of 0.14 and 0.23. In patients with chronic otitis media treated with 0.75 g 8-hourly for 6–8 days, peak concentrations in middle ear of 0.73–1.70 mg/l were reached about 2 h after the dose. In patients given 750 mg i.m. on 5 consecutive days the mean sputum concentration rose from 0.57 mg/l on the first day to 1.15 mg/l on the third.

Excretion
The parenterally administered drug is recovered in the urine within 6 h of administration, producing concentrations around 300–3000 mg/l. About 45–55% of the drug is excreted by tubular secretion, so that the administration of probenecid increases the serum peak, prolongs the plasma half-life and reduces the apparent volume of distribution and renal clearance. Renal clearance is slightly affected by the route of administration but lies between 95 and 180 l/min. Frusemide has no effect on the plasma half-life.

Cefuroxime axetil
The acetoxyethyl ester of cefuroxime. It is rapidly hydrolysed on passage through the intestinal mucosa and in the portal circulation to liberate acetaldehyde and acetic acid. No unchanged ester is detectable in the systemic circulation.

Esterification of the carboxyl group at C-4 renders the molecule more lipophilic, and in contrast to the parent substance a significant proportion is absorbed after oral administration. In a comparison between i.v. and oral doses of 1 g, the mean absolute bioavailability in male subjects was 0.35 and in female subjects 0.32, with absorption significantly better after food: 0.45 and 0.41 in the two sexes. Larger effects of food have been found in elderly subjects, in whom doses of 500 mg 2 or 3 times daily produced peak plasma levels in 1.5–2 h of 5.5 mg/l in the fasting state, rising to 7.56 20 min after the dose was administered with food. Problems of inconsistent absorption have been ameliorated by reformulation, with bioavailability after food rising to 50%. In volunteers, 500 or 600 mg produced mean peak plasma levels of 6.4–9.0 mg/l at 1.8–2.5 h, with a plasma half-life of 1.1 h. Absorption is independent of dose in the range 0.25–1 g, and there is no accumulation on repeated dosing. Binding to plasma protein in 30%. The plasma level after 500 mg given after food was raised to 7–10 mg/l at 2–3 h when administered with probenecid. A fluid:serum ratio of 0.64 in artificial blisters has been reported.

In older children given 15 or 20 mg/kg as crushed tablets a mean peak plasma level of 4.5 mg/l at 1.5–2 h was unaffected by food intake but the AUC was significantly increased when the preparation was given with milk. The plasma half-life in children (1.4 h) is similar to that in adults.

Toxicity and side-effects

It is well tolerated with little pain or phlebitis on injection. Reactions described are minor hypersensitivity manifestations and biochemical changes common to cephalosporins. There is no evidence of nephrotoxicity in patients with pre-existing renal impairment and no effect of the addition of frusemide or of tobramycin in normal doses.

The axetil ester is also well tolerated but diarrhoea and, in some cases, vomiting, accompanied by changes in the bowel flora, occasionally with the appearance of *Cl. difficile*, have been reported in about 15% of patients. Vaginitis is reported in about 2% of female patients.

Clinical use

Its uses are generally those of group 3 compounds (p. 206). It has been successfully used to treat urinary, soft-tissue and pulmonary infections and septicaemia. It has been commended as a single-dose treatment with probenecid of gonorrhoea due to β-lactamase-producing strains. Reference is made to its use in renal transplant patients, CAPD peritonitis, meningitis, impetigo and urinary tract infection. The ester is appropriate if the oral route is preferred.

CEFUROXIME
Preparations and dosage

Proprietary name: Zinacef.

Preparation: Injection.

Dosage: Adults, i.m., i.v., 750 mg every 6–8 h; 1.5 g every 6–8 h in severe infections. Children, 30–100 mg/day in 3–4 divided doses; 60 mg/kg per day in divided doses is appropriate for most infections. Neonates, 30–100 mg/kg per day in 2–3 divided doses.

Widely available.

CEFUROXIME AXETIL
Preparations and dosage

Proprietary name: Zinnat.

Preparation: Tablets, suspension.

Dosage: Adults, oral, 250–500 mg twice daily depending on severity of infection. Children over 3 months, oral, 125 mg twice daily; if necessary, dose doubled in children over 2 years with otitis media.

Widely available.

Further information

Baldwin D R, Andrews J M, Wise R, Honeybourne D 1992 Bronchoalveolar distribution of cefuroxime axetil and in-vitro efficacy of observed concentrations against respiratory pathogens. *Journal of Antimicrobial Chemotherapy* 30: 377–385

Brogden R N, Heel R C, Speight T M, Avery G S 1979 Cefuroxime: a review of its antibacterial activity, pharmacological properties and therapeutic use. *Drugs* 17: 233–266

Colaizzi P A, Goodwin S D, Poynor W J, Karnes H T, Polk R E 1987 Single dose pharmacokinetics of cefuroxime and cefamandole in healthy subjects. *Clinical Pharmacy* 6: 894–899

Dellamonica P 1994 Cefuroxime axetil. *International Journal of Antimicrobial Agents* 4: 23–36

Donn K H, James N C, Powell J R 1994 Bioavailability of cefuroxime axetil formulations. *Journal of Pharmaceutical Sciences* 83: 842–844

Edwards M S, Baker C J, Butler K M, Mason E O, Laurent J P, Cheek W R 1989 Penetration of cefuroxime into ventricular fluid in cerebrospinal fluid shunt infections. *Antimicrobial Agents and Chemotherapy* 33: 1108–1110

Emmerson A M 1988 Cefuroxime axetil. *Journal of Antimicrobial Chemotherapy* 22: 101–104

Finn A, Straughan A, Meyer M, Chubb J 1987 Effect of dose and food on the bioavailability of cefuroxime axetil. *Biopharmaceutics and Drug Disposition* 8: 519–526

Ginsburg C M, McCracken G H, Petruska M, Olson K 1985 Pharmacokinetics and bactericidal activity of cefuroxime axetil. *Antimicrobial Agents and Chemotherapy* 28: 504–507

Goddard J K, Janning S W, Gass J S, Wilson R E 1994 Cefuroxime-induced acute renal failure. *Pharmacotherapy* 14: 488–491

Gold B, Rodriguez W J 1983 Cefuroxime: mechanisms of action, antimicrobial activity, pharmacokinetics, clinical application, adverse reactions and therapeutic indications. *Pharmacotherapy* 3: 82–100

Gooch W M, McLinn S E, Aronovitz G H et al 1993 Efficacy of cefuroxime axetil suspension compared with that of penicillin V suspension in children with group A streptococcal pharyngitis. *Antimicrobial Agents and Chemotherapy* 37: 159–163

Hoddinott C, Lovering A M, Fernando H C, Dixon J H, Reeves D S 1990 Determination of bone and fat concentrations following systemic cefamandole and regional cefuroxime administration in patients undergoing knee arthroplasty. *Journal of Antimicrobial Chemotherapy* 26: 823–829

Huizinga W K J, Hirshberg A, Thomson S R, Elson K F, Salisbury R T, Brock-Utne J G 1989 Prophylactic parenteral cefuroxime: subcutaneous concentrations in laparotomy wounds. *Journal of Hospital Infection* 13: 395–398

Kaukonen J P, Tuomainen P, Makijarv J, Mokka R, Mannisto P T 1995 Intravenous cefuroxime prophylaxis. Tissue levels after one 3-gram dose in 40 cases of hip fracture. *Acta Orthopaedica Scandinavica* 66: 14–16

Leigh D A, Walsh B, Leung A, Tait S, Peatey K, Hancock P 1990 The effect of cefuroxime axetil on the faecal flora of healthy volunteers. *Journal of Antimicrobial Chemotherapy* 26: 261–268

Marx M A, Fant W K 1988 Cefuroxime axetil. *Drug Intelligence and Clinical Pharmacy* 22: 651–658

Perea E J, Ayarra J, Garcia Iglesias M C, Garcia Luque I, Loscatales J 1988 Penetration of cefuroxime and ceftazidime into human lungs. *Chemotherapy* 34: 1–7

Shah S H, Shah I S, Turnbull G, Cunningham K 1994 Cefuroxime axetil in the treatment of bronchitis: comparison with amoxycillin in a multicentre study in general practice patients. *British Journal of Clinical Practice* 48: 185–189

Williams P R, Harding S M 1984 The absolute bioavailability of oral cefuroxime axetil in male and female volunteers after fasting and after food. *Journal of Antimicrobial Chemotherapy* 13: 191–196

CEPHAMANDOLE

A semi-synthetic cephalosporin of group 3. Supplied as the nafate, an antibacterially inactive ester hydrolysed in the body to cephamandole.

Antimicrobial activity

It is active against staphylococci, including β-lactamase-producing strains. It resembles cephalothin in its resistance to staphylococcal β-lactamase. It is generally active against both aerobic and anaerobic Gram-positive rods and cocci. Neisseria, including β-lactamase-positive *N. gonorrhoeae*, are susceptible. It is highly active (MIC <1 mg/l) against capsulate *H. influenzae*, including β-lactamase-positive strains, but non-typeable strains may be much less susceptible or show marked disparity in the MBC:MIC ratio ('tolerance'). It is widely active against enterobacteria, but there is considerable strain variation in susceptibility. *Citrobacter*, *Providencia* and *Yersinia* spp. are commonly susceptible, but *Pr. vulgaris*, *Morg. morgani* and *Providencia rettgeri* are often resistant, as are *Acinetobacter*, *Serratia* and *Pseudomonas* spp. Some anaerobic Gram-negative rods are susceptible but *B. fragilis* is resistant (Table 14.3). It is stable to a number of enterobacterial β-lactamases.

Acquired resistance

Derepressed mutants of *Enterobacter* spp. elaborating chromosomal β-lactamase (p. 319), and cross-resistant to other β-lactam agents, emerge on passage in the presence of the drug in vitro and may do so in the course of treatment.

Pharmacokinetics

Following an i.m. dose of 0.5 g of the nafate, peak plasma levels of 13–15 mg/l are reached 0.75–1 h after injection. After 1 g the peak plasma level is 20–35 mg/l. Doubling the dose approximately doubles the plasma level. A few minutes after rapid i.v. administration of 1 g the plasma level is 130 mg/l; shortly after infusion of 1 or 2 g over 20–30 min, the plasma concentration is around 90 or 190 mg/l, respectively. It is not significantly metabolized; 65–80% is bound to plasma protein and the volume of distribution is 12.5–19 l. The plasma half-life is 0.7–1 h.

Distribution

It enters serous fluids, achieving levels in the synovial fluid of 30–50 mg/l following a 2 g i.v. dose. Following a dose of 1 g i.v. the mean concentration in cantharides blister fluid was 22 mg/l half an hour after administration when the plasma concentration was 50 mg/l. Therapeutically effective concentrations are found in bone of the order of 9 mg/kg following a dose of 2 g i.v. In patients given 1 g i.v. at the time of induction of anaesthesia, mean concentrations in the femoral head were 12.6 mg/l 20–70 min after the dose, giving a bone:serum ratio of 0.36.

Excretion

Excretion is mainly through the urine, by both glomerular

and tubular routes, where 75–80% of the unchanged drug is found within the first 6 h after i.v. and 65–75% in the first 8 h after i.m. administration. Concentrations of 200–400 mg/kg are found in urine after an i.m. dose of 500 mg and up to 2000 mg/kg following 1 g i.m. Renal clearance is 230–260 ml/min per 1.72 m² and declines in renal failure. Only about 5% is removed by haemodialysis.

Bile. High levels are found in T-tube bile of the order of 150–250 mg/kg following 1 g of the drug i.v., but this route of excretion accounts for less than 0.1% of the dose. In hepatobiliary disease, concentrations of 1.6–1400 mg/l have been found in gallbladder bile and 9–>2000 mg/l in common duct bile following 4–6 hourly i.v. infusions of 1 g over 15–20 min. It was absent only in complete aseptic common duct obstruction, following relief of which levels were still depressed 7 days later.

Toxicity and side-effects

Side-effects common to cephalosporins have been described: urticarial rash, eosinophilia, fever, diarrhoea, positive Coombs' test and increase in transaminase and creatinine phosphokinase. Cephamandole and analogues containing the methyltetrazole side-chain are associated with bleeding attributed to depression of vitamin-K-dependent carboxylase. Rare renal damage or enhancement of existing renal damage has been described. Thrombophlebitis on i.v. administration is relatively common.

Clinical use

Those of group 3 cephalosporins (p. 206). It has been recommended for the treatment of Gram-negative bacillary pneumonia, for enteric fever and other systemic salmonelloses. It has been used for the treatment of meningitis, particularly that due to β-lactamase-positive *H. influenzae*, but experience with it has been mixed. Failure to control *Staph. aureus* bacteraemia has been relatively common, but it has been claimed to be equally effective against methicillin-resistant and methicillin-susceptible strains. Reference is made to its use in neutropenic patients (p. 619).

Preparations and dosage

Proprietary name: Kefadol.

Preparation: Injection.

Dosage: Adults, i.m., i.v., 500 mg to 2 g every 4–8 h depending on severity of infection. Children over 1 month, 50–100 mg/kg per day in divided doses every 4–8 h; increase dose to 150 mg/kg per day in severe infections (do not exceed the maximum adult dose).

Widely available.

Further information

Colaizzi P A, Goodwin S D, Poynor W J, Karnes H T, Polk R E 1987 Single dose pharmacokinetics of cefuroxime and cefamandole in healthy subjects. *Clinical Pharmacology* 6: 894–899

Fraser D G 1979 Drug therapy reviews: antimicrobial spectrum, pharmacology and therapeutic use of cefamandole and cefoxitin. *American Journal of Hospital Pharmacy* 36: 1503–1508

Ridley P D 1990 Comparative evaluation of cefotaxime and cephamandole in the prevention of post-operative infective complications of abdominal surgery. *British Journal of Clinical Pharmacology* 44: 17–21

Townsend T R, Reitz B A, Bilker W B, Bartlett J G 1993 Clinical trial of cefamandole, cefazolin, and cefuroxime for antibiotic prophylaxis in cardiac operations. *Journal of Thoracic and Cardiovascular Surgery* 106: 664–670

Woods G L, Knapp C C, Washington J A 1987 Relationship between cefamandole and cefuroxime activity against oxacillin-resistant *Staphylococcus epidermidis* and oxacillin resistance phenotype. *Antimicrobial Agents and Chemotherapy* 31: 1332–1337

Group 4

Parenteral cephalosporins with wide-spectrum high potency antimicrobial activity and resistance to a wide range of β-lactamases. They exhibit exceptional potency against most enterobacteria, but *Acinetobacter*, *Citrobacter*, *Enterobacter* and *Serratia* spp. are often resistant. Staphylococci are only moderately susceptible, but streptococci and *Neisseria* spp. are highly susceptible; enterococci are resistant (Table 14.4). *Listeria monocytogenes* is generally resistant, although ceftizoxime and cefotaxime exhibit more activity than other compounds of this group.

CEFMENOXIME

A semi-synthetic cephalosporin of group 4 supplied as the hydrochloride. The *syn* stereoisomer is about 30 times more active than the *anti* isomer, of which commercial preparations contain less than 0.8%.

Table 14.4 *Activity of group 4 cephalosporins against common pathogenic bacteria: MIC (mg/l)*

	Cefmenoxime	Cefodizime	Cefotaxime	Ceftizoxime	Ceftriaxone	Latamoxef
Staph. aureus	2–4	2–8	2–4	2–4	4	8–16
Str. pyogenes	0.03	0.06–0.1	0.03–0.06	0.03	0.03	I
Str. pneumoniae*	0.06	0.03–0.25	0.1	0.1	0.25	I
Ent. faecalis	R	8–R	R	R	R	R
N. gonorrhoeae	<0.01–0.03	0.008	<0.01–0.03	<0.01–0.03	<0.01–0.06	0.03–0.1
N. meningitidis	<0.01	0.008	0.01	<0.01	<0.01	<0.01
H. influenzae	0.03	0.008	<0.01–0.03	0.03	<0.01–0.03	0.1
Esch. coli	0.06–0.1	0.1–1	0.03–0.1	0.03	0.06–0.1	0.1–0.25
Klebsiella spp.	0.03	0.1–2	0.03–0.1	0.01	0.03–0.06	0.1–0.25
Pr. mirabilis	0.03	0.008–0.03	0.03–0.06	0.01	<0.01–0.03	0.03–0.1
Pr. vulgaris	0.1	0.03–1	0.1–2	0.06	0.01–0.1	0.1–0.25
Morganella/Providencia	0.06–2	0.06–4	0.06–2	0.06–16	0.06–4	0.25–1
Enterobacter spp.	0.1	0.1–8	0.1–R	0.1	0.06–0.25	0.1–0.25
Salmonella spp.	0.25	0.1–1	0.03–0.5	0.25	0.6–0.25	0.1–0.25
Shigella spp.	0.25	0.1–1	0.1–0.25	0.25	0.25	0.25
Ser. marcescens	0.25	0.25–2	0.1–0.5	0.1	0.1–0.25	0.25
Citrobacter spp.	0.25	1–16	0.25	0.25	0.5	0.25
Ps. aeruginosa	16–32	R	8–32	32–64	16–32	4–16
B. fragilis	8–64	8–R	2–32	8–64	16–64	0.5–4

* Penicillin-resistant strains are often less susceptible.

Antimicrobial activity

It is active against common pathogenic bacteria with the exception of *Ps. aeruginosa* and *B. fragilis* (Table 14.4). Bactericidal synergy with gentamicin was demonstrated against all strains of *Ps. aeruginosa* tested. It is stable to β-lactamases of *Staph. aureus*, and most enterobacteria, but susceptible to some TEM enzymes (p. 316).

Pharmacokinetics

After i.m. doses of 0.25, 0.5 and 1 g the peak plasma concentrations are around 9, 15 and 27 mg/l, respectively, at about 40 min. A few minutes after administration of similar doses i.v., the plasma concentrations are around 64, 100 and 200 mg/l. The plasma half-life is around 1 h and independent of the route or dose. Binding to plasma proteins is 77% (reduced in disease) and the apparent volume of distribution is 9–14 l.

In patients with non-inflamed meninges receiving 30 mg/kg i.v. 6-hourly, CSF concentrations were 0.15–1.4 mg/l when the simultaneous serum level was 4–65 mg/l, giving a penetrance of 0.2–9%. In patients with meningitis receiving 2 g i.v. 8-hourly the mean peak CSF concentration occurred at about 4 h, falling from 5.75 mg/l on day 3 to 2.6 mg/l on days 10–12. There was 10-fold or more variation between patients, concentrations up to 15 mg/l being associated with moderate renal insufficiency.

Excretion
There is a degradation product with a long half-life (around 40 h), but 80–92% of the drug is recovered unchanged from the urine. Involvement of tubular secretion in urinary excretion is shown by the effect of probenecid, which increases peak plasma levels and extends the plasma half-life from 1.1 to 1.8 h. In patients with renal insufficiency, no significant relation was found between creatinine clearance and peak serum concentrations but there was a linear relationship with plasma half-life and total body clearance.

Bile. In patients receiving 0.5 g by i.v. infusion over 20–30 min pre-operatively, mean concentrations around 55 mg/l were found in gallbladder bile 1–3 h after the dose, around 10 times the simultaneous serum levels. About 10% of the dose appears in the faeces, mostly extensively degraded, possibly by the faecal flora.

Toxicity, side-effects and clinical use

Those common to group 4 cephalosporins (p. 206).

Further information

Campoli-Richards D M, Todd P A 1987 Cefmenoxime. A review of its antibacterial activity, pharmacokinetic properties and therapeutic use. *Drugs* 34: 188–221

Evers J, Borner K, Koeppe P 1993 Elimination of cefmenoxime during continuous hemofiltration. *European Journal of Clinical Pharmacology* 44 (suppl 1): S31–S32

Humbert G, Veyssier P, Fourtillan J B et al 1986 Penetration of cefmenoxime into cerebrospinal fluid of patients with bacterial meningitis. *Journal of Antimicrobial Chemotherapy* 18: 503–506

Konishi K 1986 Pharmacokinetics of cefmenoxime in patients with impaired renal function and in those undergoing haemodialysis. *Antimicrobial Agents and Chemotherapy* 30: 901–905

Paladino J A, Fell R E, Labrada L, Larouche M 1994 Pharmaco-economic analysis of cefmenoxime dual individualization in the treatment of nosocomial pneumonia. *Annals of Pharmacotherapy* 28: 384–389

Serieys C, Bergogne-Berezin E, Kafe H, Bryskier A 1986 Study of the diffusion of cefmenoxime into the bronchial secretions. *Chemotherapy* 32: 1–6

CEFODIZIME

A semi-synthetic cephalosporin of group 4.

Its antimicrobial activity is typical of the group (Table 14.4) but it is somewhat less active overall than cefotaxime against enterobacteria. *Moraxella catarrhalis* is inhibited by 0.5 mg/l. Acinetobacter is resistant. There has been particular interest in its immunomodulating properties which affect a number of functions.

In volunteers receiving 1 g i.m., the absolute bioavailability was >90%, i.m. injection producing mean peak plasma values around 55–60 mg/l at about 1.5 h with a terminal plasma elimination half-life of 3.5–3.7 h. Binding to plasma protein is high: around 88%. The apparent volume of distribution is 11–15 l. The dose response is linear between 0.5 and 2 g; there was no accumulation in normal volunteers on 2 g twice daily. Pharmacokinetic behaviour in the elderly is similar. In children receiving 25 mg/kg i.m., mean peak plasma concentrations around 55 mg/l were reached at about 1 h.

Penetration occurs into lung, sputum, serous fluids and prostate. Excretion in mainly renal with about 60% of the dose appearing in the urine over 12 h in adults and 80–90% in children. Elimination is inversely correlated with creatinine clearance.

It is well tolerated apart from some pain at the site of injection, mild gastro-intestinal upset and rash in a few patients. It has no effect on haemostasis.

It has been used to treat respiratory and urinary tract infection. It has some immunomodulating activity.

Further information

Andrassy K, Koderisch J, Trenk D, Jahnchen E, Iwand A 1987 Hemostasis in patients with normal and impaired renal function under treatment with cefodizime. *Infection* 15: 348–350

Barradell L B, Brogden R N 1992 Cefodizime: a review of its antibacterial activity, pharmacokinetic properties and therapeutic use. *Drugs* 44: 800–834

Conte J E 1994 Pharmacokinetics of cefodizime in volunteers with normal or impaired renal function. *Journal of Clinical Pharmacology* 34: 1066–1070

Fietta A, Bersani C, Bertoletti R, Grassi F M, Grassi G G 1988 In vitro and in vivo enhancement of non-specific phagocytosis by cefodizime. *Chemotherapy* 34: 430–436

Korting H C, Schafer-Korting M, Maass L, Klesel N, Mutschler E 1987 Cefodizime in serum and skin blister fluid after single intravenous and intramuscular doses in healthy volunteers. *Antimicrobial Agents and Chemotherapy* 31: 1822–1825

Labro M T 1992 Immunological evaluation of cefodizime: a unique molecule among cephalosporins. *Infection* 20 (suppl 1): S45–S47

Symposium 1990 Cefodizime: a third generation cephalosporin with immunomodulating properties. *Journal of Antimicrobial Chemotherapy* 26 (suppl C): 1–34

CEFOTAXIME

A semi-synthetic cephalosporin of group 4.

Antimicrobial activity

It exhibits potent activity against many Gram-negative species, including *Esch. coli, K. pneumoniae, Pr. mirabilis, H. influenzae* and *N. gonorrhoeae* (Table 14.4). *Brucella melitensis* and some strains of *N. asteroides* are also susceptible. Action is bactericidal at concentrations close to the MIC.

It is stable to most β-lactamases, but hydrolysed by variants of the TEM enzymes (p. 316) and by the chromosomal β-lactamase of *B. fragilis*.

Acquired resistance

Many enterobacteria resistant to other β-lactam agents are susceptible, but selection of resistant strains with derepressed chromosomal β-lactamases (p. 319) may occur.

Pharmacokinetics

Intramuscular injections of 0.5 g produce peak plasma levels around 10 mg/l. The plasma concentration 20 min after intravenous injection of 1 g is 40–80 mg/l. The plasma half-life is around 1 h. Plasma protein binding is around 40% and the apparent volume of distribution is 32–37 l.

Metabolism
It is metabolized by hepatic esterases to the desacetyl form of which significant concentrations are found in the serum. The desacetyl metabolite has about 10% of the activity of the parent against enterobacteria, less against *Staph. aureus* and *B. fragilis*, and none against *Ps. aeruginosa*. It may,

nonetheless, have some clinical importance because of its concentration in bile and accumulation in renal failure. Its half-life in normal subjects is around 1.5 h.

Distribution
Cefotaxime crosses inflamed serous membranes, producing levels in ascites fluid of 12–18 mg/kg following 12-hourly administration of 1 g i.v. In volunteers given 1 g i.v., the mean peak concentration in cantharides blister fluid was 7.2 mg/l at 1–2 h. The half-life in blister fluid was 3.5 times and that of the desacetyl metabolite 2.5 times that of the corresponding serum values.

In patients receiving 2 g 8-hourly, mean CSF concentrations in aseptic meningitis were 0.8 mg/l. Levels of 2–15 mg/kg can be found in the CSF in the presence of inflammation. In children treated for meningitis with 50 mg/kg by i.v. infusion over 30 min, the mean CSF concentration 1 h after dose 6 was 6.2 mg/l, giving a mean penetrance of 10%. For the desacetyl metabolite the corresponding values were 5.6 mg/l and 28.8% but penetrance of the metabolite was much more variable (0–103%). A single dose of 40 mg/kg injected into the ventricle produced levels at 2, 4 and 6 h of 6.4, 5.7 and 4.5 mg/l.

Sputum. Concentrations of 0.5–4.3 mg/l have been found in bronchial secretions following a dose of 1 g intramuscularly.

Excretion
Elimination is predominantly by the renal route, around 50% of the dose being recovered in the urine over the first 24 h, much as the desacetyl derivative, although other microbiologically inactive minor products are also found. Excretion is depressed by probenecid and declines in renal failure with accumulation of the metabolite. In patients with creatinine clearances in the range 3–10 ml/min, the plasma half-life rose to 2.6 h while that of the metabolite rose to 10.0 h.

Bile. Levels in bile of 40–80 mg/l have been found following multiple intravenous doses of 12 g.

Toxicity and side-effects

Minor haematological and dermatological side-effects common to group 4 cephalosporins have been described. Superinfection with *Ps. aeruginosa* and emergence of resistant *Ps. aeruginosa* in the course of treatment has occurred. Occasional cases of pseudomembranous colitis have been reported.

Clinical uses

Those of group 4 cephalosporins (p. 206). It is widely used in neutropenic patients, respiratory infection, meningitis, intra-abdominal sepsis, osteomyelitis, typhoid fever, urinary tract infection, neonatal sepsis and gonorrhoea.

Preparations and dosage

Proprietary name: Claforan.

Preparation: Injection.

Dosage: Adults, i.m., i.v., 1–2 g every 8 h depending on severity of infection, with a maximum dose of 12 g/day. Neonates, 50 mg/kg per day in 2–4 divided doses, increased to 150–200 mg/kg per day in severe infections; children, 100–150 mg/kg per day in 2–4 divided doses, increased to 200 mg/kg per day in severe infections. Widely available.

Further information

Aldridge K E 1995 Cefotaxime in the treatment of staphylococcal infections: comparison of in vitro and in vivo studies. *Diagnostic Microbiology and Infectious Disease* 22: 195–201

Beyssac E, Cardot J M, Colnel G, Sirot J, Aiache J M 1987 Pharmacokinetics of cefotaxime and its desacetyl metabolite in plasma and cerebrospinal fluid. *European Journal of Drug Metabolism and Pharmacokinetics* 12: 91–102

Davies A, Speller D C E (eds) 1990 Cefotaxime – recent clinical investigations. *Journal of Antimicrobial Chemotherapy* 26 (suppl A): 1–83

Fick R B Jr, Alexander M R, Prince R A, Kaslik J E 1987 Penetration of cefotaxime into respiration secretions. *Antimicrobial Agents and Chemotherapy* 11: 815–817

Helm K L, Halstenson C E, Comty C M, Affrime M B, Matzke G R 1985 Disposition of cefotaxime and desacetylcefotaxime during continuous ambulatory peritoneal dialysis. *Antimicrobial Agents and Chemotherapy* 30: 15–19

Ings R M, Reeves D S, White L O, Bax R P, Bywater M J, Holt H A 1985 The human pharmacokinetics of cefotaxime and its metabolites and the role of renal tubular secretion on their elimination. *Journal of Pharmacokinetics and Biopharmaceutics* 13: 121–142

Jacobs R F, Darville T, Parks J A, Enderlin G 1992 Safety profile and efficacy of cefotaxime for the treatment of hospitalized children. *Clinical Infectious Diseases* 14: 56–65

Nau R, Prange H W, Muth P et al 1993 Passage of cefotaxime and ceftriaxone into cerebrospinal fluid of patients with uninflamed meninges. *Antimicrobial Agents and Chemotherapy* 37: 1518–1524

Odio C M 1995 Cefotaxime for treatment of neonatal sepsis and meningitis. *Diagnostic Microbiology and Infectious Disease* 22: 111–117

Prevot M H, Andremont A, Sancho-Garnier H, Tancrede C 1986 Epidemiology of intestinal colonization by members of the family *Enterobacteriaceae* resistant to cefotaxime in a hematology–oncology unit. *Antimicrobial Agents and Chemotherapy* 30: 945–947

Raymond J, Bingen E, Doit C et al 1995 Failure of cefotaxime treatment in a patient with penicillin-resistant pneumococcal meningitis and confirmation of nosocomial spread by random amplified polymorphic DNA analysis. *Clinical Infectious Diseases* 21: 234–235

Todd P A, Brogden R N 1990 Cefotaxime: an update of its pharmacology and therapeutic use. *Drugs* 40: 608–651

CEFTIZOXIME

A semi-synthetic cephalosporin of group 4 supplied as the sodium salt. It has many similarities to cefotaxime, but is not metabolized.

Antimicrobial activity

Its activity against common pathogenic bacteria is shown in Table 14.4. It is active against a wide range of enterobacteria, including most cephazolin-resistant strains, except *Enterobacter*, *Citrobacter* and *Ps. aeruginosa*. Activity against *B. fragilis* is inoculum dependent due to its susceptibility to the chromosomal β-lactamase. The MIC_{50} for *M. avium/M. intracellulare* is 4–8 mg/l and the MIC_{90} for *Br. melitensis* is 1 mg/l.

Pharmacokinetics

In volunteers, i.m. injection of 0.5 g produced peak plasma levels around 14 mg/l. The end-infusion plasma concentration after i.v. infusion of 1.0 g over 30 min is 85–90 mg/l. It is 30% bound to plasma protein and is not significantly metabolized. The plasma half-life is 1.3–1.9 h and the apparent volume of distribution is 23–27 l.

Distribution

Its penetration into serous fluid and the CSF in meningitis is generally good, mean penetrance into peritoneal fluid being around 0.6. In patients receiving 200 mg/kg daily the mean CSF concentration was 8.5 mg/l. In children receiving 200–250 mg/kg daily as four daily doses for 14–21 days, mean CSF concentrations 2 h after a dose were 6.4 mg/l on day 2 and 3.6 mg/l on day 14. Mean subdural fluid concentrations were 12.6–25.2 mg/l. In children without meningitis penetration was much less and much more variable.

Excretion

It is excreted in the urine from which 70–90% of the dose is recovered in the first 24 h after the dose and virtually 100% after 48 h. Excretion is principally by glomerular filtration, but an element of tubular secretion is shown by the effect of probenecid, a 1 g oral dose of which increases the plasma half-life and AUC by approximately 50%.

In patients receiving 1 g i.v. over 30 min, the plasma elimination half-life rose to 35 h when the corrected creatinine clearance was <10 ml/min. After 4 h haemodialysis, the plasma concentration fell by about 50% but it was still above 10 mg/l 48 h later. In patients on CAPD who received 3 g i.v. over 12 min, peritoneal clearance contributed modestly to clearance reducing the plasma elimination half-life to 2.8 h.

Toxicity and side-effects

Reported adverse reactions are few, reversible and typical of those of agents of its class. Mention has been made of increased values in liver function tests including alkaline phosphatase, eosinophilia and thrombocytosis, mild dizziness and moderate headache.

Clinical use

Those of group 4 cephalosporins (p. 206). It has had wide use in the treatment of infections with otherwise resistant organisms, particularly in immunocompromised patients. Infections of the lower respiratory and urinary tracts and soft tissue, and intra-abdominal sepsis have all been successfully treated. Reference is made to its use in osteomyelitis and meningitis (p. 745).

Preparations and dosage

Proprietary name: Cefizox.

Preparation: Injection.

Dosage: Adult, i.m., i.v., 1–2 g every 8–12 h, increased in severe infections up to 8 g/day in 3 divided doses. Children >3 months, 30–60 mg/kg per day in 2–4 divided doses, increased in severe infections to 100–150 mg/kg per day.

Widely available.

Further information

Diez M, Ruiz B, Morales S, Morales S, Davila D 1989 Evaluation of ceftizoxime in the treatment of postoperative peritoneal infections. *Current Therapeutic Research – Clinical and Experimental* 45: 368–373

Haas D W, Stratton C W, Griffin J P, Weeks L, Alls S C 1995 Diminished activity of ceftizoxime in comparison to cefotaxime and ceftriaxone against *Streptococcus pneumoniae*. *Clinical Infectious Diseases* 20: 671–676

Richards D M, Heel R C 1985 Ceftizoxime. A review of its antibacterial activity, pharmacokinetic properties and therapeutic use. *Drugs* 29: 281–329

Vallee F, LeBel M 1991 Comparative study of pharmacokinetics and serum bactericidal activity of ceftizoxime and cefotaxime. *Antimicrobial Agents and Chemotherapy* 35: 2057–2064

Yangco B G, Baird I, Lorber B et al 1987 Comparative efficacy and safety of ceftizoxime, cefotaxime and latamoxef in the treatment of bacterial pneumonia in high risk patients. *Journal of Antimicrobial Chemotherapy* 19: 239–248

CEFTRIAXONE

A semi-synthetic cephalosporin of group 4 supplied as the disodium salt. Its main feature is the long serum elimination half-life.

Antimicrobial activity

It exhibits highly potent activity against a wide range of Gram-positive and Gram-negative organisms (Table 14.4) including most β-lactamase-producing strains. Enterococci are resistant. All enterobacteria are inhibited by about 1 mg/l. It has modest activity against *Ps. aeruginosa*. Group B streptococci are inhibited by 0.05–1 mg/l. The MIC_{90} for *Br. melitensis* is 0.5–1 and that for *Pasteurella multocida* is <0.01–0.25. Activity against *Bacteroides* spp., including *B. fragilis*, is of doubtful clinical utility.

It is bactericidal for most susceptible strains at or close to the MIC. It is stable to most plasmid-encoded β-lactamases but hydrolysed by some chromosomal enzymes, including those of *Enterobacter* and *B. fragilis*.

Acquired resistance

Derepression of chromosomal β-lactamase production (p. 319) can result in the appearance of resistance in some species in vitro and has been observed in patients.

Pharmacokinetics

In volunteers, i.m. injection of 0.5 g produced peak plasma levels of 40–85 mg/l. The use of 1% lidocaine in the place of water as diluent greatly reduced the intensity and frequency of local pain, but did not affect the plasma peak or half-life. In cancer patients receiving the same dose, a mean plasma peak around 33 mg/l was found at 2.0 h with a half-life of 10.9 h. In volunteers given i.v. injections over 5 min of 1 g 12-hourly or 2 g once-daily, the mean end-infusion concentrations after single and multiple doses were around 255 and 375 mg/l and 410 and 445 mg/l, respectively. End-infusion concentrations in patients receiving 1 g i.v. over 20–30 min 12-hourly for 5 days for various infections were 103 mg/l on day 1 and 119 mg/l on day 4 and, in cancer patients given 0.5 or 1 g i.v. over 5 min, 83 and 130 mg/l, respectively. In similar patients given 1 g 8-hourly or 2 g 12-hourly end-infusion values on days 3–4 were 154 and 262 mg/l with plasma half-lives of 5.6 and 6.3 h, respectively. The apparent volume of distribution is 6–13 l and is increased in children.

It is very highly protein bound, the free fraction in plasma being 3.3–4.4% up to 150 mg/ml, and it has a very long plasma half-life of 5.5–11 h. Effects on protein binding at higher dosage do not appear to affect pharmacokinetics within the normal therapeutic range, the dose–response curve being essentially linear at least up to 1.5 g, although in some studies there is an indication that the elimination half-life diminishes with dose, the half-life declining on 0.5 and 2 g doses from 6.5 to 5.9 h. There is an apparently unique effect on probenecid in displacing ceftriaxone from its protein sites and raising the free plasma fraction up to 75%.

In children receiving 50 mg/kg i.v. over 10–15 min, mean end-infusion concentrations were 207 mg/l; 8-hourly doses following a loading dose of 75 mg/kg produced values of 230 after the first dose and 263 after the last. In the newborn, 50 mg/kg i.v. over 15 min produced end-infusion concentrations of 136–173 mg/kg with a half-life of 5.2–8.4 h. In older children treated for various infections, the plasma half-life (4–6.3 h) appears to be shorter than that in adults.

Distribution

It penetrates well into normal body fluids and natural and experimental exudates. In children treated for meningitis with 50 or 75 mg/kg i.v. over 10–15 min, mean peak CSF concentrations have ranged from 3.2 to 10.4 mg/l, with lower values later in the disease. In patients receiving 2 g some hours before surgery, concentrations in cerebral tissue reached 0.3–12 mg/l. In patients with pleural effusions of variable aetiology given 1 g i.v. bolus, concentrations of 7–8.7 mg/l were found at 4–6 h. In patients with exacerbations of rheumatoid arthritis receiving the same dose, joint fluid contained concentrations close to those in the serum, but with wide individual variation. Tissue fluid to serum ratios have varied from around 0.05 in bone and muscle to 0.39 in cantharides blister fluid. The apparent volume of distribution is increased in patients with cirrhosis where the drug rapidly enters the ascitic fluid, but its elimination kinetics are unaffected.

It rapidly crosses the placenta, maternal doses of 2 g i.v. over 2–5 min producing mean concentrations in cord blood of 19.5 mg/l, a mean cord:maternal serum ratio of 0.18; and in amniotic fluid 3.8 mg/l a fluid:maternal serum ratio of 0.04. The plasma elimination half-life appears to be somewhat shortened in pregnancy (5–6 h).

Excretion

Only 41–59% appears in the urine over the first 48 h, almost entirely by glomerular filtration, since there is only a small effect of probenecid on the excretion of the drug. There is no increased renal clearance at high plasma concentrations, so that tubular reabsorption is not saturable in the way that it is, for example, with cephaloridine. The half-life is not linearly correlated with creatinine clearance in renal failure and, in keeping with the low free plasma fraction, it is not significantly removed by haemodialysis. The volume of distribution is not affected by renal failure. Some appears in the breast milk, the milk:serum ratio being about 0.03–0.04, secretion persisting over a long period with a half-life of 12–17 h.

Bile. Biliary excretion is very high, 10–20% of the drug appearing in the bile in unchanged form, with concentrations up to 130 mg/g in biopsied liver tissue from patients receiving 1 g i.v. over 30 min. Insoluble calcium may precipitate in the bile leading to pseudolithiasis.

Toxicity and side-effects

It is generally well tolerated, reactions being those noted with class 4 cephalosporins. Mention has been made of thrombocytopenia, thrombocytosis, leucopenia, eosinophilia abdominal pain, phlebitis, rash, fever, Antabuse-like effect and increased values in liver function tests. Diarrhoea has been commonly noted and pronounced suppression of the aerobic and anaerobic faecal flora has been associated with the appearance of resistant bacteria and yeasts.

Biliary pseudolithiasis due to concretions of insoluble calcium salt has been described in adults but principally in children. The precipitates can be detected in a high proportion of patients by ultrasonography and can occasionally cause pain, but resolve on cessation of treatment. The drug is better avoided in patients with pre-existing biliary disease, but the principal hazard appears to be misdiagnosis of gallbladder disease and unnecessary surgery.

Clinical uses

Those of group 4 cephalosporins (p. 206). A single 250 mg dose has been reported to be effective in chancroid and in uncomplicated gonorrhoea (p. 819) and in genital ulceration due to *Haemophilus ducreyi* (p. 824). It has been commended for the treatment of enteric fever (p. 711) but found to be disappointing in shigellosis (p. 713). It compares favourably with established treatment for acute bacterial meningitis (p. 745). Reference is made to its use in osteomyelitis, meningococcal carriage, impetigo and spirochaetoses.

Preparations and dosage

Proprietary name: Rocephin.

Preparation: Injection.

Dosage: Adults, i.m., i.v., 1 g/day as a single dose, 2–4 g/day as a single dose in severe infections. Children over 6 weeks, 20–50 mg/kg per day as a single dose; in severe infections, 80 mg/kg per day as a single dose. Doses over 50 mg/kg must be given as an i.v. infusion.

Widely available.

Further information

Albin H, Rignaud M, Demotes-Mainard F, Vincon G, Couzineau M, Wone C 1986 Pharmacokinetics of intravenous and intraperitoneal ceftriaxone in chronic ambulatory peritoneal dialysis. *European Journal of Clinical Pharmacology* 31: 479–483

Arvidsson A, Leijd B, Nord C E, Angelin B 1988 Interindividual variability in biliary excretion of ceftriaxone: effects on biliary lipid metabolism and on intestinal microflora. *European Journal of Clinical Investigation* 18: 261–266

Brogden R N, Ward A 1988 Ceftriaxone: a reappraisal of its antibacterial activity and pharmacokinetic properties, and an update on its therapeutic use with particular reference to once-daily administration. *Drugs* 35: 604–645

Cometta A, Gallot-Lavallee-Villars S, Iten A et al 1990 Incidence of gallbladder lithiasis after ceftriaxone treatment. *Journal of Antimicrobial Chemotherapy* 25: 689–695

Dansey R D, Jacka P J, Strachan S A, Hay M 1992 Comparison of cefotaxime with ceftriaxone given intramuscularly 12-hourly for community-acquired pneumonia. *Diagnostic Microbiology and Infectious Disease* 15: 81–84

Fraschini F, Braga P C, Scarpazza G et al 1986 Human pharmacokinetics and distribution in various tissues of ceftriaxone. *Chemotherapy* 32: 192–199

Hary L, Andrejak M, Lelu S, Orfila J, Capron J P 1989 The pharmacokinetics of ceftriaxone and cefotaxime in cirrhotic patients with ascites. *European Journal of Clinical Pharmacology* 36: 613–616

Holazo A A, Patel I H, Weinfeld R E, Konikoff J J, Parsonnet M 1986 Ceftriaxone pharmacokinetics following multiple intramuscular dosing. *European Journal of Clinical Pharmacology* 30: 109–112

Lopez A J, O'Keefe P, Morrissey M, Pickleman J 1991 Ceftriaxone-induced cholelithiasis. *Annals of Internal Medicine* 115: 712–714

Lucht F, Dorche G, Aubert G, Boissier C, Bertrand A M, Brunon J 1990 The penetration of ceftriaxone into human brain tissue. *Journal of Antimicrobial Chemotherapy* 26: 81–86

Nahata M C, Durrell D E, Barnes W J 1986 Ceftriaxone kinetics and cerebrospinal fluid penetration in infants and children with meningitis. *Chemotherapy* 32: 89–94

Paull A, Morgan J R 1986 Emergence of ceftriaxone-resistant strains of *Pseudomonas aeruginosa* in cystic fibrosis patients. *Journal of Antimicrobial Chemotherapy* 18: 635–639

Schaad V B, Tshappeler H, Lentze M J 1986 Transient formation of precipitations in the gallbladder associated with ceftriaxone therapy. *Pediatric Infectious Diseases* 5: 708–710

Spector R 1987 Ceftriaxone transport through the blood-brain barrier. *Journal of Infectious Diseases* 156: 209–211

Stoekel K, Trueb V, DuBach U C, McNamara P J 1988 Effect of probenecid on the elimination and protein binding of ceftriaxone. *European Journal of Clinical Pharmacology* 34: 151–156

Stratton C W, Anthony L B, Johnston P E 1988 A review of ceftriaxone: a long-acting cephalosporin. *American Journal of Medical Science* 296: 221–222

Yuk J H, Nightingale C H, Quintiliani R 1989 Clinical pharmacokinetics of ceftriaxone. *Clinical Pharmacokinetics* 17: 223–235

Zimmerman A E, Katona B G, Jodhka J S, Williams R B 1993 Ceftriaxone-induced acute pancreatitis. *Annals of Pharmacotherapy* 27: 36–37

LATAMOXEF
Moxalactam

A semi-synthetic 7-methoxyoxacephem, supplied as the disodium salt, classed with group 4 cephalosporins. There are two epimeric forms, (*R*) and (*S*), or which (*R*) has about twice the activity but is slightly less stable at 37°C in serum in which the mixture has a half-life in vitro of about 8 h.

Antimicrobial activity

Its activity against common pathogenic bacteria is shown in Table 14.4. *Staph. aureus* is moderately susceptible. It exhibits potent activity against enterobacteria; many otherwise multiply-resistant strains are susceptible. Most *H. influenzae*, including β-lactamase-producing strains, are inhibited by <0.1 mg/l. *Ps. aeruginosa* is moderately susceptible, including carbenicillin-resistant and multiply-resistant strains, although the MIC for such strains is often increased. Acinetobacter is moderately resistant. The MIC_{90} for *Br. melitensis* is 16 mg/l. Among *Bacteroides* spp., *B. fragilis* and *B. vulgatus* (MIC 0.25 mg/l) are more susceptible than *B. thetaiotaomicron* (MIC 2 mg/l) and *B. ovatus* (MIC 4–8 mg/l).

There is a large inoculum effect against some species, and bactericidal activity exhibited close to the MIC proceeds slowly. It is resistant to hydrolysis by a wide range of β-lactamases including those of *Staph. aureus*, various enterobacteria, *Ps. aeruginosa* and *B. fragilis*. It is a potent suicide inhibitor (p. 64) of cephalosporinases of *Ent. cloacae* and *Ps. aeruginosa* and an effective competitive inhibitor of that of *B. fragilis*.

Bactericidal synergy has been demonstrated with gentamicin against *Staph. aureus* and gentamicin-susceptible and some gentamicin-resistant strains of *Ps. aeruginosa*.

Acquired resistance

Resistance, predominantly in *Enterobacter* spp., *Ps. aeruginosa* and *Ser. marcescens* due to induction of chromosomal enzymes (p. 319), has been found in vitro and in some patients. Resistance also arises in some organisms through reduced entry into the cell due to modification of outer membrane proteins and to change in PBPs (p. 257). Resistant strains of bacteroides other than *B. fragilis* have been commonly found in some series and have emerged in occasional patients treated for anaerobic infections.

Pharmacokinetics

Intramuscular injection of 0.5 g produces mean peak plasma levels of 12–22 mg/l at about 1.2 h. The plasma elimination half-life is 2.5–2.7 h. After 1 g i.m. levels around 50 mg/l have been found at 0.5–1 h. End-infusion plasma concentrations after i.v. administration of 1.0 g over 5–20 min were around 70 mg/l and over 30 min were 60 mg/l. Following bolus administration of 0.5 or 1 g, the concentration 15 min after the dose was around 40 mg/l and 70–100 mg/l, respectively. Kinetics were linear and independent of dose over the range 0.25–1 g. No active metabolites have been detected. Binding to plasma protein is 52%. The plasma half-life by the i.v. route has generally been found to lie between 1.9 and 2.9 h. Interaction with tobramycin caused its rate of elimination to fall in normal, but not in uraemic subjects.

It is well absorbed after instillation into the peritoneal cavity in patients on CAPD. In patients receiving a loading dose of 200 mg/2 l dialysate followed by 60 mg/2 l in subse-

quent exchanges, mean serum concentrations were 2.5 mg/l after the first dialysis, rising to 10.3 mg/l. There were no adverse effects. When 1 g was instilled into the peritoneum, 60% of the dose was absorbed during the dwell time of 1 h, giving mean peak plasma concentrations around 25 mg/l with a half-life around 13 h.

In children given 50 mg/kg i.v. 8-hourly, the mean plasma concentration 5 min after the dose was around 250 mg/l with a mean half-life of 2.4 h. There was no significant accumulation. Children under 1 year had lower mean plasma levels at 30 min, larger volumes of distribution and longer half-lives. The epimers behaved similarly. In volunteers over 60 years of age, mean plasma half-lives were 2.9 h after i.v. and 3.5 h after i.m. administration.

Distribution

The apparent volume of distribution is 9–13 l. There is reasonably good penetration into serous fluids, the concentration in ascitic fluid reaching 75% and in pleural fluid 50% of the concentration simultaneously present in the serum. After 1 g i.v., the concentration in pleural fluid 4–6 h after the dose, was 9–35 mg/l with a half-life 2–5 times that of the serum. In volunteers given 1 g i.v., mean peak concentrations in cantharides blister fluid around 16 mg/l were found at 3–4 h. Levels of 5–35 mg/l or 10–20% of the corresponding plasma levels have been obtained in inflamed meninges. In adults with bacterial meningitis receiving 2 i.v. over 30–60 min 4–8 hourly, mean concentrations around 14 mg/l were found in lumbar CSF and 12 mg/l in ventricular CSF. Sputum levels are of the order of 2 mg/l following 1 g of the drug intravenously.

Tissues. In patients given 10 mg/kg by i.v. bolus preoperatively, concentrations in cancellous bone were around 2.6 mg/g, a bone:serum ratio of 0.07. In patients similarly receiving 1 g, before amputation for limb ischaemia, the mean concentration in subcutaneous fat was 4.3 mg/g and in muscle 4.8 mg/g, mean tissue:serum ratios of 0.14 and 0.15. In patients receiving two doses of 500 mg 2 h preoperatively and at the time of surgery, mean concentrations in enucleated or transurethrally resected prostate tissue were 4.0 and 5.2 mg/l with tissue:serum ratios of 0.24 and 0.31, respectively.

Excretion

Renal elimination accounts for 90% of the clearance, but significant concentrations are found in the faeces, presumably via biliary excretion. There is little tubular excretion since the effect of probenecid is negligible. Around 75% is excreted in the urine in the first 24 h after i.m. administration and 65–85% after i.v. administration. The main reason for the modest increase in plasma half-life in patients aged 60 years or more is diminished renal function, but non-renal elimination is highly variable. Excretion is depressed in renal failure, the elimination half-life rising with falling creatinine clearance to around 50 h. Binding to plasma protein is reduced to 35% in uraemic serum. Haemodialysis removes 48–51% of the drug in 4 h, a mean half-life of 18 h between dialyses falling to 2.7 h on dialysis. Peritoneal dialysis has little or no effect.

Bile. Concentrations in T-tube bile in excess of 170 mg/l 2 h after a 2 g i.v. dose and 30 mg/l 30 min after a 2 g i.m. dose have been found. In patients given 1 g i.m. at the time of premedication, mean concentrations around 2 h were 22.6 mg/l in gallbladder bile, 63.5 mg/l in common duct bile and 14.6 mg/g in gallbladder wall, but there was marked interpatient variation with bile:serum ratios of 0.02–1.2. There is some evidence of enterohepatic recirculation and mean concentrations in faeces of patients receiving three doses of 2 g at 8-hourly intervals were around 9 mg/g although in some, none could be detected.

Toxicity and side-effects

It is generally well tolerated. Overgrowth of resistant cocci, pseudomonas, yeasts and the occasional appearance of *Cl. difficile* may occur. Failure of therapy due to superinfection with *Ent. faecalis* or other resistant species, or the emergence of resistant variants particularly in patients infected with *Ps. aeruginosa* or *Ser. marcescens* has been observed.

Mention has been made of reversible neutropenia, eosinophilia and increased values in liver function tests and prothrombin time. Increased bleeding tendency associated with the methyltetrazole side-chain appears to be uncommon. In most volunteers given the large dose of 4 g 12-hourly, template bleeding times at least doubled after 7 doses. ADP-induced primary platelet aggregation was approximately halved with an increasing tendency to disaggregation. The agent is contraindicated in patients on anticoagulant therapy.

Clinical uses

These are essentially those of group 4 cephalosporins (p. 206). It was formerly used for the treatment of meningitis due to susceptible Gram-negative rods including *Bacteroides*, although some have noted the response to be slow. It is generally less successful in the treatment of infections due to Gram-positive organisms which may cause serious superinfection during treatment.

Preparations and dosage
Preparation: Injection.
Dosage: Adults, i.m., i.v., 0.5–4 g/day in 2 divided doses.
Available in continental Europe, not available in the UK.

Further information

Andritz M H, Smith R P, Baltch A L et al 1984 Pharmacokinetics of moxalactam in elderly subjects. *Antimicrobial Agents and Chemotherapy* 25: 33–36

Benno Y, Shiragami N, Uchida K, Yoshida T, Mitsuoka T 1986 Effect of moxalactam on human faecal microflora. *Antimicrobial Agents and Chemotherapy* 29: 175–178

Carmine A A, Brogden R N, Heel R C, Romankiewicz J A, Speight T M, Avery G S 1983 Moxalactam (latamoxef). A review of its antibacterial activity, pharmacokinetic properties and therapeutic use. *Drugs* 26: 279–333

Deery H G, Jones P G, Kauffman C A et al 1984 Effect of therapy with latamoxef (moxalactam) on carriage of *Clostridium difficile*. *Journal of Antimicrobial Chemotherapy* 13: 521–524

Drusand G L, Standiford H C, Fitzpatrick B et al 1984 Comparison of the pharmacokinetics of ceftazidime and moxalactam and their microbiological correlates in volunteers. *Antimicrobial Agents and Chemotherapy* 26: 388–393

Morris D L, Frabricius P J, Ambrose N S, Scammell B, Burdon D W, Keighley M R 1984 A high incidence of bleeding is observed in a trial to determine whether addition of metronidazole is needed with latamoxef for prophylaxis in colonic surgery. *Journal of Hospital Infection* 5: 398–408

Oturai P S, Hollander N H, Hansen O P et al 1993 Ceftriaxone versus latamoxef in febrile neutropenic patients: empirical monotherapy in patients with solid tumours. *European Journal of Cancer Part A: General Topics* 29: 1274–1279

Uchida K, Kakushi H, Shike T 1987 Effect of latamoxef (moxalactam) and its related compounds on platelet aggregation in vitro-structure activity relationships. *Thrombosis Research* 47: 215–222

Group 5

Oral cephalosporins with wide-spectrum high potency antimicrobial activity, although the susceptibility of *Str. pneumoniae* varies considerably (Table 14.5). They are resistant to a wide range of β-lactamases.

Table 14.5 *Activity of group 5 cephalosporins against common pathogenic bacteria: MIC (mg/l)*

	Cefdinir	Cefetamet	Cefixime	Cefpodoxime	Cefprozil	Ceftibuten
Staph. aureus	0.002–1	16–R	4–16	0.5	0.25–2	32
Str. pyogenes	<0.06–0.25	0.015–0.25	0.01–0.25	0.06	0.06–0.25	8–16
Str. pneumoniae	0.03–0.5	0.06–0.25	0.01–0.25	0.06	0.06–0.25	0.5–32
Ent. faecalis	2–R	R	R	R	8	R
N. gonorrhoeae	0.002–0.06	<0.03–0.25	0.01–0.1	<0.06	0.004–0.06	0.008–0.06
H. influenzae	0.25–1	0.06–0.25	0.06–0.25	0.06–0.12	0.004–0.06	0.01–1
Esch. coli	0.008–1	0.125–8	0.25	0.25	1–4	0.01–16
Klebsiella spp.	0.008–0.5	0.06–1	0.01–1	0.12	1–32	0.12
Pr. mirabilis	0.12–0.25	0.12–8	0.1–1	0.06	1–4	0.03
Enterobacter spp.	0.5–4	0.25–R	2–8	0.06–R	2–R	0.06–R
Salmonella spp.	0.12–2	0.5–16	0.02–0.4		1–R	0.01–0.1
Shigella spp.	0.12–0.5	0.25–2	0.1–1		1–64	0.25–4
Citrobacter spp.	0.25–R	1–R	1–R	0.01–R	0.5–8	0.01–R
Ps. aeruginosa	R	R	2–32	R	R	R
B. fragilis	R	R	R	R	R	R

CEFDINIR

An oral cephalosporin of group 5.

It is very active against staphylococci, streptococci (but not enterococci), neisseriae, *H. influenzae* and most enterobacteria. *Ps. aeruginosa* and *B. fragilis* are resistant (Table 14.5). It is poorly hydrolysed by staphylococcal or the common enterobacterial β-lactamases.

After oral administration of 200 or 400 mg to healthy volunteers, plasma concentrations of 1 and 2.15 mg/l, respectively, were achieved after about 3 h. A total of 12–20% of the dose was excreted into urine within 12 h, the renal elimination declining with increasing dose. Absorption is reduced after a fatty meal. The elimination half-life is about 1.5 h and around 60% of the drug in plasma is protein bound. Maximum concentrations in suction-induced blister fluid were achieved later than in plasma, but were more prolonged. Concentrations equal to, or higher than corresponding plasma levels were present in blister fluid 6–12 h after administration of an oral dose.

It appears to be well tolerated, although some volunteers receiving the drug experienced diarrhoea. Its uses are similar to those of cefixime and other oral cephalosporins with improved β-lactamase stability.

Further information

Cohen M A, Joannides E T, Roland G E et al 1994 In vitro evaluation of cefdinir (FK482), a new oral cephalosporin with enhanced antistaphylococcal activity and beta-lactamase stability. *Diagnostic Microbiology and Infectious Disease* 18: 31–39

Gerlach E H, Jones R N, Allen S D et al 1992 Cefdinir (FK482), an orally administered cephalosporin in vitro activity comparison against recent clinical isolates from five medical centers and determination of MIC quality control guidelines. *Diagnostic Microbiology and Infectious Disease* 15: 537–543

Labia R, Morand A Interaction of cefdinir with beta-lactamases. *Drugs under Experimental and Clinical Research* 20: 43–48

Marchese A, Saverino D, Debbia E A, Pesce A, Schito G C 1995 Antistaphylococcal activity of cefdinir, a new oral third-generation cephalosporin, alone and in combination with other antibiotics, at supra- and sub-MIC levels. *Journal of Antimicrobial Chemotherapy* 35: 53–66

Payne D J, Amyes S G B 1993 Stability of cefdinir (CI-983, FK482) to extended-spectrum plasmid-mediated β-lactamases. *Journal of Medical Microbiology* 38: 114–117

Richer M, Allard S, Manseau L, Vallee F, Pak R, LeBel M 1995 Suction-induced blister fluid penetration of cefdinir in healthy volunteers following ascending oral doses. *Antimicrobial Agents and Chemotherapy* 39: 1082–1086

Scriver S R, Willey B M, Low D E, Simor A E 1992 Comparative in vitro activity of cefdinir (CI-983; FK-482) against staphylococci, Gram-negative bacilli and respiratory tract pathogens. *European Journal of Clinical Microbiology and Infectious Diseases* 11: 646–652

Wise R, Andrews J M, Thornber D 1991 The in-vitro activity of cefdinir (FK482), a new oral cephalosporin. *Journal of Antimicrobial Chemotherapy* 28: 239–248

CEFETAMET

A semi-synthetic cephalosporin of group 5 supplied as the prodrug, cefetamet pivoxyl.

It is less active than cefaclor and cefadroxil against *Staph. aureus*, but as active against streptococci and more active against enterobacteria (Table 14.5). It is highly active against *H. influenzae* and *N. gonorrhoeae*, including β-lactamase-producing strains (MIC$_{90}$ 0.03 mg/l). *L. monocytogenes*, *Cl. difficile*, *Stenotrophomonas maltophilia* and *Burkholderia cepacia* are all resistant. There is a marked inoculum effect against enterobacteria elaborating chromosomal β-lactamase, but it is resistant to hydrolysis by common plasmid-mediated enzymes. It is active against cefaclor-resistant *Pr. vulgaris*, *Ser. marcescens* and *Ps. aeruginosa* and against enterobacteria exhibiting high production of chromosomally determined cephalosporinase. In each case, activity is related to enhanced β-lactamase stability.

The pivaloyl ester is orally absorbed and rapidly cleaved by esterases in the gut wall and hepatic circulation to liberate cefetamet to which it owes its activity. The absolute bioavailability is about 50%. After doses of 0.5–2 g, 10 min after a standard breakfast, the rate and extent of absorption declined with increase of dose, but the delay in peak (around 4–5 h) and the reduction in AUC (about 10%) were not materially different from the degree of intragroup variation. The plasma peak is delayed by food, but unaffected by fluid intake. The effect of food does not appear to be related to gastric pH: there is no effect of antacids or ranitidine. Binding to plasma protein is about 20%. The volume of distribution approximates to the extracellular water.

It is excreted by the renal route, predominantly in the glomerular filtrate, and elimination is linearly related to creatinine clearance. The normal elimination half-life is 2–2.5 h, but may reach 30 h in anuric subjects. The plasma peak concentration is elevated and delayed, but bioavailability and distribution at steady state are not altered. Cirrhosis has no effect on the bioavailability and renal and non-renal clearance are not altered.

Its safety profile is similar to that of other oral cephalosporins. It uses are similar to those of cefixime and other oral cephalosporins that exhibit improved β-lactamase stability.

Further information

Angehrn P, Hohl P, Then R L 1989 In vitro antibacterial properties of cefetamet and in vivo activity of its orally absorbable ester derivative, cefetamet pivoxil. *European Journal of Clinical Microbiology and Infectious Diseases* 8: 536–543

Bernstein-Hahn L, Valdes E, Gehanno P et al 1989 Clinical experience with 1000 patients treated with cefetamet pivoxil. *Current Medical Research and Opinion* 11: 442–452

Blouin R, Stoekel K 1993 Cefetamet pivoxil clinical pharmacokinetics. *Clinical Pharmacokinetics* 25: 172–188

Bryson H M, Brogden R N 1993 Cefetamet pivoxil. *Drugs* 45: 589–621

Hayton W L, Kneer J, Blouin R A, Stoeckel K 1990 Pharmacokinetics of intravenous cefetamet and oral cefetamet pivoxil in patients with hepatic cirrhosis. *Antimicrobial Agents and Chemotherapy* 34: 1318–1322

Hohl P, von Graevenitz A, Zollinger-Iten J 1988 Cefetamet pivoxil: bacteriostatic and bactericidal activity of the free acid against 355 Gram-negative rods. *Infection* 16: 194–198

Kneer J 1989 Pharmacokinetics of intravenous cefetamet and oral cefetamet pivoxil in patients with renal insufficiency. *Antimicrobial Agents and Chemotherapy* 33: 1952–1957

Neu H C, Chin N Y, Labthavikul P 1986 In vitro activity and β-lactamase stability of two oral cephalosporins, ceftetrame (Ro 19-5247) and cefetamet (Ro 15-8074). *Antimicrobial Agents and Chemotherapy* 30: 423–428

Stoekel K, Tam Y K, Kneer J 1989 Pharmacokinetics of oral cefetamet pivoxil (Ro 15-8075) and intravenous cefetamet (Ro 15-8074) in humans: a review. *Current Medical Research and Opinion* 11: 432–441

Tam Y K, Kneer J, Dubach U C, Stoeckel K 1989 Pharmacokinetics of cefetamet pivoxil (Ro 15-8075) with ascending oral doses in normal healthy volunteers. *Antimicrobial Agents and Chemotherapy* 33: 957–959

Tam Y K, Kneer J, Dubach U C, Stoeckel K 1990 Effects of timing and food and fluid volume on cefetamet pivoxil absorption in healthy normal volunteers. *Antimicrobial Agents and Chemotherapy* 34: 1556–1559

CEFIXIME

A semi-synthetic cephalosporin of group 5.

It is highly active against streptococci (but not enterococci), less so against *Staph. aureus*. It is active against *N. gonorrhoeae*, *M. catarrhalis* and *H. influenzae*, including β-lactamase-producing strains, and against a wide range of enterobacteria, including most strains of *Citrobacter*, *Enterobacter* and *Serratia* spp. and many ampicillin- and cephalexin-resistant strains. Its action is bactericidal at concentrations close to the MIC. It is not active against *Acinetobacter* spp., *Ps. aeruginosa* or *B. fragilis*. Its activity against common pathogenic bacteria is shown in Table 14.5. It is resistant to hydrolysis by common β-lactamases.

After an oral dose of 400 mg, mean peak plasma levels around 4–5.5 mg/l are achieved at about 4 h. Absorption is not materially affected by aluminium magnesium hydroxide. About 60% is bound to plasma protein. Penetration into cantharides blister fluid was very slow but exceeded the plasma level. The bioavailability of the drug is 40–50% and the elimination half-life is 3–4 h. Less than 20% of an oral dose is recovered from the urine over 24 h, falling to less than 5% in patients with severe renal impairment, in whom the plasma concentrations is increased.

It is well tolerated, with some reports of transient diarrhoea or hepatic enzyme disturbance, which is dose related.

Clinical use

Comparative clinical trials have shown equal efficacy to co-trimoxazole and amoxycillin in uncomplicated cystitis, and similar efficacy to cefaclor and amoxycillin in otitis media and lower respiratory tract infections.

Preparations and dosage

Proprietary name: Suprax.

Preparation: Tablets, suspension.

Dosage: Adults, oral, 200–400 mg/day as a single dose or in 2 divided doses. Children, 8 mg/kg per day as a single dose or in 2 divided doses.

Available in the UK.

Further information

Bialer M, Wu W H, Faulkner R D, Silber B M, Yacobi A 1988 In vitro protein binding interaction studies involving cefixime. *Biopharmaceutics and Drug Disposition* 9: 315–320

Brogden R N, Campoli-Richards D M 1989 Cefixime: a review of its antibacterial activity, pharmacokinetic properties and therapeutic potential. *Drugs* 38: 524–550

Counts G W, Bougher L K, Ulness B K, Hamilton D J 1988 Comparative in vitro activity of the new oral cephalosporin cefixime. *European Journal of Clinical Microbiology and Infectious Diseases* 7: 428–431

Faulkner R D, Fernandez P, Lawrence G et al 1988 Absolute bioavailability of cefixime in man. *Journal of Clinical Pharmacology* 26: 700–706

Finegold S M, Ingram-Drake L, Gee R et al 1987 Bowel flora changes in humans receiving cefixime (CL 284, 635) or cefaclor. *Antimicrobial Agents and Chemotherapy* 31: 443–446

Gremse D A, Dean P C, Farquhar D S 1994 Cefixime and antibiotic-associated colitis. *Pediatric Infectious Disease Journal* 13: 331–333

Guay D R, Meatherall R C, Harding G K, Brown G R 1986 Pharmacokinetics of cefixime (CL 284, 635; FK 027) in healthy subjects and patients with renal insufficiency. *Antimicrobial Agents and Chemotherapy* 30: 485–490

Leggett N J, Caravaggio C, Rybak M J 1990 Cefixime. *Annals of Pharmacotherapy* 24: 489–495

Leroy A, Oser B, Grise P, Humbert G 1995 Cefixime penetration in human renal parenchyma. *Antimicrobial Agents and Chemotherapy* 39: 1240–1242

Markham A, Brogden R N 1995 Cefixime. A review of its therapeutic efficacy in lower respiratory tract infections. *Drugs* 49: 1007–1022

Stone J W, Linong G, Andrews J M, Wise R 1989 Cefixime in-vitro activity, pharmacokinetics and tissue penetration. *Journal of Antimicrobial Chemotherapy* 23: 221–228

Symposium 1987 Clinical pharmacology and efficacy of cefixime. *Pediatric Infectious Disease Journal* 6: 949–1009

Wu D H A 1993 Review of the safety profile of cefixime. *Clinical Therapeutics* 15: 1108–1119

CEFPODOXIME

A semi-synthetic cephalosporin of group 5, supplied as the pro-drug, cefpodoxime proxetil:

It exhibits potent, broad activity typical of the group (Table 14.5). Among other susceptible organisms, it inhibits *M. catarrhalis* at 0.5–1 mg/l and *Acinetobacter* spp. at 2 mg/l. It is stable to a wide range of plasmid-mediated β-lactamases. It induces the chromosomal β-lactamases of *Ps. aeruginosa*, *Enterobacter* spp., *Ser. marcescens* and *Citrobacter* spp., but the increase produced is only about 1% of that resulting from exposure to cefoxitin.

The ester cefpodoxime proxetil is rapidly hydrolysed to the parent compound on oral administration, absolute bioavailability being about 50%, increasing to 65% if taken with food. A dose equivalent to 200 mg cefpodoxime produced a mean peak plasma concentration around 2.1 mg/l at about 2.9 h with a plasma elimination half-life of 2.2 h. It appears to be well distributed. About 30% of the dose appears in the urine over 24 h. Plasma protein binding is around 20% and the apparent volume of distribution is 32.3 l.

Tolerance has generally been good, the adverse reactions described, mainly gastro-intestinal disturbance, being those common to the group.

It has been used principally for the treatment of respiratory tract infection.

Preparations and dosage

Proprietary name: Orelox.

Preparation: Tablets.

Dosage: Adults, oral, 100–200 mg twice daily depending on infection being treated.

Widely available.

Further information

Borin M T, Ferry J J, Forbes K K, Hughes G S 1994 Pharmacokinetics of cefpodoxime proxetil in healthy young and elderly volunteers. *Journal of Clinical Pharmacology* 34: 774–781

Borin M T, Driver M R, Forbes K K 1995 Effect of timing of food on absorption of cefpodoxime proxetil. *Journal of Clinical Pharmacology* 35: 505–509

Green J A, Butler T, Mark Todd W 1994 Randomized double-blind trial of the comparative efficacy and safety of cefpodoxime proxetil and cefaclor in the treatment of acute community-acquired pneumonia. *Current Therapeutic Research – Clinical and Experimental* 9: 1003–1015

Knapp C C, Sierra-Madero J, Washington J A 1988 Antibacterial activities of cefpodoxime, cefixime and ceftriaxone. *Antimicrobial Agents and Chemotherapy* 32: 1896–1898

Moore E P, Speller D C E, White L O, Wilkinson P J (eds) 1990 Cefpodoxime proxetil: a third-generation oral cephalosporin. *Journal of Antimicrobial Chemotherapy* 26 (suppl E): 1–100

O'Neill P, Nye K, Douce G, Andrews J, Wise R 1990 Pharmacokinetics and inflammatory fluid penetration of cefpodoxime proxetil in volunteers. *Antimicrobial Agents and Chemotherapy* 34: 232–234

Todd W M 1994 Cefpodoxime proxetil: a comprehensive review. *International Journal of Antimicrobial Agents* 4: 37–62

Wise R, Andrews J M, Ashby J P, Thornlier D 1990 The in vitro activity of cefpodoxime: a comparison with other oral cephalosporins. *Journal of Antimicrobial Chemotherapy* 25: 541–550

CEFPROZIL

A semi-synthetic cephalosporin of group 5.

It has good activity against Gram-positive cocci and Gram-negative bacilli, although it is not as active as other agents in this group (Table 14.5). It is stable to hydrolysis by the common plasmid-mediated β-lactamases, but is hydrolysed by the chromosomal enzymes of Gram-negative bacilli (p. 319).

It is well absorbed by mouth, a 500 mg dose giving peak plasma concentrations of about 10 mg/l. The elimination half-life is between 1.6 and 2.1 h, and is prolonged in anuric patients. Binding to plasma proteins is 35–45%.

It has primarily been used to treat upper and lower respiratory tract infections, urinary tract infections and infections of skin and soft tissue. It is well tolerated.

Preparations and dosage

Proprietary name: Cefzil.

Dosage: Adults, oral, 250–500 mg once or twice daily depending on infection being treated.

Available in the USA.

Further information

Ball A P 1994 Efficacy and safety of cefprozil versus other beta-lactam antibiotics in the treatment of lower respiratory tract infections. *European Journal of Clinical Microbiology and Infectious Diseases* 13: 851–856

Gainer R B 1995 Cefprozil, a new cephalosporin: its use in various clinical trials. *Southern Medical Journal* 88: 338–346

Lowery N, Kearns G L, Young R A, Wheeler J G 1994 Serum-sickness-like reactions associated with cefprozil therapy. *Journal of Pediatrics* 125: 325–328

Nolen T 1994 Comparative studies of cefprozil in the management of skin and soft tissue infections. *European Journal of Clinical Microbiology and Infectious Diseases* 13: 866–871

Saez-Llorens X, Shyu W C, Shelton S, Kumiesz H, Nelson J 1990 Pharmacokinetics of cefprozil in infants and children. *Antimicrobial Agents and Chemotherapy* 34: 2152–2155

Shyu W C, Haddad J, Reilly J et al 1994 Penetration of cefprozil into middle ear fluid of patients with otitis media. *Antimicrobial Agents and Chemotherapy* 38: 2210–2212

Wise R 1994 Comparative microbiological activity and pharmacokinetics of cefprozil. *European Journal of Clinical Microbiology and Infectious Diseases* 13: 839–845

CEFTIBUTEN

A semi-synthetic cephalosporin of group 5.

The activity is shown in Table 14.5. It is considerably more active against Gram-negative bacilli than Gram-positive cocci. It is stable to hydrolysis by the common plasmid mediated β-lactamases such as TEM-1 and SHV-1.

It is rapidly and almost completely absorbed by mouth and has a somewhat longer elimination half-life (2.5 h) than many other oral cephalosporins. Binding to plasma proteins is 65–77%. Side-effects mostly consist of mild gastro-intestinal symptoms and mild liver function test changes.

Clinical trials have mainly been conducted in urinary tract and respiratory tract infections which, despite the poor in vitro activity against *Str. pneumoniae*, have shown ceftibuten to be as efficacious as comparator agents.

Preparations and dosage

Proprietary name: Cedax.

Preparations: Capsules, suspension.

Dosage: Adult and child over 10 years (over 45 kg), 400 mg daily as a single dose. Child over 6 months, 9 mg/kg daily as a single dose.

Further information

Andrews J M, Wise R, Baldwin D R, Honeybourne D 1995 Concentrations of ceftibuten in plasma and the respiratory tract following a single 400 mg oral dose. *International Journal of Antimicrobial Agents* 5: 141–144

Bragman S G L, Casewell M W 1990 The in-vitro activity of ceftibuten against 475 clinical isolates of Gram-negative bacilli compared with cefuroxime and cefadroxil. *Journal of Antimicrobial Chemotherapy* 25: 221–226

Kearns G L, Young R A 1994 Ceftibuten pharmacokinetics and pharmacodynamics: focus on paediatric use. *Clinical Pharmacokinetics* 26: 169–189

Lin C, Radwanski E, Affrime M, Cayen M N 1995 Multiple-dose pharmacokinetics of ceftibuten in healthy volunteers. *Antimicrobial Agents and Chemotherapy* 39: 356–358

Perrotta R, McCabe R, Rumans L, Nolen T 1994 Comparison of the efficacy and safety of ceftibuten and cefaclor in the treatment of acute bacterial bronchitis. *Infectious Diseases in Clinical Practice* 3: 270–276

Scaglione F, Triscari F, Demartini G, Arcidiacono M, Cocuzza C, Fraschini F 1995 Concentrations of ceftibuten in bronchial secretions. *Chemotherapy* 41: 229–223

Shawar R, La Rocco M, Cleary T G 1989 Comparative in vitro activity of ceftibuten (Sch 39720) against bacterial enteropathogens. *Antimicrobial Agents and Chemotherapy* 33: 781–784

Wise R, Andrews I M, Ashby J P, Thornber D 1990 Ceftibuten–in vitro activity against respiratory pathogens, β-lactamase stability and mechanism of action. *Journal of Antimicrobial Chemotherapy* 26: 209–213

Wiseman L R, Balfour J A 1994 Ceftibuten. A review of its antibacterial activity, pharmacokinetic properties and clinical efficacy. *Drugs* 47: 784–808

Group 6

Cephalosporins notable particularly for their antipseudo-monal activity. Ceftazidime has by far the widest spectrum, which generally matches that of group 4 compounds. Cefsulodin has the greatest activity against *Ps. aeruginosa*, but virtually none against other Gram-negative bacilli and little against Gram-positive cocci (Table 14.6).

CEFOPERAZONE

A semi-synthetic cephalosporin of group 6. It is unstable, losing activity on storage even at −20°C.

Staphylococci (except methicillin-resistant strains) and streptococci are susceptible, but enterococci are resistant. It is active against most enterobacteria and carbenicillin-sensitive strains of *Ps. aeruginosa*, but strains producing TEM β-lactamases are resistant (MIC 32 mg/l). Activity against *Burk. (Ps.) cepacia* and *Sten. (Xanthomonas) maltophilia* is unreliable. Some *K. pneumoniae* seem highly susceptible (MIC 0.12–0.25 mg/l) others rest much less so (MIC >4 mg/l). It is highly active against *H. influenzae* and *N. gonorrhoeae*, although β-lactamase-positive strains are less susceptible. It is active against *Achromobacter, Flavobacterium, Aeromonas* and associated non-fermenters. *Past. multocida* is extremely susceptible (MIC <0.01–0.02 mg/l). It exhibits modest activity against most Gram-negative anaerobes, but not *B. fragilis*. Its activity against common pathogenic bacteria is shown in Table 14.6.

Activity is bactericidal at 1–4 times the MIC and is little affected by the presence of 75% serum. Inoculum effects vary with the species but can be considerable.

Acquired resistance

Resistance in enterobacteria and non-fermenting Gram-negative rods is nearly always due to the production of

Table 14.6 *Activity of group 6 cephalosporins against common pathogenic bacteria: MIC (mg/l)*

	Cefoperazone	Cefpimizole	Cefpiramide	Cefsulodin	Ceftazidime
Staph. aureus	1–4	R	1	2–4	4–8
Str. pyogenes	0.1	I	0.1	2	0.1–0.25
*Str. pneumoniae**	0.1–0.25	I	0.1	4–8	0.25
Ent. faecalis	64–R	R	R	R	R
N. gonorrhoeae	0.06			4–8	0.06–0.1
N. meningitidis	0.06			4–8	<0.01
H. influenzae	0.1	0.25	0.5	32	0.1
Esch. coli	0.1–2	0.5	0.5	64–R	0.1
Klebsiella spp.	0.5–8	4	2	64–R	0.1
Pr. mirabilis	0.5–1	0.5	4	R	0.06
Pr. vulgaris	4	R	4	R	0.1
Morganella/Providencia	1–64		8–R	R	0.06–1
Enterobacter spp.	1–R	4	I	R	0.25
Salmonella spp.	0.5–1	4	I	R	0.25
Shigella spp.	0.5	2		R	0.25
Ser. marcescens	2–8	R	32	R	0.1
Citrobacter spp.	4	16	4	R	0.5
Ps. aeruginosa	4–8	8	2	2	1–4
B. fragilis	16–32	R	R	R	16–64

* Penicillin-resistant strains are often less susceptible.

β-lactamase. Hydrolysis by the cephalosporinases of _Entero-bacter_ spp., _Citrobacter_ spp., _Morg. morgani_ and _Pr. vulgaris_ is less than 10% of that of cephaloridine, but it is almost as susceptible as cephaloridine to the TEM β-lactamases and the chromosomal enzyme of _B. fragilis_. Carbenicillin and ticarcillin resistant _Ps. aeruginosa_ are often resistant due to the presence of β-lactamases. Combination with clavulanic acid or sulbactam renders many resistant strains of _Esch. coli_, klebsiella and _B. fragilis_, but not _Ps. aeruginosa_, susceptible. Sulbactam increases activity against many, but not all, enterobacteria and non-fermenters, and almost all _B. fragilis_.

Pharmacokinetics

Intramuscular injection of 0.5 g produces a peak plasma level around 25 mg/l. Plasma concentrations shortly after rapid i.v. administration of 0.5 g are 50–100 mg/l. The mean end-infusion concentrations in subjects receiving 2 g by i.v. infusions over 15–30 min were around 260 mg/l. In patients receiving 8 or 16 g per day by continuous infusion, mean steady-state serum concentrations of 80 and 153 mg/l were obtained. It is 85–95% protein bound. The plasma half-life is 1.5–2 h. As a result of the way in which the drug is excreted, the pattern alters in pregnancy where, following 2 g i.v., mean peak plasma concentrations were around 170 mg/l with a plasma half-life of 2.5 h. Percentage binding to plasma protein, 74%, was significantly lower than that in non-pregnant controls. These changes persist for some weeks into the puerperium.

In pre- and full-term infants given 50 mg/kg i.v. over 3 min, mean end-infusion concentrations at less than 33 weeks and full-term were 160 and 110 mg/l, respectively. The plasma half-life was related to gestational age, being around 5.8 h in the youngest infants.

Distribution

The volume of distribution is 10–17 l. It crosses serous membranes, producing concentrations of the order of 20–60 mg/kg in ascitic fluid. In patients given 2 g i.m. preoperatively mean concentrations in pelvic tissue were 19.8 mg/g, a tissue:serum ratio of 0.22–0.47. In patients given 2 g i.v. over 30 min pre-operatively, muscle concentrations were 17% of the simultaneous serum level with concentrations in wound drainage fluid 1–2 h after the fourth of 8-hourly 2 g doses of 55 mg/l. Concentrations of 7–25 mg/l have been found in pleural fluid 4–6 h after 2 g i.v.

It does not enter the normal CSF, but in the presence of meningitis, mean concentrations of 1.97 mg/l have been found in patients receiving 50–100 mg/kg. Levels tended to increase with the dose and protein content of the CSF, but penetration was unreliable.

Variable low levels are found in the sputum up to 1.5% of simultaneous serum levels.

Excretion

Renal clearance is only 15–25%, and the low recovery in urine (20–30%), is remarkable among currently available cephalosporins. Elimination is almost entirely by glomerular filtration and probenecid has no effect. The fate of the rest is unknown. Cefoperazone A, a degradation product with about 6% of the activity of the parent is seldom demonstrable in plasma or urine. Clearance is effectively unchanged by renal failure or dialysis.

Bile. The bile is a major route of excretion, accounting for almost 20% of the dose. In patients receiving 2 g i.v. over 15 min, very high concentrations between 500 and 6500 mg/l have been found in T-tube bile. Concentrations in gallbladder bile in patients receiving 1 g i.v. were very variable but in some exceeded 600 mg/l. Compensatory responses in the route of excretion are naturally found in the presence of renal or hepatic dysfunction.

In normal and anephric subjects receiving 3 g i.v., there was no difference in peak serum concentrations, volume of distribution or half-life. In patients with hepatic cirrhosis, given 2 g i.v. over 15 min, mean peak plasma concentrations rose to 240 mg/l, mean plasma half-life to 4.5 h, and urinary recovery to 50%. The apparent volume of distribution more than doubled probably as a result of ascites and lowered plasma protein concentration. In the presence of biliary obstruction as little as 40 mg/l was found in bile after a 2 g i.v. dose.

Administration with sulbactam

There is no significant change in the pharmacokinetics of the two agents when they are administered together apart from a reduction in sulbactam clearance of about 10%. In patients on CAPD given 2 g cefoperazone plus 1 g sulbactam intraperitoneally, the absolute bioavailability of the two agents differs markedly in renal failure: cefoperazone is virtually unaffected, whereas the elimination half-life of sulbactam is prolonged and its clearance approximately doubled by haemodialysis. In the elderly ill, handling of both components is more variable and excretion delayed.

Toxicity and side-effects

It is generally well tolerated. No increase in alanine amino peptidase or β_2-microglobulin excretion has been detected. Impaired coagulation has been observed in elderly patients, which is readily reversed by vitamin K. Diarrhoea has been notable in some studies but has been said to occur overall in 3% of patients. Marked general suppression of faecal flora has been reported, with sparing of enterococci and clostridia and the appearance of _Cl. difficile_ in some patients. There is a 5–10% incidence of mild transient increases in liver function tests.

Clinical use

That of group 6 cephalosporins (p. 207). It has been used as single dose treatment of uncomplicated and anogenital gonorrhoea. Reference is made to its use in neutropenic patients, *H. influenzae* meningitis and typhoid fever.

Preparations and dosage

Preparation: Injection.
Dosage: Adults, i.m., i.v., 2–4 g/day in 2 divided doses; in severe infections up to 12 g/day in 2–4 divided doses. Widely available, except UK.

Further information

Brogden R N, Carmine A, Heel R C, Morley P A, Speight T M, Avery G S 1981 Cefoperazone: a review of its in vitro antimicrobial activity, pharmacological properties and therapeutic efficacy. *Drugs* 22: 423–460

Fass R J, Gregory W W, D'Amato R F, Matsen J M, Wright D N, Young L S 1990 In vitro activities of cefoperazone and sulbactam singly and in combination against cefoperazone-resistant members of the family enterobacteriaceae and non-fermenters. *Antimicrobial Agents and Chemotherapy* 34: 2256–2259

Gibbs D L 1987 Worldwide study of cefoperazone susceptibility. *Clinical Therapeutics* 9: 193–200

Gonik B 1986 Pharmacokinetics of cefoperazone in the parturient. *Antimicrobial Agents and Chemotherapy* 30: 874–876

Greenberg R N, Cayavec P, Danko L S et al 1994 Comparison of cefoperazone plus sulbactam with clindamycin plus gentamicin as treatment for intra-abdominal infections. *Journal of Antimicrobial Chemotherapy* 34: 391–401

Gugliemo B J, Flaherty J F, Woods T M, La Follette G, Gambertoglio J G 1987 Pharmacokinetics of cefoperazone and tobramycin alone and in combination. *Antimicrobial Agents and Chemotherapy* 31: 264–266

Johnson C A, Zimmerman S W, Reitberg D P, Whall T J, Leggett J E, Craig W A 1988 Pharmacokinetics and pharmacodynamics of cefoperazone-sulbactam in patients on continuous ambulatory peritoneal dialysis. *Antimicrobial Agents and Chemotherapy* 32: 51–56

Meyers B R, Mendelson M H, Deeter R G, Srulevitch-Chin E, Sarni M T, Hirschman S Z 1987 Pharmacokinetics of cefoperazone in ambulatory elderly volunteers compared with young adults. *Antimicrobial Agents and Chemotherapy* 31: 925–929

Reitberg D P, Marble D A, Schultz R W, Whall T J, Schentag J 1988 Pharmacokinetics of cefoperazone (2.0 g) and sulbactam (1.0 g) coadministered to subjects with normal renal function, patients with decreased renal function and patients with end-stage renal disease on hemodialysis. *Antimicrobial Agents and Chemotherapy* 32: 503–509

Reitberg D P, Whall T J, Chung M, Blickens D, Swarz H, Arnold J 1988 Multiple-dose pharmacokinetics and toleration of intravenously administered cefoperazone and sulbactam when given as single agents and in combination. *Antimicrobial Agents and Chemotherapy* 32: 42–46

Saudek F, Moravek J, Modr Z 1989 Cefoperazone pharmacokinetics in patients with liver cirrhosis: a predictive value of the ujoviridin test. *International Journal of Clinical Pharmacology, Therapy and Toxicology* 27: 82–87

Schwartz J I, Jauregui I E, Bachmann K A, Martin M E, Reitberg D P 1988 Multiple-dose pharmacokinetics of intravenously administered cefoperazone and sulbactam when given in combination to infected, seriously ill elderly patients. *Antimicrobial Agents and Chemotherapy* 32: 730–735

Silva M, Cornick M A, Gorbach S L 1989 Suppression of colonic microflora by cefoperazone and evaluation of the drug as potential prophylaxis in bowel surgery. *Antimicrobial Agents and Chemotherapy* 33: 835–838

Symposium 1983 Evaluation of cefoperazone. *Reviews of Infectious Diseases* 5 (suppl 1): S108–S209

Welage I S, Borin M T, Wilton J H, Hejmanowski L G, Wels P B, Schentag J J 1990 Comparative evaluation of the pharmacokinetics of N-methyl-thiotetrazole following administration of cefoperazone, cefotetan, and cefmetazole. *Antimicrobial Agents and Chemotherapy* 34: 2369–2374

Wexler H M, Finegold S M 1988 In vitro activity of cefoperazone plus sulbactam compared with that of other antimicrobial agents against anaerobic bacteria. *Antimicrobial Agents and Chemotherapy* 32: 403–406

CEFPIMIZOLE

A semi-synthetic cephalosporin of group 6.

It exhibits modest activity against Gram-positive cocci, enterobacteria and *Ps. aeruginosa* (Table 14.6). Particular attention has been paid to its activity against *N. gonorrhoeae* (geometric mean MIC 0.088 mg/l). Its stability to β-lactamases resembles that of cefoperazone.In volunteers rec iving 0.1–1 g i.m. or 1, 2 or 4 g i.v. over 20 min, plas a concentrations increased proportionally, mean peak concen rations reaching 15–20 and 35–40 mg/l after 500 and 10 0 mg i.m., respectively

There was no change and no accumulation when the dose was repeated 8-hourly for 7 days. No metabolites have been detected. The plasma elimination half-life is 1.8–2.1 h. The principal route of elimination is renal, 70–80% being recovered unchanged in the urine.

Significant pain at the site of infection has been a prominent adverse effect. A single dose of 1 g, but not less, has been successful in curing urethral but not rectal or pharyngeal gonorrhoea.

Preparations

Available in Japan.

Further information

Jones R N, Ayers L W, Gavan T L, Gerlach E H, Sommers H M 1985 In vitro comparative antimicrobial activity of cefpimizole against clinical isolates from five medical centres. *Antimicrobial Agents and Chemotherapy* 27: 982–984

Lakings D B, Fries J M, Brown R J, Allen H R 1984 Pharmacokinetics of cefpimizole in normal humans after single- and multiple-dose intravenous infusions. *Antimicrobial Agents and Chemotherapy* 26: 802–806

Novak E, Lakings D B, Paxton L M 1987 Tolerance and disposition of cefpimizole in normal human volunteers after intramuscular administration. *Antimicrobial Agents and Chemotherapy* 31: 1706–1710

CEFPIRAMIDE

A semi-synthetic cephalosporin of group 6.

Its properties are typical of the group: broad range of activity (Table 14.6), synergy with selected aminoglycosides against some organisms and antagonism of its activity against *Enterobacter* spp. and *Ps. aeruginosa* by cefoxitin. The MIC$_{90}$ for *Ps. aeruginosa* is 16 mg/l and for *Acinetobacter* spp. 32 mg/l. It is active against anaerobes. It is moderately stable to most cephalosporinases but less so to penicillinases.

In volunteers given 0.5 or 1 g by i.v. bolus, the mean plasma concentration shortly after injection was around 150 or 300 mg/l, respectively. The mean plasma half-life was 4.5 h. There was no accumulation when the same doses were repeated 12 hourly for 11 doses. It is highly bound to plasma protein. Less than a quarter of the dose was recovered from the urine over 24 h. In some cases almost 40% appeared in the faeces via biliary excretion. Renal impairment has little effect on elimination in patients with normal liver function. Diarrhoea may be associated with marked suppression of gut flora resulting from biliary excretion of the drug.

Its clinical uses are those of group 6 cephalosporins (p. 207).

Preparations

Available in Japan.

Further information

Barry A L, Jones R N, Thornsberry C et al 1985 Cefpiramide: comparative in-vitro activity and β-lactamase stability. *Journal of Antimicrobial Chemotherapy* 16: 315–325

Brogard J M, Jeal F, Adloff M, Bickle J F, Montell H 1988 High hepatic excretion in humans of cefpiramide, a new cephalosporin. *Antimicrobial Agents and Chemotherapy* 32: 1360–1364

Conte J E 1987 Pharmacokinetics of cefpiramide in volunteers with normal or impaired renal function. *Antimicrobial Agents and Chemotherapy* 31: 1585–1588

Demontes-Mainard F, Vinccon G, Labat L et al 1994 Cefpiramide kinetics and plasma protein binding in cholestasis. *British Journal of Clinical Pharmacology* 37: 295–297

Matsui H, Okada T 1988 Renal tubular mechanisms for excretion of cefpiramide (SM-1 652) in association with its long-lasting pharmacokinetic properties. *Journal of Pharmaco-biodynamics* 11: 67–73

Nakagawa K, Koyama M, Matsui H et al 1984 Pharmacokinetics of cefpiramide (SM-1652) in humans. *Antimicrobial Agents and Chemotherapy* 25: 221–225

Quentin C, Noury P, Titonel M 1989 Comparative in vitro activity of cefpiramide, a new parenteral cephalosporin. *European Journal of Clinical Microbiology and Infectious Diseases* 7: 544–549

CEFSULODIN

A semi-synthetic cephalosporin of group 6 supplied as the sodium salt.

Antimicrobial activity

Notable for its activity against *Ps. aeruginosa*, most strains of which are susceptible to 4–8 mg/l, which contrasts strikingly with that against many other organisms (Table 14.6). The MIC increases little with inoculum size, but the MBC, which is close to the MIC at lower inocula, is more significantly affected. It is relatively unstable in agar. Anaerobic Gram-negative rods, Gram-positive rods and cocci are all resistant. Synergy has been demonstrated with cefoxitin against *Bacteroides* spp. and some anaerobic cocci, including some β-lactamase negative strains and with clavulanic acid against *B. fragilis*.

It is stable to many β-lactamases, including the *Ps. aeruginosa* chromosomal enzyme and is a poor substrate for the enzymes of *Enterobacter* spp. and *Morg. morganii*. It is slowly hydrolysed by TEM β-lactamases and more rapidly by the enzymes of some carbenicillin-resistant strains of *Ps. aeruginosa* with which distinct inoculum effects may be seen.

Acquired resistance

Resistant *Ps. aeruginosa* has emerged during the course of treatment. In five hospitals in Japan the MIC_{90} for *Ps. aeruginosa* rose from 12.5 mg/l in 1980 to 100 mg/l in 1983, largely due to the spread of strains also resistant to gentamicin. The increase was attributed to the use not of cefsulodin, but of group 4 cephalosporins.

Pharmacokinetics

Intramuscular injection of 0.5 g produces peak plasma levels around 15 mg/l. Plasma concentrations shortly after rapid i.v. administration of the same dose are around 70 mg/l. Immediately after a dose of 1 g by i.v. bolus, the mean plasma concentration was 146 mg/l and the elimination half-life 1.5 h. In patients with cystic fibrosis given 3 g i.v. over 30 min, the plasma half-life was not different from that in normal subjects. Plasma protein binding is 15–30% and the apparent volume of distribution is around 18 l.

There is some metabolism of the drug, but the main route of excretion is via the kidneys, most appearing in the urine

in the first 6 h but total reported recoveries over 24 h have varied from 50% to 90%. It accumulates in renal failure, but the volume of distribution is unaffected. The plasma half-life is linearly related to creatinine clearance, rising to a mean of 10–13 h in patients where clearance was <10 ml/min, falling to around 2 h on haemodialysis.

Toxicity and side-effects

It is well tolerated apart from nausea and vomiting in some subjects. There are occasional reports of vertigo that may be related to the rate of infusion.

Clinical use

It has been used in severe pseudomonas infections, usually in combination with an aminoglycoside, but treatment has been complicated on a number of occasions by the emergence of resistance or superinfection.

Preparations and dosage

Proprietary name: Monaspor.

Preparation: Injection.

Dosage: Adults, i.m., i.v., 1–4 g/day in 2–4 divided doses, increased in severe infections to 6 g/day. Children, 20–50 mg/kg per day.

Limited availability.

Further information

Bergogne-Berezin E, Bertelot G, Safran D, Even P, Kafe H 1984 Penetration of cefsulodin into bronchial secretions. *Chemotherapy* 30: 205–210

Granneman G R, Sennello L T, Sonders R C, Wynne B, Thomas E W 1982 Cefsulodin kinetics in healthy subjects after intramuscular and intravenous injection. *Clinical Pharmacology and Therapeutics* 31: 95–103

King A, Shannon K, Phillips I 1980 In vitro antibacterial activity and susceptibility of cefsulodin, an antipseudomonal cephalosporin, to beta-lactamases. *Antimicrobial Agents and Chemotherapy* 17: 165–169

Reed M D, Stern R C, Yamashita T S, Ackers I, Myers C M, Blumer J L 1984 Single-dose pharmacokinetics of cefsulodin in patients with cystic fibrosis. *Antimicrobial Agents and Chemotherapy* 25: 579–581

Wright D B 1986 Cefsulodin. *Drug Intelligence and Clinical Pharmacy* 20: 845–849

Young L S 1984 *Pseudomonas aeruginosa* – biology, immunology and therapy: a cefsulodin symposium. *Reviews of Infectious Diseases* 6 (suppl 3): S603–S776

CEFTAZIDIME

A semi-synthetic cephalosporin of group 6.

Antimicrobial activity

It is highly active against *H. influenzae*, including β-lactamase-producing strains, enterobacteria, *Ps. aeruginosa*, including almost all gentamicin-resistant strains, and *Burk. (Ps.) cepacia*. It is substantially less active against *Staph. aureus* and *B. fragilis* is resistant. Its activity against common pathogenic bacteria is shown in Table 14.6.

It is stable to a wide range of β-lactamases. Induction of chromosomal β-lactamase in vitro and in some treated patients can result in resistance to other β-lactam agents.

Pharmacokinetics

It is not absorbed when given by mouth. Intramuscular injection of 0.5 g produces peak plasma levels of 18–20 mg/l. Plasma concentrations shortly after rapid i.v. administration of 1.0 g are 80–120 mg/l. In volunteers given 2 g i.v. over 20 min, mean end-infusion values were around 185 mg/l. No accumulation was seen in subjects receiving 2 g 12-hourly over 8 days. No metabolites of the drug have been detected and its plasma protein binding is low at around 10–20%. The plasma half-life has been variously given as 1.5–1.85 h. In premature infants given 25 mg/kg twice daily, mean peak plasma concentrations were 77 mg/l after i.v. and 56 mg/l after i.m. administration with plasma elimination half-lives of 7.3 and 14.2 h, respectively. Postnatal age was the most important determinant of elimination rate, the elimination half-life being halved after 5 days. In newborn infants given 50 mg/kg i.v. over 20 min, mean peak plasma concentrations varied inversely with gestational age from 102 to 124 mg/l with half-lives of 2.9–6.7 h.

Distribution
There is ready penetration into serous fluids, the concentration reaching 50% or more of those of the simultaneous serum level. In patients given 1 g i.v. during abdominal surgery, detectable concentrations appeared within a few minutes in the peritoneal fluid reaching a peak around 67 mg/l with a half-life of 0.9 h. Following a similar i.v. dose, a mean peak of 9.4 mg/l was reached at 2 h in ascitic fluid.

Concentrations in middle ear fluid following 1 g i.v. were broadly comparable with those of the plasma: fluid:plasma ratio 0.6–1.3.

In patients with meningitis, CSF concentrations of 2–30 mg/l have been found 2–3 h after doses of 2 g i.v. over 30 min given 8-hourly for four doses. Mean concentrations in patients receiving 2 or 3 g doses were substantially less (0.8 mg/l) in the absence of meningitis than in its presence (22.6 mg/l). The same dose produced peak concentrations in cantharides blister fluid comparable with those of serum and with a similar half-life. Penetration occurred into intracranial abscesses with concentrations of around 3–27 mg/g being found in patients treated with 0.5–2 g three times daily. Concentrations around 0.4 mg/g in skin, 0.6 mg/g in muscle and 0.2 mg/g in fatty tissue have been found in patients given 2 g i.v. over 5 min preoperatively. A similar dose has produced mean prostate tissue:serum ratios of around 0.14. Effective concentrations are achieved in bone: in patients given 1 g i.v. mean bone concentrations were 14.4 mg/l at 35–40 min after the dose.

Excretion
There is secretion in breast milk, peak concentrations being around 5 mg/l at about 1 h in patients receiving 2 g i.v. 8-hourly. Elimination is almost exclusively renal, predominantly via the glomerular filtrate with 80–90% of the dose appearing in the urine in the first 24 h. A slight but significant increase in the fraction filtered has been noted on repeated dosage. Renal clearance is between 90 and 115 ml/min. Elimination half-life is inversely correlated with creatinine clearance: as the values fall to 2–12 ml/min, the mean plasma half-life rises to 16 h. In patients maintained on haemodialysis the half-life fell to 2.8 h on dialysis. No accumulation occurred over 10 days in severe renal impairment on a daily dose of 0.5–1 g.

Bile. There is some excretion in bile, concentrations of 6.6–58 mg/l being found 25–160 min after the dose at times when the mean serum concentration was 77.4 mg/l. In T-tube bile there was considerable interpatient variation, with mean concentrations of 34 mg/l at 1–2 h after the dose. No accumulation occurs in patients with impaired hepatic function, but the presence of ascites, low plasma albumin and accumulation of protein-binding inhibitors may increase the volume of distribution.

Toxicity and side-effects

It is generally well tolerated. Reactions common to cephalosporins have been observed in some patients, including positive antiglobulin tests without haemolysis, raised liver function test values, eosinophilia, rashes, leucopenia, thrombocytopenia and diarrhoea, occasionally associated with the presence of toxigenic *Cl. difficile*. Faecal enterobacterial counts may fall significantly on therapy, while anaerobes remain intact. Increase in ampicillin- and cephazolin-resistant enterobacteria after treatment is common.

Effervescence occurring with preparations containing sodium carbonate produce pain in many patients on i.m. injection sufficiently severe to require the addition of lignocaine. This was eliminated in preparations containing arginine. Failure of therapy in a number of cases has been associated with superinfection with resistant organisms, including *Staph. aureus*, enterococci and *Candida*, or emergence of resistance principally in *Ps. aeruginosa*, *Ser. marcescens* or *Enterobacter* spp. associated with induction of chromosomal β-lactamases.

Clinical use

It has been successfully used to treat severe urinary, respiratory and wound infections, mostly due to enterobacteria or *Ps. aeruginosa*, in immunocompromised (p. 619) or otherwise normal patients and in children. It has been found useful for the treatment of haemophilus (p. 745), enterobacterial or *Ps. aeruginosa* meningitis. Reference is made to its use in pneumonia, septicaemia, peritonitis, osteomyelitis, neonatal sepsis, burns and melioidosis (p. 588). In many cases, combined treatment with an aminoglycoside has been used. Concern has been expressed at the relative frequency with which failure is associated with superinfection or the emergence of resistance.

Preparations and dosage

Proprietary names: Fortum, Kefadim.

Preparation: Injection.

Dosage: Adults, i.m., i.v., 1–6 g/day in divided doses, depending on severity of infection. Neonates and children up to 2 months, 25–60 mg/kg per day in 2 divided doses; children >2 months 30–100 mg/kg per day in 2–3 divided doses.

Widely available.

Further information

Boogaerts M A, Demuynck H, Mestdagh N et al 1995 Equivalent efficacies of meropenem and ceftazidime as empirical monotherapy of febrile neutropenic patients. *Journal of Antimicrobial Chemotherapy* 36: 185–200

Brogard J M, Jehl F, Paris-Bockel D, Blickle J F, Adloff M, Monteil H 1987 Biliary elimination of ceftazidime. *Journal of Antimicrobial Chemotherapy* 19: 671–678

Burwen D R, Banerjee S N, Gaynes R P 1994 Ceftazidime resistance among selected nosocomial Gram-negative bacilli in the United States. *Journal of Infectious Diseases* 170: 1622–1625

Demotes-Mainard F, Vincon G, Ragnaud J M, Morlat P, Bannwarth B, Dangoumau J 1993 Pharmacokinetics of intravenous and intraperitoneal ceftazidime in chronic ambulatory peritoneal dialysis. *Journal of Clinical Pharmacology* 33: 475–479

De Pauw B E, Deresinski S C, Feld R, Lane Allman E F, Donnelly J P, Elahi N 1994 Ceftazidime compared with piperacillin and tobramycin for the empiric treatment of fever in neutropenic patients with cancer: a multicenter randomized trial. *Annals of Internal Medicine* 120: 834–844

Fong I N, Tomkins K B 1985 Review of *Pseudomonas aeruginosa* meningitis with special emphasis on treatment with ceftazidime. *Reviews of Infectious Diseases* 7: 604–612

Fung-Tomc J, Huczko E, Pearce M, Kessler R E 1988 Frequency of in vitro resistance of *Pseudomonas aeruginosa* to cefepime, ceftazidime and cefotaxime. *Antimicrobial Agents and Chemotherapy* 32: 1443–1445

Green H T, O'Donoghue M A T, Shaw M D M, Dowling C 1989 Pentration of ceftazidime into intracranial abscess. *Journal of Antimicrobial Chemotherapy* 24: 431–436

Heim-Duthoy K L, Bubrick M P, Cocchetto D M, Matzke G R 1988 Disposition of ceftazidime in surgical patients with intra-abdominal infection. *Antimicrobial Agents and Chemotherapy* 32: 1845–1847

Jonsson M, Walder M 1992 Pharmacokinetics of ceftazidime in acutely ill hospitalised elderly patients. *European Journal of Clinical Microbiology and Infectious Diseases* 11: 15–21

LeBel M, Barbeau G, Vallee F, Bergeron M G 1985 Pharmacokinetics of ceftazidime in elderly volunteers. *Antimicrobial Agents and Chemotherapy* 28: 713–715

Lin M S, Wang L S, Huang J D 1989 Single- and multiple-dose pharmacokinetics of ceftazidime in infected patients with varying degrees of renal function. *Journal of Clinical Pharmacology* 29: 331–337

Ljungberg B, Nilsson-Ehle I 1988 Influence of age on the pharmacokinetics of ceftazidime in acutely ill adult patients. *European Journal of Clinical Pharmacology* 34: 173–178

Norrby S R, Finch R G, Glauser M et al 1993 Monotherapy in serious hospital-acquired infections: a clinical trial of ceftazidime versus imipenem/cilastatin. *Journal of Antimicrobial Chemotherapy* 31: 927–937

O'Donoghue M A, Green H T, Mackenzie I J, Durham L, Dowling C A 1989 Ceftazidime in middle ear fluid. *Journal of Antimicrobial Chemotherapy* 23: 664–666

Ohkawa M, Nakashima T, Shoda R et al 1985 Pharmacokinetics of ceftazidime in patients with renal insufficiency and in those undergoing haemodialysis. *Chemotherapy* 31: 410–416

Perea E J, Ayarra K, Garcia-Iglesias M C, Garcia Luque I, Loscertales J 1988 Penetration of cefuroxime and ceftazidime into human lungs. *Chemotherapy* 34: 1–7

Rains C P, Bryson H M, Peters D H 1995 Ceftazidime: An update of its antibacterial activity, pharmacokinetic properties and therapeutic efficacy. *Drugs* 49: 577–617

Shiramatsu K, Hirata K, Yamada T et al 1988 Ceftazidime concentration in gallbladder tissue and excretion in bile. *Antimicrobial Agents and Chemotherapy* 32: 1588–1589

Tessin I, Trollfors B, Thiringer K, Thorn Z, Larsson P 1989 Concentrations of ceftazidime, tobramycin and ampicillin in the cerebrospinal fluid of newborn infants. *European Journal of Pediatrics* 148: 678–681

Walstad R A, Aanerud L, Thurmann-Nielsen E 1988 Pharmacokinetics and tissue concentrations of ceftazidime in burn patients. *European Journal of Clinical Pharmacology* 35: 543–549

Walstad R A, Dahl K, Hellum K B, Thurmann-Nielsen E 1988 The pharmacokinetics of ceftazidime in patients with impaired renal function and concurrent frusemide therapy. *European Journal of Clinical Pharmacology* 35: 272–279

Table 14.7 *Activity of group 7 cephalosporins against common pathogenic bacteria: MIC (mg/l)*

	Cefepime	Cefpirome
Staph. aureus	2–4	0.5–1
Str. pyogenes	0.1	0.03
Str. pneumoniae	<0.05	<0.05
Ent. faecalis	R	4–R
H. influenzae	0.1	0.03
Esch. coli	0.1–0.5	0.1–0.5
Klebsiella spp.	0.1–0.5	0.1–0.5
Pr. mirabilis	<0.2	<0.2
Enterobacter spp.	2	0.5–2
Salmonella spp.	0.1	0.1
Shigella spp.	0.1	0.1
Citrobacter spp.	2	2–8
Ps. aeruginosa	8–16	2–8
B. fragilis	R	R

Group 7

Parenteral compounds with potent activity against enterobacteria, modest activity against *Ps. aeruginosa*, enhanced β-lactamase stability and enhanced antistaphylococcal activity. They show increased potency against those strains (such as *Enterobacter* and *Serratia* spp.) which are less susceptible to group 4 and 6 compounds.

CEFEPIME

A semi-synthetic cephalosporin of group 7.

It is widely active against staphylococci, streptococci (but not enterococci), *H. influenzae*, neisseriae, enterobacteria and *Ps. aeruginosa* (Table 14.7). It is active against most *Citrobacter* spp., *Enterobacter* spp. and *Ps. aeruginosa* resistant to cefoperazone, cefotaxime and ceftazidime. It has poor activity against *L. monocytogenes* and against anaerobic organisms.

In volunteers given 2 g i.v. over 30 min, end-infusion plasma concentrations were around 190 mg/l with a plasma elimination half-life around 2 h. Virtually the whole dose appeared in the urine over 8 h. On the same dosage, penetration into the bronchial mucosa was about 60% of the plasma value. Binding to plasma proteins is low (10–19%). The apparent volume of distribution is 14–20 l.

It is indicated for the treatment of serious infection due to organisms resistant to group 4 compounds. It appears to be well tolerated.

Further information

Barbhaiya R H, Forgue S T, Gleason C R et al 1992 Pharmacokinetics of cefepime after single and multiple intravenous administrations in healthy subjects. *Antimicrobial Agents and Chemotherapy* 36: 552–557

Barradell L B, Bryson H M 1994 Cefepime: a review of its antibacterial activity, pharmacokinetic properties and therapeutic use. *Drugs* 47: 471–505

Brown E M, Finch R G, White L O (eds) 1993 Cefepime: a β-lactamase-stable extended-spectrum cephalosporin. *Journal of Antimicrobial Chemotherapy* 32 (suppl B): 1–214

Chadha D, Wise R, Baldwin D R, Andrews J M, Ashby J P, Honeybourne D 1990 Cefepime concentrations in bronchial mucosa and serum following a single 2 gram intravenous dose. *Journal of Antimicrobial Chemotherapy* 25: 959–963

Fung-Tomc J, Dougherty T J, DeOrio F J, Simich-Jacobson V, Kessler R E 1989 Activity of cefepime against ceftazidime- and cefotaxime-resistant Gram-negative bacteria and its relationship to β-lactamase levels. *Antimicrobial Agents and Chemotherapy* 33: 498–502

Fung-Tomc J, Huczko E, Pearce M, Kessler R E 1989 Frequency of in vitro resistance of *Pseudomonas aeruginosa* to cefepime, ceftazidime and cefotaxime. *Antimicrobial Agents and Chemotherapy* 32: 1443–1445

Kieft H, Hoepelman A I M, Rozenberg Arska M et al 1994 Cefepime compared with ceftazidime as initial therapy for serious bacterial infections and sepsis syndrome. *Antimicrobial Agents and Chemotherapy* 38: 415–421

Kovaric J M, ter Maaten J C, Rademaker C M A et al 1990 Pharmacokinetics of cefepime in patients with respiratory tract infections. *Antimicrobial Agents and Chemotherapy* 34: 1885–1888

Liu Y C, Huang W K, Cheng D L 1994 Antibacterial activity of cefepime in vitro. *Chemotherapy (Basel)* 40: 384–390

Okamoto M P, Nakahiro R K, Chin A, Bedikian A 1993 Cefepime clinical pharmacokinetics. *Clinical Pharmacokinetics* 25: 88–102

Saez Llorens X, Castano E, Garcia R et al 1995 Prospective randomized comparison of cefepime and cefotaxime for treatment of bacterial meningitis in infants and children. *Antimicrobial Agents and Chemotherapy* 39: 937–940

CEFPIROME

A semi-synthetic cephalosporin of group 7.

It shows wide activity typical of the group (Table 14.7). The MIC_{90} for *L. pneumophila* is 16 mg/l. *B. fragilis* is resistant. It is bactericidal at concentrations 2–4 times the MIC. Activity against enterococci fell as the inoculum was raised from 10^3 to 10^7 cfu. Synergy was demonstrated with gentamicin against most strains of *Ent. faecium* but less than half the isolates of *Ent. faecalis*. It is generally very stable to β-lactamases. There is very low affinity for the cephalosporinases of *Enterobacter* spp., *Citrobacter* spp., *Ser. marcescens* and *Pr. vulgaris*, which probably accounts for its potent activity against producer strains. Induction of β-lactamase in *Ser. marcescens* and *Pr. vulgaris* increases with concentration.

In volunteers given 1 g i.v., the plasma concentration 5 min after the end of injection was around 97 mg/l with an elimination half-life around 2.3 h. Penetration into cantharides blisters was around 12.5% with a similar half-life. About 75% of the dose appeared in the urine over 24 h. Plasma protein binding is 10%. The apparent volume of distribution is 17–26 l.

It is mainly used in the treatment of serious sepsis, particularly nosocomial chest infections. It is generally well tolerated.

Preparations and dosage

Proprietary name: Cefrom.

Preparation: Injection.

Dosage: i.v., 1–2 g every 12 h. Not recommended for children <12.

Available in the UK.

Further information

Kavi J, Andrews J M, Ashby J P, Hillman G, Wise R 1988 Pharmacokinetics and tissue penetration of cefpirome, a new cephalosporin. *Journal of Antimicrobial Chemotherapy* 22: 911–916

Kavi J, Ashby J P, Wise R, Donovan I A 1989 Intraperitoneal penetration of cefpirome. *European Journal of Clinical Microbiology and Infectious Diseases* 8: 556–558

Kearns G L, Weber W, Harnisch L et al 1995 Single-dose pharmacokinetics of cefpirome in paediatric patients. *Clinical Drug Investigation* 10: 71–78

Kobayashi S, Arai S, Hayashi S, Fujimoto K 1986 β-lactamase stability of cefpirome (HR 810) a new cephalosporin with a broad antimicrobial spectrum. *Antimicrobial Agents and Chemotherapy* 30: 713–718

Mitsukude M, Inoue M, Mitsuhashi S 1989 In vitro and in vivo antibacterial activity of the new semisynthetic cephalosporin cefpirome. *Arzneimittelforschung* 39: 26–30

Neu H C, Norrby S R (eds) 1993 Serious bacterial infections: antibiotic resistance and novel therapeutic approaches. *Scandinavian Journal of Infectious Diseases* (suppl 91): 1–59

Neu H C, Chin N X, Labthavikul P 1985 The in vitro activity and beta-lactamase stability of cefpirome (HR 810), a pyridine cephalosporin agent active against staphylococci, enterobacteriaceae and *Pseudomonas aeruginosa*. *Infection* 13: 146–155

Rubinstein E, Labs R, Reeves A 1993 A review of the adverse effects profile of cefpirome. *Drug Safety* 9: 340–345

Strenkoski L C, Nix D E 1993 Cefpirome clinical pharmacokinetics. *Clinical Pharmacokinetics* 25: 263–273

β-Lactams: penicillins

R. Sutherland

Introduction

The penicillin class of antibiotics comprises a large group of bicyclic penam compounds (p. 307) differing in the nature of the acyl side-chain attached to the fused β-lactam thiazolidine ring system. Most are semi-synthetic derivatives of the penicillin nucleus, 6-aminopenicillanic acid (6-APA), prepared by the addition by chemical synthesis of acyl side-chains at the 6-amino group:

6-Aminopenicillanic acid (6-APA)

Benzylpenicillin (penicillin G)

Discovery of penicillin as the substance responsible for the powerful antibacterial activity displayed by the mould Penicillium notatum was reported by Fleming in 1929, but it was not until 1940 that the efforts of Florey and his collaborators at Oxford resulted in the isolation of the active material. In subsequent studies into the chemical nature of penicillin it became apparent that the product derived from industrial fermentations of Penicillium chrysogenum was in fact a family of closely related compounds differing only in the nature of the acyl side-chain. These natural penicillins consisted of penicillins F (pentenylpenicillin), G (benzylpenicillin), K (heptylpenicillin) and X (p-hydroxybenzylpenicillin). From this family, benzylpenicillin (penicillin G) was selected as the penicillin of choice on the basis of biological properties and ease of commercial production.

The limitations of benzylpenicillin as an antibacterial agent soon led to efforts to produce novel penicillins with superior properties to the naturally occurring substance. An early approach was the addition to the fermentation of acidic side-chain precursors that could be assimilated by the mould during biosynthesis. The number of side-chain structures that can be introduced in this way is limited and the only penicillin produced by this approach to show any advantage over penicillin G was phenoxymethylpenicillin (penicillin V), derived from fermentations to which phenoxyacetic acid had been added as a precursor. The important properties of potent antibacterial activity combined with acid stability and improved oral absorption compared to penicillin G ensured the development of penicillin V as a clinically useful agent.

Another approach was the preparation of the first semi-synthetic penicillins by substitution by chemical means of the p-hydroxy group of the naturally occurring penicillin X (p-hydroxybenzylpenicillin), but none of the derivatives synthesized was found to be superior to penicillin G. This line of research was pursued later, also unsuccessfully, in a programme of work to prepare novel penicillins by modification of the amino group of p-aminobenzylpenicillin. Although failing in its original objective to produce semi-synthetic penicillins of clinical utility, the programme was of great significance in leading to the identification in 1957 of the penicillin nucleus in fermentations carried out in the absence of side-chain precursors. The compound, 6-aminopenicillanic acid (6-APA), was first isolated and produced as a naturally occurring substance in fermentations of P. chrysogenum but was later obtained more readily by removal of the side-chain of benzylpenicillin by microbial enzymes or by chemical means and which is now the basis of the commercial production of the material.

The significance of the discovery of 6-APA is that there is almost no limit to the number of semi-synthetic penicillins that can be prepared by the addition of acyl side-chain structures in the 6-amino group of the molecule, and since 1959 thousands of novel structures have been reported in the literature. Apart from penicillin G and penicillin V the penicillins in clinical use are all derivatives of 6-APA, which display advantages over benzylpenicillin in one or more characteristics in terms of antibacterial activity, stability to bacterial β-lactamases or pharmacokinetic properties. Substantial research programmes to develop novel penicillins by further modifications of the penicillin molecule have been disappointing, yielding only two clinically useful

Table 15.1 *Classification of penicillins on the basis of antibacterial spectra*

Group 1: Benzylpenicillin and its long-acting parenteral forms
• Benzylpenicillin
• Benethamine penicillin
• Benzathine penicillin
• Clemizole penicillin
• Procaine penicillin
Group 2: Orally absorbed penicillins similar to benzylpenicillin
• Azidocillin
Phenoxypenicillins:
• Phenethicillin
• Phenoxymethyl penicillin (penicillin V)
• Propicillin
Group 3: Anistaphylococcal β-lactamase-stable penicillins
Isoxazolyl penicillins:
• Cloxacillin
• Dicloxacillin
• Flucloxacillin
• Oxacillin
• Methicillin
• Nafcillin
Group 4: Extended-spectrum penicillins
• Ampicillin:
Ampicillin condensates
• Hetacillin
• Metampicillin
Ampicillin esters:
• Bacampicillin
• Lenampicillin
• Pivampicillin
• Talampicillin
• Amoxycillin (amoxicillin):
• Cyclacillin
• Epicillin
• Mecillinam
Mecillinam ester
• Pivmecillinam
Group 5: Penicillins active against *Pseudomonas aeruginosa*
• Apalcillin
• Aspoxicillin
Acylureidopenicillins:
• Azlocillin
• Mezlocillin
• Piperacillin
Group 6: β-Lactamase-resistant penicillins
• Temocillin

compounds: mecillinam, in which the side-chain is joined in an amidine linkage; and temocillin, in which a 6-methoxy group has been incorporated in the β-lactam ring. In recent years research emphasis in the β-lactam field has switched from penicillins to other β-lactams, notably the cephalosporins, cephamycins and carbapenems (p. 307) and the development of novel penams appears to have come to a halt.

Essentially, the objectives of early research programmes initiated following the isolation of the penicillin nucleus were three-fold:

1. Synthesis of narrow-spectrum penicillins similar to benzylpenicillin in activity but with superior oral absorption characteristics.
2. Preparation of penicillins stable to staphylococcal β-lactamase and active against penicillin-resistant staphylococci.
3. Development of penicillins with broader spectra of antibacterial activity than benzylpenicillin.

The first two objectives have been achieved to a significant extent, but less so in the case of the third, in that the extended-spectrum penicillins currently available are largely inactive against β-lactamase-producing bacteria. Despite substantial research efforts, only one compound of the many synthesized, temocillin, a modified penicillin, has displayed sufficient activity against β-lactamase-producing Gram-negative bacilli to achieve clinical use. The large number of semi-synthetic penicillins in clinical usage may be conveniently divided into five groups on the basis of their antibacterial spectra. These are listed in Table 15.1 which also includes a group comprising long-acting preparations of benzylpenicillin, making six groups in all.

Mode of action

The target sites for penicillins and other β-lactam antibiotics are cell-wall synthesizing enzymes located in the cytoplasmic membrane. The enzymes bind covalently to penicillins and are known as 'penicillin-binding proteins' or, more commonly, PBPs. All pathogenic bacteria possess PBPs and hence are potentially susceptible to penicillins depending upon the affinity of the target enzymes of the particular bacterial strain. However, other factors also come into play and the antibacterial effects displayed by a penicillin typically result from a combination of binding to PBPs, stability to β-lactamases and ability to penetrate the bacterial cell wall. PBPs are not encountered in mammalian cells, which accounts for the low toxicity of penicillins and the consequent clinical popularity of this class of antibiotics.

Gram-positive cocci, Gram-negative bacilli and Gram-positive bacilli respond to penicillins in different ways. In staphylococci exposed to concentrations exceeding the minimum inhibitory concentration (MIC), growth occurs at the normal rate until the cell wall is sufficiently weakened to succumb to osmotic lysis. The response of the population is heterogeneous. Most of the cells incur extensive cell wall damage, but others exhibit loss of cell substance without apparent major injury. Bacteria surviving exposure to penicillins, 'persisters', resume growth after a period of dormancy once the antibiotic is removed.

Concentrations around the MIC effectively halt septation in Gram-negative rods, but cell growth continues at a near-normal rate so that the bacilli are transformed into long filaments. At higher concentrations, depending on the species, cells spontaneously lyse without undergoing any obvious morphological change, or transform into sphero-plasts, which may survive as cell-wall deficient forms, or subsequently lyse depending on local osmolality and other factors. These morphological changes and their relation to binding of the drug by penicillin-binding proteins are discussed further in Chapter 2. Because of their mode of action, penicillins can facilitate the access of compounds acting on internal targets, potentiating inhibition or killing, as in classical synergy with aminoglycosides.

Acquired resistance

Bacteria may exhibit resistance to penicillins and other β-lactam antibiotics by one or more mechanisms. In most cases, the resistance of clinical isolates is due to the production of a bacterial enzyme, β-lactamase, that opens the β-lactam ring causing inactivation of the antibiotic. Another resistance mechanism of increasing importance is the production of modified target sites with reduced affinities for β-lactam antibiotics. A third means by which Gram-negative bacteria may display resistance is by modification of the cell wall creating a permeability barrier to the passage of penicillins into the bacterial cell. It is not uncommon for bacteria to display more than one resistance mechanism; one instance is that of methicillin-resistant staphylococci which typically produce β-lactamase but whose resistance is primarily due to altered target sites.

β-Lactamases and resistance

The β-lactamases are a large family of enzymes (see p. 316) produced by many Gram-positive and Gram-negative bacteria and also by legionellae, mycobacteria and nocardia. Bacterial resistance to penicillin due to β-lactamase activity was first demonstrated in a strain of *Escherichia coli* by Abraham and Chain in 1940, soon after isolation of the antibiotic (Table 15.2). The clinical significance of β-lactamase became apparent a few years later with the isolation of β-lactamase-producing clinical isolates of *Staphylococcus aureus* resistant to penicillin. At the time, the frequency of isolation of penicillin-resistant *Staph. aureus* was low, but increased rapidly, and nowadays approximately 90% of *Staph. aureus* causing infections in

Table 15.2 *Chronology of the discovery of β-lactamase-producing bacteria*

1940	*Escherichia coli*
1944	*Staphylococcus aureus*
1961–64	Enteric bacilli (chromosomal β-lactamase)
1965	Enteric bacilli (plasmid β-lactamase)
1974	*Haemophilus influenzae*
1976	*Neisseria gonorrhoeae*
1977	*Moraxella catarrhalis*
1980	*Haemophilus ducreyi*
1982	*Enterococcus faecalis*
1983	Enterobacteriaceae (extended spectrum enzymes)
1988	*Neisseria meningitidis*

community and hospital practice are β-lactamase-producing strains.

With the advent in the early 1960s of the broad-spectrum penicillins, ampicillin and carbenicillin, it became evident that the resistance of Gram-negative bacilli to these agents was most often associated with β-lactamase production. Most aerobic and anaerobic Gram-negative bacilli were discovered to produce chromosomally-mediated β-lactamases characteristic of each species, which accounted for the intrinsic resistance of organisms such as *Bacteroides fragilis*, *Klebsiella pneumoniae*, enterobacteria species and *Serratia marcescens* to benzylpenicillin and ampicillin. The discovery in 1965 that β-lactamases could be mediated by plasmids and readily transferred by conjugation among Gram-negative bacilli raised the spectre of widespread dissemination among Gram-negative bacteria including species not previously known to possess the enzyme. This prediction has been largely fulfilled, and plasmid-mediated β-lactamase-producing isolates of Gram-negative bacilli are currently a major and increasing clinical problem. For instance, when ampicillin was first developed, approximately 90% of strains of *Escherichia coli* were susceptible to the antibiotic; nowadays, 50% or more of isolates of *Esch. coli* in general practice and in hospitals possess plasmid-mediated β-lactamases conferring resistance to ampicillin and other β-lactam antibiotics. In addition, β-lactamase-producing strains of *Haemophilus influenzae*, *Haemophilus ducreyi*, *Moraxella catarrhalis* and *Neisseria gonorrhoeae*, which were unknown before the mid-1970s, are now common causes of infection. More recently, β-lactamase-producing strains of *Enterococcus faecalis* and *Neisseria meningitidis* have been described, but are as yet compara-tively uncommon.

The spread and appearance of new β-lactamases has generally followed the development and usage of novel β-lactam antibiotics, as is evidenced by the appearance of extended spectrum β-lactamases (see p. 319), variants of common plasmid-mediated β-lactamases, which have been selected as a result of the extensive usage of the third-generation cephalosporins. Novel β-lactamases conferring resistance to carbapenems have been isolated recently and may be expected to present yet another problem to the clinician.

Altered target sites

β-Lactam antibiotics function by inhibiting the terminal stages of peptidoglycan synthesis leading to the development of a weakened wall and eventual lysis of the bacterial cell. The target sites are transpeptidase and carboxypeptidase enzymes that catalyse cross-linking and the penicillins bind covalently with these PBPs. Several PBPs, frequently from four to seven in number, are present in most bacterial species and resistance to penicillins may be acquired by modifications in one or more of the PBPs, leading to a decrease in the affinity of the lethal targets for the antibiotics.

The most important clinical examples arising from modified PBPs include methicillin-resistant staphylococci, penicillin-resistant pneumococci and ampicillin-resistant enterococci, but this mechanism is responsible also for low level penicillin resistance in *H. influenzae*, *N. gonorrhoeae* and viridans streptococci. Methicillin-resistant strains of *Staph. aureus* (MRSA) are considered to be resistant to all β-lactam antibiotics and are frequently multiply-resistant strains, susceptible only to vancomycin or teicoplanin. The prevalence of MRSA is variable and is largely confined to hospitals, where its appearance can cause severe problems, including the closure of wards and units and a halt to patient transfer.

Methicillin-resistance is reported to be even higher amongst *Staphylococcus epidermidis* and other coagulase-negative staphylococci, which are now responsible for up to 25% of nosocomial bloodstream infections.

Until comparatively recently, clinical isolates of *Streptococcus pneumoniae* were considered to be uniformly susceptible to penicillin, but this perception has changed dramatically. The prevalence of pneumococci with reduced susceptibility to penicillins and other β-lactams varies world-wide, but is high in some countries and may be rising. National and international surveys reported in 1990 found the frequency of isolation of penicillin-resistant pneumococci to be 51% in Hungary, 44% in Spain and 12% in France, falling to 4% in the USA and 2% in the UK. Most isolates are deemed to show a low level of resistance (penicillin MIC 0.1–0.5 mg/l), but the frequency of isolation of pneumococci with high level resistance (penicillin MIC >1.0 mg/l) appears to be on the increase.

As was the case with the pneumococcus, enterococci were perceived always to be susceptible to ampicillin and benzylpenicillin but resistant strains are being encountered with increasing frequency. Resistance is comparatively uncommon among the most common species, *Ent. faecalis*, apart from a small number of reports describing β-lactamase-producing strains, but high level resistance to penicillins is being observed routinely among *Enterococcus faecium* the next most clinically important species. Unlike *Ent. faecalis*, the resistance of *Ent. faecium* is due to modified PBPs. As enterococci are one of the leading causes of nosocomial infection, the spread of penicillin-resistant strains represents a serious therapeutic threat.

Impermeability resistance

The penicillin-binding proteins of Gram-negative bacteria are protected by the outer membrane of the cell wall which can function as a permeability barrier. The passage of β-lactam antibiotics across the outer membrane is facilitated by porin proteins, which act as pores allowing the diffusion of small hydrophobic molecules such as the penicillins. The resistance of Gram-negative bacteria to β-lactam antibiotics may be increased by alterations in porin structure leading to decreased permeability, as can be readily demonstrated in the laboratory. The isolation of clinical porin-deficient mutants of enterobacteriaceae is low apart from a few reports implicating *Salmonella typhimurium* and, more frequently, *S. marcescens*. Impermeability resistance is undoubtedly of greater significance among *Pseudomonas aeruginosa*, which possesses a less permeable membrane, and is probably combined with a low order of chromosomally-mediated β-lactamase activity. Gram-positive bacteria lack an outer membrane and this mechanism of resistance does not apply.

Antibiotic tolerance

Penicillins are bactericidal against growing cultures of most pathogens, but a proportion of strains which are susceptible by MIC criteria are not readily lysed or lose viability at much lower rates even in the presence of high concentrations of antibiotic. The phenomenon has been called 'tolerance' as the penicillins appear to act in a bacteriostatic fashion rather than the normal bactericidal mode. Tolerance appears to be due to the presence of autolysin-defective mutants which are killed more slowly than the parent strains. The incidence among clinical isolates is not clear, but they are found among viridans streptococci, enterococci, pneumococci and staphylococci. The clinical significance of antibiotic tolerance has not been clearly established, but data from experimental endocarditis studies provide evidence showing a clear relationship between degree of tolerance and efficacy of treatment.

Toxicity and side-effects

Much the most important untoward reactions to penicillins are those resulting from hypersensitivity, benzylpenicillin being the most frequent cause of anaphylaxis. There is cross-reaction amongst penicillins (although ampicillin constitutes a special case) and the agent to which the patient reacts is not necessarily the sensitizing agent.

Several different forms of hypersensitivity reaction are described, the allergic basis of some of the rarer ones being disputed. The most severe are immediate anaphylactic reactions which develop within minutes of administration of the drug, producing collapse, nausea, vomiting, dyspnoea and coma which may rapidly end fatally. Less severe forms of the immediate reaction include pruritis, urticaria, angio-oedema, rhinitis, bronchospasm or laryngeal oedema. These may also develop as 'accelerated reactions' within 1–72 h of the administration of the drug. In some patients, there is the delayed development (7–10 days) of 'serum sickness' with urticaria, fever, polyarthralgia and, in some cases, lymphadenopathy and eosinophilia. The commonest manifestation of hypersensitivity is a variety of skin eruptions, usually maculopapular with itching but sometimes urticarial or mixed, and occasionally purpuric. Penicillins should not be applied to the skin as topical preparations are likely to lead to contact dermatitis.

Anaphylaxis is much less common with penicillins other than benzylpenicillin. Ampicillin, however, is much more likely to produce rashes, which may be severe, especially in patients with certain lymphoid disorders, notably infectious mononucleosis. It has been claimed that this propensity is not exhibited to the same degree by amoxycillin, epicillin, cyclacillin or mecillinam.

Allergens

The principal antigen responsible for these reactions is generated by opening the β-lactam ring, allowing the carbonyl group to react with the amino groups of proteins. A similar reaction may occur between penicillin molecules to produce penicillin polymers when the amino group already present (as in ampicillin), or revealed by opening the β-lactam bond of one molecule, reacts with the β-lactam carbonyl group of another molecule. A number of other reactions within and between the molecules can occur, leading to the so-called 'minor determinants' – minor components of the complex mixtures, but potentially important determinants of penicillin allergy. There is evidence that penicillins with different side chains have different sensitizing capacities and lead to different populations of antibodies in treated patients.

The traditional view has been that the antigens responsible for initiating and eliciting penicillin reactions are produced by reactive derivatives of penicillin with normal plasma proteins, but such reactions could also involve bacterial proteins or inflammatory products. Moreover, there are ample opportunities during manufacture of penicillins for reactions between derivatives of the penicillin molecule and proteins present in the fermentation process. Some success has been achieved in reducing allergic reactions by removing potential allergens from benzylpenicillin and ampicillin at the end of the manufacturing process, but there remains considerable disagreement about the relative importance of the components of these complex mixtures and of their generation outside and inside the body.

Detection and control

Many patients without a history of penicillin allergy have circulating antibodies to the drug, and their presence is of no prognostic value. The use of skin tests to detect patients likely to suffer reactions to penicillins is also far from being universally accepted as reliable. The use of benzylpenicillin itself is generally regarded as hazardous, since it may lead to a severe reaction in the highly susceptible patient and may sensitize the previously non-allergic individual. For this reason, various reagents have been developed which will detect, but not elicit, allergy. Principal amongst them is penicilloyl-polylysine in which the amino groups of an artificial peptide are virtually saturated with penicilloyl residues. As there are other antigens concerned, however, it cannot be expected that a single reagent will detect all allergic patients or that patients will react equally to various antigens. It is claimed that mixtures of benzylpenicillin and penicilloyl-polylysine will detect virtually all allergic patients, and excellent predictive performance has been claimed for penicilloyl-polylysine plus a 'minor determinant' mixture. These mixtures are valuable tools in the hands of experts but are of very limited value in ordinary practice, where the principal safeguard is careful questioning about possible penicillin allergy (p. 266).

Cross-reactions with cephalosporins

A major interest in early cephalosporins was the belief that they could be safely administered to patients allergic to penicillin. This appears to be true of the majority of patients, but those having a history of penicillin allergy are about four times as likely as those without such a history to react to cephalosporins. However, it must be added that such patients are likely to react to a variety of other drugs. It appears that about 6–9% of patients are cross-allergic to penicillins and cephalosporins, and specific allergy to cephalosporins in the absence of reactions to penicillin also occurs. Our own advice is to avoid the use of cephalosporins in patients who give a clear history of a previous severe reaction to penicillin.

Other reactions

Amongst other uncommon reactions, some may have an allergic basis, including haemolytic anaemia, thrombocytopenic purpura and Stevens–Johnson syndrome. Various other manifestations possibly of allergic origin include vasculitis, haemorrhagic disorders, nephropathies and polymyositis.

Leucopenia has occurred in patients receiving various penicillins including methicillin and piperacillin. Neutropenia in patients treated with benzylpenicillin for bacterial endocarditis was related both to high dosage (18 g/day) and to low neutrophil counts before treatment. Prolonged bleeding times due to platelet abnormalities have been noted, particularly with carboxypenicillins and, to a lesser extent, with acylureidopenicillins. Various nephrotoxic manifestations have been described with carbenicillin, dicloxacillin and methicillin, and reversible abnormalities of liver function tests with carboxypenicillins and less frequently acylureidopenicillins.

Because penicillins are given in large doses as sodium salts, sodium overload and hypokalaemia may develop, particularly with the disodium salts of extended spectrum penicillins. Large doses of penicillins, especially in patients with impaired renal function, may result in convulsions. Access to the CNS of neurotoxic concentrations is related to lipophilicity and protein binding of the compounds.

Further information

Anderson J A 1986 Cross-sensitivity to cephalosporins in patients allergic to penicillin. *Pediatric Infectious Diseases* 5: 557–561

Barrons R W, Murray K M, Richey R M 1992 Populations at risk for penicillin-induced seizures. *Annals of Pharmacotherapy* 26: 26–29

Bint A J 1980 Esters of penicillins – are they hepatoxic? *Journal of Antimicrobial Chemotherapy* 6: 697–699

Blanca M, Fernandez J, Miranda A et al 1989 Cross-reactivity between penicillins and cephalosporins: clinical and immunological studies. *Journal of Allergy and Clinical Immunology* 83: 381–385

Brenner S, Wolf R, Ruocco V 1993 Drug induced pemphigus. I. A survey. *Clinical Dermatology* 11: 501–505

Bruynzeel D P, von Blomberg-van der Flier M, Scheper R J, van Ketel W G, de Haas P 1985 Penicillin allergy and the relevance of epicutaneous tests. *Dermatologica* 171: 429–434

Cullmann W, Dick W 1989 Induction potency of various beta-lactam derivatives in Gram-negative rods. *Chemotherapy* 35: 45–53

de Haan P, Bruynzeel P, van Ketel W G 1986 Onset of penicillin rashes: relation between type of penicillin administered and type of immune reactivity. *Allergy* 41: 75–78

Derendorf H 1989 Pharmacokinetic evaluation of β-lactam antibiotics. *Journal of Antimicrobial Chemotherapy* 24: 407–413

Erffmeyer J E 1986 Penicillin allergy. *Clinical Reviews in Allergy* 4: 171–188

Fass R J, Copelan E A, Brandt J T, Moeschberger M L, Ashton J J 1987 Platelet mediated bleeding caused by broad-spectrum penicillins. *Journal of Infectious Diseases* 155: 1242–1248

Gutmann L, Williamson R, Kitzis M D, Acar J F 1986 Synergism and antagonism in double beta-lactam antibiotic combinations. *American Journal of Medicine* 80 (5C): 21–29

Jarlier V, Nicolas M H, Fournier G, Phillipon A 1988 Extended broad-spectrum beta-lactamases conferring transferable resistance to newer beta-lactam agents in Enterobacteriaceae: hospital prevalence and susceptibility patterns. *Reviews of Infectious Diseases* 10: 867–878

Kim K S 1988 Clinical perspectives on penicillin tolerance. *Journal of Pediatrics* 112: 509–514

Klugman K P 1990 Pneumococcal resistance to antibiotics. *Clinical Microbiology Reviews* 3: 171–196

Leading article 1983 Antimicrobials and haemostasis. *Lancet* i: 510–511

Leitman P S 1988 Pharmacokinetics of antimicrobial drugs in cystic fibrosis. Beta-lactam antibiotics. *Chest* 94 (2 suppl): 115S–120S

Lin R Y 1992 A perspective on penicillin allergy. *Archives of Internal Medicine* 152: 930–937

Livermore D M 1987 Clinical significance of beta-lactamase induction and stable derepression in Gram-negative rods. *European Journal of Clinical Microbiology* 6: 439–445

Livermore D M 1991 Mechanisms of resistance to β-lactam antibiotics. *Scandinavian Journal of Antibiotics* 78 (suppl): 7–16

Markowitz M 1985 Long-acting penicillins: historical perspectives. *Pediatric Infectious Diseases* 4: 570–573

Moellering R C Jr, Eliopoulos G M, Allan J D 1986 Beta-lactam/aminoglycoside combination interactions and their mechanisms. *American Journal of Medicine* 80 (5C): 30–34

Møller N E, von Wurden K 1992 Hypersensitivity to semisynthetic penicillins and cross-reactivity with penicillin. *Contact Dermatitis* 26: 351–352

Møller N E, Nielsen B, von Wurden K 1986 Contact dermatitis to semisynthetic penicillins in factory workers. *Contact Dermatitis* 14: 307–311

Moulis H, Vender R J 1994 Antibiotic-associated haemorrhagic colitis. *Journal of Clinical Gastroenterology* 18: 227–231

Mouton R P, Hermans J, Simoons-Smit A M, Hoogkamo-Korstanje J A A, Degener J E, van Klingeren B 1990 Correlations between consumption of antibiotics and methicillin resistance in coagulase negative staphylococci. *Journal of Antimicrobial Chemotherapy* 26: 573–583

Nathwani D, Wood M J 1993 Penicillins. A current review of their clinical pharmacology and therapeutic use. *Drugs* 45: 866–894

Neftel K A, Hauser S P, Muller M R 1985 Inhibition of granulopoiesis in vivo and in vitro by beta-lactam antibiotics. *Journal of Infectious Diseases* 152: 90–98

Olaison L, Alestig K 1990 A prospective study of neutropenia by high doses of β-lactam antibiotics. *Journal of Antimicrobial Chemotherapy* 25: 449–453

O'Leary M R, Smith M S 1986 Penicillin anaphylaxis. *American Journal of Emergency Medicine* 4: 241–247

River Y, Averbuch-Heller L, Weinberger M et al 1994 Antibiotic induced meningitis. *Journal of Neurology, Neurosurgery and Psychiatry* 57: 705–708

Rolinson G N 1989 Beta-lactamase induction and resistance to beta-lactam antibiotics. *Journal of Antimicrobial Chemotherapy* 23: 1–2

Sanders C C 1987 Chromosomal cephalosporinases responsible for multiple resistance to newer beta-lactam antibiotics. *Annual Review of Microbiology* 41: 573–593

Snavely S R, Hodges G R 1984 The neurotoxicity of antibacterial agents. *Annals of Internal Medicine* 101: 92–104

Sogn D D, Evans R 3rd, Shepherd G M et al 1992 Results of the National Institute of Allergy and Infectious Diseases Collaborative Clinical Trial to test the predictive value of skin testing with major and minor penicillin derivatives in hospitalised patients. *Archives of Internal Medicine* 152: 1025–1032

Sutherland R 1993 Bacterial resistance to β-lactam antibiotics; problems and solutions. *Progress in Drug Research* 41: 95–149

Symposium 1988 New developments in resistance to beta-lactam antibiotics among non-fastidious Gram-negative organisms. *Reviews of Infectious Diseases* 10: 677–914

Tipper D J 1985 Mode of action of β-lactam antibiotics. *Pharmacology and Therapeutics* 27: 1–35

Tuomanen E, Durack D T, Tomasz A 1986 Antibiotic tolerance among clinical isolates of bacteria. *Antimicrobial Agents and Chemotherapy* 30: 521–527

Weiss M E, Adkinson N F 1988 Immediate hypersensitivity reactions to penicillin and related antibiotics. *Clinical Allergy* 18: 515–540

Group 1: Benzylpenicillin and its long-acting parenteral forms

Benzylpenicillin, the first natural penicillin, is poorly absorbed by mouth and must be given by injection. The plasma half-life is short and in order to prolong its effect benzylpenicillin was first mixed with oils or waxes, so that the release of penicillin from intramuscular injection sites was retarded. Later, insoluble salts of penicillin were prepared which similarly act as intramuscular depots for the release of penicillin into the circulation. Three such repository penicillins are in common use: procaine penicillin (also available in some countries as an oily suspension with aluminium monostearate), benethamine penicillin and benzathine penicillin. Others are clemizole penicillin, designed to combine slow release with antihistaminic properties of clemizole, and penethicillin, penicillin diethylaminoethyl ester hydriodide which is no longer commercially available, but was of interest because of a particular capacity to penetrate into lung tissue.

Antimicrobial activity and systemic untoward effects of the long-acting forms are due to the liberation of benzylpenicillin. Injection, particularly of benzathine penicillin, may produce local pain or tenderness, and accidental intravascular injection of procaine penicillin may produce acute agitation, hallucinations and collapse. It should not be given intravenously.

Long-acting forms have their principal use in the treatment of gonorrhoea, syphilis, and in the follow-on treatment of patients requiring prolonged therapy after initial treatment with benzylpenicillin and in prophylaxis, particularly of rheumatic fever.

BENZYLPENICILLIN

Archetypal penicillin produced by *P. chrysogenum*; supplied as the potassium or sodium salt.

Antimicrobial activity

Benzylpenicillin is active against almost all Gram-positive pathogens, Gram-negative cocci and some other Gram-negative bacteria, but it is very labile to bacterial β-lactamases and so β-lactamase-producing strains are resistant. Aerobic and anaerobic Gram-negative bacilli are largely resistant. Its activity against common pathogenic bacteria is shown in Table 15.3.

Most species of streptococci are highly susceptible (MIC 0.03 mg/l), but group B streptococci, an important cause of neonatal infections, are about 10-fold less sensitive. Enterococci are more resistant than other Gram-positive cocci, but group D non-enterococcal streptococci are fully susceptible. Wild-type strains of *Staph. aureus* were originally highly susceptible to benzlpenicillin, but most clinical isolates are now β-lactamase-producing strains resistant to the antibiotic. Non-β-lactamase-producing strains of coagulase-negative staphylococci are susceptible, but most clinical isolates of *Staph. epidermidis* are penicillin-resistant strains. A small number of isolates of the urinary pathogen *Staphylococcus saprophyticus* display intermediate resistance, possibly as a result of β-lactamase production. Other Gram-positive organisms susceptible to benzylpenicillin include *Bacillus anthracis*, *Erysipelothrix rhusiopthiae* and *Listeria monocytogenes*. The spirochaetes *Borrelia burgdorferi* and *Treponema pallidum* are also considered to be susceptible.

The aerobic Gram-negative cocci *N. gonorrhoeae* and *N. meningitidis* are highly susceptible to benzylpenicillin, but β-lactamase-producing strains of gonococci are common. *H. influenzae* and *Moraxella (Branhamella) catarrhalis* are inhibited by relatively low concentrations but are usually regarded as being penicillin-resistant, whereas *H. ducreyi* is considered to be susceptible. *Pasteurella multocida* and *Streptobacillus moniliformis* are also susceptible; *Legionella pneumophila* is inhibited by 0.5–2.0 mg/ml, but benzylpenicillin is inactive in tests against intracellular legionellae. The Enterobacteriaceae are almost all resistant to benzylpenicillin as a result of β-lactamase production or the impermeability of the bacterial cell wall to the antibiotic. However, some strains of *Esch. coli* and many strains of *Pr. mirabilis*, *Salmonella typhi* and *Salm. paratyphi* are inhibited by 8 mg/l. Most other aerobic Gram-negative bacilli, including *Brucella* spp., *V. cholerae*, *Ps. aeruginosa* and *Stenotrophomonas (Xanthomonas) maltophilia* are also resistant. Other resistant organisms include mycobacteria, mycoplasma, *Nocardia* spp. rickettsiae, fungi and protozoa.

Anaerobic Gram-positive cocci are very susceptible, and non-sporing Gram-positive bacilli including *Actinomyces israelii* are also susceptible. Most strains of *Clostridium perfringens* and many strains of other clostridial species are susceptible, but resistance is observed. Anaerobic Gram-negative bacilli vary in their sensitivity. The *B. fragilis* group is resistant as the result of β-lactamase action, but the majority of *Prevotella melaninogenica* (*Bacteroides melaninogenicus*) and Fusobacteria are susceptible.

Benzylpenicillin is bactericidal to growing organisms, the effect being maximum at about four times the MIC, above which no increase in killing occurs. Against many strains of

Table 15.3   *Activity of benzylpenicillin and group 2 penicillins against common pathogenic bacteria: MIC (mg/l)*

	Benzylpenicillin	Azidocillin	Phenethicillin	Phenoxymethyl-penicillin
Staph. aureus	0.03	0.03	0.06	0.06
Str. pyogenes (group A)	0.01	0.01	0.06	0.03
Str. pneumoniae	0.01–0.03	0.06	0.06	0.03
Ent. faecalis	2	1	4–8	4–8
N. gonorrhoeae	0.01–0.03	0.01	0.1	0.03–0.1
N. meningitidis	0.03		0.1	0.06
H. influenzae	1.0	0.25	4–8	4–8
Esch. coli	64	64	R	R
K. pneumoniae	R	R	R	R
Pr. mirabilis	4–8	32	R	32–64
Proteus indole + spp.	R	R	R	R
Enterobacter spp.	R	R	R	R
Salm. typhi	8	32	R	64
Shigella spp.	64	32	R	R
Ser. marcescens	R	R	R	R
Citrobacter spp.	R	R	R	R
Ps. aeruginosa	R	R	R	R
B. fragilis	32			

R (resistant) MIC ≥ 128 mg/l.

Staph. aureus and *Ent. faecalis*, further increase in the concentration actually reduces the death rate, a paradoxical zone phenomenon called the 'Eagle effect' after its describer. Killing of highly susceptible Gram-positive cocci seldom proceeds to extinction, there remaining significant numbers of survivors called 'persisters' which on retesting are fully susceptible. Combination with aminoglycosides results in pronounced bacterial synergy due to the permeation effects of the penicillin on the cell wall. Some strains of staphylococci, streptococci, including group B, and pneumococci show very large numbers of survivors so that there is a large discrepancy between the MIC and MBC, the phenomenon known as 'tolerance' (p. 14).

Acquired resistance

Most strains of *Staph. aureus* isolated in general practice and in hospitals world-wide are β-lactamase-producing strains resistant to benzylpenicillin and often harbouring resistance to other antistaphylococcal antibiotics. β-Lactamase-producing strains of *Ent. faecalis* have been isolated since 1993 from various locations in the USA and South America; the β-lactamase appears to be of staphylococcal origin and raises the prospect of possible spread to streptococci. β-Lactamase production also appears to be on the increase among clostridial species formerly susceptible to penicillin.

Until comparatively recently, clinical isolates of *Str. pneumoniae* were considered to be uniformly susceptible to benzylpenicillin, and reports in 1967 and 1970 of the isolation in Australia and New Guinea of strains with reduced susceptibility to penicillin were largely disregarded. Attention was focused on this topic with the report from South Africa in 1977 of strains of pneumococci with intermediate or high-level resistance to benzylpenicillin causing serious infections including meningitis, pneumonia and septicaemia. Many of these strains were resistant to other antibiotics and some were susceptible only to rifampicin and vancomycin. The emergence of penicillin-resistant pneumococci has now been described world-wide, but the prevalence is variable from one part to another. In Hungary and Spain, 40–50% of isolates of *Str. pneumoniae* have been reported to be resistant to benzylpenicillin, whereas in the UK and USA the prevalence is of the order of 2–4%. Penicillin resistance has been found in a wide range of serotypes of *Str. pneumoniae*, but high-level and multiple resistance is restricted mainly to a few, including 6, 9, 14, 19 and 23. The resistance of pneumococci to penicillin has been shown to be associated with alterations in the specific target sites of PBPs. All strains of pneumococci resistant to penicillin also demonstrate reduced susceptibility to other β-lactams, but in some cases to a lower degree, encouraging the use of third-generation cephalosporins in treatment.

Penicillin-resistant strains of the clinically important pathogen *Ent. faecium* are being encountered with increasing frequency, and resistance is attributed to modified PBPs with reduced affinity for penicillin. Viridans group streptococci are also increasingly resistant to benzylpenicillin, and serious infections due to penicillin-resistant strains have been reported. Their resistance is associated with altered PBPs, particularly PBP 2b which has been shown to be identical to the PBP 2b of *Str. pneumoniae*, suggesting transfer between the two species.

Strains of *N. gonorrhoeae* with reduced susceptibility to benzylpenicillin appeared more than 20 years ago and the degree of resistance gradually increased from MICs of 0.06 mg/l to MICs in excess of 2 mg/l. The mechanism of resistance has been shown to be due to the production of modified PBPs with reduced sensitivity to β-lactam antibiotics. These strains became widespread, particularly in South-East Asia, and often became multiresistant. Even after the emergence of these strains with reduced susceptibility, gonorrhoea could still be treated with high doses of penicillin, but in 1976 and 1977 β-lactamase-producing strains of *N. gonorrhoeae* completely resistant to benzylpenicillin were isolated in Africa and the Philippines. These strains had acquired plasmid-mediated TEM-1 β-lactamase (p. 319) but appeared to have arisen independently, as the TEM-1 β-lactamase positive isolates from the Far East possessed a conjugative plasmid that facilitated its spread and was lacking from the strains originally isolated in Africa and Europe. The frequency of isolation of β-lactamase-producing strains of *N. gonorrhoeae* is usually reported to be lower in Europe and the USA than in other parts of the world, but this may be a misconception because of the variability of isolation. For instance, frequencies ranging from 2% to 41% isolation of β-lactamase-producing strains have been reported from different centres in the UK. In many areas of the world, benzylpenicillin can no longer be considered for empirical treatment of gonorrhoea. The same is also true for another sexually-transmitted pathogen, *H. ducreyi*, formerly susceptible to benzylpenicillin, which has acquired TEM-1 β-lactamase so that most isolates now display high level resistance. β-Lactamase-producing strains of *H. influenzae* mediating TEM-1 β-lactamases are becoming increasingly common, but great variation exists in different areas.

Some mammalian enzymes are capable of destroying penicillin and the presence of such enzymes in exudate has been claimed on occasion to be responsible for treatment failure.

Pharmacokinetics

Benzylpenicillin is unstable in acid and destroyed in the stomach. As a result, plasma concentrations obtained after oral administration are irregular and unreliable and further depressed by administration with food. Absorption may be better in the elderly due to the relative frequency of achlorhydria. Unabsorbed drug is largely degraded by colonic bacteria and very little activity remains in the faeces. After i.m. injection, absorption occurs within a few minutes to produce mean peak plasma concentrations after 0.3 and 1 MU around 2 and 12 mg/l, respectively. The plasma half-life is short, about 30 min, although there is considerable individual variation.

The mean end-infusion plasma concentration after 3 g (5 MU) by i.v. infusion over 3–5 min is around 400 mg/l. By continuous infusion over 6 h, the same dose produced steady state levels of 12–20 mg/l. Doses of 1.2 g (2 MU) 2 hourly or 1.8 g (3 MU) 3 hourly produced average values around 20 mg/l.

In the newborn, i.m. doses of 25 or 50 mg/kg produced mean peak plasma levels around 25 or 35 mg/l, respectively. The plasma half-life decreased with age, falling from 3.2 h in the first week to 1.7 h in the second and 1.4 h in the third. It is absorbed from serous cavities, joints and the subarachnoid space. It is not absorbed following applications to the skin which should, in any case, be avoided because of the likelihood of sensitization. Between 45 and 65% is bound to plasma protein. About 40% is metabolized in the liver, mainly to penicilloic acid.

Distribution

It is widely distributed, penetrating into the pleural, pericardial, peritoneal and synovial fluids. Low concentrations appear in saliva and in maternal milk. It does not enter uninflamed bone or the normal cerebrospinal fluid (CSF). Its entry is limited by its low pK_a (2.6) which results in its almost complete ionization and very low lipid/water partition coefficient at pH 7.4. What does enter the CSF is efficiently removed partly through the arachnoid villi but principally through active secretion by the choroid plexus. When the meninges are inflamed, the concentrations obtained in CSF are very variable, around 5% of the plasma level, active transport via the choroid plexus out of the CSF being depressed by meningitis. It is also reduced by probenecid, which inhibits the transport of weak acids from the CSF, giving rise to 2- to 3-fold increases in CSF concentrations – a potential cause of toxicity if large doses are given. In uraemia, accumulated organic acids may enter the CSF and compete for transport of penicillin, causing the concentration to reach convulsive levels.

About 10% of the distributed drug enters erythrocytes, where the concentration may slightly exceed that of the plasma and the lower rate of release from the cells (elimination half-life 50–60 min) helps to maintain the tail of penicillin concentration. It diffuses into wound exudates and experimental transudates when the serum level is high and persists there longer than in the serum. Average sputum levels 2 h after 1 MU are 0.3 mg/l. It enters glandular secretions and the fetal circulation, whence it is excreted in increased concentrations into the amniotic fluid.

Excretion

Concentrations 2–4 times those of the plasma are found in bile, but 60–90% is excreted in the urine, largely in the first hour, 90% by tubular secretion. This can be blocked by probenecid, with consequent doubling of the peak concentration and prolongation of the plasma half-life. Claims that this results partly from confining the drug to the vascular space have not been confirmed. Other drugs, especially organic acids, including aspirin, sulphonamides and some nonsteroidal anti-inflammatory drugs and diuretics, may prolong the half-life, which naturally increases with decrease of renal function including that which occurs with advancing age.

Toxicity and side-effects

Benzylpenicillin has almost no toxicity for man in the ordinary sense, except for the nervous system, to which it is normally denied access (p. 744), where it is one of the most active convulsants amongst the β-lactams. CSF concentrations in excess of 10 mg/l are associated with drowsiness, occasional hallucinations, hyperreflexia, loss of consciousness, and myoclonic movements progressing to focal convulsions which may proceed to coma and death. The manifestations are due to a direct effect on the cortex and usually appear 12–72 h after institution of treatment. Toxic levels may reach the CSF in three ways: (1) by intrathecal injection – and the dose should never exceed 20 000 units in the adult or 5000 units in the child as a single daily dose; (2) in the presence of meningitis where high blood levels produced by large doses can reach the CSF more readily, particularly if renal function is impaired or probenecid is administered; and (3) excessive dosage (100 MU/day or more) or more modest dosage in the presence of unidentified predisposing factors or impaired renal function.

Massive intravenous doses of the sodium or potassium salts can lead to severe electrolyte disturbance. Administration of large amounts of sodium salts produces a large load of both sodium and non-resorbable anion in the distal renal tubule which can lead to significant potassium loss. Similarly, in patients treated with large doses of potassium salt (100 MU/day or more) hyponatraemia, hyperkalaemia and metabolic acidosis can develop. The severity of these effects is determined not only by the sodium load but by the osmotic diuretic effect of the drug and its action in depressing renal tubular excretion of potassium.

Thrombocytopenia and platelet dysfunction resulting in coagulopathy and involving several different mechanisms has been described.

Large doses (40 MU per day i.v. or smaller doses given to patients with impaired renal function) may interfere with platelet function in a manner analogous to that seen with carbenicillin, with resulting coagulation defects which persist for 3–4 days after cessation of therapy.

Allergic reactions

The most dramatic untoward response is anaphylactic shock due to allergy which is discussed in relation to penicillins at large on page 260. Although serious or life-threatening reactions are rare, allergic reactions present a more serious problem with benzylpenicillin than with any other antibiotic. The most dangerous form of drug allergy is acute anaphylactic shock, which may develop within a few minutes to 30 min after administration. It is characterized by profound circulatory collapse, nausea, vomiting, abdominal pain, severe bronchospasm and coma, and may be rapidly fatal. Anaphylaxis is said to occur in 0.005–0.05% of treated patients, with a mortality rate of 10%. Some patients show other manifestations such as arthritis, lymphadenopathy and eosinophilia. If the tissue oedema affects the larynx, the patient is at risk of respiratory obstruction. In addition to these dramatic syndromes, there are much more frequent rashes which are usually maculopapular and itchy, but a wide variety of patterns is seen and some patients show a mixture of urticarial and maculopapular elements.

Rashes are said to occur in 1–7% of patient courses of penicillin. Contact dermatitis or local swelling and oedema can occur at sites of topical application. Although reactions can occur after any route of administration, the severe forms are much more common after injections than after oral administration. A serum sickness form of allergy can arise 7–10 days after first treatment (earlier in previously sensitized patients) in which fever, malaise, urticaria, joint pains, lymphadenopathy and possibly angioneurotic oedema, sometimes erythema nodosum and, rarely, Stevens–Johnson syndrome occur.

Some patients develop allergic reactions only after repeated administration of penicillin, but in others, reactions develop on the first occasion penicillin is prescribed. The history of previous antibiotic use if often uncertain but, even when a reliable account is obtainable, non-medicinal exposure to penicillin may have occurred, for example to aerosols of penicillin in the environment of patients receiving the drug, or by ingestion of penicillin in milk. Preparations for injection should always be freshly made.

Detection and control

A careful history is the main safeguard against administering penicillin to hypersensitive patients. No entirely adequate in vitro antibody or skin tests exist. Some success has been claimed for skin tests with mixtures containing benzylpeni-

cillin, penicilloate, penilloate and α-benzyl penicilloylamine but even in expert hands, reliable correlation of tests with clinical reactions is not always achieved. In general, the prevention of penicillin allergy must still depend on avoiding its use in patients who say they are allergic to penicillin, even though in many of them the evidence for this belief is tenuous and unreliable.

A significant minority of patients (6–9% has been quoted) allergic to penicillins also react to cephalosporins, which should be avoided in patients with a history of immediate-type penicillin reactions and, if possible, in all patients with a history of penicillin allergy.

The management of penicillin reactions relies on the use of antihistamines, corticosteroids and, in anaphylaxis or dangerous angio-oedema, adrenaline. Desensitization can sometimes be achieved by careful control of treatment in patients for whom penicillin is strongly indicated. Allergic patients may also sometimes be successfully treated with penicillin, where that is much the most appropriate agent, by giving concurrent corticosteroids.

In addition to the generalized allergic reactions, particular organs may be damaged by a variety of immunological mechanisms. Haemolytic anaemia occurs only in patients who have been treated with penicillin before, and again receive a prolonged course of large doses (commonly 20 MU/day) usually for bacterial endocarditis. The haemolysis is due to the action of anti-penicillin immunoglobulin G (IgG) on cells which have absorbed the antibiotic. It can be detected by direct positive antiglobulin reaction. Disruption of bystander red cells not coated with penicillin may occur from attack by liberated activated complement complexes from other cells. Rapid recovery ensues when administration is stopped. A suggestive association between penicillin therapy and the onset of polymyositis has been described. Nephritis, resulting in dysuria, pyuria, proteinuria, azotaemia and histological evidence of nephritis of allergic origin is rarely seen, usually in patients receiving large doses (20–60 MU/day). Milder forms occur in which the other manifestations are seen without azotaemia.

A few cases of neutropenia have been reported which appear to be related to total dose, usually in excess of 150 MU. It can be very severe, but in the majority of patients, recovery occurs within a few days of withdrawal of treatment. In most cases, it is associated with fever and allergic rash. As with other β-lactam-induced neutropenia, the bone marrow shows maturation arrest.

The Jarisch–Herxheimer reaction is seen almost entirely in patients with spirochaetal diseases, notably syphilis (where it occurs in up to 70% of patients, depending on the stage of the disease), leptospirosis and relapsing fever treated with penicillin but also with other agents. Fever, malaise and headache develop within a few hours of starting treatment due to the release of endotoxin from damaged spirochaetes. In patients with syphilis the reaction can be associated with exacerbation of the lesions, with potentially serious consequences when they involve the cardiovascular or nervous systems. The frequency and degree of the reaction in late syphilis has been much disputed, but it is customary to give prednisolone for a few days before initiating treatment in the unproven expectation that the reaction will be ameliorated.

Clinical use

It has been the drug of choice in many common infections with streptococci (pp. 584, 735), pneumococci (p. 748 – except in those parts of the world where resistant strains are encountered), meningococci (p. 747), penicillin-susceptible gonococci and non-penicillinase-producing staphylococci. It is not effective in eradicating pharyngeal carriage of *N. meningitidis* (p. 747). It is also the agent of choice for the treatment and prophylaxis of clostridial infection (p. 737) including the support treatment of tetanus (p. 739) and in the prophylaxis of rheumatic fever (p. 677). It has been used in the treatment of infection due to *Listeria*, but ampicillin is preferred. Its role in the treatment of gonorrhoea is discussed on page 818. In the treatment of streptococcal endocarditis it is used alone where the organism is readily killed in vitro, and otherwise in combination with an appropriate aminoglycoside (p. 701).

Because it is active against many anaerobes other than *B. fragilis*, it is effective in periodontal, Vincent's and pulmonary infections, but not in those of pelvic or large bowel origin.

Amongst rare indications are spirochaetal infections (leptospirosis (p. 887), both varieties of rat bite fever (p. 886), syphilis (p. 816) and yaws), actinomycosis (p. 739), anthrax (p. 737), and diphtheria (p. 677).

Preparations and dosage

Proprietary name: Crystapen.

Preparation: Injection.

Dosage: Adults, i.m., i.v., 60 mg to 1.2 g daily in 2–4 divided doses; adult meningitis, up to 14.4 g/day may be given in divided doses; bacterial endocarditis, 4.8 g/day or more in divided doses. Children 1 month to 12 years, 10–20 mg/kg per day in 4 divided doses; newborn infants, 30 mg/kg per day in 2 divided doses in first few days of life, then in 3–4 divided doses. Meningitis in children and neonates: neonates ≤7 days old, 60–90 mg/kg per day in 2 divided doses; neonates >7 days old, 90–120 mg/kg per day as 3 divided doses; children 1 month to 12 years, 150–300 mg/kg per day in 4–6 divided doses.

Intrathecal, see manufacturers literature.

Widely available.

Further information

de Swarte R D 1982 Penicillin allergy skin tests. *Journal of the American Medical Association* 247: 1745

Ducas J, Robson H G 1981 Cerebrospinal fluid penicillin levels during therapy for latent syphilis. *Journal of the American Medical Association* 246: 2583–2584

Farber B F, Eliopoulos G M, Ward J I, Ruoff K, Moellering R C Jr 1983 Resistance to penicillin-streptomycin synergy among clinical isolates of viridans streptococci *Antimicrobial Agents and Chemotherapy* 24: 871–875

Farber B F, Eliopoulos G M, Ward J I, Ruoff K L, Syriopoulou V, Moellering R C Jr 1983 Multiply resistant viridans streptococci: susceptibility to beta-lactam antibiotics and comparison of penicillin-binding protein patterns. *Antimicrobial Agents and Chemotherapy* 24: 702–705

Hannedouche T, Fillastre J P 1987 Penicillin-induced hypersensitivity vasculitides. *Journal of Antimicrobial Chemotherapy* 20: 3–5

Holbrook W P, Olafsdóttir D, Magnússon H B, Benediktsdottir E 1988 Penicillin tolerance among oral streptococci. *Journal of Medical Microbiology* 27: 17–22

Kim K S 1988 Clinical perspectives on penicillin tolerance. *Journal of Pediatrics* 112: 509–514

Kourtópoulos H, Holm S E, Norrby S R 1983 The effects of irradiation and probenecid on cerebrospinal fluid transport of penicillin. *Journal of Antimicrobial Chemotherapy* 11: 251–255

Neftel K A, Walti M, Spengler H, de Weck A L 1982 Effect of storage of penicillin-G solutions on sensitization to penicillin-G intravenous administration. *Lancet* i: 986–988

Nicholls P J 1980 Neurotoxicity of penicillin. *Journal of Antimicrobial Chemotherapy* 6: 161–164

Oppenheim B, Koornhof H J, Austrian R 1986 Antibiotic resistant pneumococcal disease in children at Baragwanath Hospital, Johannesburg. *Pediatric Infectious Diseases* 5: 520–524

Overbosch D, van Gulpen C, Hermans J, Mattie H 1988 The effect of probenecid on the renal tubular excretion of benzylpenicillin. *British Journal of Clinical Pharmacology* 25: 51–58

Ressler C, Mendelson L M 1987 Skin test for diagnosis of penicillin allergy – current status. *Annals of Allergy* 59: 167–170

Sáez-Nieto J A, Fontanals D, Garcia de Jalon J et al 1987 Isolation of *Neisseria meningitidis* strains with increase of penicillin minimal inhibitory concentrations. *Epidemiology and Infection* 99: 463–469

Schoth P E, Wolters E C 1987 Penicillin concentration in serum and CSF during high-dose intravenous treatment for neurosyphilis. *Neurology* 37: 1214–1216

Shenep J L, Feldman S, Thornton D 1986 Evaluation for endotoxaemia in patients receiving penicillin therapy for secondary syphilis. *Journal of the American Medical Association* 256: 388–390

Stark B J, Earl H S, Gross G N, Lumry W R, Goodman E L, Sullivan T J 1987 Acute and chronic desensitization of penicillin-allergic patients using oral penicillin. *Journal of Allergy and Clinical Immunology* 79: 523–532

Sullivan T J 1982 Cardiac disorders in penicillin-induced anaphylaxis. Association with intravenous epinephrine therapy. *Journal of the American Medical Association* 248: 2161–2162

Thin R N, Barlow D, Eykyn S, Philips I 1983 Imported penicillinase producing *Neisseria gonorrhoeae* becomes epidemic in London. *British Journal of Venereal Diseases* 59: 364–368.

Compounds liberating benzylpenicillin

These include benethamine penicillin, benzathine penicillin, clemizole penicillin and procaine penicillin.

BENETHAMINE PENICILLIN

A poorly soluble (1 : 5000 in water) derivative of benzylpenicillin for intramuscular injection: 1 g is approximately equivalent to 600 mg benzylpenicillin. Its antimicrobial activity and side-effects are those of liberated benzylpenicillin. A single dose will provide a low concentration of penicillin in the plasma sufficient to inhibit the most sensitive organisms, such as haemolytic streptococci, for 4–5 days. It is generally given in a mixture with benzylpenicillin and procaine penicillin to achieve immediate and prolonged effects. It is used in the single-dose treatment of gonorrhoea due to penicillin-susceptible strains and for the prophylaxis of rheumatic fever.

Preparations
Available in combination with other penicillins.
Limited availability, not available in the UK.

Further information

Collart P, Poitevin M, Milovanovic A, Herlin A, Durel J 1980 Kinetic study of serum penicillin concentrations after single doses of benzathine and benethamine penicillin in young and old people. *British Journal of Venereal Diseases* 56: 355–362

BENZATHINE PENICILLIN

An aqueous suspension of the poorly soluble (1 : 6000 in water) *N*, *N'*-dibenzolylethylene diamine dipenicillin salt of benzylpenicillin.

Oral and i.m. preparations together with various mixtures with benzyl- and procaine penicillins are available. It has a local anaesthetic effect comparable with that of procaine penicillin. After absorption, benzylpenicillin, to which it owes its activity and side-effects, is slowly released.

It is stable in gastric acid and when given by mouth its absorption is little affected by food, but its insolubility is such that the plasma concentrations achieved are very low. It was widely prescribed for the treatment of mild infections in children but was quickly replaced by penicillin V and oral semi-synthetic penicillins.

It is very slowly absorbed after i.m. injection, a dose of 1.2 MU producing mean plasma concentrations of 0.1 mg/l 1 week after injection, 0.02 mg/l after 2 weeks and 0.002 mg/l after 4 weeks.

It has been used in the treatment of streptococcal pharyngitis, diphtheria carriers (p. 677), syphilis (p. 816) and for the prophylaxis of rheumatic fever (p. 145). It should not be used in the treatment of gonorrhoea.

Preparations and dosage
Preparation: Injection.
Dosage: Varies according to infection being treated.
Limited availability; not available in the UK.

Further information

Ginsburg C M, McCracken G H Jr, Zweighaft T C 1982 Serum penicillin concentrations after intramuscular administration of benzathine penicillin G in children. *Pediatrics* 69: 452–454

Hagdrup H K, Lang E, Wantzin G, Secher L, Rosdahl V T 1986 Penicillin concentrations in serum following weekly injections of benzathine penicillin G. *Chemotherapy* 32: 99–101

Kaplan E L, Berrios X, Speth J, Siefferman T, Guzman B, Quesny F 1989 Pharmacokinetics of benzathine penicillin G: serum levels during the 28 days after intramuscular injection of 1 200 000 units. *Journal of Pediatrics* 115: 146–150

Peter G, Dudley M N 1985 Clinical pharmacology of benzathine penicillin G. *Pediatric Infectious Diseases* 4: 586–591

van der Valk P G, Kraai E J, van Voorst Vader P C, Haaxma-Reiche H, Snijder J A 1988 Penicillin concentrations in cerebrospinal fluid (CSF) during repository treatment regimen for syphilis. *Genitourinary Medicine* 64: 223–225

CLEMIZOLE PENICILLIN

A long-acting preparation of benzylpenicillin with the antihistamine, clemizole, given by deep intramuscular injection.

Preparations

Preparation: Injection.

Limited availability in continental Europe.

PROCAINE PENICILLIN

A poorly soluble (1 : 200 in water) equimolecular compound of penicillin and procaine, administered i.m. as a suspension of crystals which slowly dissolve at the site of the injection, liberating benzylpenicillin, to which it owes its antimicrobial activity.

Pharmacokinetics

It must not be given intravenously. Intramuscular administration produces a flat sustained plasma concentration of penicillin, which is much less than that achieved by an equivalent dose of benzylpenicillin. Following a dose of 0.6 g i.m. in adults, concentrations of 1–2 mg/l are achieved in 2–4 h. Levels are still detectable 24 h later. Free procaine is detectable in the plasma within 30 min. In infants given 50 mg/kg, levels of 7–9 mg/l were obtained at 2–4 h in those less than 1 week old and 5–6 mg/l in those who were older.

Toxicity and side-effects

Very severe and potentially fatal reactions resembling those of anaphylactic shock, but non-allergic in character, may occur, probably due to accidental entry into the vascular system at the site of injection and blockage of pulmonary and cerebral capillaries by crystals of the suspension. Some untoward reactions may be due to liberated procaine. There may be acute anxiety and angor animi without physical signs or fever, hypertension, tachycardia, vomiting, audiovisual hallucinations and acute psychotic disturbance. The most severe reactions lead to convulsions and cardiac arrest. Other reactions are those to liberated benzylpenicillin.

Clinical uses

It is used as a single injection combined with benzathine penicillin in the prophylaxis of rheumatic fever and as a combined injection with benzylpenicillin in the prophylaxis of endocarditis. It has been used in a single daily dose in the treatment of pneumococcal pneumonia (p. 685), gonorrhoea, syphilis (p. 817) and sore throat (p. 676).

Preparations and dosage

Proprietary name: Bicillin.

Preparation: Injection.

Dosage: Adults, i.m., 300 mg (plus 60 mg benzylpenicillin) every 12–24 h; primary syphilis, 900 mg (plus 180 mg benzylpenicillin) for 10 days; 14 days for secondary or latent syphilis.

Widely available.

Further information

Shann F, Linnemann V, Gratten M 1987 Serum concentration of penicillin after intramuscular administration of procaine, benzyl and benethamine penicillin in children with pneumonia. *Journal of Pediatrics* 110: 299–302

Silber T J, D'Angelo L 1985 Psychosis and seizures following the injection of penicillin G procaine. *American Journal of Diseases of Children* 139: 335–337

Group 2: Orally absorbed penicillins resembling benzylpenicillin

Early efforts to improve the oral absorption characteristics of benzylpenicillin concentrated on esterification of the C-3 carboxyl group. Simple methyl or alkyl esters were found to be ineffective since man lacks the necessary esterase to release active penicillin, but the acetoxymethyl ester, at one time available as penamecillin, is hydrolysed by non-specific esterases to yield benzylpenicillin and formaldehyde. Benzathine penicillin, the sparingly soluble long-acting parenteral salt of benzylpenicillin (p. 262), produces low plasma concentrations after oral use but has largely fallen into disuse as an oral agent.

The first natural penicillin to be identified as a true oral compound was penicillin V (phenoxymethylpenicillin) produced by addition of phenoxyacetic acid as a precursor to the fermentation. Penicillin V is significantly more acid stable than benzylpenicillin and is absorbed after oral administration producing therapeutically useful plasma antibiotic concentrations. After the discovery of the penicillin nucleus, 6-APA, a number of phenoxypenicillins, analogues of penicillin V, were developed with claims for superior oral absorption characteristics. The most important of these semi-synthetic penicillins are phenethicillin (the immediate homologue of penicillin V) and propicillin, which both enjoyed considerable clinical success. The phenoxypenicillins display an antibacterial spectrum generally similar to that of benzylpenicillin, although there are important differences against certain bacteria. Another phenoxypenicillin, phenbenicillin (phenoxybenzylpenicillin) is no longer available because its superior oral absorption was offset by very high protein binding and extensive metabolism. Generally speaking, the efficiency of absorption of the phenoxypenicillins appears to increase with increasing molecular weight.

The remaining oral narrow-spectrum penicillin in clinical use in some areas of the world is azidopenicillin, which is not a phenoxypenicillin, but which has an antibacterial spectrum essentially similar to that of benzylpenicillin.

Antimicrobial activity

The group 2 penicillins resemble benzylpenicillin in their antibacterial spectrum and lack of stability to β-lactamase. The phenoxypenicillins exhibit slightly lower activity than benzylpenicillin against Gram-positive cocci and are distinctly less active against Gram-negative bacteria. Azidocillin, an analogue of benzylpenicillin, resembles the latter in potency and range of activity.

Pharmacokinetics

The peak plasma levels obtained from the phenoxypenicillins and from azidocillin are well in excess of those required to inhibit the organisms for which benzylpenicillin is normally used.

Clinical use

They may be prescribed for many indications for which benzylpenicillin is suitable, including streptococcal pharyngitis and skin sepsis, but are not recommended for initial therapy of serious infections. They are useful for continuation therapy after initial control of the disease by parenteral benzylpenicillin where prolonged treatment is required, as in osteomyelitis due to penicillin-susceptible *Staph. aureus* or bacterial endocarditis due to fully penicillin-susceptible streptococci. In such potentially dangerous conditions, it needs to be established that the organisms are killed by the particular oral penicillin used and that bactericidal levels for the infecting organisms are achieved in the patient's plasma, because although they are much more reliably absorbed than benzylpenicillin, there are still some patients who absorb them poorly. They have been used prophylactically in recurrent pneumococcal meningitis after head injury and in rheumatic fever. They are not appropriate for respiratory infections where *H. influenzae* may be implicated, and are not recommended for the treatment of gonorrhoea, syphilis or leptospirosis; or for infections caused by Gram-negative bacilli.

AZIDOCILLIN
D-Azidobenzylpenicillin

It is as active as benzylpenicillin and more active than the phenoxypenicillins against susceptible strains of *Staph. aureus*, *Str. pyogenes* and *Str. pneumoniae* (Table 15.3). Azidocillin is also more active than benzylpenicillin against *H. influenzae*, showing activity almost equal to that of ampicillin. Other Gram-negative bacteria are not notably susceptible. The extent of protein binding (80%) is generally similar to penicillin V and phenethicillin. It is well absorbed after oral administration and produces plasma concentrations higher than those of penicillin V and comparable with phenethicillin. Urinary excretion is 68% of an oral dose and 80% of an intravenous dose, indicating about 75% absorption by the oral route. Azidocillin has been used for the treatment of upper respiratory tract infection.

Preparations and dosage
Dosage: Adult, oral, 750 mg twice daily.
Limited availability in continental Europe.

Further information
Bergan T, Sorensen G 1980 Pharmacokinetics of azidocillin in healthy adults. *Arzneimittel Forschung – Drug Research* 30: 185–191

Weiser O, Wenton H 1980 Azidocillin in acute attacks of chronic bronchitis. Comparison of b.i.d. and t.i.d. administration. *British Journal of Clinical Practice* 34: 101–106

PHENETHICILLIN
Phenoxyethylpenicillin

The immediate homologue of penicillin V and the first semi-synthetic penicillin to enter clinical use after the discovery of 6-APA. Supplied as the potassium salt.

Antimicrobial activity

Its antibacterial spectrum and activity is similar to that of penicillin V and differs slightly from that of benzylpenicillin (Table 15.3). It is slightly more stable than benzylpenicillin to staphylococcal β-lactamase, but this difference is not considered to be of clinical significance.

Pharmacokinetics

After oral administration, phenethecillin produces plasma antibiotic concentrations which are higher and more prolonged than those obtained with penicillin V. The difference in plasma concentrations between the two compounds may be the result of less extensive metabolism of phenethecillin. Absorption of phenethecillin may be erratic, with it being undetectable in the plasma of some subjects.

Mean peak plasma levels around 3.5 mg/l are produced about 1 h after a dose of 250 mg. The peak is depressed but prolonged on administration with food. Protein binding is 75%. It is well distributed into serous and synovial fluid but does not reach the normal CSF. Doses corresponding to 1 MU of benzylpenicillin produced sputum levels of 0.8–0.9 mg/l, with sustained levels after 4–5 days' treatment up to 0.7 mg/l.

The bulk of the dose appears in the urine, about 25% as penicilloic acid and 50% as unchanged penicillin. Small amounts also appear as other metabolites, some of which are biologically active.

Toxicity and side-effects

There is cross-allergy with other penicillins, but severe reactions are much less common than with benzylpenicillin. A serum-sickness-like illness has been noted relatively frequently. Haemolytic anaemia has been reported, and overdosage may result in potassium intoxication.

Clinical uses

Those of group 2 penicillins (p. 270).

Preparations and dosage

Dosage: Adults, oral, 250–500 mg every 6 h.
Limited availability, not available in the UK.

Further information

Overbosch D, Mattie H, vanFurth R 1985 Comparative pharmacodynamics and clinical pharmacokinetics of phenoxymethylpenicillin and pheneticillin. *British Journal of Clinical Pharmacology* 19: 657–668

PHENOXYMETHYLPENICILLIN
Penicillin V

A naturally occurring penicillin produced by *P. chrysogenum* in media containing phenoxyacetic acid as a precursor. It is supplied as the potassium salt.

Antimicrobial activity

The antibacterial spectrum and level of activity is generally similar to that of benzylpenicillin, although there are minor but important differences (Table 15.3). It is as active as benzylpenicillin against streptococci, slightly less active against staphylococci and 2–8 times less active against gonococci, meningococci and *H. influenzae*. Enteric Gram-negative bacilli are highly resistant.

Pharmacokinetics

Owing to acid stability, it is not destroyed in the stomach, but absorption is variable and incomplete, about 30% remaining in the faeces. Absorption is better from a rapidly disintegrating tablet and after administration in the fasting state. Following an oral dose of 250 mg, peak plasma levels around 2 mg/l are reached at about 1 h. An oral dose of 2 g produced mean peak levels in plasma of 18.6 mg/l at 0.75 h and in saliva of 0.09 mg/l. Protein binding is 80%. It is fairly extensively metabolized and degraded in the bowel. Some 60% of the dose is excreted in the urine, 25% in the unchanged form and the remainder as metabolites.

Toxicity and side-effects

Those common to penicillins (p. 259). Following treatment for 5 days, oral streptococci, *H. influenzae* and fusobacteria all fell significantly, but no penicillin-resistant strains emerged and no overgrowth with enterobacteria or enterococci occurred.

Clinical uses

Those of group 2 penicillins (p. 270).

Preparations and dosage

Preparations: Tablets, oral solution.

Dosage: Adults, oral, 250–500 mg every 6 h. Children <1 year, 62.5 mg every 6 h; children 1–5 years, 125 mg every 6 h; children 6–12 years, 250 mg every 6 h.

Further information

Josefsson K, Nord C E 1982 Effects of phenoxymethylpenicillin and erythromycin in high doses on the salivary microflora. *Journal of Antimicrobial Chemotherapy* 10: 325–333

Overbosch D, Mattie H, vanFurth R 1985 Comparative pharmacodynamics and clinical pharmacokinetics of phenoxymethyl penicillin and pheneticillin. *British Journal of Clinical Pharmacology* 19: 657–668

PROPICILLIN
Phenoxypropylpenicillin

A semi-synthetic penicillin supplied as the potassium salt. Up to 30% is excreted in the urine as biologically active metabolites. Superior absorption is offset by its protein binding (90%) and inferior activity against some organisms. Clinical uses are those of group 2 penicillins (p. 270).

Group 3: Antistaphylococcal β-lactamase-stable penicillins

The members of this group, methicillin, nafcillin and four isoxazolyl penicillins, are intrinsically less active than benzylpenicillin but are stable to staphylococcal β-lactamase and consequently display significant activity against penicillin-resistant strains of Staph. aureus. Their resistance to staphylococcal β-lactamase is caused by the side-chain structures which result in poor affinities for the enzymes.

Antimicrobial activity

The compounds are active against staphylococci, streptococci, gonococci and meningococci but have no useful

Table 15.4 *Antibacterial activity of group 3 penicillins against common pathogenic bacteria: MIC (mg/l)*

	Cloxacillin*	Methicillin	Nafcillin
Staph. aureus	0.1	1	0.1
Staph. epidermidis	0.1	1	0.1
Str. pyogenes	0.1	0.25	0.06
Str. pneumoniae	0.25	0.25	0.1
Ent. faecalis	16–32	16–32	16
N. gonorrhoeae	0.1	0.1–0.5	2
N. meningitidis	0.25	0.25	–
H. influenzae	8–16	2	4
Enterobacteriaceae	R	R	R
Ps. aeruginosa	R	R	R
B. fragilis	R	R	R

*Activities of dicloxacillin, flucloxacillin and oxacillin are similar.
R (resistant) MIC ≥ 128 mg/l.

activity against enterococci, *H. influenzae* or enterobacteria (Table 15.4). Methicillin is approximately 10 times less active than the others against *Staph. aureus* and is 100-fold less active than benzylpenicillin against penicillin-susceptible *Staph. aureus*.

Methicillin displays a very high degree of stability to staphylococcal β-lactamase but has been largely replaced in clinical practice by the isoxazolyl penicillins because of low activity, lack of oral absorption and a propensity to cause interstitial nephritis. Methicillin and nafcillin are more stable than the isoxazolyl penicillins to staphylococcal β-lactamase, but there is no evidence that this has any clinical significance. Oxacillin is rather less stable than the other isoxazole compounds, the order of stability being: methicillin > nafcillin > cloxacillin, dicloxacillin, flucloxacillin > oxacillin. Cloxacillin and flucloxacillin enjoy clinical usage in Europe and elsewhere, and nafcillin, oxacillin and dicloxacillin are preferred in North America.

Pharmacokinetics

Methicillin is the most metabolically stable and least protein bound. It is unstable in acid and not absorbed when given by mouth. Nafcillin is also relatively acid labile and poorly and irregularly absorbed by mouth. The isoxazolyl penicillins are considerably better absorbed from the gut than are methicillin or nafcillin, but differ considerably amongst themselves. The mean peak plasma levels of cloxacillin are about twice those resulting from similar doses of oxacillin and those of dicloxacillin and flucloxacillin about twice those of cloxacillin. Levels are depressed when the agents are given with food, oxacillin being the most affected.

Oxacillin is also more extensively metabolized than dicloxacillin or flucloxacillin. All are highly protein bound. Levels obtained by intravenous bolus injection of isoxazolyl penicillins are higher than those produced by the extensively metabolized nafcillin, but this advantage is offset by their greater degree of protein binding. Overall, dicloxacillin and flucloxacillin are superior to oxacillin and cloxacillin for oral administration. Flucloxacillin is better absorbed and provides more unbound drug than does dicloxacillin.

They are widely distributed in the extracellular fluid, and their plasma levels are correspondingly depressed when the extracellular volume is increased as in pregnancy or in the newborn. They are well distributed into serous fluids, but as highly protein-bound agents, their access to blister fluid is limited though their persistence there is prolonged. They do not enter normal CSF, but their entry is somewhat erratically increased by inflammation, nafcillin penetrating better than others.

Little of these drugs appears in the bile, and they are excreted principally unchanged in the urine by both glomerular filtration and tubular secretion to produce very high urinary levels. Serum half-lives are consequently prolonged by probenecid and in the newborn and with the exception of oxacillin, which is the most extensively metabolized, in renal failure. Patients with cystic fibrosis clear the drugs unusually rapidly, and allowance for this must be made in their dosage.

Toxicity and side-effects

Immediate and delayed hypersensitivity reactions and asymptomatic eosinophilia can occur with all the agents, but acute anaphylaxis is much less common than with benzylpenicillin. Rashes occur but are much less common than with ampicillin. Drug fever occurs most commonly with methicillin. Some patients develop diarrhoea, which can be sufficiently severe to require withdrawal of therapy, and pseudomembranous colitis has been reported. Amongst rare haematological disorders are reversible dose-related leucopenia and platelet abnormalities. Reversible abnormalities of liver function tests can develop, particularly with oxacillin, and cholestatic jaundice has been described. Unless excessively high doses are employed (which may produce neurological manifestations like those of benzylpenicillin (p. 265), there is no danger of electrolyte overload as the drugs contain less than 1 milliequivalent of sodium per gram. Renal damage (generally reversible) has been described, usually in patients receiving large doses, and most frequently the interstitial nephritis associated with methicillin.

Clinical use

The only, but important, therapeutic use for these agents is in the treatment of proven staphylococcal infection or, usually in combination therapy, where staphylococcal infection is suspected. The injectable forms are used in severe staphylococcal infections, including those of the bones, joints, heart valves, meninges and in brain abscess and disseminated infection. The oral drugs are valuable in the treatment of staphylococcal infections of soft tissues and as continuation therapy in infections of bone and joints. The reservations concerning oral drugs in the treatment of severe infection already discussed under group 2 penicillins (p. 270) must be considered if this form of therapy is contemplated. There has been some interest in their ability to inhibit β-lactamases and hence potentiate the activity of β-lactamases-labile agents against organisms which owe their resistance to elaboration of these enzymes (p. 320).

Isoxazolyl penicillins

Four members of this series are in clinical use, namely, oxacillin, cloxacillin, dicloxacillin and flucloxacillin. They are all closely related in chemical structure and display similar antibacterial properties but addition of halogen atoms to the phenyl ring in the side-chain results in improved oral absorption characteristics.

CLOXACILLIN

A semi-synthetic isoxazolyl penicillin supplied as the sodium salt.

Antimicrobial activity

Cloxacillin is active against most Gram-positive cocci, including *Staph. aureus*, *Staph. epidermidis*, *Str. pyogenes*, *Str. pneumoniae* and viridans streptococci, but *Ent. faecalis* is relatively resistant (Table 15.4). It shows the same order of activity against β-lactamase-producing and β-lactamase-negative strains of staphylococci (MIC 0.1–0.25 mg/l). Other susceptible bacteria include *N. gonorrhoeae*, *N. meningitidis* and Gram-positive anaerobes (MIC 0.1–0.25 mg/l). *H. influenzae* is relatively resistant, Enterobacteriaceae and *Ps. aeruginosa* are highly resistant (MIC >512 mg/l) and Gram-negative anaerobes may be moderately or highly resistant.

Cloxacillin is slightly less stable than methicillin to preparations of staphylococcal β-lactamase but this is not reflected in antibacterial tests and methicillin-susceptible β-lactamase-producing strains of *Staph. aureus* are uniformly susceptible. The compound is highly bound to serum protein and activity is substantially diminished in the presence of serum.

Acquired resistance

Cloxacillin exhibits complete cross-resistance with methicillin and other group 3 penicillins (see methicillin-resistance, p. 277). Penicillin-tolerant strains are also tolerant to cloxacillin.

Pharmacokinetics

Cloxacillin is moderately well absorbed by mouth but absorption is depressed by food. Following an oral dose of 500 mg, fasting mean peak plasma levels around 8 mg/l are obtained about 1 h after the dose. With food, only about a quarter of the fasting level is achieved. Higher blood levels are produced by intramuscular injection, mean peak plasma levels around 15 mg/l being obtained 0.5–1 h after a dose of 500 mg. Doubling the dose approximately doubles the peak level. Some inactivation occurs in the liver and about 10% of the serum content is in the form of metabolites. Protein binding is 93–95%. Being highly protein bound, it diffuses poorly into normal interstitial fluid, serous cavities and CSF, but enters pus and inflamed bones and joints. It crosses the placenta.

About 10% of an oral dose is excreted in the bile, but the main route of excretion is renal, about 30% of an oral dose and 40–60% of an i.m. dose appearing in the urine as active antibiotic with 10–20% in the form of metabolites. Excretion is by both glomerular filtration and tubular secretion and is depressed by probenecid, which elevates and prolongs the plasma concentration. Excretion is impaired in renal failure and there is some accumulation of metabolites. In patients with cystic fibrosis, tubular secretion is enhanced and elimination increased two- to three-fold.

Toxicity and side-effects

It is generally well tolerated, but there is cross-allergy with benzylpenicillin. Nausea and diarrhoea may occur on oral dosage, but are usually mild. Elevated SGOT levels have been described in some patients. As with other penicillins, large doses, especially in patients in renal failure, can be neurotoxic, and occasional neutropenia has been described.

Clinical uses

Those of Group 3 penicillins (p. 273), including staphylococcal septicaemia and lower respiratory tract infection, but particularly the prolonged oral treatment of chronic staphylococcal osteomyelitis.

Preparations and dosage

Proprietary name: Orbenin.

Preparations: Capsules, injection.

Dosage: Adults, oral, 500 mg every 6 h; i.m., i.v., 250–500 mg every 4–6 h, the dose may be doubled in severe infections. Children <2 years, all routes, quarter adult dose; children 2–10 years, all routes, half adult dose. Widely available.

Further information

Bergeron M G, Desaulnier S D, Lessard C et al 1985 Concentrations of fusidic acid, cloxacillin and cefamandole in sera and atrial appendages of patients undergoing cardiac surgery. *Antimicrobial Agents and Chemotherapy* 27: 928–932

Grimm P C, Ogborn M R, Larson A J, Crocker J F 1989 Interstitial nephritis induced by cloxacillin. *Nephron* 51: 285–286

Konikoff F, Alcalay J, Halevy J 1986 Cloxacillin-induced cholestatic jaundice. *American Journal of Gastroenterology* 81: 1082–1083

Spino M, Chai R P, Isles A F et al 1984 Cloxacillin absorption and disposition in cystic fibrosis. *Journal of Pediatrics* 105: 829–835

DICLOXACILLIN

A semi-synthetic isoxazolyl penicillin which differs from cloxacillin by an additional chlorine atom. It is supplied as the sodium monohydrate.

Antimicrobial activity

Its activities are generally similar to those of other isoxazolyl penicillins (Table 15.4) but it is slightly more active than cloxacillin and oxacillin against some strains of both penicillin-susceptible and penicillin-resistant staphylococci. It is also highly active against streptococci and pneumococci. It is very highly bound to serum protein and its activity in the presence of human serum is depressed to a greater extent than that of other isoxazolyl penicillins.

Amongst the isoxazolyl penicillins it is one of the more resistant to staphylococcal β-lactamase. There is complete cross-resistance with other penicillins of the group.

Pharmacokinetics

The concentrations attained in the blood after oral dosing exceed those of cloxacillin by two-fold and those of oxacillin by four-fold and the concentrations are better sustained. Following an oral dose of 250 mg, mean peak plasma levels around 9 mg/l are obtained at about 1 h; 500 mg i.m. produced mean peak plasma concentrations of 14–16 mg/l at 0.5–1 h. Absorption in the very young is poor and unpredictable. It is partly metabolized in the liver and about 10% of the circulating drug is in the form of metabolites. It is very highly protein bound (95–97%). Some 50–70% of a dose is excreted in the urine, about 20% as metabolites.

It is eliminated both in the glomerular filtrate and by tubular secretion, and plasma concentrations are raised by probenecid. Dicloxacillin and increased proportions of metabolites accumulate in renal failure. Elimination is increased through enhanced tubular secretion in patients with cystic fibrosis.

Toxicity and clinical use

Phlebitis is common after i.v. injection. Its toxicity and clinical uses are otherwise those of group 3 penicillins (p. 273).

Preparations and dosage

Dosage: Adults, oral, 125–250 mg, 4 times daily.

Available in continental Europe.

Further information

Bergdahl S, Eriksson M, Finkel Y 1987 Plasma concentration following oral administration of di- and flucloxacillin in infants and children. *Pharmacology and Toxicology* 60: 233–234

Kleinman M S, Presberg J E 1986 Cholestatic hepatitis after dicloxacillin-sodium therapy. *Journal of Clinical Gastroenterology* 8: 77–78

Lofgren S, Bucht G, Hermansson B, Holm S E, Winblad B, Norrby S R 1986 Single-dose pharmacokinetics of dicloxacillin in healthy subjects of young and old age. *Scandinavian Journal of Infectious Diseases* 18: 365–369

Pacifici G M, Viani A, Taddeuchi-Brunelli G, Rizzo G, Carrai M 1987 Plasma protein binding of dicloxacillin: effects of age and disease. *International Journal of Clinical Pharmacology Therapy and Toxicology* 25: 622–626

FLUCLOXACILLIN

A semi-synthetic isoxazolyl penicillin which differs from dicloxacillin by the substitution of a fluorine atom for a chlorine atom. It is supplied as the sodium salt.

Antimicrobial activity

Its antibacterial activity is almost identical with that of cloxacillin (Table 15.4). It exhibits a uniform level of activity against β-lactamase-negative and β-lactamase-positive strains of *Staph. aureus*. There is complete cross-resistance with other β-lactamase-stable penicillins.

Pharmacokinetics

It is well absorbed after oral administration, the blood levels attained being about double those produced by the same dose of cloxacillin, 250 and 500 mg producing mean peak plasma levels between 0.5 and 1 h of around 11 and 15 mg/l, respectively. Protein binding is high (95%). The plasma elimination half-life is around 2 h. It is partly metabolized in the liver and about 10% of the plasma concentration is made up of metabolites.

Distribution of flucloxacillin resembles that of other isoxazolyl penicillins, its high protein binding limiting its diffusion notably into the normal CSF. Penetration into extravascular exudates is rapid. In patients receiving 500 mg i.v. at the beginning and during operation, mean concentrations in wound fluid were 16 mg/l. In volunteers receiving 2 g by i.v. bolus injection, mean peak concentrations in lymph and suction blister fluid were 11.7 and 4.6 mg/l, respectively with mean elimination half-lives of 1.4 and 11.0 h.

It is more slowly eliminated than cloxacillin. Some appears in the bile but about 50–60% of an oral dose is recovered from the urine, about 20% as metabolites.

Toxicity and side-effects

In patients treated by i.v. infusion, about 5% developed phlebitis by the first and 15% by the second day after which the proportion rose dramatically. Side-effects are otherwise those of group 3 penicillins (p. 273).

Clinical use

The clinical uses are those of group 3 penicillins (p. 273). The clinical significance of methicillin resistance in vitro has been questioned (p. 278) and controlled trails of the treatment of burns colonized with methicillin-resistant

Staph. aureus showed that in the majority of cases the organisms were eliminated by oral flucloxacillin, whereas untreated controls remained colonized. Reference is made to its use in neutropenic patients (p. 619), pneumonia (p. 687), endocarditis (p. 703), septicaemia (p. 586), meningitis (p. 750), cystic fibrosis (p. 691), bone and joint infection (p. 761) and skin sepsis (p. 734).

Preparations and dosage

Proprietary name: Floxapen.

Preparations: Capsules, oral solution, injection.

Dosage: Adults, oral, 250 mg every 6 h; i.m., i.v., 250 mg to 1 g every 6 h, the dose may be doubled in severe infections. Children <2 years, any route, quarter adult dose; children 2–10 years, any route, half adult dose. Widely available.

Further information

Basker M J, Edmondson R A, Sutherland R 1980 Comparative stabilities of penicillins and cephalosporins to staphylococcal β-lactamase and activities against *Staph. aureus. Journal of Antimicrobial Chemotherapy* 6: 333–341

Bergan T, Engeset A, Olszewski W, Ostby N, Solberg R 1986 Extravascular penetration of highly protein-bound flucloxacillin. *Antimicrobial Agents and Chemotherapy* 30: 729–732

Farrington M, Fenn A, Phillips I 1985 Flucloxacillin concentration in serum and wound exudate during open heart surgery. *Journal of Antimicrobial Chemotherapy* 16: 253–259

Frank U, Schmidt-Eisenlohr E, Schlosser V, Spillner G, Schindler M, Daschner F D 1988 Concentrations of flucloxacillin in heart valves and subcutaneous and muscle tissues of patients undergoing open-heart surgery. *Antimicrobial Agents and Chemotherapy* 32: 930–931

Herngren L, Ehrnebo M, Broberger U 1987 Pharmacokinetics of free and total flucloxacillin in newborn infants. *European Journal of Clinical Pharmacology* 32: 403–409

Victorino R M, Maria V A, Correia A P, de Moura C 1987 Flucloxacillin-induced cholestatic hepatitis with evidence of lymphocyte sensitization. *Archives of Internal Medicine* 147: 987–989

OXACILLIN

A semi-synthetic penicillin of group 3 (p. 272) supplied as the sodium salt. The first of the isoxazolyl series of β-lactamase-resistant penicillins.

Antimicrobial activity

Its spectrum and activity are those of isoxazolyl penicillins (Table 15.4). Typical β-lactam synergy is shown with aminoglycosides, but it antagonizes the bactericidal activity of rifampicin against *Staph. aureus*. Resistant and tolerant strains show complete cross-resistance and tolerance with other group 3 penicillins. Oxacillin is slightly less stable to staphylococcal β-lactamase than other isoxazolyl penicillins.

Acquired resistance

The β-lactamase-stable antistaphylococcal penicillins are usually considered to be universally active against β-lactamase-producing *Staph. aureus* save for the methicillin-resistant strains possessing modified PBPs. However, a small proportion of methicillin-susceptible isolates of *Staph. aureus* have been reported to display reduced susceptibility to oxacillin. These BORSA strains (borderline oxacillin-resistant *Staph. aureus*) are assumed to hyperproduce β-lactamase. Oxacillin is the least stable of the isoxazolyl penicillins to staphylococcal β-lactamase, and the BORSA strains appear to be susceptible to cloxacillin, dicloxacillin and flucloxacillin. The clinical significance of these isolates is unclear.

Pharmacokinetics

Oxacillin is the least well absorbed of the isoxazolyl penicillins, with mean peak plasma levels around 4 mg/l at 0.5 h after an oral dose of 500 mg. Approximately twice the oral fasting level is produced by the same dose administered i.m. Protein binding is 92–96%. It is rapidly metabolized. It is widely distributed into interstitial fluid despite its high protein binding. Some appears in the bile, but the main route of elimination is renal, about 25% of the dose being recovered from the urine as active material and about another 25% as inactive metabolites. It is rapidly inactivated in the body and there is no accumulation in patients with end-stage kidney disease, the blood level becoming undetectable 8 h after a 1 g dose. It is still more rapidly eliminated in patients with cystic fibrosis.

Toxicity and side-effects

There is cross allergy with other penicillins and reactions are generally typical of the group. Abnormalities of liver function, especially elevation of SGOT levels, sometimes accompanied by fever, nausea, vomiting and eosinophilia occur with biopsy evidence of non-specific hepatitis. There is rapid reversal on withdrawal of treatment and the response appears to be peculiar to oxacillin in that recrudescence was not observed on subsequent administration of benzylpenicillin or nafcillin. Neurotoxicity may develop on high dosage of patients with renal failure. Agranulocytosis is rare, but reversible neutropenia has been observed in children, adults and the elderly, which may be due to depression of neutrophil maturation.

Clinical use

That of group 3 penicillins (p. 273).

Preparations and dosage

Preparations: Capsules, oral solution, injection.

Dosage: Adults, oral, 500 mg to 1 g every 6 h; i.m., i.v., 250 mg to 1 g every 4–6 h. Children (under 40 kg), 25–50 mg/kg every 4–6 h. Newborn and premature infants, 25 mg/kg per day in divided doses may be given, but used with caution.

Available widely in continental Europe, North America, S. America and Japan. Not available in the UK.

Further information

Craven D E, Reed C, Kollisch N et al 1981 A large outbreak of infections caused by a strain of *Staphylococcus aureus* resistant to oxacillin and aminoglycosides. *American Journal of Medicine* 71: 53–58

Hilty M D, Venglarcik J S, Best G K 1980 Oxacillin-tolerant staphylococcal bacteremia in children. *Journal of Pediatrics* 96: 1035–1037

Massanari R M, Pfaller M A, Wakefield D S et al 1988 Implications of acquired oxacillin resistance in the management and control of *Staphylococcus aureus* infections. *Journal of Infectious Diseases* 158: 702–709

McDougal L K, Thornsberry C 1986 The role of β-lactamase in staphylococcal resistance to penicillinase-resistant penicillins and cephalosporins. *Journal of Clinical Microbiology* 23: 832–839

Pfaller M A, Wakefield D S, Stewart B, Bale M, Hammons G T, Massanari R M 1988 Evaluation of laboratory methods for the classification of oxacillin-resistant and oxacillin-susceptible *Staphylococcus aureus. American Journal of Clinical Pathology* 89: 120–125

Schlaeffer F 1988 Oxacillin-associated hypokalemia. *Drug Intelligence and Clinical Pharmacy* 22: 695–696

METHICILLIN
2,6-Dimethoxyphenylpenicillin

The first β-lactamase-resistant semi-synthetic penicillin which initially was used widely but has since been superseded by other group 3 members.

It is supplied as the sodium salt. Aqueous solutions are unstable, particularly at low pH.

Antimicrobial activity

Methicillin is active against most Gram-positive bacteria and against *Neisseria* spp. but it is much less active than benzylpenicillin (Table 15.4) and is the least active of the group 3 penicillins. It is highly stable to staphylococcal β-lactamase and is equally active against penicillin-susceptible and β-lactamase-producing strains of *Staph. aureus*. It is actively bactericidal at concentrations close to the MIC and antibacterial activity is not affected by the presence of serum.

Acquired resistance

Methicillin-resistant strains of *Staph. aureus* which are resistant to all group 3 penicillins as a result of modified PBPs are most readily detected in susceptibility tests utilizing methicillin. Strains of *Staph. aureus* resistant to methicillin were thought at first not to exist and then to be exceedingly rare, but their prevalence rose rapidly. It has since fluctuated markedly with high isolation rates being reported in individual hospitals, particularly from Australia, France, Switzerland and Denmark with outbreaks in many hospitals in Europe, the USA and elsewhere. The strains are usually resistant to many other antibiotics and their acquisition in hospitals or nursing homes causes severe administrative and clinical problems in calling for substantial control measures. Almost all strains of methicillin-resistant staphylococci (MRSA) produce large amounts of β-lactamase, but they do not inactive methicillin and the mechanism of resistance is the acquisition of a supplementary PBP (PBP2[1] or PBP2a) with a low affinity for methicillin and other β-lactam antibiotics.

The bacterial population is highly heterogenous in its response to the agent and only a small minority of cells (10^{-6}–10^{-7}) may appear to be resistant in conventional media. The resistance of individual cells can differ by more than 100-fold and the progeny of resistant colonies are similarly heterogenous. The population can be rendered homogeneously resistant by growth either at 30°C, or in a medium containing an excess of electrolytes, such as 5% NaCl, or by lowering the pH. For the above reasons, standard susceptibility testing may not detect MRSA and the use of large inocula plus media supplemented with NaCl and/or incubation at 30°C is recommended.

Because reversion to the minority resistant state occurs readily in vitro, the therapeutic significance of MRSA has been questioned. There is, however, adequate evidence to show that patients infected with such strains may undoubtedly develop life-threatening infections which fail to respond to the anti-staphylococcal penicillins.

MRSA are considered to be resistant to all β-lactam agents including imipenem and meropenem, and many isolates are resistant also to most other antistaphylococcal antibiotics. The 6-fluoroquinolones appeared to have the desired properties to be effective against MRSA, but resistance has been reported to arise during therapy with ciprofloxacin, and 6-fluoroquinolone-resistant MRSA have been isolated in many parts of the world. Currently, vancomycin is the mainstay of treatment of serious infections and the related glycopeptide, teicoplanin appears to be an alternative.

Resistance to methicillin is very common among coagulase-negative staphylococci which are now responsible for many nosocomial bloodstream infections. *Staph. epidermidis* predominates as the resistant species most frequently isolated followed by *Staph. haemolyticus*. As is the case with MRSA, most methicillin-resistant isolates of coagulase-negative staphylococci display multiple resistance and vancomycin is often the only choice for the treatment of serious hospital-acquired infections.

Pharmacokinetics

Methicillin is not acid resistant, and must therefore be administered parenterally. The mean peak plasma concentration following a 1 g i.m. dose is around 17 mg/l at 0.5 h. By rapid i.v. infusion over 5 min the same dose produced mean end infusion concentrations around 60 mg/l. Doubling the dose approximately doubles the peak plasma concentration. In the newborn, 25 mg/kg produced mean peak plasma concentrations of 47 mg/l in the first week of life, 41 mg/l in the second, 35 mg/l in the third and 25 mg/l in the fourth. Values given for protein binding have varied widely from 17 to 45%. About 10% is metabolized, but this is enhanced in renal impairment and depressed in hepatic failure.

It is widely distributed, levels in serous fluids approximating to those in the serum, but it does not enter the CSF except, irregularly, in the presence of meningitis. Concentrations close to the simultaneous serum level have been found in infected bone.

A small amount (2–3%) appears in the bile but 60–80% is excreted in the urine by glomerular filtration and tubular secretion. Administration of probenecid significantly elevates and prolongs the plasma level. It is only slowly removed by haemodialysis.

Toxicity and side-effects

Methicillin is, in general, well tolerated, but reversible leucopenia is fairly common and agranulocytosis and thrombocytopenia are described. Acute haemorrhagic cystitis is a rare reaction, and interstitial nephritis is common in patients receiving large doses who may be slow to recover and subsequently relapse on administration of the same or another β-lactam. Nephritis appears to be a more common side-effect with methicillin than with other penicillins, and therapy with nafcillin or an isoxazolyl penicillin is preferred. Concurrent appearance of neutropenia due to maturation arrest, haematuria and renal tubular atrophy associated with intense C_3 fixation, suggests all may be of immunological origin.

Patients sensitized to benzylpenicillin usually, but not always, react. Maculopapular and urticarial rashes have been noted, particularly in children. Other reactions are those common to the group (p. 273).

Clinical use

That of group 3 penicillins (p. 273).

Preparations and dosage

Preparation: Injection.

Dosage: Adults, i.m., i.v., 1 g every 4–6 h; in severe infections up to 12 g/day may be given. Children <2 years, quarter adult dose; children 2–10 years, half the adult dose.

Limited availability.

Further information

Blumberg H M 1991 Rapid development of ciprofloxacin resistance in methicillin-susceptible and -resistant *Staphylococcus aureus*. *Journal of Infectious Disease* 163: 1279–1285

Boyce J M 1990 Increasing prevalence of methicillin-resistant *Staphylococcus aureus* in the United States. *Infection Control and Hospital Epidemiology* 11: 633–642

Boyce J M, White R L, Causey W A, Lockwood W R 1983 Burn units as a source of methicillin-resistant *Staphylococcus aureus* infections. *Journal of the American Medical Association* 249: 2803–2807

Brown D F, Yates V S 1986 Methicillin susceptibility testing of *Staphylococcus aureus* on media containing five per cent sodium chloride. *European Journal of Clinical Microbiology* 5: 726–728

Cafferkey M T, Hone R, Keane C T 1988 Sources and outcome for methicillin-resistant *Staphylococcus aureus* bacteraemia. *Journal of Hospital Infection* 11: 136–143

Casewell M W 1986 Epidemiology and control of the 'modern' methicillin-resistant *Staphylococcus aureus*. *Journal of Hospital Infection* 7 (suppl A): 1–11

Chambers H F 1988 Methicillin-resistant staphylococci. *Clinical Microbiology Reviews* 1: 173–186

Coudron P E, Jones D L, Dalton H P, Archer G L 1986 Evaluation of laboratory tests for detection of methicillin-resistant *Staphylococcus aureus* and *Staphylococcus epidermidis*. *Journal of Clinical Microbiology* 24: 764–769

Gengo F M, Schentag J J 1981 Methicillin distribution in serum and extravascular fluid and its relevance to normal and damaged heart valves. *Antimicrobial Agents and Chemotherapy* 19: 836–841

Godin M, Deshayes P, Ducastelle P, Delpech A, Leloët Y, Fillastre J P 1980 Agranulocytosis, haemorrahagic cystitis and acute interstitial nephritis during methicillin therapy. *Journal of Antimicrobial Chemotherapy* 6: 296–297

Hackbarth C J, Chambers H F 1989 Methicillin-resistant staphylococci. *Antimicrobial Agents and Chemotherapy* 33: 991–999

Jarløv J O, Rosdahl V T, Mortensen I, Bentzon M W 1988 In vitro activity and beta-lactamase stability of methicillin, isoxazolyl penicillins and cephalothin against coagulase-negative staphylococci. *Journal of Antimicrobial Chemotherapy* 22: 119–125

John J F Jr, McNeill W F 1980 Activity of cephalosporins against methicillin-susceptible and methicillin-resistant, coagulase-negative staphylococci: minimal effect of beta-lactamase. *Antimicrobial Agents and Chemotherapy* 17: 179–183

Keane C T, Cafferkey M T 1984 Re-emergence of methicillin-resistant *Staphylococcus aureus* causing severe infection. *Journal of Infection* 9: 6–16

Kline M W, Mason E O Jr, Kaplan S L 1987 Outcome of heteroresistant *Staphylococcus aureus* infections in children. *Journal of Infectious Diseases* 156: 205–208

Lacey R W 1986 The mechanism of methicillin resistance. *Journal of Antimicrobial Chemotherapy* 18: 435–436

Maple P A, Hamilton-Miller J M, Brumfitt W 1989 World-wide antibiotic resistance in methicillin-resistant *Staphylococcus aureus*. *Lancet* i: 537–540

Marples R R, Cooke E M 1988 Current problems with methicillin-resistant *Staphylococcus aureus*. *Journal of Hospital Infection* 11: 381–392

Richardson J F, Marples R R 1982 Changing resistance to antimicrobial drugs and resistance typing in clinically significant strains of *Staphylococcus epidermidis*. *Journal of Medical Microbiology* 15: 475–484

Vigeral P, Kanfer A, Kenouch S, Blanchet F, Mougenot B, Méry J P 1987 Nephrogenic diabetes insipidus and distal tubular acidosis in methicillin-induced interstitial nephritis. *Advances in Experimental Biology and Medicine* 212: 129–134

Wakefield D S, Pfaller M, Massanari R M, Hammons G T 1987 Variation in methicillin-resistant *Staphylococcus aureus* occurrence by geographic location and hospital characteristics. *Infection Control* 8: 151–157

Waldvogel F A 1986 Treatment of infection due to methicillin-resistant *Staphylococcus aureus*. *Journal of Hospital Infection* 7 (suppl A): 37–46

NAFCILLIN

A semi-synthetic penicillin supplied as the sodium salt.

Antimicrobial activity

Nafcillin has an antibacterial spectrum similar to that of the isoxazolyl penicillins but is more active than the latter against streptococci and pneumococci (Table 15.4). Activity is depressed in the presence of serum. Nafcillin bears some structural similarity to methicillin and it is as stable as methicillin and more stable than the isoxazolyl penicillins to staphylococcal β-lactamase. There is complete cross-resistance with other group 3 penicillins. Bactericidal synergy is demonstrable against *Staph. aureus* with rifampicin and aminoglycosides. Synergy is also seen with ampicillin and nafcillin against β-lactamase-negative ampicillin-resistant strains of *H. influenzae*.

Pharmacokinetics

It is poorly and irregularly absorbed after oral administration, even on an empty stomach, and absorption is further depressed if the drug is given with food. Mean peak plasma levels around 8 mg/l are obtained about 1 h after i.m. injection of 1 g. It is highly protein bound (87%). Plasma concentrations are relatively low because of wide distribution and because about 60–70% is inactivated in the liver.

In the treatment of meningitis with 3 g i.v. 4-hourly, CSF levels up to 9.5 mg/l were found. Penetration into normal meninges is low. In patients with bacterial ventriculitis, CSF concentrations ranged from 1% to 20% of the simultaneous plasma value. Penetration was inversely related to ventricular fluid glucose, but poorly correlated with pleocytosis. Nafcillin penetrates into other tissues to a similar extent as the isoxazolyl penicillins.

Only about 11% is recovered over 12 h in the urine following oral administration. Following i.m. administration, about 30% appears in the urine, producing concentrations up to 1000 mg/l. Administration of probenecid reduces the urinary excretion and raises and prolongs the plasma level. About 8% of the dose is excreted in the bile.

Toxicity and side-effects

There is cross-allergy with other penicillins, and reappearance of methicillin-induced nephropathy on treatment with nafcillin has been described. Reversible neutropenia may occur. Abnormal platelet aggregation responses with normal platelet counts and morphology have been associated with bleeding in some cases.

Clinical uses

Those of group 3 penicillins (p. 273), but it has been particularly commended for the treatment of staphylococcal meningitis. Reference is made to its use in osteomyelitis (p. 761).

Preparations and dosage

Preparations: Injection, tablets.
Dosage: Adults, oral, 250 mg to 1 g every 4–6 h. Children 6.25–12.5 mg/kg 4 times daily; neonates, 10 mg/kg 3–4 times daily. Adults, i.m., i.v., 0.5–1 g every 4–6 h. Children, 25 mg/kg twice a day; neonates, 10 mg/kg twice a day. Available in USA.

Further information

Alexander D P, Russo M E, Fohrman D E, Rothstein G 1983 Nafcillin-induced platelet dysfunction and bleeding. *Antimicrobial Agents and Chemotherapy* 23: 59–62

Arthur J D, Bass J W, Keiser J F, Harden L B, Brown S L 1982 Nafcillin-tolerant *Staphylococcus epidermidis* endocarditis. *Journal of the American Medical Association* 247: 487–488

Banner W Jr, Gooch W M, Burckart G, Korones S B 1980 Pharmacokinetics of nafcillin in infants with low birth weights. *Antimicrobial Agents and Chemotherapy* 17: 691–694

Fraser G L, Miller M, Kane K 1989 Warfarin resistance associated with nafcillin therapy. *American Journal of Medicine* 87: 237–238

Tilden S J, Craft J C, Cano R, Daum R S 1980 Cutaneous necrosis associated with intravenous nafcillin therapy. *American Journal of Diseases of Children* 134: 1046–1048

Yogev R, Schultz W E, Rosenman S B 1981 Penetrance of nafcillin into human ventricular fluid: correlation with ventricular pleocytosis and glucose levels. *Antimicrobial Agents and Chemotherapy* 19: 545–548

Zenk K E, Dungy C I, Greene G R 1981 Nafcillin extravasation injury. *American Journal of Diseases of Children* 135: 1113–1114

Group 4: Extended-spectrum penicillins

The introduction of an amino group in the α-position of the side-chain of benzylpenicillin confers a high degree of acid stability together with enhanced activity against Gram-negative bacteria. Ampicillin, the first of the aminopenicillins to be developed, retains the activity of benzylpenicillin against Gram-positive cocci but exhibits increased activity against H. influenzae and certain Gram-negative bacilli, notably Esch. coli, Salmonella and Shigella spp. and Pr. mirabilis. The aminopenicillins lack stability to β-lactamases and are readily inactivated by β-lactamase-producing bacteria; but in combination with β-lactamase inhibitors (p. 320) they display enhanced activity against many β-lactamase-producing isolates.

The clinical success of ampicillin resulted in the development of a number of modified aminopenicillins with claims for superior properties. Compounds closely related structurally to ampicillin include amoxycillin, epicillin and cyclacillin. Amoxycillin differs from ampicillin in possessing a p-hydroxy group in the benzene ring of the side-chain and has an essentially identical spectrum of activity to ampicillin, but is bactericidal to susceptible Gram-negative bacilli at rather lower concentrations. Also, amoxycillin has superior oral absorption characteristics and the combination of improved antibacterial and pharmacokinetic properties has resulted in the newer compound largely displacing ampicillin.

In epicillin, the benzene ring is partially saturated and its antibacterial activity is virtually identical to that of ampicillin. Cyclacillin has a greater variation in structure in that the benzene ring is completely saturated and the amino substituent is attached directly to it instead of being linked to an adjacent carbon atom. The antibacterial activity of cyclacillin is substantially less than that of ampicillin.

Four esters of ampicillin (bacampicillin, lenampicillin, pivampicillin, talampicillin) have been developed as pro-drugs with superior oral absorption characteristics to the parent penicillin. The esters are lipophilic compounds that are devoid of antibacterial activity in their own right but are hydrolysed by tissue esterates during absorption to liberate ampicillin. Two condensation products, hetacillin and metampicillin, formed by combination of ampicillin with acetone and formaldehyde respectively, hydrolyse spontaneously to release ampicillin. The antibacterial activity of all these compounds is due solely to the ampicillin liberated.

Two other group 4 penicillins, mecillinam and its pro-drug pivmecillinam, are amidinopenicillins which are quite different structurally from the aminopenicillins. Like other semi-synthetic penicillins they are derived from 6-APA but differ in being 6-α-amidinopenicillanates rather than 6-α-acylaminopenicillanates. This is reflected in the antibacterial spectrum of mecillinam, which is atypical of the penicillins in displaying high activity against Gram-negative bacteria but poor activity against Gram-positive cocci. The mechanism of action of mecillinam differs from that of other penicillins in binding almost exclusively to PBP2 (p. 13) in Gram-negative bacteria.

Pharmacokinetics

The aminopenicillins are acid stable and can be given by mouth. Ampicillin is the least well absorbed, about one-third of the dose appearing in the urine as active drug, and absorption is further reduced by food. The esters and amoxycillin are substantially better absorbed and not significantly affected by food, peak plasma levels generally being at least twice those achieved by equivalent doses of ampicillin. The condensates and epicillin offer no material advantage compared with ampicillin in terms of absorption, whereas cyclacillin is more similar to amoxycillin in producing high plasma antibiotic concentrations. Plasma elimination half-lives are generally around 1 h and plasma protein binding is low (around 20%). Excretion is primarily renal, resulting in high concentrations of active antibiotic in urine; a proportion of an oral dose (10–20%) is metabolized in the liver and small amounts are found in the bile. With metampicillin, comparatively high biliary concentrations of ampicillin appear after parenteral administration. The aminopenicillins and the condensates may be administered by parenteral routes, but the esters are given by mouth

only. Mecillinam is not absorbed by mouth but its pivaloyloxymethyl ester, pivmecillinam, is relatively well absorbed by the oral route, about 40% of the dose being recovered as mecillinam in the urine.

Toxicity and side-effects

Ampicillin appears to be less likely than benzylpenicillin to elicit true allergic reactions, but much more likely to give rise to rashes which appear not to be of allergic origin. Rashes occur with almost diagnostic frequency (95%) in patients with infectious mononucleosis and are also more common in patients with other lymphoid disorders. It was originally thought that the prevalence of rashes was lower in patients treated with amoxycillin, but this appears not to be so. Ampicillin esters naturally have the same potential to give rise to rashes, but it has been claimed that they are less common after epicillin, cyclacillin and mecillinam.

Gastrointestinal side-effects are relatively common in patients treated with oral ampicillin. Ampicillin esters and the ester of mecillinam are more likely to cause upper abdominal discomfort, nausea and vomiting, but are less likely, being better absorbed (as are amoxycillin and cyclacillin) to cause diarrhoea. Upper abdominal symptoms are substantially ameliorated if the esters are taken with food. There has been concern about the potential toxicity of esters on the grounds that unhydrolysed ester may reach and damage the liver and the liberated ester moiety may itself be toxic. Caution has been advocated in the use of these agents, but the available evidence is that these esters are very rapidly degraded and no toxic manifestation has been traced to the various degradation products. Liver function should be monitored in patients receiving prolonged courses, or in those in whom renal or hepatic function is impaired.

Clinical use

Aminopenicillins are all recommended for the wide range of infections that made ampicillin one of the most commonly prescribed agents, notably urinary and respiratory infections. However, the increasing frequency of isolation of β-lactamase-producing pathogens has resulted in a reduction of the usefulness of the aminopenicillins and often relegation to second-line treatment in these areas. This difficulty is overcome by combining ampicillin or amoxycillin with β-lactamase inhibitors (p. 321). Ampicillin and amoxycillin also have an important place in the treatment of severe infections, including endocarditis, meningitis and septicaemia, often in combination with other antibacterial agents, particularly aminoglycosides. The amidinopenicillins are suitable only for infections involving Gram-negative bacteria and should not be used where Gram-positive organisms may be implicated.

AMPICILLIN

A semi-synthetic penicillin administered orally as the free acid, which is soluble only to the extent of about 10% in water, and parenterally as the soluble sodium salt.

Antimicrobial activity

Ampicillin is slightly less active than benzylpenicillin against most Gram-positive bacteria but is more active against *Ent. faecalis*. It is destroyed by staphylococcal β-lactamase so that most clinical isolates of *Staph. aureus* and *Staph. epidermidis* are resistant. Some strains of *Str. pneumoniae* with reduced susceptibility to benzylpenicillin may be more susceptible to ampicillin, but strains with high-level resistance to penicillin are resistant. Most group D streptococci, anaerobic Gram-positive cocci and bacilli including *L. monocytogenes*, *Actinomyces* spp. and *Arachnia* spp. are susceptible. Mycobacteria and nocardia are resistant.

Ampicillin is slightly less active than benzylpenicillin against *N. gonorrhoeae* and *N. meningitidis*, slightly more active against *M. catarrhalis*, and 2–4 times more active against *H. influenzae*. It is 4–8 times more active than benzylpenicillin against *Esch. coli*, *Pr. mirabilis*, *Salmonella* spp. and *Shigella* spp. but β-lactamase-producing strains are resistant. Most other Enterobacteriaceae including *Citrobacter*, *Enterobacter*, *Hafnia*, *Klebsiella*, indole-positive *Proteus*, *Providencia* and *Yersinia* spp. are resistant by virtue of β-lactamase production. *Pseudomonas* spp. are resistant. *Bordetella*, *Brucella* and *Legionella* spp. are susceptible and *Campylobacter* spp. are frequently so. Certain Gram-negative anaerobes such as *Prevotella melaninogenica* (*B. melaninogenicus*) and *Fusobacteria* spp. are susceptible, but *B. fragilis* is resistant, as are mycoplasma and rickettsiae. Its activity against common pathogenic bacteria is shown in Table 15.5.

The activity of ampicillin against β-lactamase-producing strains of staphylococci, gonococci, *H. influenzae*, *M. catarrhalis*, certain Enterobacteriaceae and *B. fragilis* is enhanced by the presence of the β-lactamase inhibitors, clavulanic acid, sulbactam and tazobactam.

Its bactericidal activity resembles that of benzylpenicillin (pp. 13, 264). Bactericidal synergy occurs with aminoglycosides against *Ent. faecalis* and many enterobacteria, and with mecillinam against a proportion of ampicillin-resistant

Table 15.5 Activity of group 4 penicillins against common pathogenic bacteria: MIC (mg/l)

	Ampicillin	Amoxycillin	Cyclacillin	Epicillin	Mecillinam
Staph. aureus	0.06–1	0.1	1	0.1	128
Str. pyogenes (group A)	0.03	0.01	0.5	0.03	2
Str. pneumoniae	0.03–0.06	0.03	0.5		2
Ent. faecalis	1	0.5	2	1	R
N. gonorrhoeae	0.03–0.06	0.1	0.06	0.06	0.1
N. meningitidis	0.03–0.06	0.06			
H. influenzae	0.25	0.5	4	0.25	16
Esch. coli	4	4	64	4	0.25
K. pneumoniae	R	R	R	R	1
Pr. mirabilis	1	1	32	2	32
Proteus (indole +)	R	R	R	R	R
Enterobacter spp.	R	R	R	R	1
Salm. typhi	0.5–1	1	32	2	1
Shigella spp.	2	2	32	2	8
Ser. marcescens	R	R	R	R	128
Citrobacter spp.	R	R			
Ps. aeruginosa	R	R	R	R	R
B. fragilis	32	32	32	32	R

R (resistant) MIC ≥ 128 mg/l.

Enterobacteriaceae. Its bactericidal activity against group B streptococci, *H. influenzae* and *L. monocytogenes* is antagonized by chloramphenicol.

Acquired resistance

Most (90%) clinical isolates of *Staph. aureus* in both community and hospital practice are β-lactamase-producing strains resistant to ampicillin, as is now the case with the respiratory pathogen *M. catarrhalis*. The prevalence of penicillin-resistant strains of *Str. pneumoniae* is increasing in many parts of the world, being low in the UK (2.0%) and the USA (3.8%), but ranging as high as 44% in Spain to 51% in Hungary. All penicillin-resistant pneumococci show reduced susceptibility to ampicillin, and strains with higher levels of resistance (benzylpenicillin MIC >1.0 mg/l) are considered to be resistant to ampicillin. Strains of *N. gonorrhoeae* and *H. influenzae* with altered penicillin-binding proteins may be moderately susceptible to ampicillin, but increasing numbers have acquired TEM plasmid-mediated β-lactamases (p. 319), rendering them fully resistant. The incidence of β-lactamase-producing gonococci varies greatly between different centres and locations, and frequencies ranging from 2% to 41% have been reported in the UK. β-Lactamase-producing strains of *H. influenzae* have been isolated with increasing frequency in the UK, from 1.6% of strains in 1977 to 8.6% in 1992. β-Lactamase production is much higher among capsulate type B strains than in non-capsulate strains; in the UK in 1992 the resistance of type B strains was reported to be 21% compared with 8.3% among non-capsulate strains. This observation has been confirmed in European and US surveys. Resistance to ampicillin among *H. influenzae* is often linked with resistance to chloramphenicol, erythromycin or tetracycline. The frequency of isolation of ampicillin-resistant, β-lactamase-negative strains of *H. influenzae* is reported to be increasing, but remains substantially lower than that of β-lactamase-producing strains. The acquisition of β-lactamases by *M. catarrhalis* has been even more striking; such strains were unknown before 1977, whereas 90% of current isolates are β-lactamase-producing strains. Most strains of the sexually transmitted pathogen *H. ducreyi* have acquired TEM plasmid-mediated β-lactamases and are resistant to ampicillin.

The widespread usage of ampicillin and other aminopenicillins has led to resistance becoming common in formerly susceptible species of enteric bacilli as a result of the widespread dissemination of plasmid-mediated β-lactamases. Approximately 50% of isolates of *Esch. coli* in domicilary practice and in hospitals in the UK are now resistant to ampicillin, and similar figures or higher are reported world-wide. β-Lactamase-producing strains of salmonellae, notably *Salm. typhimurium*, are commonly isolated, and strains resistant to ampicillin and other antibiotics including aminoglycosides, chloramphenicol, sulphonamides and tetracyclines present a serious problem in Africa, Asia and South America. In contrast, most strains of *Salm. typhi* remain susceptible to ampicillin. Multiply resistant strains of shigellae also predominate in many parts of the world.

Pharmacokinetics

Ampicillin is highly stable to acid; in 2 h at pH 2 and 37°C only 5% of activity is lost. It is relatively well absorbed when given by mouth, peak plasma concentrations of 0.8–3.5 and 0.6–6 mg/l being produced by doses of 250 and 500 g around 1 and 2 h after administration, respectively. Absorption is impaired when it is given with meals, but is not affected by administration of antacids or cimetidine.

It is given parenterally as the sodium salt. Peak plasma concentrations 1 h after 500 mg i.m. are around 5–15 mg/l and following a similar dose by i.v. infusion, around 12–29 mg/l. Doubling the dose approximately doubles the peak level. The plasma half-life is 1–1.5 h.

In pregnancy, the peak plasma concentration is reduced due to increased extracellular water volume and increased renal clearance. In newborn and premature infants given 10 or 25 mg/kg, mean peak plasma concentrations were 20 and 60 mg/l, respectively, with mean plasma elimination half-lives in the first, second and third weeks of life of 4.0, 2.8 and 1.7 h, respectively. About 20% is bound to plasma protein. Only a small proportion is converted to penicilloic acid.

Distribution

Ampicillin is distributed in the extracellular fluid. Adequate concentrations are obtained in serous effusions. Effective CSF levels are obtained only in the presence of inflammation and then irregularly, peak concentrations around 3 mg/l being found in the first 3 days of treatment in patients receiving 150 mg/kg per day.

It accumulates and persists in the amniotic fluid, evidently in consequence of renal excretion by the fetus, the levels generally exceeding 2.5 mg/l after three maternal doses of 500 mg, with corresponding cord blood levels of 0.2–2 mg/l.

Excretion

About 30% of an oral dose and 60–80% of i.m. or i.v. doses are recoverable from the urine where concentrations around 250–1000 mg/l appear. Excretion is partly in the glomerular filtrate and partly by tubular secretion, which can be blocked by probenecid. Impairment of renal function reduces the rate of excretion, the plasma half-life rising to 8–9 h in anuric patients. Haemodialysis reduces the blood level, removing about 40% of the dose in 6 h, but peritoneal dialysis is without significant effect.

Bile. Although excretion is mainly renal, fairly high concentrations are attained in the bile, up to 50 times the corresponding serum level. There are wide variations among patients with normal biliary tracts, and in those with obstructive lesions concentrations are very low or nil. There is a degree of enterohepatic recirculation and significant quantities appear in the faeces. Bioavailability may be affected in severe liver disease.

Toxicity and side-effects

It appears generally free from severe toxicity, and apart from gastrointestinal intolerance, the only significant side-effects seen have been rashes. In common with other semi-synthetic penicillins, it appears to be less likely than benzylpenicillin to elicit true allergic reactions. On the other hand, it is much more likely to give rise to rashes, which are found in 5–10% of treated patients. They may be of toxic rather than allergic origin and there is some evidence of dose relation, since they occur more frequently in patients receiving large doses or in renal failure. Rashes occur with almost diagnostic frequency (95%) in patients with infectious mononucleosis. This unusual susceptibility disappears when the disease resolves. Rashes are also more common in patients with other lymphoid disorders, including lymphatic leukaemia. The eruption, which is usually maculopapular, typically appears 4–5 days after beginning treatment. In keeping with a toxic rather than an allergic origin, skin tests to ampicillin and to mixed allergen moieties of benzylpenicillin are negative.

There have been much the same arguments about the nature of the toxic products responsible for the rashes as there have been about penicillin allergens (p. 260). Polymer-free ampicillin produced fewer rashes when given to patients with lymphatic disorders than did commercial ampicillin. Since the typical maculopapular rash of ampicillin does not have an allergic origin, its development does not indicate penicillin allergy and is not a contraindication to the use of other penicillins.

Gastrointestinal side effects are relatively common (around 10%) in patients treated with oral ampicillin, and occur in 2–3% of patients given the drug parenterally, presumably as a result of drug entering the gut through the bile. The very young and the old are most likely to suffer. Diarrhoea can be sufficiently severe to require withdrawal of treatment and pseudomembranous colitis occurs, rates of 0.3–0.7% being quoted. Interference with the bowel flora, which is presumably implicated in diarrhoea, can also affect enterohepatic recirculation of steroids, and the derangement can be sufficient to impair the absorption of oral

contraceptives and affect the interpretation of oestriol levels.

Other rare toxic manifestations typical of penicillins have been described, particularly in those receiving high doses, including leukopenia, thrombocytopenia, haemolytic anaemia, interstitial nephritis and epileptiform seizures, though these are less frequent than with benzylpenicillin.

Clinical use

It has been widely and successfully used for the treatment of acute and chronic urinary tract infection and may be given safely in pregnancy, but its value in these infections is threatened by the advancing prevalence of resistant strains. The other common use of the agent is in the treatment of respiratory tract infection, including the control of exacerbations of chronic bronchitis (p. 690). It should not be used in acute upper respiratory tract infections; they are commonly of viral origin and where sore throat is due to infectious mononucleosis, rashes are frequent and can be severe. In the young child, where otitis media is commonly due to *H. influenzae*, ampicillin is a drug of choice. It is not effective in brucellosis. Single dose treatment is effective in gonorrhoea due to ampicillin-susceptible strains.

It is used in the treatment of meningitis (pp. 747, 749, 751) and is the drug of choice when infection is due to *L. monocytogenes* (p. 752). Its spectrum is not adequate to permit its use alone for the treatment of patients suffering from severe undiagnosed bacterial infection. The combination with an aminoglycoside, notably gentamicin, provides activity against the great majority of neonatal pathogens (p. 811), including streptococci, Listeria, enterobacteria and pseudomonas. Because it is more active than benzyl-penicillin against *Ent. faecalis*, its combination with an aminoglycoside (commonly streptomycin or gentamicin) has been recommended for the treatment (and prophylaxis) of endocarditis due to that organism (p. 703). It may be useful in enteric fever and other septicaemic salmonelloses, including infection due to chloramphenicol-resistant strains. It is ineffective in the eradication of the carrier state. It has also been used in shigellosis, infantile gastroenteritis, intra-abdominal and pelvic sepsis, bone and joint infection, non-specific urethritis, plague (p. 885) and leptospirosis.

Preparations and dosage

Proprietary name: Penbritin.

Preparations: Capsules, syrup, injection.

Dosage: Adults, oral, 250 mg to 1 g every 6 h; i.m., i.v., 500 mg every 4–6 h. Children under 10 years, any route, half the adult dose.

Widely available.

Further information

Campoli-Richards D M, Brogden R N 1987 Sulbactam/ampicillin; a review of its antibacterial activity, pharmacokinetic properties and therapeutic use. *Drugs* 33: 577–609

Cohen M L 1992 Epidemiology of drug resistance; implications for a post-antibiotic era. *Science* 257: 1050–1055

Feder H M Jr 1982 Comparative tolerability of ampicillin, amoxicillin and trimethoprim-sulfamethoxazole suspensions in children with otitis media. *Antimicrobial Agents and Chemotherapy* 21: 426–427

Givner L B, Abramson J S, Wasilauskas B 1989 Meningitis due to *Haemophilus influenzae* type B resistant to ampicillin and chloramphenicol. *Reviews of Infectious Diseases* 11: 329–334

Kovatch A L, Wald E R, Michaels R 1983 β-Lactamase-producing *Branhamella catarrhalis* causing otitis media in children. *Journal of Pediatrics* 102: 261–264

Loria R C, Jadidi S, Wedner H J 1987 Anaphylactic reaction to ampicillin in a patient with common variable immunodeficiency syndrome desensitised to penicillin. *Annals of Allergy* 59: 15–16, 34–38

Mendelman P M, Chaffin D O, Stull T L, Rubens C E, Mack K D, Smith A L 1984 Characterization of non-beta-lactamase-mediated ampicillin resistance in *Haemophilus influenzae*. *Antimicrobial Agents and Chemotherapy* 26: 235–244

Mikhail I A, Sippel J F, Girgis N I, Yassin M W 1981 Cerebrospinal fluid and serum ampicillin levels in bacterial meningitis patients after intravenous and intramuscular administration. *Scandinavian Journal of Infectious Diseases* 13: 237–238

Overturf G D, Cable D, Ward J 1987 Ampicillin-chloramphenicol-resistant *Haemophilus influenzae*: plasmid-mediated resistance in bacterial meningitis. *Pediatric Research* 22: 438–441

Powell M, Fah Y S, Seymour A, Juan M, Williams J D 1992 Antimicrobial resistance in *Haemophilus influenzae* from England and Scotland in 1991. *Journal of Antimicrobial Chemotherapy* 29: 832–839

Rogers H J, James C A, Morrison P J, Bradbrook I D 1980 Effect of cimetidine on oral absorption of ampicillin and co-trimoxazole. *Journal of Antimicrobial Chemotherapy* 6: 297–300

Rupar D G, Fischer M C, Fletcher H, Mortensen J 1989 Emergence of isolates resistant to ampicillin. *American Journal of Diseases of Children* 143: 1033–1037

Sapico F L, Canawat H N, Ginunas V J et al 1989 Enterococci highly resistant to penicillin and ampicillin: an emerging clinical problem? *Journal of Clinical Microbiology* 27: 2091–2095

Sutherland R 1993 Bacterial resistance to β-lactam antibiotics. *Progress in Drug Research* 41: 95–149

Tessin I, Trollfors B, Thiringer K, Thorn Z, Larsson P 1989 Concentrations of ceftazidime, tobramycin and ampicillin in the cerebrospinal fluid of newborn infants. *European Journal of Pediatrics* 147: 679–681

Trottier S, Bergeron M G 1981 Intrarenal concentrations of ampicillin in acute pyelonephritis. *Antimicrobial Agents and Chemotherapy* 19: 761–765

Ampicillin esters

These include bacampicillin, lenampicillin, pivampicillin and talampicillin.

BACAMPICILLIN

Ethoxycarbonyloxyethyl ester of ampicillin.

There is near-complete oral absorption and rapid hydrolysis of the ester by tissue esterases with liberation of ampicillin, to which it owes its antibacterial activity.

Average peak plasma levels are 2–3 times those produced by equivalent doses of ampicillin: following oral doses of 200 and 800 mg, around 12 and 40 mg/l, respectively. Mean absorption differed considerably amongst hospitalized patients and was less than in volunteers. In young children receiving 10 mg/kg, mean peak plasma levels of 7 mg/l were obtained after 0.5–1 h.

Mean concentrations of 2.7 mg/l in pleural fluid and 4.7 mg/l in lymph were found after doses of 1600 and 800 mg, respectively.

Clinical uses are those of ampicillin (p. 284).

Preparations and dosage

Proprietary name: Ambaxin.

Preparation: Tablets.

Dosage: Adults, oral, 400 mg, 2–3 times daily; dose doubled in severe infections. Children over 5 years, 200 mg three times daily.

Widely available.

Further information

Bergan T 1978 Pharmacokinetic comparison of oral bacampicillin and parenteral ampicillin. *Antimicrobial Agents and Chemotherapy* 13: 971–974

Daschner F D, Gier E, Lentzen H, Kaiser D, Bamberg P 1981 Penetration into the pleural fluid after bacampicillin and amoxycillin. *Journal of Antimicrobial Chemotherapy* 7: 585–588

Ginsburg C M, McCracken G H Jr, Clahsen J C, Zweighaft T C 1981 Comparative pharmacokinetics of bacampicillin and ampicillin suspensions in infants and children. *Reviews of Infectious Diseases* 3: 117–120

Neu H C 1981 The pharmacokinetics of bacampicillin. *Reviews of Infectious Diseases* 3: 110–116

Schonwald S, Beus I, Car V et al 1988 Bacampicillin, amoxycillin and talampicillin concentrations in bronchial secretions. *International Journal of Clinical Pharmacology Research* 8: 263–266

Sjovall J 1981 Tissue levels after administration of bacampicillin, a pro-drug of ampicillin and comparisons with other aminopenicillins: a review. *Journal of Antimicrobial Chemotherapy* 8 (suppl C): 41–58

LENAMPICILLIN
KBT-1585

The daloxate ester of ampicillin metabolized to ampicillin and acetoin. In volunteers receiving 400 mg orally, peak concentrations were around 6.0 mg/l at about 1 h: about double those produced by an equimolecular dose (250 mg) of ampicillin. The peak plasma concentration is slightly depressed and delayed by food, but the area under the curve (AUC) is unaltered. Urinary excretion is blocked by probenecid.

Preparations
Available in Japan.

Further information

Saito A, Nakashima M 1986 Pharmacokinetic study of lenampicillin (KBT-1585) in healthy volunteers. *Antimicrobial Agents and Chemotherapy* 29: 948–950

Sum Z M, Sefton A M, Jepson A P, Williams J D 1989 Comparative pharmacokinetic study between lenampicillin, bacampicillin and amoxycillin. *Journal of Antimicrobial Chemotherapy* 23: 861–868

PIVAMPICILLIN

The pivaloyloxymethyl ester of ampicillin.

Its antimicrobial activity is that of liberated ampicillin. Its absorption is considerably better than that of the parent ampicillin and less affected by food. In its passage through the gut it is rapidly hydrolysed to pivalic acid and an unstable hydroxymethyl ester which decomposes to ampicillin. More than 99% conversion to ampicillin is achieved in less than 15 min and not more than 2% of the unchanged ester can be detected in the peripheral blood. Plasma levels rise more rapidly to 2–3 times those produced by corresponding doses of ampicillin: mean peak concentrations around 10 mg/l being obtained 1–2 h after an oral dose of 700 mg (equivalent to 500 mg ampicillin). Relative excretions in the urine as a measure of degree of absorption are: ampicillin 30–45%, pivampicillin 55–75%.

Clinical uses are those of ampicillin (p. 284).

Preparations and dosage
Proprietary names: Pondocillin, Miraxid.
Preparations: Tablets, suspension.
Dosage: Adults, oral, 500 mg every 12 h; dose doubled in severe infection. Children, 6–10 years, 525–700 mg/day in 2–3 divided doses; children 1–5 years, 350–525 mg/day in 2–3 divided doses; children up to 1 year, 40–60 mg/kg per day in 2–3 divided doses; the doses may be doubled in severe infections.
Widely available.

Further information

Hamilton-Miller J M T, Kosmidis J, Brumfitt W 1974 Pharmacokinetic studies with a new pivampicillin: the free base. *Infection* 2: 193–195

Roholt K, Nielsen B, Kristensen E 1974 Clinical pharmacology of pivampicillin. *Antimicrobial Agents and Chemotherapy* 6: 563–571

Verbist L 1974 Triple crossover study on absorption and excretion of ampicillin, pivampicillin and amoxycillin. *Antimicrobial Agents and Chemotherapy* 6: 588–593

TALAMPICILLIN

The phthalidyl thiazolidine carboxylic ester of ampicillin.

Its antimicrobial activity is that of liberated ampicillin. It is well absorbed when administered by mouth, doses of 250 or 500 mg producing mean peak plasma levels around 4 or 11 mg/l, respectively, about 2 h after the dose. Administration with food delays and depresses the peak concentration but the AUC is unaffected.

It is generally well tolerated. Diarrhoea is infrequent and as the compound is antibacterially inactive, there is no effect from any unabsorbed residue on the gut flora.

Clinical uses are those of ampicillin (p. 284).

Preparations and dosage

Dosage: Adults, oral, 250–500 mg three times daily.
Limited availability.

Further information

Jones K H, Langley P F, Lees L J 1979 Bioavailability and metabolism of talampicillin. *Chemotherapy* 24: 217–226

Symonds J, Georg R H 1978 The effect of talampicillin on faecal flora. *Journal of Antimicrobial Chemotherapy* 4: 92–94

Ampicillin condensates

HETACILLIN

A condensation product of ampicillin and acetone. It is disputed whether it has any antibacterial action distinct from that of ampicillin, but any such activity is of no therapeutic significance since it hydrolyses rapidly in the body to liberate ampicillin, leaving only trace amounts of the parent compound detectable in the plasma for about 90 min. Although there is disagreement, in general it appears that absorption, peak levels and excretion are all rather lower than those for ampicillin.

Preparations and dosage

Dosage: Adults, oral, 250–500 mg four times daily.
Very limited availability.

Further information

Kahrimanis R, Pierpaoli P 1971 Hetacillin vs ampicillin. *New England Journal of Medicine* 285: 236–237

METAMPICILLIN

A condensation product of ampicillin with formaldehyde. It hydrolyses sufficiently rapidly to ampicillin for there to be no unchanged drug detectable in the plasma after oral dosage. When high levels are produced by parenteral administration, the drug bound to protein is more slowly hydrolysed at the neutral pH of the plasma and unchanged compound is detectable and is excreted, in part in the bile, where it may give elevated free ampicillin levels.

Preparations and dosage

Dosage: Adults, oral, 2 g/day in 2–4 divided doses.
Available in Spain.

Further information

DeVecchi Pellati M, Falqune F, Perraro F 1970 La metampicillina nella patologia delle vie biliari entraepatiche. Eliminazione biliare e profilassi operatoria e post-operatoria. *Minerva Medicine* 61: 946–952

Lande M 1970 L'elimination biliare de la métampicilline. *Presse Medicale* 78: 805–806

Sutherland R, Elson S, Croydon E A 1972 Metampicillin: antibacterial activity and absorption and excretion in man. *Chemotherapy* 17: 145–160

Ampicillin-like aminopenicillins

AMOXYCILLIN
Amoxicillin; p-hydroxy ampicillin

Antimicrobial activity

Its antibacterial spectrum is identical to that of ampicillin and there are few differences in the antibacterial activities of the two aminopenicillins (Table 15.5). Amoxycillin is two-fold more active against *Ent. faecalis* and some *Salmonella* species and is slightly less active against *H. influenzae*. Amoxycillin is unstable to β-lactamases and significant protection is afforded by β-lactamase inhibitors against β-lactamase-producing bacteria. The clinically-available combination of amoxycillin with clavulanic acid (p. 321) provides enhanced activity against Gram-negative bacteria possessing the plasmid encoded enzymes TEM 1 and 2, SHV 1, OXA 1, 2 and 3 and PSE-1-4, and against *B. fragilis, K. pneumoniae* and *Pr. mirabilis* the chromosomally-mediated β-lactamases of which are highly susceptible to clavulanic acid. β-Lactamase-producing strains of *Staph. aureus* are also readily inhibited by the combination. Amoxycillin produces more rapid bactericidal effects than ampicillin against Gram-negative bacilli at concentrations close to MIC values as a consequence of higher affinity for PBPs leading to the development of spheroplasts that lyse readily.

Acquired resistance

There is complete cross-resistance with ampicillin. Its action against many strains which owe their resistance to elaboration of β-lactamases can be restored by co-administration with β-lactamase inhibitors.

In volunteers receiving a single 3 g oral dose, there was a rapid fall in oral streptococci which had mostly recovered within 48 h and no resistance emerged. Treatment with 2–3 g at weekly intervals up to five doses produced highly resistant *Str. sanguis*, some of which were also resistant to erythromycin. Most had disappeared by 6 weeks and all by 13 weeks.

Pharmacokinetics

Oral absorption is comparable with that of the ampicillin esters, producing around 2.5 times the peak concentration resulting from comparable doses of ampicillin. Mean peak concentrations of 2.7 mg/l after a dose of 125 mg are obtained, the peak concentrations doubling with doubling of the dose up to 1 g. Following a single oral dose of 3 g, plasma concentrations were around 16 mg/l at 2 h, 8.5 mg/l at 4 h and still detectable at 14 h. Absorption is unaffected by food. Protein binding is similar to that of ampicillin: 17–20%.

In patients receiving 500 mg 8-hourly for 10 days concentrations in mucoid and purulent sputum were 0–1.2 (mean 0.2) mg/l and 0–3.0 (mean 1.0) mg/l, respectively. In patients receiving 750 mg, mean concentrations of 1.56 mg/l were achieved in pleural fluid. Levels of 84% of those in the serum were found in the peritoneal fluid of patients given 1 g by i.v. bolus. In children with chronic serous otitis media, given 15 mg/kg, variable peak concentrations up to those in the serum were found in middle ear fluid at 2–3 h when the mean serum concentration was 5.8 mg/l. Peak concentrations in interstitial fluid as determined by the skin window method are also twice those produced by equivalent doses of ampicillin. Some 10–25% is converted to the penicilloic acid. Between 50 and 70% of unchanged drug is recovered in the urine in the first 6 h after a dose of 250 mg. Plasma levels are elevated and prolonged by the administration of probenecid.

Toxicity and side-effects

It is generally well tolerated, side-effects, including rashes,

being those common to group 4 penicillins. Being well absorbed, diarrhoea is generally infrequent and rarely sufficiently severe to require withdrawal of treatment.

Clinical use

Its uses are those of ampicillin (p. 284). A single 3 g dose is effective in the treatment of acute, uncomplicated urinary tract infection. It has been used for the treatment of typhoid fever (p. 711) and is more effective than ampicillin, though still not entirely so, in eradicating *Salmonella* carriers (p. 712). It is commended for the prophylactic use in those at risk from subacute bacterial endocarditis (p. 706).

Preparations and dosage

Proprietary names: Amoxil, Flemoxin, Solutab.

Preparations: Capsules, suspension, injection, dispersable tablets.

Dosage: Adults, oral, 250–500 mg every 8 h; high dose therapy, 3 g twice daily; short course therapy, simple acute urinary tract infection, two 3 g doses with 10–12 h between doses; dental abscess, two 3 g doses, with 8 h between doses; gonorrhoea, single 3 g dose. i.m., i.v., 500 mg every 8 h, the dose may be increased to 1 g i.v. every 6 h in severe infections. Children up to 10 years, oral, 125–250 mg 3 times daily. In severe otitis media, 750 mg twice daily for 2 days may be used in children 3–10 years, i.m., i.v., 50–100 mg/kg per day in divided doses. Widely available.

Further information

Blanca M, Perez E, Garcia J et al 1988 Anaphylaxis to amoxycillin but good tolerance for benzylpenicillin. In vivo and in vitro studies of specific IgE antibodies. *Allergy* 43: 508–510

Brogden R N, Speight T M, Avery G S 1975 Amoxycillin: a review of its antibacterial and pharmacokinetic properties and therapeutic use. *Drugs* 9: 88–140

Brun Y, Forey F, Gamondes J P, Tebib A, Brune K, Fleurette J 1981 Levels of erythromycin in pulmonary tissue and bronchial mucus compared to those of amoxycillin. *Journal of Antimicrobial Chemotherapy* 8: 459–466

Cannon P D, Black H J, Kitson K 1987 Serum concentrations of amoxycillin in children following an oral loading dose prior to general anaesthesia: relevance for the prophylaxis of infective endocarditis. *Journal of Antimicrobial Chemotherapy* 19: 795–797

Chopra R, Roberts J, Warrington R J 1989 Severe delayed onset hypersensitivity reaction to amoxycillin in children. *Canadian Medical Association Journal* 140: 921–923

Clumeck N, Thys J P, Vanhoof R, Vanderlinden M P, Butzler J P, Yourassowsky E 1978 Amoxicillin entry into human cerebro-spinal fluid: comparison with ampicillin. *Antimicrobial Agents and Chemotherapy* 14: 531–532

Feder H M Jr 1982 Comparative tolerability of ampicillin, amoxicillin and trimethoprim–sulfamethoxazole suspensions in children with otitis media. *Antimicrobial Agents and Chemotherapy* 21: 426–427

Gmur J, Walti M, Neftel K A 1985 Amoxicillin-induced immune haemolysis. *Acta Haematologica (Basle)* 74: 230–233

Levine L R 1985 Quantitative comparison of adverse reactions to cefaclor vs. amoxicillin in a surveillance study. *Pediatric Infectious Diseases* 4: 358–361

MacGregor A J, Hart P 1986 The effect of a single large dose of amoxycillin on oral streptococci. *Journal of Antimicrobial Chemotherapy* 18: 113–117

Mattie H, Van der Voet G B 1981 The relative potency of amoxicillin and ampicillin in vitro and in vivo. *Scandinavian Journal of Infectious Diseases* 13: 291–296

Shah P M 1981 Bactericidal activity of ampicillin and amoxicillin. *Journal of Antimicrobial Chemotherapy* 8 (suppl C): 93–99

Sjovall J, Alvan G, Huitfeldt B 1986 Intra- and inter-individual variation in pharmacokinetics of intravenously infused amoxicillin and ampicillin to elderly volunteers. *British Journal of Clinical Pharmacology* 21: 171–181

Todd P A, Benfield P 1990 Amoxicillin/clavulanic acid; an update of its antibacterial activity, pharmacokinetic properties and clinical use. *Drugs* 39: 264–307

CYCLACILLIN
Ciclacillin

The antibacterial activity of cyclacillin against most Gram-positive and Gram-negative bacteria is relatively low compared with that of ampicillin (Table 15.5). It is some 10–20 times less active against staphylococci, streptococci and *H. influenzae* and is only active against susceptible Gram-negative bacilli at concentrations of 32 mg/l or greater.

It is rapidly and completely absorbed by mouth, peak plasma levels of 10–18 mg/l being reached 30–60 min after a 500 mg oral dose. Following a 3 g oral dose, peak plasma levels around 115 mg/l were found at about 45 min. In infants given 15 or 25 mg/kg, peak plasma concentrations around 15 and 25 mg/l, respectively, were found at about 30 min. Absorption is not depressed by administration with food. Protein binding is low (20%). Its distribution resembles that of ampicillin. It is rapidly eliminated with a plasma half-life of 0.5–0.8 h. While some appears in the bile, the bulk of the dose can be recovered unchanged from the urine. Plasma and urine concentrations are not materially affected by administration of probenecid.

Side-effects, which resemble those of ampicillin, are mild: principally nausea, epigastric discomfort and diarrhoea. Coupled with lower antibacterial activity, this tends to the possibility of less gut disturbance through the effect of unabsorbed agent. Its uses resemble those of ampicillin (p. 284).

Preparations and dosage
Dosage: Adults, oral, 250–500 mg four times daily.
Very limited availability.

Further information

Bone M, Symonds J, Dougan P 1986 Penetration of ciclacillin into bronchial secretions. *Chemioterapia* 5: 105–108

Ginsburg C M, McCracken G H Jr, Zweighaft T C, Clahsen J C 1981 Comparative pharmacokinetics of cyclacillin and amoxicillin in infants and children. *Antimicrobial Agents and Chemotherapy* 19: 1086–1088

Gonzaga A J, Antonio-Velmonte M, Tupasi T E 1974 Cyclacillin: a clinical and in vitro profile. *Journal of Infectious Diseases* 129: 545–551

Wagner K F, Blair A D, Counts G W, Holmes K K 1980 Pharmacological and in vitro evaluation of cyclacillin: assessment as potential single dose therapy for treatment of *Neisseria gonorrhoeae* infection. *Antimicrobial Agents and Chemotherapy* 17: 89–91

EPICILLIN

It closely resembles ampicillin in antibacterial properties; it is somewhat more active against *Ps. aeruginosa*, but this is of no therapeutic significance (Table 15.5). It is moderately well absorbed, a 500 mg oral dose producing mean peak plasma levels around 2–3 mg/l. Its behaviour on i.m. injection, distribution, excretion, toxicity and uses resemble those of ampicillin.

Preparations

Available fairly widely in continental Europe, and in Argentina and South Africa.

Further information

Gadebusch H, Miraglia G, Pansy F 1971 Epicillin: experimental chemotherapy, pharmacodynamics and susceptibility testing. *Infection and Immunity* 4: 50–53

MECILLINAM
Amdinocillin

6-β-Amidinopenicillin. Available as the hydrochloride dihydrate.

Antimicrobial activity

The antibacterial spectrum of mecillinam differs greatly from that of the aminopenicillins in that the compound displays high activity against many Gram-negative bacteria but only low activity against Gram-positive organisms. It is very active against many Enterobacteriaceae including *Esch. coli*, *Citrobacter*, *Enterobacter*, *Klebsiella*, *Salmonella*, *Shigella* and *Yersinia* spp. The susceptibility of *Proteus* and *Providencia* spp. is variable: *Pr. vulgaris* is usually susceptible as are some strains of *Pr. mirabilis*, but *Morganella* and *Providencia* spp. are often resistant. *H. influenzae* is relatively resistant and *Acinetobacter* spp., *B. fragilis* and *Ps. aeruginosa* are resistant. Its activity against common pathogenic bacteria is shown in Table 15.5. The activity of mecillinam is greatly reduced in media with high osmolality and in tests employing large inocula.

Mecillinam is readily inactivated by many β-lactamases, although it is more stable than ampicillin. Its activity against certain β-lactamase-producing bacteria is attributed to its poor affinity for the enzymes, coupled with rapid penetration of the bacterial cell. Combination with the β-lactamase inhibitors, clavulanic acid or sulbactam results in increased activity against many β-lactamase-producing strains of *Esch. coli* and other Enterobacteriaceae.

Mecillinam differs from other penicillins in having a high affinity for PBP2, the penicillin binding protein responsible for cell shape. Inhibition of PBP2 by mecillinam results in the formation of osmotically stable round bodies that are relatively slow to lyse. As a consequence, bactericidal activity is slow, inoculum dependent and varies inversely with NaCl, other salts and sucrose content of the medium. Synergic effects may be observed with *H. influenzae*, *Esch. coli* and other Enterobacteriaceae when mecillinam is combined with β-lactams that bind preferentially to penicillin binding proteins other than PBP2. These agents include ampicillin, amoxycillin, carbenicillin and cephalosporins.

Acquired resistance

Mecillinam does not prevent cell division and the round forms generated after exposure to the drug can continue to grow and divide in spheroplast-like forms. These variants are phenotypically resistant in that they can grow in high concentrations of mecillinam, but growth is relatively slow and their therapeutic significance has been questioned.

However, mecillinam resistance has emerged during therapy of urinary tract infection and of *Salmonella* carriers. The mecillinam-resistant variants were round shaped, grew slowly and were generally unstable, reverting readily to normal bacillary form. The spherical variants have been shown to be relatively resistant to phagocytosis and killing by PMN.

Intrinsic resistance in susceptible species of enterobacteria is uncommon and many ampicillin-resistant Enterobacteriaceae are susceptible to mecillinam. Bacteria that are resistant to both ampicillin and mecillinam are usually those producing large amounts of β-lactamase, most commonly plasmid-mediated enzymes.

Pharmacokinetics

Absorption by mouth is very poor, conventional doses producing plasma levels of less than 1 mg/l and recovery of only about 5% in the urine. The pivaloyl ester, pivmecillinam, is relatively well absorbed.

After i.v. injection of 200 mg, the mean peak plasma concentration at 5 min is around 12 mg/l. A similar dose given i.m. produces peak levels around 6 mg/l at 30 min. Doubling the dose approximately doubles the peak plasma concentration. Administration of 10 mg/kg i.v. over 15 min produces mean peak plasma concentrations close to 50 mg/l with a plasma elimination half-life around 50 min. No accumulation occurred on a 4-hourly schedule. A similar dose i.m. produced a peak around 26 mg/l with a plasma elimination half-life close to 1 h. It is widely distributed in the body water. Protein binding is only 5–10%.

The bulk of the dose, about 60%, is excreted unchanged in the urine in the first 6 h, producing concentrations in excess of 1 mg/l. Plasma clearance and creatinine clearance are linearly related. Haemodialysis removes up to 70% but peritoneal dialysis has little effect. The concentration in bile exceeds that in the serum reaching 40 or 50 mg/l in patients with normally functioning gallbladders treated with 800 mg i.m.

Toxicity and side-effects

It is generally well tolerated, but is assumed to show cross-allergy with penicillins.

Clinical uses

It has been used with some success in the treatment of urinary tract infections due to *Escherichia*, *Enterobacter*, some *Klebsiella* and *Proteus*; in enteric fever, shigellosis and usually in combination with other agents, in some other *Salmonella* septicaemias and in exacerbations of chronic bronchitis.

Preparations and dosage

Preparation: Injection.
Dosage: Adults, 5–10 mg/kg every 6–8 h depending on the severity of the infection.
Limited availability.

Further information

Bornemann L D, Castellano S, Lin A H, Enthoven D, Patel I H 1988 Influence of food on bioavailability of amdinocillin pivoxil. *Antimicrobial Agents and Chemotherapy* 32: 592–594

Eng R H, Liu R, Smith S M, Johnson E S, Cherubin C E 1988 Amidinocillin-interaction with other beta-lactam antibiotics for Gram-negative bacteria. *Chemotherapy* 34: 18–26

Geddes A M, Wise R 1977 Mecillinam. *Journal of Antimicrobial Chemotherapy* 3 (suppl B): 1–160

Hares M M, Hegarty A, Tomkyns J, Burdon D W, Keighley M R B 1982 A study of the biliary excretion of mecillinam in patients with biliary disease. *Journal of Antimicrobial Chemotherapy* 9: 217–222

Moukhtar I, Nawishy S, Sabbour M 1987 Pharmacokinetics of mecillinam after a single intravenous dose in patients with impaired renal function. *International Journal of Clinical Pharmacological Research* 7: 59–62

Neu H C 1982 Synergistic activity of mecillinam in combination with the beta-lactamase inhibitors clavulanic acid and sulbactam. *Antimicrobial Agents and Chemotherapy* 22: 518–519

Patel I H, Bornemann L D, Brocks V M, Fang L S T, Tolkoff-Rubin N E, Rubin R H 1985 Pharmacokinetics of intravenous amdinocillin in healthy subjects and patients with renal insufficiency. *Antimicrobial Agents and Chemotherapy* 28: 46–50

Symposium 1983 An international review of amdinocillin: a new beta-lactam antibiotic. *American Journal of Medicine* 75 (suppl): 1–138

Whelton A, Spilman P S, Stout R L, Delgado F A 1987 The influence of renal functional changes on the intrarenal distribution and urinary kinetics of amdinocillin. *Renal Failure* 10: 101–106

PIVMECILLINAM

The pivaloyloxymethyl ester of mecillinam.

Its effect is due to the liberation of mecillinam in vivo. It is relatively well, but variably, absorbed. Mean peak concentrations are 2–5 mg/l, 1–1.5 h after a 400 mg (273 mg mecillinam) dose. Administration with food has little or no effect on its absorption. The plasma half-life is around 1 h. Urinary recovery falls from around 50% after 200 mg to 30% after 800 mg, suggesting an absorption threshold. Elevated and prolonged levels are obtained after probenecid. Four metabolites account for about 20% of the drug in the urine, of which three are biologically inactive.

It is generally well tolerated, although nausea, upper abdominal discomfort and vomiting, which may be persistent, occur with diarrhoea in some patients. Its clinical uses are those of mecillinam.

Preparations and dosage

Preparations: Suspension, tablets.
Dosage: Adults, oral, 200–400 mg 3–4 times daily.
Available in continental Europe.

Further information

Holme E 1989 Carnitine deficiency induced by pivampicillin and pivmecillinam therapy. *Lancet* ii: 469–473

Roholt K 1977 Pharmacokinetic studies with mecillinam and pivmecillinam. *Journal of Antimicrobial Chemotherapy* 3 (suppl B): 71–81

Group 5: Penicillins active against *Ps. aeruginosa*

Activity against Ps. aeruginosa is not a property usually associated with ampicillin or benzylpenicillin, but certain derivatives of these penicillins display useful activity against

Gram-positive and Gram-negative bacteria including Ps. aeruginosa. *Three derivatives of benzylpenicillin possessing an acidic group in the acyl side-chain are in clinical use: carbenicillin and ticarcillin, are α-carboxypenicillins, and the third, sulbenicillin, possesses a sulphanic acid group in the side-chain. The acyl derivatives of ampicillin active against* Ps. aeruginosa *include the clinically important group of acylureidopenicillins: azlocillin, mezlocillin and piperacillin. Apalcillin and aspoxicillin are also acylaminopenicillins, with properties generally similar to the ureidopenicillins, but lack the ureido group in the side-chain.*

In addition, two pro-drug forms of carbenicillin are available for oral use: the phenyl ester, carfecillin, and the indanyl ester, carindacillin. Unlike ampicillin esters, these compounds are esterified at the side-chain carboxyl group and, since the carboxyl of the penicillin nucleus is free, they exhibit antibacterial activity in vitro which differs in some respects from that of the parent compound. This is of academic interest only since in the body they are rapidly hydrolysed to carbenicillin, to which they owe their therapeutic activity. Carbenicillin and ticarcillin exist as pairs of diasterioisomers (R and S epimers), which interconvert in aqueous solutions at rates that depend on temperature, pH and ionic strength. The epimers show differences in detail in their antimicrobial activity and pharmacokinetic behaviour, but this is considered not to influence the clinical efficacy of the mixtures.

Antimicrobial activity

The acylureidopenicillins and the carboxypenicillins display similar antibacterial spectra, but the ureidopenicillins are notably more active than the latter against streptococci and enterococci (Table 15.6). Both groups are as active as ampicillin against susceptible Gram-negative bacteria and exhibit moderate to good activity against many ampicillin-resistant strains of Enterobacteriaceae possessing class 1 chromosomally-mediated β-lactamases (p. 319). These include nosocomial pathogens such as *Citrobacter*, *Enterobacter*, *Morganella*, *Providencia* and *Serratia* spp., but strains producing elevated amounts of β-lactamase ('derepressed mutants'), are resistant. Particular interest in these penicillins lies in their activity against *Ps. aeruginosa*, apalcillin and the ureidopenicillins generally being more active than the carboxypenicillins in conventional tests. However, the ureidopenicillins are less stable to the chromosomally mediated β-lactamase of *Ps. aeruginosa*, and activity is greatly reduced in tests against large inocula. The superior activity of the ureidopenicillins against *Ps. aeruginosa* may be due to a combination of better penetration characteristics and greater affinity for PBPs. Although the activity of the compounds against anaerobes is not high, considerable attention has been paid to this aspect of their antibacterial spectrum.

Acquired resistance

These penicillins are readily inactivated by plasmid-mediated β-lactamases and, consequently, increasing numbers of clinical isolates are resistant. Activity can be largely restored by combination with β-lactamase inhibitors and fixed combinations of ticarcillin with clavulanic acid (p. 323) and piperacillin with tazobactam (p. 326) have been developed for clinical use.

Pharmacokinetics

None of the compounds is absorbed by mouth, but two esters of carbenicillin are available for oral use. After parenteral administration the plasma half-lives of carbenicillin and ticarcillin are approximately 1 h and the compounds are predominately excreted unchanged by tubular secretion, only small amounts appearing in the bile.

The acylureidopenicillins produce peak plasma levels which are lower than those obtained with the carboxypenicillins. The half-lives and volumes of distribution of the ureidopenicillins are generally similar and increase with larger doses. Elimination from the body is largely by the renal route and most of the drug appears unchanged in the urine, but comparatively high concentrations appear in bile.

Apalcillin differs from the ureidopenicillins in being largely eliminated via the liver; this is related to high molecular weight and high protein binding, and only about 20% of the drug appears in the urine, some in the form of penicilloic acid.

Clinical use

The principal role of these compounds is the treatment of established pseudomonas infection, but they are also active against some other Gram-negative bacilli resistant to other penicillins including *Enterobacter* spp., indole-positive *Proteus* and *Morganella* spp. They are also used in the treatment and prophylaxis of anaerobic and mixed infections. A special role has been claimed, particularly for the acylureidopenicillins in providing broad prophylactic cover, notably in bowel surgery (p. 596). The clinical performance of ticarcillin, piperacillin and mezlocillin appears generally comparable. A major advantage claimed for acylureido-penicillins over carboxypenicillins is that they are mono- rather than disodium salts. They therefore present substantially less sodium load, but the clinical importance of this has not been established.

There is no reason to believe that these compounds are adequate when used alone for the treatment of patients with severe undiagnosed sepsis. In neutropenic patients they need to be combined with an aminoglycoside, but it should be noted that penicillins and aminoglycosides should not be mixed in infusion fluids because of the possibility of mutual degradation (p. 170).

The results of treatment with piperacillin or ticarcillin when combined with amikacin appear comparable. Combined therapy with an aminoglycoside is also required in *Ps. aeruginosa* pneumonia, although the penicillins alone are more effective than aminoglycosides alone. Soft tissue and burn wound infections usually respond, but infections requiring treatment with these agents generally arise in patients with underlying disorders, and suppression rather than eradication of infection is often the best result obtainable. Good examples of such 'control' are provided by cystic fibrosis (where accelerated elimination of the drugs requires high dosage), osteomyelitis, urinary tract infection and the grave necrotizing otitis externa of diabetes. With all these agents, failure may be due to the emergence of resistant variants during treatment.

Acylaminopenicillins

These include apalcillin and aspoxicillin.

APALCILLIN

A semi-synthetic penicillin supplied as the sodium salt.

Antimicrobial activity

The antibacterial spectrum of apalcillin is similar to that of the acylureidopenicillins and the compound is active against *Ps. aeruginosa* and a wide range of Gram-positive and Gram-negative bacteria. It displays a high level of activity against streptococci, *H. influenzae* and *Neisseria* spp., but *Ent. faecalis* is less susceptible and β-lactamase-producing *Staph. aureus* are resistant. Apalcillin is as active as mezlocillin and slightly less active than piperacillin against ampicillin-susceptible and certain ampicillin-resistant Enterobacteriaceae. It exhibits good activity against *Ps. aeruginosa* and other *Pseudomonas* spp. (MIC 1–2 mg/l), including some strains moderately resistant to carbenicillin. *B. fragilis* and many other anaerobes are susceptible. It is relatively labile to many β-lactamases and is readily inactivated by the common TEM plasmid-mediated enzyme.

It is highly bound to plasma protein and its activity is reduced in the presence of plasma. Its activity against common pathogenic bacteria is shown in Table 15.6.

Pharmacokinetics

Mean end-infusion concentrations in patients receiving 30 mg/kg i.v. over 30 min were around 87 mg/l (continuous infusion produced steady-state levels around 30 mg/l) and in volunteers receiving 2 g i.v. over 15 min, 220 mg/l. The elimination half-life has been variously found to be 1.1–2.4 h, longer in patients than in volunteers, probably due to impaired renal elimination. Plasma protein binding is high (80–90%).

It causes concentration- and time-dependent degradation of aminoglycosides, amikacin being the most stable (95% remaining after 36 h) and tobramycin the least (58% after 8 h). Mean concentrations in bronchial secretions in patients receiving 3 g i.v. were 5.8 mg/l. Following similar doses, concentrations in normal CSF did not exceed 1.75 mg/l, but in the presence of inflammation reached 5–30 mg/l.

Only 20% of the dose appears in the urine, mostly as two inactive penicilloic acids. It is mainly eliminated via the liver, concentrations of active drug in the common duct bile reaching 2–4 g/l accounting for about 12% of the dose. The remainder is eliminated as metabolites; there is no significant enterohepatic recirculation.

Toxicity and side-effects

It is generally well tolerated but maculopapular rashes which resolve on cessation of treatment are relatively common. In volunteers receiving 75–225 mg/kg, abnormal platelet aggregation developed and there was a consistent and major fall in antithrombin III activity but plasma coagulation and fibrinogen were not affected.

Clinical uses

Those of group 5 penicillins (p. 292).

Preparations and dosage

Dosage: Adults, i.v., 2–3 g three times daily.

Available in Germany.

Further information

Bergogne-Berezin E, Pierre J, Chastre J, Gilbert C, Heinzel G, Akbaraly J P 1984 Pharmacokinetics of apalcillin in intensive-care patients: study of penetration into the respiratory tract. *Journal of Antimicrobial Chemotherapy* 14: 67–73

Brogard J M, Arnaud J P, Blickle J F, Dorner M, Lautier F 1986 Biliary elimination of apalcillin: an experimental and clinical study. *International Journal of Clinical Pharmacology, Therapy and Toxicology* 24: 180–187

Gentry L O, Wood B A, Natelson E A 1985 Effect of apalcillin on platelet function in normal volunteers. *Antimicrobial Agents and Chemotherapy* 27: 683–684

Hoffler U 1986 Efficacy of apalcillin alone and in combination with four aminoglycoside antibiotics against *Pseudomonas aeruginosa*. *Chemotherapy* 32: 255–259

Neu H C, Labthavikul P 1982 In vitro activity of apalcillin compared with that of other new penicillins and anti-pseudomonas cephalosporins. *Antimicrobial Agents and Chemotherapy* 21: 906–911

Raoult D, Gallias H, Casanova P, Bedjaoui A, Akbaraly R, Auzerie J 1985 Meningeal penetration of apalcillin in man. *Journal of Antimicrobial Chemotherapy* 15: 123–125

Weler H, Carter W T, Harris B, Finegold S M 1984 Comparative in vitro activities of cefpiramide and apalcillin against anaerobic bacteria. *Antimicrobial Agents and Chemotherapy* 25: 162–164

ASPOXICILLIN
TA 058

Unlike the other acylaminopenicillins, which are derivatives of ampicillin, aspoxicillin is synthesized from amoxicillin. It has been studied extensively in Japan where it is available.

Aspoxicillin has a broad antibacterial spectrum against Gram-positive and Gram-negative aerobes and anaerobes. It is twice as active as carbenicillin against *Ps. aeruginosa* and is less active than piperacillin against *Staph. aureus, H. influenzae, Esch. coli, K. pneumoniae* and *Ps. aeruginosa*. It is not absorbed by mouth; the plasma half-life is 87 min after i.v. infusion.

It is reported to be more efficacious against experimental infections than would be predicted from its in vitro activity. It has been reported to be effective in the treatment of respiratory, skin and soft tissue and urinary infections in adults and children, and, in combination with aminoglycosides, against gynaecological infections and infections in patients with haematological disorders.

Further information

Geyer J, Hoffler D, Koeppe P 1988 Pharmacokinetics of aspoxicillin in subjects with normal and impaired renal function. *Arzneimittel Forschung* 11: 1635–1639

Wagatsuma M, Seto M, Miyagishima T, Kawazu M, Yamagushi T, Ohshima S 1983 Synthesis and antibacterial activity of asparagine derivates of aminobenzylpenicillin. *Journal of Antibiotics* 36: 147–154

Acylureidopenicillins

These include azlocillin, mezlocillin and piperacillin.

AZLOCILLIN

A semi-synthetic penicillin supplied as the sodium salt.

Antimicrobial activity

It is distinguished mainly by its activity against *Ps. aeruginosa* (Table 15.6), being as active as piperacillin; most strains are inhibited by 4–8 mg/l, although activity is inoculum dependent. Activity is retained against certain carbenicillin-resistant strains of this organism. It is active against a wide range of Gram-negative bacteria other than *Ps. aeruginosa*, including Enterobacter spp., indole-positive *Proteus* and *Ser. marcescens*, but is less active than mezlocillin and piperacillin against most Enterobacteriaceae. *B. fragilis* and other anaerobes are susceptible. Azlocillin is as active as the other ureidopenicillins against Gram-positive cocci, *H. influenzae* and *N. gonorrhoeae*. It is labile to most β-lactamases and many β-lactamase-producing isolates are resistant.

Pharmacokinetics

Typical mean peak serum levels are 250 and 400 mg/l following 30 and 80 mg/kg, respectively, and there is evidence of dose-dependent pharmacokinetics. The plasma elimination half-life is 0.9–1.1 h. Binding to plasma protein is 20–30%.

Concentrations of 0.5–4 mg/kg were detected in the sputum of about a third of patients receiving 40 mg/kg i.v.

Table 15.6   *Activity of group 5 and 6 penicillins against common pathogenic bacteria: MIC (mg/l)*

	Apalcillin	Azlocillin	Mezlocillin	Piperacillin	Carbenicillin	Ticarcillin	Sulbenicillin	Temocillin
Staph. aureus	1	1	1	0.5	1	1	2	R
Str. pyogenes (group A)	0.03	0.03	0.06	0.03	0.5	0.25	0.5	R
Str. pneumoniae	0.03	0.03	0.03	0.03	1	0.5	1	R
Ent. faecalis	4	2	2	2	16–32	32	32	R
N. gonorrhoeae	<0.01	<0.01	<0.01	<0.01	0.06–0.1	0.06	0.1	0.01–1
N. meningitidis			0.03	0.06	0.06	0.06		
H. influenzae	0.06	0.06	0.1	0.03	0.25–0.5	0.5		0.1–2
Esch. coli	4	16	4	2	4–8	4	4	1–8
K. pneumoniae	16	64	32	16	R	R	R	1–16
Pr. mirabilis	1	4	1	0.5	1–2	1	1	0.5–8
Proteus (indole +)	4	16	4	2	4–8	8	8	1–16
Enterobacter spp.	4	32	4	2	4–8	4	4	1–8
Salm. typhi	4	4	4	4	16	8	4	4–8
Shigella spp.	4	4	4	4	16	8	8	4–8
Ser. marcescens	4	16	4	2	16	8		1–16
Citrobacter spp.	4	8	4	4	16	8		1–16
Ps. aeruginosa	2	4	32	2	64	16–32	32	R
B. fragilis	16	8	16	8	16	16		R

R (resistant) MIC ≥ 128 mg/l.

over 10 min, 4-hourly. Concentrations in amniotic fluid and cord serum were 2.9–7.6 and 12–18 mg/l respectively when the maternal serum concentrations following 2 g by i.v. bolus were 48–69 mg/l.

Up to 60% of the dose is recoverable from the urine and the plasma half-life rises to 6 h when the creatinine clearance is less than 10 ml/3 min.

Toxicity and side-effects

Reactions similar to those associated with carboxypenicillins occur, including hypersensitivity, increase of bleeding time and abnormalities of liver enzymes. Reversible neutropenia has been encountered relatively frequently in patients treated for more than 2 weeks. A mean fall in serum uric acid from 6.4 to 2.3 mg/dl has been observed in treated patients, indicating a probenecid-like effect.

Clinical uses

Those of group 5 penicillins (p. 292).

Preparations and dosage
Proprietary name: Securopen.
Preparation: Injection.

Dosage: Adults, 2–5 g every 8 h depending on severity of infection. Children 1–14 years, 75 mg/kg every 8 h. Premature infants, 50 mg/kg every 12 h; neonates, 100 mg/kg every 12 h; infants 7 days to 1 year, 100 mg/kg every 8 h.
Widely available.

Further information

Bosso J A, Saxon B A, Herbst J T, Matsen J M 1984 Azlocillin pharmacokinetics in patients with cystic fibrosis. *Antimicrobial Agents and Chemotherapy* 25: 630–632

Dijkmans B A C, van der Meer J W M, Boekhout-Mussert M J, Zaal-de Jong M, Mattie H 1980 Prolonged bleeding time during azlocillin therapy. *Journal of Antimicrobial Chemotherapy* 6: 554–555

Jacobs J Y, Livermore D M, Davy K W M 1984 *Pseudomonas aeruginosa* beta-lactamase as a defence against azlocillin, mezlocillin and piperacillin. *Journal of Antimicrobial Chemotherapy* 14: 221–229

Kefetzis D A, Brater D C, Fanourgakis J E 1983 Materno-fetal transfer of azlocillin. *Journal of Antimicrobial Chemotherapy* 12: 157–162

Lander R D, Henderson R P, Pyszcynski D R 1989 Pharmacokinetic comparison of 5 g of azlocillin every 8 h and 4 g every 6 h in healthy volunteers. *Antimicrobial Agents and Chemotherapy* 33: 710–713

Parry M F 1985 The safety and tolerance of azlocillin. *Arzneimittelforschung* 35: 1292–1294

Symposium 1983 Azlocillin – an antipseudomonas penicillin. *Journal of Antimicrobial Chemotherapy* 11 (suppl B): 1–239

Wenk M, Follath F 1986 Azlocillin serum levels on repetitive dosage in patients with normal and abnormal renal function. *Chemotherapy* 32: 205–208

White A R, Comber K R, Sutherland R 1980 Comparative bactericidal effects of azlocillin and ticarcillin against *Pseudomonas aeruginosa*. *Antimicrobial Agents and Chemotherapy* 18: 182–189

Williams R J, Linridge M A, Said A A, Livermore D M, Williams J D 1984 National Survey of antibiotic resistance in *Pseudomonas aeruginosa*. *Journal of Antimicrobial Chemotherapy* 14: 9–16

MEZLOCILLIN

A semi-synthetic penicillin supplied as the sodium salt.

Antimicrobial activity

Mezlocillin is active against Gram-positive cocci and many Gram-negative bacilli including *Esch. coli*, *K. pneumoniae*, *Enterobacter* spp. and *Ser. marcescens* (Table 15.6). *H. influenzae* is very susceptible, but strains encoding TEM β-lactamase are resistant. *Neisseria* spp. are also susceptible, including strains of *N. gonorrhoeae* relatively resistant to benzylpenicillin; β-lactamase-producing strains of the organism are resistant. Mezlocillin is less active than azlocillin and piperacillin against *Ps. aeruginosa* and its activity is inoculum dependent. Activity against *B. fragilis* is variable and the drug is readily hydrolysed by the β-lactamases of this species. Mezlocillin is labile to many β-lactamases, particularly the common TEM plasmid-mediated enzyme.

It exhibits typical β-lactam synergy with aminoglycosides against many strains of *Ps. aeruginosa* and enterobacteria, and synergy is produced with both mezlocillin-susceptible and mezlocillin-resistant strains. In combination with cefoxitin, antagonism was observed in tests against *Enterobacter*, *Serratia* and *Pseudomonas* spp. as a result of β-lactamase induction by cefoxitin.

Pharmacokinetics

Typical mean levels are 55, 150 and 350 mg/l 15 min after i.v. doses of 1, 2 and 5 g, respectively. There is a loss of dose linearity at higher doses, probably due to saturation of non-renal clearance. The plasma elimination half-life is 1.2 h. Plasma peak concentrations and half-life in children are similar to those in adults. In the newborn infant the plasma half-life was 4.5 h, falling to 1.8 h at 7 days.

Up to 60% is recoverable unchanged from the urine. The elimination half-life rises with decline in renal function and urinary excretion falls to 5% or less, but non-renal clearance is appreciable and no change in dosage is indicated until the glomerular filtration rate (GFR) falls to less than 10%. The plasma half-life falls to around 1.5 h on haemodialysis. Up to 2.5% is excreted in the bile producing concentrations around 300 mg/l following 1 g i.v. In patients with alcoholic liver disease, mean end infusion plasma levels following 3 g i.v. were around 140 mg/l with a half-life of 2 h. Plasma clearance was inversely related to serum alkaline phosphatase and total bilirubin.

Toxicity and side-effects

It is generally well tolerated. Untoward reactions are similar to those associated with carboxypenicillins, including hypersensitivity, prolongation of bleeding time (less than with carbenicillin), reversible neutropenia and abnormalities of liver enzymes. False reactions for urinary protein may occur.

Clinical use

Those of group 5 penicillins (p. 292). It is not recommended for single agent treatment of immunocompromised cancer patients. It is commended for the prophylaxis of postoperative sepsis following bowel or pelvic surgery, where both Gram-negative aerobes and anaerobes are likely to be implicated.

Preparations and dosage

Preparation: Injection.

Dosage: Adults, i.v., 2–4 g every 6 h depending on severity of infection; maximum daily dose 24 g.

Limited availability.

Further information

Adelman R D, Wirth R, Rubio T 1987 A controlled study of the nephrotoxicity of mezlocillin and amikacin in the neonate. *American Journal of Diseases of Children* 14: 1175–1178

Brogard J-M, Kopferschmitt J, Arnaud J-P, Dorner M, Lavillaureix J 1980 Biliary elimination of mezlocillin: an experimental and clinical study. *Antimicrobial Agents and Chemotherapy* 18: 69–76

Colaizzi P A, Coniglio A A, Poynor W J, Vishniavsky N, Karnes H T, Polk R E 1986 Comparative pharmacokinetics of two multiple-dose mezlocillin regimens in normal volunteers. *Antimicrobial Agents and Chemotherapy* 30: 675–678

Cushner H M, Copley J B, Bauman J, Hill S C 1985 Acute interstitial nephritis associated with mezlocillin, nafcillin and gentamicin treatment for *Pseudomonas* infection. *Archives of Internal Medicine* 145: 1204–1207

Drusano G L, Schimpff S C, Hewitt W L 1984 The acylampicillins: mezlocillin, piperacillin and azlocillin. *Reviews of Infectious Diseases* 6: 13–32

Esposito S, Galante D, Barba D 1986 In vitro microbiological properties of mezlocillin compared with four cephalosporins. *Chemioterapia* 5: 273–277

Flaherty J F, Barriere S L, Mordenti J, Gambertoglio J G 1987 Effect of dose on pharmacokinetics and serum bactericidal activity of mezlocillin. *Antimicrobial Agents and Chemotherapy* 31: 895–898

Janicke D M, Mangione A, Schultz R W, Jusko W J 1981 Mezlocillin disposition in chronic hemodialysis patients. *Antimicrobial Agents and Chemotherapy* 20: 590–594

Meyers B R, Srulevitch E S, Sacks H S et al 1987 Pharmacokinetic of mezlocillin in patients with hepatobiliary dysfunction. *Journal of Antimicrobial Chemotherapy* 18: 709–713

Odio C, Threlkeld M, Thomas M L, McCracken G H Jr 1984 Pharmacokinetic properties of mezlocillin in new-born infants. *Antimicrobial Agents and Chemotherapy* 25: 556–559

Symposium 1983 Mezlocillin – a broad spectrum penicillin. An update. *Journal of Antimicrobial Chemotherapy* 11 (suppl C): 1–108

PIPERACILLIN

A semi-synthetic penicillin supplied as the sodium salt.

Antimicrobial activity

Piperacillin displays good activity against streptococci, *Ent. faecalis* and penicillin-susceptible strains of *Staph. aureus*. It is highly active against ampicillin-susceptible *H. influenzae* and penicillin-susceptible strains of *N. gonorrhoeae* (Table 15.6). Gonococci resistant to benzylpenicillin due to modified PBPs are also susceptible to piperacillin, but β-lactamase-producing strains are resistant. Piperacillin is the most active of the commonly used antipseudomonal penicillins against *Ps. aeruginosa* and many strains of *Ps. cepacia*, *Ps. maltophila* and *Ps. fluorescens*. It is active against most Enterobacteriaceae, including ampicillin-resistant species such as *Citrobacter*, *Enterobacter*, *Morganella*, *Providencia* and *Ser. marcescens*. *B. fragilis* and many other anaerobes are susceptible, but differences between MIC_{50} and MIC_{90} values can be considerable.

There is complete cross-resistance with apalcillin and other ureidopenicillins, but strains of *Ps. aeruginosa* moderately resistant to carbenicillin and ticarcillin are often susceptible. It is only slowly bactericidal and there may be wide divergence between the MIC and the MBC, some susceptible strains not being killed by 256 mg/l. Synergy with amikacin, gentamicin and tobramycin has been demonstrated against many strains of Enterobacteriaceae and *Ps. aeruginosa*.

Piperacillin is rapidly hydrolysed by most β-lactamases, and many β-lactamase-producing isolates are resistant, particularly those possessing TEM- or other plasmid-encoded enzymes. The penicillin is protected by β-lactamase inhibitors from inactivation by β-lactamase-producing bacteria and the clinically available combination of piperacillin plus tazobactam (p. 326) has been shown to be active against a high proportion of piperacillin-resistant strains of *Staph. aureus*, *H. influenzae*, *N. gonorrhoeae*, *Esch. coli*, *K. pneumoniae* and *B. fragilis*. The inhibitor does not enhance the activity of piperacillin against resistant strains of *Ps. aeruginosa*.

Acquired resistance

Monotherapy of *Ps. aeruginosa* infections with piperacillin has resulted in the development of resistance during treatment. In some cases resistance to piperacillin was due to changes in penicillin-binding proteins, and in others to the production of elevated amounts of chromosomal β-lactamase. Piperacillin-resistant strains of *B. fragilis* and other *Bacteroides* spp. quickly appeared. The spread of plasmid-mediated β-lactamases amongst Gram-negative bacilli has led to increased resistance to piperacillin and corresponding interest in the combination of piperacillin and the β-lactamase inhibitor, tazobactam.

Pharmacokinetics

The mean peak plasma concentration following rapid i.v.

administration of 30 mg/kg is around 200 mg/l. Mean end-infusion concentrations in volunteers receiving 2 g i.v. over 15 min were around 300 mg/l. The elimination half-life is 1 h. In children, peak plasma concentrations are similar but the half-life is shorter, around 35 min. There are no significant dose-dependent effects on the pharmacokinetics. In the presence of meningitis, mean penetrance around 30% has been found.

The urine is the principal route of excretion, 50–70% of the dose appearing over 12 h, most in the first 4 h. Most is excreted via the tubules, 75–90% in active form. The half-life is prolonged in renal failure but much less than is the case with carboxypenicillins. Neither serum half-life nor clearance are correlated with creatinine clearance, indicating significant non-renal elimination. There is substantial biliary excretion, levels in common duct bile following 1 g i.v., commonly reaching 500 mg/l or more. During haemodialysis the plasma half-life remains elevated and only 10–15% of the dose is removed.

Toxicity and side-effects

It is generally well tolerated, with mild to moderate pain on injection, thrombophlebitis and diarrhoea in some patients. It otherwise exhibits side effects common to the group, including leucopenia and abnormalities of platelet aggregation without coagulation defect except on prolonged treatment.

Clinical uses

Those of group 5 penicillins (p. 292). As with related agents, failure of therapy, particularly in pseudomonas infection, may be due to the emergence of resistance and its use as single agent therapy for severe Gram-negative sepsis is questioned.

Preparations and dosage

Proprietary names: Pipril, Tazocin (with tazobactam).

Preparation: Injection.

Dosage: Piperacillin, adults, i.m., i.v., 100–150 mg/kg per day in divided doses, increased to 200–300 mg/kg per day in severe infections; in life-threatening infections a dose of not less than 16 g/day is recommended. Children 2 months–12 years, 100–300 mg/kg per day in 3–4 divided doses; neonates and infants <2 months, 100–300 mg/kg per day in 2 equally divided doses. Piperacillin with tazobactam, adults and children >12 years, i.v., 2.25–4.5 g every 6–8 h.

Widely available.

Further information

Daschner F D, Just M, Spillner G, Schlosser V 1982 Penetration of piperacillin into cardiac valves, subcutaneous and muscle tissue of patients undergoing open-heart surgery. *Journal of Antimicrobial Chemotherapy* 9: 489–492

Dickinson G M, Droller D G, Greenman R L, Hoffman T A 1981 Clinical evaluation of piperacillin with observation on penetrability into cerebrospinal fluid. *Antimicrobial Agents and Chemotherapy* 20: 481–486

Giron J A, Meyers B R, Hirschmann S Z 1981 Biliary concentration of piperacillin in patients undergoing cholecystectomy. *Antimicrobial Agents of Chemotherapy* 19: 309–311

Holmes B, Richards D M, Brogdeb R N, Heel R C 1984 Piperacillin. A review of its antibacterial activity, pharmacokinetic properties and therapeutic use. *Drugs* 28: 375–425

Lau A, Lee M, Flascha S, Prasad R, Sharifi R 1983 Effect of piperacillin on tobramycin pharmacokinetics in patients with normal renal function. *Antimicrobial Agents and Chemotherapy* 24: 533–537

Lee M, Stobnicki M, Sharifi R 1986 Haemorrhagic complications of piperacillin therapy. *Journal of Urology* 136: 454–455

Mandell G L 1985 In vitro microbiology and pharmacokinetics of piperacillin. *Clinical Therapeutics* 7 (suppl A): 37–44

Stefani S, Russo G, Nicolosi V M, Nicoletti G 1987 Enterococci and aminoglycosides: evaluation of susceptibility and synergism of their combination with piperacillin. *Chemioterapia* 6: 12–16

Sutherland R 1993 Bacterial resistance to β-lactam antibiotics; problems and solutions. *Progress in Drug Research* 41: 95–149

Symposium 1982 From penicillin to piperacillin. *Journal of Antimicrobial Chemotherapy* 9 (suppl B): 1–101

Symposium 1993 Piperacillin/tazobactam; a new β-lactam/β-lactamase inhibitor combination. *Journal of Antimicrobial Chemotherapy* 31 (suppl A): 1–124

Tartaglione T A, Nye I, Vishniavsky N, Poynor W, Polk R E 1986 Multiple dose pharmacokinetics of piperacillin and azlocillin in 12 healthy volunteers. *Clinical Pharmacology* 5: 911–916

Thrumoorthi M C, Asmar B I, Buckley J A, Bollinger R O, Kauffman E, Dajani A S 1983 Pharmacokinetics of intravenously administered piperacillin in pre-adolescent children. *Journal of Pediatrics* 102: 941–946

Tipper D J 1985 Mode of action of β-lactam antibiotics. *Pharmacology and Therapeutics* 27: 1–35

Warrington R J, Silviu-Dan F, Magro C 1993 Accelerated cell-mediated immune reactions in penicillin allergy. *Journal of Allergy and Clinical Immunology* 94: 626–628

Welling P G, Craig W A, Buntzen R W, Kwok F W, Gerber A U, Matsen P O 1983 Pharmacokinetics of piperacillin in subjects with various degrees of renal failure. *Antimicrobial Agents and Chemotherapy* 23: 881–887

Carboxypenicillins

These include carbenicillin, carfecillin, carindacillin and ticarcillin.

CARBENICILLIN
α-Carboxybenzylpenicillin

A semi-synthetic penicillin supplied as the disodium salt.

Antimicrobial activity

The first of the antipseudomonal penicillins to be developed, carbenicillin displays a relatively low order of activity against *Ps. aeruginosa* (MIC 64 mg/l) and is the least active of the group 5 agents (Table 15.6). Most Enterobacteriaceae are susceptible, including some ampicillin-resistant species producing class I chromosomal β-lactamases (p. 319) such as *Enterobacter*, indole-positive *Proteus*, *Providencia* spp. and *Ser. marcescens*. *Klebsiella* spp. are almost invariably resistant, as are many strains of *Acinetobacter* spp. Carbenicillin shows good activity against β-lactamase-negative strains of *H. influenzae* and *N. gonorrhoeae*. Introduction of the acidic group into the side-chain has resulted in a notable reduction in activity against Gram-positive cocci compared to benzylpenicillin, but staphylococci, streptococci and anaerobic Gram-positive bacteria are susceptible. *Ent. faecalis* and β-lactamase-producing strains of *Staph. aureus* are resistant. Many strains of *B. fragilis* are moderately susceptible, and other *Bacteroides* and *Fusobacteria* spp. are highly susceptible.

Carbenicillin is labile to staphylococcal β-lactamase and is readily hydrolysed by plasmid-mediated β-lactamases, including the TEM enzyme responsible for the resistance of many clinical isolates of Gram-negative bacteria. It is, however, comparatively stable to the class I chromosomal β-lactamases of Enterobacteriaceae and *Ps. aeruginosa*.

It is bactericidal in action and synergy is demonstrable with aminoglycosides, notably gentamicin and tobramycin, against *Ps. aeruginosa* and other Gram-negative bacteria.

Acquired resistance

Resistant strains of *Ps. aeruginosa* may emerge during therapy with carbenicillin alone. Cystic fibrosis patients have been shown to be infected with heterogenous populations of *Ps. aeruginosa* containing cells hypersusceptible, susceptible and resistant to carbenicillin. Resistance may be due to the selection of strains with reduced cell-wall permeability, modified penicillin-binding proteins, or to the acquisition of plasmid-mediated β-lactamases. In some strains highly resistant to carbenicillin all three mechanisms of resistance have been shown to be involved. The frequency of isolation of *Ps. aeruginosa* with plasmid-mediated β-lactamase varies, but most surveys have reported 25% or less of carbenicillin-resistant strains to produce the enzymes.

In most hospitals, 80–90% of stains of *Ps. aeruginosa* are susceptible and resistance is usually confined to special areas such as intensive care or burns units where the agent is used extensively.

Pharmacokinetics

It is not absorbed by mouth. Following 1 g i.m., mean peak plasma concentrations of 20–30 mg/l are found 0.5–1.5 h after injection. End injection concentrations following a similar dose i.v. are around 150 mg/l. Doubling the dose approximately doubles the mean peak concentration. Steady state levels on continuous i.v. infusion of 0.5 or 1 g/h were 70–80 and 150–170 mg/l, respectively. The half-life is around 1 h. Protein binding is 50–60%.

It is distributed in the extracellular fluid and plasma levels are reduced when the extracellular volume is increased. It enters the serous fluids, providing concentrations up to 60% of those of the plasma. Concentrations can reach 25% of those of the plasma in skin window and blister fluid and in sputum, but in patients with cystic fibrosis these may not reach inhibitory levels for *Ps. aeruginosa*. It does not cross the normal meninges but levels of up to 50% of those of the plasma can be found in meningitis.

Some is excreted in the bile, producing levels 2–3 times those in the plasma, but the main route of excretion is through the kidneys, around 80% of the dose appearing principally as unchanged drug in the urine, producing very high levels, 2–4000 mg/l. Excretion is by both glomerular filtration and tubular secretion, which accounts for about 40%. Some is metabolized and up to 5% is excreted as penicilloic acid. Peak plasma levels are elevated by about

50% and prolonged by probenecid and the half-life is prolonged in the newborn and in renal failure. Some further prolongation occurs in the presence of hepatic failure. Significant reduction in the half-life can be obtained with haemodialysis, but peritoneal dialysis is much less efficient. It is more rapidly disposed of in patients with cystic fibrosis.

Toxicity and side-effects

It is generally free from toxicity, except for pain on i.m. injection and a liability of high blood levels to cause a coagulation defect manifested by prolonged bleeding time due to an action on platelets. Purpura and mucosal bleeding has occasionally progressed to life threatening bleeding. The effect is dose dependent and most likely to be seen in patients with impaired excretion on receiving 500 mg/kg per day or more. Coagulopathy due to depression of fibrinogen levels has also been described.

Hypersensitivity reactions occur, but are much less frequent and severe than those associated with benzylpenicillin. Rashes and eosinophilia occur, and reversible neutropenia and interstitial nephritis are rarely encountered. Reversible abnormalities of liver function can occur, apparently more commonly than with other antipseudomonal penicillins. Since large doses of the drug have to be used, convulsions can occur as with other penicillins (p. 261), and being administered as the disodium salt, electrolyte disturbances can result from the sodium load and from the loss of potassium due to large amounts of non-absorbable ion in the distal tubules.

Clinical use

Its primary use is in the treatment of established generalized infections, endocarditis or meningitis due to *Ps. aeruginosa*, but it is also effective against *Enterobacter*, indole-positive *Proteus* and *Morganella*. It is often combined with aminoglycosides, with which synergy is demonstrable in vitro. It is used in pulmonary infections due to *Pseudomonas* and enterobacteria, but in cystic fibrosis, concentrations in bronchial secretions are commonly insufficient to inhibit the more resistant mucoid strains of *Pseudomonas* involved. It is effective in the treatment of pelvic and abdominal infections due to mixed aerobic and anaerobic Gram-negative rods.

Preparations and dosage

Proprietary name: Pyopen.

Preparation: Injection.

Dosage: Adults, i.v., 5 g every 4–6 h; i.m., 2 g every 6 h. Children, i.v., 250–400 mg/kg per day in divided doses; i.m., 50–100 mg/kg per day in divided doses.

Widely available.

Further information

Godfrey A J, Bryan L E, Rabin H R 1981 Beta-lactam-resistant *Pseudomonas aeruginosa* with modified penicillin-binding protein emerging during cystic fibrosis treatment. *Antimicrobial Agents and Chemotherapy* 19: 705–711

Rodriguez-Tebar A, Rojo F, Dámaso D, Vazquez D 1982 Carbenicillin resistance of *Pseudomonas aeruginosa*. *Antimicrobial Agents and Chemotherapy* 22: 255–261

Sattler F R, Weitekamp M R, Sayegh A, Ballard J O 1988 Impaired hemostasis caused by beta-lactam antibiotics. *American Journal of Surgery* 155 (5A): 30–39

Symposium 1970 Symposium on carbenicillin: a clinical profile. *Journal of Infectious Diseases* 122 (suppl): S1–S116

Tirado M, Roy C, Segura C, Reig R, Hermida M, Fox A 1986 Incidence of strains producing plasmid determined beta-lactamases among carbenicillin resistant *Pseudomonas aeruginosa*. *Journal of Antimicrobial Chemotherapy* 18: 453–458

Williams R J, Lindridge M A, Said A A, Livermore D M, Williams J D 1984 National survey of antibiotic resistance in *Pseudomonas aeruginosa*. *Journal of Antimicrobial Chemotherapy* 14: 9–16

CARFECILLIN

The carboxyphenyl ester of carbenicillin.

Antimicrobial activity

It is esterified on the side-chain and, because the carboxyl group of the nucleus is free, it exhibits greater activity in vitro than carbenicillin against Gram-positive cocci. In vivo it is rapidly de-esterified and all activity is due to liberated carbenicillin.

Pharmacokinetics

It is acid stable and well absorbed when given orally. It is subsequently de-esterified, only trace amounts of the esters being found in the serum, to yield carbenicillin and phenol which is rapidly detoxified by conjugation and excreted in the urine. Single oral doses of 500 and 1000 mg produce blood levels which vary widely, but the peak, reached at 1–2 h, is around 3 and 5 mg/l respectively, levels which are too low to permit the treatment of systemic infection. Following a 1 g intramuscular injection mean peak plasma levels around 25 mg/l are obtained.

About 30–35% of the dose is excreted over 6 h in the urine, producing concentrations following an oral dose of 1 h around 500–1000 mg/l. The liberated phenol moiety is excreted as glucuronide and sulphate.

Toxicity and side-effects

Tolerance is generally good, with no after-taste, but nausea, and occasional mild diarrhoea occur in some patients.

Clinical use

Its sole use is in the treatment of urinary tract infection due to *Pseudomonas*, *Enterobacter* or indole-positive *Proteus*. Fear that its widespread use might encourage the emergence of carbenicillin-resistant strains and threaten the place of carboxypenicillins in the systemic treatment of grave infections has led to recommendations that its use be restricted to infections due to organisms resistant to other agents. Because of its antibacterial activity, unabsorbed ester may affect the gut flora.

Preparations and dosage

Preparation: Tablets.

Dosage: Adults, oral, 0.5–1 g three times daily. Children 2–10 years, half the adult dose.

Limited availability.

Further information

O'Grady F (ed) 1979 Carfecillin. International Congress Series No. 467. Excerpta Medica, Oxford

---

CARINDACILLIN

The indanyl ester of carbenicillin supplied as the sodium salt. As with carfecillin, it shows activity independent of that of carbenicillin in vitro but not in vivo.

It is acid stable, and after absorption is rapidly hydrolysed to carbenicillin and indanol, which is excreted in the urine. The peak blood level after a dose of 1 g is only about 10 mg/l, but high concentrations are attained in the urine. A bitter after-taste and sometimes vomiting occur and doses adequate to achieve a systemic effect are impracticable.

Strictures on its widespread use are those applied to carfecillin and its only indications are urinary infections due to Pseudomonas and enterobacteria, notably indole-positive Proteus, sensitive only to carbenicillin. Because it possesses independent antibacterial activity, unabsorbed product can affect the gut flora.

Preparations and dosage

Preparation: Tablets.

Dosage: 382–764 mg four times daily.

Limited availability.

Further information

English A R, Retsema J A, Ray V A, Lynch J E 1972 Carbenicillin indanyl sodium, an orally active derivative of carbenicillin. *Antimicrobial Agents and Chemotherapy* 1: 185–191

Knirsch A K, Hobbs D C, Korst J J 1973 Pharmacokinetics, toleration and safety of indanyl carbenicillin in man. *Journal of Infectious Diseases* 127 (suppl): S105–S110

TICARCILLIN

α-Carboxy-3-thienylmethyl penicillin; supplied as the disodium salt.

Antimicrobial activity

The antibacterial activity of ticarcillin is similar to that of carbenicillin, except that ticarcillin is 2–4 times more active against *Ps. aeruginosa* (Table 15.6). Ticarcillin displays good activity against Enterobacteriaceae, including ampicillin-resistant species such as *Citrobacter*, *Enterobacter*, indole-positive *Proteus* and *Ser. marcescens*. β-Lactamase-negative strains of *H. influenzae* and *N. gonorrhoeae* are highly susceptible. Most aerobic and anaerobic Gram-positive cocci and bacilli are susceptible, with the exception of *Ent. faecalis* and β-lactamase-producing *Staph. aureus*. Anaerobic Gram-negative bacteria including *B. fragilis* are usually susceptible. Bactericidal synergy with aminoglycosides is demonstrable against *Ps. aeruginosa* and enterobacteria.

Ticarcillin is comparatively stable to the class I chromosomally-mediated β-lactamases of Gram-negative bacilli, but is rapidly hydrolysed by most other chromosomally- and plasmid-mediated enzymes. There is complete cross-resistance with carbenicillin. The activity of ticarcillin against β-lactamase-producing bacteria is enhanced by β-lactamase inhibitors and a combination of ticarcillin plus clavulanic acid has been developed for clinical use (p. 323). Ticarcillin/clavulanic acid is active against many ticarcillin-resistant strains of *Staph. aureus*, *H. influenzae*, *Esch. coli*, *K. pneumoniae*, *Pr. mirabilis* and *B. fragilis*. Ticarcillin-resistant strains of *Ps. aeruginosa* are not susceptible to the combination.

Acquired resistance

There is complete cross-resistance with carbenicillin. The increasing prevalence of bacteria possessing plasmid-mediated β-lactamases has resulted in extensive clinical use of ticarcillin/clavulanic acid combinations.

Pharmacokinetics

It is not absorbed by mouth. By i.m. injection, 1 g produced an average peak plasma level of 35 mg/l at 1 h. The same dose infused i.v. over 5 min produced a concentration of 257 mg/l at 15 min. Infused over 90–120 min 4-hourly, the same dose produced a mean peak concentration of 240 mg/l. Infusion of 5 g i.v. over 30 min produced end-infusion concentrations around 450 mg/l. The plasma half-life is around 1.3 h. On co-administration with gentamicin, the plasma concentration of ticarcillin is unaffected, but the concentration of gentamicin is lowered. Doubling the dose approximately doubles the mean peak concentration. There is no evidence of dose-dependent pharmacokinetics at doses between 50 and 80 mg/kg. Protein binding is 50–60%.

It is distributed in the extracellular fluid and plasma levels are reduced when the extracellular volume is increased. It enters the serous fluids, providing concentrations up to 60% of those of the plasma. Concentrations can reach 25% of those of the plasma in sputum and in skin window fluid. It does not cross the normal meninges but levels of up to 50% of those of the plasma can be found in meningitis. On co-administration with clavulanic acid, there is preservation of the ratio to serum concentration in lymph and in peritoneal fluid with peak concentrations of 70% and 67% of the plasma concentrations of ticarcillin and clavulanic acid, respectively, declining in parallel with the plasma concentrations.

Some is excreted in the bile, producing levels 2–3 times those in the plasma but the main route of excretion is through the kidneys, 80%, principally as unchanged drug, appearing in the urine in the first 6 h, producing concentrations of 650–2500 mg/l after doses of 3 g i.v. Some is metabolized and the fraction excreted as penicilloic acid is higher for ticarcillin (up to 15%) than for carbenicillin (up to 5%). Peak plasma levels are elevated and prolonged by probenecid and the half-life is prolonged in the newborn and in renal failure. Some further prolongation occurs in the presence of hepatic failure. Significant reduction in the half-life can be obtained by haemodialysis, but peritoneal dialysis is much less efficient. It is more rapidly disposed of in children with cystic fibrosis.

Toxicity and side-effects

There is cross-allergy with other penicillins, but hypersensitivity reactions are much less frequent and severe than those associated with benzylpenicillin. Rashes and eosinophilia occur and reversible neutropenia, dose-related platelet abnormalities, occasionally leading to haemorrhage, and interstitial nephritis are rarely encountered. In volunteers receiving 100–300 mg/kg per day for 3–10 days coagulation was unaffected, but platelet function was impaired, and in patients with impaired renal function who received normal dosages, petechiae, echymoses and epistaxis have occurred. Reversible abnormalities of liver function can occur. Since large doses of the drug have to be used, convulsions can occur, as with other penicillins, and being a disodium salt, electrolyte disturbances can result from the sodium load and from loss of potassium.

Clinical use

Its principal use is in the treatment of proven pseudomonas infection, notably in neutropenic patients and in cystic fibrosis. It may be preferred to carbenicillin because its greater activity permits lower dosage. It is also effective against *Enterobacter*, indole-positive *Proteus*, *Morganella* and *Serratia* spp. It is also active against many anaerobes and is said to be as effective as the combination of chloramphenicol or clindamycin with gentamicin in the treatment of polymicrobial abdominal and female genital sepsis.

Preparations and dosage

Proprietary names: Ticar; Timentin (with clavulanic acid).
Preparation: Injection.

Dosage: Ticarcillin, adults, i.v., 15–20 g/day in divided doses. Children, 200–300 mg/kg per day in divided doses. Ticarcillin with clavulanic acid, adults, i.v., 3.2 g every 6–8 h increased to every 4 h in more severe infections. Children, 80 mg/kg every 6–8 h; neonates, 80 mg/kg every 12 h. Widely available.

Further information

Brogden R N, Heel R C, Speight T M, Avery G S 1980 Ticarcillin: a review of its pharmacological properties and therapeutic efficacy. *Drugs* 20: 325–352

Daschner F D, Thoma G, Langmaack H, Dalhoff A 1980 Ticarcillin concentrations in serum, muscle and fat after a single intravenous injection. *Antimicrobial Agents and Chemotherapy* 17: 738–739

Graft D F, Chesney P J 1982 Use of ticarcillin following carbenicillin-associated hepatotoxicity. *Journal of Pediatrics* 100: 497–499

Guenthner S H, Chao H P, Wenzel R P 1986 Synergy between amikacin and ticarcillin or mezlocillin against nosocomial blood-stream isolates. *Journal of Antimicrobial Chemotherapy* 18: 550–552

Gugliemo B J, Flaherty J F, Batman R, Barriere S L, Gambertoglio J G 1986 Comparative pharmacokinetics of low- and high-dose ticarcillin. *Antimicrobial Agents and Chemotherapy* 30: 359–360

Konishi H, Goto M, Nakamoto Y, Yamamoto I, Yamashina H 1983 Tobramycin inactivation by carbenicillin, ticarcillin and piperacillin. *Antimicrobial Agents and Chemotherapy* 23: 653–657

Leigh D A, Phillips I, Wise R 1986 Ticarcillin plus clavulanic acid. A laboratory and clinical perspective. *Journal of Antimicrobial Chemotherapy* 17 (suppl C): 1–240

Symposium 1978 Ticarcillin (BRL 2288). International Congress Series No. 445. Excerpta Medica, Oxford, p 3–163

SULBENICILLIN
α-Sulphobenzylpenicillin

A semi-synthetic penicillin supplied as the disodium salt.

Its antimicrobial spectrum and potency closely resemble those of carbenicillin (Table 15.6) as does its pharmaco-kinetic behaviour. Following i.v. administration of 4 g, the mean plasma concentration at 1 h was around 160 mg/l, with a plasma elimination half-life around 70 min. Following 2 g i.m. in parturition, the mean peak maternal blood concentration was 109 mg/l at 55 min, while that in umbilical cord blood was around 25 mg/l at 1–3 h and in amniotic fluid around 27 mg/l at 7.5 h. It is largely excreted in the urine, around 80% of the dose appearing in the first 24 h, less than 5% as the penicilloic acid. There is an inverse correlation between creatinine clearance and plasma half-life.

It has been noted that the penicilloic acid causes much stronger platelet aggregation than the parent substance.

The 6-α-methoxy derivative exhibits poor activity against Gram-positive organisms, but its Gram-negative range includes *Ps. aeruginosa* resistant to ticarcillin and piperacillin.

Preparations and dosage
Preparation: Injection.
Dosage: Adults, i.m., i.v., 2–4 g/day in divided doses.
Very limited availability.

Further information

Debbia E, Pesce A, Schito G C 1987 Evaluation of the minimum bactericidal time (MBT) of sulbenicillin against multiresistant pathogens. *Chemioterapia* 6: 85–87

Eftimiadi C, DeLeo C, Schito G C 1985 Antibacterial activity in vitro of sulbenicillin against mucoid and non-mucoid strains of *Pseudomonas aeruginosa, Drugs under Experimental and Clinical Research* 11: 241–245

Fraschini F, Scaglione F, Bichisao E et al 1987 Comparison between sulbenicillin and piperacillin levels in serum and in bronchial secretions – a pharmacokinetic study. *International Journal of Clinical Pharmacology, Therapeutics and Toxicology* 25: 638–642

Hansen I, Jacobsen E, Weiss J 1975 Pharmacokinetics of sulbenicillin, a new broad-spectrum semisynthetic penicillin. *Clinical Pharmacology and Therapeutics* 17: 339–347

Ikeda Y, Kikuchi M, Matsuda S et al 1978 Inhibition of platelet function by sulbenicillin and its metabolite. *Antimicrobial Agents and Chemotherapy* 13: 881–883

Miyakawi I, Taniyama K, Inoue H, Chan Lee H, Mori N 1982 Placental transfer of disodium sulbenicillin. *Antimicrobial Agents and Chemotherapy* 21: 838–839

Group 6: β-lactamase-resistant penicillins

The introduction of substituents into the 6-α-position of the penicillin nucleus generally results in loss of antibacterial activity, but the 6-α-methoxylpenicillin, temocillin (a derivative of ticarcillin), possesses useful antibacterial and pharmacokinetic properties and has attained clinical status. It is highly resistant to most bacterial β-lactamases, analogous to the cephamycin antibiotics which contain a 7-α-methoxy group in the nucleus. It has a long serum half-life after parenteral administration. Temocillin is not absorbed by the oral route but the o-methylphenyl ester has been reported to produce substantial serum concentrations after oral dosing to human volunteers. The compound has not progressed to clinical trial.

A second substituted penicillin, foramidocillin, has a formamido (NHCHO) group in the 6-α-position and also shows pronounced resistance to bacterial β-lactamases. The compound exhibits very potent antibacterial activity against most aerobic enteric bacilli, including Ps. aeruginosa *and is active against many bacteria resistant to other penicillins and cephalosporins. Its potent activity is due to the fact that the compound contains an iron-sequestering catechol moiety which enables it to enter bacterial cells via iron transport* systems in the same way as naturally occurring siderophores. Foramidocillin has been evaluated in pharmacokinetic studies in human volunteers but has not been developed further for clinical use.

Further information

Basker M J, Edmondson R A, Knowles S J, Ponsford R J, Slocombe B, White S J 1984 In vitro antibacterial properties of BRL 36650, a novel 6-alpha-substituted penicillin. *Antimicrobial Agents and Chemotherapy* 26: 734–740

Critchley A 1990 Catecholic β-lactams: facilitated transport. *Journal of Antimicrobial Chemotherapy* 26: 733–737

TEMOCILLIN

A semi-synthetic penicillin available as the disodium salt.

Antimicrobial activity

It is widely active against Enterobacteriaceae (MIC 1–8 mg/l) *H. influenzae* and *M. catarrhalis*. β-Lactamase-producing strains are generally as susceptible as are β-lactamase-negative strains. In contrast to the related penicillin, ticarcillin, temocillin is inactive against *Ps. aeruginosa*, but *Ps. cepacia* and *Ps. acidovorans* are susceptible (MIC 4 mg/l) as are *Aeromonas* spp. Most *Acinetobacter* spp. are resistant, and *Ser. marcescens* exhibits variable susceptibility. The introduction of the 6-α-methoxy group has resulted in loss of activity against Gram-positive cocci and anaerobic Gram-negative bacilli (Table 15.6).

It is bactericidal at concentrations 2–4 times the MIC, filaments formed at lower concentrations slowly lysing at higher concentrations. Temocillin consists of diastereo-isomers and the *R* epimer (which predominates in the natural mixture) is more rapidly bactericidal than the *S* epimer. It is highly resistant to most bacterial β-lactamases, including the extended-spectrum β-lactamases that confer resistance to third-generation cephalosporins (p. 319) and, as a result, there is no inoculum effect with the majority of β-lactamase-producing bacteria. It is lysed by the β-lactamases produced by Flavobacterium spp. and slowly by those of *Bacteroides* spp.

Pharmacokinetics

It is not absorbed when administered by mouth, but produces high and prolonged concentrations in plasma following an intramuscular or intravenous injection. A pro-drug, (the *o*-phenyl ester), has been reported to be well absorbed by the oral route, but has not progressed beyond pharmacokinetic studies in healthy subjects.

Doses of temocillin of 250, 500 or 1000 mg given by rapid i.v. infusion produced mean plasma concentrations at 5 min of 40, 74 and 172 mg/l, respectively, and by intramuscular injection gave mean peak plasma concentrations of 25, 48 and 70 mg/l. The plasma elimination half-life is 4.3–5.4 h. Binding to plasma protein is around 85%, and this, together with its distribution in a volume less than the extracellular fluid, accounts for its relatively low renal clearance. In artificial blister fluid and peritoneal fluid concentrations reach some 50% of the peak plasma level, and in lymph concentrations reach 25–60% of the simultaneous plasma level, with a similar half-life.

Elimination is principally in the glomerular filtrate, with 80% of the dose appearing in the urine in the first 24 h. A small amount is disposed of in the bile and by degradation. Following a 2 g dose, concentrations in the bile of 300–1200 mg/l have been found. Elimination declines in parallel with renal function, the half-life reaching 30 h in patients with creatinine clearance below 5%.

The *R* epimer differs from the *S* epimer in less protein binding, a 25% greater volume of distribution and a 60% shorter half-life.

Toxicity and side-effects

It is generally well tolerated and administration of 4 g i.v. 12-hourly produced no significant effect on template bleeding time, prothrombin time or ADP-induced platelet aggregation.

Clinical use

Its properties encourage its use in clinical conditions where β-lactamase-producing Gram-negative bacteria would be expected to predominate. It has been shown to be safe and effective in the treatment of severe urinary and respiratory infections, peritonitis and septicaemia. Its activity against bacteria possessing extended spectrum β-lactamases suggest wider application should these enzymes become more prevalent.

Preparations and dosage

Proprietary name: Temopen.

Preparation: Injection.

Dosage: Adults, i.m., i.v., 1–2 g every 12 h.

Available in the UK.

Further information

Basker M J, Merrikin D J, Ponsford R J, Slocombe B, Tasker T C 1986 BRL 20330, an oral prodrug of temocillin, bioavailability studies in man. *Journal of Antimicrobial Chemotherapy* 18: 399–405

Bergan T, Engeset A, Olszewski W 1983 Temocillin in peripheral lymph. *Journal of Antimicrobial Chemotherapy* 12: 59–63

Brown R M, Wise R, Andrews J M 1982 Temocillin, in-vitro activity and the pharmacokinetics and tissue penetration in healthy volunteers. *Journal of Antimicrobial Chemotherapy* 10: 295–302

Clarke A M, Zemcov S J V 1983 Comparative in vitro activity of temocillin (BRL 17421) a new penicillin. *Journal of Antimicrobial Chemotherapy* 11: 319–324

Guest E A, Horton R, Mellows G, Slocombe B, Swaisland A J, Tasker T C G 1985 Human pharmacokinetics of temocillin (BRL 17421) side chain epimers. *Journal of Antimicrobial Chemotherapy* 15: 327–336

Jules K, Neu H C 1982 Antibacterial activity and beta-lactamase stability of temocillin. *Antimicrobial Agents and Chemotherapy* 22: 453–460

Leroy A, Humbert G, Fillastre J-P, Borsa F, Godin M 1983 Pharmacokinetics of temocillin (BRL 17241) in subjects with normal and impaired renal function. *Journal of Antimicrobial Chemotherapy* 12: 47–58

Lode H, Verbist L, Williams J D, Richards D M 1985 First international workshop on temocillin. *Drugs* 29 (suppl 5): 1–243

Nunn B, Baird A, Chamberlain P D 1985 Effect of temocillin and moxalactam on platelet responsiveness and bleeding time in normal volunteers. *Antimicrobial Agents and Chemotherapy* 27: 858–862

Spencer R C 1990 Temocillin. *Journal of Antimicrobial Chemotherapy* 26: 735–737

Wise R, Donovan I A, Drumm J, Dyas A, Cross C 1983 The intraperitoneal penetration of temocillin. *Journal of Antimicrobial Chemotherapy* 12: 93–96

16

Other β-lactams

K. Bush

Introduction

In the penicillins and cephalosporins, the β-lactam ring is fused to a five- and six-membered ring, respectively, but monocyclic and tricyclic β-lactam compounds also exist. Indeed, the situation has become so complicated that it is now necessary to group them according to their chemical structure. There are nine chemical skeletons which support the agents that have current or potential therapeutic use:

SKELETON

Penam

Penem

Carbapenam

Carbapenem

EXAMPLE

Sulbactam

SUN 5555

Thienamycins

Cephem

Cephalosporins

Cephamycins

Carbacephem

Loracarbef

Oxacephem

Latamoxef

Oxapenam

Clavulanic acid

Azetidinone

Monobactams

Tribactam

GV104326

Penams

Penicillins are N-acylated derivatives of 6-β-aminopenicillanic acid. In these compounds the β-lactam ring is fused with a saturated five-membered thiazolidine ring containing sulphur. The sulphur can be oxidized synthetically to a sulphone to yield β-lactamase inhibitors such as sulbactam or tazobactam.

Penems

These differ from penams by the presence of a double bond between C-2 and C-3. No natural penems have so far been described, but many have been synthesized.

Carbapenams and carbapenems

These compounds differ from penams and penems in the substitution of CH_2 for sulphur in the five-membered ring. Many natural and synthetic members of the group have been described, of which the most interesting therapeutically are thienamycin and its analogues.

Cephems

Cephalosporins are N-acylated derivatives of 7-β-amino-cephalosporanic acid. In these compounds, the β-lactam ring is fused with a six-membered dihydrothiazine ring containing sulphur and a double bond. Closely related are cephamycins, which are substituted at the 7-position with an α-methoxy group, oxacephems, notably latamoxef, in which the sulphur of cephalosporins is replaced by oxygen, and carbacephems, including loracarbef, in which the sulphur is replaced by carbon.

Clavams

The only notable member of this group at present is clavulanic acid, a compound which has little antibacterial activity and owes its therapeutic place to its ability to inhibit bacterial β-lactamases. The skeleton differs from penams in the substitution of oxygen for sulphur.

Monobactams

The monocyclic β-lactams are most prominently represented by aztreonam and carumonam, but the group also contains the nocardicins.

Tribactams

The fused tricyclic skeleton of the tribactams is closely related to the carbapenems. This type of molecule is currently under development to provide a broad-spectrum orally active β-lactam agent.

The penicillins are considered in Chapter 15, and the cephalosporins and their close relatives, the cephamycins, oxacephems and carbacephems, in Chapter 14. This chapter deals with the remaining agents: the carbapenems, monobactams and tribactams, which are notable for their antibacterial activity; and clavulanic acid, and the penicillanic acid sulphones, which are primarily of interest as inhibitors of β-lactamases.

Further information

Allan J D, Eliopoulos G M, Moellering R C Jr 1986 The expanding spectrum of β-lactam antibiotics. *Advances in Internal Medicine* 31: 119–146

Demain A L, Solomon N A (eds) 1983 Antibiotics containing the β-lactam structure. Handbook of experimental pharmacology 67. Springer, Berlin, Vols 1, 2

Di Modugno E, Erbetti I, Ferrari L, Galassi G, Hammond S M, Xerri L 1994 In vitro activity of the tribactam GV 104236 against Gram-positive, Gram-negative, and anaerobic bacteria. *Antimicrobial Agents and Chemotherapy* 38: 2362–2368

Donowitz G R, Mandell, G L 1988 Beta-lactam antibiotics. *New England Journal of Medicine* 318: 490–500

Frere J M, Joris B, Varetto L, Crine M 1988 Structure–activity relationships in the β-lactam family: an impossible dream. *Biochemical Pharmacology* 37: 125–132

McCombie S W, Gangully A K 1988 Synthesis and in vitro activity of the penem antibiotics. *Medical Research Review* 8: 393–440

Neu H C 1986 β-lactam antibiotics: structural relationships affecting in vitro activity and pharmacologic properties. *Reviews of Infectious Diseases* 8 (suppl 3): S237–S259

Nishino T, Maeda Y, Ohtsu E, Koizuka S 1989 Studies on penem antibiotics. II. In vitro activity of SUN5555, a new oral penem. *Journal of Antibiotics* 42: 977–988

Norrby S R, Bergan T, Holm S E, Normark S 1986 Evaluation of new β-lactam antibiotics. *Reviews of Infectious Diseases* 8 (suppl 3): S235–S370

Rohl F, Rabenhorst J, Zahner H 1987 Biological properties and mode of action of clavams. *Archives of Microbiology* 147: 315–320

Rolinson G N 1986 β-lactam antibiotics. *Journal of Antimicrobial Chemotherapy* 17: 5–36

Sykes R B, Bonner D P, Swabb E A 1985 Modern β-lactam antibiotics. *Pharmacology and Therapeutics* 29: 321–352

Turck M 1988 Clinical application of the newer β-lactam antibiotics. *Journal of Antimicrobial Chemotherapy* 22 (suppl A): 45–62

Carbapenems

More than 40 carbapenems have been isolated from fermentation products of various streptomycetes. Their nomenclature has been complicated by the use of multiple generic names to describe the same class of compounds, including, thienamycins, olivanic acids, carpetimycins, asparenomycins and pluracidomycins. Their interest lies in their potent activity against a broad range of Gram-positive and Gram-negative bacteria and in their resistance to hydrolysis by β-lactamases. Some are also β-lactamase inhibitors. Unfortunately, the naturally occurring carbapenems are chemically unstable and the concentration-related instability of thienamycin, the most active of the natural compounds, precludes its clinical use.

A search for more stable derivatives which retain potent antibacterial activity led to the development of *N*-formimidoyl-thienamycin, imipenem. This compound is stable to practically all bacterial β-lactamases other than the metallo-enzymes, but it is rapidly degraded by the mammalian renal dipeptidase, dehydropeptidase I. This enzyme hydrolyses carbapenems and penems but not aztreonam, benzyl-penicillin or cephaloridine. Various potential inhibitors of dehydropeptidase have been investigated for co-administration with imipenem and one of these, cilastatin, is included in therapeutic formulations.

Addition of a 1-β-methyl substituent on the carbapenem ring confers stability to hydrolysis by dehydropeptidase. As a result semi-synthetic carbapenems such as meropenem and biapenem, have been developed. These compounds retain broad-spectrum antimicrobial activity and β-lactamase stability, and do not need to be administered with a dehydropeptidase inhibitor.

Further information

Basker M J 1982 The carbapenem family. *Journal of Antimicrobial Chemotherapy* 10: 4–7

Drusano, G L (ed) 1994 The emerging role of carbapenems in the empirical treatment of infections. *Current Opinion in Infectious Diseases* 7 (suppl 1): S1–S45

Nakamura Y, Ono E, Kohda T, Shibai H 1989 Highly targeted screening system for carbapenem antibiotics. *Journal of Antibiotics* 42: 73–83

Wise R 1986 In vitro and pharmacokinetic properties of the carbapenems. *Antimicrobial Agents and Chemotherapy* 30: 343–349

BIAPENEM

This semi-synthetic carbapenem with a 2-substituted triazolium moiety has broad-spectrum activity against most aerobic and anaerobic Gram-positive and Gram-negative organisms. It is equivalent to or slightly more active than imipenem against Gram-negative aerobic bacteria and slightly less active than imipenem against Gram-positive organisms. The methyl group at C-1 confers stability to hydrolysis by dehydropeptidase from various sources, including human kidney. Efficacy in animal infections is equivalent to, or better than, that of imipenem plus cilastatin. It is not hydrolysed by most serine β-lactamases, but like all carbapenems and penems is readily hydrolysed by metallo-β-lactamases. The potential for neurotoxicity is less than that for imipenem.

Further information

Hikida M, Kawashima K, Nishiki K et al 1992 Renal dehydropeptidase-I stability of LJC 10,627, a new carbapenem antibiotic. *Antimicrobial Agents and Chemotherapy* 36: 481–483

Hikida M, Masukawa Y, Nishiki K, Inomata N 1993 Low neurotoxicity of LJC 10,627, a novel 1β-methyl carbapenem antibiotic: inhibition of γ-aminobutyric acid$_A$, benzodiazepine, and glycine receptor binding in relation to lack of central nervous system toxicity in rats. *Antimicrobial Agents and Chemotherapy* 37: 199–202

Petersen P J, Jacobus N V, Weiss W J, Testa R T 1991 In vitro and in vivo activities of LJC10,627, a new carbapenem with stability to dehydropeptidase I. *Antimicrobial Agents and Chemotherapy* 35: 203–207

Ubukata K, Hikida M, Yoshida M et al 1990 In vitro activity of LJC10,627, a new carbapenem antibiotic with high stability to dehydropeptidase I. *Antimicrobial Agents and Chemotherapy* 34: 994–1000

IMIPENEM

Semi-synthetic *N*-formimidoylthienamycin.

The parent thienamycin is very unstable, but imipenem is stable in the solid state for 6 months at 37°C. In aqueous solution at room temperature it decays at 10%/h.

Antimicrobial activity

It shows potent activity against a very wide range of Gram-positive and Gram-negative aerobes and anaerobes, including many resistant to other agents. Its activity against common pathogenic organisms is shown in Table 16.1. Concentrations (mg/l) inhibiting 50% and 90%, respectively, of strains of other oragnisms are: *Brucella melitensis*, 1 and 2; *Listeria monocytogenes*, 0.03 and 0.25; *Legionella pneumophila*, 0.03 and 0.25; *Enterococcus faecium*, 4 and 32; *Norcardia asteroides*, 2 and 4; *Yersinia* spp., 0.06 and 0.1. *Mycobacterium fortuitum* is inhibited by 6.25 mg/l. It is active against all *Pseudomonas* species, but not *Stenotrophomonas (Xanthomonas) maltophilia*. It is active against most anaerobes, with the exception of *Clostridium*

Table 16.1 *Activity of aztreonam, imipenem and meropenem against common bacterial pathogens:* MIC_{50} *and* MIC_{90} *(mg/l)*

Organism	Aztreonam		Imipenem		Meropenem	
	MIC_{50}	MIC_{90}	MIC_{50}	MIC_{90}	MIC_{50}	MIC_{90}
Staph. aureus (MSSA)	64–>128	>128	≤0.015–0.03	0.03	0.06–0.12	0.12
Staph. aureus (MRSA)	>128	>128	0.5	4.0	2.0	8.0
Str. pyogenes	8	8	ND	ND	<0.01	0.01
Str. pneumoniae						
penicillin-susceptible	8–>128	8–>128	0.008	0.016	0.008	0.008
penicillin-resistant	ND	ND	0.03	0.12	0.12	0.25
Ent. faecalis	>128	>128	1.0–2.0	1.0–2.0	4.0	4.0–8.0
Clostridium spp.	64	>128	0.5	1.0–4.0	≤0.06–0.25	0.12–1.0
N. gonorrhoeae	0.025–0.06	0.25	0.12–0.25	0.12–0.5	0.008–0.03	0.016–0.5
N. meningitidis	0.012	0.025	0.03	0.03	≤0.004	0.015
H. influenzae	0.03–0.05	0.12	0.12–2.0	0.25–4.0	0.015–0.12	0.03–0.5
Esch. coli	≤0.03–0.1	0.12–1.0	0.12–0.25	0.25–0.5	0.016–0.03	0.03
Klebsiella spp.	≤0.03–0.06	0.12–8.0	0.12–0.5	0.5–1.0	0.03	0.03–0.06
Enterobacter spp.	≤0.03–0.25	0.25–25	0.5–1.0	1.0–2.0	0.03	0.03–0.25
Pr. mirabilis	≤0.015–0.06	0.03–0.12	2.0–4.0	4.0	0.12	0.12–0.25
Pr. vulgaris/providencia	≤0.015	≤0.015–0.03	2.0	2.0–4.0	0.12	0.12–0.25
Salmonella spp.	0.03–0.05	0.06–0.2	0.12–0.5	0.12–0.5	0.015–0.03	0.015–0.03
Shigella spp.	0.06–0.25	0.06–0.1	0.12	0.12–0.25	0.03	0.03–0.06
Ser. marcescens	0.12–0.5	0.25–3.1	0.5–1.0	1.0–2.0	0.06	0.12–0.25
Citrobacter spp.	≤0.03–0.25	0.06–0.4	0.12–0.5	0.12–1.0	0.03	0.03–0.06
Ps. aeruginosa	4–8	4–25	1.0	2.0–4.0	0.5–1.0	2.0–4.0
B. fragilis	16–32	64–>128	0.25	0.5–1.0	0.12	0.25–0.5

ND, not determined.

perfringens which is only moderately susceptible. There is usually little effect of inoculum size up to 10^7 cfu/ml, of pH up to 8, or the presence of serum, but marked inoculum effects have been described with *Haemophilus influenzae*, *Enterococcus faecalis* and methicillin-resistant *Staphylococcus aureus*, organisms in which resistance to β-lactam antibiotics is due to poor affinity of specific target penicillin-binding proteins. It is bactericidal at 2–4 times the minimum inhibitory concentration (MIC) for most species, but some strains of *L. monocytogenes* and *Staph. aureus* exhibit 'tolerance' (see p. 259). Bactericidal synergy with aminoglycosides, glycopeptides, fosfomycin and rifampicin has been observed against many strains of *Staph. aureus* and enterococci.

It is stable to hydrolysis by most serine β-lactamases, including the group 2a penicillinases from *Staph. aureus* and the common group 2e cephalosporinases of *Bacteroides*

fragilis (see p. 317 for the basis of β-lactamase classification). It is a potent inhibitor of group 1 β-lactamase from *Pseudomonas aeruginosa* and the group 2a penicillinase from *Bacillus cereus*, acting like a poor substrate that is released slowly. It can be hydrolysed by the TEM-1 and TEM-2 β-lactamases, but so slowly that organisms elaborating the enzymes remain susceptible. β-lactamase-producing strains of *H. influenzae* and *N. gonorrhoeae* are as susceptible, or only slightly more resistant than β-lactamase-negative strains. The MIC for *Escherichia coli* strains elaborating non-extended spectrum TEM, SHV and OXA β-lactamases is about 0.25 mg/l. Strains of *B. fragilis* and *Sten. maltophilia* can produce metallo-β-lactamases that hydrolyse the drug rapidly. These strains, in addition to rare strains of Enterobacteriaceae, show variable resistance to imipenem depending upon the level of carbapenem-hydrolysing activity.

Acquired resistance

Some strains of *Citrobacter, Enterobacter, Proteus vulgaris, Providencia, Ps. aeruginosa* and *Serratia* spp. that elaborate high levels of β-lactamases may be resistant to imipenem and other β-lactam agents, often because stably derepressed mutants expressing high levels of group 1 β-lactamases have been selected. These cephalosporinases hydrolyse imipenem and extended-spectrum cephalosporins such as cefotaxime very slowly, but the mutants also exhibit decreased permeability; they are resistance to all β-lactams, but imipenem is usually affected less than expanded-spectrum cephalosporins and aztreonam. Induction of class I β-lactams by imipenem in strains of *Aeromonas, Pseudomonas* and *Serratia* spp. is responsible for antagonism of β-lactamase-labile β-lactam agents in vitro. Resistance in *Ps. aeruginosa* has also been documented following selection by imipenem of mutants that hyper-produce the group 1 cephalosporinase and that are also deficient in an outer membrane protein (OprD or D2) which specifically transports imipenem and other carbapenems, but not cephalosporins or monobactams.

Pharmacokinetics

Imipenem is slowly hydrolysed with a half-life of 0.7 h in serum in vitro; at the end of intravenous (i.v.) infusion over 20 min, about 9% of the labelled drug is in the form of the open-ring metabolite. Most destruction, however, occurs in the kidney and only about 5–40% of the drug is recovered in the urine, where 80–90% is in the open-ring form. This can be substantially overcome by administration with the dehydropeptidase I inhibitor, cilastatin. Protein binding of imipenem is low (about 25%).

IMIPENEM–CILASTATIN

The combination is commercially available as a 1 : 1 mixture.

Pharmacokinetics

When imipenem is administered with the dehydropeptidase I inhibitor, cilastatin, in a 1 : 1 ratio, urinary recovery of imipenem rises to 65–75% with only 20% in the open-ring form. Renal excretion of cilastatin closely follows that of imipenem, 75% being excreted unchanged in the urine over 6 h with about 12% as the *N*-acetyl metabolite.

In volunteers receiving 2 g of the mixture i.v. over 30 min, every 6 h for 40 doses, serum concentrations of imipenem at the end of infusion were around 19 mg/l after the first dose and 23 mg/l after the last. Corresponding half-lives were 0.9 and 0.8 h and renal excretion was 55–60%.

In newborn infants receiving each component at a dosage of 10, 15 or 20 mg/kg over 60 min, the plasma concentration of cilastatin was consistently higher because of its smaller volume of distribution. Plasma half-lives were: imipenem 1.7–2.4 h and cilastatin 3.9–6.3 h. In patients with bacterial meningitis receiving 1 mg/kg i.v. over 20 min, cerebrospinal fluid (CSF) concentrations of 0.5–11 mg/l have been found. The plasma clearance of cilastatin was about one-quarter that of imipenem but its urinary concentration was approximately double. There was marked intersubject variation, especially in the handling of cilastatin.

One source of intersubject variation also described in adults may be in the ability to metabolize the drug. The inhibitor has more effect in 'high metabolizers' – those in whom less than 16% of the dose appears in the urine. Probenecid has little effect on the plasma half-life, but markedly increases urinary recovery.

In patients with chronic renal failure, about 75% of the mixture was eliminated by 3 h haemofiltration. The half-lives of the two components differed markedly: around 3.4 h for imipenem and 16 h for cilastatin.

Toxicity and side-effects

It is generally well tolerated, reactions being those common to β-lactam compounds. There is an extensive cross-reactivity with penicillins and the same precautions are necessary in instituting treatment in patients allergic to penicillins (p. 260). Seizures have been observed in patients with renal failure. Transient changes can occur in some liver function tests.

Other reactions include nausea (which may be controlled by reducing the dose or rate of infusion), diarrhoea (including antibiotic-associated colitis), rash, pruritis, eosinophilia, thrombocytopenia and positive Coombs' reaction without haemolysis. No profound changes have been found in the bowel flora, but the concentrations of enterococci and candida have tended to rise. Superinfection with *Aspergillus, Candida* and resistant *Pseudomonas* spp. have been described.

Clinical use

It has been successfully used to treat septicaemia due to Gram-negative rods (p. 589), although resistant *Pseudomonas* has emerged in some cases and regularly in patients with cystic fibrosis in whom the drug, in combination with tobramycin, failed to eradicate *Ps. aeruginosa*. It has also been used in infections of the urinary and respiratory tracts, of skin, soft tissues, bone and joints, and in abdominal (including gynaecological) sepsis. Reference is also made to its use in neutropenic patients, endocarditis, meningitis, legionellosis and gonorrhoea.

Preparations and dosage

Proprietary names: Primaxin.

Preparation: Injection.

Dosage: Adults, deep i.m. injection, 500–750 mg every 12 h depending on the severity of the infection; gonococcal urethritis or cervicitis, 500 mg as a single dose. Adults, i.v., 1–2 g/day in 3–4 equally divided doses; the dose is determined by the severity of the infection and the condition of the patient. Children, ≥ 3 months (< 40 kg body weight) 15 mg/kg in four divided doses, with a maximum daily dose of 60 mg/kg.

Widely available.

Further information

Alarabi A A, Cars O, Danielson B G, Salmonson T, Wikstrom B 1990 Pharmacokinetics of intravenous imipenem/cilastatin during intermittent haemofiltration. *Journal of Antimicrobial Chemotherapy* 26: 91–98

Bint A J, Speller D C E, Williams R J (eds) 1986 Imipenem – assessing its clinical role. *Journal of Antimicrobial Chemotherapy* 18 (suppl E): 1–210

Clissold S P, Todd P A, Campoli-Richards D M 1987 Imipenem/cilastatin: a review of its antibacterial activity, pharmacokinetic properties and therapeutic efficacy. *Drugs* 33: 183–241

Geddes A M, Stille W (eds) 1985 Imipenem: the first thienamycin antibiotic. *Reviews of Infectious Diseases* 7 (suppl 3): S353–S356

Janmohamed R M I 1990 Pharmacokinetics of imipenem/cilastatin in neutropenic patients with haematological malignancies. *Journal of Antimicrobial Chemotherapy* 25: 407–412

Livermore D 1992 Interplay of impermeability and chromosomal β-lactamase activity in imipenem-resistant *Pseudomonas aeruginosa*. *Antimicrobial Agents and Chemotherapy* 36: 2046–2048

Luthy R, Neu H C, Phillips I (eds) 1983 A perspective of imipenem. *Journal of Antimicrobial Chemotherapy* 12 (suppl D): 1–153

Remington J S (ed) 1985 Carbapenems: a new class of antibiotics (Symposium on imipenem – cilastatin). *American Journal of Medicine* 78 (suppl 6A): 1–167

Saxon A, Adelman D C, Patel A, Hajdu R, Calandra G B 1988 Imipenem cross-reactivity with penicillin in humans. *Journal of Allergy and Clinical Immunology* 82: 213–217

Trias J, Nikaido, H 1990 Outer membrane protein D2 catalyzes facilitated diffusion of carbapenems and penems through the outer membrane of *Pseudomonas aeruginosa*. *Antimicrobial Agents and Chemotherapy* 34: 52–57

MEROPENEM

A carbapenem differing from imipenem in a unique side-chain at C-2 which is associated with increased activity against Gram-negative bacteria, including *Ps. aeruginosa*, and a methyl group at C-1 which confers increased stability to hydrolysis by mammalian dehydropeptidase I. It is slightly less active than imipenem against Gram-positive organisms. It is quite active against anaerobes and more active against some strains which are moderately resistant (but not those that are fully resistant) to imipenem. Its excellent activity against Gram-negative organisms is due to high affinity for multiple penicillin-binding proteins (PBPs). Activity is little affected by inoculum size or the presence of serum. It is bactericidal at concentrations close to the MIC.

Stability to β-lactamases is similar to that of other carbapenems: it is highly resistant to most serine β-lactamases, including extended-spectrum enzymes, but can be hydrolysed by metallo-β-lactamases and by rare carbapenem-hydrolysing group 2f serine β-lactamases. It induces, but is not degraded by, chromosomally-mediated group 1 enzymes (see p. 319).

It is stable to dehydropeptidase I (other than that of rodents) and does not need to be administered with an enzyme inhibitor.

Pharmacokinetics

After a dose of 0.25, 0.5 or 1.0 g given by i.v. infusion over 30 min, maximum serum concentrations were 12.1, 25.6 and 55.4 mg/l, respectively. The elimination half-life was 1.0 h.

Co-administration with probenecid significantly prolonged the half-life by 33% and increased the area under the curve (AUC) by 55%, but peak concentrations were not greatly affected.

Plasma protein binding of meropenem is extremely low (<10%). Renal excretion is greater than 70% of the plasma clearance. The mean recovery of unchanged meropenem is 65–79%, attesting to its stability to human dehydropeptidase. The remainder of the material was identified as the open-ring form, produced either by chemical hydrolysis, by the action of dehydropeptidase or other metabolic enzymes.

In patients with inflamed meninges it achieved CSF levels of 0.9–6.5 mg/l after a single i.v. infusion over 30 min, or a 5 min bolus. Dosing in one group was 20 mg/kg for patients who weighed ≤50 kg or 1 g for patients weighing >50 kg; dosing in a second group was 40 mg/kg if they weighed ≤50 kg or 2 g if their weight was >50 kg. CSF concentrations are directly related to the degree of meningeal inflammation. The CSF:plasma concentration ratio is 0.02 –0.5. CSF levels are above the MIC_{90} for most organisms causing community-acquired bacterial meningitis.

Toxicity and side-effects

Adverse effects are similar to those of other β-lactam antibiotics. A low incidence of nausea and vomiting (0.9%) is reported (maximum dose of 6 g/day). It can be administered by bolus injection without inducing nasuea or vomiting. Thirteen seizures were reported from a patient population of 3357 (0.4%) with only one patient classified as having a meropenem-related event. Little or no nephrotoxicity is seen. Reversible elevation of the liver enzymes aspartate aminotransferase/alanine aminotransferase and, to a lesser extent, alkaline phosphatase is seen in 4–5% of patients. Cross-reactivity with penicillins should be assumed and appropriate precautions taken for penicillin-allergic patients.

Clinical use

It has been efficacious in treating abdominal infections, meningitis and lower respiratory tract infections. It is being evaluated as monotherapy to treat febrile neutropenic patients.

Further information

Conference 1989 Meropenem (SM 7338) – a new carbapenem. *Journal of Antimicrobial Chemotherapy* 24 (suppl A): 1–320

Cornaglia G, Guan L, Fontana R, Satta G 1992 Diffusion of meropenem and imipenem through the outer membrane of *Escherichia coli* K-12 and correlation with their antibacterial activities. *Antimicrobial Agents and Chemotherapy* 36: 1902–1908

Dagan R, Velghe L, Rodda J L, Klugman K P 1994 Penetration of meropenem into the cerebrospinal fluid of patients with inflamed meninges. *Journal of Antimicrobial Chemotherapy* 34: 175–179

Davey P, Davies A, Livermore D, Speller D, Daly P J (eds) 1989 Meropenem (SM7338) – a new carbapenem. *Journal of Antimicrobial Chemotherapy* 24 (suppl A): 1–320

Fukasawa M, Sumita Y, Harabe E T et al 1992 Stability of meropenem and effect of 1β-methyl substitution on its stability in the presence of renal dehydropeptidase I. *Antimicrobial Agents and Chemotherapy* 36: 1577–1579

Wise R 1990 Meropenem pharmacokinetics and penetration into an inflammatory exudate. *Antimicrobial Agents and Chemotherapy* 34: 1515–1517

PANIPENEM

A 3-acetimidoylpyrrolidinyl-substituted carbapenem with no methyl group at the C-1 position. It has broad-spectrum antibacterial activity against Gram-positive and Gram-negative organisms. It is co-administered with betamipron (*N*-benzoyl-β-alanine) in a ratio of 1 : 1. Betamipron is a renal anion transport inhibitor that decreases nephrotoxicity caused by high doses of the carbapenem by inhibiting its accumulation in the renal cortex. Panipenem is slightly more stable to hydrolysis by dehydropeptidase than imipenem, but not as stable as meropenem or biapenem. It is also hydrolysed by metallo-β-lactamases.

Following i.v. infusion in children, the half-life of panipenem was about 0.8–1 h; the half-life of betamipron was about 0.5 h.

The combination has been used parenterally in Japan to treat paediatric infections, including respiratory infections, otitis media and sepsis. It has also shown efficacy in urinary tract infections, skin and soft-tissue infections, and surgical infections in adults. Side-effects were minor and included occasional transient elevations of transaminases.

Further information

Kurihara A, Naganuma H, Hisaoka M, Tokiwa H, Kawahara Y 1992 Prediction of human pharmacokinetics of panipenem–betamipron, a new carbapenem, from animal data. *Antimicrobial Agents and Chemotherapy* 36: 1810–1816

Panipenem/betamipron 1991 In: *Chemotherapy (Tokyo)* S–3: 1–813

Shimada K 1994 Panipenem/betamipron. *Japanese Journal of Antibiotics* 47: 219–244

Monobactams

Study of the structural basis of activity of β-lactam compounds led to the expectation that compounds in which the β-lactam ring was not strained by fusion to another ring would be inactive as antimicrobial agents. It came as a surprise, therefore, to find active natural monocyclic β-lactams, nocardicins and monobactams. Nocardicin A, the most potent of the seven nocardicin analogues, attracted interest principally for its activity against *Ps. aeruginosa* and for an apparently beneficial interaction with host defences, but it has been overtaken by more active compounds and has not been made commercially available.

The antibacterial monocyclic β-lactam-1-sulphonic acids, originally called 'sulphazecins' and later 'monobactams', are produced by bacteria, in contrast to penicillins and cephalosporins which are commonly produced by fungi and actinomycetes. In the naturally occurring monobactams the β-lactam ring may carry an α-methoxy group, a feature which is responsible for β-lactamase stability in cephamycins. Because of their simplicity of structure, they can be obtained by total synthesis. The compound which first came into therapeutic use, aztreonam, incorporates an unnatural aminothiazoleoxime substituent in the 3-position.

Monobactams exhibit no useful activity against Gram-positive organisms or strict anaerobes because of poor binding to PBPs. Activity against Gram-negative bacteria, including *Ps. aeruginosa* is due to tight binding to PBP3 in *Esch. coli* and analogous PBPs in other Gram-negative organisms. They are hydrolysed poorly by many serine β-lactamases and all metallo-β-lactamases tested to date, but can be hydrolysed by the extended-spectrum β-lactamases. Group 1 cephalosporinases have high affinities for non-methoxylated monobactams, whereas group 2 β-lactamases generally bind aztreonam poorly. They are generally not inducers of the group 1 chromosomal cephalosporinases of Gram-negative bacteria.

Further information

Bush K, Sykes R B 1982 Interaction of new β-lactams with β-lactamases and β-lactamase-producing Gram-negative rods. In: Neu H C (ed) New beta-lactam antibiotics: a review from chemistry to clinical efficacy of the new cephalosporins. *College of Physicians of Philadelphia*, p 47–63

Bush K, Liu F Y, Smith S A 1987 Interactions of monobactams with bacterial enzymes. *Journal of Industrial Microbiology* 27 (suppl 1): 153–164

Parker W L, O'Sullivan J, Sykes R B 1986 Naturally occurring monobactams. *Advances in Applied Microbiology* 31: 181–205

Sykes R B, Koster W H, Bonner D P 1988 The new monobactams: chemistry and biology. *Journal of Clinical Pharmacology* 28: 113–119

AZTREONAM

A synthetic 3-desmethoxy monobactam.

Antimicrobial activity

It is active against a wide range of aerobic Gram-negative organisms, including many strains resistant to other agents. It has no useful activity against Gram-positive organisms or strict anaerobes. Its activity against common pathogenic organisms is shown in Table 16.1. Concentrations (mg/l) inhibiting 50% and 90%, respectively, of other organisms are: *Aeromonas* spp., 0.1 and 0.1; *Acinetobacter* spp., 16 and 64; *Moraxella (Branhamella) catarrhalis*, 0.1 and 4; *Burkholderia (Ps.) cepacia*, 2 and 16; *Sten. maltophilia*, 128 and 256; and *Yersinia* spp., 0.1 and 0.1. An inoculum effect may be observed in Enterobacteriaceae when tested at 10^3 colony forming units (cfu), but not at lower inocula (10^4–10^6 cfu), perhaps due to selection of variants exhibiting de-repressed production of chromosomal cephalosporinases together with the development of permeability barriers. Synergy has been shown with gentamicin, tobramycin and amikacin against 52–89% of strains of *Ps. aeruginosa* and gentamicin-resistant Gram-negative bacteria.

Pharmacokinetics

Oral bioavailability is less than 1%; doses of 500 mg as solution or capsules produce average peak plasma levels of <0.2 mg/l. In volunteers receiving 0.5, 1 or 2 g i.v. over 3 min, concentrations at 5 min were 58, 125 and 242 mg/l, respectively; when the same doses were given i.v. over 30 min, peak levels were 54, 90 and 204, respectively. After i.m. administration of 0.5 and 1.0 g doses, average peak concentrations achieved after 1 h were 22 and 46 mg/l respectively. Plasma protein binding is about 50%.

Bioavailability by the i.m. route is 100%. The elimination half-life is similar on i.v. or i.m. administration: 1.5–2 h (mean 1.7 h). There is no accumulation when 1 g is administered 8-hourly. In the elderly, the half-life is slightly prolonged, values of 2.7 h being reported. In children given 30 mg/kg as i.v. bolus, plasma concentrations were around 100 mg/l at 15 min at all ages (<7 days, premature infants – 83 mg/l; <7 days, full-term – 98 mg/l; 1 week to 1 month – 97 mg/l; 1 month to 2 years – 118 mg/l). Elimination half-lives were directly related to age and reached adult values at 2 years (<7 days, premature – 5.7 h; <7 days, full-term – 2.6 h; week to 1 month – 2.4 h; 1 month to 12 years – 1.7 h). It is not accumulated in adults with normal renal clearance.

Aztreonam does not inactivate and is not inactivated by gentamicin.

Distribution

In patients receiving 2 g i.v. over 5 min, concentrations in the CSF in the absence of inflammation were 0.5–0.9 mg/l at 1.2–8 h; in the presence of inflammation 2.0–3.2 mg/l and in patients with bacterial meningitis 0.8–16 mg/l. In children receiving 30 mg/kg i.v. in a single dose, CSF concentrations of 2–20 mg/l were found, depending on the time of sampling and disease state. In patients receiving 1 or 2 g i.v., concentrations in the aqueous humour were 2.1–12.5 mg/l.

Sputum. In patients receiving 1 or 2 g i.m., concentrations in sputum were 1.3 and 2.5 mg/l when the corresponding serum concentrations were 37 and 55 mg/l, respectively. In critically ill intubated patients receiving 2 g i.v. over 3 min, concentrations in bronchial secretion ranged from 4.8 to 18.7 mg/l with a peak within the first 2 h, but there was much individual variation.

Serous fluids and exudates. In volunteers given 1 g by i.v. bolus, concentrations in cantharides blister fluid rose rapidly to a mean maximum of 25 mg/l at 1.8 h. Good penetration has been reported into synovial fluid and bone. In patients undergoing joint replacement given 2 g i.v. over 5 min preoperatively, concentrations around 83 mg/l in synovial fluid (a simultaneous serum ratio of 0.99) and 16 mg/g in cancellous bone (a simultaneous serum ratio of 0.2) were found. In patients receiving 1 g i.m. preoperatively, the concentration in prostate tissue 50–180 min after dosing was, on average, 8 mg/kg.

It is not extensively metabolized, the most prominent product, that which results from opening the β-lactam ring, being scarcely detectable in the serum and accounting for about 7% of the dose in the urine and 3% in the faeces. Its half-life is much longer than that of the parent compound. However, hepatic handling of the drug is sufficient to influence the elimination half-life in liver derangement. In patients with alcoholic cirrhosis, the average half-life was found to be 3.2 h and in biliary cirrhosis 2.2 versus 1.9 h in normal subjects.

Excretion

It is predominantly eliminated in the urine, where 58–72% appears within 24 h. The mean plasma clearance correlates well with creatinine clearance corrected for sex and age, the elimination half-life rising to 6 h in severe renal failure, with recovery in the urine falling to 1.4%.

Less than 1% is eliminated unchanged in the faeces, suggesting low biliary excretion. In patients given 1 g by i.v. bolus, concentrations in T-tube bile reached a mean peak around 34 mg/l, with mean concentrations of 42 mg/l in common duct bile and 30 mg/l in gallbladder bile.

Toxicity and side-effects

It is well tolerated, with a few patients developing mild rashes, diarrhoea, eosinophilia, rapidly reversible leucopenia, and fever. Increase in prothrombin time without bleeding, discomfort at the i.m. injection site have been reported. There were no reactions in patients with immunoglobulin E (IgE) antibodies to benzylpenicillin or penicillin moieties.

Clinical use

It has been successfully used to treat respiratory and urinary infections and severe sepsis including osteomyelitis and meningitis due to Gram-negative organisms. It has been used in combination with other agents including gentamicin or other aminoglycoside in severe pseudomonas infection. A single 1 g i.m. dose has been satisfactory for the treatment of uncomplicated gonorrhoea, including rectal and cervical infections. When co-administered with clindamycin or metronidazole it can clear intra-abdominal infections caused by mixed populations of aerobic Gram-negative organisms and anaerobes. Reference is made to its use in neutropenic patients and necrotizing soft tissue infection.

There is little effect on the throat flora and variable effect on that of the faeces, but superinfection with Gram-positive organisms may cause therapeutic failure. In patients treated for acute purulent exacerbations of chronic bronchitis, almost a third needed treatment for emergent pneumococcal infection; in patients with urinary infection or Gram-negative bacillary septicaemia, enterococcal superinfection has occurred. Emergence of candida and staphylococci has also been observed in some patients. Treatment failure can occur if infections are caused by Enterobacteriaceae that produce extended-spectrum β-lactamases.

Preparations and dosage

Proprietary name: Azactam.

Preparation: Injection.

Dosage: Adults, i.m., i.v., i.v. infusion, 1–8 g/day in equally divided doses. The route and dose is determined by the severity of the infection and the condition of the patient. Children >1 week, i.v., i.v. infusion, 30 mg/kg every 6–8 h; children ≥2 years, 50 mg/kg every 6–8 h; the total daily dose should not exceed 8 g.

Available in the UK and the USA.

Further information

Acar J F, Neu H C (eds) 1985 Gram-negative aerobic bacterial infections: a focus on directed therapy with special reference to aztreonam. *Reviews of Infectious Diseases* 7 (suppl 4): S537–S843

Bocazzi A, Langer M, Mandelli M, Ranzi A M, Urso R 1989 The pharmacokinetics of aztreonam and penetration into the bronchial secretions of critically ill patients. *Journal of Antimicrobial Chemotherapy* 23: 401–407

Brogden R N, Heel R C 1986 Aztreonam: a review of its antibacterial activity, pharmacokinetic properties and therapeutic use. *Drugs* 31: 96–130

Likitnukul S, McCracken J H, Threlkeld N, Darabi A, Olsen K 1987 Pharmacokinetics and plasma bactericidal activity of aztreonam in low-birth-weight infants. *Antimicrobial Agents and Chemotherapy* 31: 81–83

Neu H C (ed) 1985 Aztreonam: a monocyclic β-lactam antibiotic. *American Journal of Medicine* 78 (suppl 2A): 1–80

Swabb E A 1985 Review of the clinical pharmacology of the monobactam antibiotic aztreonam. *American Journal of Medicine* 78 (2A): 11–18

Sykes R B, Phillips I (eds) 1981 Azthreonam, a synthetic monobactam. *Journal of Antimicrobial Chemotherapy* 8 (suppl E): 1–146

CARUMONAM

A synthetic monobactam.

Antimicrobial activity

Its activity against common pathogenic organisms is similar to that of aztreonam: MICs generally differ no more than two-fold, except for strains of klebsiella that produce an aztreonam-hydrolysing enzyme. As with aztreonam, the principal biochemical target is PBP3 of Gram-negative bacteria and the effect is exerted predominantly through conversion of the organisms to filaments which slowly lyse.

It is resistant to hydrolysis by the common plasmid and chromosomal β-lactamases, but it can be hydrolysed by extended spectrum β-lactamases. It inhibits but does not induce chromosomal cephalosporinases.

Pharmacokinetics

In volunteers receiving 0.5, 1 or 2 g i.v. over 20 min, levels at the end of infusion were 36, 78 and 150 mg/l, respectively. Binding to plasma protein is 18–28%. A linear correlation has been found between the dose and AUC. The mean half-life is 1.7 h. In blister fluid a peak concentration

of 61 mg/l was found 1.5 h after a dose of 2 g i.v. over 20 min, with a half-life identical to that in serum.

Excretion

It is almost entirely eliminated in the glomerular filtrate, probenecid having no effect on excretion; 96% of labelled compound is found in the urine, with 3% in the faeces. Between 68% and 91% of the dose appears in the urine within 24 h. In patients with renal failure whose creatinine clearance was less than 10 ml/min the half-life rose to 11 h.

Clinical use

It is not used in Europe or the USA. It has been approved for use in Japan. It is effective against appropriate respiratory and urinary tract infections.

Further information

Imada A, Kondo M, Okonogi K, Yukishige K, Kuno M 1985 In vitro and in vivo antibacterial activities of carumonam (AMA-1080), a new *N*-sulfonated monocyclic β-lactam antibiotic. *Antimicrobial Agents and Chemotherapy* 27: 821–827

McNulty C A, Garden G M, Ashby J, Wise R 1985 Pharmacokinetics and tissue penetration of carumonam, a new synthetic monobactam. *Antimicrobial Agents and Chemotherapy* 28: 425–427

Neu H C, Chin N X, Labthavikul P 1986 The in vitro activity and β-lactamase stability of carumonam. *Journal of Antimicrobial Chemotherapy* 18: 35–44

Patel J H, Soni P P, Portmann R, Suter K, Banken L, Weidekamm E 1989 Multiple intravenous dose pharmacokinetic study of carumonam in healthy subjects. *Journal of Antimicrobial Chemotherapy* 23: 107–111

β-Lactamases

Even before penicillin was widely used clinically, it was learned that bacteria, particularly *Staph. aureus*, could easily develop resistance to benzylpenicillin, not as a result of a reduction in their intrinsic susceptibility to the agent, but as the result of the ability to degrade it. The bacterial enzyme shown to open the β-lactam ring was initially called 'penicillinase', and penicillinase-producing *Staph. aureus* became of great importance in outbreaks of hospital infection in the 1950s. Since that time, similar enzymes have become increasingly important as a cause of resistance in Gram-negative bacteria. Because of their collective ability to degrade a wide range of β-lactam agents, the enzymes have been renamed β-lactamases. In the case of the penicillins, the products are stable penicilloates, but in the case of cephalosporins the 'cephalosporoates' rapidly undergo further degradation, liberating a variety of fragments depending on the C-3 substituent. Virtually every β-lactam can be inactivated by an appropriate β-lactamase.

β-Lactam antibiotics can be attacked at other sites by microbial acylases and esterases, but these enzymes, which have important uses in semi-synthetic processes, are of no significance as a cause of clinical resistance. The presence of esterases in mammalian tissues is exploited in the cleavage of oral pro-drug esters of penicillins and cephalosporins with liberation of the active parent compound. Some penems and carbapenems are hydrolysed by mammalian dehydropeptidases (see above).

Bacterial β-lactamases may be plasmid-mediated, or chromosomal with inducible or constitutive production. Those found in Gram-positive organisms are often extracellular enzymes, but Gram-negative β-lactamases are almost invariably confined to the periplasmic space. Because the outer cell membrane of Gram-negative bacteria generally restricts transport of large molecules, little β-lactamase activity is detected extracellularly. Quantitative measurement of β-lactamase activity in intact cells can be difficult, depending upon the permeability properties of the specific outer membrane of an organism, so that the enzymes are usually studied after liberation by disruption of the cell.

Classification

The enzymes are usually characterized on the basis of one of two properties: molecular characteristics, which now frequently include a full nucleotide or amino acid sequence; or functional characteristics, including substrate and inhibition profiles (Table 16.2). Numerous classification schemes have been proposed. The three most cited schemes are: that of Ambler, who proposed a classification based upon molecular structure; that of Richmond and Sykes, who divided the β-lactamases produced by Gram-negative bacteria according to functional properties; and that of Bush who combined the functional properties with the known molecular sequences of β-lactamases from both Gram-positive and Gram-negative bacteria. The latter scheme has been expanded to include 190 unique β-lactamases in a functional classification that has been correlated with their classification by molecular sequence.

Hydrolytic activity is customarily defined by comparison with benzylpenicillin or cephaloridine, with rates of hydrolysis normalized to 100 for the reference compound (Table 16.3). Inhibition properties deemed to be significant include inhibition by clavulanic acid, a good inhibitor of many

Table 16.2 *Classification schemes for bacterial β-lactamases*

Functional group	Richmond–Sykes class	Molecular class	Preferred substrates	Inhibited by CA	Inhibited by EDTA	Representative enzymes
I	Ia, Ib, Id	C	Cephalosporins	−	−	Amp C, chromosomal enzymes from Gram-negatives
2a	Not included	A	Penicillins	+	−	Penicillinases from Gram-positives
2b	III	A	Penicillins, cephalosporins	+	−	TEM-1, TEM-2, SHV-1
2be	Not included except K1 in class IV	A	Penicillins, narrow- and extended-spectrum cephalosporins, monobactams	+	−	TEM-3 ...TEM-26; SHV-2 ... SHV-7 K. oxytoca K1
2br	Not included	A	Penicillins	+/−	−	TEM 30-37 (IRT 1-4)
2c	II	A	Penicillins, carbenicillin	+	−	PSE-1, PSE-3, PSE-4
2d	V	D	Penicillins, cloxacillin	+	−	OXA-1 ...OXA-12, PSE-2 (OXA-10)
2e	Ic	A	Cephalosporins	+	−	Inducible cephalosporinases from Pr. vulgaris
2f	Not included	A	Cephalosporins, penicillins, carbapenems	+	−	NMC-A from Ent. cloacae Sme-1 from Ser. marcescens
3	Not included	B	Most β-lactams, including carbapenems	−	+	L1 from X. maltophilia, CfiA/CcrA from B. fragilis
4	Not included	ND	Penicillins	−	?	Penicillinase from Burk. cepacia

ª Based on Bush K, Jacoby G A, Medeiros A A 1995 *Antimicrobial Agents and Chemotherapy* 39: 1211–1233.
CA, clavulanic acid; EDTA, ethylenediaminetetraacetic acid.

Table 16.3 *Characteristics of selected bacterial β-lactamases[a]*

β-Lactamase	Hydrolysis relative to benzylpenicillin as 100					IC$_{50}$ (μM)* Clavulanic acid	Molecular mass (kDa)	pI	Molecular class	Functional class
	Ampicillin	Cephaloridine	Cefotaxime	Ceftazidime	Imipenem					
Ent. cloacae P99	1.3	6,700	<7	<0.7	<0.7	>100	39	8.2	C	1
Esch. coli AmpC	9.1	290	0.37	ND	<0.03	190	40	8.5	C	1
Staph. aureus PC1	180	1.1	ND	ND	ND	0.03	27	10.1	A	2a
TEM-1	110	140	0.07	0.01	<0.01	0.09	29	5.4	A	2b
TEM-3	110	120	170	8.3	0.01	0.03	29	6.3	A	2be
TEM-10	130	77	1.6	68	<0.02	0.03	29	5.6	A	2be
SHV-1	150	48	0.18	0.02	<0.01	0.03	29	7.6	A	2b
SHV-4	200	320	120	52	<0.01	0.03	29	7.8	A	2be
Klebsiella K1	61	36	1.8	0.01	<0.01	0.007	27	6.5	A	2be
TEM-31 (IRT-1)	250	13	<1	<1	<1	9.4	29	5.2	A	2br
PSE-4 (Dalgleish)	88	40	0.02	0.02	0.01	0.15	32	5.3	A	2c
OXA-10 (PSE-2)	270	32	1	0.12	0.05	0.81	28	6.1	D	2d
Pr. vulgaris	100	3 000	13	0.17	ND	0.35	28	8.3	A	2e
Ser. marcescens Sme-1	1 300	1 200	18	ND	310	0.28	29	9.7	A	2f
B. fragilis CcrA[b]	98	22	51	68	100	>500	26	5.2	B	3
Ps. paucimobilis	62	3.9	ND	<0.1	<0.1	19	30	4.6	ND	4

ND, not determined.
[a] Data from Bush K, Jacoby G A, Medeiros A A 1995 *Antimicrobial Agents and Chemotherapy* 39: 1211–1233.
[b] Inhibited by EDTA.

β-lactamases that contain an active site serine, and inhibition by the chelating agent, ethylenediaminetetraacetic acid (EDTA) which is used to identify the zinc-containing metallo-β-lactamases. Characteristics of representative β-lactamases from each class are shown in Table 16.3.

Bush groups are identified according to inhibitory properties based primarily upon clavulanic acid and EDTA. Additional subgroups are identified according to substrate hydrolysis profiles. The easiest group to identify are the group 3 metallo-β-lactamases, which were not included in earlier functional classification schemes. These enzymes are readily distinguished from all other β-lactamases because they can hydrolyse carbapenems, are not inhibited by clavulanic acid, but are inhibited by chelators such as EDTA or 1,10-*o*-phenanthroline.

Former Richmond and Sykes class I β-lactamases generally belong to the Bush group 1 cephalosporinases, enzymes which include the chromosomal β-lactamases from Enterobacteriaceae that are not inhibited well by clavulanic acid. The class Ic cephalosporinases were segregated into group 2e because of their high affinity for clavulanic acid. Some of the Richmond and Sykes class Ic cephalosporinases have now been sequenced and found to belong to molecular class A like most group 2 β-lactamases, whereas the Bush group 1 enzymes belong to molecular class C.

Other group 2 enzymes are generally inhibited by clavulanate, with the exception of the rare TEM-1 β-lactamase derivatives which have reduced affinities for the inhibitor. Group 2a enzymes are penicillinases; group 2b enzymes have a broader spectrum of activity, hydrolysing penicillins and cephalosporins almost equally well. Group 2be enzymes are often derived from group 2b enzymes, but exhibit enhanced hydrolytic properties that enable them to hydrolyse expanded-spectrum cephalosporins and mono-bactams. Group 2c enzymes hydrolyse carbenicillin, and group 2d enzymes hydrolyse the isoxazoylpenicillins such as cloxacillin or oxacillin. The 2d enzymes are the only β-lactamases in group 2 that belong to molecular class D rather than class A. The 2f enzymes are carbapenem-hydrolysing enzymes that are class A serine β-lactamases rather than metallo-enzymes.

The genes for β-lactamases are located on the chromosome or on plasmids, and may be translocated from or into the chromosome or into another plasmid by transposons (Ch. 3). Transfer within and between species or genera explains the successful spread of resistance mediated by these enzymes. For instance, the TEM-1 β-lactamase has been identified in virtually every genus of Enterobacteriaceae. Some of the chromosomal cephalosporinases from enterobacteria have begun to appear as plasmid-mediated enzymes; most seriously, plasmid-encoded metallo-β-lactamases are now being identified that are capable of hydrolysing almost all classes of β-lactam agent and that are refractory to inhibition by commercially available β-lactamase inhibitors.

STAPH. AUREUS β-LACTAMASE

The enzyme occurs in four serologically distinct forms that are closely related on a molecular level. Production may be plasmid-mediated or chromosomal. The chromosomal enzymes can be induced by penicillins such as methicillin or by the β-lactamase inhibitor sulbactam. The enzymes are predominantly active against penicillins, but can be differentiated on the basis of hydrolysis of cephalosporins including cephaloridine, nitrocefin and cefazolin.

CHROMOSOMAL CEPHALOSPORINASES OF GRAM-NEGATIVE BACTERIA

Virtually all Gram-negative bacteria elaborate chromosomally mediated enzymes, most of which fall into group 1. These hydrolyse cephalosporins up to 1000 times more rapidly than penicillins, some of which (e.g. cloxacillin) may inhibit them. Traditional β-lactamase-inhibitors work poorly against these enzymes.

In some species, including *Acinetobacter, Citrobacter, Enterobacter, Morganella, Pseudomonas* and *Serratia*, they are inducible and often species specific. Plasmid-mediated forms of these enzymes, such as those designated FOX-1, LAT-1, MIR-1 and MOX-1, have appeared, particularly in *Klebsiella pneumoniae* strains that have an additional chromosomal β-lactamase. Sequence data indicate high homology with the AmpC cephalosporinases from *Ps. aeruginosa, Ser. marcescens, Ent. cloacae* and *Citrobacter freundii*. Induction is a clinically relevant phenomenon when the inducing molecule is a substrate that can be hydrolysed by the enzyme, such as ampicillin or amoxycillin. Many good inducers, such as cefoxitin and imipenem, are not good substrates for these enzymes, and pose problems only if they are co-administered with a second β-lactam agent. Because induction is a transient event, the producing organisms revert to their original low basal production of β-lactamase on removal of the inducer. A more serious problem occurs if there is selection for a permanently altered organism with derepressed production of the chromosomal β-lactamase. Strains that hyperproduce group 1 cephalosporinases are responsible for a number of clinical failures of cephalosporins among the Enterobacteriaceae. Interestingly, β-lactam compounds that are good inducers rarely select for derepressed hyperproducing mutants.

PLASMID-MEDIATED β-LACTAMASES

Plasmid-mediated enzymes account for the most important β-lactamase-related resistance mechanisms. The most common β-lactamase in Gram-negative organisms is the TEM-1 β-lactamase, responsible for transferable ampicillin resistance among Enterobacteriaceae world-wide. In *Klebsiella*, a broad-spectrum SHV-1 β-lactamase predominates. Other important families of plasmid-mediated β-lactamases include the OXA enzymes which hydrolyse oxacillin, and the PSE enzymes, a group originally believed to be confined to pseudomonas.

In the mid-1980s, plasmid-mediated β-lactamases that conferred resistance to oxyimino β-lactams, notably cefotaxime, ceftazidime and aztreonam, began to appear in central Europe. These enzymes are related to TEM-1 and SHV-1 and are now numbered through at least TEM-28 and SHV-7. Organisms elaborating these extended-spectrum β-lactamases generally remain susceptible to cefoxitin and imipenem, and the enzymes are readily inhibited by clavulanic acid, sulbactam or tazobactam. They differ from their parent TEM and SHV enzymes by selected point mutations. They have spread rapidly within localized metropolitan areas to cause hospital outbreaks and colonization in nursing homes. Several TEM mutants that are resistant to β-lactamase inhibitors have become a community problem in Spain and France. These inhibitor-resistant TEM β-lactamases have been assigned TEM numbers from TEM-30 to TEM-41. Infections caused by organisms producing these enzymes do not respond to available β-lactamase inhibitor combinations.

METALLO-β-LACTAMASES

Perhaps the most formidable β-lactamases known are the metallo-β-lactamases, which rapidly hydrolyse most β-lactam agents, including the carbapenems. They are resistant to β-lactamase inhibitors. These enzymes were originally confined to a few isolated strains of *B. fragilis* and *Bac. cereus* as chromosomal enzymes, but have been identified in Japan on plasmids carried by *B. fragilis, Ser. marcescens, K. pneumoniae* and *Ps. aeruginosa*. Such strains appear to be confined to localized areas, but they have the potential for widespread dissemination.

Further information

Ambler R P 1980 The structure of β-lactamases. *Philosophical Transactions of the Royal Society of London, Series B* 289: 321–331

Bush K, Sykes R B 1986 Methodology for the study of β-lactamases. *Antimicrobial Agents and Chemotherapy* 30: 6–10

Bush K, Jacoby G A, Medeiros A A 1995 A functional classification scheme for β-lactamases and its correlation with molecular structure. *Antimicrobial Agents and Chemotherapy* 39: 1211–1233

Jacoby G A, Carreras L 1990 Activities of β-lactam antibiotics against *Escherichia coli* strains producing extended-spectrum β-lactamases. *Antimicrobial Agents and Chemotherapy* 34: 858–862

Michira-Hamzepour M, Pechère J-C 1989 How predictable is development of resistance after β-lactam therapy in *Enterobacter cloacae* infection? *Journal of Antimicrobial Chemotherapy* 24: 387–395

Nikaido H 1985 Role of permeability barriers in resistance to β-lactam antibiotics. *Pharmacology and Therapeutics* 27: 197–231

Payne D J 1993 Metallo-β-lactamases – a new therapeutic challenge. *Journal of Medical Microbiology* 39: 93–99

Philippon A, Labia R, Jacoby G 1989 Extended-spectrum β-lactamases. *Antimicrobial Agents and Chemotherapy* 33: 1131–1136

Sanders C C 1987 Chromosomal cephalosporinases responsible for multiple resistance to newer β-lactam antibiotics. *Annual Review of Microbiology* 41: 573–593

Symposium 1988 New developments in resistance to β-lactam antibiotics among non-fastidious Gram-negative organisms. *Reviews of Infectious Diseases* 10: 677–912

Wiedemann B, Kliebe C, Kresken M 1989 The epidemiology of β-lactamases. *Journal of Antimicrobial Chemotherapy* 24 (suppl B): 1–22

Zygmunt D J, Stratton C W, Kernodle D S 1992 Characterization of four β-lactamases produced by *Staphylococcus aureus*. *Antimicrobial Agents and Chemotherapy* 36: 440–445

β-Lactamase inhibitors

As β-lactamase production is the predominant cause of clinically important resistance to β-lactams in most species, an attractive approach to the therapy of infections caused by such organisms is to co-administer with the labile antibiotic an agent capable of inhibiting the enzyme. Implicit in this approach, however, are some demanding requirements: the inhibitor must be active against a wide range of β-lactamases, since tests for differential activity as a guide to therapy are not practicable in the diagnostic laboratory; the absorption, distribution and excretion characteristics of the inhibitor must match closely those of the β-lactam agent with which it is to be paired; and its use must not add materially to the toxicity.

The ability of certain natural and semi-synthetic β-lactam agents to inhibit selected β-lactamases has been known for a long time. Cephalosporin C, some semisynthetic cephalosporins and isoxazolyl penicillins all show limited inhibitory activity against a relatively narrow range of enzymes. A wide search for more potent compounds resulted in the discovery of carbapenems and clavulanic acid from natural products, and the subsequent synthesis of the sulphones, sulbactam and tazobactam. The β-lactamase inhibitors in therapeutic use have poor antimicrobial activity and act synergistically in combination with β-lactamase-labile penicillins. None is effective against metallo-β-lactamases. In some organisms these inhibitors may act as inducers of β-lactamse activity.

The penicillins, cephalosporins and monobactams are primarily competitive inhibitors, or, more specifically, competitive substrates. Their action is often reversible, leaving the enzyme intact, because they simply act as poor substrates that are bound tightly to the β-lactamase and are hydrolysed slowly. The most effective inhibitors that have been developed commercially are irreversible, the enzyme and inhibitor interacting competitively initially and then progressively forming a complex in which both enzyme and inhibitor are inactivated: progressive or 'suicide' inhibitors. Inactivation usually occurs after a fixed amount of inhibitor has been hydrolysed like a normal substrate. Clavulanic acid, sulbactam, and tazobactam are all of this form, although the precise nature, rate and degree of inactivation differ considerably among the various agents and enzymes.

Further information

Bush K 1988 β-Lactamase inhibitors from laboratory to clinic. *Clinical Microbiology Reviews* 1: 109–123

Farmer T H, Reading C 1988 The effects of clavulanic acid and sulbactam on β-lactamase biosynthesis. *Journal of Antimicrobial Chemotherapy* 22: 105–111

Knowles J R 1985 Penicillin resistance: the chemistry of β-lactamase inhibition. *Accounts of Chemical Research* 18: 97–104

Muratani T, Yokota E, Nakane T, Inoue E, Mitsuhashi S 1993 In-vitro evaluation of the four β-lactamase inhibitors: BRL-42715, clavulanic acid, sulbactam, and tazobactam. *Journal of Antimicrobial Chemotherapy* 32: 421–429

Payne D J, Cramp R, Winstanley D J, Knowles D J C 1994 Comparative activities of clavulanic acid, sulbactam, and tazobactam against clinically important β-lactamases. *Antimicrobial Agents and Chemotherapy* 38: 767–772

Sirot D, Chanal C, Henquell C, Labia R, Sirot J, Cluzel R 1994 Clinical isolates of *Escherichia coli* producing multiple TEM mutants resistant to β-lactamase inhibitors. *Journal of Antimicrobial Chemotherapy* 33: 1117–1126

Sorg T B, Cynamon M H 1987 Comparison of four β-lactamase inhibitors in combination with ampicillin against *Mycobacterium tuberculosis*. *Journal of Antimicrobial Chemotherapy* 19: 59–64

Symposium 1988 β-Lactamase inhibition: therapeutic implications in obstetrics and gynecology. *Journal of Reproductive Medicine* 33 (suppl 6): 565–606

Weber D A, Sanders C C 1990 Diverse potential of (b-lactamase inhibitors to induce class I enzymes. *Antimicrobial Agents and Chemotherapy* 34: 156–158

Wexler H M, Molitoris E, Finegold S M 1991 Effect of β-lactamase inhibitors on the activities of various b-lactam agents against anaerobic bacteria. *Antimicrobial Agents and Chemotherapy* 35: 1219–1224

Zhou X Y, Bordon F, Sirot D, Kitzis M-D, Gutmann L 1994 Emergence of clinical isolates of *Escherichia coli* producing TEM-1 derivatives or an OXA-1 β-lactamase conferring resistance to β-lactamase inhibitors. *Antimicrobial Agents and Chemotherapy* 38: 1085–1089

CLAVULANIC ACID

An oxapenam produced by *Streptomyces clavuligerus*.

It is used to inhibit β-lactamase destruction of labile β-lactam agents. Available for therapeutic use in fixed-ratio combinations with amoxycillin or with ticarcillin.

Antimicrobial activity

It exhibits broad-spectrum but low intrinsic activity, most MICs being in the range 16–128 mg/l. Enterobacteriaceae and *Staph. aureus* are at the lower end of the range and *Ps. aeruginosa* at the upper. MICs of 8 mg/l against *H. influenzae* and 0.1–4 mg/l for penicillinase-producing *N. gonorrhoeae* are notable.

It is a potent, progressive inhibitor of most group 2 β-lactamases, with the exception of some TEM variants. It is particularly active against many of the plasmid-mediated enzymes that include TEM-1 to TEM-26, SHV-1 to SHV-7, PSE-2, and PSE-4. It is very active against *Klebsiella* K1 (group 2be) enzyme, the group 2e chromosomal enzymes produced by *Pr. vulgaris* and *B. fragilis*, both enzymes produced by *Moraxella catarrhalis* and the group 2a penicillinases from *Staph. aureus*. It does not effectively inhibit the group 1 chromosomal cephalosporinases from Enterobacteriaceae or the group 3 metallo-β-lactamases.

In the presence of low concentrations of clavulanic acid (0.5–1 mg/l) the MICs of amoxycillin for β-lactamase-producing *Staph. aureus*, *M. catarrhalis*, *N. gonorrhoeae*, *H. influenzae*, enterobacteria and *Bact. fragilis* are reduced 8- to 64-fold (Table 16.4). Both inhibitory and bactericidal activity are enhanced. MICs of *M. fortuitum* and *Nocardia asteroides* are reduced two- to four-fold. In *B. fragilis* strains resistant to penicillin, the addition of clavulanic acid renders most of the strains susceptible to amoxycillin or ticarcillin.

AMOXYCILLIN–CLAVULANIC ACID

Co-amoxiclav

The ratio of clavulanic acid to amoxycillin in the commercially available oral preparations is generally 1 : 2 or 1 : 4; it is 1 : 5 in the i.v. formulation.

Pharmacokinetics

Peak plasma levels of clavulanic acid in fasting subjects receiving a single oral dose of 125 mg plus 250 mg amoxycillin range from 4 to 6 mg/l. There is little effect on the pharmacokinetics of each agent from the presence of the other, although clavulanic acid is marginally better absorbed in the presence of amoxycillin. There is no significant effect of food on absorption. The terminal plasma half-lives range from 0.9 to 1.1 h. Bioavailability by the oral route is around 60%, with wide individual variation from 30–99%.

Children
In fasting children aged 3–14 years given 25 mg/kg of a syrup formulation containing amoxycillin and clavulanic acid in the ratio 4 : 1 the average peak plasma concentration of clavulanic acid was 2 mg/l at 1–1.5 h with a half-life of 1 h. In children given 5 mg clavulanate/kg plus 25 mg amoxycillin/kg by i.v. bolus, the mean concentrations at 5 min were around 20 mg clavulanic acid/l and 90 mg amoxycillin/l, with terminal half-lives of 0.8 and 1.2 h, respectively. Average concentrations of 3 mg amoxycillin/l and 0.5 mg clavulanate/l of were measured in middle ear

Table 16.4 *Activity of β-lactam antibiotics tested in combinations with β-lactamase-inhibitors (clavulanic acid 2 mg/l; sulbactam and tazobactam 4 mg/l) against common bacterial pathogens: MIC$_{90}$ (mg/l)*

Organism	Amoxycillin (+ clavulanate)	Ticarcillin (+ clavulanate)	Ampicillin (+ sulbactam)	Piperacillin (+ tazobactam)
Staph. aureus (MSSA)	0.5	4.0	0.5	2.0
Str. pneumoniae				
penicillin-susceptible	0.12	2.0	0.13	≤0.06
penicillin-resistant	1.0	128	4.0	4.0
H. influenzae	0.5	≤1	≤1	≤1
M. catarrhalis	0.12	≤1	≤1	≤1
Esch. coli	8.0	32	64	16
Klebsiella spp.	16	16	64	16
Enterobacter spp.	128	128	64	128
Pr. mirabilis	2.0	2.0	8.0	2.0
Pr. vulgaris/Providencia	8.0	32	32	2.0
Ser. marcescens	128	32	128	32
Citrobacter spp.	128	>256	64	128
Ps. aeruginosa	>64	128	>256	64
B. fragilis	4.0	8.0	4.0	4.0

MSSA, methicillin-sensitive *Staph. aureus.*

fluid 2 h after fasting children were given 35 mg/kg of a clavulanic acid/amoxycillin suspension orally.

In sick children given 50 mg amoxycillin/kg plus 5 mg clavulanic acid/kg, mean end-infusion plasma concentrations were around 120 and 12 mg/l, respectively. The mean plasma elimination half-lives were around 0.9 h for amoxycillin and 0.8 h for clavulanic acid, but high plasma clearance in some individuals can call for more frequent dosage.

Distribution

In patients with bacterial meningitis receiving 0.2 g clavulanate plus 2 g amoxycillin by i.v. infusion over 30 min, concentrations of the drugs in the CSF were highest in patients with moderate to severe inflammation: around 0.25 mg/l for clavulanate and over 2 mg/l for amoxycillin at about 2 h. Total penetration into the CSF was 8% and 6% of the corresponding plasma values for clavulanate and amoxycillin, respectively.

Penetration into peritoneal fluid is 66% (the half-life similar to that in serum), 55% into cantharides blister fluid, and 46–91% into pleural fluid. Effective levels are found in bile, middle ear fluid, tonsil tissue, wound pus and amniotic fluid. In cirrhotic patients, receiving 1 g amoxycillin plus 0.2 g clavulanic acid, ascites fluid:serum ratios were around 1.4 for amoxycillin and 1.0 for clavulanic acid. The plasma elimination half-lives were considerably prolonged (to >45 h for amoxycillin and >3 h for clavulanic acid), probably due

to low elution from ascitic fluid. Clavulanate penetrates poorly into sputum after oral dosing.

Metabolism and excretion

Binding of clavulanic acid and amoxycillin to plasma proteins is low (about 30% and 20%, respectively.) Clavulanic acid appears to be metabolized extensively, with metabolites eliminated via the urine, bile, faeces and lungs. Variation in bioavailability may be related to differences in first-pass effects through those organs.

Only 25–40% of the administered clavulanic acid is recovered from the urine. After a dose of 125 mg plus 250 mg amoxycillin the mean recovery was 37%, falling to 30% when the mixture was taken with food, while that of amoxycillin was 70%. Most renal excretion occurs in the first 6 h and is unaffected by probenecid, although probenecid prolongs the renal excretion of amoxycillin. In renal failure, following oral or i.v. administration the volume of distribution and systemic availability are unaffected, but clearance is progressively depressed with renal function. Amoxycillin is more affected than clavulanic acid, as shown by the relative ratios of AUC: in patients with glomerular filtration rates of 75 ml/min the mean ratio was 4.9, while in patients requiring haemodialysis it was 14.7.

Toxicity and side-effects

The commonest side-effects of treatment with the combination are diarrhoea (9%), nausea (3%), rashes (3%) and vomiting (1%), all of which are transient. Symptomatic vaginal candidiasis and pseudomembranous colitis caused by *Clostridium difficile* have been reported, as has superinfection with *Ps. aeruginosa*. Mild increased transaminase levels have been noted. Experience of changes in the faecal flora have been variable, with some observers noting an increase in the proportion of amoxycillin-resistant enterobacteria. Some cases of jaundice and hepatic dysfunction are described, with a cholestatic or mixed cholestatic–hepatocellular rather than pure hepatocellular picture, but in some the occurrence of fever and eosinophilia have suggested an allergic origin. All have resolved on withdrawal of therapy.

Clinical use

The combination has been most widely and successfully used in the treatment of urinary infection and otitis media but has also been particularly commended in the management of infection with β-lactamase-producing *H. influenzae* and *B. catarrhalis*. Reference is made to its use in gonorrhoea, pelvic inflammatory disease, chancroid, lower respiratory tract infection, sinusitis, wound infection and surgical prophylaxis.

Preparations and dosage

Proprietary name: Augmentin.

Preparations: Tablets, suspension, injection.

Dosage: Adults, oral, 250–500 mg every 8 h. Children, the dose varies according to age and severity of infection. Adults, i.v., 1 g every 6–8 h depending on severity of infection. Infants ≤ 3 months, 25 mg/kg every 8 h (every 12 h in the perinatal period and premature infants); children 3 months to 12 years, 25 mg/kg every 6–8 h depending on severity of infection.

Widely available.

TICARCILLIN–CLAVULANIC ACID

The ratio of clavulanic acid to ticarcillin in the parenteral mixture is 1 : 15 or 1 : 30. Resistance to ticarcillin–clavulanic acid is generally due to decreased antimicrobial activity of ticarcillin rather than resistance of the β-lactamase to clavulanic acid. Specifically implicated in documented resistance are the chromosomal cephalosporinases of Enterobacteriaceae, the PSE-1 group 2d β-lactamase and hyperproduction of the TEM-1 or SHV-1 enzymes.

In patients receiving 0.2 g clavulanic acid plus 3 g ticarcillin i.v. over 15 min, end-infusion values were around 16 and 340 mg/l, respectively. The plasma elimination half-lives were similar (around 65 min). Co-administration resulted in limited changes in the pharmacokinetics of both agents.

In patients receiving 3 g ticarcillin and 0.5 g clavulanic acid as an i.v. bolus pre-operatively, rapid penetration into peritoneal fluid produced concentrations around 70% of the simultaneous plasma level of both agents. Elimination half-lives from peritoneum and plasma were similar. Ratios in blister fluid were significantly lower than those in serum.

Mean urinary recovery over the first 24 h is around 45%. Clearance of both components of the ticarcillin/clavulanic acid mixture is inversely related to creatinine clearance. At steady state, the volume of distribution approximates that of the extracellular fluid, irrespective of creatinine clearance. In advanced renal failure, the plasma elimination half-life of ticarcillin rises to around 6.5 h and that of clavulanic acid to around 4.5 h. The combination is generally well tolerated, with occasional patients exhibiting skin rash, oral candidiasis, eosinophilia, reactions at the injection site, hypersensitivity, nausea, vomiting and diarrhoea. As with other penicillins, the potential to cause central nervous system reactions is documented. The combination has been successfully used in a variety of acute infections, predominantly those of the urinary tract, but also in patients with complicating neoplastic disease, osteomyelitis, pneumonia, soft-tissue infections and abdominal sepsis. Treatment failure or superinfection by a non-susceptible organism has been reported, especially when used as empiric therapy.

Preparations and dosage

Proprietary name: Timentin.

Preparation: Injection.

Dosage: Adults, i.v. infusion, 3.2 g every 6–8 h increased to every 4 h in more severe infections. Children, 80 mg/kg every 6–8 h (every 12 h in neonates).

Available in the UK and the USA.

Further information

Allen G D, Coates P E, Davies B E 1988 On the absorption of clavulanic acid. *Biopharmaceutics and Drug Disposition* 9: 127–136

Bakken J S, Bruun J N, Gaustad P, Tasker T C 1986 Penetration of amoxicillin and potassium clavulanate into the cerebrospinal fluid of patients with inflamed meninges. *Antimicrobial Agents and Chemotherapy* 30: 481–484

Bolton G C, Allen G D, Davies B E, Filer C W, Jeffery D J 1986 The disposition of clavulanic acid in man. *Xenobiotica* 16: 853–863

Davies B E, Coates P E, Clarke J G, Thawley A R, Sutton J A 1985 Bioavailability and pharmacokinetics of clavulanic acid in healthy subjects. *International Journal of Clinical Pharmacology, Therapy and Toxicology* 23: 70–73

Davies B E, Boon R, Horton R, Reubi F C, Descoeedres C E 1988 Pharmacokinetics of amoxicillin and clavulanic acid in haemodialysis patients following intravenous administration of Augmentin. *British Journal of Clinical Pharmacology* 26: 385–390

Ferslew K E, Daigneault G A, Aten R M, Roseman R M 1984 Pharmacokinetics and urinary excretion of clavulanic acid after oral administration of amoxicillin and potassium clavulanate. *Journal of Clinical Pharmacology* 24: 452–456

Jones A E, Barnes N D, Tasker T C G, Horton R 1989 Pharmacokinetics of intravenous amoxicillin and potassium clavulanate in seriously ill children. *Journal of Antimicrobial Chemotherapy* 25: 269–274

Leigh D A, Robinson O P W (eds) 1982 Augmentin: clavulanate–potentiated amoxycillin. Excerpta Medica, Amsterdam, p 1–244

Leigh D A, Phillips I, Wise R (eds) 1986 Timentin–ticarcillin plus clavulanic acid: a laboratory and clinical perspective. *Journal of Antimicrobial Chemotherapy* 17 (suppl C): 1–240

Manek N, Wise R, Donovan I A 1987 Intraperitoneal penetration of ticarcillin/clavulanic acid (Timentin). *Journal of Antimicrobial Chemotherapy* 19: 363–366

Neu H C 1985 β-lactamase inhibition: therapeutic advances (Symposium on ticarcillin–clavulanate). *American Journal of Medicine* 79 (suppl 5B): 1–196

Sanders C C, Jaconis J P, Bodey G P, Samonis G 1988 Resistance to ticarcillin–potassium clavulanate among clinical isolates of the family Enterobacteriaceae: the role of PSE-1 β-lactamase and high levels of TEM-1 and SHV-1 and problems with false susceptibility in dose diffusion tests. *Antimicrobial Agents and Chemotherapy* 32: 1365–1369

Speller D C E, White L O, Wilkinson P J (eds) 1989 Clavulanate/β-lactam antibiotics: further experience. *Journal of Antimicrobial Chemotherapy* 24 (suppl B): 1–226

SULBACTAM

Penicillanic acid sulphone.

Antimicrobial activity

It has very weak antimicrobial activity against most Gram-negative rods, anaerobes and Gram-positive bacteria. Its only notable activity is against *N. gonorrhoeae* and *N. meningitidis* and *Acinetobacter baumanii*. It inhibits a wide range of group 2 β-lactamases, including those from *Staph. aureus*, klebsiella and bacteroides. It is a good inhibitor of the TEM enzymes of groups 2b and 2be but has little effect on SHV-1, group 1, group 2br or group 3 β-lactamases. It does not induce the activity of cephalosporinases from Gram-negative bacteria but is a weak inducer of penicillinases from *Staph. aureus*. Inhibitory effects are dependent upon the amount of enzyme in the organism, so increased β-lactamase production results in lower efficacy for sulbactam-β-lactam combinations.

Clinical use

It is usually combined with ampicillin, but the combination with cefoperazone is available in some countries. Sulbactam has been used alone in the treatment of uncomplicated gonorrhoea for which it is not satisfactory. Ampicillin–sulbactam was successfully used in an outbreak of infection with *A. baumanii* in which the inhibitor was shown to be responsible for the antimicrobial activity of the combination.

Preparations

Preparation: Injection.

Not available in the UK.

AMPICILLIN–SULBACTAM

The ratio of ampicillin to sulbactam in the commercially available product is 2:1. The combination inhibits β-lactamase-producing *Staph. aureus, H. influenzae, M. catarrhalis, Pr. mirabilis* and *B. fragilis* (Table 16.4), but there is a large inoculum effect. The combination is bactericidal at concentrations that are usually no more than two-fold higher than MICs.

Pharmacokinetics

The sodium salt of sulbactam is poorly absorbed orally, but oral bioavailability of a methylene-linked double ester pro-drug of ampicillin–sulbactam, sultamicillin, is >80% for both drugs. It undergoes first-pass hydrolysis to liberate equimolecular proportions of the components. In volunteers given 750 mg, mean peak plasma levels at 1 h were ampicillin 9.1 mg/l and sulbactam 8.9 mg/l. Bioavailability of both drugs was more than 80%. The plasma elimination half-life of each component was around 1 h.

In volunteers, i.v. infusions over 30 min of sulbactam 125, 500 or 1000 mg gives mean end-infusion concentrations of around 12, 31 and 64 mg/l, respectively. Mean urinary excretion is 76%. Elimination half-life is approximately 1 h. It is completely bioavailable from intramuscular (i.m.) injection, doses of 0.5 and 1 g producing mean peak plasma levels around 13 and 28 mg/l, respectively. Co-administration with ampicillin, benzylpenicillin or cefoperazone has no effect on the pharmacokinetics of either agent. When the ampicillin–sulbactam combination in a 2 : 1 ratio (by weight) was given to healthy subjects over 15 min by i.v. infusion, mean peak serum concentrations were 120 and 60 mg/l, respectively. About 75–85% of each drug is excreted in the urine within 8 h of administration of the combination.

In infants and children given 42.5 mg/kg, mean peak plasma levels were: sulbactam 11.4 mg/l at 1 h and ampicillin 6.9 mg/l at 1.5 h. Half-lives of both ampicillin and sulbactam are increased to 9.4 and 7.9 h, respectively, in premature neonates; the half-life of sulbactam in infected children (2–14 years) is 3.7 h.

Sulbactam is not metabolized. It enters the CSF (mean peak concentration 17.3 mg/l) and sputum, crosses the placenta and appears in maternal milk. A small amount is eliminated in the bile and faeces, but it is principally excreted through the kidneys by both glomerular filtration and tubular secretion. Probenecid and renal impairment increase the plasma elimination half-life and reduce the urinary concentration.

Toxicity and side-effects

In patients treated for respiratory infections, including sinusitis and infections due to *H. influenzae*, diarrhoea has been reported, but usually affecting less than 10% of the patients. In a few patients this has been severe enough to require cessation of treatment or, when associated with *Cl. difficile* toxin, vancomycin therapy. Diarrhoea seems particularly common with the linked ester, sultamicillin. It is otherwise generally well tolerated apart from local pain on i.m. injection (which can be controlled by lignocaine) and thrombophlebitis on i.v. administration. Transient changes in some liver function tests may occur, but it was well tolerated in patients with chronic liver disease. Elevated aspartate aminotransferase, serum alanine aminotransferase and lactic dehydrogenase levels have also been reported. Superinfection with resistant organisms may occur.

Clinical use

The combination with ampicillin has been used for the treatment of infections of the urinary and respiratory tracts,

of skin, bones and joints, for gonorrhoea and in intra-abdominal, including gynaecological, sepsis. It has also been used in meningitis caused by β-lactamase-producing *H. influenzae* and in surgical prophylaxis.

Further information

Benson J M, Nahata M C 1988 Sulbactam/ampicillin, a new β-lactamase inhibitor/β-lactam antibiotic combination. *Drug Intelligence and Clinical Pharmacy* 22: 534–541

Blum R A, Kohli R K, Harrison N J, Schentag J J 1989 Pharmacokinetics of ampicillin (2.0 grams) and sulbactam (1.0 gram) coadministered to subjects with normal and abnormal renal function with end stage renal disease on haemodialysis. *Antimicrobial Agents and Chemotherapy* 33: 1470–1476

Campoli-Richards D M, Brogden R N 1987 Sulbactam/ampicillin. A review of its antibacterial activity, pharmacokinetic properties and therapeutic use. *Drugs* 33: 577–609

Foulds G, McBride T J, Knirsch A K, Rodriguez W J, Khan W N 1987 Penetration of sulbactam and ampicillin into cerebrospinal fluid of infants and young children with meningitis. *Antimicrobial Agents and Chemotherapy* 31: 1703–1705

Frieder H A, Campoli-Richards D M, Goa K L 1989 Sultamicillin. A review of its antibacterial activity, pharmacokinetic properties and therapeutic use. *Drugs* 37: 491–522

Symposium 1986 Enzyme-mediated resistance to β-lactam antibiotics. A symposium on sulbactam/ampicillin. *Reviews of Infectious Diseases* 8 (suppl 5): S465–S650

Symposium 1988 Sulbactam–ampicillin in clinical practice. *Drugs* 35 (suppl 7): 1–94

Urban C, Go E, Mariano N et al 1993 Effect of sulbactam on infections caused by imipenem-resistant *Acinetobacter calcoaceticus* biotype *anitratus*. *Journal of Infectious Diseases* 167: 448–451

TAZOBACTAM

It exhibits little useful antimicrobial activity, although activity against *Acinetobacter* spp. and *Borrelia burgdorferi* is reported. It inhibits a wide range of β-lactamases, including the group 2 penicillinases from *Staph. aureus*, the broad-spectrum TEM and SHV-1 ß-lactamases, most extended-spectrum enzymes in the TEM and SHV families, and the common group 2e cephalosporinases of *B. fragilis*. Against the group 1 cephalosporinases, activity is strongly influenced by the amount of enzyme produced. Diminished inhibition of the inhibitor-resistant group 2br TEM β-lactamases is seen; group 3 metallo-β-lactamases are not inhibited at clinically useful levels. It is a poor inducer of β-lactamases of Gram-positive and Gram-negative organisms.

When administered as a 500 mg dose i.v. over 30 min in healthy volunteers, the peak concentration was 24 mg/l, with mean plasma levels of 0.6 mg/l at 4 h. The elimination half-life was 1.1 h. Mean urinary recoveries over 24 h were 64%. It is metabolized to a ring-opened compound which further degrades to a butanoic acid derivative known as M1, devoid of pharmacological activity.

PIPERACILLIN–TAZOBACTAM

The ratio of piperacillin to tazobactam in the commercially available product is 8 : 1. Tazobactam at a concentration of 4 mg/l markedly reduces the MICs and enhances the bactericidal activity of piperacillin against most β-lactamase-producing organisms, but only moderately against those elaborating group 1 cephalosporinases. It enhances labile β-lactam activity against β-lactamase-producing *Staph. aureus, H. influenzae, M. catarrhalis,* most of the *B. fragilis* group, *Acinetobacter* spp., many Enterobacteriaceae, especially *Pr. mirabilis* and *Morganella morganii,* and occasional *Enterobacter* spp. and *C. freundii* (Table 16.4). The activity of piperacillin against *Ps. aeruginosa* is not enhanced.

Pharmacokinetics

Co-administration of tazobactam does not affect the pharmacokinetics of piperacillin. After a dose of 4.0 g piperacillin and 0.5 g tazobactam given as an i.v. infusion over 30 min, the maximum serum concentration of piperacillin was 224 mg/l; the half-life was 1 h. Pharmacokinetics of tazobactam, however, are altered when administered with piperacillin: peak serum concentrations after an i.v. dose of 0.5 g increased from 24 mg/l to 27 mg/l when piperacillin was given simultaneously; the mean serum level at 4 h doubled from 0.6 to 1.2 mg/l. The half-life was not affected, but a decrease in renal clearance of tazobactam from 279 to 164 ml/min was seen when it was co-administered with piperacillin. Pharmacokinetic properties of piperacillin and tazobactam were altered less than 14% when given with tobramycin. Co-administration of piperacillin and tazobactam with vancomycin resulted in a <7% increase in AUC for piperacillin, and no other change in pharmacokinetic properties. A decrease in systemic clearance of the two agents is seen in cirrhotic subjects.

The combination has good tissue distribution as judged by penetration into blister fluid. Mean maximum concentrations of tazobactam in the inflammatory exudate were 6.4 mg/l

when 0.5 g was given alone and 11.3 mg/l when administered with piperacillin. Both agents are found in most tissues, including bronchial secretions, prostatic secretions and tissue in elderly patients, and in uterine, ovarian and fallopian tube tissue.

Clinical use

The combination is effective in appendicitis (complicated by rupture or abscess) and peritonitis, uncomplicated and complicated skin and skin structure infections, postpartum endometritis or pelvic inflammatory disease, and community-acquired pneumonia. It has been used for urinary tract infections and in combination with amikacin as empiric therapy in the treatment of febrile neutropenic patients.

Toxicity and side-effects

Adverse effects are usually not severe. The most common side-effects are diarrhoea and allergic skin reactions. In clinical trials with 944 subjects treated with piperacillin–tazobactam 3.8% reported drug-related diarrhoea and 2.2% reported rashes. In a population also treated with an aminoglycoside 13% reported diarrhoea and 2.4% had rashes. Liver function tests can be affected by treatment with the piperacillin/tazobactam combination, with <6% of the patients having significant drug-related increases in alkaline phosphatase, serum glutamic oxaloacetic transaminase and serum glutamic pyruvic transaminase. The percentage of patients with abnormal liver function increased slightly (to *ca.*7%) in those additionally treated with an aminoglycoside.

Preparations and dosage

Proprietary name: Tazocin.

Preparation: Injection.

Dosage: Adults and children over 12 years, by i.v. injection over 3–5 min or by i.v. infusion, 2.25–4.5 g every 6–8 h, usually 4.5 g every 8 h.

Further information

Bush K, Macalintal C, Rasmussen B A, Lee V J, Yang Y 1993 Kinetic interactions of tazobactam with β-lactamases from all major structural classes. *Antimicrobial Agents and Chemotherapy* 37: 851–858

Chen H Y, Bonfiglio G, Allen M et al 1993 Multicentre survey of the comparative in-vitro activity of piperacillin/tazobactam against bacteria from hospitalized patients in the British Isles. *Journal of Antimicrobial Chemotherapy* 32: 247–266

Cometta A, Zinner S, De Bock R et al 1995 Piperacillin–tazobactam plus amikacin versus ceftazidime plus amikacin as empiric therapy for fever in granulocytopenic patients with cancer. *Antimicrobial Agents and Chemotherapy* 39: 445–452

Greenwood D, Finch R G (eds) 1993 Piperacillin/tazobactam: a new β-lactam/β-lactamase inhibitor combination. *Journal of Antimicrobial Chemotherapy* 31 (suppl A): 1–124

Kuck N A, Jacobus N V, Petersen P J, Weiss W J, Testa R T 1989 Comparative in vitro and in vivo activities of piperacillin combined with the β-lactamase inhibitors tazobactam, clavulanic acid, and sulbactam. *Antimicrobial Agents and Chemotherapy* 33: 1964–1969

Kuye O Teal J, DeVries V G, Morrow C A, Tally F P 1993 Safety profile of piperacillin/tazobactam in phase I and III clinical studies. *Journal of Antimicrobial Chemotherapy* 31 (suppl A): 113–124

Lathia C, Sia L, Lanc R et al 1991 Pharmacokinetics of piperacillin/tazobactam (PIP/TAZ) IV with and without tobramycin IV in healthy adult male volunteers. *Pharmaceutical Research* 8: S303

Murray P R, Cantrell H F, Lankford R B, In vitro Susceptibility Surveillance Group 1994 Multicenter evaluation of the in vitro activity of piperacillin–tazobactam compared with eleven selected β-lactam antibiotics and ciprofloxacin against more than 42,000 aerobic Gram-positive and Gram-negative bacteria. *Diagnostic Microbiology and Infectious Disease* 19: 111–120

Polk H C Jr, Fink M P, Laverdiere M et al 1993 Prospective randomized study of piperacillin/tazobactam therapy of surgically treated intra-abdominal infection. *American Surgeon* 59: 598–605

Shlaes D M, Baughman R, Boylen C T et al 1994 Piperacillin/tazobactam compared with ticarcillin/clavulanate in community-acquired bacterial lower respiratory tract infection. *Journal of Antimicrobial Chemotherapy* 34: 565–577

Tan J S, Wishnow R M, Talan D A, Duncanson F P, Norden C W 1993 Treatment of hospitalized patients with complicated skin and skin structure infections: double-blind, randomized, multicenter study of piperacillin–tazobactam versus ticarcillin–clavulanate. *Antimicrobial Agents and Chemotherapy* 37: 1580–1586

Wise R, Logan M, Cooper M, Andrews J M 1991 Pharmacokinetics and tissue penetration of tazobactam administered alone and with piperacillin. *Antimicrobial Agents and Chemotherapy* 35: 1081–1084

17

Chloramphenicol and thiamphenicol

M. H. Wilcox

Introduction

Chloramphenicol was the first broad-spectrum antibiotic to be discovered. It was isolated independently from streptomycetes from soil in Venezuela and a compost heap in Illinois. The commercial product is manufactured synthetically. There are four isomers of chloramphenicol, all of which have been synthesized, but none has greater activity than the natural compound. The major drawback of chloramphenicol is a rare, idiosyncratic, often fatal aplastic anaemia, and numerous attempts have been made to manufacture related agents which retain the spectrum of activity and pharmacokinetics of the parent compound but not the toxicity. The only derivative to come into commercial use in which this is believed to have been achieved is thiamphenicol, in which the nitro group of chloramphenicol is replaced by a sulphomethyl group. However, compounds in which the nitro group is replaced are all less active than the parent compound.

Substitution of fluorine for chlorine or the 3'-OH group has produced analogues of both chloramphenicol and thiamphenicol that are active against strains of Escherichia coli, Klebsiella *spp.,* Enterobacter *spp. and* Haemophilus influenzae *that owe their resistance to chloramphenicol acetylation, but not against organisms with reduced permeability. Fluorinated derivatives are not marketed for human use, but florfenicol is available as a veterinary product in some countries.*

Further information

Baumelou E, Najean Y 1983 Why still prescribe chloramphenicol in 1983? Comparison of the clinical and biological haematologic effects of chloramphenicol and thiamphenicol. *Blut* 47: 317–320

Fuglesang J, Bergan T 1982 Chloramphenicol and thiamphenicol. *Antibiotics and Chemotherapy* 31: 1–21

Graham R, Palmer D, Pratt B C, Hart C A 1988 In vitro activity of florphenical. *European Journal of Clinical Microbiology and Infectious Diseases* 7: 691–694

Skolimowski I M, Knight R C, Edwards D I 1983 Molecular basis of chloramphenicol and thiamphenicol toxicity to DNA in vitro. *Journal of Antimicrobial Chemotherapy* 12: 535–542

CHLORAMPHENICOL

A fermentation product of *Streptomyces venezualae*. Commercially manufactured synthetically. Aqueous solutions are extremely stable, but some hydrolysis occurs on autoclaving.

Antimicrobial activity

It is active against a very wide range of organisms. The susceptibility of common pathogenic bacteria is shown in Table 17.1. Minimum inhibitory concentrations (MICs) (mg/l) for other organisms are: *Staphylococcus epidermidis*, 1–8; *Corynebacterium diphtheriae*, 0.5–2; *Bacillus anthracis*, 1–4; *Clostridium perfringens*, 2–8; *Mycobacterium tuberculosis*, 8–32; *Legionella pneumophila*, 0.5–1; *Bordetella pertussis*, 0.25–4; *Brucella abortus*, 1–4; *Campylobacter fetus*, 2–4; *Pasteurella* spp., 0.25–4; *Serratia marcescens*, 2–8; *Burkholderia pseudomallei*, 4–8; *Actinomyces israeli*, 1–4; *Peptococcus* spp., 0.1–8; and *Fusobacterium* spp., 0.5–2. Most Gram-negative bacilli are susceptible, but *Pseudomonas aeruginosa* is resistant.

Table 17.1 *Activity of chloramphenicol and thiamphenicol: MIC (mg/l)*

	Chloramphenicol	Thiamphenicol
Staph. aureus	2–8	4–32
Str. pyogenes	2–4	1–2
Str. pneumoniae	1–4	2–4
Ent. faecalis	4–16	8–32
N. gonorrhoeae	0.5–2	0.5–2
N. meningitidis	0.5–2	0.5–2
H. influenzae	0.25–0.5	0.1–2
Esch. coli	2–8	4–64
Klebsiella spp.	0.5–32	4–32
Enterobacter spp.	0.5–64	16–128
Pr. mirabilis	2–8	2–16
Pr. vulgaris/providencia	4–32	8–32
Salmonella spp.	0.5–8	0.5–8
Shigella spp.	1–8	2–8
Ps. aeruginosa	32–128	16–128
Bacteroides spp.	1–8	0.5–32

Leptospira spp., *Treponema pallidum*, chlamydiae, mycoplasmas and rickettsiae are all susceptible, but *Nocardia* spp. are resistant. It is widely active against anaerobes, but *Bacteroides fragilis* is only moderately susceptible (MIC about 8 mg/l).

It is strictly bacteriostatic against almost all bacterial species, but exerts a bactericidal effect at 2–4 times the MIC against some strains of Gram-positive cocci, *H. influenzae* and *Neisseria* spp. The minimum bactericidal concentrations (MBCs) of chloramphenicol for penicillin-resistant pneumococci are often significantly higher than those for penicillin-susceptible strains, although this cannot be detected by conventional disc susceptibility testing or MIC determination. Its bacteriostatic effect may inhibit the action of penicillins and other β-lactam antibiotics against *Klebsiella pneumoniae* and other enterobacteria in vitro, but the clinical significance of this is doubtful. The presence of ampicillin does not affect the bactericidal effect of chloramphenicol on *H. influenzae*.

Acquired resistance

Resistance has been seen in many wild strains of both Gram-positive and Gram-negative organisms and the prevalence of resistant strains has often reflected the usage of the antibiotic. Over-the-counter sales of the antibiotic are believed to have compounded the problem in some countries. For example, chloramphenicol has long been the drug of choice for the treatment of typhoid and paratyphoid, but its widespread use has led to a high prevalence of resistant *Salmonella typhi*. Outbreaks of infection caused by chlor-

amphenicol-resistant *Salm. typhi* have been seen since the early 1970s. The prescription of alternative antibiotics, such as co-trimoxazole and fluoroquinolones, has in turn resulted in a decline in chloramphenicol resistance in some typhoid endemic areas. Many hospital outbreaks caused by multiply resistant strains of enterobacteria, notably *Enterobacter, Klebsiella* and *Serratia* spp. have been described.

Plasmid-borne resistance was first noted in shigellae in Japan and subsequently spread widely in Central America to Mexico, where *Salm. typhi* acquired the same resistance and was responsible for a huge outbreak. Strains of *Salm. typhi* resistant to multiple antibiotics including chloramphenicol are now particularly common in the Indian subcontinent. Resistance in shigella is also relatively common in some parts of the world. Resistant strains of *Neisseria meningitidis, H. influenzae* (some also resistant to ampicillin), *Staph. aureus* and *Str. pyogenes* are also encountered. Chloramphenicol resistance in *H. influenzae* is particularly common in Spain. Resistant strains of *Enterococcus faecalis* are relatively common, and resistance to chloramphenicol is found in the multiple resistance of some South African strains of pneumococci. Chloramphenicol-resistant *Staph. aureus* owe their resistance to inactivation of the enzyme by an inducible acetylase. In *Esch. coli*, the capacity to acetylate choramphenicol (at least three enzymes are involved) is carried by R factors. Replacement of the OH group, which is the target of acetylation, accounts for the activity of fluorinated analogues against strains resistant to chloramphenicol and thiamphenicol. The resistance of *B. fragilis* and some strains of *H. influenzae* is also due to elaboration of a plasmid-encoded acetylating enzyme; in others it is due to reduced permeability resulting from loss of an outer membrane protein. Some resistant bacteria reduce the nitro group or hydrolyse the amide linkage. Resistance of *Ps. aeruginosa* is partly enzymic and partly due to impermeability.

Pharmacokinetics

It is rapidly absorbed by the oral route, a dose of 0.5 g producing peak plasma levels of 10–13 mg/l at 1–2 h after the dose. The plasma half-life is 1.5–3.5 h. The plasma concentration achieved is proportional to the dose administered. Suspensions for oral administration to children contain chloramphenicol palmitate, a tasteless and bacteriologically inert compound which is hydrolysed in the gut to liberate chloramphenicol. Following a dose of 25 mg/kg peak plasma levels around 6–12 mg/l are obtained, but there is much individual variation. Pancreatic lipase is deficient in neonates and, because of poor hydrolysis, the palmitate should be avoided. In very young infants, deficient ability to form glucuronides and low glomerular and tubular excretion ability greatly prolong the plasma half-life. For parenteral use, chloramphenicol sodium succinate, which is freely soluble and undergoes hydrolysis in the tissues with the liberation of chloramphenicol, can be injected intravenously or in small volumes intramuscularly. The plasma concentrations of antibiotic after administration by these routes are unpredictable, and approximate to only 30–70% of those obtained after the same dose by the oral route. About 25–60% of chloramphenicol in the plasma is bound to protein. Binding is reduced in cirrhotic patients and neonates, with correspondingly elevated concentrations of free drug.

Free diffusion occurs into serous effusions. Penetration occurs into all parts of the eye, the therapeutic levels in the aqueous humour being obtained even after local application of 0.5% ophthalmic solution. Concentrations obtained in cerebrospinal fluid (CSF) in the absence of meningitis are 30–50% those of the blood and greater in brain. It crosses the placenta into the fetal circulation and appears in breast milk. It is largely inactivated in the liver by conjugation with glucuronic acid or by reduction to inactive arylamines; clearance of the drug in patients with impaired liver function is depressed in relation to the plasma bilirubin level. It has been suggested that genetically determined variance of hepatic glucuronyl transferase may determine the disposition and toxicity of the drug. Induction of liver microsomal enzymes, for example by phenobarbitone or rifampicin, diminishes blood levels of chloramphenicol and, conversely, chloramphenicol, which inhibits hepatic microsomal oxidases, potentiates the activity of dicoumerol, phenytoin, tolbutamide and those barbiturates which are eliminated by metabolism. It also depresses the action of cyclophosphamide, which depends for its cytotoxicity on transformation into active metabolites. It is uncertain whether this interaction may lead to a clinically significant level of inhibition of the activity of cyclophosphamide. The half-life of chloramphenicol is considerably prolonged if paracetamol is given concurrently, and co-administration of these drugs should therefore be avoided.

It is excreted in the glomerular filtrate and in the newborn its elimination may be impaired by the concomitant administration of benzylpenicillin, which is handled early in life by the same route. Its inactive derivatives are eliminated partly in the glomerular filtrate and partly by active tubular secretion. Over 24 h, 75–90% of the dose appears in the urine, 5–10% in the biologically active forms and the rest as metabolites, chiefly a glucuronide conjugate. Excretion diminishes linearly with renal function and at a creatinine clearance of less than 20 ml/min, maximum concentrations are 10–20 mg/l of urine rather than the 150–200 mg/l found in normal subjects. Because of metabolism, blood levels of active chloramphenicol are only marginally elevated in renal failure, but microbiologically inactive metabolites accumulate. The plasma half-life of the products in the anuric patient is around 100 h, and little is removed by peritoneal or haemodialysis. Dosage modification is normally unnecessary in renal failure as the metabolites are less toxic than the

active parent compound. About 3% of the administered dose is excreted in the bile, but only 1% appears in the faeces, and this mostly in inactive forms.

Toxicity and side-effects

Glossitis, associated with overgrowth of *Candida albicans,* is fairly common if the course of treatment exceeds 1 week. Stomatitis, nausea, vomiting and diarrhoea may occur, but are uncommon. Hypersensitivity reactions are very uncommon. Jarisch–Herxheimer-like reactions have been described in patients treated for brucellosis, enteric fever and syphilis.

It exerts a dose-related but reversible depressant effect on the marrow of all those treated resulting in vacuolization of erythroid and myeloid cells, reticulocytopenia and ferrokinetic changes indicative of decreased erythropoiesis. Evidence of bone-marrow depression is regularly seen if the plasma concentration exceeds 25 mg/l, and leucopenia and thrombocytopenia may be severe. There is no evidence that this common marrow depression is the precursor of potentially fatal aplasia, which differs in that it is fortunately rare, late in onset, usually irreversible and may follow the smallest dose. Aplasia can follow systemic, oral and even ophthalmic administration and may be potentiated by cimetidine. Liver disease, uraemia and pre-existing bone-marrow dysfunction may increase the risk. It is unusual for manifestations to appear during treatment, and the interval between cessation of treatment and onset of dyscrasia can be months. A few patients survive with protracted aplasia, and myeloblastic leukaemia then often supervenes.

It is thought that the toxic agent is not chloramphenicol itself but an as yet unidentified metabolite. Studies in infants and children indicate that chloramphenicol is partially metabolized by a number of pathways to produce oxidized, reduced and conjugated products. The toxic metabolite may be a short-lived product of reduction of the nitro group which damages DNA by helix destabilization and strand breakage. Predisposition to aplasia may be explained by genetically determined differences in metabolism of the agent. Risk of fatal aplastic anaemia has been estimated to increase 13-fold on average treatment with 4 g of chloramphenicol. Corresponding increases are 10-fold in patients treated with mepacrine and 4-fold in patients treated with oxyphenbutazone.

Infants given large doses of chloramphenicol may develop exceedingly high plasma levels of the drug because of their immature conjugation and excretion mechanisms. A life-threatening disorder called the 'grey baby syndrome', characterized by vomiting, refusal to suck and abdominal distension followed by circulatory collapse, may appear when the plasma concentration exceeds 20 mg/l. If concentrations reach 200 mg/l, the disorder can develop in older children or even adults. Optic neuritis has been described in children with cystic fibrosis receiving prolonged chloramphenicol treatment for pulmonary infection. Most improve when the drug is discontinued, but central visual acuity can be permanently impaired. There is some experimental evidence that ear drops containing 5% chloramphenicol sodium succinate can damage hearing. One study identified an increased risk of acute leukaemia following childhood administration of chloramphenicol, particularly for durations exceeding 10 days.

Clinical use

Chloramphenicol should never be given systemically for minor infections. Topical application is widely used for the treatment of eye infections. It is still a useful drug for typhoid fever and other severe infections due to salmonellae (depending on the country of origin, see above) and rickettsiae. Some authorities take the view that these are the only indications. The least contested of other indications are meningitis, invasive infection caused by *H. influenzae* and destructive lung lesions involving anaerobes. Meningitis caused by penicillin-resistant pneumococci has been found to respond poorly to treatment with chloramphenicol, and this appears to be due to the failure to achieve bactericidal concentrations of the antibiotic in CSF. Metronidazole in combination with β-lactam antibiotics are now usually preferred to chloramphenicol for the treatment of brain abscesses. Severe pertussis at an early age may be an indication if treatment can be initiated quickly. Reference is made to its use in cholera (p. 711), cellulitis (p. 737), plague and tularaemia (p. 885), bartonellosis and melioidosis (p. 886), Whipple's disease (p. 714), relapsing fever (p. 889) and rickettsioses (pp. 889 et seq). Treatment for other serious infections should be restricted to those organisms (now very uncommon) which are resistant or much less susceptible to other antibiotics.

Both the daily dose (usually not exceeding 2 g) and the duration of the course (e.g. 10 days) should be limited. Although patients may show toxic manifestations after receiving very little of the drug, the danger is almost certainly increased by excessive or repeated dosage or by the treatment of patients with impaired hepatic or renal function, including those at the extremes of life. The wide pharmacokinetic variability of the antibiotic in neonates makes monitoring of serum concentrations advisable. Determination of full blood counts should be carried out twice weekly.

Preparations and dosage

Proprietary names: Chloromycetin, Kemicetine.

Preparations: Capsules, suspension, injection.

Dosage: Adults, oral, i.v., 50 mg/kg per day in 4 divided doses; the dose may be doubled for severe infections and reduced as soon as clinically indicated.
Children, 50–100 mg/kg per day in divided doses; infants <2 weeks, 25 mg/kg per day in 4 divided doses; infants 2 weeks to 1 year, 50 mg/kg per day in 4 divided doses.
Widely available.

Further information

Ambrose P J 1984 Clinical pharmacokinetics of chloramphenicol and chloramphenicol succinate. *Clinical Pharmacokinetics* 9: 222–238

Friedland I R, Klugman K P 1992 Failure of chloramphenicol therapy in penicillin-resistant pneumococcal meningitis. *Lancet* 339: 405–408

Friedland I R, Shelton S, McCracken G H 1992 Chloramphenicol in penicillin-resistant pneumococcal meningitis. *Lancet* 342: 240–241

Givner L B, Abramson J S, Wasilauskas B 1989 Meningitis due to *Haemophilus influenzae* type b resistant to ampicillin and chloramphenicol. *Reviews of Infectious Diseases* 11: 329–334

Holt D E, Hurley R, Harvey D 1995 A reappraisal of chloramphenicol metabolism: detection and quantification of metabolites in the sera of children. *Journal of Antimicrobial Chemotherapy* 35: 115–127

Kumana C R, Li K Y, Chau P Y 1988 Worldwide variation in chloramphenicol utilization: should it cause concern? *Journal of Clinical Pharmacology* 28: 1071–1075

Mirza S H, Beeching N J, Hark C A 1996 Multi-drug resistant typhoid: a global problem. *Journal of Medical Microbiology* 44: 317–319

Nahata M C 1987 Serum concentrations and adverse effects of chloramphenicol in pediatric patients. *Chemotherapy* 33: 322–327

Ramilo O, Kinane B T, McCracken G H Jr 1988 Chloramphenicol neurotoxicity. *Pediatric Infectious Diseases Journal* 7: 358–359

Ristuccia A M 1985 Chloramphenicol clinical pharmacology in pediatrics. *Therapeutic Drug Monitoring* 7: 159–167

Wallace R J Jr, Steele L C, Brooks D L et al 1988 Ampicillin, tetracycline and chloramphenicol resistant *Haemophilus influenzae* in adults with chronic lung disease. Relationship of resistance to prior antimicrobial therapy. *American Review of Respiratory Diseases* 137: 695–699

West B C, De Vault G A Jr, Clement J C, Williams D M 1988 Aplastic anemia associated with parenteral chloramphenicol: review of 10 cases, including the second case of possible increased risk with cimetidine. *Reviews of Infectious Diseases* 10: 1048–1051

Yunis A A 1988 Chloramphenicol: relation of structure to activity and toxicity. *Annual Review of Pharmacology and Toxicology* 28: 83–100

THIAMPHENICOL

A chloramphenicol analogue in which a sulphomethyl group is substituted for the *p*-nitro group. Also available as the glycinate hydrochloride (1.26 g approximately equivalent to 1 g thiamphenicol). Aqueous solutions are very stable.

Antimicrobial activity

It is generally less active than chloramphenicol against both Gram-positive and Gram-negative bacteria, but the two compounds are equally active against *Str. pyogenes, Str. pneumoniae, H. influenzae* and *N. meningitidis*, including some strains resistant to chloramphenicol (Table 17.1). It is more actively bactericidal against *Haemophilus* and *Neisseria* spp.

Acquired resistance

There is complete cross-resistance with chloramphenicol in those bacteria which elaborate acetyltransferase, although the affinity of the enzyme for thiamphenicol is lower. Organisms which owe their resistance to other mechanisms may be susceptible.

Pharmacokinetics

Thiamphenicol is absorbed by the oral route, a dose of 500 mg producing a peak plasma level of 3–6 mg/l after about 2 h. The plasma half-life is 2.6–3.5 h. It is said to reach the bronchial lumen in concentrations sufficient to exert a bactericidal effect on *H. influenzae*. Disposal of the drug is different from that of chloramphenicol: thiamphenicol is not a substrate for hepatic glucuronyl transferase, it is not eliminated by conjugation and its half-life is not affected by phenobarbitone induction.

It is excreted in the urine in the active form, about 50% of the dose being recovered after the first 8 h and 70% over 24 h. The drug is correspondingly retained in the presence of renal failure, and in anuric patients the plasma half-life has been reported to be 9 h, a value not significantly affected by peritoneal dialysis. Biliary excretion is believed to account for removal of the antibiotic in anuric patients. The plasma concentration is elevated and half-life prolonged in patients with hepatitis or cirrhosis.

Toxicity and side-effects

There are no reports of irreversible bone-marrow toxicity following the use of thiamphenicol. This has been related to the absence of the nitro group, and hence its reduction products, and differences in the detail of the biochemical effects of thiamphenicol and chloramphenicol on mammalian cells. Thiamphenicol induces dose-dependent reversible depression of haemopoiesis and immunogenesis to a greater extent than does chloramphenicol, and has been used for its immunosuppressive effect. Therapeutic doses (1–1.5 g) are likely to depress erythropoiesis in the elderly or others with impaired renal function.

Clinical use

In Europe the drug has been widely administered for a variety of conditions suggested by its broad antimicrobial spectrum.

Preparations and dosage

Preparations: Oral, injection.

Dosage: Adults, oral, 1.5–3 g/day in divided doses depending on severity of infection.

Limited availability in continental Europe. Not available in the UK.

Further information

Franceschinis R (ed) 1984 International symposium on thiamphenicol and sexually transmitted diseases. *Sexually Transmitted Diseases* 11 (suppl 4): 333–469

Goris H, Loeffler M, Bungart B, Schmitz S, Nijhof W 1989 Hemopoiesis during thiamphenicol treatment. *Experimental Hematology* 17: 957–961, 962–967

Ravizzola G 1984 In vitro antibacterial activity of thiamphenicol. *Chemioterapia* 3: 163–166

Coumarins

F. O'Grady

Introduction

A small group of naturally occurring antibiotics based on a substituted coumarin nucleus:

They are chemically related to the coumarin group of anticoagulants. The best known is novobiocin, but a few naturally occurring coumermycins and some semi-synthetic derivatives have been studied. They share a narrow range of antimicrobial activity largely directed against aerobic Gram-positive organisms.

The principle reason for revived interest in them is activity against methicillin-resistant Staphylococcus aureus, *against which the minimum inhibitory concentration of coumermycins is 0.004–0.01 mg/l. There is, however, a marked inoculum effect. Activity against* Staph. aureus *is bactericidal at, or close to, the minimum inhibitory concentration (MIC). Other Gram-positive organisms are similarly susceptible, with MIC values of <0.06 mg/l for coagulase-negative staphylococci, including methicillin-resistant strains, and <0.1 mg/l for streptococci (except* Enterococcus faecalis*), corynebacteria and listeria, including cephalosporin-resistant strains. Multiply-resistant strains of* Streptococcus pneumoniae *are inhibited by 0.25–1 mg/l. There is no useful activity against enterobacteria or pseudomonads and there is no cross-resistance with aminoglycosides or β-lactam antibiotics.*

Antimicrobial coumermycins bind to the B subunit of DNA gyrase and inhibit supercoiling by blocking ATPase activity. The bactericidal activity of quinolones, which bind to A

subunits, is inhibited by coumermycins. In additional to activity against certain protozoa, fungi and viruses, they eliminate some plasmids, and may influence DNA replication in the cells of mammalian species, including man. Calanolides are novel HIV-inhibiting coumermycins derived from a tropical rain forest tree.

Further information

Althaus I W, Dolak L, Reusser F 1988 Coumarins as inhibitors of bacterial DNA gyrase. *Journal of Antibiotics* 41: 373–376

Dresler S L, Robinson-Hill R M 1987 Direct inhibition of UV-induced DNA excision repair in human cells by novobiocin, coumermycin and nalidixic acid. *Carcinogenesis* 8: 813–817

Gilbert E J, Maxwell A 1994 The 24 kDa N-terminal subdomain of the DNA gyrase B protein binds coumarin drugs. *Molecular Microbiology* 12: 365–373

Howard B M, Pinney R J, Smith J T 1994 Antagonism between bactericidal activities of 4-quinolones and coumarins gives insight into 4-quinolone killing mechanisms. *Microbios* 77: 121–131

Kashman Y, Gustafson K R, Fuller R W et al 1992 The calanolides, a novel HIV-inhibitory class of coumarin derivatives from the tropical rainforest tree. *Journal of Medicinal Chemistry* 35: 2735–2743

Maxwell A 1993 The interaction between coumarin drugs and DNA gyrase. *Molecular Microbiology* 9: 681–686

NOVOBIOCIN
Cathomycin; streptonivicin

A fermentation product of *Streptomyces spheroides* and *Streptomyces niveus*, usually supplied as the calcium or the much more soluble monosodium salt.

Antimicrobial activity

It is active against *Staph. aureus*, including β-lactamase-producing and methicillin-resistant strains, *Str. pneumoniae*, *Corynebacterium diphtheriae*, *Haemophilus influenzae*, *Neisseria gonorrhoeae* and *Neisseria meningitidis*.

Resistance to it has been used to distinguish *Staphylococcus saprophyticus* from other staphylococci (but the specificity of this has been questioned), and peptococci from peptostreptococci.

Most enterobacteria are resistant, it was thought because of impermeability, but the mechanism is more complex. Some strains of *Pasteurella*, *Citrobacter* and *Proteus*, particularly *Proteus vulgaris*, are susceptible to moderate concentrations. Concentrations 2–8 times the MIC are slowly bactericidal. The MIC is 8 or more times greater at pH 8.0 than at pH 5.4, and markedly increased by the presence of 10% or more serum, or by increase in the magnesium or nutrient content of the medium. Tetracyclines may enhance its effect by chelating magnesium ions, and this may be the basis of the bactericidal synergy claimed between them.

It has been claimed that novobiocin enhances the activity of idoxuridine against herpes simplex and vaccinia viruses in vitro. It is a potent inhibitor of DNA gyrase subunit A and eliminates plasmids at concentrations two- to eight-fold less than the MIC.

Its activity against common pathogenic bacteria is shown in Table 18.1.

Acquired resistance

Increase in the resistance of staphylococci may occur in vitro or during treatment. 'Synergy' with rifampicin against *Staph. aureus* may be due to prevention of emergent resistance. There is no cross-resistance with other common antibiotics.

Pharmacokinetics

It is well absorbed from the gut, producing peak plasma levels around 11 and 19 mg/l at 1–4 h after doses of 250 and 500 mg, respectively. The plasma half-life is 1.7–4 h.

Table 18.1 *Activity of novobiocin against common pathogenic bacteria: MIC (mg/l)*

	MIC (mg/l)		MIC (mg/l)
Staph. aureus	0.1–2	H. influenzae	0.5–1
Str. pyogenes	0.5–4	N. meningitidis	0.5–4
Str. pneumoniae	0.2–2	N. gonorrhoeae	4
Ent. faecalis	1–16	Past. multocida	2–16
Coryn. diphtheriae	0.5	Pr. vulgaris	2–64
Cl. perfringens	1	Pr. mirabilis	8–128
B. anthracis	1	M. morgani	16–>128
L. monocytogenes	2	Escherichia, Klebsiella,	>128
A. israeli	2	Salmonella, Shigella,	R
M. tuberculosis	R	Pseudomonas spp.	R

R, resistant.

After repeated doses, serum levels of 50 to over 100 mg/l may be reached. About 90% is reversibly bound to serum protein.

Concentrations rather lower than those in the blood are found in serous effusions, but cerebrospinal fluid contains little or none. Less than 3% of the dose appears in the urine. It is excreted mainly in the bile, in which the concentration is high. There is extensive biliary recirculation and high concentrations are found in the faeces.

Toxicity and side-effects

Nausea, abdominal pain and diarrhoea are fairly common. Maculopapular, morbilliform or urticarial skin eruptions with or without fever are common, often developing about the ninth day. Stevens–Johnson syndrome and haemorrhagic rashes have been encountered. Rashes usually disappear on stopping the drug, but may promptly reappear on readministration together with a prompt and profound fall in circulating basophils indicative of sensitization. Allergic myocarditis and pneumonitis have been described. It may displace other substances from protein binding sites and can lower the plasma-bound iodine by displacing thyroxine.

Eosinophilia and moderate transient leucopenia are occasionally seen. Thrombocytopenia, which may be severe, and haemolytic anaemia have also been reported.

It gives rise to a yellow metabolite which may give an indirect positive van den Bergh reaction, but in addition exerts a profound effect on hepatic excretory function by interfering with the uptake of various compounds by hepatic cells, inhibiting glucuronyl transferase and suppressing excretion of conjugates into the bile. Particularly severe effects may occur in the newborn, where glucuronide formation is imperfectly developed. It exerts a different depressant effect on the biliary excretion of different compounds and on the excretion of the same conjugate when this is produced endogenously or infused.

Clinical use

Its principle use has been as an antistaphylococcal agent, particularly in combination with sodium fusidate or rifampicin, in the treatment of the infection due to methicillin-resistant strains. The combination with rifampicin has been commended for the elimination of methicillin-resistant staphylococci from the noses of carriers.

There has been considerable interest in the ability of novobiocin to inhibit various malignant cells and to potentiate the effects of anticancer agents and cisplatin.

Preparations

Very limited availability, not available in the UK.

Further information

Drusano G L, Townsend R J, Walsh T J, Forrest A, Antal E J, Standiford H C 1986 Steady-state serum pharmacokinetics of rifampicin alone and in combination. *Antimicrobial Agents and Chemotherapy* 30: 42–45

Ellis G K, Crowley J, Livingston R B, Goodwin J W, Hutchins L, Allen A 1991 Cisplatin and novobiocin in the treatment of

non-small cell lung cancer. A Southwest Oncology Group Study. *Cancer* 67: 2969–2973

French P, Venuti E, Fraimow H S 1993 In vitro activity of novobiocin against multiresistant strains of *Enterococcus faecium*. *Antimicrobial Agents and Chemotherapy* 37: 2736–2739

McTaggart L A, Elliott T S 1989 Is resistance to novobiocin a reliable test for confirmation of the identity of *Staphylococcus saprophyticus? Medical Microbiology* 30: 253–266

Nordenberg J, Albukrek D, Hadar T et al 1992 Novobiocin-induced anti-proliferative and differentiating effects in melanoma. *British Journal of Cancer* 65: 183–188

Rappa G, Lorico A, Sartorelli A C 1992 Potentiation by novobiocin of the cytotoxic activity of etoposide (VP-16) and teniposide (VM-26). *International Journal of Cancer* 51: 780–787

Rius C, Zorrilla A R, Cabanas C, Mata F, Bernabeu C, Aller P 1991 Differentiation of human pro-monocytic leukaemia U-937 cells with DNA topoisomerase II inhibitors: induction of vimentin gene expression. *Molecular Pharmacology* 39: 442–448

Walsh T J, Auger F, Tatem B A, Hansen S L, Standiford H C 1986 Novobiocin and rifampicin in combination against methicillin-resistant *Staphylococcus aureus*: an in-vitro comparison with vancomycin plus rifampicin. *Journal of Antimicrobial Chemotherapy* 17: 75–82

CHAPTER 19

Cyclic peptides

F. O'Grady and D. Greenwood

Introduction

These compounds marked the beginning of the era of isolation and purification of potent antibiotics from natural sources. The recovery of tyrothricin from Bacillus brevis was reported in 1939 and its separation into gramicidin and tyrocidine in 1941. The almost simultaneous discovery of polymyxin B in the USA as a product of Bacillus polymyxa and in the UK as a product of Bacillus aerosporus followed in 1947.

Among the huge number of antibiotics subsequently discovered, they remain rarities in their bacterial origin, their chemical nature, their disruptive activity on the cell membrane (to which they owe their mammalian toxicity), and the infrequency of acquired resistance. Toxicity has limited their therapeutic use, but their transmembrane effects have excited some interest in their use (or that of analogues) to facilitate the access of other antimicrobial agents to their intracellular targets.

Daptomycin, a semi-synthetic lipopeptide, resembles the polymyxins structurally (consisting of a cyclic peptide with a lipophilic tail) but is derived from a fermentation product of Streptomyces roseosporus and has an apparently novel mode of action involving an early stage of cell wall synthesis. Its useful activity is restricted to Gram-positive cocci, and its chief attraction is that it retains activity against glycopeptide-resistant organisms, including enterococci (see p. 364). Its activity in vitro is greatly potentiated by the presence of calcium (but not magnesium) ions and in these conditions it is more potently bactericidal than the glycopeptides. Development has been hampered by reports of neurotoxicity and it seems unlikely that it will be marketed.

With rapid growth in the numbers and variety of alternative agents, cyclic peptides are now virtually restricted to local therapeutic uses, but the polymyxins, notably as colistin sulphomethate, are still occasionally used systemically, against otherwise resistant organisms.

Further information

Benson C A, Beaudette F, Trenholm G 1987 Comparative in vitro activity of LY 146032, a new peptolide with vancomycin and eight other agents against Gram-positive organisms. Journal of Antimicrobial Chemotherapy 20: 191–196

de la Maza L, Ruoff K L, Ferraro M J 1989 In vitro activity of daptomycin and other antimicrobial agents against vancomycin-resistant Gram-positive bacteria. Antimicrobial Agents and Chemotherapy 33: 1383–1384.

BACITRACIN

A mixture of peptides produced by *Bacillus licheniformis*. The commercial product is a mixture of bacitracins A, B and C and contains at least 13 minor components derived from bacitracins A and F. Also supplied as the more stable zinc salt. Bacitracin A has the structure:

Antimicrobial activity

It is highly active against many Gram-positive bacteria and the pathogenic neisseriae. Although strains of *Staphylococcus aureus* are usually susceptible, they are rather less so than most other Gram-positive bacteria. Haemolytic streptococci of Lancefield's group A are so much more susceptible than streptococci of other groups, notably B, C and G, that bacitracin susceptibility is used as a screening test for the identification of group A streptococci. *Actinomyces* spp. are susceptible, but *Nocardia* spp. are resistant. Amongst other susceptible organisms are *Haemophilus influenzae* and fusobacteria but enterobacteria and *Pseudomonas* spp. are resistant. Synergy is exhibited with rifampicin against *Clostridium difficile*. *Entamoeba histolytica* is inhibited by 0.6–10 mg/l.

Acquired resistance is rare, but has been detected in *Staph. aureus* following topical treatment.

Pharmacokinetics

The bacitracins are not absorbed by mouth. Absorption may occur from application to ulcerated areas.

Toxicity and side-effects

All bacitracins are nephrotoxic when given parenterally and depression of renal function may persist for weeks. Although some absorption may occur, local applications do not appear to produce systemic toxicity, but occasional anaphylaxis, associated with raised serum histamine and IgE, has been described, particularly in women with stasis dermatitis ulcers. A potent 5-HT agonist exerting a contractile effect on smooth muscle may be derived from bacitracin A by renal transformation.

Several important molecules, e.g. insulin and diphtheria toxin, exist as disulphide-linked heterodimer precursors that need to be cleaved to exert their biological effects. The thiol-activated proteases responsible for this cleavage are blocked by bacitracin.

Clinical use

Bacitracin is included in some preparations for local application and has been used orally for the suppression of gut flora, including *Cl. difficile*.

Preparations

Ointment and ophthalmic ointments.

Various preparations with polymyxin, neomycin and corticosteroids.

Widely available.

Further information

Andrews B J, Bjorvatn B 1994 Chemotherapy of *Entamoeba histolytica*: studies in vitro with bacitracin and its zinc salt. *Transactions of the Royal Society of Tropical Medicine and Hygiene* 88: 98–100

Bacon A E, McGrath S, Fekety R, Holloway W J 1991 In vitro synergy studies with *Clostridium difficile*. *Antimicrobial Agents and Chemotherapy* 35: 582–583

Dahl D C, Tsaot, Duckworth W C, Frank B H, Rabkin R 1990 Effect of bacitracin on retroendocytosis and degradation of insulin in cultured kidney epithelial cell line. *Diabetes* 39: 339–346

deBlois D, Bouthillier J, Marceau F 1990 Bacitracin USP contains a factor that stimulates receptors for 5-hydroxytryptamine on rabbit aortic strips. *Life Sciences* 47: 103–108

Eedy D J, McMillan J C, Bingham E A 1990 Anaphylactic reactions to topical antibiotic combinations. *Postgraduate Medical Journal* 66: 858–859

Ikai Y, Oka H, Hayakawa J, Harada K I, Suzuki M 1992 Structural characteristics of bacitracin components by Frit-fast atom bombardment (FAB) liquid chromatography/mass spectrometry (LC/MS). *Journal of Antibiotics (Tokyo)* 45: 1325–1334

Katz B E, Fisher A A 1987 Bacitracin: a unique topical antibiotic sensitiser. *Journal of the American Academy of Dermatology* 17: 1016–1024

Mandel R, Ryser H J, Ghani F, Wu M, Peak D 1993 Inhibition of a reductive function of the plasma membrane by bacitracin and antibodies against protein disulphide isomerase. *Proceedings of the National Academy of Science USA* 90: 4112–4116

Sprung J, Schedewie H K, Kampine J P 1990 Intraoperative anaphylactic shock after bacitracin irrigation. *Anesthesia and Analgesia* 71: 430–433

GRAMICIDIN

A product of *B. brevis*. The commercial mixture contains at least four gramicidins. Gramicidin S (Soviet), also produced by a strain of *B. brevis*, was developed commercially in the former Soviet Union. 1-L-Valine gramicidin A, the major component of gramicidin A has the structure:

L–Val–L–Orn–L–Leu–D–Phe–L–Pro
| |
L–Pro–D–Phe–L–Leu–L–Orn–L–Val

It is active against most species of aerobic and anaerobic Gram-positive bacteria, including mycobacteria. Synergic activity with amphotericin B has been demonstrated against *Candida* spp. and toxicity of the combined agents has been reduced by incorporation into liposomes, Gram-negative bacilli are completely insensitive, probably due to the presence of surface phospholipids which inhibit the action of gramicidin. Trp-*N*-formylated gramicidin is taken up specifically by infected cells to inhibit the growth of *Plasmodium falciparum*.

Gramicidin A is the most widely studied ion channel molecule because of its relatively simple structure and the ease with which the pure congener can be separated from the readily available commercial mixture. Much effort has been devoted to elucidating the precise structure of the ion conducting unit, but the exact conformation in vivo remains difficult to determine.

By intravenous injection, gramicidin is highly toxic to erythrocytes, liver and kidney, and it is not used therapeutically except for its inclusion in mixtures for local application. It has been widely used in the former Soviet Union as a spermicide with antiviral properties.

Preparations

Topical applications with neomycin and other mixtures. Widely available.

Further information

Bourinbaiar A S, Krasinski K, Borkowsky W 1994 Anti-HIV effect of gramicidin in vitro: potential for spermicide use. *Life Sciences* 54: PL5-9

Henkel T, Mittler S, Pfeiffer W, Rotzer H, Apell H J, Knoll W 1989 Lateral order in mixed lipid biolayers and its influence on ion translocation by gramicidin: a model for the structure–function relationships in membranes. *Biochemie* 71: 89–98

Hopfer R L, Mehta R, Lopez-Berenstein G 1987 Synergistic antifungal activity and reduced toxicity of liposomal amphotericin B combined with gramicidin S or NF. *Antimicrobial Agents and Chemotherapy* 31: 1978–1981

Moll G N, Van dem Eertwegh V, Tournois H, Roelofsen B, Op den Kamp J A, VanDeenen L L 1991 Growth inhibition of *Plasmodium falciparum* in in vitro cultures by selective action of tryptophan-*N*-formylated gramicidin incorporated in lipid vesicles. *Biochimica Biophysica Acta* 1062: 206–210

Pascal S M, Cross T A 1992 Structure of an isolated gramicidin A double helical species by high-resolution nuclear magnetic resonance. *Journal of Molecular Biology* 226: 1101–1109

Stankovic C J, Delfino T M, Schreiber S L 1990 Purification of gramicidin A. *Analytical Biochemistry* 184: 100–103

POLYMYXINS

A group of basic polypeptide antibiotics with a side-chain terminated by characteristic fatty acids. Five polymyxins, A, B, C, D and E, were originally isolated and characterized and others have since been added. Polymyxin B and colistin (polymyxin E) sulphates have been commercially developed. By treatment with formalin and sodium bisulphite, some or all of the five amino groups of the polymyxins can be replaced by sulphomethyl groups. Sulphomethyl polymyxins differ considerably in their properties from the parent antibiotics. They are less active antibacterially, relatively painless on injection, more rapidly excreted by the kidney and less toxic. They consist of undefined mixtures of the mono-, di-, tri-, tetra- and penta-substituted polymyxins and differences in the toxicity of the colistin sulphomethate commercially available in America from that available in the UK suggest that the two compounds probably differ in their degree of sulphomethylation.

Their antibacterial activity increases progressively on incubation until it approaches that of the parent polymyxin. It has been argued from this and other evidence that the sulphomethyl derivatives are relatively non-toxic, inactive compounds which owe their effect to the liberation of the parent polymyxin, but other evidence suggests that the less substituted compounds must possess some intrinsic antibacterial activity of their own. Only colistin sulphomethate is now commercially available.

Antimicrobial activity

All the polymyxins have a similar antibacterial spectrum, although there are slight quantitative differences in their activity in vitro. They are inactive against Gram-positive organisms, but nearly all enterobacteria, excluding *Proteus* spp. and *Serratia marcescens*, are highly susceptible, as are *H. influenzae*, *Bordetella pertussis* and *Pseudomonas aeruginosa*. *Bacteroides fragilis* is resistant, but other *Bacteroides* spp. and fusobacteria are susceptible. The pathogenic neisseriae and nearly all species of Gram-positive bacteria and fungi are resistant. Their action is inhibited by the presence of calcium and magnesium ions in the medium. The sulphates are generally 4–8 times more active than the sulphomethyl derivatives.

Acquired resistance

There is complete cross-resistance between the polymyxins, but stable acquired resistance in normally susceptible species is very rare. Adaptive resistance, probably due to changes in cell wall permeability, is readily achieved by passage of a variety of enterobacteria in the presence of the agents in vitro.

Pharmacokinetics

They are not absorbed from the alimentary tract, from mucosal surfaces or even from inflamed surfaces or burns. After parenteral administration of the sulphates, blood levels are usually low. Substantially higher plasma levels are obtained from intramuscular injections of sulphomethyl polymyxins.

As a result of binding to mammalian cell membranes, they persist in the tissues, where they accumulate on repeated dosage, although they disappear from the serum. The sulphates are excreted mainly by the kidney, but after a considerable lag, while the sulphomethyl derivatives are much more rapidly excreted, accounting for their shorter half-lives.

Toxicity and side-effects

Pain (and tissue injury) can occur at the site of injection of the sulphates but less so with the sulphomethyl derivatives. Neurological symptoms such as paraesthesiae with typical numbness and tingling around the mouth, dizziness and weakness are relatively common, and neuromuscular blockade, sometimes severe enough to impede respiration, occurs.

Polymyxins bind specifically to the lipid A region of lipopolysaccharide with neutralization of its biological effects, notably endotoxin shock. In attempts to separate this desirable therapeutic property from the toxicity of the molecule, the lipid tail has been removed to leave the corresponding nonapeptide. Unfortunately, as in the case of the sulphomethates, activity and toxicity have generally altered in parallel. Polymyxins liberate histamine and serotonin from mast cells and acute respiratory distress on inhalation has been attributed to histamine liberation. Hypersensitivity has been rarely reported.

Clinical use

Should systemic therapy with polymyxins be contemplated, the relative painlessness on intramuscular injection and lower toxicity of colistin sulphomethate makes it preferable. For oral and local applications, the more active polymyxin sulphates should be used. Oral polymyxins have been used for the treatment of gastro-intestinal infection and, in combination with other agents, for the suppression of bowel flora in leukaemic patients and preoperatively.

Since the development of resistance has not been a problem, topical preparations are used to treat superficial infections with *Ps. aeruginosa* and to prevent the colonization of burns.

COLISTIN SULPHATE

A mixture of peptide sulphates produced by strains of *B. polymyxa var. colistinus*.

$$L-DAB \cdot NH_2 - D-Leu-L-Leu-L-DAB \cdot NH_2$$
$$|$$
$$L-DAB-L-Thr-L-DAB \cdot NH_2 \longrightarrow |$$
$$|$$
$$L-DAB \cdot NH_2 - L-Thr-L-DAB \cdot NH_2 - 6-Me-octanoyl$$

Antimicrobial activity

Its antimicrobial activity (Table 19.1), pharmacokinetic behaviour, toxicity and clinical uses are for practical purposes identical with those of polymyxin B sulphate. It inhibits *Mycobacterium avium* at around 4 mg/l but the minimum bactericidal concentration (MBC) is much greater. Attempts to use its membrane breaching effect to facilitate the entry of erythromycin did not result in synergy against *Ser. marcescens*. Its marked differential activity against Gram-positive and Gram-negative organisms has led to its use in several selective media. The nonapeptide, liberated by removing the lipid tail of the molecule, which it was hoped could be used to neutralize circulating endotoxins, is less effective than the parent molecule. The specificity of its inhibitory action on the classical complement cascade may make it a useful tool.

Table 19.1 *Activity of polymyxins against common pathogenic bacteria: MIC (mg/l)*

	Colistin sulphate	Colistin sulphomethate	Polymyxin B sulphate
Staph. aureus	64–R	R	64–R
Str. pyogenes	32	32	16–R
Viridans streptococci	32–R	32–R	32–R
Ent. faecalis	R	R	R
H. influenzae	0.5–1		0.03
Esch. coli	0.01–32	0.05–R	0.03
K. pneumoniae	0.01–1	0.01–4	0.03–0.5
Enterobacter spp.	0.03–32	0.5–R	0.03–16
Proteus spp.	R	R	R
Salmonella spp.	0.01–1	0.03–0.5	0.01–1
Shigella spp.	0.01–1	0.1–0.25	0.01–1
Ps. aeruginosa	0.03–4	2–32	0.03–4

R, resistant.

Further information

Asghar S S, DeKoster A, van der Helm H J 1986 In vitro inhibition of the classical pathway of human complement by a natural microbial product, colistin sulphate. *Biochemical Pharmacology* 35: 2917–2921

Hartenauer U, Thülig B, Diemer W et al 1991 Effect of selective flora suppression on colonization, infection and mortality in critically ill patients: a one-year prospective consecutive study. *Critical Care Medicine* 19: 463–473

Warren H S, Kania S A, Siber G R 1985 Binding and neutralization of bacterial lipopolysaccharide by colistin nonapeptide. *Antimicrobial Agents and Chemotherapy* 28: 107–112

COLISTIN SULPHOMETHATE

Produced from colistin by treatment with formaldehyde and sodium bisulphite.

Antimicrobial activity

It is significantly less active than colistin sulphate but its activity is difficult to measure precisely, being composed of the activities of various hydrolysis products (p. 338).

Pharmacokinetics

In adults receiving 3 MU (≈150 mg) intramuscularly (i.m.), mean peak plasma concentrations around 6–15 mg/l were obtained at 2–3 h. On doubling the dose, the corresponding values were 17–25 mg/l at 3–5 h. There is some accumulation in patients receiving 120 mg 8-hourly. In patients treated intravenously (i.v.) with a priming dose of 1.5–2.5 mg/kg followed by continuous infusion of 4.8–6.0 mg/h for 20–30 h, steady state levels were around 5–10 mg/l.

The initial half-life is 2–3 h with a terminal phase extending to 12 h; in the neonate it is 9 h falling to 2–3 h after 3–4 days.

It diffuses poorly into the tissue fluids and does not enter the cerebrospinal fluid. The tissue binding which is a feature of polymyxins is through the amino groups and consequently does not occur with colistin sulphomethate, in which the amino groups are occluded. It crosses the placenta, but the levels achieved are low. Following a maternal dose of 150 mg i.v., none could be detected in amniotic fluid after 3 h and mean plasma concentrations less than 0.5 mg/l were found in infants born 6–20 h later. Some appears in the breast milk.

It is much more rapidly excreted than the sulphate, up to 75% appearing in the urine over 24 h with concentrations reaching around 100–300 mg/l at 2 h. Excretion is still more rapid in children. Other mechanisms than renal are evidently involved in the disposition of the drug and plasma levels are not augmented by probenecid; but there is some accumulation in renal failure. It is not removed by peritoneal dialysis. It is not detectable in the bile.

Because it is less toxic than the sulphate, it has been investigated as a possible neutralizer of circulating endotoxin but it is less effective, some have found much less effective, as is the nonapeptide, than the parent compound.

Toxicity and side-effects

Although less toxic than the sulphate, it is not innocuous and untoward effects have been observed in up to a quarter of those treated. Evidence of nephrotoxicity is the most common (increase in urea and creatinine is almost invariable over the first few days of treatment) and potentially most serious, with acute tubular necrosis being heralded by the appearance of proteinuria, haematuria and casts, sometimes without prior evidence of functional impairment. Renal damage usually continues to progress for up to 2 weeks after withdrawal of therapy. Renal damage is likely to increase with the dose and with the simultaneous administration of other potentially nephrotoxic agents.

Manifestations of central and peripheral neurotoxicity are similar to those seen with polymyxin B (p. 342), and occur particularly in patients with impaired renal function. Neuromuscular blockade is seen principally in patients also receiving anaesthetics or other agents which impair neuromuscular transmission. Complete flaccid paralysis with respiratory arrest and subsequent complete recovery has been seen in a patient with myaesthenia gravis. Allergy is occasionally seen, and nebulized colistin has caused bronchial hyperreactivity with tightness in the chest in adults with cystic fibrosis. Application of colistin ear drops can lead to ototoxicity.

Clinical uses

It is used systemically, rarely nowadays, and usually in combination, for the treatment of infections due to organisms resistant to less toxic agents. It is used in mixtures of various agents, including tobramycin, amphotericin B and trimethoprim, for selective decontamination of the gut (p. 147) and as a paste for control of upper respiratory tract colonization in patients on prolonged mechanical ventilation. It has been used as inhalation therapy for pseudomonas infection in cystic fibrosis.

Further information

Antonelli M, Cicconetti F, Vivino G, Gasparetto A 1991 Closure of a tracheoesophageal fistula by bronchoscopic application of fibrin glue and decontamination of the oral cavity. *Chest* 100: 578–579

Arning M, Wolf H H, Auc C, Heyll A, Scharf R E, Scheider W 1990 Infection prophylaxis in neutropenic patients with acute leukaemia – a randomised, comparative study with ofloxacin, ciprofloxacin and co-trimoxazole/colistin. *Journal of Antimicrobial Chemotherapy* 26 (suppl D): 137–142

Maddison J, Dodd M, Webb A K 1994 Nebulised colistin causes chest tightness in adults with cystic fibrosis. *Respiratory Medicine* 88: 145–147

Rogers M J, Cohen J 1986 Comparison of the binding of Gram-negative bacterial endotoxin by polymyxin B sulphate, colistin sulphate and colistin sulphomethate sodium. *Infection* 14: 79–81

Vazquez C, Municio M, Corera M, Gaztelurrutia L, Sojo A, Vitoria J C 1993 Early treatment of *Pseudomonas aeruginosa* colonization in cystic fibrosis. *Acta Paediatrica* 82: 308–309

POLYMYXIN B SULPHATE

```
    L–DAB·NH₂–D–Phe–L–Leu–L–DAB·NH₂
        |
    L–DAB–L–Thr–L–DAB–NH₂ ──────┐
        |                        |
    L–DAB·NH₂–L–Thr–L–DAB–NH₂–6–Me–octanoyl
```

A mixture of sulphates of polypeptides produced by strains of *B. polymyxa* (1 unit = 0.0119 μg).

Antimicrobial activity

It exhibits potent bactericidal activity against almost all Gram-negative aerobes, including *Ps. aeruginosa,* with the notable exception of *Proteus* spp. (Table 19.1). Resistance of *Vibrio cholerae* eltor to polymyxin B distinguishes it from the classical vibrio. The pathogenic neisseriae and nearly all species of Gram-positive bacteria, anaerobes and fungi are moderately or completely resistant. *Candida tropicalis* is exceptional in that its susceptibility to 30–75 mg/l can be used as a screening test for its identification. *Coccidioides immitis* is even more susceptible, being inhibited by concentrations of 5–10 mg/l.

The nonapeptide prepared by enzymic removal of the fatty acid moiety is 2–64 times less inhibitory than the parent compound, depending on the bacterial species, and about 100 times less toxic to cells in tissue culture. Polymyxin B displaces the cations linking lipopolysaccharide (LPS) molecules, making the membrane more permeable. The nonapeptide differs in binding only to the surface of the cell envelope, but this serves to obstruct the access of *Escherichia coli* fimbriae to receptor sites and to facilitate the passage of a number of compounds which do not ordinarily enter the cell. Deacyl polymyxin B is less effective than hepta- and octapeptides (which are potent permeabilizing agents) in increasing the susceptibility of *Esch. coli* to hydrophobic antibiotics, but it is effective in releasing heat-labile endotoxin from *Esch. coli.*

Through its disruptive effect on the cell membrane, polymyxin B can evidently admit hydrophilic compounds, including sulphonamides and trimethoprim, to the cell, producing significant synergy. Synergy with ciprofloxacin is also described. Hepta- and octapeptides derived from polymyxin B exert similar effects in increasing the susceptibility of *Esch. coli* to rifampicin and other hydrophobic antibiotics. Because of its wide activity against Gram-negative organisms, it has been used in a number of selective media and in combination with nalidixic acid, for the selective isolation of group B streptococci. Calcium ions exert a strong pH-dependent competition for membrane binding sites, and the presence of calcium and magnesium ions in certain media adversely affects its bactericidal activity, notably against *Ps. aeruginosa.*

Acquired resistance

Stable acquired resistance in susceptible species remains extremely rare, but adaptive resistance to growth in high concentrations is readily achieved in a variety of enterobacteria by passage in the presence of the drug. Aerosolized contaminated solutions of the drug can spread resistant organisms.

Pharmacokinetics

It is not absorbed from the alimentary tract or from uninflamed skin or mucosal surfaces, but can be absorbed from denuded areas or large burns. After parenteral administration, blood levels are very variable and often low, reaching 1–8 mg/l after a dose of 50 mg (~500 000 units) i.m. On 2.5 mg/kg (~25 000 units/day), the drug accumulates over 1 week to reach levels around 15 mg/l. Somewhat higher levels are obtained from corresponding doses in children.

Very little enters serous effusions, the cerebrospinal fluid or exudates. As a result of binding to cell membranes, it persists in the liver, kidneys, heart, muscle, lungs and notably in brain, where it accumulates on repeated dosage. Binding to plasma protein is low.

Excretion is mainly via the kidneys, but is delayed: only about 0.1% of the dose appears in the first 12 h but subsequently up to 100% can be recovered, giving urinary concentrations up to 400 mg/l from 24 h onwards. It accumulates in renal failure, the plasma elimination half-life rising in anuria to 2–3 days, although it may sometimes be much shorter because of the mobilization of non-renal mechanisms of elimination. Removal by haemodialysis is very limited. It is not detectable in the bile. Of oral doses, about 25 mg/g is reversibly bound to faeces, mostly to non-bacterial content, except at low pH.

Like other cationic amphiphiles, polymyxin B exerts charge-mediated effects, including prevention of ATP-depletion-induced calcium leak from myocardial cells and multiple blocking actions on ATP-sensitive potassium channels in insulin-secreting cells. It inhibits insulin-stimulated glucose transformation and transport (which it also inhibits directly) depressing glucose uptake into contracting muscle and its incorporation into lipid. LPS mimics the effects of hyperinsulinism and part of the ameliorating influence of polymyxin B on endotoxin shock may be through carbohydrate homeostasis, perhaps involving protein kinase, of which polymyxin B is also a potent indirect inhibitor. Since polymyxin B inhibits insulin stimulated glucose transformation it may be a useful tool in elucidating details of insulin's action.

Toxicity and side-effects

In keeping with its poor local absorption, there are no systemic reactions from applications to intact skin or mucous membranes, but rare allergy is described.

Pain (and tissue injury) can occur at the site of injection. Neurological symptoms such as paraesthesiae with typical numbness and tingling around the mouth, dizziness and weakness are relatively common and peripheral neuropathy, confusion, psychosis and coma are described. Of all antibiotics, polymyxin B is the most potent neuromuscular blocking agent. Its action is incompletely reversed by calcium ions or anticholinesterase inhibitors and appears to be due largely to endplate channel blockade. The effect is likely to be most severe in patients with impaired renal function or those receiving muscle relaxants or anaesthetics or suffering from impaired neuromuscular activity.

Evidence of nephrotoxicity is common, being observed in about 20% of patients, with proteinuria, haematuria and urinary casts heralding acute tubular necrosis in about 2%. Damage is more likely in patients with preexisting renal disease.

The appearance of any evidence of deterioration of renal function or of neuromuscular blockade calls for immediate cessation of treatment. All the toxic manifestations appear to be reversible, but complete recovery may be slow.

Polymyxin B liberates histamine and serotonin from mast cells and anaphylaxis has been described. Severe acute respiratory distress observed in some patients receiving the drug by inhalation has been attributed not to neuromuscular blockade but to airways obstruction resulting from histamine release. Ototoxicity may result from local instillation into the ear.

Severe hypocalcaemia with depression of K^+ and Na^+ and elevation of blood nitrogen may occur on prolonged treatment.

It exhibits a variety of interesting interactions. Those with lipids affect ionic conductance, surface receptor turnover and catabolism of low-density lipoprotein. In particular, it binds specifically to the lipid A region of LPS, thereby inhibiting its biological effects, notably endotoxin shock due to LPS of *Esch. coli*. However, LPS of *N. meningitidis* is unaffected.

Clinical uses

Since the development of resistance has not been a problem, and it does not appear to damage healing wounds, it can be used as a spray, powder or cream, for the treatment of any superficial infection with *Ps. aeruginosa* such as superficial wounds, ulcers or otitis externa. A cream containing 1 mg/g has had considerable success in preventing burns becoming colonized by *Ps. aeruginosa*. It has been used prophylactically as an aerosol in an attempt to control respiratory colonization and infection in intensive care patients.

Oral preparations have been used for the treatment of gastro-intestinal infection and in combination with other agents for the suppression of bowel flora in leukaemic patients and preoperatively.

Where systemic polymyxin therapy is indicated, relative painlessness on intramuscular injection and lower toxicity have caused colistin sulphomethate to be used generally.

Preparations and dosage

Proprietary name: Aerosporin.

Preparations: Injection, ear and eye drops and ointment. Also in multi-ingredient topical preparations.

Dosage: Adults, i.v., 1.5–2.5 mg/kg per day.

Topical preparations widely available.

Further information

Brown R B, Phillips D, Barker M J et al 1989 Outbreak of nosocomial *Flavobacterium meningosepticum* respiratory infection associated with the use of aerosolised polymyxin B. *American Journal of Infection Control* 17: 121–125

Duwe A K, Rupar C A, Horsman G B, Vas S I 1986 In vitro cytotoxicity and antibiotic activity of polymyxin B nonapeptide. *Antimicrobial Agents and Chemotherapy* 30: 340–341

Gremeux T, Tanti J F, Van Obberghen E, LeMarchand-Brustel Y 1987 Polymyxin B selectively inhibits insulin effects on transport in isolated muscle. *American Journal of Physiology* 252: E248–254

Gurski P, Rozniecki J, Kuziminska B, Grzegorczyk J 1985 Bronchial and basophilic reaction to polymyxin B in asthmatic subjects. *Allergy* 40: 70–72

Hanasawa K, Tani T, Kodama M 1989 New approach to endotoxic and septic shock by means of polymyxin B immobilised fibre. *Surgery, Gynecology and Obstetrics* 168: 323–331

Kubesch P, Roggs J, Luciano L, Maas G, Tummler B 1987 Interaction of polymyxin B nonapeptide with anionic phospholipids. *Biochemistry* 26: 2139–2149

Morizono T, Tono T, Sano N 1992 Repeated measurements of compound action potential: evaluation of the ototoxicity of otic drops. *Acta Otolaryngologica* 493 (suppl): 77–80

Qu Z H, Boesman-Finkelstein M, Finkelstein R A 1991 Urea-inducated release of heat-labile enterotoxin from *Escherichia coli. Journal of Clinical Microbiology* 29: 773–777

Richards R M, Xing D K 1993 Investigation of synergism between combinations of ciprofloxacin, polymyxin, sulphadiazine and p-aminobenzoic acid. *Journal of Pharmacy and Pharmacology* 45: 171–175

20

Cycloserine, amino acid analogues and oligopeptides

F. O'Grady

Introduction

Anomalous amino acids and oligopeptides are prominent amongst antibiotics in therapeutic use. All the β-lactam agents fall into this group: the penicillin nucleus can be viewed as a dipeptide condensation product of L-cysteine and D-valine. Amino acids play such a crucial part in the structure and function of the bacterial cell that the processes that handle them are natural targets for antimicrobial action. Attention has particularly focused on D-alanine and the ubiquitous cell wall peptide D-ala D-ala, for the supply and utilization of which the cell depends on enzymes which are the targets of penicillins, cephalosporins and cycloserine. Several successful mimetics of D-alanine, notably alafosfalin and D-fluoroalanine, have been synthesized but none has so far come into therapeutic use.

Short peptide molecules with antimicrobial activity are virtually ubiquitous throughout the natural world and are thought to play a part in native defences against infection. Such peptides include, among many others, the cecropins (originally described in insects, but now known to be more widely distributed), magainins (from the skin of the toad, Xenopus laevis), lantibiotics (lanthionine-containing peptides, like nisin, from bacteria) and the defensins (from mammalian phagocytes). Many of these compounds interfere with membrane integrity and exhibit differential activity against various species. Synthetic oligopeptides are also under investigation as potential antimicrobial agents.

Cycloserine is a naturally occurring amino acid and is the only one, so far, to come into therapeutic use. All these compounds, unlike β-lactam agents, are antagonized in vitro by the presence of certain amino acids and peptides in the medium.

Further information

Boman H G, Marsh J, Goode J A (eds) 1994 *Antimicrobial peptides* (Ciba Foundation Symposium 186). John Wiley, Chichester

Dickinson J M, Mitchison D A 1985 Activity of the combination of fluoroalanine and cycloserine against mycobacteria in vitro. *Tubercle* 66: 109–115

Ringrose P S 1985 Warhead delivery and suicide substrates as concepts in antimicrobial drug design. In: Greenwood D, O'Grady F (eds) *The scientific basis of antimicrobial chemotherapy.* Symposium of the Society of General Microbiology. Cambridge University Press, Cambridge, p 219–266

CYCLOSERINE

A fermentation product of *Streptomyces orchidaceus* and other organisms. Commercially produced synthetically. Aqueous solutions are stable at pH 7.8 but rapidly destroyed in acid conditions.

Antimicrobial activity

It is active against a wide range of Gram-negative and Gram-positive bacteria, including *Staphylococcus aureus*, streptococci, including *Enterococcus faecalis*, a variety of enterobacteria, *Nocardia* and *Chlamydia* spp. *Mycobacterium tuberculosis*, including streptomycin- and isoniazid-resistant strains, is inhibited by 8–16 mg/l. 'Atypical' mycobacteria, including *Mycobacterium avium*, are also susceptible. Its action is specifically antagonized by D-alanine, from which media for in vitro tests should be free.

Acquired resistance

Primary resistance in *M. tuberculosis* is rare and develops only slowly in patients treated with cycloserine alone. Its inclusion in combinations deters the development of resistance to other drugs. There is no cross-resistance with other therapeutic antibiotics.

Pharmacokinetics

It is almost completely absorbed after oral administration, attaining high and well sustained concentrations in the blood. Following an oral dose of 250 mg, average peak plasma concentrations around 10 mg/l are obtained 3–4 h after the dose. Doubling the dose approximately doubles the plasma level. Some accumulation occurs over the first 3 or 4 days of treatment. In children receiving 20 mg/kg orally, plasma levels of 20–35 mg/l have been found. Terizidone, a Schiff's base incorporating two molecules of cycloserine, and pentizidone are pro-drugs which are rapidly hydrolysed after oral absorption to produce improved plasma concentrations of cycloserine. It is widely distributed throughout the body fluids, including the cerebrospinal fluid (CSF). About 50% is excreted unchanged in the glomerular filtrate over 24 h and 65–70% over the subsequent 2 days. The remainder is metabolized. There is no tubular secretion and no effect of probenecid. It accumulates in renal failure, reaching toxic levels if dosage is uncontrolled. It can be removed by haemodialysis.

Toxicity and side-effects

Rarely, rashes, drug fever and cardiac arrhythmia occur. Evidence of central nervous system (CNS) toxicity may develop over the first 2 weeks of treatment and disappear on its withdrawal. Effects include headache, somnolence, vertigo, visual disturbances, confusional states, depression, acute psychotic reactions, hyperreflexia, pareses, tremors and dysarthria. Treatment should be stopped promptly if any mental or neurological signs develop. Convulsions are said to occur in about 50% of patients when the plasma concentration exceeds 20–25 mg/l, but the relationship to dose is not particularly close. No permanent damage

appears to be caused. It is believed the effects may be exacerbated by alcohol and associated with reduced levels of Mg^{2+} and Ca^{2+} in the CSF. Cycloserine inhibits mammalian transaminases and this and the convulsant effects of the drug have been attributed to a metabolite, amino-oxyalanine. The drug should be avoided in patients with previous fits or other neurological or psychiatric abnormalities. Peripheral neuritis has been rarely encountered.

Clinical use

It has been used for urinary tract infection but its principle use is in the combination treatment of tuberculosis due to organisms resistant to preferred agents. It has a place in the treatment of nontuberculous mycobacterioses.

It appears to act as a partial agonist of the glycine site on the *N*-methyl-D-aspartate receptor ionophore complex and has been proposed as a cognitive enhancer, especially in Alzheimer's disease.

Preparations and dosage

Proprietary name: Cycloserine.

Preparation: Capsules.

Dosage: Adults, oral, 250 mg every 12 h for 2 weeks, with a maximum of 50 mg every 12 h. Children, initially 10 mg/kg per day, adjusted according to blood levels and response.

Limited availability; available in the UK.

Further information

Chessell I P, Proctor A W, Francis P T, Bowen D M 1991 D-Cycloserine, a putative cognitive enhancer facilitates activation of the *N*-methyl-D-aspartate receptor–ionophore complex in Alzheimer brain. *Brain Research* 565: 145–148

Flood J F, Morley J E, Lanthorn T H 1992 Effect on memory processing by D-cycloserine, an agonist of the NMDA/glycine receptor. *European Journal of Pharmacology* 221: 249–254

Kaltenis P 1986 Cycloserine as a urinary tract antiseptic. *International Urology and Nephrology* 18: 125–130

Thompson L T, Moskal J R, Disterhoft J F 1992 Hippocampus-dependent learning facilitated by a monoclonal antibody or D-cycloserine. *Nature* 359: 638–641

Diaminopyrimidines

D. T. D. Hughes

Introduction

A group of agents based on the structure 2,4-diaminopyrimidine:

They owe their activity to interference with folate formation through species-specific inhibition of dihydrofolate reductase. The group includes: the antiprotozoal agents pyrimethamine and cycloguanil (the active metabolite of proguanil, p. 532); the antibacterial agents trimethoprim, tetroxoprim and brodimoprim; the antineoplastic agent methotrexate; and trimetrexate, which is in use as an antipneumocystis agent.

For the synthesis of protein and nucleic acids, all living cells require folate intermediates. Dihydrofolate reductase is a key enzyme in their generation, and the safety and efficacy of the antimicrobial diaminopyrimidines used therapeutically (except in the special case of trimetrexate) depends on differential affinities for human and parasite enzymes. In the case of trimethoprim, its affinity for the bacterial enzyme exceeds that for the corresponding mammalian enzyme many thousand-fold. Interference with human folate metabolism may be encountered in the course of treatment, but only if dosage is grossly excessive or the patient's folate status is already depressed for other reasons.

Because sulphonamides inhibit the incorporation by bacteria of p-aminobenzoate into dihydrofolate, the reduction of which is inhibited by trimethoprim, the two agents act sequentially in the same metabolic pathway. The result (though the reasons are more complex) is that their combined action is strongly synergic, there being about a 10-fold increase in activity when they are used together.

This is so striking that when trimethoprim first became available for therapy it was generally assumed that the synergic interaction which is so easily demonstrable in the laboratory would contribute materially to therapeutic efficacy and that trimethoprim and sulphonamide would regularly be used together. The use of trimethoprim alone at that time was not contemplated, and the issue was the selection of a sulphonamide that matched the pharmacokinetic behaviour of trimethoprim sufficiently closely to ensure that the optimum ratio of concentration of the two drugs was delivered to the site of infection. Differing views about the most appropriate partner have produced combinations with sulphamethoxazole (co-trimoxazole), sulphadiazine (co-trimazine) and sulphamoxole (co-trifamole), among others.

The view of trimethoprim, and consequently of its analogues, purely as a co-drug for sulphonamide has come to be questioned on several grounds. The first is that bacteristatic synergy is, by definition, demonstrable only when the concentration of each component is in itself insufficient to exert a bacteristatic effect. In fact, the peak concentrations of each agent exceed the minimum inhibitory concentrations (MICs) of sensitive organisms in the plasma and greatly exceed them in the urine. After a single dose, inhibitory concentrations of trimethoprim can frequently be detected in the urine for several days, and as the drug is usually given twice a day it is hard to see a role for synergic enhancement of its effect by the simultaneous presence of sulphonamide. There may be an opportunity for synergic interaction in plasma as the concentration falls, but infected sites are separated from the plasma concentrations by barriers which are not equally permeable to the two components. Although the plasma profiles of the two drugs show reasonable concordance, their distribution is markedly different, diaminopyrimidines reaching many sites relatively inaccessible to sulphonamide. The second ground for questioning the use of the combination was concern about the proportion of patients in whom untoward reactions can be attributed to the sulphonamide component. A substantial part of the skin and haematological toxicity was typical of sulphonamides.

The third ground was growing scepticism about the validity of the belief that the combination had a second valuable antimicrobial property in addition to synergy: control of the emergence of resistance. The reasons for this scepticism were first, that sulphonamide resistance in relevant bacteria was already widespread and hence sulphonamide could not modify the emergence of resistance to trimethoprim, and second, that the plasmids responsible for the transfer of resistance to trimethoprim also commonly conferred resistance to sulphonamide – among other assorted agents. The weight of these combined arguments – the irrelevance of synergy, the inefficacy of resistance control and enhanced toxicity – was sufficient to split the combination and release trimethoprim for use alone. Despite the logic of the grounds for separation, concern has persisted that the effect has been to accelerate the rate of accumulation of trimethoprim-resistant strains.

Evidence that trimethoprim alone is effective in most clinical situations in which co-trimoxazole has been used, together with concerns about the unnecessary risks associated with the combined formulation, have persuaded the Medicines Control Agency in the UK to limit the licensed indications of co-trimoxazole to the treatment and prophylaxis of Pneumocystis carinii pneumonitis and certain other circumstances in which there are good grounds for preferring the combination over trimethoprim alone.

The success of trimethoprim has naturally led to attempts to synthesize congeners with improved properties. Some adverse effects of trimethoprim appear not to be related to its antifolate activity, and those effects might therefore be reduced without loss of activity.

Tetroxoprim, in which one methoxy group of trimethoprim is replaced by $O \cdot CH_2 \cdot CH_2 \cdot O \cdot CH_3$, is generally at least four-fold less active than trimethoprim, but there is much variation among strains and species, some of which are more susceptible. It was concluded that its pharmacokinetics match most closely those of sulphadiazine and in that combination it has been marketed as co-tetroxazine. Brodimoprim and metioprim, in which one methoxy group of trimethoprim is replaced by bromine and a thiomethyl group, respectively, have generally similar activity to trimethoprim. The latest congener to be described, epiroprim, is more active than trimethoprim against Gram-positive cocci, but less active against enterobacteria.

Further information

Anonymous 1986 Co-trimoxazole, or just trimethoprim? *Drug and Therapeutics Bulletin* 24: 17–19

Anonymous 1995 Co-trimoxazole use restricted. *Drug and Therapeutics Bulletin* 33: 92–93

Bowden K, Harris N V, Watson C A 1993 Structure–activity relationships of dihydrofolate reductase inhibitors. *Journal of Chemotherapy* 5: 377–388

Committee on the Safety of Medicine/Medicines Control Agency 1995 Revised indications for co-trimoxazole (Septrin, Bactrim, various generic preparations). *Current Problems in Pharmacovigilance* 21: 6

Garg S K, Ghosh S S, Mathur V S 1986 Comparative pharmacokinetic study of four different sulfonamides in combination with trimethoprim in human volunteers. *International Journal of Clinical Pharmacology, Therapy and Toxicology* 24: 23–25

Hartman P G 1993 Molecular aspects and mechanism of action of dihydrofolate reductase inhibitors. *Journal of Chemotherapy* 5: 369–376

Locher H H, Schlunegger H, Hartman P G et al 1996 Antibacterial activities of epiroprim, a new dihydrofolate reductase inhibitor, alone and in combination with dapsone. *Antimicrobial Agents and Chemotherapy* 40: 1376–1381

Then R L, Hartman P G, Kompis I, Santi D 1993 Selective inhibition of dihydrofolate reductase from problem human pathogens. *Advances in Experimental Medicine and Biology* 338: 533–536

BRODIMOPRIM

A synthetic diaminopyrimidine closely related to trimethoprim.

Antimicrobial activity

Its antibacterial activity is very similar to that of trimethoprim (Table 21.1), although activity against some anaerobic bacteria, including *Bacteroides fragilis*, *Clostridium* spp. and *Fusobacterium* spp., is somewhat better. MICs for *Nocardia* spp. are 4–16 mg/l and for *Moraxella (Branhamella) catarrhalis* are ≥8 mg/l. Like trimethoprim and other diaminopyrimidines, it interacts synergically with sulphonamides in vitro.

Acquired resistance

There is complete cross-resistance with strains resistant to trimethoprim (p. 350).

Table 21.1 *Activity of trimethoprim and brodimoprim against common pathogenic bacteria: MIC (mg/l)*

	Trimethoprim	Brodimoprim
Staph. aureus	0.2–1	1
Str. pyogenes	0.5–1	2
Str. pneumoniae	0.5–2	1
Viridans streptococci	0.25	
Ent. faecalis	0.25–0.5	0.4
Coryn. diphtheriae	0.5	
Cl. perfringens	0.2–>64	0.4–>64
Myc. tuberculosis	R	
N. gonorrhoeae	8–128	8–>64
N. meningitidis	8	32
H. influenzae	0.12–1	0.03–0.25
Bord. pertussis	4	
Esch. coli	0.01–1	0.04–1
K. pneumoniae	0.5–2	0.5–1
E. aerogenes	1–4	1
Proteus spp.	1–4	0.5–4
Salmonella spp.	0.01–0.5	0.5
Shigella spp.	0.5	0.5
Ps. aeruginosa	R	R
B. fragilis	8–16	1–16

Pharmacokinetics

Bioavailability after oral administration is 80–90%. Maximum plasma concentrations after a single oral dose of 400 or 600 mg were 3.3 and 6.2 mg/l, respectively. The apparent volume of distribution was about 1.5 l/kg and the postdistribution phase elimination half-life was 32–35 h. Concentrations achieved in suction-induced skin blisters were about one-third of the simultaneous plasma level. Excretion is predominantly by the renal route, but less than 10% is in the form of unchanged drug, the remainder being accounted for by several metabolites, some of which may retain partial antibacterial activity.

Toxicity and side-effects

On the basis of the limited information presently available, brodimoprim appears to share the safety profile of trimethoprim, the main problem relating to potential interference with folate levels.

Clinical use

Its uses are similar to those of trimethoprim, but the long plasma half-life allows a once daily, or even less frequent dosing interval.

Preparations

Available in Italy.

Further information

Kalager T, Digranes A, Salveson A, Bergan T 1985 Pharmacokinetics of brodimoprim in serum and blister fluid. *Chemotherapy* 31: 405–409

Periti P 1995 Brodimoprim, a new bacterial dihydrofolate reductase inhibitor: a mini review. *Journal of Chemotherapy* 7: 221–223

Salmi H A, Lehtomaki K, Kylmamaa T 1986 Comparison of brodimoprim and doxycycline in acute respiratory tract infections. A double blind clinical trial. *Drugs Under Experimental and Clinical Research* 12: 349–353

Then R C, Hermann F 1984 Properties of brodimoprim as an inhibitor of dihydrofolate reductases. *Chemotherapy* 30: 18–25

Then R L, Böhni E, Angehrn P, Plozza-Nottebrock H, Stoekel K 1982 New analogues of trimethoprim. *Reviews of Infectious Diseases* 4: 372–377

Various authors 1993 Seminar on bacterial dihydrofolate reductase inhibitors in antimicrobial chemotherapy. *Journal of Chemotherapy* 5: 357–566

PYRIMETHAMINE

A synthetic diaminopyrimidine.

Also available as fixed ratio combinations with dapsone (Maloprim) and sulfadoxine (Fansidar).

Antimicrobial activity

Most notable activity is against *Plasmodium* spp., *Pneum. carinii* and *Toxoplasma gondii*. Slow-growing bradyzoite forms of *Tox. gondii* in tissue cysts are less sensitive than the intracellular tachyzoites. Its activity against plasmodial dihydrofolate reductase is about 1000 times that against the human enzyme. It is much less active against the bacterial enzyme. Synergy with sulphonamides is such that the ED_{50} and clinically curative dose of the mixture is about one-tenth that of the individual components.

Acquired resistance

Resistant plasmodia emerge rapidly when there is mass treatment or prophylaxis with pyrimethamine alone, but much less so with the combinations. Many strains are cross-resistant to other agents but, surprisingly, cross-resistance with the related antifolate drug, proguanil (p. 532), is incomplete.

Pharmacokinetics

It is well absorbed by mouth, 25 or 50 mg producing peak plasma concentrations around 0.1–0.25 and 0.4 mg/l, respectively, at around 5 (2–8) h. The plasma half-life is very long, around 90 (45–150) h. It is highly protein bound (87%) and cleared principally by hepatic metabolism. Levels in cerebrospinal fluid (CSF) are around 10–25% of the simultaneous plasma level. A substantial part of the dose appears in maternal milk, the ratio of milk:serum area under the curve (AUC) being 0.46–0.66, so that the infant might ingest almost half the maternal dose over 9 days.

It is excreted in the urine partly unchanged, but also as several metabolites.

Toxicity and side-effects

Rashes, some severe, occur, but the principal toxic effect is on the bone marrow, particularly on prolonged administration. This is the basis for its therapeutic use in polycythaemia rubra vera and leukaemia. Large doses may lead to megaloblastic anaemia, leucocytopenia, thrombocytopenia or pancytopenia. Very large doses in children have produced vomiting, convulsions, respiratory failure and death. Aggravation of subclinical folate deficiency may be alleviated by folinic acid. Fetal abnormalities have been demonstrated in animals, but administration for malaria prophylaxis is not contra-indicated in pregnancy.

Combinations with dapsone or sulphonamides (sulfadoxine or sulfalene) are more toxic; an incidence of agranulocytosis of 1 in 2000 has been reported with the combination of pyrimethamine with dapsone (Maloprim), and Stevens–Johnson syndrome is an uncommon, but serious hazard of the combination with sulfadoxine (Fansidar).

Clinical use

It is not used alone because of resistance and the combinations with dapsone or sulphonamides are no longer recommended for antimalarial prophylaxis because of the unacceptable frequency of serious side-effects. Combinations with sulfadoxine or sulfalene (sulfametopyrazine) have a useful place in the therapy of falciparum malaria in Africa,

where resistance is less prevalent. It is also used in combination with a sulphonamide (usually sulphadiazine) in toxoplasmosis (Ch. 63) and in combination with dapsone in pneumocystis pneumonia, notably in patients with acquired immunodeficiency syndrome (Ch. 46).

Preparations and dosage

Proprietary names: Fansidar (with sulfadoxine), Maloprim (with dapsone).

Preparation: Tablets.

Dosage: The dose is dependent on malaria prophylaxis recommendations.

Widely available in combinations; limited availability of pyrimethamine as a single agent.

Further information

Bowcock S J, Linch D C, Machin S J, Stewart J W 1987 Pyrimethamine in the myeloproliferative disorders: a forgotten treatment. *Clinical and Laboratory Haematology* 9: 129–136

Cook I F, Cochrane J P, Edstein M D 1986 Race-linked differences in serum concentrations of dapsone, mono-acetyldapsone and pyrimethamine during malaria prophylaxis. *Transactions of the Royal Society of Tropical Medicine and Hygiene* 80: 897–901

Edstein M D 1987 Pharmacokinetics of sulfadoxine and pyrimethamine after Fansidar administration in man. *Chemotherapy* 33: 229–233

Edstein M D, Veenendaal J R, Newman K, Hyslop R 1986 Excretion of chloroquine, dapsone and pyrimethamine in human milk. *British Journal of Clinical Pharmacology* 22: 733–735

Girard P M, Landman R, Gaudebout C et al 1993 Dapsone-pyrimethamine compared with aerosolized pentamidine as primary prophylaxis against *Pneumocystis carinii* pneumonia and toxoplasmosis in HIV infection. *New England Journal of Medicine* 328: 1514–1520

Hutchinson D B, Whiteman P D, Farquar J A 1986 Granulocytosis associated with maloprim: review of cases. *Human Toxicology* 5: 221–227

Lee P S , Lau E Y 1988 Risk of acute non-specific upper respiratory tract infections in healthy men taking dapsone–pyrimethamine for prophylaxis against malaria. *British Medical Journal* 296: 893–895

Newton C R J C, Winstanley P A, Watkins W M et al 1993 A single dose of intramuscular sulfadoxine–pyrimethamine as an adjunct to quinine in the treatment of severe malaria: pharmacokinetics and efficacy. *Transactions of the Royal Society of Tropical Medicine and Hygiene* 87: 207–210

Pearson R D, Hewlett E L 1987 Use of pyrimethamine-sulfadoxine (Fansidar) in prophylaxis against chloroquine-resistant *Plasmodium falciparum* and *Pneumocystis carinii*. *Annals of Internal Medicine* 106: 714–718

Petersen E 1987 In vitro susceptibility of *Plasmodium falciparum* to pyrimethamine, sulfadoxine, trimethoprim and sulfamethoxazole singly and in combination. *Transactions of the Royal Society of Tropical Medicine and Hygiene* 81: 238–241

Weiss L M, Harris C, Berger M, Tanowitz H B, Wittner M 1988 Pyrimethamine concentrations in serum and cerebrospinal fluid during treatment of acute *Toxoplasma* encephalitis in patients with AIDS. *Journal of Infectious Diseases* 157: 580–583

Winstanley P A, Watkins W M, Newton C R J C et al 1992 The disposition of oral and intramuscular pyrimethamine/sulphadoxine in Kenyan children with high parasitaemia but clinically non-severe falciparum malaria. *British Journal of Clinical Pharmacology* 33: 143–148

TRIMETHOPRIM

A synthetic diaminopyrimidine.

Antimicrobial activity

Its activity against common pathogenic bacteria is shown in Table 21.1. It is active against aerobic Gram-positive bacilli and cocci including *Staphylococcus aureus*, irrespective of β-lactamase production or methicillin resistance, and *Enterococcus faecalis*, although *Ent. faecalis* is unusual in being able to utilize preformed folinic acid, thymine and thymidine. As a result, mean MICs of trimethoprim and sulphamethoxazole for *Ent. faecalis* of 0.13 and 0.32 mg/l rose to 3.3 and 5.5 mg/l, respectively, in the presence of folinic acid and 1.6–50 mg/l in urine – a result sharply reversed by the presence of the folate analogue, methotrexate. *Mycobacterium tuberculosis* is resistant, but *Mycobacterium marinum* is susceptible, as are *Listeria* spp. Nocardiae are relatively resistant. *Haemophilus influenzae*, including β-lactamase-producing strains and *Haemophilus ducreyi* (MIC 0.03–0.6 mg/l), are susceptible, but Neisseria and *Brucella* spp. are moderately resistant. The MIC_{90} for *Brucella melitensis* is 0.25 mg/l.

Most enterobacteria are susceptible, as are *Bordetella*, *Legionella*, *Pasteurella* and *Vibrio* spp. Pseudomonads, with the exception of *Burkholderia (Pseudomonas) cepacia*, are resistant. Anaerobes are resistant, as are *Chlamydia*, *Coxiella*, *Leptospira*, *Mycoplasma*, *Rickettsia* and *Treponema* spp. Among non-bacterial organisms, *Naegleria* spp., *Plasmodium* spp., *Pneum. carinii* and *Tox. gondii* are susceptible. Its differential activity is such that it is used in selective media for the isolation of *Neisseria gonorrhoeae* and group A streptococci. It is predominantly bacteriostatic, but bactericidal against some strains.

Acquired resistance

Resistance is due to a variety of mechanisms. Chromosomal mutations can result in overproduction or modification of the target enzyme, alterations in metabolic pathway or reduced permeability to the drug. These mechanisms generally confer moderate degrees of resistance. Plasmid-encoded resistance results in the synthesis of mutant enzyme which is highly resistant to the action of the drug. The number of distinct types of these enzymes is growing steadily. The first to be described, type I, which is still the most prevalent, and its immediate successors confer very high level resistance which appeared to be the hallmark of plasmid-encoded resistance. Some later types, however, confer only moderate resistance. Increasingly, high level resistance is due to chromosomal location of the responsible transposon.

Following the introduction of co-trimoxazole, the prevalence of resistance, notably in *Escherichia coli*, increased slowly, but in the early 1980s rapid increase in resistance was noted in many countries associated with great diversification of resistance mechanisms, variety and number of plasmids involved, the resistances transferred and the species involved.

The prevalence and predominant mechanism varies markedly among species and countries, particularly high levels being encountered in developing countries. For example, 75% or more salmonellae are resistant in some areas of South America. Originally, with the exception of some species (for example *Proteus mirabilis*), resistant strains were almost invariably also resistant to sulphonamide; however strains resistant to trimethoprim, but susceptible to sulphonamide, are now encountered.

The prevalence of resistance in common urinary pathogens has several times been thought to have reached a plateau around 5% and later around 12–15%, but further increases have occurred and changes originally manifest in hospital have relatively quickly spread into the community. There is no convincing evidence that the use of trimethoprim alone (rather than co-trimoxazole) has materially influenced the prevalence of resistance.

Since thymine can supply the metabolic requirement imposed by trimethoprim, thymine-requiring mutant bacteria are trimethoprim resistant. Such organisms have rarely been implicated in infection, probably because tissues generally fail to provide the necessary thymine. Infection with trimethoprim-resistant, thymine-requiring mutants has occasionally been observed in patients treated for prolonged periods with co-trimoxazole. Such organisms do not grow on media used for susceptibility testing, which are made deficient in thymine or thymidine. Although the concentrations of thymine and thymidine are extremely low in normal human blood or urine, in pathological states sufficient thymine-like compounds (possibly derived from the breakdown of neutrophils) may be present and can be detected in the urine of patients infected with such strains.

Pharmacokinetics

Trimethoprim is rapidly absorbed from the gut, giving peak plasma levels of about 0.9–1.2 mg/l at 1.5–3.5 h after a dose of 100 mg, and 2.2–3.2 mg/l after 250 mg. At these concentrations, 42–46% of the drug is protein bound. Increasing the dose up to 12-fold produces a proportionate increase in the mean peak plasma concentration, but the mean plasma half-life increases from 13 to 17 h. Because it is almost insoluble in water and has a pK_a of 7.2, it was postulated that its absorption might be increased in an alkaline medium, but cimetidine was without effect.

A dose of 100 mg by intravenous (i.v.) bolus produced a mean plasma concentration of 5 mg after the injection of 1.4 mg/l with a half-life of 11–12 h.

Distribution
See co-trimoxazole (p. 354).

Excretion
Elimination is almost wholly via the urine, giving levels of 50–100 mg/l, of which less than 8% is in conjugated, inactive forms. About 70% is excreted in the first 24 h, but detectable levels are present in the urine for 4–5 days, during which time about 90% of the dose can be recovered.

The renal clearance of trimethoprim in the normal subject is 19–148 ml/min, the wide variation being accounted for to a large extent by the influence of pH. Trimethoprim is a weak base, and urinary excretion rises sharply with falling pH as the drug ionizes and non-ionic back-diffusion in the tubules decreases. Trimethoprim clearance declines with renal function, but less rapidly than that of creatinine, so that at the poorest function levels, trimethoprim clearance exceeds that of creatinine (supporting other evidence that the drug is partly excreted by active tubular secretion) and therapeutic concentrations of the drug are still found in urine.

Toxicity and side-effects

The most serious foreseeable toxic effect of trimethoprim is the induction of folate deficiency, although the affinity of the drug for the mammalian enzyme is very low and any depressant effect can be offset by feeding folate supplements, which cannot be utilized by the parasite. Transient early falls in folate levels may occur with little haematological change, except in patients in poor nutritional state. Experimentally, some immunosuppressive effects can be demonstrated, but their clinical significance, if any, is not clear. Megaloblastic anaemia, which responded very poorly to haematinics, and transient erythroid hypoplasia have been described. Haematological changes are most likely in patients whose folate metabolism is deranged for some other reason. Renal impairment ascribed to trimethoprim in patients treated with co-trimoxazole has probably been due to the sulphonamide or to changes in creatinine excretion. A quarter of patients treated with 160 mg twice daily for urinary tract infection developed significantly raised serum creatinine, but there was no effect on β_2-microglobulin excretion. The absence of any effect on glomerular flow rate as measured by $[^{51}Cr]EDTA$ supports the view that the effect is due not to reduction in renal function, but to competitive inhibition of tubular secretion of creatinine. Development of aseptic meningitis has been described.

Clinical use

The main use of trimethoprim alone is in the treatment of urinary infections (Ch. 56). Because trimethoprim, but not sulphamethoxazole, is concentrated in sputum, some authors have recommended it in preference to co-trimoxazole in chest infections, but this practice is not widespread. Topical preparations have been used in the treatment of burns and, combined with polymyxin, as eye drops to treat infective conjunctivitis. It is successful in the treatment of enteric fever (p. 711) and the control of infection in neutropenic patients. It is not effective in the treatment of chancroid and the relapse rate in brucellosis is unacceptably high.

Preparation and dosage

Proprietary names: Ipral, Monotrim, Trimopan.

Preparations: Tablets, suspension, injection.

Dosage: Adults, oral, 200 mg every 12 h; chronic infections and prophylaxis 100 mg at night. Children 2–5 months, 25 mg twice daily; 6 months to 5 years, 50 mg twice daily , 6–12 years, 100 mg twice daily; chronic infections and prophylaxis, 1–2 mg/kg at night. Adults, i.v., 150–250 mg every 12 h; children <12 years, 6–9 mg/kg per day in 2–3 divided doses.

Widely available.

Further information

Brogden R N, Carmine A A, Heel R C, Speight T M, Avery G S 1982 Trimethoprim: a review of its antibacterial activity, pharmacokinetics and therapeutic use in urinary tract infections. *Drugs* 23: 405–430

Derbes S J 1984 Trimethoprim-induced aseptic meningitis. *Journal of the American Medical Association* 252: 2865–2866

Goldstein F W, Papadopoulou B, Acar J F 1986 The changing pattern of trimethoprim resistance in Paris, with a review of world-wide experience. *Reviews of Infectious Diseases* 8: 725–737

Gross R J, Threlfall E J, Ward L R, Rowe B 1984 Drug resistance in *Shigella dysenteriae, S. flexneri* and *S. boydii* in England and Wales: increasing incidence of resistance to trimethoprim. *British Medical Journal* 288: 784–786

Hamilton-Miller J M T 1988 Reversal of activity of trimethoprim against Gram-positive cocci by thymidine, thymine and 'folates'. *Journal of Antimicrobial Chemotherapy* 22: 35–39

Hamilton-Miller J M T, Purvis D 1986 Enterococci and antifolate antibiotics. *European Journal of Clinical Microbiology* 5: 391–394

Hoppu K 1987 Age differences in trimethoprim pharmacokinetics: need for revised dosing in children? *Clinical Pharmacology and Therapeutics* 41: 336–343

Hoppu K 1989 Changes in trimethoprim pharmacokinetics after the newborn period. *Archives of Diseases in Childhood* 64: 343–345

Hughes B R, Holt P J, Marks R 1987 Trimethoprim associated fixed drug eruption. *British Journal of Dermatology* 116: 241–242

Huovinen P 1987 Trimethoprim resistance. *Antimicrobial Agents and Chemotherapy* 31: 1451–1456

Myre S A, McCann J, First M R, Cluston R J Jr 1987 Effect of trimethoprim on serum creatinine in healthy and chronic renal failure volunteers. *Therapeutic Drug Monitoring* 9: 161–165

Rylance G W, George R H, Healing D E, Robert D G 1985 Single dose pharmacokinetics of trimethoprim. *Archives of Diseases in Childhood* 60: 29–33

Towner K J 1992 Resistance to antifolate antibacterial agents. *Journal of Medical Microbiology* 36: 4–6

TRIMETREXATE

A synthetic diaminoquinazoline related to the anticancer drug, methotrexate. Formulated as the glucuronate.

Antimicrobial activity

It is a non-specific inhibitor of dihydrofolate reductase, which has attracted attention as a potential anticancer compound, but also exhibits useful activity against *Pneum. carinii*. Concentrations of 3–54 μM inhibited growth of *Pneum. carinii* trophozoites in cultures of human embryonic lung fibroblasts in vitro. Unlike methotrexate, trimetrexate is lipid soluble and penetrates into pneumocystis cells. It is a much more potent inhibitor of the pneumocystis (and mammalian) dihydrofolate reductase than trimethoprim: the 50% inhibitory concentration for *Pneum. carinii* dihydrofolate reductase is 26 nM, compared with 39 600 nM for trimethoprim. Despite high affinity for the mammalian enzyme, serious toxicity can be avoided by concurrent administration of leucovorin (folinic acid), which *Pneum. carinii* lacks the ability to take up.

Pharmacokinetics

After intravenous infusion of 30 mg/m^2 to adult patients with acquired immune deficiency syndrome (AIDS), concentrations of trimetrexate were around 2 μM at 4 h. The elimination half-life varied from 6 to 16 h. Although the drug is usually administered by i.v. infusion, oral bioavailability is about 44% and concentrations comparable to those achieved by an i.v. infusion of 30 mg/m^2 were achieved after 2 h of an oral dose of 60 mg/m^2. Protein binding is >95%. Excretion is largely by the renal route, but since the urinary recovery measured by high pressure liquid chromatography (around 10% of the dose) was much lower than that indicated by a dihydrofolate reductase inhibition assay (40% of the dose), it is assumed that a substantial proportion of the dose is excreted as metabolites that retain inhibitory activity. The influence of renal or hepatic impairment on pharmacokinetic properties is presently unknown.

Toxicity and side-effects

As might be expected from its anticancer activity, it is extremely toxic unless administered with leucovorin (see above). Important side-effects include bone marrow suppression, ulceration of the oral and gastric mucosa, and impairment of hepatic and renal function. Administration of leucovorin should be continued for 72 h after the last dose of trimetrexate in order to minimize these complications.

Clinical use

Trimetrexate glucuronate (with leucovorin) is indicated in moderate to severe *Pneum. carinii* pneumonia in patients who are intolerant of, or refractory to, co-trimoxazole, or those in whom co-trimoxazole is contra-indicated. It has also been used in cerebral toxoplasmosis in patients with AIDS, but results have not been encouraging.

Preparations and dosage

Proprietary name: Neutrexin.

Dosage: 45 mg/m² once daily by i.v. infusion over 60–90 min. Leucovorin, 20 mg/m² i.v. over 5–10 min, or orally, every 6 h. Leucovorin must be continued for 72 h after the last dose of trimetrexate. Recommended course of therapy 21 days (24 days of leucovorin).

Available in the USA. Not available in the UK.

Further information

Allegra C J, Chabner B A, Tuazon C U et al 1987 Trimetrexate for the treatment of *Pneumocystis carinii* pneumonia in patients with acquired immunodeficiency syndrome. *New England Journal of Medicine* 317: 978–986

Allegra C J, Kovacs J A, Drake J C, Swan J C, Chabner B A, Masur H 1987 Activity of antifolates against *Pneumocystis carinii* dihydrofolate reductase and identification of a potent new agent. *Journal of Experimental Medicine* 165: 926–931

Amsden G W, Kowalsky S F, Morse G D 1992 Trimetrexate for *Pneumocystis carinii* pneumonia in patients with AIDS. *Annals of Pharmacotherapy* 26: 218–226

Freij B J, Wientzen R L, Hayek G, Whitfield L R 1993 Pharmacokinetics of trimetrexate glucuronate in infants with AIDS and *Pneumocystis carinii* pneumonia. *Annals of the New York Academy of Sciences* 693: 302–305

Fulton B, Wagstaff A J, McTavish D 1995 Trimetrexate: a review of its pharmacodynamic and pharmacokinetic properties and therapeutic potential in the treatment of *Pneumocystis carinii* pneumonia. *Drugs* 49: 563–576

Marshall J L, DeLap R J 1994 Clinical pharmacokinetics and pharmacology of trimetrexate. *Clinical Pharmacokinetics* 26: 190–200

Masur H, Polis M A, Tuazon C U et al 1993 Salvage trial of trimetrexate–leucovorin for the treatment of cerebral toxoplasmosis in patients with AIDS. *Journal of Infectious Diseases* 167: 1422–1426

Rogers P, Allegra C J, Murphy R F et al 1988 The bioavailability of oral trimetrexate in patients with acquired immunodeficiency syndrome. *Antimicrobial Agents and Chemotherapy* 32: 324–326

Sattler F R, Frame P, Davis R et al 1994 Trimetrexate with leucovorin versus trimethoprim-sulfamethoxazole for moderate to severe episodes of *Pneumocystis carinii* pneumonia in patients with AIDS: a prospective, controlled multicenter investigation of the AIDS clinical trials group protocol 029/031. *Journal of Infectious Diseases* 170: 165–172

DIAMINOPYRIMIDINE–SULPHONAMIDE COMBINATIONS

As well as the formulations of pyrimethamine with sulphones or sulphonamides (p. 349), various other combinations of diaminopyrimidines and sulphonamides have come into use; co-trimoxazole, a 1 : 5 mixture of trimethoprim and sulphamethoxazole, is much the most commonly used combination. Others include co-trimazine, a 1 : 5 mixture of trimethoprim and sulphadiazine, and co-teroxazine, a 1 : 2.5 mixture of tetroxoprim and sulphadiazine. In addition, combinations of trimethoprim with sulphamoxole (co-trifamole), sulfametopyrazine, sulfametrole or sulphamethoxypyridazine are available in some countries. The components of the mixtures are so similar that it comes as no surprise that no clear differences have emerged in their therapeutic utility or benefit.

They exhibit the activity of, and synergic interaction between, the two components and may additionally cross-suppress the emergence of resistance. The pharmacokinetic behaviour of the mixture is that of the components, there being no significant interaction between them. The extent to which the two components diverge from perfect match in absorption, metabolism, distribution and excretion characteristics and the effect on those properties of such factors as protein binding and pH determines the deviation from the optimum synergic ratio at the site of infection.

Maximum potentiation occurs when the drugs are present in the ratio of their MICs. For example, an organism susceptible to 1 mg trimethoprim/l and 20 mg sulphonamide/l will show maximum inhibition when exposed to a 1 : 20 mixture. This is the optimum ratio for many organisms, but for others proportionately more trimethoprim is required. Some (neisseriae are important examples) are more susceptible to sulphonamide than trimethoprim, and for optimum synergy the mixture must contain more trimethoprim than sulphonamide. In addition to lowering the concentration required to inhibit growth, the mixture may be bactericidal where either drug alone is bacteristatic. In some cases, synergy may be so marked that it can be demonstrated with organisms which would be conventionally regarded as resistant to one or other agent. In other cases, some degree of susceptibility to both agents must be demonstrable.

Rifampicin and polymyxin also act synergically with both sulphonamides and trimethoprim against Gram-negative bacilli. Formulations of trimethoprim with polymyxin B are widely available for topical use in eye drops and ointment. The triple mixture of sulphamethoxazole, trimethoprim and colistin may be more active than any pair of these agents against some organisms, including multiply-resistant *Serratia*.

CO-TRIMAZINE

A fixed ratio (1 : 5) combination of trimethoprim and sulphadiazine.

Its antimicrobial activity is that of its components and synergic interaction between them.

Following a dose of 1 g, mean peak serum concentrations were around 25 mg/l at 3 h with a plasma elimination half-life of 9.3 h.

Untoward effects resemble those of co-trimoxazole, and its clinical uses are similar.

Preparation and dosage

Preparation: Tablets.

Dosage: Adult, oral, 1 g/day.

Limited availability; not available in the UK.

Further information

Bergan T, Allgulander S, Fellner H 1986 Pharmacokinetics of co-trimazine (sulfadiazine plus trimethoprim) in geriatric patients. *Chemotherapy* 32: 478–485

Bergan T, Ortengan B, Westerlund D 1986 Clinical pharmacokinetics of co-trimazine. *Clinical Pharmacokinetics* 11: 372–386

Leone N, Barzaghi N, Monteleone M, Perucca E, Cerutti R, Crema A 1987 Pharmacokinetics of co-trimazine after single and multiple doses. *Arzneimittelforschung* 37: 70–74

CO-TRIMOXAZOLE

A fixed-ratio (1 : 5) combination of trimethoprim with sulphamethoxazole.

Antimicrobial activity

Its activity is that of the components, enhanced when the concentrations are appropriate, by synergic interaction.

Acquired resistance

Resistance has increased over the years in a complex way, further complicated by the effects of the release of trimethoprim for use as a single agent (p. 351). Resistance has emerged in the course of treatment of patients infected with *H. influenzae*, enterobacteria and *Vibrio cholerae*.

Pharmacokinetics

After a single large dose (nine tablets) intended for the treatment of gonorrhoea, plasma levels after 2 h were 4–11 mg trimethoprim and 50–150 mg sulphamethoxazole/l. Mean plasma levels were still around 2.2 mg trimethoprim and 32 mg sulphamethoxazole/l after 24 h. Intravenous infusion of 160 mg trimethoprim and 800 mg sulphamethoxazole over 1 h, every 8 h, maintained serum levels in excess of 30 mg free sulphamethoxazole/l and 2 mg trimethoprim/l. Relatively little difference was found in maximum plasma concentrations of trimethoprim and sulphamethoxazole at 4 h which were around 1.2 and 54 mg/l, respectively.

In children, a significant increase in plasma levels has been found between the third and sixth days, suggesting that the steady state had not been reached by the third day as it is in adults. Metabolic disposition of sulphamethoxazole in children and adults appears to be similar.

Distribution

The volume of distribution of trimethoprim is greater than that of the total body water, indicating concentration at one or more sites, while that of sulphamethoxazole is only about 20% of the body water – a volume corresponding to the extracellular fluid. This difference in distribution accounts for the fact that the ratio of sulphamethoxazole to trimethoprim is 20 : 1 in plasma, while that in the administered mixture is 5 : 1.

Cerebrospinal fluid. Following 30 mg of the mixture by i.v. infusion over 2 h, mean peak concentrations in uninflamed meninges were around 1.0 mg trimethoprim/l (at 1 h postinfusion) and around 14 mg sulphamethoxazole/l (at 4 h postinfusion), respectively, giving CSF:serum ratios of 0.23–0.53 for trimethoprim and 0.20–0.36 for sulphamethoxazole. In patients given 5 mg trimethoprim + 25 mg sulphamethoxazole by i.v. infusion over 1 h up to 8 h before craniotomy, concentrations of trimethoprim in ventricular fluid in the absence of meningeal inflammation were 0.5–3.2 mg/l. In patients receiving 960 mg of the mixture twice daily, concentrations in cerebral abscess pus were 1.5–6 mg/l.

Serous fluid and exudates. Concentrations of trimethoprim in non-infected synovial fluid following two doses of two tablets were around 1.6 mg/l. In volunteers receiving four tablets followed by two tablets twice daily for 4 days, the mean peak blister:serum ratios on day 4 were trimethoprim 0.89 and sulphamethoxazole 0.54. In children with chronic serous otitis media given 24 mg/kg of the mixture up to a maximum of 160 mg of trimethoprim, peak concentrations in middle ear fluid around 1.9 mg/l were found at 1.5–2 h when the serum concentration was around 1.6 mg/l.

In patients receiving a single dose of four tablets of co-trimoxazole, prostatic levels of 1.7–9.8 mg trimethoprim with simultaneous plasma levels of 0.3–5 mg per kg were found, although the difference in the mean values (3.6 and 3 mg/kg) was not significant. Corresponding levels of free sulphamethoxazole were <1–13.3 mg/kg in the prostate and 17.5–142 mg/l in plasma. In patients who had completed a week's treatment, the prostatic levels of trimethoprim were 0.8–15.9 mg/kg with plasma levels of 0.9–6 mg/l, while the free sulphamethoxazole levels in the prostate were 6.1–27 mg/kg with corresponding plasma levels of 15–78 mg/l.

Vaginal secretion concentrations of trimethoprim were 0.15–2.25 mg/l in patients receiving low-dose prophylaxis and 0.9–10 mg/l in patients on conventional dosage – in most cases substantially above the corresponding serum levels – while the sulphamethoxazole levels were very low.

In patients undergoing cataract extraction who were given conventional doses of co-trimoxazole on the morning of surgery and on the evening before, concentrations in the aqueous humour were 0.14–0.4 mg trimethoprim/l and 10–29 mg sulphamethoxazole/l.

Fetus. The concentrations of trimethoprim in maternal and fetal serum and amniotic fluid have been found to be similar, while those of sulphamethoxazole were lower in fetal than in maternal serum and still lower in amniotic fluid. Sulphonamide to trimethoprim ratios were: 100 in cord blood, 10 in liver, 9 in placenta and 5 in lung.

Excretion

Both components are excreted in the urine, the non-ionic back-diffusion of trimethoprim being affected by urinary pH. The excretion of sulphamethoxazole (p. 461) is mainly in the form of acetylated metabolites and the ratio of the two components is markedly effected by pH. The excretion of trimethoprim increases in acid urine, while that of the sulphonamide is unchanged; in alkaline urine the excretion of trimethoprim is depressed and that of sulphamethoxazole enhanced. As a result, the ratio of the urinary concentrations of active sulphonamide to trimethoprim is around 1 in acid urine and around 5 in alkaline urine.

Biliary levels are about 50% of the corresponding plasma level at 4 h, rising to approximate to plasma levels at 24 h.

At 12 h after a single conventional dose, the biliary concentration of active sulphamethoxazole was 8–14 mg/l and that of trimethoprim 0.4–1.0 mg/l.

Toxicity and side-effects

Serious toxicity is uncommon, but the increased risks of co-trimoxazole compared with trimethoprim alone, particularly in the elderly, have been sufficient to limit the licensed indications for the combination.

Haematological abnormalities in patients whose folate status is already impaired can result from the trimethoprim component. Erythema multiforme and Stevens–Johnson syndrome are rare, but the risk is higher with co-trimoxazole than with trimethoprim alone. Deterioration of renal function in patients with renal disease treated with co-trimoxazole and a number of other untoward reactions (especially in patients suffering from AIDS) including rashes, leucopenia, thrombocytopenia (commoner in the elderly) and rare hepatic disturbance can probably be attributed to the sulphonamide component (p. 462). Several cases of aseptic meningitis have been described. Nausea, vomiting (occasionally severe enough to require withdrawal of treatment) and skin rashes have occurred in some patients.

Administration of the mixture (or trimethoprim alone) results in marked depression of faecal enterobacteria with little or no effect on faecal anaerobes. Corresponding clearance of the perianal and introital areas of enterobacteria is believed to be an important feature of the drug's value in the control of recurrent urinary tract infection (Ch. 56). Emergence of resistance in the course of treatment has generally not been a problem, and while intrinsically resistant species, including *Pseudomonas aeruginosa*, have naturally persisted, major overgrowth has not been a troublesome feature. Diarrhoea may be severe enough in some patients to require withdrawal of treatment.

In the rat, doses greater than 200 mg/kg daily were teratogenic, but complete protection was afforded by folinic acid or dietary folate supplements. No abnormalities were produced in the rabbit or infants born to treated mothers, but use of the drug in pregnancy is not recommended.

Clinical use

Co-trimoxazole has been used for infections as diverse as acne, listeriosis, nocardiasis, gonorrhoea, brucellosis, endocarditis, severe enterobacterial infections, including enteric fever and cholera, plague, meningitis (since both components penetrate well into the CSF), chancroid, melioidosis, Whipple's disease and granuloma inguinale. However, licensed indications in the UK are now restricted to the treatment and prophylaxis of *Pneum. carinii* pneumonitis and toxoplasmosis, the treatment of nocardiasis and the treatment of certain other conditions (urinary tract infections; acute exacerbations of chronic bronchitis; acute otitis media in children) where there is microbiological evidence of sensitivity to the combination and good reason to prefer the combination to trimethoprim alone.

Co-trimoxazole has some activity against protozoa. It has been used in malaria and toxoplasmosis, but is much inferior to pyrimethamine combinations. It is recommended for treatment of *Isospora belli* and *Cyclospora* infections in man.

Preparations and dosage

Proprietary names: Bactrim, Septrin.

Preparations: Tablets, injections, suspension.

Dosage: Adults, oral 960 mg every 12 h increased to 1.44 g in severe infections. Children >12 years, as for adults; 6 weeks to 5 months, 120 mg every 12 h; 6 months to 5 years, 240 mg every 12 h; 6–12 years, 480 mg every 12 h. High dose therapy for *Pneumocystis carinii* infections, 120 mg/kg per day in divided doses for 14 days. Adults, i.m., i.v. infusion, 960 mg every 12 h increased to 1.44 g every 12 h in severe infections. Children, i.v. infusion, 36 mg/kg per day in 2 divided doses, increased to 54 mg/kg per day in severe infections.

Widely available.

Further information

Bjornson B H, McIntyre A P, Harvey J M, Tauber A I 1986 Studies of the effects of trimethoprim and sulfamethoxazole on human granulopoiesis. *American Journal of Haematology* 23: 1–7

Burman L G 1986 The antimicrobial activities of trimethoprim and sulphonamides. *Scandinavian Journal of Infectious Diseases* 18: 3–13

Burman L G 1986 Significance of the sulphonamide component for the clinical efficacy of trimethoprim–sulphonamide combination. *Scandinavian Journal of Infectious Diseases* 18: 89–99

Gordin F M, Simon G C, Wofsy C B, Mills J 1984 Adverse reactions to trimethoprim–sulfamethoxazole in patients with the acquired immunodeficiency syndrome. *Annals of Internal Medicine* 100: 495–499

Gutman L T 1984 The use of trimethoprim–sulfamethoxazole in children: a review of adverse reactions and indications. *Pediatric Infectious Diseases* 3: 349–357

Halstenson C E, Blevins R B, Salem N G, Matzke G R 1984 Trimethoprim-sulfamethoxazole pharmacokinetics during continuous ambulatory peritoneal dialysis. *Clinical Nephrology* 22: 239–243

Jick H, Derby L E 1995 A large population-based follow-up study of trimethoprim-sulphamethoxazole, trimethoprim and cephalexin for uncommon serious drug toxicity. *Pharmacotherapy* 15: 428–432

Joffe A M, Farley J D, Linden A, Goldsand G 1980 Trimethoprim-sulfamethoxazole-associated aseptic meningitis: case reports and a review of the literature. *American Journal of Medicine* 87: 332–338

Lee B L, Medina I, Benowitz N L, Jacob P, Wofsy C B, Mills J 1989 Dapsone, trimethoprim and sulfamethoxazole plasma levels during treatment of Pneumocystis pneumonia in patients with the acquired immunodeficiency syndrome (AIDS). Evidence of drug interactions. *Annals of Internal Medicine* 110: 606–611

Nissenson A R, Wilson C, Holazo A 1987 Pharmacokinetics of intravenous trimethoprim–sulfamethoxazole during hemodialysis. *American Journal of Nephrology* 7: 270–274

Nowak A, Klimowicz A, Kadydow M 1985 Distribution of trimethoprim and sulfamethoxazole in blood during treatment with co-trimoxazole. *European Journal of Clinical Pharmacology* 29: 231–234

Remington J S (ed) 1987 Update and advances in intravenous therapy with trimethoprim–sulfamethoxazole. *Reviews of Infectious Diseases* 9 (suppl 2): S153–S229

Symposium 1987 Benefits and risk of co-trimoxazole (Bactrim) therapy. *Infection* 15 (suppl 5): S333–S266

Van der Ven A J M, Koopmans P P, Vree T B, van der Meer J W M 1994 Drug intolerance in HIV disease. *Journal of Antimicrobial Chemotherapy* 34: 1–5

Varoquaux O O, Lajoie D, Gobert C et al 1985 Pharmacokinetics of the trimethoprim–sulphamethoxazole combination in the elderly. *British Journal of Clinical Pharmacology* 20: 575–581

White M V, Haddad Z H, Brunner E, Sainz C 1989 Desensitization to trimethoprim–sulfamethoxazole in patients with acquired immune deficiency syndrome and *Pneumocystis carinii* pneumonia. *Annals of Allergy* 62: 177–179

Fosfomycin and fosmidomycin

D. Greenwood

Introduction

These organic phosphonates interfere with bacterial cell-wall synthesis. Fosfomycin inhibits phosphoenolpyruvate transferase and fosmidomycin probably acts in a similar manner. Both enter the bacterial cell via active transport mechanisms for α-glycerophosphate or hexose phosphate. In many Gram-negative bacteria, notably Escherichia coli, *the hexose phosphate pathway is induced by glucose 6-phosphate (G-6P) and this greatly potentiates the activity of these antibiotics in vitro. G-6P is present in places where glycolysis takes place, but the tissue content generally is low and located intracellularly. It is not present in the serum or cerebrospinal fluid (CSF) and is probably suboptimal at sites of infection, since the efficacy of the agents in experimental infection is increased by co-administration of G-6P. Nonetheless, the correlation between their in vivo and in vitro activity is better when tested in the presence of G-6P.*

As with other agents which interfere with cell-wall synthesis, synergy has been demonstrated against some organisms with aminoglycosides and with other agents which act in the cell-wall synthetic sequence, notably β-lactam antibiotics.

Resistant mutants, typically exhibiting loss of the G-6P-induced hexose phosphate transport system, arise in vitro with relatively high frequency (10^{-4}–10^{-5}). Resistance that emerges in vivo is generally associated with deletion of the α-glycerophosphate transport mechanism. Plasmid encoded resistance to fosfomycin also occurs in some species and such strains may remain susceptible to fosmidomycin.

Further information

Neuman M 1984 Recent developments in the field of phosphonic acid antibiotics. *Journal of Antimicrobial Chemotherapy* 14: 309–311

FOSFOMYCIN

Phosphonomycin; *cis*-1,2-epoxypropylphosphonic acid

A fermentation product of *Streptomyces fradae, Streptomyces viridochromogenes* and *Streptomyces wedmorensis*. Commercially produced synthetically. The calcium salt, which is relatively insoluble, and a much more soluble salt, fosfomycin trometamol, are used in oral preparations and the very soluble sodium salt in the parenteral form of the drug.

Antimicrobial activity

It is moderately active against a wide range of pathogens, but its activity in vitro is reduced at an alkaline pH and by the presence of glucose, phosphates or sodium chloride in the culture medium. Consequently, different results may be obtained depending on the medium used: thus, inhibitory concentrations observed in simple nutrient broth or agar are usually lower than those in Mueller–Hinton medium. Addition of glucose 6-phosphate (25 mg/l) to the medium enhances the activity of the drug against most enterobacteria. Its activity against common pathogens is shown in Table 22.1. It is, in general, more active against Gram-negative bacilli than Gram-positive cocci, although most strains of *Staphylococcus aureus* (including methicillin-resistant strains) are susceptible and *Pseudomonas aeruginosa* is usually resistant. Synergy with a variety of β-lactam antibiotics, aminoglycosides and other agents has been exhibited against a proportion of enterococci, methicillin-resistant *Staph. aureus* and enterobacteria.

Table 22.1 *Activity of fosfomycin and fosmidomycin, in the presence of G-6P against common pathogenic bacteria: MIC (mg/l)*

	Fosfomycin	Fosmidomycin
Staph. aureus	2–32	R
Str. pyogenes	8–64	R
Str. pneumoniae	8–64	R
Ent. faecalis	64	R
H. influenzae	4	–
Esch. coli	1–4	1
Klebsiella spp.	2–64	0.5
Pr. mirabilis	1–32	2
Pr. vulgaris/providencia	2–R	8–R
Enterobacter spp.	2–R	0.1
Salmonella spp.	1–8	1
Shigella spp.	1–8	1
Ps. aeruginosa	4–R	2–R
B. fragilis	R	R

R, resistant.

Trometamol (syn. tromethamine; tris(hydroxymethyl)amino-methane) has a molecular weight similar to that of fosfomycin itself, and the trometamol salt consequently exhibits half the activity of other derivatives in tests in vitro.

Acquired resistance

Bacterial populations contain variants which are highly resistant to the drug, but these are said not to have become prevalent in those countries in which the drug is used therapeutically. There is no cross-resistance with important antibiotics, and the agent is active against many strains resistant to other agents. A type of enzyme-mediated resistance in which the epoxide ring is opened in the presence of glutathione is transferred by plasmids and may be associated with multidrug resistance.

Pharmacokinetics

The sodium salt causes gastric irritation and is used only for parenteral administration. About 30–40% of the calcium salt is absorbed orally, producing peak plasma levels about 4 h after 1 g doses of around 7 mg/l. The trometamol salt is considerably better absorbed: in volunteers receiving 50 mg/kg, mean peak plasma levels were about 32 mg/l after 2 h.

Comparison with intravenous (i.v.) administration gave bioavailability of about 60%. Absorption is dose dependent, the fraction recovered from the urine falling from about a half after 2 g to a fifth after 5 g. The effect of food is variable, but generally depresses absorption. Peak blood levels occur about 1 h after intramuscular injection and are 3–5 times higher than those produced by the oral route, average values being 17 and 28 mg/l after 0.5 and 1 g doses. There is some accumulation after repeated doses given 6-hourly. In volunteers given 20 or 40 mg/kg i.v. end-injection levels were 130 and 260 mg/l, respectively. Constant i.v. infusion of 500 mg/h produced a steady-state blood level of about 60 mg/l. The mean plasma half-life was 2.2 h.

It is not bound to plasma protein. The large volume of distribution (20–22 l) indicates free diffusion into interstitial fluid and tissues. In patients with acute meningitis, CSF levels were 10.9 mg/l when the serum level was 65.2 mg/l. In patients with pleural effusions given 30 mg/kg as an i.v. bolus, average peak concentrations in pleural fluid around 43 mg/l were found at 3.7 h. Clearance from the fluid was slower than from plasma. Relatively high concentrations have been found in fetal blood (17.6 mg/l) and amniotic fluid (45 mg/l).

The drug is excreted by glomerular filtration, almost entirely unchanged; recovery over the first 24 h was 80% of an i.v. dose, but less than 20% of an oral dose of the calcium salt. Urinary levels in excess of 1000 mg/l are found after a parenteral dose or 300–500 mg/l after an oral dose. Following 50 mg/kg of the trometamol salt, concentrations in the urine exceed 2000 mg/l and remain above 1000 mg/l for 12 h.

Toxicity and side-effects

Adverse reactions have been observed in about 10–17% of patients, mostly slight gastro-intestinal disorders, although there has been some rise in transaminase levels. Fosfomycin prevents lysosomal accumulation of aminoglycosides when given at the same time but not later, and exerts competitive but not curative protection against their nephrotoxicity. Similar protection has been demonstrated against ototoxicity and against the corresponding toxic effects of cisplatin.

Clinical use

It has been used for a wide variety of conditions including respiratory, gastro-intestinal, generalized and genito-urinary infections. The trometamol salt has been particularly commended for the single-dose treatment of urinary tract infection and is also licensed in the UK for prophylaxis in transurethral surgery.

Preparations and dosage

Proprietary name: Monuril.

Preparation: Granules as fosfomycin trometamol.

Dosage: Adults, oral, 3 g as a single dose. Children, >5 years, 2 g as a single dose.

Widely available.

Further information

Bergan T 1993 Pharmacokinetic profile of fosfomycin trometamol. *Chemotherapy* 39: 297–301

Chin N X, Neu N M, Neu H C 1986 Synergy of fosfomycin with β-lactam antibiotics against staphylococci and aerobic Gram-negative bacilli. *Drugs under Experimental and Clinical Research* 12: 943–947

Greenwood D 1994 Fosfomycin trometamol and the single-dose treatment of cystitis. *Journal of Medical Microbiology* 41: 293–294

Greenwood D, Jones A, Eley A 1986 Factors influencing the activity of the trometamol salt of fosfomycin. *European Journal of Clinical Microbiology* 5: 29–34

Kuhnen E, Pfeifer G, Frenkel C 1987 Penetration of fosfomycin into cerebrospinal fluid across non-inflamed and inflamed meninges. *Infection* 15: 422–424

Lau W Y, Teoh-Chan C H, Fan S T, Lau K F 1986 In vitro and in vivo study of fosfomycin in methicillin-resistant *Staphylococcus aureus* septicaemia. *Journal of Hygiene* 96: 419–423

Mayama T, Yokota M, Shimatani I, Ohyagi H 1993 Analysis of oral fosfomycin calcium (Fosmicin) side-effects after marketing. *International Journal of Clinical Pharmacology, Therapy and Toxicology* 31: 77–82

Naber K G 1992 Fosfomycin trometamol in treatment of uncomplicated lower urinary tract infection in women – an overview. *Infection* 20 (suppl 4): S310–S312

Reeves D S 1994 Fosfomycin trometamol. *Journal of Antimicrobial Chemotherapy* 34: 853–858

Suárez J E, Mendoza M C 1991 Plasmid-encoded fosfomycin resistance. *Antimicrobial Agents and Chemotherapy* 35: 791–795

FOSMIDOMYCIN

Sodium hydrogen-3(*N*-hydroxyformamido)propyl phosphate.

$$\underset{\underset{O}{\|}}{HC}\,N\,CH_2CH_2CH_2\,\underset{\underset{ONa}{|}}{\overset{\overset{O}{\|}}{P}}\!-OH \quad (OH)$$

It is active against a broad range of enterobacteria. It is not active against Gram-positive organisms or anaerobes. Its activity is much affected by medium composition and enhanced by the presence of glucose 6-phosphate or fructose 6-phosphate, but not of glycerol phosphate. Its activity against common pathogenic organisms, in the presence of glucose 6-phosphate, is shown in Table 22.1. It is bactericidal at concentrations close to the minimum inhibitory concentration and shows synergy with a variety of aminoglycosides and β-lactam antibiotics. Bacteria resistant to fosfomycin are usually, but not always cross-resistant to fosmidomycin.

Only about a quarter of the dose is absorbed by mouth. In volunteers given 500 mg orally, mean peak plasma concentrations were 2.3 mg/l at about 2.4 h. In those given 7.5 mg/kg intramuscularly (i.m.), corresponding values were 11 mg/l at 1 h. In volunteers receiving 30 mg/kg i.v. the mean plasma concentration at 0.25 h after the end of the dose was around 160 mg/kg. Plasma protein binding was <5%. Mean plasma elimination half-lives after oral and parenteral administration were 1.8 and 1.6 h, respectively. There was no accumulation after 1 or 2 g i.v. 6-hourly. It is not metabolized to a significant extent and elimination is almost entirely renal, mean urinary recoveries in the first 24 h after oral, i.m. and i.v. administration being around 25%, 65% and 85%, respectively.

It appears to be well tolerated, and anticipated uses are similar to those of fosfomycin against Gram-negative organisms.

Preparations

Available in Japan.

Further information

Kuemmerle H P, Murakawa T, De Santis F 1987 Pharmacokinetic evaluation of fosmidomycin, a new phosphonic acid antibiotic. *Chemiotherapia* 6: 113–119

Neu H C, Kamimura T 1982 Synergy of fosmidomycin (FR-31564) and other antimicrobial agents. *Antimicrobial Agents and Chemotherapy* 22: 560–563

Fusidanes

D. Greenwood

Introduction

A group of naturally occurring antibiotics with a basic cyclopentenophenanthrene structure. Their stereochemistry differs from that of metabolically active steroids and they do not exert any hormonal or anti-inflammatory activity. The group includes cephalosporin P₁, helvolic acid and fusidic acid. They inhibit bacterial protein synthesis and have in common a narrow antibacterial range, synergic activity with penicillin and some other agents, and ready emergence of resistant mutants on passage in vitro. Fusidic acid is about 10 times as active as the others, and is the only one commercially available. Its principal interest lies in activity against β-lactamase-producing and methicillin-resistant staphylococci.

FUSIDIC ACID

A fermentation product of *Fusidium coccineum*.

Supplied as the sodium salt which is readily soluble in water. The diethanolamine salt in phosphate/citrate buffer is used for intravenous infusion. Several preparations are available for topical application.

Antimicrobial activity

It is active against most Gram-positive bacteria and the Gram-negative cocci. Nearly all strains of *Staphylococcus aureus* and *Staphylococcus epidermidis*, including β-lactamase-producing and methicillin-resistant strains, are susceptible, but *Staphylococcus saprophyticus* is considerably less so (minimum inhibitory concentration (MIC) 8 mg/l). Streptococci and pneumococci are much less susceptible than staphylococci, and all aerobic Gram-negative bacilli and fungi are highly resistant. *Bacteroides fragilis* (MIC 2 mg/l), *Nocardia asteroides* (MIC 0.5–4 mg/l), some *Corynebacterium diphtheriae* (MIC <0.01 mg/l), and many strains of clostridia (MIC 0.01–0.5 mg/l) are also susceptible. Its activity against common pathogenic bacteria is shown in Table 23.1.

Among mycobacteria, *Mycobacterium tuberculosis*, *Mycobacterium bovis* and *Mycobacterium malmoense* are moderately susceptible, and good activity against *Mycobacterium leprae* has been reported; other mycobacteria are resistant. Fusidic acid shows some activity against certain protozoa, including *Giardia lamblia* and *Plasmodium falciparum*.

High concentrations have been shown to inhibit the growth of several viruses, including human immunodeficiency virus (HIV), in vitro, but hope that it may be of value in HIV infection has not been sustained. Antiviral activity in vitro may be due to a surfactant effect. In 50% serum, the MIC may double and it is slightly more effective at pH 6–7 than at pH 8. It is bactericidal for many strains in

Table 23.1 *Activity of sodium fusidate against some common pathogenic bacteria: MIC (mg/l)*

Species	MIC (mg/l)
Staph. aureus	0.03–0.1
Str. pyogenes	4–16
Str. pneumoniae	2–16
Ent. faecalis	1–4
N. gonorrhoeae	0.03–1
N. meningitidis	0.06–0.25
Enterobacteria	R
Ps. aeruginosa	R
B. fragilis	2
M. tuberculosis	8–32

R, resistant.

concentrations close to the MIC, but for 90% of methicillin-resistant *Staph. aureus* the MBC/MIC ratio was >4.

Interaction with penicillins is complex, and three distinct patterns of interaction have been described. In the commonest, there is two-way antagonism: more staphylococci survived overnight incubation in the presence of fusidic acid and a penicillin than in the presence of either agent alone. In the second kind, fewest survivors were recovered after incubation with a penicillin alone, more from the mixture and most from fusidic acid. In this case there was one-way antagonism of penicillin by fusidic acid. The remaining strains showed 'indifference' in that the effect of the more bactericidal agent (which against some strains was fusidic acid) prevailed. No synergy was found with rifampicin or vancomycin.

In addition to its antibacterial activity, fusidic acid is said to posses immunosuppressive properties by stimulation of T-cells and production of γ-interferon.

Acquired resistance

Large inocula of most strains of *Staph. aureus* contain a small number of resistant mutants which emerge rapidly in vitro and sometimes during therapy. As with other agents, topical applications are liable to facilitate the emergence of resistant mutants. The growth rate, coagulase, haemolysin and β-lactamase production of these mutants appear to be unimpaired. Despite the ease of emergence of resistance in vitro, resistance remains rare in clinical isolates (1–2%) and mostly plasmid mediated. Even extensive use of the drug on the skin seems not to have added significantly to the pool of resistant strains.

Plasmid-mediated resistance appears to be due to drug exclusion and may be associated with chloramphenicol acetyl transferase, to which it binds avidly. Genes for β-

lactamase and sodium fusidate resistance are commonly carried on the same plasmid. Resistance may also be due to chromosomal mutation, which results in a change at the target site (elongation factor G).

Antistaphylococcal penicillins prevent the emergence of fusidic-acid-resistant mutants even in strains of *Staph. aureus* in which the penicillin antagonizes the effect of fusidic acid against the bulk of the population. In addition, a peculiar form of 'synergy' may be seen in which penicillin kills any emergent resistant mutants, while fusidic acid prevents generation of sufficient β-lactamase to destroy penicillin. Addition of rifampicin failed to prevent the emergence of resistant variants of *Enterococcus faecalis* in vitro.

Pharmacokinetics

It is well absorbed after oral administration in the adult. In children absorption is more rapid. Milk appears to delay absorption, peak concentrations not being reached for 4–8 h. Considerable intersubject variation occurred in the concentrations obtained when 500 mg doses were given orally or by infusion to volunteers, but there was little difference when 100 mg was given by rapid intravenous (i.v.) injection. The mean peak concentrations obtained were 31 mg/l from the oral capsules, 23 mg/l from the suspension and 43 mg/l from the infusion. The areas under the serum concentration curves showed that only about 70% of the suspension was assimilated as compared with the capsule from which the drug was virtually completely absorbed. A new film-coated tablet produced peak plasma levels of around 33 mg/l at about 2 h; absolute bioavailability was 90% and the plasma elimination half-life about 9 h.

Because of slow elimination, considerable accumulation of the drug occurs on repeated administration of doses above 250 mg: 500 mg three times daily for 4 days produced plasma concentrations of 11–41 mg/l after 24 h and 30–144 mg/l after 96 h. Some accumulation occurred on i.v. infusion of sodium fusidate every 8 h over 3 days, the end-infusion levels after the first and last doses being around 50 and 120 mg/l, respectively. On doses of 3 g/day (40 mg/kg) plasma levels can reach 200 mg/l. Relative concentrations in plasma and pus (2 and 17 mg/l) correspond to the ratio of their protein contents. The extravascular albumen pool and protein in oedema fluid and exudate constitute an important depot of the drug. About 95–97.5% is reversibly bound to plasma protein.

Sodium fusidate is well distributed in the tissues and most organs of the body. The volume of distribution is about 12 l. It does not reach the cerebrospinal fluid but penetrates into cerebral abscesses. Inhibitory levels are obtained in muscle, kidney, lungs and pleural exudate. Bone concentrations in samples taken at operation from patients with chronic osteomyelitis treated for at least 5 days were 1.7–14.9 mg/g in patients receiving 1.5 g/day and 3.4–14.8 mg/g in patients receiving 3 g/day.

Levels in excess of 7 mg/l have been demonstrated in aspirated synovial fluid from patients with osteo- or rheumatoid arthritis after 3–7 days' treatment with 0.75 or 1.5 g/day. The drug has been detected in brain, milk and placenta, which it crosses to reach the fetus. In patients treated with 1.5 g/day, levels of 0.08–0.84 mg/l were found in the aqueous humour after 1 day and 1.2–2.0 mg/l after 3 days' treatment. In the postdistribution phase, about half of the drug is in the peripheral compartment, in keeping with the known ability of sodium fusidate to penetrate into tissues including bone.

It is extensively metabolized in the liver and is excreted in the bile in the form of glucuronides and various other metabolites. Only about 2% of the administered dose can be recovered in active form in the faeces. Less than 1% of active antibiotic is excreted in the urine, producing concentrations of only 0.8 mg/l after 4 days' treatment. Very little of the drug is removed by dialysis.

Toxicity and side-effects

Oral sodium fusidate has been administered for prolonged periods for the control of chronic staphylococcal sepsis without mishap. Mild gastro-intestinal disturbance and occasional rashes have been reported. Some patients develop abnormalities in liver function tests and jaundice which resolve on withdrawal of therapy. Jaundice is less common with oral than with parenteral therapy. Rapid infusion of diethanolamine fusidate may lead to venospasm or thrombosis, and occasionally to hypocalcaemia, possibly as an effect of the buffer.

Clinical use

Sodium fusidate has been used for the treatment of a variety of severe staphylococcal infections, particularly bone and joint infections, in both the acute and intractable chronic forms of the disease (p. 762). It has commonly been given in combination with penicillins or erythromycin and also with clindamycin. The mixture with erythromycin has been used to treat patients with prosthetic valve endocarditis due to 'diphtheroids'. Reference is made to its use in cystic fibrosis (p. 691), and in actinomycosis (p. 739). It has been commended (unconvincingly) as an alternative to vancomycin in the control of *Clostridium-difficile*-associated colitis. Because jaundice has developed in some patients it is not recommended in hepatic insufficiency.

Local therapy has been successfully used for a number of skin infections, principally those involving staphylococci, but including erythrasma (p. 738). A formulation that liquefies on contact with lacrimal fluid is used for acute conjunctivitis. Topical use may be associated with the emergence of resistant variants.

Discovery of the immunosuppressive properties of fusidic acid has led to the suggestion that it might be of value in the treatment of several non-bacterial conditions, including Crohn's disease and autoimmune diabetes.

Preparations and dosage

Proprietary name: Fucidin.

Preparations: Tablets, suspension, injection, topical preparations.

Dosage: Adults, oral, 500 mg every 8 h, doubled for severe infections. Children (as fusidic acid) ≤1 year, 50 mg/kg per day in 3 divided doses; 1–5 years, 250 mg every 8 h; 5–12 years, 500 mg every 8 h.

i.v. infusion (as diethanolamine fusidate), adults >50 kg, 500 mg three times daily; adult <50 kg and children, 6–7 mg/kg three times daily.

Widely available.

Further information

Franzblau S G, Biswas A N, Harris E B 1992 Fusidic acid is highly active against extracellular and intracellular *Mycobacterium leprae. Antimicrobial Agents and Chemotherapy* 36: 92–94

Lloyd G, Atkinson T, Sutton P M 1988 Effect of bile salts and fusidic acid on HIV-1 infection of cultured cells. *Lancet* i: 1418–1421

MacGowan A P, Greig M A, Andrew J M, Reeves D S, Wise R 1989 Pharmacokinetics and tolerance of a new film-coated tablet of sodium fusidate administered as a single oral dose to healthy volunteers. *Journal of Antimicrobial Chemotherapy* 23: 409–415

Maehlen T, Degre M 1989 Lack of activity of fusidic acid against human immunodeficiency virus in monocytes. *Antimicrobial Agents and Chemotherapy* 33: 680–683

Nicoletti F, Di Marco R, Morrone S et al 1994 Reduction of spontaneous autoimmune diabetes in diabetes-prone BB rats with the novel immunosuppressant fusidic acid. Effect on T-cell proliferation and production of γ-interferon. *Immunology* 81: 317–321

Reeves D S 1987 The pharmacokinetics of fusidic acid. *Journal of Antimicrobial Chemotherapy* 20: 467–476

Symposium 1990 Fusidic acid: a reappraisal. *Journal of Antimicrobial Chemotherapy* 25 (suppl B): 1–60

CHAPTER 24

Glycopeptides

D. Felmingham

Introduction

The glycopeptides are a group of chemically complex antibacterial compounds obtained originally from various species of the soil actinomycetes. They all contain a core heptapeptide with a high degree of homology in aromatic amino acids 4 to 7. Variation in amino acids 1 to 3, which can be either aromatic or aliphatic, is seen in different subclasses of the glycopeptides, and individual compounds are characterized further by the sugar moieties attached to the amino acid residues, some of which are unique. Vancomycin and ristocetin were discovered in the mid-1950s. Both were developed for the treatment of patients with serious infection caused by Gram-positive bacteria, particularly Staphylococcus aureus. However, ristocetin was withdrawn from human systemic use soon afterwards because of significant bone marrow and platelet toxicity.

Vancomycin was the only available glycopeptide until the development of teicoplanin in the 1980s. This compound is now licensed for systemic therapeutic use in many parts of the world. Among other glycopeptides, avoparcin and actaplanin have been developed for use as animal-feed additives, while actinoidin, like ristocetin, has been used as an investigational aid in the diagnosis of von Willebrand's disease and platelet aggregation dysfunction. A lipoglycodepsipeptide, ramoplanin, shares many of the microbiological properties of vancomycin and teicoplanin (but is 4–8 times more active against staphylococci). It is, however, chemically distinct and may have a different mode of action. It is under investigation as a topical agent, as a component of gut decontamination regimens, and for the oral therapy of antibiotic associated colitis.

A more detailed understanding of structure–activity relationships among the glycopeptides has been made possible by the antibacterial characterization of naturally occurring and chemically derived analogues of vancomycin.

These include: the synmonicins, orienticins, chloro-orienticins, eremomycin and various others described by their laboratory codes. Particularly interesting is the observation that N-alkylization of vancomycin both increases potency and imparts activity against vancomycin-resistant strains of enterococci. Semi-synthetic derivatives of the teicoplanin complex have also been produced. The amide derivatives of the teicoplanin complex and the A2-2 component are 2–4 times more active than teicoplanin against most Gram-positive organisms, and 16–32 times more active against the more resistant isolates of coagulase-negative staphylococci.

Antimicrobial activity

The activity of glycopeptides is essentially restricted to Gram-positive organisms, notably staphylococci and streptococci of all kinds. However, Lactobacillus, Leuconostoc, Pediococcus and Erysipelothrix spp. are inherently resistant. With rare exceptions (e.g. Neisseria spp. and some Prevotella and Porphyromonas spp.) they are inactive against Gram-negative bacteria.

Glycopeptides inhibit the second stage of peptidoglycan synthesis in which UDP-N-acetylmuramyl pentapeptide is added to the N-acetylglucosamine terminus of a lengthening peptidoglycan strand. They bind to the acyl-D-alanyl-D-alanine carboxy terminus of the pentapeptide side-chain on N-acetylmuramic acid and the transglycosylase enzyme responsible for transfer of the peptidoglycan precursor to the growing glycan polymer is inhibited by steric hindrance. Transpeptidase and carboxypeptidase activity may also be inhibited.

Acquired resistance

Resistance to vancomycin and teicoplanin (VanA resistance)

or vancomycin alone (VanB and VanC resistance), has now been studied extensively in *Enterococcus* spp., especially *Enterococcus faecium*. VanA resistance is associated with an alteration in the acyl-D-alanyl-D-alanine carboxy terminus of the pentapeptide side-chain of *N*-acetymuramic acid to D-alanyl-D-lactate, with a consequent loss of binding affinity for both vancomycin and teicoplanin. The modification is inducible and is brought about by the functioning of a cluster of genes which are on a transposable element and may be present on a transferable plasmid. VanB resistance, resulting in loss of susceptibility to vancomycin but not teicoplanin, is also inducible but usually chromosomally mediated and generally not transferable. VanC resistance is observed in virtually all isolates of *Enterococcus gallinarum*; it is chromosomally mediated, constitutively expressed and is characterized by low-level resistance to vancomycin alone. The precise mechanism of VanB and VanC resistance is at present unclear.

Acquired resistance has been demonstrated in laboratory derivatives of *Staph. aureus* and is associated with the production of a 39 kDa cell-wall protein which shows poor homology with a similar-sized molecule produced by enterococci exhibiting VanA resistance. Low-level resistance (MIC 8–32 mg/l) is described in clinical isolates of coagulase-negative staphylococci, notably *Staphylococcus epidermidis* and *Staphylococcus haemolyticus*. Such resistance has been variously attributed to alterations in cell-wall structure, overproduction of the cell-wall peptidoglycan and binding to cell-wall sites other than the primary target. Subtle differences may exist in the modes of action of various glycopeptides, and further work is necessary to elucidate fully the mechanisms of resistance among the different phenotypes.

Further information

Arthur M, Courvalin P 1993 Genetics and mechanisms of glycopeptide resistance in enterococci. *Antimicrobial Agents and Chemotherapy* 37: 1563–1571

Felmingham D 1993 Towards the ideal glycopeptide. *Journal of Antimicrobial Chemotherapy* 32: 663–666

Felmingham G, Solomonides K, O'Hare M D, Wilson A P R, Grüneberg R N 1987 The effect of medium and inoculum on the activity of vancomycin and teicoplanin against coagulase-negative staphylococci. *Journal of Antimicrobial Chemotherapy* 20: 609–610

O'Hare M D, Felmingham D, Grüneberg R N 1989 The bactericidal activity of vancomycin and teicoplanin against methicillin-resistant strains of coagulase-negative *Staphylococcus* spp. *Journal of Antimicrobial Chemotherapy* 23: 800–802

Quintiliani R, Evers S, Courvalin P 1993 The *van B* gene confers various levels of self transferable resistance to vancomycin in enterococci. *Journal of Infectious Diseases* 167: 1220–1223

Woodford N, Johnson A P, Morrison D, Speller D C E 1995 Current perspectives on glycopeptide resistance *Clinical Microbiology Reviews* 8: 585–615

VANCOMYCIN

A tricyclic glycopeptide isolated from the fermentation products of the actinomycete, *Amycolatopsis orientalis*. Two chlorinated β-hydroxytyrosine molecules, three substituted phenylglycine systems, *N*-methylleucine and aspartic acid amide form the basic heptapeptide chain. A disaccharide, made up of glucose and the unique amino sugar, vancosamine, is attached to one of the phenylglycine residues.

Antimicrobial activity

The antibacterial activity is essentially restricted to Gram-positive species (Table 24.1); isolates inhibited by ≤4 mg/l are considered clinically susceptible. It is slowly bactericidal for most susceptible bacteria (≥99.9% reduction in viability after 6–12 h exposure of the inoculum to 8 times the minimum inhibitory concentration). However, against isolates of *Enterococcus* spp., some viridans streptococci (e.g. *Str. sanguis*) and *Staph. haemolyticus*, vancomycin is effectively bacteriostatic.

Pharmacokinetics

It is very poorly absorbed from the gastro-intestinal tract and large concentrations of unaltered drug are found in the faeces. Rapid infusion or bolus administration is dangerous (see below). The intramuscular (i.m.) route of administration causes pain and necrosis and is not used. Following slow intravenous (i.v.) infusion over at least 1 h, it is distributed widely reaching therapeutic concentrations in most body compartments. It does not penetrate appreciably into the cerebrospinal fluid (CSF) of subjects with normal meninges, although levels in patients with meningitis may approach therapeutic concentrations.

After administration of 0.5 g (7.5 mg/kg) and 1 g (15 mg/kg body weight), peak concentrations of 10–25 and 20–50 mg/l, respectively, are achieved 1 h after the end of the infusion; an ideal peak is considered to lie between 25 and 40 mg/l. Dose intervals should be adjusted to give trough concentrations of 5–10 mg/l, immediately prior to the next dose. Protein binding is about 55%.

It is removed from the body almost exclusively by glomerular filtration without significant tubular secretion or reabsorption. The elimination half-life in patients with normal renal function is usually 6–8 h (range 3–13 h). The half-life is altered substantially in patients with impaired renal function necessitating modification to dosage which can be predicted to some extent by creatinine clearance values, but adequately optimized only by monitoring plasma concentrations. Renal clearance may be more rapid in intravenous-drug abusers and children (with the exception

Table 24.1 *Comparative in vitro activity of glycopeptides against some common pathogenic bacteria: MIC (mg/l)*

Species	Vancomycin	Teicoplanin
Staph. aureus (methicillin-sensitive)	1–2	0.12–1
Staph. aureus (methicillin-resistant)	1–2	0.5–1
Coagulase-negative staphylococci	1–4	0.25–32
Haemolytic streptococci (Lancefield groups A–C and G)	0.12–0.25	0.03–0.12
Viridans streptococci	0.25–2	0.06–2
Str. pneumoniae	0.12–0.25	0.03–0.12
Ent. faecalis	1–4	0.12–0.5
L. monocytogenes	0.25–0.5	0.25–0.5
Coryn. diphtheriae	0.06–0.25	0.06–0.5
Coryn. jeikeium	0.5–2	0.5–1
Propionibacterium acnes	0.5–1	0.06–2
Peptostreptococcus spp.	0.12–0.5	0.12–0.25
Cl. perfringens	0.12–0.5	0.03–0.12
Cl. difficile	0.06–1	0.03–0.25
Enterobacteriaceae	R	R
Ps. aeruginosa	R	R
B. fragilis group	R	R

R, resistant.

of neonates in whom the half-life may be prolonged), and plasma monitoring is indicated in such patients, particularly when receiving therapy for endocarditis or other life-threatening sepsis. A prolonged half-life has been observed in some patients with hepatic failure. Plasma monitoring is also indicated in these patients.

It is not removed efficiently by haemodialysis or haemofiltration. Patients undergoing these procedures should be given an appropriate loading dose and the frequency and size of further doses determined by monitoring plasma concentrations. It crosses the peritoneal membrane in both directions with a transfer half-life of about 3 h resulting in about 75% equilibration over a 6 h dialysis period. Because of the large dilution effect, many exchanges may be required before the plasma concentration reaches that of the dialysate and to achieve rapid equilibration, a loading dose of about three times the maintenance dose has been suggested. Thus, in patients on continuous ambulatory peritoneal dialysis (CAPD), incorporation of 50 mg vancomycin/l of dialysate eventually produces plasma concentrations of 5–20 mg/l. Alternatively, a loading dose of 0.5 g vancomycin, administered by i.v. infusion, followed by 7.5 mg/l dialysate with 4–6 hourly exchange, produces plasma concentrations of 6.5–37 mg/l.

Toxicity and side-effects

Rapid i.v. administration (<60 min) may result in release of histamine from basophils and mast cells leading to the so-called 'red-man' or 'red-neck' syndrome characterized by one or more of: pruritis, erythema, flushing of the upper torso, anaphylactoid reaction, angio-oedema and, rarely, cardiovascular depression and collapse.

It is potentially nephrotoxic and ototoxic, although both risks may be overstated in view of the highly purified drug preparations in current use, and the relative ease of plasma monitoring. Increase risk of nephrotoxicity has been associated with treatment for longer than 3 weeks, trough plasma concentrations continually in excess of 10 mg/l, and concurrent therapy with an aminoglycoside or a loop diuretic. When it was first used, often in excessive doses, vancomycin was associated with ototoxicity, particularly in the elderly and in patients with levels in excess of 80 mg/l. Deafness, when it occurs, progresses after withdrawal of treatment and is often irreversible. However, a study of 98 patients treated with the more highly purified preparations of vancomycin between 1974 and 1981 failed to find evidence of ototoxicity. The risk of ototoxicity is minimized if the peak serum level is kept below 50 mg/l and is very unusual if the level is less than 30 mg/l, unless the patient has prior auditory nerve damage or is receiving another potentially ototoxic drug. Reversible neutropenia and/or thrombocytopenia, which can be profound, may occur, notably in patients with renal impairment.

Clinical use

It is used in the treatment of serious infections caused by *Staph. aureus* and other Gram-positive pathogens. It is appropriate for patients in whom penicillins and cephalosporins are contra-indicated because of hypersensitivity, and for those infected with methicillin-resistant staphylococci. It has an important role in the treatment of i.v. catheter or device-related infection caused by coagulase-negative staphylococci (p. 650). It is also used for the treatment and prophylaxis of endocarditis caused by Gram-positive species, often in combination with an aminoglycoside (Ch. 49). Oral vancomycin is used for antibiotic-associated *Clostridium difficile* (pseudomembranous) colitis (p. 714), for staphylococcal enterocolitis, and, in combination with other agents, for the suppression of bowel flora in neutropenic patients.

Preparations and dosage

Proprietary name: Vancocin.

Preparations: Injection, capsules.

Dosage: Adults, oral, 125 mg every 6 h for 7–10 days; i.v., 500 mg every 6 h or 1 g every 12 h. Children, oral, 5 mg/kg every 6 h; >5 years, half the adult dose. Children, i.v., >1 month 10 mg/kg every 6 h; infants 1–4 weeks, 15 mg/kg initially then 10 mg/kg every 8 h; neonates up to 1 week, 15 mg/kg initially then 10 mg/kg every 12 h.

Widely available.

Further information

Falcoz C, Ferry N, Pozet N, Cuisinaud G, Zech P Y, Sassard J 1987 Pharmacokinetics of teicoplanin in renal failure. *Antimicrobial Agents and Chemotherapy* 31: 1255–1262

Rotschafer J C, Crossley K, Zaske D E, Mead K, Sawchuk R J, Solem L D 1982 Pharmacokinetics of vancomycin: observations in 28 patients and dosage recommendations. *Antimicrobial Agents and Chemotherapy* 22: 391–394

Rybak M J, Albrecht L M, Berman J R, Warbasse L H, Svensson C K 1990 Vancomycin pharmacokinetics in burn patients and intravenous drug abusers. *Antimicrobial Agents and Chemotherapy* 34: 792–795

Rybak M J, Albrecht L M, Boike S C, Chandreesekar P H 1990 Nephrotoxicity of vancomycin, alone and with an aminoglycoside. *Journal of Antimicrobial Chemotherapy* 25: 679–687

TEICOPLANIN *

A fermentation product of *Actinoplanes teichomyceticus*. It is a complex of several molecules of similar antibiotic potency, each possessing the same aglycone backbone: a linear heptapeptide of linked aromatic amino acids substituted with the two sugars, D-mannose and N-acetyl glucosamine. The five components (A2-1, A2-2, A2-3, A2-4 and A2-5), are differentiated from each other by the acylaliphatic side-chain substitutions present on the additional sugar.

Antimicrobial activity

The antibacterial spectrum is similar, but not identical to that of vancomycin (Table 24.1).

In general, teicoplanin is 2–4 times more active than vancomycin against susceptible strains. However, against some coagulase-negative staphylococci, especially Staph. *haemolyticus*, teicoplanin may be less active (minimum inhibitory concentration (MIC) 16–64 mg/l compared with ≤4 mg vancomycin/l). For these strains, the MIC of teicoplanin, but not vancomycin, is greatly affected by the composition of the medium, including the presence of lysed horse blood, and the bacterial inoculum density. An MIC ≤8 mg/l is generally used to separate susceptible isolates from those considered to be of intermediate susceptibility (MIC 16 mg/l) or resistant (MIC ≥32 mg/l). This 'breakpoint' is based on experience with use of teicoplanin at a daily maintenance dose of 400 mg following two 400 mg doses 12 h apart during the first 24 h of treatment. A 'breakpoint' of 4 mg/l may be more appropriate if a lower dose is used. Bactericidal activity is similar to that of vancomycin.

Pharmacokinetics

It is very poorly absorbed from the gastro-intestinal tract but, unlike vancomycin, it can be safely administered by the i.m. route or as a rapid i.v. bolus injection. A peak serum concentration of about 25–40 mg/l is seen 1 h after a 400 mg i.v. dose. The peak concentration is achieved about 3 h after i.m. administration, and may be considerably less than the concentration found with the same dose intravenously. However, the area under the time curve (AUC) is similar for both routes of administration.

The elimination half-life ranges from 33 to 190 h or longer, depending upon the pharmacokinetic model used for analysis and the last sampling time. This allows once-daily maintenance dosing following the administration of two doses 12 h apart during the first 24 h of treatment. A daily dose of 400 mg, or 6 mg/kg body weight, is appropriate for most infections. Protein binding is >90%. The pharmacokinetics may be altered in children, in whom some, but not all investigators have found a shorter elimination half-life. A daily dose of 6 mg/kg body weight produced a mean trough concentration of 4.6 mg/l and a peak concentration of 19.1 mg/l. After a dose of 10 mg/kg the corresponding concentrations were 15.8 and 36.9 mg/l, respectively.

It is removed from the body almost entirely by glomerular filtration. The elimination half-life is substantially altered in patients with renal failure (and the elderly), and adjustment of dosage may be necessary. It is not removed during haemodialysis or haemofiltration and clearance by peritoneal dialysis is less than 20% of total body clearance. In all three procedures, management of plasma concentration is best achieved by giving a loading dose followed by monitoring at appropriate intervals.

Toxicity and side-effects

Unlike vancomycin, it does not cause significant histamine release and the 'red-man' syndrome is very seldom seen. Doses of 200 mg or less can be administered without problem by the i.m. route, but pharmacokinetic parameters are altered (see above). Nephrotoxicity is uncommon and, when it does occur, is not related to dose, plasma concentration or concomitant therapy with an amino-glycoside. Accidental overdosing in two children in whom plasma levels in excess of 300 mg/l were found, was not associated with symptoms or laboratory abnormalities. Ototoxicity has been reported rarely and is not dose related.

Other, reversible adverse effects include allergy, local intolerance, fever and altered liver function. Thrombo-cytopenia has been seen in patients with raised trough levels (about 60 mg/l). None of these effects occur with a frequency greater than 3%.

Clinical use

It is an alternative to vancomycin in virtually all clinical situations in which the latter compound is indicated, with the advantage of less frequent dosing and less potential for nephro- and ototoxicity.

Preparations and dosage

Proprietary name: Targocid.

Preparation: Injection.

Dosage: Adults, i.v., 400 mg initial loading dose on day 1 then 200 mg/day; severe infections, 400 mg loading dose every 12 h for the first 3 doses, then 400 mg/day. Children ≥2 months, 10 mg/kg every 12 h for 3 doses then 6 mg/kg daily; severe infections, 10 mg/kg every 12 h for 3 doses, then 10 mg/kg daily. Neonates, 16 mg/kg initial loading dose on day 1, subsequently 8 mg/kg daily.

Widely available.

Further information

Assandri A, Bernareggi A 1987 Binding of teicoplanin to human serum albumin. *European Journal of Pharmacology* 33: 191–195

Campoli-Richards D M, Brogden R N, Faulds D 1990 Teicoplanin. A review of its antibacterial activity, pharmacokinetic properties and therapeutic potential. *Drugs* 40: 449–486

Kureishi A, Jewesson P J, Rubinger M et al 1991 Double-blind comparison of teicoplanin versus vancomycin in febrile neutropenic patients receiving concomitant tobramycin and piperacillin: effect on cyclosporin A-associated nephrotoxicity. *Antimicrobial Agents and Chemotherapy* 35: 2246–2252

Rybak M J, Lerner S A, Levine D P et al 1991 Teicoplanin pharmacokinetics in intravenous drug abusers being treated for bacterial endocarditis. *Antimicrobial Agents and Chemotherapy* 35: 696–700

Stahl J P, Croize J, Wolff M. et al 1987 Poor penetration of teicoplanin into cerebrospinal fluid in patients with bacterial meningitis. *Journal of Antimicrobial Chemotherapy* 20: 141–142

Wilson A P R, Grüneberg R N, Neu H 1994 A critical review of the dosage of teicoplanin in Europe and the USA. *International Journal of Antimicrobial Agents* 4 (suppl 1): S1–S30

Hexamine

F. O'Grady

Introduction

Hexamine has no intrinsic antimicrobial activity and owes its effect to decomposition in acid conditions to formaldehyde, to which all microorganisms are susceptible (minimum inhibitory concentration (MIC) about 20 mg/l). Decomposition is slow, equilibrium concentrations being reached only after 3–4 h, and highly pH dependent, the extent of breakdown being zero at pH 7.0, 5% at pH 6.0 and 20% at pH 5.0. Such acidity is found normally: in the stomach, where the preparations must be protected by enteric coating; on the skin, where topical preparations have been used to control hyperhydrosis; in some cells, where liberation of toxic products can lead to cell death; and in the urine. To facilitate acidification of the urine, hexamine is generally in the form of its salts with organic acids, which exert some antibacterial effect in their own right and reduce the urinary pH to the low levels necessary for the liberation of formaldehyde. Two salts are generally available: hexamine mandelate and hexamine hippurate. The hippurate appears to give higher urinary formaldehyde levels. Mandelic acid is sometimes given alone as a urinary antiseptic, usually as the calcium or ammonium salt. Effective levels of formaldehyde are unlikely to be produced by conventional dosage of hexamine unless the urinary pH is less than 5.8. Breakdown does not occur in the blood and there is neither systemic toxicity nor antimicrobial effect.

Bacterial resistance to formaldehyde has been described but is rare and has not limited long-term therapy.

HEXAMINE
Methenamine; hexamethylenetetramine

Also available as the salts of hippuric and mandelic acids.

Its antimicrobial activity is due to liberation of formaldehyde in acid conditions. Urinary infection with urea-splitting organisms such as *Proteus* spp. causes the urine to become alkaline, and hexamine is unsuitable for these infections.

Pharmacokinetics

It is absorbed from the gut and mainly excreted unchanged in the urine. Unless it is given in enteric-coated tablets, formaldehyde is liberated in the acid of the stomach, with gastro-intestinal distress. It is widely distributed, but at physiological pH there is little breakdown in the blood and no systemic effect or toxicity. It is almost quantitatively excreted into the urine, producing formaldehyde concentrations around 2–60 mg/l. Hexamine hippurate is rapidly and well absorbed on an empty stomach, mean peak plasma concentrations reaching about 30 mg/l, with a half-life of around 14 h. No accumulation occurred in subjects receiving 1 g twice daily. It is widely distributed in a volume which approximates to the total body water and almost 90% appears in the urine in the first 12 h, giving concentrations in excess of 150 mg/l. Little hydrolysis occurs at pH 6.0, and unless the lower urinary pH can be maintained, even at these concentrations, insufficient formaldehyde will be liberated to exert a useful antimicrobial effect.

The odour of sweat is partly due to the action of skin bacteria, and hexamine is included in some deodorant preparations, where on contact with acid sweat it liberates formaldehyde which inhibits bacterial activity and reduces sweating to a sufficient degree for local applications to have been used in the control of hyperhydrosis.

Toxicity and side-effects

Some patients complain of gastro-intestinal upset or frequent and burning micturition. If side-effects are controlled by giving alkali, as is sometimes recommended, the increase in urinary pH abolishes the antibacterial effect of the drug. Contact dermatitis and anterior uveitis have occasionally been encountered. Prolonged administration or high dosage may produce proteinuria, haematuria and bladder changes. Fears about the potential carcinogenicity of formaldehyde have led to warnings about the use of agents which act through its liberation. Large quantities of hexamine are used in diverse industrial processes, where excessive exposure may cause dermatitis and respiratory distress.

Since accumulation does not lead to systemic liberation of toxic products, renal insufficiency is not a contraindication to its use, but it should not be given to patients with acidosis or gout. Because of ammonia liberation in the gut, it is contraindicated in patients with hepatic insufficiency. Hexamine produces a positive Ames' test, but the genetic risk appears to be low.

Clinical use

Hexamine and its salts are not suitable for the treatment of acute urinary tract infection and their main use, now largely supplanted by other agents, has been in long-term prophylaxis or chronic suppressive treatment. Excessive fluid intake lowers the urinary formaldehyde concentration to subeffective levels. Treatment is inapplicable to urea-splitting organisms unless gross alkalinization of the urine is controlled; administration of acetohydroxamic acid, a potent inhibitor of bacterial urease, has been used for this purpose.

Preparations and dosage

Proprietary name: Hiprex (hexamine hippurate).

Preparation: Tablets.

Dosage: Adults, oral 1 g every 12 h; children 6–12 years, 500 mg every 12 h.

Widely available.

Further information

Dreyfors J M, Jones S B, Sayed Y 1989 Hexamethylene-tetramine – a review. *American Industrial Hygiene Association Journal* 50: 579–585

Kolker R J 1991 Medication-induced bilateral anterior ureitis. *Archives of Ophthalmology* 109: 1343

Marren P, deBerker D, Dawber R P, Powell S 1991 Occupational contact dermatitis due to quaternium 15 presenting as nail dystrophy. *Contact Dermatitis* 25: 253–255

Reitz M, Jaeger K H 1989 Effects of methenamine on mouse lymphoma cells. *Arzneimittelforschung* 39: 1411–1412

Introduction

A small group of agents based on a novel structure unlike that of any other antibiotic.

The naturally occurring members of the group are lincomycin and celesticetin, which has only 25% of the activity of lincomycin in vitro, falling to about 5% in vivo, presumably as a result of degradation. Semi-synthetic derivatives of lincomycin have been prepared in the hope of improving on its properties. They have proved to be less active, with the important exception of the chlorinated derivative, clindamycin. Pirlimycin, a clindamycin analogue in which the substituted pyrrolidine moiety is replaced by ethylpiperic acid, is generally less active, but appears to be less extensively metabolized.

They share an unusual antimicrobial spectrum, being active against only Gram-positive and not Gram-negative aerobes, but widely and potently active against anaerobes. They are also active against some mycoplasmas and protozoa.

There are wide geographical variations in the frequency with which resistant staphylococci are found: up to 20% in some areas, while in others they are uncommon. There are reports from various parts of the world of lincosamide-resistant haemolytic streptococci and pneumococci, and these strains are commonly also resistant to erythromycin. Resistance in Bacteroides spp. was originally very rare, but has been increasingly reported from various countries.

They are moderately well absorbed when administered by mouth and distributed widely to tissues, including penetration into cells and bone. Little appears in the urine and the liver is an important route of excretion. Several metabolites have been identified.

They are generally well tolerated, except for the relative frequency with which they have been associated with severe diarrhoea, including Clostridium difficile-associated pseudo-membranous colitis. Diarrhoea is more common in women, and in patients over 60 years of age. In about 40%, diarrhoea abates while treatment is continued. There are no consistent associated changes in bowel flora. A small proportion of patients suffer persistent gastro-intestinal symptoms after cessation of therapy.

Their principal therapeutic indications are penicillin susceptible infections in allergic patients, staphylococcal infections, particularly of bones and joints, and anaerobic infections, including mixed infections for which they must be combined with an agent exhibiting potent activity against aerobic Gram-negative bacilli.

Further information

Phillips I, Wise R (eds) 1985 Macrolides–lincosamides–streptogramins. *Journal of Antimicrobial Chemotherapy* 16 (suppl A): 1–226

CLINDAMYCIN

Semi-synthetic chloro-7-deoxylincomycin supplied as the hydrochloride.

Aqueous solutions are very stable at pH 3.5. It has a very bitter taste, detectable in concentrations as low as 8 mg/l water, which is absent from the ester, clindamycin palmitate. Clindamycin hydrochloride is poorly soluble at neutral pH and too irritating for parenteral use, so clindamycin phosphate is used for this purpose. Capsules of clindamycin contain microbiologically active clindamycin hydrochloride, but the syrup contains clindamycin palmitate and the injectable form clindamycin phosphate, both of which are inactive in vitro and must be hydrolysed to free clindamycin.

Antimicrobial activity

Its spectrum closely resembles that of lincomycin, but it is generally more potent (Table 26.1). It is active against most, but not all, strains of methicillin-resistant *Staphylococcus aureus*. Anaerobic bacteria are generally highly susceptible. Typical minimum inhibitory concentrations (MICs) are: *Prevotella* and *Porphyromonas* spp., 0.1–2 mg/l; *Fusobacterium* spp., <0.5 mg/l; and *Peptostreptococcus* spp., 0.1–0.5 mg/l. It is active against *Toxoplasma gondii* and *Plasmodium falciparum*. The MIC_{90} for *Chlamydia trachomatis* is 16 mg/l, that for *Mobiluncus* spp. is 0.5 mg/l, and that for *Gardnerella vaginalis* is 0.03 mg/l.

It inhibits the bactericidal action of aminoglycosides in vitro against enterobacteria, *Staph. aureus* and *Streptococcus mutans*. In contrast, synergy has been said to occur against some viridans streptococci and, after 24–48 h incubation, against *Staph. aureus*. Synergy with ceftazidime has been demonstrated against a variety of aerobic and anaerobic organisms. The combination with primaquine showed enhanced activity in experimental infections with *Pneumocystis carinii*.

Acquired resistance

Resistance in streptococci, including pneumococci, and *Staph. aureus* follows the pattern for lincomycin with which there is complete cross resistance. Clinically encountered,

Table 26.1 Susceptibility of common pathogenic bacteria: MIC (mg/l)

	Lincomycin	Clindamycin
Staph. aureus	0.5–2	0.1–1
Str. pyogenes	0.05–1	0.01–0.25
Str. pneumoniae	0.1–1	0.05
Ent. faecalis	2–64	0.05–64
N. gonorrhoeae	8–64	0.5–4
N. meningitidis	>32	4
H. influenzae	4–16	0.5–16
Enterobacteria	R	R
B. fragilis	2–4	0.02–2

R, resistant.

including epidemic, strains may exhibit the inducible form of resistance which also involves macrolides and streptogramins. Resistance in faecal *Bacteroides* spp. is increasing. *Bacteroides fragilis* has been divided into three groups: highly susceptible (MIC <0.25 mg/l); susceptible (MIC 0.25–4 mg/l) and resistant (MIC ≥8 mg/l). About 10% of *B. fragilis* strains (rather more in other species) have been found resistant in the USA. Prevalence of resistance varies from negligible levels in some parts of Europe to 25% in others. Most strains are also resistant to erythromycin, but susceptible to other unrelated drugs. Resistance arises readily in vitro and resistant strains can be recovered from the faeces of treated patients.

Pharmacokinetics

Oral doses of 150, 300 and 600 mg of the hydrochloride produce peak plasma concentrations close to 2, 4 and 8 mg/l, respectively, at 1–2 h (Table 26.2). Plasma levels in

Table 26.2 Plasma concentrations following administration of lincosamides

Agent	Route	Dose (mg)	Peak Hour	Peak mg/l	Half-life (h)
Lincomycin hydrochloride	Oral	500	4	2–7	4–6
	i.m.	200		3.5–4.2	
		600	1–2	8.0–18.0	4–6
	i.v.	300	0	8.0–22.0	3.5–5
Clindamycin hydrochloride	Oral	300	1–2	3.6	2–3
Clindamycin palmitate	Oral	300	1	1.4–4.2	
Clindamycin phosphate	i.m.	300	4	3.8	1.5–4
	i.v.	300	0	4.3–6.6	
		600		7.9–8.7	

pregnant women following a single oral dose of 450 mg (3.4–9 mg/l) were similar to those found in non-pregnant women. Binding to plasma protein is high at 94%. Behaviour of the palmitate, which is rapidly hydrolysed in the gut before absorption, is similar. The presence of food does not depress or delay oral absorption. No free ester has been detected in human serum after a 600 mg dose.

In contrast, clindamycin phosphate is absorbed intact after intramuscular (i.m.) injection and relatively slowly hydrolysed by alkaline phosphatases. A substantial amount of unhydrolysed clindamycin phosphate (1–2 mg/l) has been detected in the serum at 30–60 min and up to 10% of the dose may still be present as phosphate after 8 h. The bioavailability in relation to dose was linear, but not proportional; that is to say, the plasma concentration was not doubled when the dose was doubled. Following a dose of 300 mg i.m., mean peak plasma concentrations of 5–6 mg/l were attained only after 2.5–3 h. The mean plasma concentration 15 min after the same dose i.v. was 15 mg/l. The plasma half-life is significantly longer in premature than in term infants (8.7 and 3.6 h, respectively).

After intravaginal administration of 5 ml of 2% clindamycin phosphate cream (= 100 mg) to healthy women and women suffering from bacterial vaginosis, less than 5% of the dose was subsequently found in the plasma.

Distribution

After hydrolysis in the serum, clindamycin phosphate is rapidly and widely distributed, but in at least four different forms: the phosphate itself, clindamycin base, clindamycose and the demethyl and sulphoxide derivatives. Demethyl clindamycin is as active, but the sulphoxide less active than the base.

Levels in the CSF are low: 0.14–0.46 mg/l, following a single dose of 150 mg. Levels in brain are low or absent. An intrathecal dose of 1–2 mg has been recommended as being safe and efficacious in producing cerebrospinal fluid (CSF) levels in excess of 6 mg/l. Following an oral dose of 300 mg, mean peak concentrations in ventricular fluid approximated to those in the serum but were more persistent.

In patients undergoing caesarean section, mean peak fetal plasma concentrations of about 3 mg/l (46% maternal level) have been found after a 600 mg intravenous (i.v.) dose of clindamycin phosphate.

In patients receiving three similar 8-hourly injections, the last immediately before operation, the mean concentrations in both cancellous and cortical bone were around 3.8 mg/l. The ratio of tissue to serum concentration has been found to be 1.0 in bone marrow, 0.5–0.75 in spongy and 0–0.15 in compact bone. Hydroxyapatite binds clindamycin and probably also the ester. Levels of the phosphate may exceed those of the base in bone and soft tissue and be considerably higher than the simultaneous serum level.

A similar situation may develop in leucocytes. Uptake into neutrophils is rapid, temperature dependent, saturable and depressed by acid pH. Clindamycin is accumulated by lysosomes to active concentrations around 40 times those of the extracellular fluid. After an initially high rate of hydrolysis, which may be accompanied by an increase in intracellular alkaline phosphatase, enzyme activity declines, presumably as a result of the rising concentration of inorganic phosphate, and after 4 h, around half of the drug is still unhydrolysed. Similar product inhibition may prevent the complete hydrolysis of the phosphate in pus where alkaline phosphatase is liberated from neutrophils. Clindamycin hydrochloride does not penetrate neutrophils.

Excretion

Only about 13% of an oral dose can be recovered from the urine, although levels are considerably higher after multiple (80–800 mg/l) than after single doses (50–250 mg/l). Less than 10% of a parenteral dose of clindamycin phosphate is excreted unchanged in the urine. Bioactivity persists in the urine for up to 4 days, suggesting slow release of the drug from tissues or body fluids. In patients with severe renal disease, plasma levels were 3–4 times normal and high levels persisted for over 24 h, but this has been said to result from the loss of normally important renal binding sites. Orally administered clindamycin is excreted in patients with renal insufficiency, although urinary recovery of the drug, already low in normal subjects, can fall below 1% in severe renal failure.

Clindamycin is not removed by haemodialysis. In uraemic patients given a 30 min i.v. infusion of 300 mg of the more diversely handled phosphate, the average level immediately after the end of the infusion (12.8 mg/l) was considerably higher than that observed in normal subjects (5.4 mg/l); elimination was also greatly prolonged, possibly as a result of changes in the disposition or degradation of the drug.

Liver. The liver plays a significant part in the elimination of clindamycin phosphate, which may be slowly converted to the base in patients with hepatic impairment. After 600 mg infused intravenously over 2 h, the bile at 1 h contained 67 mg/l. Most of the activity was due to the desmethyl metabolite. Patients with proven hepatic cirrhosis show significant impairment of clindamycin elimination. The plasma half-life varied from 0.6 to 4.7 h in patients with liver disease without ascites or biliary obstruction. The volume of distribution and serum protein binding (79%) was similar to that in normal subjects.

In patients with patent common ducts undergoing biliary tract surgery, the concentrations in gallbladder bile, common duct bile, gallbladder wall and liver were 2–3 times those in serum. Where the common duct was obstructed, none could be detected in bile and the level was lower in gallbladder wall, but the concentration in liver was slightly higher than in those without obstruction. The ranges found when the serum concentration was 10–30 mg/l were: gallbladder bile 8–100 mg/l, common duct bile 15–170 mg/l and gallbladder wall 5–45 mg/kg. Less than 5% of an oral dose can be recovered from the faeces.

Toxicity and side-effects

Rashes occur in about 10% of patients but severe eruptions are rare. Drug fever and eosinophilia also occur. Granulocytopenia and thrombocytopenia have been noted. Diarrhoea has developed in 10–30% of patients and pseudomembranous colitis in 1–2%. Parenteral administration can cause elevation of transaminases and serum alkaline phosphatase, but there has not generally been accompanying hyperbilirubinaemia and other evidence of hepatotoxicity is rare. The changes may be due to muscle damage or to interference with the tests. Intravenous administration may be complicated by thrombophlebitis.

Isolated episodes of toxic epidermal necrolysis have been reported with oral clindamycin and there is a single report of prolonged neuromuscular blockade after an accidental i.v. overdose (2.4 g instead of 600 mg).

Clinical use

Clindamycin has been successfully used for the treatment of staphylococcal infection, including that due to methicillin-resistant strains, particularly of bones and joints (p. 761). In some cases of endocarditis, failure has been due to emergence of resistance. It has been used as a penicillin substitute in allergic patients for the treatment of streptococcal, including pneumococcal, infection but its use in respiratory infection may be unsuccessful because of the persistence or emergence of *H. influenzae*. It is said to be suitable for the treatment of diphtheria (p. 676) and carriers. It has not been reliably effective in the treatment of infection due to *Mycoplasma pneumoniae*. It is an effective adjunct treatment in chloroquine-resistant falciparum malaria.

It is effective for the prophylaxis and treatment of anaerobic infections (pp. 588, 736, 739) and is indicated where *B. fragilis* is suspected, as in intra-abdominal sepsis and infections of the female genito-urinary tract, including bacterial vaginosis (p. 806). It has been successfully used in aspiration lung abscess (p. 689). It is not recommended for the treatment of infections of the central nervous system or for infections with peptococci. It should be supplemented with penicillin G where there are anaerobes likely to be resistant to clindamycin and with appropriate agents where the infection is likely to include aerobic Gram-negative rods. It should be noted that clostridia and enterococci are resistant to aminoglycosides and superinfection can arise in patients receiving the combination. Reference is made to its use in treatment of pneumonia (p. 685), sore throat

(p. 677), actinomycosis (p. 739), acne (p. 740) and toxoplasmosis (p. 670). It has been used in combination with quinine in babesiosis.

Preparations and dosage

Proprietary names: Dalacin C, Dalacin T.

Preparations: Capsules, suspension, injection.

Dosage: Adults, oral, 150–300 mg every 6 h, increased to 450 mg every 6 h for severe infections. Children, oral, 3–6 mg/kg every 6 h. Adults, i.m., i.v., 600 mg to 1.2 g daily in 2–4 equal doses; more severe infections, 1.2–2.7 g/day in 2–4 equal doses. Children >1 month, i.m., i.v., 15–25 mg/kg per day in 3–4 divided doses; severe infections, 25–40 mg/kg in 3–4 divided doses; in severe infections it is recommended that children are given no less than 300 mg/day, regardless of body weight.

Widely available.

Further information

Ahmed Jushuf I H, Shahmanesh M, Arya O P 1995 The treatment of bacterial vaginosis with a 3 day course of 2% clindamycin cream: results of a multicentre, double blind, placebo controlled trial. *Genitourinary Medicine* 71: 254–256

Al Ahdal O, Bevan D R 1995 Clindamycin-induced neuromuscular blockade. *Canadian Journal of Anaesthesia* 42: 614–617

Bell M J, Shackelford P, Smith R, Schroeder K 1984 Pharmacokinetics of clindamycin phosphate in the first year of life. *Journal of Paediatrics* 105: 482–486

Blais J, Tardif C, Chamberland S 1993 Effect of clindamycin on intracellular replication, protein synthesis, and infectivity of *Toxoplasma gondii*. *Antimicrobial Agents and Chemotherapy* 37: 2571–2577

Borin M T, Powley G W, Tackwell K R, Batts D H 1995 Absorption of clindamycin after intravaginal application of clindamycin phosphate 2% cream. *Journal of Antimicrobial Chemotherapy* 35: 833–841

Easmon C S, Crane J P 1984 Cellular uptake of clindamycin and lincomycin. *British Journal of Experimental Pathology* 65: 725–730

Falagas M E, Gorbach S L 1995 Clindamycin and metronidazole. *Medical Clinics of North America* 79: 845–867

Fischbach F, Petersen E E, Weissenbacher E R, Martius J, Hosmann J, Mayer H O 1993 Efficacy of clindamycin vaginal cream versus oral metronidazole in the treatment of bacterial vaginosis. *Obstetrics and Gynecology* 82: 405–410

Goldstein E J C, Citron D M, Cherubin C E, Hillier S L 1993 Comparative susceptibility of the *Bacteroides fragilis* group species and other anaerobic bacteria to meropenem, imipenem, piperacillin, cefoxitin, ampicillin/sulbactam, clindamycin and metronidazole. *Journal of Antimicrobial Chemotherapy* 31: 363–372

Klainer A S 1987 Clindamycin. *Medical Clinics of North America* 71: 1169–1175

Kremsner P G, Radloff P, Metzger W et al 1995 Quinine plus clindamycin improves chemotherapy of severe malaria in children. *Antimicrobial Agents and Chemotherapy* 39: 1603–1605

Mann H J 1987 Decreased hepatic clearance of clindamycin in critically ill patients with sepsis. *Clinical Pharmacy* 6: 154–159

Oleske J M, Phillips I (eds) 1983 Clindamycin:bacterial virulence and host defence. *Journal of Antimicrobial Chemotherapy* 12 (suppl C): 1–122

Paquet P, Schaaf-Lafontaine N, Piérard G E 1995 Toxic epidermal necrolysis following clindamycin treatment. *British Journal of Dermatology* 132: 665–666

Plaisance K I, Drusano G L, Forrest A, Townsend R J, Standiford H C 1989 Pharmacokinetic evaluation of two dosage regimens of clindamycin phosphate. *Antimicrobial Agents and Chemotherapy* 33: 618–620

Rolston K V 1988 Clindamycin in cerebral toxoplasmosis. *American Journal of Medicine* 85: 285

Townsend R J, Baker R P 1987 Pharmacokinetic comparison of three clindamycin phosphate dosing schedules. *Drug Intelligence and Clinical Pharmacy* 21: 279–281

LINCOMYCIN

A fermentation product of *Streptomyces lincolnensis* var. *lincolnensis* supplied as the hydrochloride. The dry crystalline hydrochloride is very stable.

Antimicrobial activity

It is active against Gram-positive organisms, notably staphylococci, haemolytic streptococci and pneumococci (Table 26.1). *Corynebacterium diphtheriae*, *Bacillus anthracis* and *Nocardia asteroides* are all susceptible, but mycobacteria are resistant. Most streptococci (except enterococci) are inhibited by <1 mg/l. Enterobacteria, *Haemophilus* spp. and *Neisseria* spp. are resistant. It is active against anaerobic bacteria, including anaerobic cocci and Gram-negative rods. Clostridia are more resistant than other anaerobes, although *Clostridium perfringens* is generally susceptible (MIC 0.5–2 mg/l). *Mycoplasma hominis* is susceptible (MIC 0.4–1.6 mg/l), but ureaplasmas are resistant. Leptospira are susceptible.

Acquired resistance

There is complete cross-resistance between clindamycin and lincomycin. Resistance is relatively easily produced in vitro, particularly in erythromycin-resistant strains. Lincomycin shares cross-resistance with erythromycin and streptogramins in strains showing inducible resistance (p. 383). Plasmid-mediated resistance in streptococci and *Staph. aureus* due to lincomycin inactivation has also been described. In some streptococci, inducible or constitutive cross resistance is plasmid encoded. Resistance of the oral viridans streptococci to both erythromycin and lincomycin has been seen to emerge in patients treated with lincomycin for as little as 3 days.

Pharmacokinetics

It is readily absorbed when given by mouth. Following a dose of 0.5 g mean peak plasma levels of 2–3 mg/l have been found at 2–4 h (Table 26.2). Food significantly delays and decreases absorption, the mean peak plasma level from a dose given immediately after a meal being only about half the fasting levels. It is also promptly and completely absorbed from intramuscular sites, mean peak plasma levels of 9–10 mg/l being found 0.5 h after a dose of 0.6 g. Following the same dose by rapid i.v. infusion, the plasma concentration was 18–20 mg/l. The mean end-infusion value following i.v. infusion of 2.1 g over 2 h was 37 mg/l. Constant, near maximum levels can be maintained on 4–6-hourly schedules. Much the same results have been obtained in children. It is 72% bound to plasma protein.

Distribution

It is widely distributed in a volume approximating to the total body water, but levels in normal CSF are low. In the presence of inflammation, ratios of CSF to serum concentration around 0.4 have been found; penetration occurs into cerebral abscesses. Concentrations in saliva and sputum approximate to the simultaneous serum level. Levels of 1.5–6.9 mg lincomycin/l of cord serum or amniotic fluid have been found after the mother received 600 mg i.m. and

0.5–2.4 mg/l in human milk after the second of two maternal 0.5 g doses.

In patients undergoing total hip replacement and given 600 mg lincomycin i.m. 6 h preoperatively, and again perioperatively by i.v. infusion, mean concentrations in capsule were 9.4 mg/kg, synovial fluid 5.4 mg/l, cancellous bone 7.2 mg/kg and cortical bone 5.4 mg/kg.

Peak concentrations of 30–135 mg/l were found in the aqueous humour 1–2 h after subconjunctival injection of 75 mg in all but one case, with plasma levels of the order of 2–3 mg/l within 10 min of subconjunctival injection.

Excretion

Urinary concentrations are generally low except after i.v. injection. Only 3–4% of the dose appears in the urine over 24 h after an oral dose, but up to 60% after i.v. administration, mostly in the first 4 h.

It appears to be virtually non-dialysable, since its plasma half-life in dialysed and undialysed azotaemic patients is approximately the same.

The liver is an important route of elimination and the proportion of the dose appearing in the urine increases in patients with severe hepatic dysfunction. About 40% of an oral dose can be recovered from the faeces, some 5–15% as metabolites probably eliminated in the bile.

Concentrations up to 7 and 10 mg/kg have been found in faeces after oral doses of 1.5 and 4 g. In patients with liver disease, the plasma half-life is approximately doubled.

Toxicity and side-effects

Nausea, vomiting and abdominal cramps may occur, but most authors have reported no side-effects apart from diarrhoea, which has commonly affected about 10% of patients – more in some series. It can occur after oral or parenteral administration and is more common in older patients and uncommon in children. It is more related to dosage than duration of treatment. It usually begins within a few days of the institution of therapy, but may develop after treatment has stopped. It usually persists for 1–2 weeks but may continue for months.

The spectrum of intestinal responses extends from bloodless watery diarrhoea without fever or leucocytosis to severe, often bloody, diarrhoea, with abdominal pain progressing to profound shock and dehydration with high mortality, despite vigorous treatment of *Cl. difficile* infection.

Hypersensitivity reactions are rare. Transient changes occur in liver function tests which are generally due to interference with the tests, since abnormalities in specific enzyme tests and clinical evidence of hepatic dysfunction are rare.

In some patients receiving large doses by rapid i.v. injection, the blood pressure has fallen precipitately with nausea, vomiting, arrhythmias and, exceptionally, cardiac arrest. These cardiac effects may be due to structural similarity to quinine. It can transiently depress neuromuscular transmission and might depress respiration after anaesthesia, but the effect is much weaker than that of neomycin.

Infants born to mothers treated in pregnancy have shown no abnormalities.

Clinical use

It has been used for the treatment of streptococcal pharyngitis, Gram-positive coccal otitis media, pneumonia and pyoderma in adults and children. It is a suitable substitute for penicillin in Gram-positive coccal infections where penicillin is contraindicated. Clindamycin is now generally used in preference to lincomycin for these indications.

Preparations and dosage

Preparations: Capsules, syrup, injection.

Dosage: Adults, oral, 500 mg, 3–4 times daily; i.m., 600 mg, 1–2 times daily; i.v. infusion, 600 mg to 1 g, 2–3 times daily. Children >1 month, oral, 30–60 mg/kg per day in divided doses; i.m., i.v., 10–20 mg/kg per day in divided doses.

Limited availability, not available in the UK.

Further information

Gwilt P R, Smith R B 1986 Protein binding and pharmacokinetics of lincomycin following intravenous administration of high doses. *Journal of Clinical Pharmacology* 26: 87–90

Mickal A, Panzer J D 1975 The safety of lincomycin in pregnancy. *American Journal of Obstetrics and Gynecology* 121: 1071–1074

Nielsen M L, Hansen I, Nielsen J B 1976 The penetration of lincomycin into normal human bone. *Acta Orthopaedica Scandinavica* 47: 267–270

Parsons R L, Beavis J P, Hossack G A, Paddock G M 1977 Plasma, bone, hip capsule synovial and drain fluid concentration of lincomycin during total hip replacement. *British Journal of Clinical Pharmacology* 4: 433–437

Smith R B, Lummis W L, Monovich R E, DeSante K A 1981 Lincomycin serum and saliva concentrations after intramuscular injection of high doses. *Journal of Clinical Pharmacology* 21: 411–417

Macrolides

A. Bryskier and J. P. Butzler

Introduction

The macrolides form a large group of closely similar naturally occurring antibiotics produced mostly by streptomyces. They consist of a macrocyclic lactone ring (to which they owe their generic name) to which typically two sugars, one an amino sugar, are attached. Interest in the group has been greatly stimulated by the activity of older compounds, notably erythromycin, against a number of newer emergent pathogens, including some encountered in immunocompromised patients, and Campylobacter and Legionella. Focusing on erythromycin has emphasized both its desirable properties and its deficiencies, and stimulated the search for analogues with extended antimicrobial range, notably against Gram-negative pathogens, improved pharmacokinetic properties, notably increased acid resistance, and reduced gastro-intestinal intolerance.

A rapidly growing number of compounds has been synthesized. The groups of macrolides which contain the most important therapeutic agents are characterized by 14-, 15- or 16-membered-ring macrolides. In the group that includes erythromycin and oleandomycin, the large lactone ring contains 14 atoms and one or two sugar groups are attached by α- or β-glycosidic linkages to the aglycone. Macrolides commercially available or in clinical development include 14-, 15- and 16-membered lactone ring compounds. Some newer derivatives of erythromycin A (14-membered-ring macrolides) are roxithromycin, dirithromycin, flurithromycin and clarithromycin and the azalide azithromycin.

In the other group of which josamycin is typical, the large ring contains 16 atoms and the two sugars are linked together and attached to the ring through the amino sugar. The natural 16-membered-ring macrolides include josamycin, kitasamycin, spiramycin and midecamycin, and there are two semi-synthetic derivatives: rokitamycin and miokamycin.

Insertion of a methyl-substituted nitrogen into the lactone ring of erythromycin A has produced a 15-membered ring macrolide, azithromycin, which belongs to the chemical class also known as azalides. It exhibits increased potency against Gram-negative bacteria, improved oral absorption, more extensive distribution and a longer half-life than the parent macrolide. Chemically, azalides are not macrolides – even though they are semi-synthetic erythromycin A derivatives – but they share the same antibacterial spectrum as typical macrolides with expansion to Gram-negative rods. It therefore seems reasonable to separate azalides as a subgroup within macrolides rather than to create a new chemical group. Azalides share the main clinical indications of macrolide antibiotics. Azithromycin is the first azalide to reach clinical use.

Antimicrobial activity

There are no major systematic differences in antimicrobial activity between the 14-, 15- and 16-membered-ring macrolides, which share the same antibacterial spectrum including most Gram-positive organisms, *Neisseria* spp., *Haemophilus* spp., *Bordetella pertussis* and both Gram-positive and Gram-negative anaerobes (Table 27.1). Except for azithromycin, other available macrolides exhibit poor activity against enterobacteria.

The new macrolides and azalides are active against *Streptococcus pneumoniae*, *Streptococcus pyogenes*, *Streptococcus agalactiae*, *Moraxella catarrhalis*, *Bordetella pertussis*, *Neisseria gonorrhoeae*, *Campylobacter jejuni*, *Rhodococcus equi*, *Haemophilus ducreyi*, *Gardnerella vaginalis*, *Mobiluncus* spp., *Propionibacterium acnes*, *Borrelia burgdorferi* and *Treponema pallidum*. Activity against *Staphylococcus aureus* is variable. The new oral compounds do not provide a significant advantage over erythromycin A against staphylococci and streptococci, and they are poorly active against enterococci. The minimum inhibitory concentrations (MICs) for *Haemophilus influenzae* range from 0.25

Table 27.1 *Susceptibility (MIC: mg/l) of common pathogenic bacteria to macrolides*

	Azithro-mycin	Erythro-mycin	Josa-mycin	Mideka-mycin	Mioca-mycin	Oleando-mycin	Rosara-mycin	Roxithro-mycin	Spira-mycin
Staph. aureus	0.25–1	0.1–1	0.25–4	0.5–2	0.5–1	0.25–4	0.1–2	0.1–2	0.25–1
Strep. pyogenes	0.03–0.1	0.01–0.25	0.06–0.5	0.1–2	0.5–2	0.1–1	0.1–0.5	0.06–0.25	0.1–2
Strep. pneumoniae	0.03–0.25	0.01–0.25	0.03–0.5	0.1–0.5		0.1–2	0.1–0.25	0.03–16	0.01–4
E. faecalis	0.5–R	0.5–4	0.5–4	1–4	0.5–R	2–4	0.25–4	0.5–8	2–4
N. gonorrhoeae	0.03–2	0.03–0.5	0.5–2			2–4	0.01–0.1	0.03–2	2–4
N. meningitidis		0.25–2				2–4	0.06–0.5	0.03–2	
H. influenzae	0.25–2	0.5–8	2–16	1–4	0.25–32	0.1–2	0.1–2	0.5–16	2–8
Esch. coli	0.5–2	8–32						32	
Salmonella	2–16	32–128	R	R	R	R	16–32	R	R
Shigella	0.5–4	16–64							
B. fragilis	0.5–16	0.1–16	0.06–1	2–32	0.5–2		0.5–8	0.25–64	

to 8 mg/l, azithromycin being the most active. The 14-OH metabolite of clarithromycin acts synergistically in vitro with clarithromycin. Variable susceptibilities are reported for *B. bronchiseptica, Listeria monocytogenes, Corynebacterium jeikeium, E. corrodens, Pasteurella multocida, Bacteroides fragilis, Prevotella melaninogenicus, Fusobacterium* spp. and *Clostridium perfringens.* Activity against respiratory pathogens is shown in Table 27.2.

The new macrolides and azalides exert important activity against intracellular pathogens, including: *Chlamydia trachomatis* (MICs being clarithromycin 0.007 mg/l, azithromycin 0.125 mg/l and roxithromycin, 0.06 mg/l) *Ureaplasma urealyticum, Mycoplasma pneumoniae, Legionella pneumophila* and other *Legionella* spp. (MICs being clarithromycin 0.03–0.06 mg/l, azithromycin and roxithromycin 0.03–0.05 mg/l); *Mycobacterium avium* complex (MICs being clarithromycin 0.25–4.0 mg/l,

Table 27.2 *In vitro activity of macrolides against respiratory pathogens: MIC$_{50}$ (mg/l)^a*

	Erythro-mycin	Azithro-mycin	Clarithro-mycin	Dirithro-mycin	Roxithro-mycin
Strep. pneumoniae	0.03	0.06	0.015	0.06	0.03
Strep. pyogenes	0.03	0.12	0.015	0.12	0.06
H. influenzae	4.00	0.25	4.00	8.00	4.00
Mor. catarrhalis	0.12	0.03	0.06	0.12	0.25
M. pneumoniae	0.01	0.01	0.01	0.03	0.03
C. pneumoniae	0.06	0.06	0.25	0.50	0.05
L. pneumophila	1.00	0.50	0.12	1.00	0.25

^{a}Adapted from Bryskier A, Labro M 1994 Macrolides, nouvelles perspectives thérapeutiques. *Presse Médicale* 23: 1762–1766.

azithromycin and roxithromycin 4–32 mg/l); and *M. lepra* and *Rickettsia* spp. (MICs being 1–2 mg/l). Azithromycin appears to be the most active of the compounds against *Brucella melitensis.*

Acquired resistance

Widespread use of the older agents has led to the emergence of resistance notably in *Staph. aureus* and later in group A streptococci. Resistance to erythromycin A is of both chromosomal and plasmid origin, and can be inducible or constitutive. Intrinsic resistance of Gram-negative bacilli to macrolides is probably due to the relative impermeability of the cellular outer membrane to the hydrophobic compounds. However, in azithromycin, the nitrogen inserted into the lactone ring contributes to improved activity against Gram-negative bacteria – in particular *Haemophilus* spp.

Acquired resistance to macrolides involves three mechanisms: modification of the target, drug inactivation and active efflux of the antibiotics. In the first type of resistance, a single alteration in 23 S ribosomal RNA confers broad cross-resistance to macrolides, azalides, lincosamides and streptogramin-B-type antibiotics (the so-called MLS phenotype), whereas the two other types confer resistance to structurally related antibiotics only.

Pharmacokinetics

Erythromycin, the first available macrolide antibiotic, is characterized by poor water solubility and rapid inactivation by stomach acid, which results in widely varying bioavailability after oral administration. Minor structural alterations of erythromycin have resulted in improved pharmacokinetic properties, including bioavailability, gastro intestinal tolerance, higher peak serum levels, longer apparent elimination serum half-lives and improved tissue concentrations. Macrolides are given by mouth, but oral absorption and bioavailability vary from one drug to the next, partly reflected in differences in daily dosage. Oral absorption is rapid, with plasma peaks varying between 0.4 mg/l (azithromycin) and 11.0 mg/l (roxithromycin). Maximum concentrations are reached between 0.5 hours (rokitamycin) and 3.0 h (clarithromycin) and are dose dependent.

Erythromycin and oleandomycin (14-membered-ring macrolides) induce hepatic microsomal enzymes and interfere via the cytochrome P450 system with clearance of such drugs as theophylline, antipyrine and carbamazepine, with a resultant increase in their blood levels. The induced isoenzymes of cytochrome P450 rapidly demethylate and oxidize macrolides to nitrosoalkanes, which combine with the iron of the enzymes, thereby inactivating them. The 16-membered-ring macrolides such as josamycin and spiramycin have no such effect. Erythromycin base, estolate and stearate and a metabolite of triacetyloleandomycin all form stable complexes with cytochrome P450; josamycin base forms an unstable complex, and josamycin propionate, spiramycin base and adipate do not bind.

The apparent elimination half-life varies from 1 h (miokamycin) to 44 hours (dirithromycin); the absolute bioavailability varies between 10% (dirithromycin) and 55–60% (roxithromycin, clarithromycin). The absolute bioavailability of azithromycin is about 37%. The main elimination route is via the bile and faeces; a proportion of clarithomycin is excreted via the intestinal mucosa. A substantial part of the administered dose of clarithomycin is eliminated in urine. The long elimination half-lives of roxithromycin, azithromycin and dirithromycin allow them to be administered as single daily oral doses.

Toxicity and side-effects

Macrolides are generally safe drugs and serious adverse events are rare. A notable exception is erythromycin estolate, which has considerable hepatotoxicity and may cause severe hepatitis, probably as a result of the mixture of lauryl sulphate and the 2'-propionyl ester. Gastro-intestinal complaints (nausea, vomiting, abdominal pain or, more infrequently, diarrhoea) are the most common side-effects reported with macrolide therapy. These reactions present a problem mainly when erythromycin doses higher than normal are used (e.g. for treatment of infections caused by pathogens with reduced susceptibility). These gastro-intestinal effects are partly due to the hemiketal degradation product which acts on motilin.

Structural modification renders the newer macrolides more acid stable, with fewer side-effects as compared with erythromycin. Some macrolides, depending on their structures, interact with several other drugs, markedly changing their pharmacokinetics (p. 104).

Clinical use

The new macrolides retain the classic clinical applications of the older compounds, including activity against intracellular pathogens (e.g. *Legionella, Chlamydia, Rickettsia* spp.). Their improved pharmacokinetic properties and tissue distribution may prove useful in more unusual settings such as infections due to mycobacteria and protozoa (e.g. *Toxoplasma gondii, Entamoeba histolytica, Plasmodium falciparum*). Other potential target infections are chronic gastritis (*Helicobacter pylori*) and borreliosis (*Borrelia burgdorferi*).

Further information

Bryskier A 1992 Newer macrolides and their potential target organisms. *Current Opinion in Infectious Diseases* 5: 764–772

Bryskier A, Agouridas C 1993 Azalides, a new medicinal chemical entity? *Current Opinion and Investigational Drugs* 2: 687–694

Bryskier A, Labro M T 1994 Macrolides – Nouvelles perspectives thérapeutiques. *Presse Médicale* 23: 1762–1766

Butzler J P, Kobayashi H 1985 Macrolides: a review without outlook on future development. Excerpta Medica, Amsterdam, p 157

Bryskier A, Butzler J P, Neu H C, Tulkens P M (eds) 1993 Macrolides, chemistry, pharmacology and clinical uses. Blackwell-Arnette, Paris, p 698

Hardy D J, Hensey D M, Beyer J M, Vojkko C, McDonald E J, Fernandes P B 1988 Comparative in vitro activity of new 14-, 15-, and 16-membered macrolides. *Antimicrobial Agents and Chemotherapy* 32: 1710–1719

Kirst H A 1992 New macrolides: expanded horizons for an old class of antibiotic. *Journal of Antimicrobial Chemotherapy* 28: 787–790

Kirst H A, Sides G D 1989 New directions for macrolide antibiotics: pharmacokinetics and clinical efficacy. *Antimicrobial Agents and Chemotherapy* 33: 1419–1422

Neu H C, Young L S, Zinner S H 1993 The new macrolides, azalides and streptogramins. In: Pharmacology and clinical applications. Marcel Dekker, New York, p 228

Phillips I, Williams J D 1985 Macrolides, lincosamides, streptogramins. *Journal of Antimicrobial and Chemotherapy* 16 (suppl A)

Williams J D, Sefton A M 1993 Comparison of macrolide antibiotics. *Journal of Antimicrobial and Chemotherapy* (suppl C): 11–26

AZITHROMYCIN

A 15-membered-ring azalide.

Antimicrobial activity

Its activity against common pathogenic bacteria is shown in Table 27.2. It is less potent than erythromycin against Gram-positive isolates but is more active against Gram-negative bacteria. It is four times more potent than erythromycin against *H. influenzae*, *N. gonorrhoeae* and *Campylobacter* spp. It is twice as active as erythromycin against *Mor. catarrhalis* and β-lactamase-producing *Neisseria* spp. In comparison with erythromycin, it exhibits superior potency against all of the *Enterobacteriaceae*, notably *Esch. coli* and *Salmonella* spp. and *Shigella* spp. It is also active against *Mycobacteria*, notably *M. avium* complex. It is active against intracellular micro-organisms such as *Legionella* spp. and *Chlamydia* spp. Its activity against common pathogens is shown in Tables 27.1 and 27.2.

Pharmacokinetics

Chemical modification of erythromycin to give azithromycin blocks the internal dehydrogenation pathway and markedly improves acid stability. At pH 2, loss of 10% activity occurred in less than 4 s with erythromycin, but took 20 min with azithromycin. A 500 mg oral dose is around 37% bioavailable, giving mean peak plasma levels around 0.4 mg/l at about 6 h. The area under the curve (AUC) at 0–2 h is 3.39 mg/h per litre. The level is only slightly increased on repeated dosing.

Binding to plasma protein varies with the concentration, from around 50% at 0.05 mg/l to 7.1% at 1 mg/l. The apparent elimination half-life is dependent upon sampling interval: between 8 and 24 h it ranged from 11 to 14 h; between 24 h and 72 h it was 35–40 h. Azithromycin rapidly penetrates the tissues, reaching levels which approach or, in some cases, exceed the simultaneous plasma levels and persist for 2–3 days. Only about 6% of the dose was recovered from the urine in the first 24 h.

Toxicity and side-effects

It is well tolerated with little gastro-intestinal disturbance.

Clinical use

The clinical efficacy of azithromycin has been demonstrated in the treatment of lower and upper respiratory tract infections (including those in children), skin and soft-tissue infections (including those in children), and in uncomplicated urethritis/cervicitis associated with *N. gonorrhoeae*, *Chl. trachomatis* or *U. urealyticum*.

Preparations and dosage

Proprietary name: Zithromax.

Preparations: Capsules, suspension.

Dosage: Adults, oral, 500 mg/day for 3 days. Children >6 months, 10 mg/kg once daily for 3 days; or, children, body weight 15–25 kg, 200 mg/day for 3 days; body weight 26–35 kg, 300 mg/day for 3 days; body weight 36–45 kg, 400 mg/day for 3 days.

Available in Europe and the USA.

Further information

Leigh D A, Ridgway G L, Leeming J P, Speller D C E 1990 Azithromycin (CP 62,993): the first azalide antimicrobial agent. *Journal of Antimicrobial and Chemotherapy* 25 (suppl A)

CLARITHROMYCIN

A 14-membered-ring semi-synthetic macrolide obtained from erythromycin A (6-*O*-methylerythromycin A).

Antimicrobial activity

Against macrolide-susceptible common pathogens, the MIC values are 10-fold less than the MIC of erythromycin. Clarithromycin inhibits most of the respiratory pathogens at a concentration of $\leq$0.25 mg/l, with the exception of *H. influenzae* (MIC 1–8 mg/l) (Table 27.2). It is twice as active as erythromycin against *Str. pyogenes* (MIC$_{90}$ 0.015 mg/l) and the 14-OH metabolite is equivalent in activity to erythromycin (MIC$_{90}$ 0.03 mg/l). Similar activity is found against *Str. pneumoniae*. It inhibits *Mycoplasma pneumoniae* at $\leq$0.008 mg/l and *M. catarrhalis* at 0.25 mg/l. It is eight-fold more active than erythromycin against *Legionella* spp. and *C. trachomatis*. Against anaerobic species activity is similar. Against *H. influenzae* it has half the activity of erythromycin with MIC$_{90}$ values of 8 mg/l, but the 14-hydroxy metabolite is more active (MIC 4 mg/l) and bactericidal at concentrations close to the MIC, an action which appears to be potentiated by the presence of the parent compound.

Pharmacokinetics

It is stable to gastric acid and rapidly absorbed orally giving 55% bioavailability. Its absorption is not affected by food. Following doses of 250 or 500 mg, mean peak plasma levels are around 1–2.5 mg/l at 1–2 h with a plasma elimination half-life of 3.5–5 h. The half-life of the main 14-hydroxy metabolite is longer (around 7 h). It penetrates the tissue of the respiratory tract, giving concentrations in tonsil and lung which exceed the simultaneous plasma level two-fold and four-fold, respectively.

The primary metabolic pathway of clarithromycin in humans is *N*-demethylation and stereospecific hydroxylation at the 14-position of the aglycone. Metabolism of clarithromycin to the 14-hydroxy derivative is saturable after 800 mg.

By macrolide standards, a large proportion of the dose (around 20–40%) appears in the urine. The drug and its principal metabolite are retained in renal failure, their plasma elimination half-lives in patients whose creatinine clearance was less than 30 ml/min exceeding 30 and 45 h, respectively.

Toxicity and side-effects

It is well tolerated, producing little gastro-intestinal disturbance and some transient changes in liver function tests.

Clinical use

It has been used principally to treat infections of the skin and soft tissues and infections of the respiratory tract, including streptococcal pharyngitis, sinusitis, exacerbations of chronic bronchitis and community-acquired pneumonia.

Further information

Finch R G, Speller D C E, Daly P J 1991 Clarithromycin: new approaches to the treatment of respiratory tract infections. *Journal of Antimicrobial Chemotherapy* 27 (suppl A)

DIRITHROMYCIN

A pro-drug of erythromycylamine, a 14-membered-ring macrolide.

Antimicrobial activity

Dirithromycin and erythromycylamine share the same antibacterial spectrum as other 14-membered-ring macrolides, but are far less active than erythromycin. The MIC of dirithromycin for Gram-positive bacteria was the same or twice that of erythromycylamine, which is usually 4- to 8-fold less active than erythromycin against *H. influenzae*, *Str. pneumoniae*, *M. catarrhalis* and *Str. agalactiae*. Against *Bord. pertussis*, *H. pylori* and *C. jejuni*, dirithromycin and erythromycylamine show the same antibacterial activity. Dirithromycin is poorly active against anaerobes, the MIC values being: *C. trachomatis* 4 mg/l, *L. pneumophila* 8 mg/l and *M. pneumoniae* 0.1 mg/l. Its activity against respiratory pathogens is shown in Table 27.2.

The intracellular/extracellular ratio in PMN of dirithromycin and erythromycylamine is time dependent, reaching 34.5 after 120 min.

Pharmacokinetics

Dirithromycin has a long elimination half-life enabling once-daily administration. Compared with erythromycin it achieves a greater cellular/extracellular concentration ratio and a higher concentration in some tissues.

Dirithromycin is rapidly hydrolysed to erythromycylamine: 60–90% of a dose is converted to the active metabolite within 35 min after intravenous (i.v.) administration. After oral administration of single doses of 500, 750 and 1000 mg to volunteers, the C_{max} values ranged between 0.29 and 0.64 mg/l and were reached 4–5 h after administration. The AUC values were 3.37–6.45 mg/h per litre, with an apparent elimination half-life of 30–44 h. The total clearance was 250–500 ml/min. Between 62% and 81% of an oral dose and 81–97% of an i.v. dose were eliminated in the faeces, predominantly as erythromycylamine. Urinary recovery accounted for 1.2–2.9% of the orally administered dose.

The absolute bioavailability of dirithromycin after oral administration is about 10% of the given dose. After a 500 mg single oral dose, the mean peak biliary concentration was 139 mg/l. In elderly patients, there was a trend toward an increase in AUC but not in C_{max}. Renal and non-renal clearance was decreased in patients with biliary disease compared with other patients or healthy volunteers.

Dosage adjustments do not appear necessary in patients with mild or moderate hepatic, biliary or renal impairment. Negligible amounts of the drug were removed during haemodialysis.

Toxicity and side-effects

The frequency and nature of adverse events reported with dirithromycin were similar to those experienced by patients receiving comparator macrolides. Gastro-intestinal events were most common, and included abdominal pain (5.6% and 4.7% of patients receiving dirithromycin and comparators, respectively), diarrhoea (5.0% and 5.5%) and nausea (4.9% and 5.1%).

Clinical use

Dirithromycin 500 mg once-daily for 5 or 7 days was effective in clinical trials in patients with community-acquired infections of the lower respiratory tract, or skin or soft-tissue infections. Dirithromycin treatment should be continued for 10 days in patients with tonsillitis/pharyngitis caused by β-haemolytic streptococci.

Further information

Brogden R N, Peters D H 1994 Dirithromycin – a review of its antimicrobial activity, pharmacokinetic properties and therapeutic efficacy. *Drugs* 48: 599–616

Finch R G, Hamilton-Miller J M T, Lovering A M, Daly P J 1993 Dirithromycin: a new once-daily macrolide. *Journal of Antimicrobial Chemotherapy* 31 (suppl C)

ERYTHROMYCIN

A 14-membered-ring macrolide.

Erythromycins are produced as a complex of six components (A to F) by *Saccharopolyspora erythreaus*. Only erythromycin A has been developed for clinical use.

Erythromycin is currently available in a large number of forms such as the base compound coated to prevent destruction by gastric acidity, esters (2'-propionate, 2'-ethylsuccinate), salt (stearate), salts of 2'-esters (estolate, acistrate) and parenteral preparations such as lactobionate or glucceptate. 2'-esters of the erythromycin and their salts are used because of their favourable pharmacokinetic and pharmaceutical properties and less bitter taste compared with erythromycin.

Antimicrobial activity

It is highly active against *Str. pyogenes* and *Str. pneumoniae* and rather less so against *Staph. aureus*, including β-lactamase-producing strains. Gram-positive rods including *Clostridium* (MIC 0.1–1 mg/l), *Corynebacterium diphtheriae*

MIC 0.1–1 mg/l), *L. monocytogenes* (MIC 0.1–0.3 mg/l) and *B. anthracis* are also generally susceptible. Most strains of *Mycobacterium scrofulaceae* and *Mycobacterium kansasii* are susceptible (MIC 0.5–2 mg/l), but *Mycobacterium intracellulare* is often and *Mycobacterium fortuitum* regularly resistant. Many strains of *Nocardia* are susceptible. *Neisseria meningitidis* (MIC 0.12 mg/l) and *N. gonorrhoeae* (MIC 0.03–4 mg/l), *H. influenzae, H. ducreyi, Bord. pertussis* (MIC 0.03–0.25 mg/l), some *Brucella, Flavobacteria, Legionella* (MIC 0.1–0.5 mg/l) and *Pasteurella* spp. are susceptible. Many anaerobic bacteria, including *Actinomyces* and *Arachnia* spp., are susceptible; *H. pylori* (MIC 0.06–0.25 mg/l) is susceptible; *C. jejuni* is mostly susceptible, but some *Campylobacter* spp., as *Esch. coli*, may be resistant. Most Gram-negative anaerobes are susceptible or moderately so, but *B. fragilis* and *Fusobacterium* spp. are resistant. *T. pallidum* and *Borrelia* spp. are susceptible. *Chlamydia* spp. (MIC $\geq$0.25 mg/l), *M. pneumoniae* and *Rickettsia* spp. are all susceptible, *Mycoplasma hominis* and *Ureaplasma* spp. are resistant. *Enterobacteria* spp. are generally resistant, although some strains of *Escherichia* are inhibited and killed by as little as 8 mg/l. Its activity against common pathogenic bacteria is shown in Table 27.2.

Inoculum size or the presence of serum has only a small effect on the MIC, but activity increases with increasing pH up to 8.5. In the presence of CO_2 the MIC for *H. influenzae* rises from 0.5–8 to 4–32 mg/l, and that for *B. fragilis* also rises steeply. Its action is predominantly bacteriostatic, but higher concentrations are slowly bactericidal. Erythromycin antagonizes the action in vitro of ampicillin and some cephalosporins against some strains of *Staph. aureus* and *H. influenzae*.

Acquired resistance

Increased resistance is not often observed to develop during successful short-term treatment, but during more prolonged treatment of infections due to *Staph. aureus*, such as endocarditis, it is common. The emergence of resistance during treatment has also been observed in patients treated for *M. pneumoniae* infection.

In volunteers receiving two 500 mg doses of erythromycin stearate at weekly intervals, all oral streptococci including *Streptococcus sanguis* and *Streptococcus mitior* had increased MICs (1–4 mg/l), and in almost half the isolates very resistant variants (MIC 16–256 mg/l; MBC $\geq$128 mg/l) were encountered and persisted for many weeks.

Resistant staphylococci emerged and spread rapidly in some hospitals where the use of erythromycin was extensive. At first, uncomplicated resistance to erythromycin emerged, but soon most clinical isolates exhibited inducible MLS_B resistance (p. 378) in which the majority of cells are susceptible to erythromycin, but growth on a medium containing the antibiotic produces a uniform population resistant not only to erythromycin but also to other macrolides, lincomycin and group B streptogramins. Reversion to susceptibility is complete within 90 min of growth in antibiotic-free medium. Resistant strains of pneumococci and of haemolytic streptococci of groups A, B and C have been widely encountered.

The majority of resistant strains of *Str. pyogenes* exhibit another form of cross-resistance called 'zonal resistance', in which induction, typically by lincomycin, occurs only within a restricted zone of concentrations. Under the same selection pressure, MLS_B resistance emerged much later in streptococci than in staphylococci and the prevalence, except in *Enterococcus faecalis*, remains low. The degree of resistance to the individual agents varies considerably amongst strains which exhibit a spectrum of unstable shared resistance with extreme strains resistant to only one agent.

Some strains of *Cl. perfringens* are resistant and the MIC for some isolates of β-lactamase-producing *N. gonorrhoeae* is 0.5 mg/l. Resistance (MIC $\geq$128 mg/l) occurs in both *Esch. coli* and *C. jejuni*, but is considerably more common in the former. MLS_B resistance is also encountered in *C. diphtheriae* and *B. fragilis*.

Pharmacokinetics

The acid lability of erythromycin base necessitates administration in a form giving protection from gastric acid. In acid media it is rapidly degraded (10% loss of activity at pH 2 in less than 4 s) by intramolecular dehydrogenation to a hemiketal and hence to anhydroerythromycin, neither of which exert antimicrobial activity. Both enteric and film-coated tablets are available commercially. Delayed and incomplete absorption is obtained from coated tablets and there is a good deal of individual variation, adequate levels not being attained at all in a few subjects. Food delays absorption of the erythromycin base, which achieves peak plasma levels of 0.3–0.4 mg/l and 0.3–1.9 mg/l about 4 h after doses of 250 and 500 mg respectively. After 500 mg of the 2'-ethylsuccinyl ester, mean peak plasma levels at 1–2 h were 1.5 mg/l. In subjects given 1 g of the ethylsuccinate 12-hourly for seven doses, the mean plasma concentration 1 h after the last dose was around 1.4 mg/l. Intra- and intersubject variation and delayed and depressed absorption in the presence of food has not yet been eliminated by new formulations. Improved 500 mg preparations of erythromycin stearate are claimed to produce peak plasma levels of <1–14 mg/l which are relatively little affected, beyond being delayed, by the presence of food. The serum levels obtained after single doses of various preparations are given in Table 27.3. 2'-Esters of erythromycin are partially hydrolysed to erythromycin; 2'-acetyl erythromycin is hydrolysed more rapidly than the 2'-propionyl ester, but more slowly than the 2'-ethyl succinate.

Table 27.3 *Erythromycin plasma concentrations following administration of various preparations*

Preparation	Dose (mg)	Route	T_{max} (h)	C_{max} (mg/l)	Half-life (h)	AUC (mg/h per l)
Base	250	Oral	3–4	1.29	1.6	1.6
	500		2–4	2.0	2.0	2.0
	1000		4	1.30–1.50		
Stearate						
Fasting	250	Oral	2.2	0.88	1.6	3
	500		2–4	2.4	1.9	8.8
After food	500		2–4	0.10–0.40	2–4	
2'-Propionate						
Fasting	500	Oral	2–4	0.40–1.90	3–5	
After food	500		4	0.30–0.50	3–4	
2'-Estolate						
Fasting	250	Oral	2–4	0.36–3.00		
	500		1–2	1.40–5.00	2–4	
After food	250			1.10–2.90		
	500		2–4	1.80–5.20		
Lactobionate	500	i.v.	0	11.5–30.0	1–2	
Gluceptate	250	i.v.	0	3.50–10.7		

Conversion to the stearate does not adequately protect erythromycin from acid degradation. After an oral dose of erythromycin stearate, equivalent concentrations of erythromycin and its main degradation product, anhydroerythromycin, could be detected.

Doses of 10 mg/kg produced mean peak plasma concentrations around 1.8 mg/l in infants weighing 1.5–2 kg and 1.2 mg/l in those weighing 2–2.5 kg. In infants less than 4 months old, 6-hourly doses of the ethyl succinate of 10 mg/kg produced steady state plasma levels of around 1.3 mg/l. The plasma half-life was 2.5 h. In children given 12.5 mg/kg of erythromycin ethyl succinate 6-hourly, the concentration in the serum 2 h after the fourth dose was around 0.5–2.5 mg/l.

Protein binding of the base is 70% and that of the propionate >90%. Interaction with the hepatic metabolism of other drugs can result in clinically significant potentiation of the action of carbamazepine, cyclosporin, methylprednisolone, theophylline and warfarin and in adverse responses to digoxin, terfendadine and ergot alkaloids. Potentiation of the effects of digoxin has been attributed in part to action on the faecal flora affecting metabolism.

Distribution

Erythromycin is distributed throughout the body water, but tends to be retained longer in the liver and spleen than in the blood. Only very low levels are obtained in cerebrospinal fluid (CSF), even in the presence of meningeal inflammation, and are not raised to therapeutic levels by parenteral administration of the drug. Levels of 0.1 mg/l in aqueous humour were found when the serum level was 0.36 mg/l, but there was no penetration into the vitreous. In children with otitis media given 12.5 mg/kg of erythromycin ethylsuccinate 6-hourly, concentrations in middle ear exudate were 0.25–1 mg/l. In those with chronic serous otitis media given 12.5 mg/kg up to a maximum of 500 mg, none was detected in middle ear fluid, but on continued treatment levels up to 1.2 mg/l have been described. Penetration also occurs into peritoneal and pleural exudates. In patients receiving 1 g erythromycin ethylsuccinate 12-hourly or 0.5 g erythromycin lactobionate i.v., the healthy lung tissue/serum concentration ratios were 5.5 and 4.6, respectively. Mean concentrations of 2.6 mg/l have been found in sputum in patients receiving 1 g of the lactobionate i.v. 12-hourly and 0.2–2.0 mg/l in those receiving an oral stearate formulation. Levels in prostatic fluid are about 40% of those in the plasma. Salivary levels of around 4 mg/l were found in subjects receiving 0.5 g doses 8-hourly at 5 h after a dose when the plasma concentration was around 5.5 mg/l. Intracellular/extracellular ratios of 15 have been found in neutrophils. Concentrations of radiolabelled agent up to 24 times the extracellular level have been described, but leakage of unaltered drug is rapid after removal of the agent.

Fetal tissue levels are considerably higher after multiple doses; when the mean peak maternal serum level was 4.94 (0.66–8) mg/l, the mean fetal concentrations were: blood 0.06 (0–0.12) mg/l and amniotic fluid 0.36 (0.32–0.39) mg/l. Concentrations were more than 0.3 mg/l in most other fetal tissues, but the concentrations were variable and unmeasurable in some. It appears to be concentrated by fetal liver.

Excretion

It is excreted both in urine and in the bile but only a fraction of the dose can be accounted for in this way. Only about 2.5% of an oral dose or 15% of an intravenous dose is recovered unchanged in the urine. Urinary concentrations in patients receiving 1 g/day of erythromycin base have been reported to be 13–46 mg/l. It is not removed to any significant extent by peritoneal dialysis or haemodialysis. Reported changes in half-life in renal failure may be related to the saturable nature of protein binding. Fairly high concentrations of 50–250 mg/l are found in the bile, the bile/serum concentration ratio in those receiving the base being about 30. In patients with alcoholic liver disease receiving 500 mg of the base, higher and earlier peak plasma levels were obtained compared with normal subjects (2.0 and 1.5 mg/l at 4.6 and 6.3 h, respectively). Elimination was found to be biphasic, the two half-lives being 1.3 and 6.6 h. It is possible that the smaller excretion of the 2'-propionyl ester in the bile by comparison with the base accounts in part for its better maintained serum levels. There is some biliary recirculation, but some of the dose is lost in the faeces, producing concentrations of around 0.5 mg/g; some is deactivated by methylation but the fate of the rest is unknown.

Toxicity and side-effects

Oral administration, especially of large doses, commonly causes epigastric distress, nausea and vomiting, which may be severe. Solutions are very irritant: i.v. infusions almost invariably produce thrombophlebitis. Cholestatic hepatitis occurs rarely. Transient auditory disturbances have been described after i.v. administration of the lactobionate, and occasionally in patients with renal and hepatic impairment in whom oral dosage has produced high plasma levels. Sensorineural hearing impairment can occur and, although this is usually a reversible effect which occurs at high dosage, can be permanent. Prolongation of the elimination half-life of carbamazepine, due to inhibition of its conversion to the epoxide, usually results in central nervous system (CNS) disturbances. Nightmares are troublesome in occasional patients. Allergic effects occur in about 0.5% of patients.

Clinical use

Erythromycin is effective in pneumococcal, streptococcal and mycoplasmal infections and in those due to actinomyces and clostridia, where it is a natural second choice for patients allergic to penicillin.

Erythromycin appears to be as effective as penicillin in the treatment of diphtheria (p. 676) and is regarded by some as the drug of choice in the treatment of carriers.

Because of common cross-resistance between them, erythromycin and lincomycin should not be used together or sequentially. Concentrations found in middle ear exudate are more than sufficient to inhibit *Str. pyogenes* and the pneumococcus, but are unlikely to be sufficient to inhibit many strains of *H. influenzae*, which is a common cause of otitis media in young children. It has been used in the prophylaxis of whooping cough. It has often been used in combination, for example, with rifampicin, both in an attempt to stem the emergence of resistant staphylococci and to secure synergy in some cases of bacterial endocarditis. It has been used prophylactically for its efficacy against anaerobic bowel flora in combination with neomycin in preoperative bowel preparation. It is recommended as the drug of choice in infection with *Campylobacter* and *Legionella* and for the treatment of early syphilis in penicillin allergic patients.

It is used in the treatment of erythrasma and regarded as a drug of choice in relapsing fever due to *B. recurrentis*.

Preparations and dosage

Proprietary names: Erythrocin, Erymax, Erythroped, Erythromid, Erythroped A.

Preparations: Tablets film coated (as ethyl succinate and stearate), suspension (as ethyl succinate), injection (as lactobionate).

Dosage: Adults and children >8 years, oral, 250–500 mg every 6 h or 0.5–1 g every 12 h, up to 4 g/day for severe infections. Children ≤2 years, 125 mg every 6 h; 2–8 years, 250 mg every 6 h; doses doubled for severe infection. Adults, children, i.v., 50 mg/kg per day by continuous i.v. infusion or in divided doses every 6 h for severe infections; 25 mg/kg per day for mild infections when oral treatment is not possible.

Widely available.

Further information

Barre J, Mallatt A, Roseumbaum J, Deforges L, Houin G, Dhumeaux D et al 1987 Pharmacokinetics of erythromycin in patients with severe cirrhosis. Respective influence of decreased serum binding and impaired liver metabolic capacity. *British Journal of Clinical Pharmacology* 23: 753–757

Barzaghi N, Gatti G, Crema F, Monteleone M, Amione C, Leone L et al 1987 Inhibition by erythromycin of the conversion of carbamazepine to its active 10,11-epoxide metabolite. *British Journal of Clinical Pharmacology* 24: 836–838

Brummett R E, Fox K E 1989 Vancomycin- and erythromycin-induced hearing loss in humans. *Antimicrobial Agents and Chemotherapy* 33: 791–796

Carter B L, Woodhead J C, Cole K J, Milavetz G 1987 Gastrointestinal side effects with erythromycin preparations. *Drug Intelligence and Clinical Pharmacy* 21: 734–738

Davey P, Williams R 1988 Erythromycin acistrate: pharmacological and clinical studies. *Journal of Antimicrobial Chemotherapy* 21 (suppl D)

Descotes J, Andre P, Evreux J C 1985 Pharmacokinetic drug interactions with macrolide antibiotics. *Journal of Antimicrobial Chemotherapy* 15: 659–664

Eady E A, Ross J J, Cove J H 1990 Multiple mechanisms of erythromycin resistance. *Journal of Antimicrobial Chemotherapy* 26: 461–465

Gupta S K, Bakran A, Johnson R W, Rowland M 1989 Cyclosporin–erythromycin interaction in renal transplant patients. *British Journal of Clinical Pharmacology* 27: 475–481

Kanfer A, Stamatakis G, Torlotin J C, Fredt G, Kenouch S, Mery J P 1987 Changes in erythromycin pharmacokinetics induced by renal failure. *Clinical Nephrology* 27: 147–150

Larrey D, Funck-Bretano C, Brell P, Vitaux J, Theodore C, Babany G et al 1983 Effects of erythromycin on hepatic drug metabolising enzymes in humans. *Biochemical Pharmacology* 32: 1063–1068

Malmborg A S 1986 The renaissance of erythromycin. *Journal of Antimicrobial Chemotherapy* 18: 293–296

Miles M V, Tennison M B 1989 Erythromycin effects on multiple-dose carbamazepine kinetics. *Therapeutic Drug Monitoring* 11: 47–52

Paulsen O, Hoglund P, Nilsson L G, Bengtsson H I 1987 The interaction of erythromycin with theophylline. *European Journal of Clinical Pharmacology* 32: 493–498

Peeters T, Matthijs G, Depoortere I, Cachet T, Hoogmartens J, Vantrappen G 1989 Erythromycin is a motilin receptor agonist. *American Journal of Physiology* 257: G470–474

Scott R J, Naidoo J, Lightfoot N F, George R C 1989 A community outbreak of group A beta haemolytic streptococci with transferable resistance to erythromycin. *Epidemiology and Infection* 102: 85–91

Umstead G S, Neumann K H 1986 Erythromycin ototoxicity and acute psychotic reaction in cancer patients with hepatic dysfunction. *Archives of Internal Medicine* 146: 897–899

Weisblum B 1984 Inducible erythromycin resistance in bacteria. *British Medical Bulletin* 40: 47–53

ERYTHROMYCIN ACISTRATE
2'-Acetylerythromycin A stearate

It is partially hydrolysed to erythromycin A to which it owes its antimicrobial activity. The total level of drug (erythromycin A plus erythromycin acistrate), following administration of the salt preparation, in plasma and tonsillar tissue exceeds that produced by erythromycin stearate several fold, with much reduced intersubject variation.

Further information

Gordin A, Mannistö P T, Antikainen R, Savolainen S, Ylikoski J, Kokkonen P et al 1988 Concentrations of erythromycin, 2'-acetyl erythromycin, and their anhydro forms in plasma and tonsillar tissue after repeated dosage of erythromycin stearate and erythromycin acistrate. *Antimicrobial Agents and Chemotherapy* 32: 1019–1024

Ricevuti G, Pasotti D, Mazzone A, Gazzani G, Fregnan G B 1988 Serum, sputum and bronchial concentrations of erythromycin in chronic bronchitis after single and multiple treatment with either propionate-N-acetylcysteinate or stearate erythromycin. *Chemotherapy* 34: 374–379

ERYTHROMYCIN ESTOLATE

The 2'-propionyl ester of erythromycin lauryl sulphate.

It is microbiologically inactive and must be hydrolysed in the body to the active base, although it has been suggested that in some cases the estolate may enter the bacterial cell and be activated there by bacterial esterases.

Pharmacokinetics

It is tasteless and more resistant to gastric acid than erythromycin. It is absorbed as the 2'-propionyl ester. Initial rapid hydrolysis affects relatively little of the drug and is followed by a period of slow breakdown, during which the ratio of active to inactive compounds remains fairly constant. Determination of the concentration of circulating active agent by microbiological assay is complicated by the possibility of further active drug being liberated from ester in the serum by hydrolysis during the period of incubation.

Mean peak plasma concentrations following doses of 0.25 and 0.5 g are around 1.5 and 2–4 mg/l, respectively, of which the free base accounts for about 20–35%. The plasma half-life is about 1.5 h.

In pregnant women admitted for therapeutic abortion, doses equivalent to 500 mg of the base produced peak serum levels of 0.29–7.2 mg/l at 2 h after the dose. Levels were still detectable after 24 h. The peak levels after the last of multiple doses were 2.5–7 mg/l. The proportion of patients exhibiting low peak levels of the drug was greater than that previously reported in non-pregnant women.

It is eliminated through both the urine and the bile, but much of the drug is metabolically degraded. In the urine, peak concentrations of 7–15 mg/l have been found 3–4 h after doses of 250 mg. In pregnant women receiving doses equivalent to 500 mg of the base, mean urinary concentrations were around 20 mg/l after one dose and 85 mg/l after multiple doses. The bile/serum concentration ratio is around 4, but only about 0.2% of the dose appears in the bile over the first 8 h.

Toxicity and side-effects

It may give rise to signs of liver damage. These consist of upper abdominal pain, fever, hepatic enlargement, a raised serum bilirubin, with or without actual jaundice, pale stools and dark urine and eosinophilia. The condition, which is rare and usually seen 10–20 days after the initiation of treatment, may mimic viral hepatitis, cholecystitis, pancreatitis or cardiac infarction. There have been no deaths, and on stopping the drug recovery has been complete. Once patients have recovered, recurrence of symptoms can be induced by giving the estolate but not by giving the base or stearate. There is evidence that erythromycin estolate is more toxic to isolated liver cells than is the propionate or the base, and it is suggested that the essential molecular feature responsible for toxicity is the propionyl–ester linkage. The relative frequency of the reaction and its rapidity of onset (within hours) after second courses of the drug, peripheral eosinophilia and other evidence of hypersensitivity and the histological appearance suggest a mixture of hepatic cholestasis, liver cell necrosis and hypersensitivity. Abnormal liver function tests in patients receiving the estolate must be interpreted with caution, since increased SGOT is often the only abnormality and some metabolite of the estolate interferes with the measurement commonly used. Elevated levels of SGOT return to normal after cessation of treatment. Serum bilirubin is generally unchanged in these patients, but γ-glutamyl transpeptidase may also be affected. Gastro-intestinal disturbances have been found in 2% of patients treated with the estolate. Nausea and vomiting are said to be more common with the propionate, and diarrhoea with the estolate. Allergic effects occur in about 0.5% of patients.

Clinical use

The estolate is used for the same purposes as erythromycin base and its salts. Because of its effect on the liver the estolate should not be used if the patient is known to have been treated with it before. It should not be given for more than 10 days.

Preparations and dosage

Proprietary name: Ilosone.

Preparations: Capsules, tablets, suspension.

Dosage: As for erythromycin.

Widely available.

Further information

Bérubé D, Kirouac D, Croteau D, Bergeron M G, Lebel M 1988 Plasma bactericidal activity after administration of erythromycin estolate and erythromycin ethylsuccinate to healthy volunteers. *Antimicrobial Agents and Chemotherapy* 32: 1227–1230

Inman W A W, Rawson N S B 1983 Erythromycin estolate and jaundice. *British Medical Journal* 286(1): 1954–1957

Phillips I, Wise R 1985 Macrolides–lincosamides–streptogramins. *Journal of Antimicrobial Chemotherapy* 16 (suppl A): 1–226

Stubbs C, Kanfer I 1989 Variability in the absorption and disposition of erythromycin estolate in humans. *Journal of Pharmaceutical Sciences* 78: 635–638

FLURITHROMYCIN

A semi-synthetic 14-membered-ring macrolide.

First isolated when (*S*)-8-fluoroerythronolide A was added to the fermentation broth of a blocked mutant of an erythromycin-producing strain of *S. erythreus*. Also obtained by fluorination of 8,9-anhydroerythromycin-6,8-hemiketal N-oxide.

Antimicrobial activity

It is active against *Str. pneumoniae*, *Str. viridans*, *Str. pyogenes* and *M. catarrhalis*. It has little or no activity against *H. influenzae*. It is active against *Str. agalactiae* (MIC 0.03 mg/l) and *N. gonorrhoeae* (MIC 0.04 mg/l); *C. trachomatis* (MIC 0.06–0.125 mg/l), *M. genitalium* (MIC 0.007 mg/l), and *U. urealyticum* (MIC 0.03 mg/l). It is inactive against *M. hominis* (MIC >128 mg/l). Flurithromycin shows similar activity against anaerobes to that of erythromycin; a provisional breakpoint of 2 mg/l has been recommended.

It displays cross-resistance with erythromycin A.

Pharmacokinetics

With administration of a single 500 mg dose orally, flurithromycin achieved a mean C_{max} of 1.2–2 mg/l. The T_{max} was 1–2 h and the AUC was 16.2 mg/h per litre. The half-life was 8 h and the volume of distribution 5.5 l/kg. With multiple-dose administration (500 mg orally three times daily for 10 doses), plasma concentrations were 0.72 mg/l immediately before and 0.67 mg/l at 4 h after the last dose. Absorption is not significantly affected by food. After administration of a single 375 mg tablet of flurithromycin ethylsuccinate, the mean serum levels at 0.5 h were 0.43 ± 0.35 mg/l. The mean peak serum concentration (1.41 ± 0.49 mg/l) was achieved at 1 h. At 8 and 12 h, the serum levels were 0.14 ± 0.05 and 0.04 ± 0.04 mg/l, respectively. The elimination half-life is 3.94 ± 1.42 h.

Flurithromycin is stable at acid pH due to the presence of the fluorine atom at C-8. The half-life in artificial gastric juice was about 40 min.

Toxicity and side-effects

It is generally well tolerated.

Clinical use

It has been used successfully for the treatment of lower respiratory tract infections.

Further information

Bariffi F, Clini V, Ginesu F, Mangiarotti P, Romoli L, Gialdroni-Grassi G 1994 Flurithromycin ethylsuccinate in the treatment of lower respiratory tract bacterial infections. *Infection* 22: 226–230

Benonl G, Cuzzolin L, Leone R et al 1988 Pharmacokinetics and human tissue distribution of flurithromycin. *Antimicrobial Agents and Chemotherapy* 32: 1875–1878

Cocuza C E, Mattina R, Lanzafame A, Romoli L, Lepore A M 1994 Serum levels of flurithromycin ethylsuccinate in healthy volunteers. *Chemotherapy* 40: 157–160

Nord C E, Lindmark A, Persson I 1988 Comparative antimicrobial activity of the new macrolide flurithromycin against respiratory pathogens. *European Journal of Clinical Microbiology and Infectious Diseases* 7: 71–73

JOSAMYCIN

A 16-membered-ring macrolide.

A relative of leucomycin A_3 it is produced by *Streptomyces narvonensis* var. *josamyceticus*.

Antimicrobial activity

Its spectrum of activity is similar to that of erythromycin, susceptible organisms being inhibited by 2 mg/l or less. *Leg. pneumophila* is inhibited by 0.06–0.25 mg/l. *N. gonorrhoeae*, including β-lactamase-producing strains, is susceptible. Many Gram-positive and Gram-negative anaerobes are susceptible, including *Peptococcus* spp., *Peptostreptococcus*, *Propionibacterium*, *Eubacterium* and *Bacteroides* spp. Clostridia are moderately resistant, and resistant strains of fusobacteria are common. Its activity against common pathogenic organisms is shown in Table 27.1.

Acquired resistance

In volunteers given 1.5 g plus 0.5 g 6-hourly, as prophylaxis for endocarditis, the low initial level of resistant oral streptococci rose substantially within 48 h, 17% being resistant to 4 mg/l and 6% to 64 mg/l; the level had declined but was still raised 3 months later. The resistant strains, mostly *Str. sanguis* and *Str. mitis*, were also resistant to clindamycin and all other macrolides tested, but not to pristinamycin.

Pharmacokinetics

After a single oral dose of 1000 mg josamycin, the peak serum concentration of 2.74 mg/l was achieved 0.75 h after dosing. The AUC was 4.2 mg/h per litre, and the apparent elimination half-life was 1.5 h. Several inactive metabolites could be detected. It penetrates into saliva, tears and sweat, and achieves high levels in bile and lungs. It is mostly metabolized and excreted in the bile in an inactive form. Less than 20% of the dose appears in the urine, producing levels of around 50 mg/l.

Toxicity and side-effects

It is generally well tolerated, producing only mild gastrointestinal disturbance.

Clinical use

It has been recommended for the treatment of lower respiratory tract infections, including those due to *M. pneumoniae*. Its uses are otherwise similar to those of erythromycin.

Preparations and dosage

Dosage: Adults, oral, 1–2 g/day in 2 or more divided doses.

Available in continental Europe and Japan.

Further information

Chabbert Y A, Modai J 1985 Perspectives josamycine – Symposium International du 16–18 mai 1985, Lisbones. *Médicine Mal Infect* (suppl)

Maskell J P, Sefton A M, Cannell H et al 1990 Predominance of resistant oral streptococci in saliva and the effect of a single course of josamycin or erythromycin. *Journal of Antimicrobial Chemotherapy* 26: 539–548

MIDECAMYCIN

A 16-membered-ring macrolide.

A fermentation product of *Streptomyces mycarofaciens*.

It has a similar spectrum but less activity than erythromycin. Its activity against common pathogenic bacteria is shown in Table 27.1. It is inactive against erythomycin-resistant strains. It is rapidly and extensively metabolized and is said to exhibit less toxicity than earlier macrolides.

Preparations and dosage

Dosage: Adults, oral, 0.8–1.6 g/day in divided doses.

Available in Japan, Italy and France.

Further information

Neu H C 1983 In vitro activity of midecamycin, a new macrolide antibiotic. *Antimicrobial Agents and Chemotherapy* 24: 443–444

MIOKAMYCIN

A 16-membered-ring macrolide.

A semi-synthetic diacetyl derivative of midecamycin.

It exhibits a bimodal distribution of MICs for *H. influenzae* and *Ent. faecalis* (Table 27.2). It is inactive against erythromycin-resistant strains.

It is rapidly and extensively metabolized and is said to exhibit less toxicity than earlier macrolides. Attention has been paid to its interaction with theophylline, which resembles that of other macrolides.

Absorption of dry formulations of miokamycin is unaffected by food, whereas absorption of the oral suspension is delayed. In various studies the peak plasma concentration was 1.65, 1.31–3 and 1.3–2.7 mg/l after doses of 400, 600 and 800 mg, respectively.

Preparations and dosage

Dosage: Adults, oral, 0.9–1.8 g/day in 2 or 3 divided doses. Available in Italy and Spain.

Further information

Lacey R W, Lord V L, Howson G L 1984 In vitro evaluation of miokamycin bactericidal activity against streptococci. *Journal of Antimicrobial Chemotherapy* 13: 5–13

Principi N, Onorato J, Giuliani M G, Vigano A 1987 Effect of miokamycin on theophylline levels in children. *European Journal of Clinical Pharmacology* 31: 701–704

Rimoldi R, Bandera M, Fioretti M, Giorcelli R 1986 Miokamycin and theophylline blood levels. *Chemiotherapia* 5: 213–216

Obadia L 1985 Results obtained with miocamycin in the treatment of pyodermas in children. *Recent Advances in Chemotherapy* 2: 1461–1462

OLEANDOMYCIN

A 14-membered-ring macrolide produce by *Streptomyces antibioticus*. It is stable in acid conditions.

Antimicrobial activity

Its in vitro activity is less than that of erythromycin A, but four times greater than that of spiramycin (Table 27.1). Several attempts have been made to improve its potency by chemical modification while retaining its relative acid stability.

Pharmacokinetics

It is incompletely absorbed, but an ester, triacetyloleando-mycin, gives improved blood levels. Following doses of 0.5 g, mean peak serum levels around 0.8 mg/l were produced by the base and 2.0 mg/l by the triacetyl ester. A single oral dose of 1 g of the ester produced a mean plasma oleando-mycin concentration of 4.0 mg/l at 1 h after dosing, with an AUC of 14 mg/h per litre. The apparent elimination half-life was 4.2 h. Significant quantities of mostly inactivated drug are eliminated in the bile. About 10% of the dose appears in the urine after administration of the base and about 20% after the ester.

Toxicity and side-effects

Nausea, vomiting and diarrhoea are common. Like erythro-mycin estolate, triacetyloleandomycin can cause liver damage. Abnormal liver function tests were found in about a third of patients treated for 2 weeks. This may be due in part to interference with the SGOT test, but 5% of affected patients became jaundiced. Hepatic dysfunction resolved when treatment was discontinued. The action of drugs eliminated via the cytochrome P450 system may be potentiated.

Clinical use

Its uses are identical with those of erythromycin. Extensive use was at one time made of a 1 : 2 mixture with tetracycline (Sigmamycin) for which synergic properties were claimed.

Further information

Koch R, Asay L D 1958 Oleandomycin, a laboratory and clinical evaluation. *Journal of Pediatrics* 53: 676–682

Ticktin H E, Zimmerman H J 1962 Hepatic dysfunction and jaundice in patients receiving triacetyloleandomycin. *New England Journal of Medicine* 267: 964–968

ROKITAMYCIN
3″-Propionyl leucomycin A₅

A semi-synthetic 16-membered-ring macrolide. Unstable in acid media.

Antimicrobial activity

It shows an identical spectrum to that of erythromycin, but is less active against Gram-positive cocci. It is active against *Staph. aureus* (MIC 0.5 mg/l), *Str. pyogenes* (MIC <0.05 mg/l), *Str. pneumoniae* (MIC 0.25 mg/l) and *Ent. faecalis* (MIC 0.5 mg/l). It is poorly active against *H. influenzae* (MIC 8 mg/l) and *M. catarrhalis* (MIC 4 mg/l). It displays good activity against *Campylobacter* spp. (MIC 0.1 mg/l), *L. pneumophila* (MIC 0.1 mg/l) and *M. pneumoniae* (MIC ≤0.003 mg/l). It is active against anaerobes, including *Peptostreptococcus* spp. (MIC <0.05 mg/l) and some species of the *Bacteroides* group (MIC <0.05 mg/l).

Pharmacokinetics

After a single oral dose of 600 mg, the peak serum concentration was 1.9 mg/l at 0.58 h after dosing. The AUC is 3.72 mg/h per litre with an apparent elimination half-life of 2.0 h.

It is mainly eliminated in the bile. Little appears in the urine (about 2%).

Its major metabolites are leucomycin A_7, 10"-OH-rokitamycin and leucomycin V. The first two metabolites show some antimicrobial activity. In healthy adults, the proportions of rokitamycin and its metabolites in serum 30 min after a single oral dose of 1200 mg were: leucomycin A_7 18%, 10"-OH-rokitamycin 33% and leucomycin V 9%. The pharmacokinetics of rokitamycin given to children and adults are summarized in Tables 27.4 and 27.5.

The pharmacokinetic behaviour of rokitamycin is not altered in patients with liver cirrhosis.

Further information

Akita H, Sunakawa K, Fujii R 1988 The usefulness of rokitamycin drug syrup in the treatment of chlamydia infections in neonates, premature babies and infants. 28th Interscience Conference of Antimicrobial Agents and Chemotherapy, Los Angeles, abstr 914

ROXITHROMYCIN

A semi-synthetic 14-membered-ring macrolide derived from erythromycin A.

Table 27.4 *Pharmacokinetics of rokitamycin following oral syrup in children*

Dose (mg)	C_{max} (mg/l)	T_{max} (h)	AUC (mg/h per l)	$t_{1/2}$ (h)
5	0.26	0.37	0.69	2.18
10	0.55	0.47	1.16	1.97
15	0.79	0.39	1.52	2.00

Table 27.5 *Pharmacokinetics of macrolides following oral dosage in adults*

	Dose (mg)	C_{max} (mg/l)	T_{max} (h)	AUC (mg/h per l)	$t_{1/2}$ (h)
Roxithromycin	150	7.90	1.0	81.0	10.5
	300	10.80	1.5	132.0	11.9
Clarithromycin	250	0.75	1.7	4.2	2.7
	500	1.65	2.0	16.2	3.5
Azithromycin	250	0.17	2.2	0.5	13.8
	500	0.38	2.0	4.5	41.0
Dirithromycin	500	0.48	4.0	3.8	44.0
Rokitamycin	200	0.49	0.6	0.9	2.1
	600	1.90	0.6	3.7	2.0
	1200	3.75	0.6	7.1	2.4
Miokamycin	600	3.01	2.0	3.0	1.0

Antimicrobial activity

It has variable activity against methicillin-susceptible *Staph. aureus* but methicillin-resistant *Staph. aureus*, as well as *Staph. epidermidis*, *Staph. haemolyticus* and *Staph. hominis*, are moderately susceptible. *Str. pyogenes* and other β-haemolytic streptococci and *Str. pneumoniae* are inhibited by <0.25 mg/l. It is generally inactive against Lancefield group G *Streptococcus* and enterococci. It is inactive against erythromycin-resistant coagulase-negative staphylococci and against Enterobacteriaceae and *Pseudomonas* spp. It is active against *L. monocytogenes*, *M. catarrhalis*, *C. jejuni*, *H. ducreyi*, *G. vaginalis*, *Bord. pertussis*, *C. diphtheriae*,

B. burgdorferi, H. pylori, the *M. avium* complex, *Legionella* spp., *M. pneumoniae, Chlamydia* spp., and *U. urealyticum*. Its activity against common pathogenic bacteria is shown in Table 27.1 and its activity against respiratory pathogens is shown in Table 27.2.

Pharmacokinetics

Mean plasma concentrations of 6.6–7.9 mg/l are achieved within 2 h of a single oral 150 mg dose. In a direct comparison, the AUC produced by 150 mg roxithromycin was 16.2-fold greater than that produced by 250 mg erythromycin A. Multiple doses produced similar differences. Behaviour in children is broadly similar, repeated doses of 2.5 mg/kg producing age-independent mean peak plasma concentrations around 10 mg/l at 1–2 h, but the apparent elimination half-life was longer (around 20 h). Absorption is not affected by food. Oral administration with antacids or H_2-receptor antagonists does not significantly affect bioavailability.

The drug is strongly, specifically and saturably bound to α_1-acid glycoprotein in plasma. The plasma clearance of roxithromycin appears to be dose dependent or plasma concentration dependent.

It is widely distributed, but does not reach the CSF. Concentrations close to the simultaneous serum level have been found in tonsillar, lung and prostatic tissue, myometrium, endometrium and synovial fluid. It achieves high levels in skin. In patients receiving 300 mg followed by three 20-hourly doses of 150 mg, the peak skin/plasma ratio at around 4 h was around 9.7.

Less than 5% of the administered dose is eliminated as degradation products. Rather more than half the dose appears in the faeces and only 7–10% (including metabolites) in the urine; up to 15% is eliminated via the lungs. Renal clearance increased in volunteers as the dose was raised from 150 to 450 mg, and is decreased in elderly subjects. In patients in whom the creatinine clearance was <10 ml/min, the apparent elimination half-life rose to around 15.5 h and total body clearance was significantly reduced. The half-life was somewhat increased in patients with hepatic cirrhosis.

Toxicity and side-effects

It is generally well tolerated, adverse effects being described in 3–4% of patients, mostly gastro-intestinal disturbance, notably abdominal pain, nausea and diarrhoea. Severe headache, weakness, dizziness, rash and reversible changes in liver function tests and blood glucose, lymphopenia and increased eosinophils and platelets have also been described.

The half-life of simultaneously administered theophylline is increased (around 10%), but there is no effect on that of

carbamazepine and no interaction with warfarin or cyclosporin.

Clinical use

It has been successfully used in the treatment of upper and lower respiratory tract infections, skin and soft-tissue infections, urogenital infections and orodental infections. The drug has also shown promise in a variety of more specialized indications, including opportunistic infections in HIV-positive patients and as part of a *H. pylori* eradication regimen.

Preparations and dosage

Proprietary name: Rulid.

Dosage: Adults, oral, 150 mg twice daily.

Available in continental Europe, Japan and Latin America.

Further information

Phillips I, Péchère J-C, Speller D 1987 Roxithromycin: a new macrolide. *Journal of Antimicrobial Chemotherapy* 21 (suppl B)

Young L S, Lode H 1995 Roxithromycin: first of a new generation of macrolides: update and perspectives. *Infection* 23 (suppl 1)

SPIRAMYCIN

A family of 16-membered ring macrolides. The spiramycin complex, composed of six components, is a fermentation product of *Streptomyces ambofaciens*. Spiramycins are relatively stable in acid conditions.

Antimicrobial activity

It is active against *Staph. aureus* (MIC 4–16 mg/l), *Str. pyogenes* and *Str. pneumoniae* (MIC 0.25–1 mg/l), *Ent. faecalis* (MIC 1–4 mg/l) and *Neisseria* spp. (MIC 0.5–4 mg/l), and poorly active against *H. influenzae* (MIC 16–32 mg/l). *L. pneumophila* is inhibited by 1–4 mg/l and

Campylobacter spp. by 0.5–16 mg/l. Enterobacteria are resistant. Many anaerobic species are susceptible, including *Actinomyces israelii* (MIC 2–4 mg/l), *C. perfringens* (MIC 2–8 mg/l) and *Bacteroides* (MIC 4–14 mg/l). It is also active against *Toxoplasma gondii*. Its activity against common pathogenic bacteria is shown in Table 27.1. It is active against some strains of *Staph. aureus* and *Str. pyogenes* resistant to erythromycin.

Pharmacokinetics

In volunteers given 2 g orally followed by 1 g 6-hourly, peak plasma levels were 1.0–6.7 mg/l. The plasma half-life is 4–8 h. After 1 g orally, a mean peak plasma concentration of 2.8 mg/l was achieved 2.6 h after dosing; the AUC was 10.8 mg/h per litre, with an apparent elimination half-life of 2.8 h. It is widely distributed in the tissues. It does not reach the CSF. Levels 12 h after a dose of 1 g were 0.25 mg/l in serum, 5.3 mg/l in bone and 6.9 mg/l in pus. Levels of 10.6 mg/l have been found 4 h after dosing in saliva, and concentrations at least equal to those in the serum are found in bronchial secretions. High levels (27 mg/g) were found in prostate after repeated dosage. Only about 5–15% is recovered from the urine. Most are metabolized, but significant quantities are eliminated via the bile in which concentrations up to 40 times those in the serum may be found.

Toxicity and side-effects

It is generally well tolerated, the most common adverse reactions being gastro-intestinal disturbance, notably abdominal pain, nausea and vomiting. Rashes and sensitization following contact or industrial exposure have been described.

Clinical use

It has been successfully used principally for the treatment of staphylococcal, streptococcal and pneumococcal infections. It is used as an alternative to pyrimethamine–sulphonamide for the treatment of toxoplasmosis, especially in pregnancy, and is claimed to be effective in cryptosporidiosis in non-immunocompromised patients.

Preparations and dosage

Proprietary name: Rovamycin.

Dosage: Adults, oral, 2–4 g/day in 2 divided doses. Children, oral, 50 mg/kg per day in divided doses.

Limited availability, not available in the UK.

Further information

Davey P, Speller D, Daly P J 1988 Spiramycin reassessed. *Journal of Antimicrobial Chemotherapy* 22 (suppl B)

Shah P, Simon C 1990 Neue Makrolide. *Forts Antimicrob Antineopl Chemother* (suppl): 9–1

Symposium 1988 Spiramycin reassessed. *Journal of Antimicrobial Chemotherapy* 22 (suppl B): 1–210

Vernillet L, Bertault-Peres P, Berland Y, Barradas J, Durand A, Olmer M 1989 Lack of effect of spiramycin on cyclosporin pharmacokinetics. *British Journal of Clinical Pharmacology* 27: 789–794

Mupirocin

M. W. Casewell

Introduction

A fermentation product of Pseudomonas fluorescens *formerly called 'pseudomonic acid'. It is supplied as the lithium, sodium or calcium salt. It is structurally unlike any other antimicrobial agent, and contains a unique hydroxynonanoic moiety linked to monic acid.*

There are four pseudomonic acids (A, B, C and D) of which that available commercially is A:

Antimicrobial activity

Mupirocin binds irreversibly to isoleucyl t-RNA synthetase, inhibiting isoleucyl incorporation and hence protein synthesis.

It exhibits potent slow bactericidal activity against staphylococci, including methicillin-resistant *Staphylococcus aureus* (MRSA), aerobic streptococci and certain Gram-negative bacteria but not *Pseudomonas aeruginosa* (Table 28.1). *Neisseria gonorrhoeae, Haemophilus influenzae* and *Mycoplasma* spp. are all susceptible. *Enterococcus faecium* is usually susceptible in contrast to *Enterococcus faecalis* which is resistant. Its activity against *Staph. aureus* is much affected by inoculum size and pH, with enhanced activity at the acid pH (5.5) of the skin. In the anterior nares its antistaphylococcal activity is not decreased by nasal secretions.

Acquired resistance

Before the introduction of mupirocin, naturally resistant

Table 28.1 *Activity of mupirocin against some common pathogenic bacteria: MIC (mg/l)*

Species	MIC (mg/l)
Staph. aureus (including MRSA)	0.01–0.25
Coagulase-negative staphylococci	0.01–4.0
Str. pyogenes	0.06–0.5
Str. pneumoniae	0.06–0.5
Ent. faecalis	16–≥64
Ent. faecium	1.0–4.0
N. gonorrhoeae	0.03–0.25
N. meningitidis	0.03–0.25
H. influenzae	0.003–0.25
Enterobacter	R
Ps. aeruginosa	R
B. fragilis	R

R, resistant.

strains of *Staph. aureus* were rare, occurring in most studies with a frequency of 10^{-9}. Low-level resistance (minimum inhibitory concentration (MIC) 16–64 mg/l) in *Staph. aureus* can be produced in vitro by passage in the presence of mupirocin and in patients with prolonged topical treatment of the anterior nares during MRSA outbreaks. High-level transferable resistance (MIC > 512 mg/l), for which coagulase-negative staphylococci may be the source, has been observed following prolonged topical use for dermatological conditions or, more recently but rarely, its nasal application in prolonged hospital outbreaks of MRSA.

Pharmacokinetics

On parenteral injection, it is rapidly de-esterified by non-specific esterases (possibly in renal or liver tissues since it is reasonably stable in blood) to inactive monic acid and its conjugates. It is strongly bound to protein. About 0.25% is absorbed from intact skin. The skin formulation contains polyethylene glycol which may be absorbed significantly when applied to open wounds or to damaged skin such as burns.

Toxicity and side-effects

Topical applications are well tolerated. It may cause irritation if applied to the conjunctiva which is therefore contraindicated. Trivial complaints of irritation and taste have been recorded for very few patients following nasal application. Polyethylene glycol from the ointment base may, if absorbed from application to open wounds or damaged skin, cause nephrotoxicity.

Clinical use

The nasal ointment has proved invaluable for the elimination of nasal carriage of MRSA by hospital patients and staff in successfully controlled outbreaks and this use is recommended in the most universally applied published guidelines for the control of MRSA. The only other regimen shown to have produced such effective clearance of MRSA is topical fusidic acid plus systemic trimethoprim and rifampicin (for MRSA sensitive to these three agents). Topical application to the insertion site of central venous lines in cardiothoracic surgery patients reduces the catheter colonization rate from 25% to 5%, but an appropriate formulation for this use is not commercially available.

Intermittent treatment of the anterior nares of haemodialysis patients to eliminate carriage of *Staph. aureus* reduces the incidence of bacteraemia caused by *Staph. aureus*. It has been proposed that preoperative elimination of nasal *Staph. aureus* with mupirocin might reduce the rate of staphylococcal infection in clean surgery, but this hypothesis has still to be tested.

Mupirocin has been recommended for staphylococcal and streptococcal infection of the skin, notably impetigo, and to control infected eczema, wounds and burns. As these indications are increasingly associated with the emergence of high-level resistance, prolonged use is best avoided.

Preparations and dosage

Proprietary name: Bactroban.

Preparations: Ointment, nasal ointment.

Dosage: Topical application, up to 3 times daily for a maximum of 10 days. Nasal application, up to 3 times daily for 3–5 days.

Widely available.

Further information

Casewell M W, Hill R L R 1985 In-vitro activity of mupirocin ('pseudomonic acid') against clinical isolates of *Staphylococcus aureus*. *Journal of Antimicrobial Chemotherapy* 15: 523–531

Cookson B D 1990 Mupirocin resistance in staphylococci. *Journal of Antimicrobial Chemotherapy* 25: 497–503

Gilbart J, Perry C R, Slocombe B 1993 High level mupirocin resistance in *Staphylococcus aureus*: evidence for two distinct isoleucyl-tRNA synthetases. *Antimicrobial Agents and Chemotherapy* 37: 3238

Hill R L R, Duckworth G D, Casewell M W 1988 Elimination of nasal carriage of methicillin-resistant *Staphylococcus aureus* with mupirocin during a hospital outbreak. *Journal of Antimicrobial Chemotherapy* 22: 377–384

Hill R L R, Fisher A P, Ware R J, Wilson S, Casewell M W 1990 Mupirocin for the reduction of colonization of internal jugular cannulae – a randomised controlled trial. *Journal of Hospital Infection* 15: 311–321

Hudson I 1994 The efficacy of mupirocin in the prevention of staphylococcal infections: a review of recent experience. *Journal of Hospital Infection* 27: 81–98

Layton M C, Perez M, Heald P, Patterson J E 1993 An outbreak of mupirocin-resistant *Staphylococcus aureus* on a dermatology ward associated with an environmental reservoir. *Infection Control and Hospital Epidemiology* 14: 369–375

Neu H C 1990 The use of mupirocin in controlling methicillin-resistant *Staphylococcus aureus*. *Infection Control and Hospital Epidemiology* 11: 11–12

Working Party Report 1990 Revised guidelines for the control of epidemic methicillin-resistant *Staphylococcus aureus*. *Journal of Hospital Infection* 16: 351–377

Nitrofurans

J. M. T. Hamilton-Miller

Introduction

The antimicrobial activity of the nitrofurans was first appreciated in the early 1940s as a result of chemical synthesis and microbiological testing in the USA and Germany. These early findings encouraged pharmaceutical companies to produce thousands of variations on the nitrofuran theme. Several of these were introduced into clinical practice, and 20 years ago four were available in the UK: nitrofurantoin, nitrofurazone, nifuratel and furazolidone. Now, however, only nitrofurantoin is available in the UK, although others (e.g. nifuroxime, nifurtoinol, nitrovin, nifurtimox) are used in different countries. The recent decline in popularity has been due to a lack of interest rather than any problems of treatment failure or adverse events resembling those that surrounded the withdrawal of furaltadone 35 years ago.

Chemistry

Antimicrobial nitrofurans are based on the 5-nitro-2-furaldehyde molecule:

$$O_2N \quad \overset{O}{\diagdown} \quad CHO$$

As 2-furaldehyde has the trivial name furfural, these compounds can also be described as 5-nitrofurfuryl derivatives. Antimicrobial activity per se requires the 5-nitro group, while substitutions may be made on the aldehyde, producing a large number of different compounds with varying degrees of activity and pharmacokinetic properties. Many are aldimines (Schiff's bases), and most contain a nitrogen heterocycle (hydantoin, oxazolidinone,

thiazine). They are yellow compounds, relatively easy to synthesize, and are poorly soluble in water but often dissolve well in aprotic solvents such as dimethylsulphoxide or dimethylformamide. Nitrofurans should be protected from light.

Antimicrobial activity

Nitrofurans are active in vitro against a wide range of bacteria. Sensitive species include: *Staphylococcus aureus*, coagulase-negative staphylococci, *Streptococcus pyogenes*, pneumococci, *Corynebacterium diphtheriae*, Clostridia, *Escherichia coli*, *Salmonella* spp., *Shigella* spp., *Bacteroides* spp. and *Neisseria* spp. The Gram-negative rods, *Klebsiella* spp., *Enterobacter* spp. and *Serratia marcescens* are less sensitive, while members of the Proteae family and *Pseudomonas aeruginosa* are resistant. It has been thought that the lack of activity against Proteae may be due to the alkaline conditions produced when such organisms grow; however, this is gainsaid by the facts that the non-ionizable nitrofurans (such as nitrofurazone) are also inactive, that when growing on sensitivity-test media in vitro Proteae do not create alkaline conditions, and also that *Providencia stuartii*, a non-producer of urease, is also resistant. Staphylococci are considerably more sensitive to nitrofurans than are micrococci, and this forms the basis of a useful laboratory test to differentiate these genera. A 100 µg disk of furazolidone is used for this purpose.

Furazolidone is the most active of the four nitrofurans listed in Table 29.1. Nifuratel has some activity against yeasts, *Trichomonas vaginalis* and *Giardia lamblia*.

While nitrofurazone and furazolidone appear to be unaffected by pH changes, nitrofurantoin, and presumably its close chemical analogue nitrofurtoinol, is much more active under acid conditions, suggesting that it is the un-ionized form in which antimicrobial activity resides.

Table 29.1 *Activity of nitrofurans against common pathogenic bacteria (MIC:mg/l)*

	Furazolidone	Nitrofurazone	Nitrofurantoin
Staph. auerus	2 – 8	8 – 16	4 – 32
Strep. pyogenes	4 – 8	8 – 64	4 – 16
Ent. faecalis	8 – 32	32 – 128	4 – 128
N. gonorrhoeae		0.1 – 8	0.25 – 2
Esch. coli	<0.5 – 4	4 – 16	0.5 – R
Proteus spp.	32 – 128	8 – 128	8 – R
Klebsiella	2 – 8	8 – 128	32 – R
Salmonella	0.25 – 2	4 – 16	4 – 128
Shigella	0.25 – 4	4 – 32	4 – 128
Ps. aeruginosa	R	R	R
B. fragilis	8 – 16	4 – 32	8 – 16

Mode of action

The mode of action of nitrofurans is complex and not fully understood. Nitrofurans are converted within bacterial cells by reductases to highly reactive intermediates, some of which have very short lives, and superoxide (Fig. 29.1). Ultimately, the nitro substituent is reduced to an amino group. The way(s) in which the intermediates bring about inhibition of bacterial growth and cell death, and their relative activity, have not been clarified; it now appears that unreduced nitrofurans exert significant antimicrobial activity.

Many candidates for the metabolic target of the nitrofurans have been put forward over the years; for example, preferential inhibition of the synthesis of inducible enzymes, damage to DNA, inhibition of acetyl coenzyme A (CoA) formation, or inhibition of enzymes involved with glycolysis and the citric acid cycle. Recent work indicates that all these suggestions may be correct, as nitrofurantoin has multiple modes of action: its highly reactive reduction products bind non-specifically to bacterial ribosomal proteins, halting all protein synthesis. At concentrations close to the minimum inhibitory concentration (MIC), nitrofurantoin may disrupt codon–anticodon interactions and thus prevent mRNA translation.

Acquired resistance

There has been very little acquisition of resistance to the nitrofurans over some 40 years of usage, in contrast with all other chemical classes of antibacterial agents. Resistance has been found rarely in *Esch. coli* and *Klebsiella pneumoniae*. R-factor-mediated resistance to nitrofurantoin has been reported at least twice, but these reports remain unconfirmed, and the phenomenon seems to be extremely rare.

It is difficult to understand why acquired resistance to the nitrofurans should be so unusual. They do not act like antiseptics, as intrinsically resistant species, such as pseudomonads, exist. Prima facie, resistance could be acquired by loss of reductase activity or by excluding the molecule from the bacterial cytoplasm. An explanation for the rarity of resistance would be if the reductase is an essential enzyme, so that its loss would usually be a lethal mutation, or if preventing the entry of a nitrofuran also limited entry of vital nutrilites.

Pharmacokinetics

The pharmacokinetics of the nitrofurans are, in general, poorly documented, and contradictions abound in the literature. This is for at least three reasons: firstly, many of them are 'old' drugs, introduced before the importance of pharmacokinetics was fully appreciated; secondly, interpretive difficulties arise because they are often heavily metabolized; and, thirdly, there are several assay techniques that may give different results when applied to the same set of specimens.

Many metabolites are produced in vivo in different animal species, and not all have been well characterized. It seems probable that they are devoid of antimicrobial activity, but that they may be responsible in part for some of the adverse events associated with therapy. Metabolites that have undergone reduction (see Fig. 29.1) and those that have been oxidized (e.g. hydroxy compounds) have been identified.

Toxicity and side-effects

Compounds available at present are, in general, free of serious toxic effects. The full spectrum of toxicity inherent in the group was graphically shown by furaltadone, which was withdrawn from clinical use in 1961, shortly after its introduction. Perhaps as a result of this experience, the

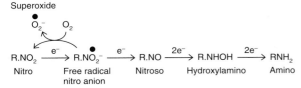

Fig. 29.1 *Step-wise reduction of nitrofurans, yielding biologically active entities.*

three nitrofurans in widest use (nitrofurantoin, nitrofurazone, furazolidone) have been subject to intensive postmarketing surveillance. Thus, probably more is known about the adverse-event profile of nitrofurans than for any other group of antibiotics. The commonest adverse event is on the upper gastro-intestinal tract, where nausea, vomiting or anorexia may occur. Skin reactions are unusual. Serious adverse events (described in more detail for specific compounds below) are very rare and may be due to hypersensitivity reactions.

Mutagenicity

Many nitrofurans have been shown to be mutagenic by a variety of tests, and some are said to be carcinogenic. Had these findings been available at the time the therapeutically useful members of this group were being developed, further work on them would doubtless have been stopped, or at least suspended. However, therapeutic use over many years has shown no evidence of any long-term harmful effects of nitrofurans.

Clinical use

Nitrofurans are now used predominantly as urinary antiseptics. Compounds used for other purposes include nifurtimox, an antitrypanosomal agent, furazolidone, used for intestinal infections, and nitrofurazone, for topical use. Nitrofurans are also employed in veterinary practice, both for treating and preventing infections, and as food additives.

Further information

Aoki T, Egusa S, Arai T 1975 Reduced nitrofuran sensitivity conferred by R factors. *Japanese Journal of Microbiology* 19: 327–329

Chamberlain R E 1976 Chemotherapeutic properties of prominent nitrofurans. *Journal of Antimicrobial Chemotherapy* 2: 325–336

Debnath A K, Hansch C, Kim K H, Martin Y C 1993 Mechanistic interpretation of the genotoxicity of nitrofurans (antibacterial agents) using quantitative structure–activity relationships and comparative molecular field analysis. *Journal of Medicinal Chemistry* 36: 1007–1016

Editorial 1961 Furaltadone condemned. *British Medical Journal* i: 264–265

Streeter A J, Krueger T R, Hoener B-A 1988 Oxidative metabolites of 5-nitrofurans. *Pharmacology* 36: 283–288

Tazima Y, Kada T, Murakami A 1975 Mutagenicity of nitrofuran derivatives, including furylfuramide, a food preservative. *Mutation Research* 32: 55–80

FURAZOLIDONE

Antimicrobial activity

This non-ionic nitrofuran has activity against a wide range of enteric pathogens. Susceptible bacteria include *Salmonella* spp., *Shigella* spp., enterotoxigenic *Esch. coli*, *Campylobacter jejuni*, *Aeromonas hydrophila*, *Plesiomonas shigelloides* and *Vibrio parahaemolyticus*, but not *Yersinia enterocolitica*. *G. lamblia* and trichomonads are also susceptible.

Pharmacokinetics

Inaccurate statements in the literature have given rise to the misconception that the drug is poorly absorbed from the intestine. There is substantial (65–75%) absorption following oral administration, but the drug is heavily metabolized to 5-amino and 4-hydroxy derivatives as well as open-chain forms, so that only about 5% of the material excreted is microbiologically active. However, intact furazolidone can be detected in various body fluids in concentrations that approximate to the MIC for various intestinal pathogens.

Toxicity and side-effects

Adverse events have been reviewed from a database of 191 clinical studies involving over 10 000 patients. Overall, 8.3% of patients reported at least one adverse event, most commonly affecting the gastro-intestinal tract (8% of patients) and characterized by nausea with or without vomiting. Neurological events (usually headache) occurred in 1.34% of patients, systemic reactions (mainly fever) in 0.56% and dermatological problems in 0.54%.

A metabolite of furazolidone (but not the unchanged molecule) is known to be an inhibitor of monoamine oxidase, but this does not seem to have given rise to significant adverse events. A disulphiram-like reaction has been reported, and alcohol should be avoided while taking the drug.

Clinical use

Furazolidone has been used extensively by mouth for the treatment and prevention of gastro-intestinal infections, including typhoid, shigellosis, salmonellosis, cholera, bacterial gastro-enteritis, travellers' diarrhoea, and giardiasis. It has also been used topically in combination with nifuroxime.

Recently, there has been a suggestion that furazolidone, or a related compound, may be useful in infections caused by *Pneumocystis carinii*.

Preparations and dosage

Dosage: Oral 100 mg, 4 times daily for 7–10 days.
Children, 1.25 mg/kg, 4 times daily.

Further information

Abraham R T, Knapp J E, Minnigh M B, Wong L K, Zemaitis M A, Alvin J D 1984 Reductive metabolism of furazolidone by *Escherichia coli* and rat liver in vitro. *Drug Metabolism and Disposition* 12: 732–741

DuPont H L (ed) 1980 Recent developments in the use of furazolidone and other antimicrobial agents in typhoid fever and infectious diarrheal diseases. *Scandinavian Journal of Gastroenterology* 24 (suppl 169): 1–80

Phillips K F, Hailey F J 1986 The use of furoxone: a perspective. *Journal of International Medical Research* 14: 19–29

Walzer P D, Kim C K, Foy J, Zhang J 1991 Furazolidone and nitrofurantoin in the treatment of experimental *Pneumocystis carinii* pneumonia. *Antimicrobial Agents and Chemotherapy* 35: 158–163

NIFURATEL

Antimicrobial activity

Nifuratel combines an in vitro antibacterial activity superior to that of nitrofurantoin (especially against anaerobes) with useful action against *T. vaginalis* (MIC $\leq$1 mg/l). Its activity against *Candida albicans* is greater than that of other commonly used nitrofurans, and although only modest in vitro (MIC $\geq$50 mg/l) its activity is sufficient to render it clinically useful.

Pharmacokinetics

There are few published data on the pharmacokinetics of nifuratel in man. Data on file from Poli Industria Chimica show that very low serum levels (<0.1 µg/l) are found following oral administration of 200 mg, and that the half-

life is about 3 h. Urine levels of the intact molecule are also very low. This pattern is consistent with that found in animals, where metabolism is rapid and extensive. It is considered likely that the antibacterial activity of nifuratel in human urine is due to the presence of active metabolites.

Plasma levels of nifuratel following use of a 250 mg vaginal suppository were even lower than those found after oral administration.

Toxicity and side-effects

Side-effects associated with nifuratel are said to be 'minimal', and mostly referable to the upper gastro-intestinal tract, but contact dermatitis has been described.

Clinical use

Because of its broad antimicrobial spectrum, nifuratel became popular in continental Europe for treating vaginitis. Its use then extended to the treatment of urinary infections including candiduria. It showed promise initially, but was withdrawn in the UK.

Preparations and dosage

Preparations: Tablets, vaginal preparations.
Dosage: Adults, oral, 200–400 mg, 3 times daily.
Available in France and Italy.

Further information

Cusano F, Caposi M, di Guilio P, Errico G 1987 Contact dermatitis from nifuratel. *Contact Dermatitis* 16: 37

Davies B I D, Mummery R V, Brumfitt W 1975 Ampicillin, carbenicillin indanyl ester and nifuratel in the treatment of urinary infection in domiciliary practice. *British Journal of Urology* 47: 335–341

Gruneberg R N, Leakey A 1976 Treatment of candidal urinary tract infection with nifuratel. *British Medical Journal* ii: 908–910

NIFUROXIME

This compound has the unusual property among nitrofurans of being active against fungi. The *anti* geometric isomer is available in the USA as a topical agent, and also in combination with furazolidone for treating vaginal infections of various aetiologies.

Preparations

Available in multi-ingredient preparations for vaginal use.

NIFURTIMOX

Antimicrobial activity

This nitrofuran exhibits antibacterial activity typical of the group; it is as active as metronidazole against anaerobes. A useful property is its activity against trypanosomes. It is particularly effective against *Trypanosoma cruzi* (MIC about 0.3 mg/l), perhaps because this species lacks catalase and has only low levels of reduced glutathione, a combination that renders it especially susceptible to attack by free radicals (see Fig. 29.1).

Pharmacokinetics

Nifurtimox is absorbed by mouth, a dose of 15 mg/kg giving a peak level at 4 h of 0.8 mg/l. It is rapidly and extensively metabolized, so that little of the intact molecule (about 0.5% of the dose) is found in urine. The half-life is about 3 h, and is not significantly altered even when the creatinine clearance is <10 ml/min.

Toxicity and side-effects

Of patients taking nifurtimox, 40–70% experience some form of adverse event, often relating to the gastro-intestinal tract (e.g. vomiting, abdominal pain, loss of appetite leading to weight loss), and/or the central nervous system (e.g. restlessness, disorientation, insomnia). Children tolerate the drug better than adults.

Clinical use

Until recently, this compound was drug of choice for acute Chagas' disease, but its use is discouraged by reason of a disappointing cure rate, the long period of treatment needed (120 days) and the high incidence of adverse events.

Preparations and dosage

Dosage: Adults, 8–10 mg/kg per day. Children 1–10 years, 15–20 mg/kg per day; 11–16 years, 12.5–15 mg/kg per day. The drug is given for 90 days.

Not available in the UK.

Further information

Gonzales-Martin G, Thambo S, Paulos C, Vasquez I, Paredes J 1992 The pharmacokinetics of nifurtimox in chronic renal failure. *European Journal of Clinical Pharmacology* 42: 671–673

Hof H 1989 Antibacterial activities of the antiparasitic drugs nifurtimox and benznidazole. *Antimicrobial Agents and Chemotherapy* 33: 404–405

Paulos C, Paredes J, Vasquez I, Thambo S, Arancibia A, Gonzales-Martin G 1989 Pharmacokinetics of a nitrofuran compound, nifurtimox, in healthy volunteers. *International Journal of Clinical Pharmacology, Therapy and Toxicology* 27: 454–457

NITROFURTOINOL

The *N*-hydroxymethyl derivative of nitrofurantoin, nitrofurtoinol is said to be more rapidly absorbed, and excreted into the urine to a greater extent, than is nitrofurantoin. It is available in some European countries for the treatment of urinary infections.

Preparations and dosage

Dosage: Adults, oral, up to 240 mg/day in divided doses.

Available in continental Europe.

NITROFURANTOIN

Antimicrobial activity

Nitrofurantoin has a pK_a of about 7.2, and is therefore more soluble in water under alkaline conditions. On the other hand, as its microbiological activity is dependent on the presence of the undissociated form (see above structure), nitrofurantoin is more active in acid media. The bacterial species that cause most urinary infections, *Esch. coli, Staph. saprophyticus* and enterococci, are susceptible, but members of the Proteae tribe (*Proteus, Providencia, Morganella* spp.) and *Ps. aeruginosa,* are uniformly resistant, and the Klebsielleae (*Klebsiella, Enterobacter* and *Serratia* spp.) are less sensitive.

Testing for susceptibility to nitrofurantoin in the laboratory is not entirely straightforward, as different disk strengths are recommended in the UK (50 µg) and the USA (300 µg), and the only recommendations for breakpoints are those provided by the National Committee for Clinical Laboratory Standards: ≤32 µg/ml for susceptibility and ≥128 µg/ml for resistance. There is poor correlation between the MIC and the zone size, so that it has been suggested that the presence of any zone of inhibition be regarded as indicating susceptibility. On the other hand, members of the Proteae family may display zones of inhibition but, since nitrofurantoin is inactive in the alkaline environment produced by such organisms in the urine, all strains of this family should be reported as resistant. Acquired resistance to nitrofurantoin is rare.

Pharmacokinetics

Nitrofurantoin is virtually only administered by the oral route. In the past, nitrofurantoin was given parenterally, at first in a toxic vehicle (polyethylene glycol), and later as sodium nitrofurantoin. The latter formulation is still occasionally used. Nitrofurantoin is well absorbed by mouth, mainly from the proximal small intestine, but the rate of absorption is dependent upon its crystalline state. Larger crystals, as in the formulation Macrodantin, are absorbed more slowly and cause less vomiting than microcrystalline varieties. It is not easy to manufacture the larger crystal form and there may be significant variation in bioavailability from different generic brands of nitrofurantoin. Such differences do not always became apparent using conventional pharmaceutical quality-control techniques, such as standardized disintegration–dissolution tests, and nitrofurantoin brands should not be substituted unless therapeutic equivalence has been formally established.

A delayed-release formulation, Macrobid, has recently been made available. This consists of capsules containing 25% macrocrystalline nitrofurantoin and 75% nitrofurantoin monohydrate blended in a dual delivery system. No pharmacokinetic data have been published. Microencapsulation of nitrofurantoin also alters its rate of excretion into the urine.

There are conflicting opinions in the literature concerning the effect of taking the drug with food (as is the recommended practice). According to various sources, taking with food either doubles or makes no difference to the bioavailability of nitrofurantoin. Protein binding is low (about 25%).

Early reports suggested a half-life for nitrofurantoin of about 30 min, but more recently flaws have been pointed out in these analyses, and a figure of 1–1.5 h now seems accurate. It is metabolized in vivo and rapidly concentrated in the urine, where about one-third of the administered dose can be recovered unchanged. Following a 100 mg dose, although blood levels peak at only about 1 mg/l, concentrations in the urine are > 32 mg/l for at least 4 h (and, according to one report, for 7 h). Tissue concentrations following oral administration are thought to be inadequate for a sustained antibacterial effect sufficient to treat a systemic infection, although intravenous use was reported to cure pyelonephritis and septicaemia.

Renal handling of nitrofurantoin involves glomerular filtration and active tubular secretion. Clearance is lower in acid urine. There appears to be significant excretion of nitrofurantoin in the bile.

Toxicity and side-effects

The most common adverse event associated with nitrofurantoin use is nausea, which may be combined with anorexia and/or vomiting. This is found in about 30% of patients taking the microcrystalline form, and requires premature cessation of therapy in about 10%. The frequency of nausea is approximately halved by the use of the macrocrystalline formulation. It is now thought to be caused by a direct effect on the vomiting centre, rather than, as originally thought, to 'gastric irritation'. It tends to occur early in a therapeutic course, and the incidence can be lessened by taking the medication with food or milk.

Serious adverse events arising during treatment with nitrofurantoin have been studied extensively. From 128 million courses of treatment prescribed world-wide, the incidences of major adverse events have been estimated as: pulmonary reactions 0.001%, hepatic reactions 0.0003%, neurological reactions 0.0007% and haematological reactions 0.0004%. Many of these events have the characteristics of hypersensitivity reactions. Fatalities have been extremely rare. Members of Nordic races appear to have a predisposition to adverse reaction.

Results of smaller surveys tend to suggest higher incidences than those cited above: haematological reactions 1.7% and liver injury 0.035%.

Pulmonary reactions seem to be of two kinds. Acute reactions are the more common, starting within 5–10 days of the first treatment with nitrofurantoin, or within a few hours on re-challenge. Symptoms may resemble those found in asthma, tracheobronchitis or pneumonia, and usually resolve within 2 days without chronicity developing. They appear to be due to a hypersensitivity reaction, and may be accompanied by eosinophilia. The subacute, or chronic, type, often referred to as 'pneumonitis', has a more gradual onset, and resolves only slowly when treatment is withdrawn. Prolonged dyspnoea and cough may be accompanied by fibrosis. It is not clear whether it is due to an immunological phenomenon or a direct toxic effect; if the former, the mechanism is different from that causing acute reactions.

Hepatic reactions to nitrofurantoin are more commonly chronic than acute, and manifest as chronic active hepatitis, sometimes with cirrhosis. These follow prolonged usage of the drug. Prognosis is good, but recovery may take many months. Immunological phenomena seem to be implicated.

Peripheral neuropathy has been reported mainly in patients with pre-existing impaired renal function. The prognosis depends upon the severity of the symptoms. It has been attributed to a direct toxic effect of either the drug itself, its metabolites or the superoxide generated in vivo (see Fig. 29.1).

Nitrofurantoin may cause haemolysis in patients whose erythrocytes lack glucose-6-phosphate dehydrogenase. As noted above, acute pulmonary reactions are accompanied by eosinophilia. More serious blood dyscrasias have been reported only in association with other drugs.

Nitrofurantoin is contraindicated in renal impairment: renal excretion is reduced if the creatinine clearance falls below 60 ml/min, and virtually ceases if creatinine clearance is less than about 20 ml/min. Thus, there is risk of accumulation and of failure to attain therapeutic concentrations in the urine. Otherwise, it is suitable for use in the elderly.

Clinical use

Nitrofurantoin is used exclusively to treat or prevent urinary infections. The range of its antimicrobial activity and the fact that as yet resistance has increased only marginally with the passing years makes it a strong contender as treatment of choice for 'blind' therapy of acute dysuria and/or frequency with infection in the domiciliary situation. It is also often useful for nosocomial urinary infections. Nitrofurantoin is of particular value in treating bacteriuria in pregnancy, as the safety database in this indication is extensive.

Nitrofurantoin is useful, in a dosage of 100 or 50 mg taken at night, in preventing recurrent attacks of infection in women prone to this condition. It may be given for periods of up to 12 months continuously, and is regarded by some as the gold standard in this indication. The presence of radiological abnormalities within the urinary tract is not a contraindication for this type of prophylaxis, provided there

is no obstruction. While some patients may experience nausea at first, this usually disappears after the first month, so patients should be encouraged to persist. Where urinary infections are directly triggered by sexual intercourse, some practitioners prefer to recommend nitrofurantoin to be used intermittently, following each 'at risk' event.

Preparations and dosage

Proprietary names: Furadantin, Macrodantin, Macrobid.

Preparations: Tablets, capsules, suspension.

Dosage: Adults, oral, therapeutic, 50–100 mg, 4 times daily for 7 days; prophylaxis, 50–100 mg at night. Children >3 months, 3 mg/kg per day in 4 divided doses.

Widely available.

Further information

Anonymous 1990 Nitrofurantoin. *IARC Monographs* 50: 211–231

Cunha B A 1988 Nitrofurantoin – bioavailability and therapeutic equivalence. *Advances in Therapy* 5: 54–63

D'Arcy P F 1985 Nitrofurantoin. *Drug Intelligence and Clinical Pharmacy* 19: 540–547

Ertan G, Karasulu E, Abou-Nada M, Tosun M, Ozer A 1994 Sustained-release dosage form of nitrofurantoin. Part 2. In vivo urinary excretion in man. *Journal of Microencapsulation* 11: 137–140

Gruneberg R N 1994 Changes in urinary pathogens and their antibiotic sensitivities 1971–1992. *Journal of Antimicrobial Chemotherapy* 33 (suppl A): 1–8

Holmberg L, Boman G, Bottiger L E, Eriksson B, Spross R, Wessling A 1980 Adverse reactions to nitrofurantoin. Analysis of 921 reports. *American Journal of Medicine* 69: 733–738

McOsker C C, Fitzpatrick P M 1994 Nitrofurantoin: mechanism of action and implications for resistance development in common uropathogens. *Journal of Antimicrobial Chemotherapy* 33 (suppl A): 23–30

Meyer M C, Wood G C, Straughn A B 1989 In vitro and in vivo evaluation of seven 50 mg and 100 mg nitrofurantoin tablets. *Biopharmaceutics and Drug Disposition* 10: 321–329

Pelletier L L, Michalak D P, Carter J Z et al 1992 A comparison of Macrobid (nitrofurantoin monohydrate/macrocrystals) and Macrodantin (nitrofurantoin macrocrystals) in the treatment of acute episodes of uncomplicated lower urinary tract infections. *Advances in Therapy* 9: 33–45

Westphal J F, Vetter D, Brogard J M 1994 Hepatic side-effects of antibiotics. *Journal of Antimicrobial Chemotherapy* 33: 387–401

NITROFURAZONE

Antimicrobial activity

The activity of this compound is not as great as that of furazolidone (Table 29.1), but it is sufficient both qualitatively and quantitatively, in topical use, to cover most of the pathogens commonly causing infections of wounds and burns, with the important exception of *Ps. aeruginosa*.

The antibacterial activity of nitrofurazone is affected neither by the presence of blood or serum, nor, as it is non-ionic, by pH changes.

Pharmacokinetics

Although it is absorbed from the gut following oral administration, nitrofurazone has been used exclusively as a topical agent. Absorption through burned skin has been estimated to amount to no more than 5%. Nitrofurazone is reported to penetrate well into eschar resulting from burns.

Toxicity and side-effects

The only important adverse effects have been skin reactions, which were reported in 1.1% of 18 249 patients involved in 136 clinical trials published between 1945 and 1970. Some formulations of nitrofurazone contain a polyethylene glycol vehicle, and these should be used with caution in patients with renal impairment.

Clinical use

Nitrofurazone was the first nitrofuran to make a major clinical impact, being used on a large scale to treat and prevent wound infections during World War II. Although there are few controlled trials of its efficacy, 'nitrofurazone soluble dressing' and nitrofurazone cream and ointment continue to be used in the treatment of burns and wounds. Nitrofurazone solution has also been used as a bladder washout. It has recently been suggested that incorporating nitrofurazone into catheter material may help to prevent catheter-associated urinary infections.

Preparations

Topical.
Very limited availability in continental Europe.

Further information

Anonymous 1990 Nitrofural (nitrofurazone). *IARC Monographs* 50: 195–209

Coffey R P, Rice T L, Thomson P D 1991 Effect of blood and serum on in vitro antibacterial activity of nitrofurazone. *American Journal of Hospital Pharmacy* 48: 1496–1499

Johnson J R, Berggren T, Conway A J 1993 Activity of a nitrofurazone matrix catheter against catheter-associated uropathogens. *Antimicrobial Agents and Chemotherapy* 37: 2033–2036

Nitroimidazoles

D. J. Edwards

Introduction and history

The history of the nitroimidazoles as agents for clinical disease began with the recognition in 1953 that vaginitis was caused by the protozoan Trichomonas vaginalis. This led to an intensive search for a drug that would provide effective treatment.

In 1955, at the research laboratories of Rhone Poulenc, Paris, a crude extract of a streptomycete isolated from a soil sample collected from the island of Reunion in the Indian Ocean was found to produce three antibiotics, one of which had activity against Trichomonas vaginalis. The active compound was subsequently found to be azomycin (2-nitroimidazole), an antibiotic discovered by Japanese researchers 2 years earlier. This led to the synthesis of several hundred related compounds, one of which had optimal activity against the parasite and acceptable animal toxicity. This compound, first synthesized in 1957, was called metronidazole.

The results of the first clinical trial were reported in 1959 and the drug entered the French and UK markets for trichomonal vaginitis in 1960. Other indications for the drug quickly followed, including acute ulcerative gingivitis (Vincent's stomatitis), anaerobic bacterial infections and postoperative sepsis. The drug also became widely used for the treatment of other protozoal infections, including giardiasis, amoebic dysentery and amoebic liver disease, and balantidiasis. It has also been used to treat Guinea worm and Leishmania mexicana infections. More recently, there has been described a synergistic effect between metronidazole, its hydroxy metabolite and amoxycillin against the capnophilic Gram-negative bacillus Actinobacillus actinomycetemcomitans, which plays a major role in the aetiology of periodontal disease. Both metronidazole and ornidazole have been found to act synergistically with fleroxacin in mixed anaerobe–aerobic

cultures, but it remains to be established whether this is a general property of the nitroimidazole group of drugs.

The imidazole ring is an important feature of many natural compounds having a wide range of biological activities including the amino acid L-histidine, purine nucleotides adenine and guanine, essential chiral components of DNA and RNA, in the phosphate esters ATP, ADP and cyclic AMP. The ring also appears as part of a much larger structure in the vitamin biotin and in the antitumour antibiotics of the bleomycin group.

Nitration of imidazoles was first reported in 1892 and subsequently in 1909, but the first patent application for a nitroimidazole was filed in 1961. Since 1963, thousands of nitroimidazoles have been synthesized, including 2-nitroimidazoles, later principally developed as radiosensitizers, and 4- and 5-nitroimidazoles. More recently, halogenated-, dinitro- and aziridine nitroimidazole derivatives have been examined for possible use combined with radiotherapy for the treatment of hypoxic tumours. In general, the nitration of imidazole by conventional methods leads the nitro group into the 4- or 5-position. These are equivalent if the imine nitrogen (N-1) is unsubstituted but, if substituted, isomers are formed and the nitro group can enter either the 4- or 5-position, although those in the 4-position predominate. All nitroimidazoles are capable of being photodegraded and should be protected from light.

Antimicrobial activity

Nitroimidazole drugs have an unusual spectrum of activity which transcends those taxonomic boundaries typical of other antibiotics. No other range of compounds has useful activity against bacteria, protozoa, some helminths, or potential as drugs for the treatment of hypoxic tumours. No other group of drugs has the property of being able to kill all organisms which inhabit a low redox environment and are thus capable of anaerobic metabolism. Table 30.1 lists the

Table 30.1   *Activity of nitroimidazoles against anaerobes: MIC (mg/l)*

	Metronidazole	Ornidazole	Tinidazole
B. fragilis	0.25–4	<0.1–4	0.1–4
B. melaninogenicus	<0.1	<0.1	<0.1
Fusobacterium spp.	<0.1–1	<0.1–1	0.1–2
C. perfringens	0.25–2	0.25–2	0.25–2
Peptococcus and			
Peptostreptococcus spp.	<0.1–4	<0.1–2	<0.1–2
Veillonella spp.	1–2	0.5–1	0.5–2
Eubacterium spp.	0.5–2	0.5–1	0.5–2
Propionibacterium spp.	R	R	R

R, resistant.

activity of three nitroimidazoles against anaerobic bacteria. Since the introduction of metronidazole, other drugs have appeared; of these tinidazole and ornidazole are in widespread clinical use and others include secnidazole, carnidazole and nimorazole. Other nitroimidazoles used experimentally, including flexnidazole, panidazole and satranidazole, are not marketed.

Mode of action

All nitroimidazole drugs exert their antimicrobial effect via reduction of the nitro group. The 5-nitroimidazole groups are reduced at reduction potentials which are only generated in anaerobes. Reduction of the nitro group to the amine requires six electrons

$$R-NO_2 \xrightarrow{1e^-} R-NO_2\cdot^- \xrightarrow{1e^-} R-NO \xrightarrow{2e^-} R-NHOH \xrightarrow{2e^-} R-NH_2$$
$$(30.1)$$

but reduction beyond the hydroxylamine is rare and the amine is never formed. The reduction process is complicated by the decomposition of the nitro radical anion ($R-NO_2\cdot^-$) to nitrite (NO_2^-) and the imidazole radical ($R\cdot$) and, at high reduction rates, by the disproportionation of the nitro radical anion to the parent drug and the nitroso derivative

$$2R-NO_2\cdot^- + 2H^+ \rightarrow R-NO_2 + R-NO + H_2O \quad (30.2)$$

Tinidazole gives about 23% nitrite and metronidazole and ornidazole about 30%. This explains why, in many cases, the electron stoichiometry is less than 4.

Reduction by typical anaerobes, including *Clostridium*, *Bacteroides* and *Trichomonas* spp., is carried out by the pyruvate:ferredoxin oxidoreductase complex where the drugs are preferentially reduced by electrons from ferredoxin and also hydrogenase. It is the nitro radical anion, probably in its protonated form, which is the damaging species. This can react with DNA, oxidizing it and causing

strand breaks and destabilization of the helix. The effect on DNA and the accompanying cell death is very rapid. With *Clostridium pasteurianum*, 10 mg/l metronidazole kills 99.9% of the bacteria in 5 min. The precise nature of the DNA damage is not fully known. Certainly the DNA SOS repair system is induced by nitroimidazoles, but the uvrABC excinuclease repair system which repairs adducts is not involved, indicating that the drugs do not bind to the DNA. More recently, the repair enzymes exonuclease III and endonuclease III have been implicated in the repair of nitroimidazole-induced damage. These enzymes primarily repair oxidative damage to pyrimidines.

Pharmacokinetics

Nitroimidazoles are generally well absorbed and widely distributed in body tissues. Binding to proteins is low. They give peak plasma levels 1–2 h after oral dosing. The decay from the peak is exponential, with the rate depending on the half-life of the drug (Table 30.2).

Metabolism

5-Nitroimidazoles with a 2-methyl group (benznidazole and nimorazole are exceptions) are metabolized to the corresponding methoxy derivative and those with an alcohol side-chain are metabolized to the corresponding acid metabolite. All can form glucuronide conjugates and, occasionally, the ethereal sulphate conjugate. The nitro group of benznidazole, a 2-nitroimidazole, undergoes reduction to the amine and hydrolysis to the hydroxy derivative.

Toxicity and side-effects

These are not generally a problem, although some degree of gastro-intestinal disturbance is fairly common, as is a metallic taste in the mouth. Nitroimidazoles may interact with alcohol to give an antabuse-like effect. Prolonged or high doses, particularly when used to eradicate hypoxic cells in tumours, may give peripheral and central neurotoxicity. Although concern has been expressed about their long-term safety, particularly since their mechanism of action has DNA

Table 30.2   *Plasma half-lives of nitroimidazole drugs*

Drug	Half-life (h)	
	Range	Average
Metronidazole	5.6–11.4	8.5
Benznidazole	10.5–13.6	12
Ornidazole	12–14	13
Tinidazole	11.6–13.3	12.6
Secnidazole	–	18

as a major target, there is no evidence that they are carcinogenic in man.

Clinical use

These drugs are used in infections due to *Entamoeba histolytica*, *Giardia intestinalis*, *Balantidium* spp. and in mixed anaerobic infections such as are found in Vincent's stomatitis, Melaney's gangrene and synergistic and necrotizing fasciitis. They are routinely used to prevent postoperative sepsis and, more recently, metronidazole and tinidazole have been used in the treatment of gastroduodenal ulcers caused by the microaerophile *Helicobacter pylori*. Benznidazole (a 2-nitroimidazole) is used for the treatment of *Trypanosoma cruzi* infections, Chagas' disease and for the experimental treatment of radioresistant hypoxic tumours.

In veterinary medicine, dimetridazole is used to prevent histomoniasis or blackhead in turkeys and poultry caused by *Histomonas melagreadis* and for the control of swine fever. Ipronidazole is frequently used for the treatment of turkey blackhead, and ronidazole is used for treating turkey enterohepatitis, swine dysentery and bovine trichomoniasis. Carnidazole and dimetridazole are used for the treatment and control of trichomoniasis in pigeons.

Recently, nitroimidazole drugs have been used in the treatment of bacterial vaginosis or non-specific vaginitis caused by the microaerophile *Gardnerella vaginalis*. Even single-dose therapy appears to allow the vaginal lactobacilli to recolonize, thus restoring the normal vaginal pH. In this system the hydroxy metabolite of metronidazole appears to exert just as effective an antimicrobial effect as the parent drug.

Further information

Aldridge K E, Schiro D D 1990 *In vitro* study of potential synergy of fleroxacin and metronidazole against mixed aerobes and anaerobes. Proceedings of the 3rd International Symposium on New Quinolones, p 15–17

Borsch G, Mai U, Opferkuch W 1988 Oral triple therapy (OTT) may effectively eradicate *Campylobacter pyloridis* in man: a pilot study. *Gastroenterology* 94: A44

Chapman J D, Lee J, Meeker B E 1989 Cellular reduction of nitroimidazole drugs: potential for selective chemotherapy and diagnosis of hypoxic cells. *International Journal of Radiation Oncology Biology and Physics* 16: 911–917

Fredricsson B, Hagstrom B, Moller A K, Nord C E 1986 Bacterial vaginosis treated with metronidazole. Effects on the vaginal microbiology by a single dose versus a five day regimen. *Zentralblatt fur Gynaecologie* 108: 799–804

Garcia-Rodriguez J A, Garcia Sanchez J E, Trujillano I, Sanchez de San Lorenzo A 1990 Fleroxacin plus metronidazole and fleroxacin plus ornidazole against *Bacteroides fragilis* group and *Escherichia coli*. Proceedings of the 3rd International Symposium on New Quinolones, p 18–19

McFadzean J A 1986 Flagyl. The story of a pharmaceutical discovery. Parthenon, Camforth

Mohanty K C, Deighton R 1985 Comparison of two different metronidazole regimens in the treatment of *Gardnerella vaginalis* infection with or without trichomoniasis. *Journal of Antimicrobial Chemotherapy* 16: 799–803

Pavicic M J A M P, van Winkelhoff A J, de Graaff J 1991 Synergistic effects between amoxicillin, metronidazole and the hydroxy metabolite of metronidazole against *Actinobacillus actinomycetemcomitans*. *Antimicrobial Agents and Chemotherapy* 35: 961–966

BENZNIDAZOLE

A 2-nitroimidazole.

Antimicrobial activity

Benznidazole exhibits antiprotozoal activity, particularly against *Trypanosoma cruzi*.

Pharmacokinetics

When given by mouth in a single 100 mg tablet, benznidazole was absorbed from the gastro-intestinal tract and gave peak plasma concentrations of 2.22–2.81 mg/l at 3–4 h after administration. The elimination half-life ranged from 10.5 to 13.6 (average 12) h and the drug was about 44% bound to plasma proteins.

Metabolic studies have revealed an amine and hydroxy metabolite, both in the C-2 position, indicating reduction of the nitro group and hydrolysis or an oxidative deamination of the amine metabolite.

Toxicity and side-effects

Adverse effects include nausea, vomiting, abdominal pain, peripheral neuropathy and severe skin reactions. A trial involving 20 cases of the chronic form of South American trypanosomiasis, or Chagas' disease, was stopped because of the high incidence of skin rashes and neurological side-effects.

Clinical use

Benznidazole is used almost exclusively for the treatment of the early acute stages of Chagas' disease. The drug appears to have doubtful use in the intermediate or chronic phases of the disease. Efficacy of treatment varies from country to country and this may be related to the relative sensitivities of the various strains of *T. cruzi*. In one study the drug was effective in curing 80% of chronic and acute cases of South American trypanosomiasis. There has been a single report of the effectiveness of benznidazole in American mucocutaneous leishmaniasis, but the trial was conducted with only six patients.

Preparations and dosage

Dosage: Adults, oral, 5 mg/kg per day, for 30–60 days.
Children, oral, 10 mg/kg per day, for 30–60 days.

Further information

Apt W 1986 Clinical trial of benznidazole and an immunopotentiator against Chagas' disease in Chile. *Transactions of the Royal Society of Tropical Medicine and Hygiene* 80: 1010

Gutteridge G E 1985 Existing chemotherapy and its limitations. *British Medical Bulletin* 41: 162–168

WHO 1991 Control of Chagas disease: report of a WHO expert committee. WHO Technical Report Series No 811. Geneva: WHO

METRONIDAZOLE

A 5-nitroimidazole.

Antimicrobial activity

Metronidazole is a potent inhibitor of obligate anaerobic bacteria, and protozoa (Table 30.1), but not of any organism which is aerobic or incapable of anaerobic metabolism. Susceptible protozoa include *T. vaginalis*, *G. intestinalis*, *E. histolytica*, *Balantidium coli* and *Blastocystis hominis*, which are inhibited by concentrations of 0.2–0.25 mg/l. Metronidazole is also active against obligate anaerobic bacteria, including *Clostridium* spp. and *Bacteroides* spp. at concentrations of 0.1–8.0 mg/l. The drug also has activity against the facultative anaerobic (microaerophilic) *H. pylori* and *G. vaginalis*. The minimum inhibitory concentration (MIC) for *H. pylori* is <0.1 to >32 mg/l, indicating the occurrence of naturally resistant strains. The MIC for susceptible strains is <1–2 mg/l. The metronidazole 2-methoxy metabolite is more active (MIC about 0.3 mg/l), but the acid metabolite shows less activity than the parent drug (MIC about 3 mg/l). *G. vaginalis* shows similar susceptibility (MIC of metronidazole 1 to >128 mg/l), but susceptible strains are killed at <8 mg/l. The methoxy metabolite is more active (MIC 0.02–2 mg/l). Organisms with MICs ≤16 mg/l may be regarded as susceptible; an MIC >16 mg/l is regarded as resistant and indicates that the infecting organism is not likely to respond to metronidazole therapy. Although metronidazole is inactive against aerobes, a recent report indicates that the drug is bactericidal to dormant cells of *Mycobacterium tuberculosis*, indicating that the dormant phase is primarily an anaerobic one.

Acquired resistance

Trichomonas vaginalis and *Giardia intestinalis*

Although resistance rates of *T. vaginalis* are low, with 150 million cases reported each year, the number of treatment failures due to resistance is significant. The MIC for metronidazole for *T. vaginalis* from refractory vaginitis is frequently 3–8 times the value for susceptible strains. In *Trichomonas* spp., resistance to metronidazole and other nitroimidazoles is characterized by a tolerance to oxygen which results in decreased susceptibility under both anaerobic and aerobic conditions, suggesting that the organism is resistant to oxygen in the environment. Until recently, *T. vaginalis* was considered a typical anaerobe, but its behaviour is now recognized as more typical of a microaerophile rather than an aerotolerant anaerobe.

The mechanisms of metronidazole resistance have been best studied in *T. vaginalis* where an anaerobic and aerobic resistance is known. Aerobic resistance is found clinically and anaerobic resistance has been generated in vitro and in vivo. The earliest studies on clinical failure of trichomonal vaginitis treated with metronidazole revealed the presence of Trichomonas fully susceptible to the drug. This led subsequently to the observation that the vaginal aerobic or microaerophilic bacteria were capable of 'absorbing' the drug without loss of viability, thus decreasing the drug concentration available to kill the protozoan. In susceptible cells, metronidazole is reduced by an intracellular pyruvate ferredoxin oxidoreductase (PFOR) system unique to anaerobes. In resistant Trichomonas there is a decrease in the PFOR system and in fully resistant strains in vitro the PFOR system is absent. The consequences of this are that pyruvate oxidation in the hydrogenosome is diverted to non-

PFOR-linked pathways and instead favour the formation of lactate (in *T. vaginalis*) or ethanol (in *Trichomonas fetus*). This mechanism of resistance appears to dominate both in resistant organisms cultured anaerobically or micro-aerophilically. The 'aerobic' resistance is shown by some strains which occur clinically. Trichomonads, now regarded as microaerophiles rather than anaerobes, have evolved at least four oxidases capable of scavenging oxygen. In aerobically resistant strains, the hydrogenosomal oxidases are defective and have a much reduced affinity for oxygen. Thus more is available to futile cycle (a process whereby the nitro group of the drug is reduced radical, re-forming the original parent drug) with reduced metronidazole. More recently, it has been reported that a decreased transcription of the ferredoxin gene resulting in decreased levels of a functional PFOR system can lead to metronidazole resistance in Trichomonas.

Rare resistance in *G. intestinalis* is also due to decreased levels of the PFOR system.

Bacteroides *and* Clostridium *spp.*

A number of strains of *B. fragilis* have been isolated with reduced susceptibility to metronidazole and other nitro-imidazoles, and resistance has also been described in *Bacteroides distasonis* and *Bacteroides bivius*. In those strains where the resistance mechanism has been studied, decreased levels of the PFOR system have been found. There have been reports that the gene(s) for resistance are borne on a 7.7 kb plasmid and transferable by conjugation, but the gene product in this case is not known.

Metronidazole resistant strains of Clostridia have not been reported clinically, but a laboratory strain of *Clostridium perfringens* made resistant by mutation possessed decreased levels of PFOR.

Mobiluncus *and* Helicobacter

In one study, all isolates of *Mobiluncus curtisii* were resistant to metronidazole and to its hydroxy metabolite. About half of all strains of *Mobiluncus mulieris* were resistant and about 20% were also resistant to the hydroxy metabolite. Acquired resistance in *Mobiluncus* spp. does not appear to be a problem at present.

Failures of treatment of *H. pylori* infections are associated with resistance to metronidazole. Neither the mechanism of action nor the mechanism of resistance is known. It has been suggested that resistance could arise by an increase in futile cycling (see above), leading to increased levels of superoxide dismutase and catalase, but the probability is that resistance in *Helicobacter* spp. is not acquired but a consequence of the environment, since all strains are susceptible when cultured anaerobically. The amount of metronidazole taken up by *Helicobacter* spp. depends on the oxygen tension and cell density; thus high levels of microaerophilia decrease the rate of drug entry into the cell and hence the amount available to kill the cell, resulting in apparent resistance.

Pharmacokinetics

Polarographic, spectrophotometric and bioassay methods all fail to detect some metabolites and the recommended procedure is high performance liquid chromatography (HPLC) in which the system can be calibrated with known reference compounds.

Absorption

Metronidazole in tablet form is rapidly and almost completely absorbed, giving peak plasma concentrations after 20 min to 3 h which are proportional to the dose. Oral administration of 250, 500 or 2000 mg produces peak plasma levels of 6, 12 and 40 mg/l, respectively. There is no difference between the bioavailability of the drug in males and females, but because of weight differences plasma levels in males are usually lower than those in females. In patients treated with intravenous metronidazole using a loading dose of 15 mg/kg followed by 7.5 mg/kg every 6 h, peak steady-state plasma concentrations averaged 25 mg/l with minimum trough concentrations averaging 18 mg/l.

The bioavailability of metronidazole in suppositories is 60–80%. Effective blood concentrations occur 5–12 h after the first suppository and are maintained by an 8 h regimen.

Metronidazole passes through the placenta and reaches concentrations in placenta and fetal tissue related to the corresponding plasma levels (Table 30.3). The drug appears in breast milk.

A study which did not distinguish between metronidazole and its metabolites indicated that, in the elderly, serum concentrations following a single 500 mg oral dose were significantly higher than those in younger healthy subjects and that the area under the curve (AUC) for plasma was almost doubled. A subsequent study has shown that plasma clearance, distribution volume and half-life did not differ in

Table 30.3 *Levels of metronidazole and tinidazole in placental and fetal tissue*

Drug	Drug concentration		
	Serum (µg/ml)	Placenta (µg/mg)	Fetus (µg/mg)
Tinidazole	13.2	4.9	7.6
Metronidazole	13.5	3.5	9.0

the young and elderly and that there was no requirement for a decreased dosage for the elderly, unless there was overt renal insufficiency.

Metabolism

Metronidazole is metabolized in the human liver by side-chain oxidation and glucuronide formation, although some dispute this because the metabolic pattern is not changed in cirrhosis. There are two principal oxidative metabolites: the acid and hydroxy derivatives. The acid metabolite is produced by oxidation of the N-1 ethanol side-chain to the corresponding acetic derivative. This metabolite is microbiologically inactive and appears in the urine because of its high water solubility. The hydroxy derivative is formed by oxidation of the methyl group on C-2 of the imidazole ring first to the hydroxymethyl derivative and subsequently, and less significantly, to the carboxylic acid. Significantly, the hydroxymethyl derivative (the hydroxy) metabolite is as active as the parent drug against *G. vaginalis*. Similar effects have been seen with niridazole in *Gardnerella* and in *H. pylori*. Both metronidazole itself and the hydroxymethyl metabolite are capable of forming sulphate or glucuronide conjugates, and the acid metabolite may be excreted as the glycine conjugate.

Small amounts of metabolites derived from reduction of the nitro group, notably the oxamic acid and acetamide, have been detected in urine and are assumed to be formed by the intestinal flora. This is indicative of fragmentation of the imidazole ring. There is no evidence for the reduction of the nitro group to the amine, which is known to be highly unstable (p. 405).

Distribution

Metronidazole is widely distributed in body tissues. The elimination half-life is 8.5 ± 2.9 h. Distribution is similar for both oral and intravenous forms. Less than 20% of the parent drug is bound to plasma proteins. It appears about 90 min after an oral dose in cerebrospinal fluid (CSF), saliva and breast milk in concentrations similar to those found in plasma, and in vaginal secretions, pleural and prostatic fluid at levels about 40% of those of the plasma. In patients receiving 500 mg twice daily or 1 g 6-hourly, CSF levels of up to 2 and 8 mg/l, respectively, have been found. Bactericidal concentrations of metronidazole have been found in pus from hepatic abscesses.

Excretion

The major route of elimination is renal with 60–80% of the dose appearing in the urine; faecal excretion accounts for 6–15%. The hydroxy metabolite and the acid metabolite are also excreted in the urine. Conjugation of the unchanged drug with glucuronide accounts for approximately 20% of

the total. Renal clearance is approximately 10 ml/min per 1.73 m^2. Decreased renal function does not alter the single-dose kinetics, but plasma clearance is decreased in patients with impaired liver function. In one study, newborn infants appeared to possess a decreased capacity to eliminate metronidazole. The elimination half-life measured during the first 3 days of life was inversely related to gestational age. In infants whose gestational ages were between 28 and 40 weeks, the corresponding half-life elimination rates ranged from 10.9 to 22.5 h.

Toxicity and side-effects

Metronidazole hydrochloride for intravenous use is incompatible with a number of agents and it is generally recommended that other drugs should not be added to solutions of metronidazole hydrochloride.

Precautions

Alcohol should not be taken during metronidazole therapy and for 48 h after because of a possible disulfuram (antabuse-like) reaction; neither should the drug be combined with formulations containing alcohol. Metronidazole should not be given in cases of known hypersensitivity to nitroimidazoles. Metronidazole enhances the anti-coagulant effect of warfarin and may impair the clearance of phenytoin and lithium. The former may increase the metabolism of metronidazole. Plasma concentrations are decreased by the concomitant administration of pheno-barbitone with a consequent decrease in the efficacy of metronidazole. The drug may also mask the immunological response of untreated early syphilis cases because metronidazole has antitreponemal activity.

Metronidazole should be used with care in patients with blood dyscrasias or with any central nervous system (CNS) disease. If any peripheral neuropathy or CNS toxicity occurs, which is more likely in those patients treated for 10 days or more, treatment should be discontinued. The co-administration of cimetidine increases plasma levels of metronidazole and may increase the risk of neurological side-effects.

Metronidazole crosses the placenta to the fetus, and the drug should be avoided especially during the first trimester of pregnancy and particularly if high doses are being administered. Use during the second and third trimesters may be acceptable if alternative therapies for trichomoniasis have failed, but single-dose (2 g oral) therapy should be avoided. The drug is efficiently excreted in breast milk and may cause the milk to taste bitter. Breast feeding should be discontinued until 24 h after the last dose to allow excretion of the drug. Metronidazole appears safe when given to nursing mothers at doses of up to 400 mg three times daily.

Adverse effects

The adverse effects of metronidazole are dose related.

Nervous system. There have been two serious convulsive seizures and peripheral neuropathy in patients treated with the intravenous metronidazole preparation. Use of the intravenous preparation has also caused headache, dizziness, syncope, ataxia and confusion. Convulsive seizures, peripheral neuropathy, dizziness, vertigo, incoordination, ataxia, confusion, irritability, depression, weakness and insomnia have been reported in association with oral preparations.

Sensory. Peripheral neuropathy was found in 11 of 13 patients aged 12–22 years treated for Crohn's disease. The symptoms disappeared when the dose was discontinued or markedly reduced. A patient receiving 2 g daily for 50 days, again for Crohn's disease, developed persistent peripheral neuropathy.

Gastro-intestinal. Gastro-intestinal disturbances, include nausea, vomiting, abdominal discomfort and diarrhoea, have been noted with both intravenous and oral preparations. Pseudomembranous colitis associated with metronidazole administration is also reported, but with its increasing use in the treatment of gastroduodenal ulcer it is perhaps surprising that more reports are not known.

Haematopoietic. Reversible neutropenia (leukopenia) has been reported after administration of both intravenous and oral preparations of metronidazole. Reversible thrombocytopenia has also been reported, but the condition is rare. Bone-marrow aplasia has been noted in one case of a 74-year-old man given 200 mg metronidazole three times a day for 7 days before and 10 days after operation, and in two patients who had previously received metronidazole. A haemolytic–uraemic syndrome was reported in 6 children who had been given metronidazole for non-specific diarrhoea or for prophylaxis after bowel surgery.

Mouth. An unpleasant sharp, metallic taste is not unusual. Furry tongue, glossitis and stomatitis have occurred; the latter may be associated with overgrowth of *Candida* spp. during treatment.

Dermatological. Erythematous rash and pruritis have been reported after use of the intravenous preparation, as has thrombophlebitis. The latter can be minimized by avoiding prolonged indwelling catheters for intravenous infusion.

Other reactions. Flattening of the T-wave may be seen in electrocardiographic tracings. A number of cases of deafness associated with metronidazole have been reported. Myopia related to treatment for trichomoniasis occurred in a woman treated for 11 days with oral metronidazole. The condition disappeared 4 days after treatment was stopped, but returned when treatment was resumed. There have been two reports of pancreatitis associated with metronidazole administration. Gynaecomastia occurred in a 36-year-old man who took metronidazole for about a month for ulcerative colitis.

Mutagenicity and carcinogenicity

Metronidazole has been shown to be weakly mutagenic using the Ames histidine reversion test in some strains of bacteria, and some metabolites in human urine have also been shown to be positive in the Ames test. However, some doubt was thrown on these results when it was demonstrated that metronidazole was not mutagenic in a properly conducted aerobic Ames test, but only when conditions were anaerobic or microaerophilic and led to the reduction of the nitro group, an essential prerequisite for its bactericidal mode of action. The microsomal fraction added to activate drugs in the Ames test has a high oxygen demand and can rapidly deplete the preparation of oxygen, resulting in the creation of anaerobiosis in a seemingly aerobic environment.

In other mutagenic and genotoxicity studies metronidazole has proved negative in the dominant lethal test in rats, the micronucleus test in mice and human cells *in vitro*, in studies of unscheduled DNA synthesis *in vitro* in human lymphocytes and fibroblasts, mitotic indices in human lymphocytes and in chromosome aberration frequency tests.

Reports of metronidazole-induced carcinogenicity are conflicting and confused. Some studies indicated that metronidazole caused lung tumours at high-dose levels in mice and lymphoreticular neoplasms in female mice only and hepatomas and mammary tumours in rats also at high doses. Other studies show lung tumours in male mice only, or in both sexes, while in the female rat one study proved negative and another non-significant. Two studies in hamsters have shown negative carcinogenicity. Some of these studies have been criticised on the grounds that overfeeding of animals is known to lead to the development of cancers typical of those seen in several studies.

Human carcinogenicity studies have shown that metronidazole did not increase the incidence of cancer in a retrospective study of 771 patients given metronidazole for trichomoniasis, or in a subsequent study involving 2460 patients. A subsequent 15–25 year follow-up study reporting to 1984 also showed no increase in cancers or cancer-related morbidity or mortality.

Clinical use

Infections treated with metronidazole include trichomonal vaginitis, bacterial vaginosis (non-specific vaginitis), acute necrotizing ulcerative gingivitis (Vincent's disease, Vincent's stomatitis) and pseudomembranous colitis. Gastroduodenal ulcers caused by *H. pylori* are treated with metronidazole, as are infections due to *Clostridium* or *Bacteroides* spp. The drug is also used for the amelioration of malodorous tumours where anaerobic bacteria are the cause. Metronidazole is also used in rosacea and Guinea worm infection. It is not indicated in cases of inflammatory bowel disease (Crohn's disease), despite reports of its success in treating the condition and claims that this may indicate an anaerobic

Table 30.4 *Treatment of metronidazole-resistant* T. vaginalis: *relationship between the in vitro aerobic susceptibility (expressed as the minimum lethal concentration (MLC)), the approximate level of clinical resistance and a suggested treatment regimen**

Aerobic MLC (mg/l)	Resistance level	Total daily oral dose (g)	Duration of treatment (days)
<50	Susceptible	2	1
50	Marginal	2	3
100	Mild	2	3–5
200	Moderate	2–2.5	7–10
>200	Severe	3–3.5	14†

* From Lossick (1988).
† Concomitant intravaginal treatment with a 500–1000 mg tablet daily may be helpful.

infection as a major factor or cause of the disease. Metronidazole has been used as an adjunct to radiotherapy of hypoxic tumours, but its use is limited by toxicity at the doses necessary.

Many cases of *T. vaginalis* resistance may have been curable with a regimen designed to take account of the oxygen sensitivity of the isolate. It is realized that few hospitals or clinics have the laboratory facilities to screen *T. vaginalis* isolates for their oxygen sensitivities, and consequently treatment regimens for resistant or intractable cases have always involved increased dosage ranging from 6 to 52 g over a 3- to 4-day period. Many successful treatments involve the additional intravaginal insertion of a 500 mg tablet of metronidazole daily. The treatment regimen for metronidazole-resistant *T. vaginalis* designed by Lossick is shown in Table 30.4. The table has been constructed from experience with a large number of refractory cases and the regimen has a cure rate of 87%. It should be noted, however, that dosages of metronidazole which exceed 2 g/day for 1–2 weeks often produce significant side-effects, including nausea, metallic taste, headache and sensorium changes. Treatment in which dosages exceed 3 g/day for more than 5 days may produce mild peripheral neurotoxicity. If susceptibility testing for *T. vaginalis* is unavailable, a recommended dose of 2 g/day for 3–5 days should clear most mildly resistant infections.

Preparations and dosage

Proprietary names: Flagyl, Zadstat, Metrotop, Metrogel, Metrolyl.
Preparations: Tablets, suppositories, topical gel, i.v. infusion, oral suspension.
Dosage: The indications are so varied that dosages are given with the uses in individual chapters.
Widely available.

Further information

Anonymous 1991 Drug-induced ototoxicity. *WHO Drug Information* 5: 12–16

Barnes A R 1990 Chemical stabilities of cefuroxime sodium and metronidazole in an admixture for intravenous infusion. *Journal of Clinical Pharmacology and Therapeutics* 15: 187–196

Beard C M 1988 Cancer after exposure to metronidazole. *Mayo Clinic Proceedings* 63: 147–153

Breuil J, Dublanchet A, Truffaut N, Sebald M 1989 Transferable 5-nitroimidazole resistance in the *Bacteroides fragilis* group. *Plasmid* 21: 151–154

Briggs G C 1990 Drugs in pregnancy and lactation, 3rd edn. Williams & Wilkins, Baltimore

Cederbrant G, Kahlmeter G, Ljungh A 1992 Proposed mechanisms for metronidazole resistance in *Helicobacter pylori*. *Journal of Antimicrobial Chemotherapy* 29: 115–120

Cerkasovova A, Cerkasov, Kulda J 1988 Resistance of Trichomonads to metronidazole. *Acta Universitatis Carolinae – Biologica* 30: 485–503

Edwards D I 1993 Nitroimidazole drugs – action and resistance mechanisms. I. Mechanisms of action. *Journal of Antimicrobial Chemotherapy* 31: 9–20

Edwards D I 1993 Nitroimidazole drugs – action and resistance mechanisms. II. Mechanisms of resistance. *Journal of Antimicrobial Chemotherapy* 31: 201–210

Ellis J E, Cole D, Lloyd D 1992 Influence of oxygen on the fermentative metabolism of metronidazole-sensitive and resistant strains of *Trichomonas vaginalis*. *Molecular and Biochemical Parasitology* 56: 79–88

Friedman G D, Selby J V 1989 Metronidazole and cancer. *Journal of the American Medical Association* 261: 866–872

Johnson P J 1993 Metronidazole and drug resistance. *Parasitology Today* 9: 183–186

Lacey S L, Moss S F, Taylor G W 1993 Metronidazole uptake by sensitive and resistant isolates of *Helicobacter pylori*. *Journal of Antimicrobial Chemotherapy* 32: 393–400

Lloyd D, Yarlett N, Yarlett C, Pedersen J Z, Kristensen B 1988 Metronidazole resistant clinical isolates of *Trichomonas vaginalis* maintain low intracellular metronidazole radical anion levels as a consequence of defective oxygen scavenging. *Acta Universitatis Carolinae – Biologica* 30: 533–545

Lossick J 1988 Chemotherapy of nitroimidazole-resistant vaginal trichomoniasis. *Acta Universitatis Carolinae – Biologica* 30: 533–545

Lossick J, Muller M, Gorrell T E 1986 *In vitro* drug susceptibility and doses of metronidazole required for cure in cases of refractory vaginal trichomoniasis. *Journal of Infectious Diseases* 12 (suppl 6): S665–S681

Lossick J G 1990 Treatment of sexually transmitted vaginosis/vaginitis. *Reviews of Infectious Diseases* 12 (suppl 6): S665–S681

Narikawa S, Suzuki T, Yamamoto M, Nakamura M 1991 Lactate dehydrogenase activity as a cause of metronidazole resistance in *Bacteroides fragilis* NTCT 11295. *Journal of Antimicrobial Chemotherapy* 28: 47–53

Paget T A, Lloyd D 1990 *Trichomonas vaginalis* requires traces of oxygen and high concentrations of carbon dioxide for optimal growth. *Molecular and Biochemical Parasitology* 41: 65–72

Plaisance K I, Quintiliani R, Nightingale C H 1988 The pharmacokinetics of metronidazole and its metabolites in critically ill patients. *Journal of Antimicrobial Chemotherapy* 21: 195–200

Quon D V K, D'Oliveira C E, Johnson P J 1992 Reduced transcription of the ferredoxin gene in metronidazole-resistant *Trichomonas vaginalis*. *Proceedings of the National Academy of Sciences USA* 89: 4402

Tachezy J, Kulda K, Tomkova E 1993 Aerobic resistance of *Trichomonas vaginalis* to metronidazole induced in vitro. *Parasitology* 106: 31–37

Uccellini D A, Morgan D J, Raymond K 1986 Relationships among duration of infusion, dose, dosing interval and steady state plasma concentrations during intermittent intravenous infusions: studies with metronidazole. *Journal of Pharmacokinetics and Biopharmaceutics* 14: 95–106

Wayne L G, Sramek H 1994 Metronidazole is bactericidal to dormant cells of *Mycobacterium tuberculosis*. *Antimicrobial Agents and Chemotherapy* 38: 2054–2058

NIMORAZOLE
Nitrimidazine
A 5-nitroimidazole.

Antimicrobial activity

It is active against *T. vaginalis, G. intestinalis* and *E. histolytica*. The drug also is active against the mixed anaerobic infection that characterizes Vincent's disease and against *Gard. vaginalis*. Nimorazole was about three times less active than metronidazole against *B. fragilis* and *Fusobacterium* spp. in one study, with a mean MIC of 1.05 mg/l, but another showed it to have identical activity against *B. fragilis* with a median MIC of 0.25 mg/l.

Nimorazole is absorbed from the intestine. A peak blood concentration of about 32 mg/l occurs within 2 h after a 500 mg oral dose. High concentrations of the drug also occur in saliva and vaginal secretions. Excretion is principally via the urine where the drug appears as metabolites which also display antimicrobial and antiprotozoal activity, but less so than that of the parent drug. Nimorazole is generally well tolerated even at the high doses required in conjunction with radiotherapy for the treatment of head and neck tumours. Antabuse-like reactions appear to be rare.

Clinical use

It is used for the single-dose (2 g oral) treatment of trichomonal vaginitis for which it is as effective as metronidazole and tinidazole. It is also used for giardiasis, intestinal amoebiasis and for Vincent's stomatitis and in the conjunctive therapy of hypoxic tumours.

Preparations and dosage
Preparation: Tablets.
Dosage: Adults, oral, trichomoniasis, 2 g as a single dose, and sexual partners should be treated concomitantly. Giardiasis or amoebiasis, adults, oral, 500 mg twice daily for 5 days. Children >10 kg body weight, 500 mg/day for 5 days. Children <10 kg body weight, 250 mg/day for 5 days.
Available in continental Europe and South Africa.

Further information
Mohanty K C, Deighton R 1987 Comparison of 2 g single dose of metronidazole, nimorazole and tinidazole in the treatment of vaginitis associated with *Gardnerella vaginalis*. *Journal of Antimicrobial Chemotherapy* 19: 393–399

Overgaard J, Hansen H S, Lindelov B et al 1991 Nimorazole as a hypoxic radiosensitizer in the treatment of supraglottic larynx and pharynx carcinoma. First report from the Danish Head and Neck Cancer Study (DAHANCA) protocol 5-85. *Radiotherapy and Oncology* 20 (suppl): 143–149

Pamba H O 1990 Comparative study of aminosidine etophamide and nimorazole alone or in combination in the treatment of intestinal amoebiasis in Kenya. *European Journal of Clinical Pharmacology* 39: 353–357

ORNIDAZOLE

A 5-nitroimidazole

Antimicrobial activity

Its activity closely parallels that of metronidazole and tinidazole (Table 30.1).

Pharmacokinetics

Ornidazole is readily absorbed from the intestinal tract; peak plasma levels reach 30 mg/l within 2 h of a single oral dose of 1.5 g. After a 750 mg oral dose, peak plasma concentrations reach 11 mg/l at 2–4 h. The half-life of the drug is 12–14 h. It is also well absorbed from the vagina, with peak plasma concentrations of 5 mg/l being reached 12 h after the insertion of a 500 mg vaginal pessary. After a single 1 g intravenous infusion for colorectal surgery, serum levels reached about 24 mg/l after 15 min and about 6 mg/l after 24 h.

Metabolism of the drug occurs in the liver. The plasma clearance rate decreases in hepatic failure because of reduced liver metabolism and decreased biliary elimination. About 60% of an oral dose is recovered in the urine and 20% in the faeces. During haemodialysis, ornidazole is removed and there is no clear indication as to whether the drug should be given before or after such dialysis.

It has wide tissue distribution including CSF.

Toxicity and side-effects

These are similar to those of metronidazole and tinidazole.

Clinical use

Ornidazole is a useful drug in the treatment of anaerobic protozoal infections, including trichomonal vaginitis, giardiasis, intestinal amoebiasis and amoebic liver abscess. It is also useful for the treatment and prophylaxis of anaerobic bacterial infections, including postoperative anaerobic infections, vaginosis and mixed aerobe–anaerobe infections.

Preparations

Tablets, vaginal pessary, i.v. infusion.
Available widely. Not in UK.

Further information

Bourget P 1988 Ornidazole pharmacokinetics in several hepatic diseases. *Journal de Pharmacologie Clinique* 7: 25–32

Horber F F, Maurer O, Probst P J, Heizman E, Frey F J 1989 High haemodialysis clearance of ornidazole in the presence of a negligible renal clearance. *European Journal of Clinical Pharmacology* 36: 389–393

Martin C, Bruguerolle B, Mallet M N, Condomines M, Sastre B, Gouin F 1990 Pharmacokinetics and tissue penetration of a single dose of ornidazole (1000 milligrams intravenously) for antibiotic prophylaxis in colorectal surgery. *Antimicrobial Agents and Chemotherapy* 34: 1921–1924

Meech R J, Loutit J 1985 Non-specific vaginitis: diagnostic features and response to imidazole therapy (metronidazole, ornidazole). *New Zealand Medical Journal* 98: 389–391

Merjian H, Baumelou A, Diquet B, Chick O, Singlas E 1985 Pharmacokinetics of ornidazole in patients with renal insufficiency: influence of haemodialysis and peritoneal dialysis. *British Journal of Clinical Pharmacology* 19: 211–217

Taburet A M, Delion F, Attali P, Thebault J J, Singlas E 1986 Pharmacokinetics of ornidazole in patients with severe liver cirrhosis. *Clinical Pharmacology and Therapeutics* 40: 359–364

Taburet A M, Attili P, Bourget P, Etienne J P, Singlas E 1989 Pharmacokinetics of ornidazole in patients with acute viral hepatitis, alcoholic cirrhosis and extrahepatic cholestasis. *Clinical Pharmacology and Therapeutics* 45: 373–379

Turcant A, Granry J C, Allain P, Cavellat M 1987 Pharmacokinetics of ornidazole in neonates and infants after a single intravenous infusion. *European Journal of Clinical Pharmacology* 32: 111–113

SECNIDAZOLE

A 5-nitroimidazole.

Its properties are similar to those of metronidazole, but it is distinguished by having the longest plasma half-life (18 h) of clinically used nitroimidazole drugs. It is used in the treatment of intestinal amoebiasis and giardiasis, and has been used in trichomoniasis.

Preparations

Available in France.

Further information

Soedin K 1985 Comparison between the efficacy of a single dose of secnidazole with a 5-day course of tetracycline and clioquinol in the treatment of acute intestinal amoebiasis. *Pharmatherapeutica* 4: 251–254

Develoux M 1990 Traitment de la giardiase par une dose unique de 30 mg/kg de secnidazole. *Medecine d'Africa Noire* 37: 412–413

TINIDAZOLE

A 5-nitroimidazole.

Antimicrobial activity

Its antibacterial and antiprotozoal activity is similar to that of metronidazole. The drug is active against *Bacteroides, Fusobacterium, Clostridium, Peptococcus, Peptostreptococcus, Gardnerella* and *Veillonella* spp. (Table 30.1). The MIC for most anaerobic bacteria is less than 4 mg/l. *H. pylori* is inhibited by 0.5 mg/l. It inhibits *T. vaginalis* and *T. fetus* at 2.5 mg/l; and *E. histolytica* at about 0.3–2.5 mg/l.

Pharmacokinetics

The pharmacokinetics of tinidazole are similar to those of metronidazole but tinidazole has a longer half-life, similar to that of ornidazole (see Table 30.2).

After a single oral 2 g dose, peak plasma concentrations of 40 mg/l are reached after 2 h. This falls to about 10 mg/l at 24 h and 2.5 mg/l at 48 h. Daily doses of 1 g will maintain plasma levels in excess of 8 mg/l, irrespective of whether the dose is oral or intravenous. Tinidazole has a low level of protein binding (12%). Six minutes after the end of infusion of 800 mg over 30 min, the mean plasma concentration was 12 mg/l.

Distribution

Tissue distribution is widespread, with concentrations similar to those reached in plasma being found in bile, CSF, breast milk and saliva. The drug readily crosses the placenta. Placental transfer of tinidazole or metronidazole into fetal and placental tissues did not differ significantly after a single 20 min intravenous infusion of 500 mg of either drug. A study in 21 women undergoing a first-trimester abortion showed significant tinidazole concentrations 1 h after the start of the infusion (Table 30.3).

Metabolism

Metabolism in mammals forms the 2-hydroxymethyl derivative, its glucuronide and two minor and unidentified metabolites. In urine about half the drug remains unmetabolized.

Excretion

Tinidazole and its metabolites are excreted primarily in the urine and to a minor extent in the faeces. The clearance rate is about 0.73 ml/min per kg and the urinary excretion as a percentage of the dose is about 21%. Total clearance of the drug is 51 ml/min, renal clearance 10 ml/min, volume of distribution 50 l and half-life 11.6 h. In healthy volunteers given an intravenous infusion of 800 mg [^{14}C]tinidazole over 30 min, a mean of 44% of the dose was excreted in the urine during the first 24 h. This increased to 63% of the dose during 5 days. Only 12% of the dose appeared in the faeces, indicating a possible role for biliary excretion. Unchanged tinidazole comprised 32% of urinary ^{14}C in 0–120 h urine. In the 0–12 h urine about 30% of the ^{14}C comprised a metabolite in which the nitro group had migrated from the 5-position of the imidazole ring to the 4-position, and the 5-position had become hydroxylated. This metabolite also appeared in the faeces. A 2-hydroxymethyl metabolite accounted for about 9% of the urinary ^{14}C and was also present in plasma.

In renal failure the pharmacokinetics of tinidazole are not significantly changed in comparison with healthy individuals, but because the drug is rapidly removed by haemodialysis it is recommended that the normal dosage be given after each dialysis, or that if treatment precedes dialysis a half dose be infused after the end of haemodialysis.

Tinidazole is sometimes given prophylactically intravenously before caesarian section and is secreted in breast milk. Consequently it is recommended that breast feeding should not be initiated until 3 days after such treatment.

Toxicity and side-effects

It is generally well tolerated, but infrequent and transient effects include nausea, vomiting, diarrhoea and a metallic taste. Disulfiram-like reactions may occur and rare neurological disturbances and transient leucopenia have been described. Rash, which may be severe, urticaria and angioneurotic oedema can occur.

Clinical use

Tinidazole is as effective as nimorazole or metronidazole in the treatment of *Gardnerella* vaginosis, where the MIC is about 0.2–2 mg/l. This may be because the hydroxy metabolite of tinidazole is significantly more active than that of metronidazole against *Gardnerella* spp. In Scandinavia the drug is widely used with doxycycline to provide antibiotic cover for abdominal surgery. The use of the drug for non-invasive amoebiasis is improved by the co-administration of diloxanide furoate (p. 914). High cure rates of about 94% have been demonstrated for the treatment of amoebic liver abscess. Tinidazole can be given as a single 2 g oral dose for giardiasis and for vaginosis. It has also been used as an alternative to metronidazole in the treatment of *H. pylori*-induced gastroduodenal ulcers.

Preparations and dosage

Proprietary names: Fasigyn, Simplotan, Tricolam, Sorquetan.

Preparation: Tablets.

Dosage: The indications are so varied that dosages are given with the uses in individual chapters.

Available widely in continental Europe, including the UK.

Further information

Anonymous 1988 Critical care requirements after elective surgery of the alimentary tract. *Current Medical Research Opinions* 11: 196–204

Bannatyne R M, Jackowski J, Karmali M A 1987 Susceptibility of *Campylobacter* species to metronidazole, its bioactive metabolites and tinidazole. *Infection* 15: 457–458

Boreham P F L, Philips R E, Shepherd R W A 1985 A comparison of the in-vitro activity of some 5-nitroimidazoles and other compounds against *Giardia intestinalis*. *Journal of Antimicrobial Chemotherapy* 16: 589–595

Edwards D I 1993 Nitroimidazole drugs – action and resistance mechanisms. I. Mechanisms of action. *Journal of Antimicrobial Chemotherapy* 31: 9–20

Edwards D I 1993 Nitroimidazole drugs – action and resistance mechanisms. II. Mechanisms of resistance. *Journal of Antimicrobial Chemotherapy* 31: 201–210

Evaldson G R, Lindgren S, Nord C E, Rane A T 1985 Tinidazole milk excretion and pharmacokinetics in lactating women. *British Journal of Clinical Pharmacology* 13: 503–507

Lossick J G 1990 Treatment of sexually transmitted vaginosis/vaginitis. *Reviews of Infectious Diseases* 12 (suppl 6): S665–S681

Lossick J G, Kent H L 1991 Trichomoniasis: trends in diagnosis and management. *American Journal of Obstetrics and Gynecology* 165: 1217–1222

Speelman P 1985 Single dose tinidazole for the treatment of giardiasis. *Antimicrobial Agents and Chemotherapy* 27: 227–229

Wood S G, John B A, Chasseaud L F et al 1986 Pharmacokinetics and metabolism of ^{14}C-tinidazole in humans. *Journal of Antimicrobial Chemotherapy* 17: 801–809

Streptogramins

J. C. Pechere

Introduction

Streptogramins are a very large group of natural cyclic peptides. They are unique in that they consist of two groups (A and B) of structurally unrelated molecules which act synergistically against susceptible bacterial isolates. Group A streptogramins are polyunsaturated macrolactones which contain lactam and lactone linkages and incorporate an oxazole ring. The main compounds of this group are pristinamycin II_A, virginiamycin M_I, madumycin and griseoviridin. Group B molecules are cyclic hexadepsipeptides, the two principal products being pristinamycin I_A and virginiamycin S_{10}. Group B components share in the plasmid-borne variety of resistance to macrolides and lincomycins which is induced by erythromycin (p. 383).

Both the groups A and B inhibit protein synthesis by acting on the peptidyltransferase domain of the 50s ribosomal subunits. Synergistic activities of these compounds render the combination bactericidal to a wide variety of Gram-positive bacteria and reduce the number of resistant strains. Typically, the in vitro antibacterial activity of the mixture of A and B compounds is at least 10-fold greater than the sum of the activities of the individual components.

In spite of their antibacterial potency, the streptogramins have not been much used in clinical practice. In particular, unavailability of a parenteral form has meant that streptogramins could not be used to treat the most severe infections. Until recently, only two oral drugs were developed commercially: virginiamycin (which is also used as an animal feed additive) and pristinamycin, which has been used almost exclusively for the oral treatment (2–3 g/day in divided doses) of staphylococcal infections. Intensive work has recently resulted in the synthesis of water-soluble derivatives of the two groups and the development of an injectable semi-synthetic streptogramin, RP 59500.

Further information

Barrière J C, Bouanchaud D H, Desnottes J F, Paris J M 1994 Streptogramin analogues. *Expert Opinion on Investigational Drugs* 3: 115–131

PRISTINAMYCIN

A naturally occurring antibiotic, isolated from *Streptomyces pristinaespiralis*. It includes two major components: pristinamycin I_A and pristinamycin I_B. RP 59500 is a new semi-synthetic injectable antibiotic made from a 30 : 70 mixture of two purified water-soluble compounds, identified as I (RP 57669) and II (RP 54476), derived from natural pristinamycin I_A and II_B, respectively.

Antimicrobial activity

Pristinamycin and RP 59500 exhibit similar inhibitory potency against a wide range of aerobic and anaerobic Gram-positive organisms and against a limited number of Gram-negative bacteria (Table 31.1). RP 59500 exerts rapid bactericidal activity against the majority of susceptible strains; it is as active at pH 6 as at pH 7 and there is no appreciable inoculum effect. A postantibiotic effect (2.4 h at the minimum inhibitory concentration (MIC), more than 5 h at 10 × MIC) has been observed against *Staphylococcus aureus* and enterococci.

Pristinamycin and RP 59500 are not affected by most mechanisms of staphylococcal resistance to macrolides, including those of target modification (genotypes *ermA* and *ermC*), active efflux (*erpA* or *msrA*) and lincosamide

Table 31.1 *Susceptibility of common pathogenic bacteria to RP 59500: MIC (mg/l)*

	MIC (mg/l)
Staph. aureus	
Methicillin susceptible	0.03–2
Methicillin resistant	0.03–4
Erythromycin susceptible	0.06–1
Erythromycin resistant	0.12–2
Staph. epidermidis	
Methicillin susceptible	0.03–4
Methicillin resistant	0.03–4
Ent. faecalis	1–8
Ent. faecium	0.25–8
Str. pyogenes	0.06–0.5
Str. agalactiae	0.03–0.5
Str. pneumoniae	
Erythromycin susceptible	0.12–0.5
Erythromycin resistant	0.25–1
Viridans streptococci	0.25–1
L. monocytogenes	2–16
Gram-positive anaerobic bacteria	0.125–0.5
H. influenzae	1–8
N. gonorrhoeae	0.25–1
N. meningitidis	≤0.12–1
B. catarrhalis	≤0.12–1
Leg. pneumophila	0.03–3

nucleotidylation (*linA* and *linA'*). However, activity is reduced against staphylococci-producing streptogramin A acetylase or streptogramin B hydrolase.

Pharmacokinetics

Following an oral dose of 2 g pristinamycin, peak plasma concentrations of the main components, pristinamycin I_A and II_B, were around 0.8 and 0.6 mg/l, respectively, at about 3 h. The plasma elimination half-lives of the two components were around 4 and 3 h, respectively.

In healthy volunteers, doses of RP 59500 from 1.4 to 29.4 mg/kg administrated as a 1 h infusion, produced peak plasma concentrations ranging from 0.95 to 24.2 mg/l, with an apparent elimination half-life of 1.27–1.53 h. The two components penetrate and accumulate in macrophages, the cellular/extracellular concentration ratios in vitro being 34 and 50, respectively. In cardiac vegetations of experimental endocarditis, component I was homogeneously distributed, whereas component II showed a gradient of concentration, the diffusion of component I being approximately 2–4 times that of component II.

Toxicity and side-effects

Pristinamycin is generally well tolerated, but shared allergy to streptogramins has been encountered. It should not be used where meningitis is suspected.

Clinical use

Virginiamycin and pristinamycin have been used for upper respiratory, dental, bronchopulmonary, skin, genital and bone infections caused by susceptible organisms.

Preparations and dosage

Dosage: Adults 2–3 g/day, in three equal doses, with meals. Children, 50 mg/kg per day in three equal doses, with meals.

Further information

Desnottes J F, Diallo N 1992 Cellular uptake and intracellular bactericidal activity of RP 59500 in murine macrophages. *Journal of Antimicrobial Chemotherapy* 30 (suppl A): 25–28

Fantin B, Leclercq R, Ottaviani M et al 1994 In vitro activities and penetration of the two component of the streptogramin RP 59500 in cardiac vegetation of experimental endocarditis. *Antimicrobial Agents and Chemotherapy* 38: 432–437

Koechlin C, Kempf J-F, Jehl F, Monteil H 1990 Single oral dose pharmacokinetics of the two main components of pristinamycin in humans. *Journal of Antimicrobial Chemotherapy* 25: 651–656

Leclercq R, Nantas L, Soussy C J, Duval J 1992 Activity of RP 59500, a new parenteral semisynthetic streptogramin, against staphylococci with various mechanisms of resistance to macrolide–linocomycin–streptogramin antibiotics. *Journal of Antimicrobial Chemotherapy* 30 (suppl A): 67–75

Neu H C, Chin N X, Gu J W 1992 The in-vitro activity of new streptogramins RP 59500, RP 57669 and RP 54476, alone and in combination. *Journal of Antimicrobial Chemotherapy* 30 (suppl A): 83–94

Nougayrede A, Berthaud N, Bouanchaud D H 1992 Post-antibiotic effects or RP 59500 with *Staphylococcus aureus*. *Journal of Antimicrobial Chemotherapy* 30 (suppl A): 101–106

Pankuch G A, Jacobs M R, Appelbaum P C 1994 Study of comparative antipneumococcal activities of penicillin G, RP 59500, erythromycin, sparfloxacin, ciprofloxacin, and vancomycin by using time-kill methodology. *Antimicrobial Agents and Chemotherapy* 38: 2065–2072

Pechère J-C 1992 In-vitro activity of RP 59500, a semisynthetic streptogramin, against staphylococci and streptococci. *Journal of Antimicrobial Chemotherapy* 30 (suppl A): 15–18

Verbist L, Verhaegen J 1992 Comparative activity of RP 59500. *Journal of Antimicrobial Chemotherapy* 30 (suppl A): 39–44

Quinolones

E. M. Brown and D. S. Reeves

Introduction

The quinolones comprise a relatively large and rapidly expanding group of synthetic compounds based on the 4-quinolone nucleus:

All such compounds are characterized by a dual-ring structure with a nitrogen at position 1, a carbonyl group at position 4 and a carboxyl group attached to the carbon at position 3 of the first ring. X may be CH or N and ring closure can occur between R_1/R_2 and R_3/R_4, thereby giving rise to compounds which are structurally diverse, but in which the properties of the quinolone nucleus are preserved and, indeed, may be enhanced. The quinolones themselves have a carbon atom at position 8 of the second ring, while the naphthyridines contain a nitrogen atom at the same position.

It is probable that the use of the original quinolones would have declined because of increasing resistance and the relative frequency and severity of central nervous system (CNS) side-effects. However, persistent efforts have been made over the years to produce congeners with superior properties. This incentive received considerable impetus with the discovery that the introduction of fluorine into the 6-position of the molecule endowed it with substantially greater potency and an expanded spectrum of activity. As a result, there are now two families of compounds – the original 4-quinolones and their successors the fluoro-quinolones, although all derivatives are commonly referred to as 'quinolones'.

The first of the 4-quinolones was nalidixic acid, a 1,8-naphthyridine, which was introduced for clinical use in 1962. This was followed by oxolinic acid, cinoxacin, piromidic and pipemidic acids and, more recently, acrosoxacin.

The fluoroquinolones themselves can be divided into four groups. The first consists of monofluoro compounds, of which the best studied is the 6-fluoroquinolone, flumequine; this agent differs from its predecessors principally in terms of its activity against Pseudomonas aeruginosa. The second and largest group includes the 6-fluoro-7-piperazinyl compounds, of which the best known are ciprofloxacin, enoxacin, norfloxacin, ofloxacin and pefloxacin, although the group also contains difloxacin, levofloxacin (the L- isomer of ofloxacin), lomefloxacin, rufloxacin, sparfloxacin and numerous others. The third group comprises polyfluorinated compounds, the most extensively studied being fleroxacin. The fourth group consists of naphthyridine derivatives which contain a pyrrolidinyl substituent at position 7 (clinafloxacin and tosufloxacin).

Recently, attempts have been made to link quinolones chemically to cephalosporins. Desacetylcefotaxime has been successfully fused by various linkages to the 3-carboxyl groups of fleroxacin and ciprofloxacin and to the piperazine group of ciprofloxacin. These linkages have produced compounds with in vitro activities characteristic of both constituent classes of antibiotic; of particular note is the greatly enhanced activity of the combinations against Streptococcus pneumoniae (including strains with reduced susceptibilities to penicillin) compared with that of either ciprofloxacin or fleroxacin.

Antimicrobial activity

The 4-quinolones exhibit relatively potent activity against a wide range of Enterobacteriaceae, as well as *Haemophilus influenzae* and *Neisseria* spp. They have little or no activity against the non-fermenting aerobic Gram-negative bacilli (AGNB) such as *Ps. aeruginosa* and *Acinetobacter* spp., anaerobes and Gram-positive bacteria. Their in vitro activities against common pathogens are compared in Table 32.1.

Manipulation of the chemical structure of the 4-quinolones imbued successive compounds with both greater potencies and much broader spectra of activity. The MICs of the 6-fluoroquinolones are up to 100-fold lower than those of the 4-quinolones for the Enterobacteriaceae, *Aeromonas* spp., *Campylobacter* spp., *Yersinia* spp., *H. influenzae*, *Neisseria* spp. and *Moraxella catarrhalis*. Unlike most of the non-fluorinated quinolones, they are also active against *Ps. aeruginosa*, although other non-fermenting AGNB, such as non-aeruginosa *Pseudomonas* spp., *Acinetobacter* spp. and

Stenotrophomonas (*Xanthomonas*) *maltophilia*, are generally less susceptible. Fluoroquinolones have good activity against both methicillin-resistant and methicillin-susceptible strains of *Staphylococcus aureus* and *Staphylococcus epidermidis*, but most currently available agents are less active against other Gram-positive bacteria, such as *Streptococcus* spp. (including *Str. pneumoniae*), *Enterococcus* spp. and *Listeria monocytogenes*, the MIC_{90} values for all these organisms being close to, or exceeding, achievable peak serum concentrations.

Several important intracellular pathogens, including *Legionella* spp., *Mycoplasma pneumoniae*, *Mycoplasma hominis*, *Ureaplasma urealyticum*, *Chlamydia pneumoniae*, *Chlamydia trachomatis*, *Coxiella burnettii* and *Brucella* spp., are susceptible to a number of fluoroquinolones. Some of the compounds belonging to this group are also active

Table 32.1 *Activity of 4-quinolones against common pathogenic bacteria: MIC_{90} (mg/l)*

Species	Acrosoxacin	Cinoxacin	Nalidixic acid	Oxolinic acid	Pipemidic acid
Staph. aureus	8–16	64–R	R	4–16	R
Coagulase-negative staphylococci	R		R		R
Str. pyogenes	R	R	R	R	R
Str. pneumoniae	R	R	R	R	R
Ent. faecalis	4	R	R	R	R
N. gonorrhoeae	0.06–0.1		I		
N. meningitidis		2	0.5	0.06–0.25	I
H. influenzae	≤0.06	I	I		2
Mor. catarrhalis			2		
Legionella spp.			I		
Esch. coli	4–8	1–4	4–8	0.25–2	2
Klebsiella spp.	0.25–2	2–32	8–16	0.5–2	
Citrobacter spp.	0.25–1		4–16		
Enterobacter spp.	0.5–1		8		16
Ser. marcescens	0.25–8	4–8	R		R
Pr. mirabilis	0.5–2		8		8
Proteus spp. (indole +)	0.5–32	1–16	8–16	0.5–1	4–8
Salmonella spp.		4	2–4	I	2–4
Shigella spp.		2–4	8	0.5–1	0.25–2
Ps. aeruginosa	1–32	R	R	R	8–32
Acinetobacter spp.			R		R
Camp. jejuni			8		
B. fragilis		R	R	R	32–R
C. trachomatis			R		

R, resistant.

Table 32.2   *Activity of fluoroquinolones against common pathogenic bacteria: MIC$_{90}$ (mg/l)*

	Ciprofloxacin	Clinafloxacin	Difloxacin	Enoxacin	Fleroxacin	Flumequine	Levofloxacin
Staph. aureus	0.25–1	<0.06	0.12–0.5	2	1–2	16–64	0.25
Coagulase-negative staphylococci	0.25–1	<0.06	0.5	2	1–4		1
Str. pyogenes	0.5–2	0.06	0.25–2	8–16	4–16		0.5
Str. pneumoniae	1–4	0.12	2	8–16	4–16		2
Ent. faecalis	0.5–2	0.12	<0.06–8	≥8	4–16	16–R	2
N. gonorrhoeae	≤0.06	<0.06	<0.06–0.5	0.12	<0.06–0.5		<0.06
N. meningitidis	≤0.06	<0.06	≤0.06	≤0.06	≤0.06		<0.06
H. influenzae	≤0.06	<0.06	<0.06–0.12	0.12	<0.06–0.25		<0.06
M. catarrhalis	<0.06–0.25	<0.06	0.06	0.12	0.25		0.06
Legionella spp.	≤0.06	<0.06	0.25	≤0.06			
Esch. coli	≤0.06	<0.06	<0.06–0.25	0.25	0.12–0.5	1–8	0.25
Klebsiella spp.	0.06–0.25	0.06	0.06–0.5	0.25	0.12–2	1–16	0.5
Citrobacter spp.	<0.06–0.25	0.12	<0.06–4	0.25	0.06–1		0.12
Enterobacter spp.	0.06–0.25	0.06	0.06–1	0.5	0.06–2		0.12
Ser. marcescens	0.12–2	0.06	0.5–4	2	0.5		0.25
Pr. mirabilis	0.12	<0.06	0.25–2	0.5	0.12–0.5		0.12
Proteus spp. (indole +)	<0.06–0.5	<0.06	0.25–1	0.5–1	0.25–2	1–16	0.12
Salmonella spp.	<0.06–0.12	0.06	0.06–0.5	0.25	0.06–0.5		0.12
Shigella spp.	≤0.06	<0.06	<0.06–4	0.25	0.12		0.12
Ps. aeruginosa	0.25–2	0.5	<0.06–16	2–8	1–8	2–32	1
Acinetobacter spp.	0.25–1	0.06	0.12	2–4	0.5–4		8
Camp. jejuni	0.12			0.5	0.5		
B. fragilis	4–16	0.12	4–8	≥32	8–64	4–128	1
C. trachomatis	0.5–2		2–8	0.5–2			0.25–1
M. tuberculosis	0.25–4	0.25	>4	>4	>4		0.25
MAC	2–>8	>8	>8	>8	>8		>8

	Lomefloxacin	Norfloxacin	Ofloxacin	Pefloxacin	Rufloxacin	Sparfloxacin	Tosufloxacin
Staph. aureus	1–2	1	0.12–1	0.5–1	2	<0.06–0.25	<0.06–0.12
Coagulase-negative staphylococci	2	2	0.5–1	1	2	0.06–0.25	0.06–0.12
Str. pyogenes	4–8	4	2	4–8	16	0.25–0.5	0.12–0.25
Str. pneumoniae	2–8	8	1–4	8	32	0.12–0.5	0.25–0.5
Ent. faecalis	8–16	8	2–4	4	32	0.25–1	1
N. gonorrhoeae	<0.06–0.12	≤0.06	≤0.06	≤0.06	0.12	≤0.06	≤0.06
N. meningitidis	≤0.06	≤0.06	≤0.06	≤0.06	0.12	≤0.06	≤0.06
H. influenzae	≤0.06–0.25	≤0.06	≤0.06	≤0.06	0.5	≤0.06	≤0.06
M. catarrhalis	0.25–1	0.5	0.12–0.5	0.25	1	<0.06–0.12	≤0.06
Legionella spp.	≤0.06	0.5	≤0.06	0.06		≤0.06	≤0.06
Esch. coli	0.25	0.25	0.06–0.25	0.25	2	<0.06–0.25	0.06–0.5

Table 32.2 *Cont'd*

	Lomefloxacin	Norfloxacin	Ofloxacin	Pefloxacin	Rufloxacin	Sparfloxacin	Tosufloxacin
Klebsiella spp.	0.25	0.5	0.25	0.5	32	<0.06–0.5	0.5
Citrobacter spp.	0.12–1	0.5	0.25	0.5–1	1	0.5	<0.06–0.12
Enterobacter spp.	0.5	0.12–1	0.25–1	0.25	64	0.5	0.12
Ser. marcescens	2	1–2	0.25–2	1	32	0.25–8	0.5
Pr. mirabilis	0.12–1	0.25	0.25	0.25	4	0.12–0.5	0.25
Proteus spp. (indole +)	0.25–4	0.5	0.12–1	0.25	2	0.25–4	0.25
Salmonella spp.	<0.06–0.5	0.06–0.25	0.06–0.25	0.25	1	<0.06–0.12	≤0.06
Shigella spp.	<0.06–0.25	0.06–0.25	0.06–0.25	0.12	0.5	≤0.06	<0.06
Ps. aeruginosa	0.25–4	1–2	2–4	2–4	8	1–4	0.06–8
Acinetobacter spp.	4	≥8	0.25–1	4	4	0.12–0.5	0.06–0.12
Camp. jejuni	0.25	0.25	0.12	0.5	32	0.12	≤0.06
B. fragilis	8–64	8–32	8	16	32	1–4	2
C. trachomatis	0.5–2	4–16	0.5–2	2–8	4–8	<0.06–0.12	0.06–0.25
M. tuberculosis	>4	2–8	0.5–2	>4		<0.06–0.5	2–>8
MAC	>8	>8	>8	>8		2–>8	>8

R, resistant.

against *Mycobacterium tuberculosis, Mycobacterium kansasii, Mycobacterium fortuitum, Mycobacterium xenopi* and some strains of *Mycobacterium chelonae*; the activities of all agents against *Mycobacterium avium/Mycobacterium intracellulare* (*M. avium* complex: MAC) strains are generally poor. Most quinolones exhibit minimal activities against anaerobic bacteria and have no antifungal activities, but *Plasmodium falciparum* has been shown to be susceptible in vitro. The minimum inhibitory concentrations (MICs) of the currently available fluoroquinolones are summarized in Table 32.2. Ciprofloxacin appears to be the most potent agent overall against Gram-negative bacteria, while sparfloxacin is the most active against Gram-positive organisms, anaerobes and *Mycobacterium* spp.

The quinolones are rapidly bactericidal against most susceptible species, the minimum bactericidal concentrations (MBCs) typically exceeding the corresponding MICs by no more than four-fold. However, the mechanism of cidal activity appears to be biphasic, i.e. the drugs exhibit a single concentration at which they are maximally bactericidal and concentrations which are either greater or lesser than this result in diminished bactericidal effects.

Mode of action

All quinolones act by inhibiting the enzyme activity of bacterial DNA gyrase (topoisomerase) which mediates the negative supercoiling of double-stranded DNA, thereby inhibiting DNA replication; the comparable mammalian enzyme is insusceptible to the actions of these compounds. At high concentrations of quinolones (which inhibit RNA synthesis) and in the presence of inhibitors of either RNA or protein synthesis, the bactericidal activity of some quinolones is reduced, although inhibition of DNA synthesis by these agents is not affected. This suggests that inhibition of DNA synthesis alone does not bring about cell death. Indeed, three independent mechanisms have been identified to account for the bactericidal activities of the quinolones. Mechanism A, the first to be recognized, is common to all compounds and is the sole mechanism exhibited by older quinolones such as nalidixic and oxolinic acids. This effect is dependent on cell division and both RNA and protein synthesis and is therefore abolished by the addition of rifampicin or chloramphenicol. Mechanism B is unique to ciprofloxacin and ofloxacin and is not abolished in the presence of chloramphenicol or rifampicin, suggesting that it is independent of cell division and RNA/protein synthesis. The third mechanism, mechanism C, which was first identified in studies involving norfloxacin, also operates in non-dividing bacteria, but is dependent on protein and RNA synthesis for bactericidal activity and is therefore abolished by the addition of chloramphenicol or rifampicin. The possession of multiple mechanisms of killing may explain why members of the newer generation of quinolones are more potent than the original compounds which have only one mechanism of action.

Quinolones have been shown to produce prolonged postantibiotic effects (PAE) at concentrations ranging from $1 \times MIC$ to $10 \times MIC$. The durations of the PAEs for Gram-negative bacteria tend to be greater than those for Gram-positive bacteria (up to 4 and 2 h, respectively). However, the duration has been shown to vary significantly according to the concentration of antibiotic tested, the length of antibiotic exposure, the bacterial species and the method of determining the PAE.

Antimicrobial interactions

In vitro interactions between quinolones and other agents have been studied extensively. Combining a quinolone with either a β-lactam or an aminoglycoside usually produces an additive or indifferent effect. Synergy has been observed only occasionally, the exceptions being combinations of ciprofloxacin with imipenem or azlocillin (which were shown in various studies to be synergistic against up to 50% of the strains of *Ps. aeruginosa* tested) or fosfomycin. Antagonism between quinolones and other agents is rare, although both rifampicin and fusidic acid have been demonstrated to antagonize the bactericidal activities of ciprofloxacin and pefloxacin against strains of *Staph. aureus*. However, these observations must be viewed with caution as conflicting results have been obtained with different in vitro methods and with in vivo tests. In animal models, for example, aminoglycosides combined with quinolones have not produced better results than quinolones alone. On the other hand, combining a quinolone with a β-lactam or an aminoglycoside in most cases has minimized the emergence of resistant strains.

Interactions with host defences

The fluoroquinolones have been shown to interact with various aspects of host defences and this may have therapeutic implications. The compounds rapidly accumulate in phagocytes (both polymorphs and mononuclear cells), at least in part because of their lipid solubility. The ratio of cellular to extracellular concentrations range from 2 : 1 to 10 : 1, depending on the drug, the cell type and the bacterial species. Quinolones are also active intracellularly, exhibiting intraphagocytic cidal activities against a number of pathogens. They have no effect on chemotaxis, but preincubation of some pathogens in the presence of subinhibitory concentrations results in enhanced phagocytic killing. Subinhibitory concentrations of quinolones have also been shown to antagonize the adherence of both Gram-positive and Gram-negative bacteria to eukaryotic cells (buccal and urinary tract epithelium) and to fibrin–platelet matrices; this may be attributed to diminished production of bacterial adhesins, alterations to outer membrane proteins or changes in the surface properties of the host cells.

Acquired resistance

Mechanisms

Spontaneous, single-step mutations to quinolone resistance tend to occur at low frequencies and lead to only small (two- to eight-fold) increases in MICs which are not clinically detectable. Therefore, the species which are most likely to become resistant in a single mutational step are those with MICs which are already high, albeit still within the susceptible range (e.g. *Ps. aeruginosa*, *Serratia* spp., *Acinetobacter* spp., *Staphylococcus* spp.). On the other hand, organisms which are highly susceptible to the quinolones remain susceptible after single-step mutations and require multiple mutations before resistance becomes apparent, as demonstrated following serial exposure to increasing drug concentrations. In general, Gram-positive bacteria mutate to quinolone resistance at higher frequencies than Gram-negative organisms. Furthermore, the frequencies at which bacteria develop resistance to the quinolones are much lower for the fluoroquinolones (10^{-12}) than for non-fluorinated compounds such as nalidixic acid (10^{-8}), possibly because the former have two distinct bactericidal mechanisms while the latter have only one. Nonetheless, mutational resistance to one quinolone tends to confer at least some degree of resistance to all the other drugs in this group.

With the exception of two reports in which the authors claimed to have identified plasmid-mediated nalidixic acid resistance in strains of *Shigella dysenteriae*, without actually demonstrating that this resistance was transferable, neither plasmid- nor transposon-mediated resistance to the 4-quinolones has been described to date in clinical isolates; indeed, these drugs have been used as plasmid-curing agents.

The only other way in which bacteria are able to become resistant to these compounds is by chromosomal mutation. This can arise by one of three mechanisms. The first involves alterations to DNA gyrase which results in inefficient binding of the quinolones to the target enzyme. Mutations in the genes encoding this enzyme confer high-level cross-resistance to all 4-quinolones but are not normally associated with resistance to unrelated groups of antibiotics.

The second mechanism involves mutations which affect the permeability of the quinolones, thereby leading to reduced uptake into the bacterial cell. This may be the result of diminished production of outer membrane proteins (OMPs), particularly OmpF, alterations to the composition and structure of the OMPs, the synthesis of novel OMPs or decreased diffusion of the drugs through the phospholipid bilayer of the outer membrane, caused by alterations to either its structure or lipopolysaccharide content. Impermeability mutants have so far been identified only in Gram-negative bacteria or Gram-positive bacteria lacking an outer membrane. This mechanism of resistance is of particular concern because the mutations also lead to decreased permeability (and hence cross-resistance) to structurally unrelated antibiotics, including β-lactams, aminoglycosides, chloramphenicol and tetracyclines.

A third mechanism, which also prevents effective intracellular concentrations of the quinolones from being attained, involves an active efflux system at the inner membrane. This mechanism has been identified in both Gram-positive and Gram-negative bacteria, but it may not affect all 4-quinolones. Furthermore, the observation that drug efflux does not invariably operate at a sufficiently high level to confer resistance to these agents (although it can still be detected in quinolone-resistant bacteria) suggests that it is not the only resistance mechanism exhibited by these organisms. Rather it appears that it acts in conjunction with a second mechanism, possibly one causing reduced diffusion across the outer membrane. To date, no quinolone-inactivating or -degrading enzymes have been implicated as a basis of resistance.

Epidemiology

There is very little published information regarding changes in susceptibility to the original 4-quinolones with time. In a UK study which extended over a 22-year period, the percentage of urinary pathogens isolated from patients in the community which were susceptible to nalidixic acid fell from 90.7 in 1971 to 77.9 in 1992; the corresponding percentages for hospital isolates were 84.8 and 63.3. In Spain, the rate of resistance to pipemidic acid amongst *Escherichia coli* strains causing urinary tract infections increased from ≤6% before 1989 to 18% in 1992.

In contrast, several large-scale epidemiological studies have monitored changes in the susceptibilities of bacterial pathogens to the modern quinolones since they were first introduced. In general, these surveys have not detected significant increases in the levels of resistance among organisms which have previously been considered to be highly susceptible, despite the extensive use of these agents. Nonetheless, there is no room for complacency in the light of increasing numbers of reports describing the isolation of resistant strains of *Salmonella* and *Campylobacter* spp. (both related to the use of quinolones in veterinary practice and to the addition of these drugs to animal feeds), *Esch. coli* and other Enterobacteriaceae. A small number of strains of *Neisseria gonorrhoeae* with reduced susceptibilities, although not completely resistant, to these agents has also been isolated. However, the bacterial species that have exhibited the greatest propensity for developing clinically significant resistance to the quinolones have been those with high initial MICs, including *Ps. aeruginosa*, *Staph. aureus* (particularly methicillin-resistant strains, for which resistance rates of up to 80% have been reported), coagulase-negative staphylococci and *Acinetobacter* spp.

Effect of treatment

The emergence of resistance during treatment with quinolones is most likely to occur where large numbers of organisms are present at the sites of infection and/or where antibiotic concentrations at these sites are subinhibitory, either because of inadequate dosage or because antibiotic penetration is impaired. Such situations arise during prolonged or repeated courses of treatment in patients with chronic infections (e.g. acute exacerbations in patients with cystic fibrosis), when vascularity is compromised (e.g. infected leg ulcers), when large numbers of pathogens are sequestered in tissues where antibiotic penetration is poor (e.g. inadequately drained abscesses and osteomyelitis) and in the presence of foreign bodies. Strategies to minimize the likelihood of resistance developing during therapy include the use of higher dosages (thereby ensuring inhibitory concentrations at the site of infection), limiting the duration of therapy, rotating antibiotics and combining the quinolones with other unrelated agents. Another effective technique is to administer one or more other antibiotics to which the pathogen is susceptible for the first 2–5 days and to follow this with a quinolone for the remainder of the course, thereby allowing the quinolone to act on a significantly reduced bacterial load. Undoubtedly, however, the most effective strategy is to promote appropriate prescribing of these agents (see Ch. 12). The emergence and spread of resistant strains have been shown to reflect the selective pressures of excessive use, hospitals in which fluoroquinolone prescribing is restricted reporting lower rates of resistance than those in which it is uncontrolled.

Pharmacokinetics

Absorption

The quinolones differ in the details of their pharmacokinetic behaviour (Table 32.3), but the earlier drugs are generally rapidly and largely absorbed when given by mouth, although there can be considerable individual variation. Absorption of the fluoroquinolones is variable, being efficient in some (e.g. ofloxacin) and rather poor in others (e.g. norfloxacin). It is also depressed by co-administration with most antacids containing divalent metals, such as magnesium, with which they form insoluble chelates. Some of the fluoroquinolones are available for administration by the intravenous (i.v.) route and their pharmacokinetic behaviour when given in this way is similar to that following oral administration. The earlier quinolones have short plasma half-lives, but some of the fluoroquinolones, particularly the later trifluorinated cogeners, tend to have long half-lives.

Distribution

Protein binding of fluoroquinolones is generally low and they are widely dispersed into large volumes of distribution. Concentrations approximating those in the plasma are found

Table 32.3 Pharmacokinetic parameters of quinolones

Parameter	Acrosoxacin	Cinoxacin	Ciprofloxacin		Difloxacin	Enoxacin		Fleroxacin		Flumequine	Levofloxacin
			Oral	i.v.		Oral	i.v.	Oral	i.v.		
Dose (mg)	300	500	500	200	400	400	200	400	100	800	200
t_{max} (h)	2–4	1–3	1–2		5.2	1–2		1–2		2	3
C_{max} (mg/l)	4–5	5–25	1.5–2.5	3.5	4.0	2–3	5.5	6–7		24	2.5
C_{th} (mg/l)				1.0			1.8				
Bioavailability (%)	60–70	60–70	60–80			80		90–100			
$t_{1/2}$ β (h)	6.6	1–1.5	3–4	3–4	25–30	3–6	3–4	9–12	9	7	3–4
$t_{1/2}$ β (h) (renal failure)		12	5–10	5–10		>20		30	10		11
$AUC_{0 \to inf}$ (mg.h/l)			6–10		28	16–25	5.4	92	10		
V_d (l per 70 kg)		20	300	200–300	98	170	203	100	105	30–40	40–55
Cl_{TOT} (l/h)				25	41	24	38	5.0	10	2.5	
Cl_{REN} (l/h)				12–18	4.3	12	20	2.6	6	0.3	
Protein binding (%)	70	63	20–40		42	35		30		70	
Elimination (%) Urine	50 (2% unchanged; 28% N-oxide; 20% glucuronide)	40–60 unchanged; 40 metabs	30–40	75	<25 (10 unchanged)	40–60	46	50		60 (30 conjugated; 6 unchanged; remainder other metabolites)	
Faeces	3–13		15			20	21	3			
Urinary conc. (mg/l)	100–500	100–200	100–200		12–24	150–300				100	

Table 32.3 Cont'd

Parameter	Lomefloxacin	Nalidixic acid	Norfloxacin	Ofloxacin Oral	Ofloxacin i.v.	Oxolinic acid	Pefloxacin Oral	Pefloxacin i.v.	Pipemidic acid	Rufloxacin	Sparfloxacin	Tosufloxacin
Dose (mg)	400	1000	400	400	200	250	400	400	500	400	400	300
t_{max} (h)	1–1.5	1–2	1–2	1–1.5		2–4	1–1.5		1–2	2–4	4–5	4
C_{max} (mg/l)	3–5	25	1.5	3–5	5.2	2–4	4.5–6	5.8	3–4	3.5–4.5	1–1.5	1
C_{th} (mg/l)					1.8							
Bioavailability (%)	>95		70	85–95		V. variable	90–100		>90			
$t_{1/2}$ β (h)	7–8	1.5	3–4	5–7	4.3	4–15	8.5–13	10	3.5	30–45	15–20	6–7
$t_{1/2}$ β (h) (renal failure)	44	21	6–8	30–50			11–15			27	30–40	
$AUC_{0 \to \inf}$ (mg.h/l)	35–50		5.5	30	14		55	47	27	154	30–40	10–15
V_d (l per 70 kg)	168		100	170	90		130	133	70–140	100	350	
Cl_{TOT} (l/h)	13–15		18	14	14		9	8	5.5	2.7	10–15	12
Cl_{REN} (l/h)	8–12		11	11	11		0.6	1	3	1	1.3	
Protein binding (%)		93	14	25		70–90	20–30		15–40	57	37	37
Elimination (%) Urine	50–70 (+ 5–10 glucuronide)	2–3 unchanged; 13 OH-metab; >80 conjugates	30 unchanged 10 metab	80–90		50 (2–20 unconjugated)	60–70 (10 unchanged)	85 (5 unchanged)	50–85 (<2 inactive metabolites)	32	5–10 unchanged; 28–34 glucuronide	30–35
Faeces		4	30			16–20	25				50–60	
Urinary conc. (mg/l)	150–250	2–400	100–400	150–250		15–155			200–400	30–50	10–50	

t_{max} – time at which C_{max} achieved.
C_{max} – maximum blood concentration following a dose.
C_{th} – concentration in blood 1 h after a dose.
$t_{1/2}$ β – half-life in blood during elimination phase.
$t_{1/2}$ β – half-life in blood during elimination phase in presence of severe renal failure.
$AUC_{0 \to \inf}$ – area under blood concentration/time curve from time of dosing extrapolated to infinity time.
V_d – fictive volume of distribution.
Cl_{TOT} – total clearance from blood.
Cl_{REN} – renal clearance.
Protein binding – extent of binding to plasma proteins.
Elimination in urine (%) – proportion of dose eliminated in the urine intact and/or as metabolite.
Elimination in faeces (%) – proportion of dose eliminated in the urine intact and/or as metabolite.
Urinary conc. – typical maximum urinary concentrations following the dose stated.

in tissue fluid and there is relatively free penetration into bone and prostate. Concentrations in the bronchial mucosa and lung epithelial lining fluid are usually higher than those in plasma, in some cases considerably so. Concentrations in alveolar macrophages are also high and the fluoroquinolones tend to be active against susceptible organisms when they are taken up by neutrophils and macrophages.

When the meninges are not inflamed, the concentrations of many quinolones in cerebrospinal fluid (CSF) are lower (about a third to a half) than those in plasma and, on the basis of the limited published data, the presence of inflammation does not appear to enhance CSF concentrations significantly. Concentrations of ciprofloxacin in the CSF have been reported as being low.

Elimination
The earlier quinolones are mostly extensively metabolized, but the complexity of the products and the degree to which they retain microbiological activity differs considerably. They are very largely excreted in the urine, producing high concentrations, partly of unchanged drug and partly of metabolites and conjugates. Consequently, they accumulate in renal failure, but as a result of continuing, and possibly enhanced, metabolism, there is little change in the elimination of unchanged drug. Significant concentrations can be found in the faeces, partly as a result of incomplete absorption and partly from biliary excretion, which may dramatically reduce the numbers of faecal Entero-bacteriaceae.

The fluoroquinolones differ widely in the degree to which they are eliminated by metabolic transformation or renal excretion. Ofloxacin is minimally metabolized and almost entirely eliminated unchanged in the urine. In contrast, pefloxacin is extensively converted to derivatives with reduced microbiological activities. Ciprofloxacin and norfloxacin are eliminated partly by metabolism and partly by renal excretion. This difference appears to be reflected in the effect of cimetidine (although not more recent H_2-receptor antagonists) which, through its effect on hepatic metabolism, affects the plasma concentration of pefloxacin, but not that of ciprofloxacin. In patients with mild to moderate hepatic failure, the pharmacokinetics of ofloxacin are unaltered, while those of ciprofloxacin are only slightly modified and those of pefloxacin significantly modified, with an increased plasma half-life and excretion which is unchanged in the urine.

Excretion in the urine, partly as metabolites, is principally by renal tubular secretion and can be depressed by probenecid. About 90% of a dose of ofloxacin, which is little metabolized, appears unchanged in the urine, compared with only about 10% of pefloxacin which is extensively metabolized. Conversely, in the presence of renal failure, ofloxacin accumulates unchanged while most other drugs are eliminated by metabolism.

Changes in pharmacokinetics in the elderly are variable and usually small. Dosage modification is therefore not usually needed on the basis of age alone.

There is some excretion in the bile and high concentrations are found in the faeces with resulting marked suppression of the aerobic Gram-negative flora; this is observed most prominently with ciprofloxacin and ofloxacin. Effects on the Gram-positive flora are both variable and minimal and the anaerobic flora is unaffected. Despite a marked reduction in the numbers of Enterobacteriaceae, there is no substitution with resistant species and the flora returns to normal after a week or two. Effects on the oropharyngeal flora are minimal, only *Neisseria* spp. being noticeably affected.

Toxicity and side-effects

Overall, the frequency of adverse events in patients receiving quinolone antibacterials is comparable to that seen with other commonly used antibacterials. Rates of 6–10% have been described, with less than 1% of adverse events being recorded as serious. Although the frequency and severity of the various types of adverse events vary between individual quinolones, the nature of the events is similar for all congeners. Adverse events related to the gastro-intestinal tract (nausea, vomiting, diarrhoea) are by far the most common (about 5%), while those related to the CNS (anxiety, nightmares, hallucinations: about 1–2%) and the skin (rash, pruritis, urticaria: 0.5–1.5%) are less frequent. The large majority of adverse events resolve without sequelae on stopping the drug.

Gastro-intestinal symptoms
Adverse events include nausea, diarrhoea, dyspepsia, abdominal pain and anorexia; vomiting has been reported less frequently. Pseudomembranous colitis or the asymptomatic excretion of *Clostridium difficile* toxin has been described with both ciprofloxacin and norfloxacin as sole therapy.

Central nervous system
Benign intracranial hypertension has been well described with nalidixic acid and has also been reported with pipemidic acid and ciprofloxacin. Sleep disturbances are associated with all quinolones, but are particularly marked with fleroxacin. Organic psychoses, manifest as delusions or hallucinations, have been reported rarely with a wide variety of quinolones. The mechanism of CNS effects is thought to be the blockade of synaptic inhibition by γ-aminobutyric acid (GABA). Convulsions or dyskinesia are rarely associated with fluoroquinolones and usually occur in patients with a history of previous or concurrent CNS abnormality (for example, epilepsy), or in renal failure. The risk/benefit ratio

of quinolone therapy in such patients always requires careful consideration.

Skin reactions

A rash is the most common skin reaction. Very rarely it can be due to hypersensitivity vasculitis and can also occur locally at the site of i.v. administration. Phototoxicity is well recognized and appears to be often photoallergic in origin because it can occur up to several weeks after stopping therapy and is unrelated to dosage. A high rate of photosensitivity reactions has been reported with the trifluorinated quinolone fleroxacin, and it is possible that the 6,8-difluoroquinolones may be more phototoxic than their 6-fluoro counterparts.

Haematological system

Thrombocytopenia has been described with nalidixic acid and fluoroquinolones, in the latter instance in association with leucopenia. Leucopenia has been associated with norfloxacin and ciprofloxacin. In one patient given norfloxacin, a leucoagglutinin was detected, implying an immunological mechanism. An immunological mechanism has been ascribed to the haemolytic anaemia rarely seen with nalidixic acid.

General immunological reactions

Adverse effects have included the very rare anaphylactoid reaction (including hypotension, bronchospasm, angio-oedema) seen with quinolones and fluoroquinolones. Onset is virtually immediate, suggesting a pre-existing allergy, and thus, if possible, the use of quinolones should be avoided in patients with a history of allergy to any quinolone. Patients with HIV infection appear to be particularly prone to such reactions.

Nephrotoxicity

Renal failure has been associated with norfloxacin and ciprofloxacin, particularly in elderly patients. In some instances there seemed to be internal nephritis; these lesions resolved on stopping therapy. Crystalluria is a feature of fluoroquinolone therapy, but since it appears to be benign, acidification of the urine is not recommended because this will adversely affect the antimicrobial activity of the quinolone.

Arthropathy

This has been described in adolescents being treated with pefloxacin or ciprofloxacin but, unlike the joint damage seen in young dogs, the lesions resolved on stopping treatment. Arthropathy has been described in older patients given nalidixic acid or norfloxacin. More recently, achilles tendinitis, amounting to rupture in some cases, has been associated with fluoroquinolone therapy in renal transplant recipients.

Drug interactions

Some interactions with quinolones are of clinical importance. The metabolized compounds can depress the hepatic cytochrome P_{450} enzyme system, resulting in reduced elimination of drugs which are handled similarly; particular attention has been paid to potentiation of methylxanthines. Inhibition of the metabolism of theophylline and other xanthine derivatives increases their blood concentrations to toxic levels if dosage is not moderated. Serious manifestations of toxicity have included hallucinations, seizures, supraventricular tachycardia and atrial fibrillation. Since it is thought that the metabolic interference is caused by fluoroquinolone metabolites, it is unsurprising that largely unmetabolized congeners (e.g. ofloxacin) have little or no effect on theophylline metabolism. The corresponding effect on caffeine does not appear to give rise to clinical problems.

Antacids containing magnesium or calcium interfere with the absorption of all fluoroquinolones, probably by the formation of insoluble complexes. Antacids should therefore not be given 6 h before or 2 h after oral doses of fluoroquinolones. Nalidixic acid and some fluoroquinolones have been found to increase the prothrombin time in patients on warfarin, although the mechanism for this is unclear. Other interactions have included reduced absorption of some fluoroquinolones with sucralfate and ferrous sulphate, increased plasma half-life with cimetidine, and the possible potentiation of their epileptogenic potential by non-steroidal anti-inflammatory drugs.

Clinical use

The spectra and pharmacokinetic profiles of the original quinolones have virtually restricted their use to the treatment of patients with urinary tract infections and, to a lesser extent, patients with infections of the gastro-intestinal tract, particularly those caused by *Shigella* spp. Their use as therapy of urinary tract infections is limited by their lack of activity against *Enterococcus* spp. and *Ps. aeruginosa*, while their long-term or prophylactic use in recurrent infection is limited by the relatively rapid emergence of resistance, although this may be usefully offset by their capacity to maintain low numbers of uropathogenic Enterobacteriaceae in the gut, and hence in the introitus. There is little scope for the use of quinolones in infections caused by *H. influenzae*, despite their potent activity against the organism in vitro. This is because they penetrate poorly to the relevant sites of infection and because of the natural resistance of Gram-positive cocci which are commonly implicated as co-pathogens. Interest has, however, been shown in their potent activity against *N. gonorrhoeae*, and the most recent addition to the group, acrosoxacin, has been promoted specifically for the treatment of infections caused by this pathogen, including those due to β-lactamase-producing strains.

On the other hand, the very broad spectra of activity, potencies, pharmacokinetic properties and safety of the fluoroquinolones make them suitable for therapy of infections of almost every organ system. They have the added advantage of being available in both oral and parenteral formulations.

Urinary tract infections

In clinical trials, quinolones have been shown to be effective as therapy for patients with uncomplicated urinary tract infections (where cure rates as high as 100% have been reported), pyelonephritis or complicated urinary tract infections (including those caused by multiresistant strains) and as long-term, low-dosage prophylaxis. Whilst single oral doses of these drugs have produced cure rates equivalent to those achieved with 3-day regimens in patients with infections caused by *Esch. coli*, the failure rates for those caused by *Staphylococcus saprophyticus* have been unacceptably high.

Despite the overwhelming success of the quinolones in the treatment of urinary tract infections of all complexities, for the time being they should be reserved for those infections caused by organisms which are resistant to standard therapeutic agents. Even then, special attention should be paid to the emergence of resistant strains.

In a limited number of studies, fluoroquinolones, administered for 4–6 weeks, have been demonstrated to be effective treatment for episodes of prostatitis caused by *Esch. coli* and other Enterobacteriaceae. However, the numbers of treatment failures in patients infected with *Ps. aeruginosa*, enterococci, staphylococci and *C. trachomatis* have been high.

Sexually transmitted diseases

The administration of single oral doses of most fluoroquinolones to patients with uncomplicated gonococcal infections has produced cure rates in excess of 97%. Although single-dose regimens have not been as effective in patients with infections caused by *C. trachomatis*, 7-day courses of ofloxacin, fleroxacin or sparfloxacin have been associated with response rates of 97–100%, comparable to those achieved with doxycycline; in contrast, the failure rates with norfloxacin, enoxacin, pefloxacin and ciprofloxacin have been unacceptably high. Three-day courses of ciprofloxacin, ofloxacin, enoxacin or fleroxacin have been highly successful as treatment of patients with chancroid.

Respiratory tract infections

Fluoroquinolones have been evaluated in large numbers of open and comparative studies involving patients with purulent bronchitis, acute exacerbations of chronic obstructive airways disease, pneumonia (both community- and hospital-acquired) or bronchiectasis and been shown to produce clinical response rates equivalent or superior to those achieved with established agents. Remarkably high bacteriological eradication rates have been reported for *H. influenzae*, *M. catarrhalis* and Enterobacteriaceae, but there have been failures in patients infected with *Str. pneumoniae* or *Ps. aeruginosa*. In addition, persistence, recurrence or reinfection has been documented in patients with primary pneumococcal infection, and bacteriological eradication rates have been significantly lower than clinical response rates. In particular, patients with pneumococcal pneumonia have frequently failed to respond and, even more worrying, some have developed life-threatening pneumococcal complications while receiving quinolones for pneumonia or other infections. It would be prudent therefore to avoid using one of these agents when pneumococcal pneumonia is suspected. Sparfloxacin may merit further trials as it is significantly more active in vitro against pneumococci than other fluoroquinolones and has been shown in a small number of studies to be effective in patients with community-acquired pneumonia caused by *Str. pneumoniae*.

Novel quinolones have not been shown convincingly to be superior to conventional agents and cannot therefore be considered drugs of first choice for patients with purulent bronchitis, bronchopneumonia or acute exacerbations of chronic bronchitis. On the other hand, they would be appropriate alternatives in patients who have failed to respond, or who are allergic, to standard antibiotics. Fluoroquinolones should not be used as initial empirical therapy of patients with community-acquired pneumonia and their poor anaerobic cover makes them unsuitable as monotherapy of patients with aspiration pneumonia. For nosocomial pneumonia caused by AGNB, intravenous followed by oral quinolones have been effective, but patients with infections caused by *Ps. aeruginosa* may not respond and resistance can be expected to arise in a high percentage of strains.

In vitro activity against *Ps. aeruginosa* has enabled oral quinolones to be used to treat pulmonary exacerbations in cystic fibrosis patients. In a number of clinical trials, these drugs have been shown to be at least as effective as traditional combination therapy with intravenous antipseudomonal β-lactams and aminoglycosides in improving pulmonary function and a sense of well-being, but, in common with other regimens, have been unsuccessful in eradicating *Ps. aeruginosa* from sputum. In view of the significant potential for resistance to develop and the need to administer repeated courses of antibiotics to these patients, it would be sensible to alternate quinolones with other appropriate agents, or combinations of agents, and to limit their use to the treatment of acute exacerbations.

In a small number of studies, ciprofloxacin has been shown to be effective therapy of patients with proven legionella infections, including those who were unresponsive to erythromycin. However, treatment failures have also been reported and, for the time being, the use of these agents should be confined to patients who have not responded to standard therapy.

Some quinolones (sparfloxacin, ciprofloxacin, ofloxacin), as part of multidrug regimens, have been shown to produce clinical and bacteriological cures in AIDS and non-AIDS patients infected with multidrug-resistant strains of *Myc. tuberculosis* (MDR-TB) and in those with disseminated infections caused by MAC strains (see Ch. 59).

Skin and soft-tissue infections

Quinolones have been shown to be effective in a diversity of skin and soft-tissue infections, including cellulitis, subcutaneous abscesses, postoperative and post-traumatic wound infections, infected decubitus, ischaemic and diabetic ulcers, polymicrobial deep foot infections and infected burns. Not surprisingly, infections caused by anaerobic bacteria frequently failed to respond to therapy with these agents and, particularly in diabetic patients, there has been relatively frequent persistence or recurrence of *Ps. aeruginosa*, some strains having become resistant during courses of therapy.

Both clinical and bacteriological response rates have been lower for infections caused by *Staph. aureus* and β-haemolytic streptococci than for those caused by AGNB. However, most studies have compared quinolones with third-generation cephalosporins which also have reduced activities against Gram-positive bacteria; there have been few comparisons with first-line antistaphylococcal and antistreptococcal drugs. In patients colonized or infected with methicillin-resistant *Staph. aureus* (MRSA), quinolone treatment has resulted in low rates of eradication, high rates of recolonization and frequent emergence of quinolone-resistant strains.

As therapy for a wide range of skin and soft-tissue infections, quinolones represent a significant advance. However, where anaerobic bacteria might be present, these drugs should not be used as monotherapy and their suitability as first-line, empirical therapy for infections caused by *Staph. aureus* and β-haemolytic streptococci must be in doubt. Unless conventional antistaphylococcal agents are contraindicated, quinolones should not be administered as treatment of MRSA infections or to eradicate colonization with this organism, except possibly in combination with rifampicin in an attempt to prevent the development of resistance.

Osteomyelitis and septic arthritis

In patients with acute or chronic osteomyelitis caused by single or multiple pathogens and with or without foreign implants, clinical and bacteriological cure rates achieved by quinolones have been similar to, or better than, those following standard parenteral therapy. The emergence of resistant strains during courses of therapy has been observed most notably for *Ps. aeruginosa* and has been almost invariably associated with the presence of a prosthesis. This may be limited by administering a β-lactam and/or an aminoglycoside for a brief initial period. Until quinolones can be confirmed to be at least as effective as standard antistaphylococcal drugs, they should not be prescribed for bone infections caused by this pathogen.

Enteric infections

A number of studies have evaluated the efficacies of quinolones as treatment of infections caused by *Salmonella typhi* and *Salmonella paratyphi*. Overall, clinical cure rates as high as 100%, have been superior to those produced by all other regimens. Owing to the high concentrations attainable in the liver, bile and gallbladder, these drugs have also been more effective than conventional therapy at eradicating chronic faecal carriage of *Salm. typhi* (see p. 712).

Most studies of patients with diarrhoea caused by salmonellae, shigellae or campylobacters have shown a fluoroquinolone to be significantly better than placebo or older antibiotics in terms of shortening the durations of fever and diarrhoea, as well as eradicating pathogens from faeces. These agents, administered for periods as short as 3 days, are as effective (both clinically and microbiologically) as tetracycline in the treatment of patients with moderate to severe cholera.

In patients with travellers' diarrhoea, a number of quinolones have been shown to reduce both the duration of diarrhoea (by 1–3 days) and the intensity of the illness when compared with a placebo. Quinolones, in particular ciprofloxacin, have also been used successfully to eliminate salmonella carriage in institutional outbreaks where there are high risks of person-to-person spread. However, both persistence and relapse have been described, particularly in patients with AIDS, despite prolonged administration.

Reports of the emergence of resistant strains of enteric pathogens (other than *Campylobacter* spp.) during therapy have been rare and experience to date suggests that a fluoroquinolone should be considered the drug of first choice for the treatment of severely ill patients with gastroenteritis of suspected or proven bacterial aetiology or where eradication of faecal carriage of an enteropathogen is deemed necessary.

Infection in the neutropenic patient

In neutropenic patients receiving cytotoxic therapy, the administration of some quinolones (ciprofloxacin, ofloxacin, pefloxacin) has been associated with reductions in the incidence of bacteraemia caused by AGNB, but has had no impact on the incidence of infections caused by Gram-positive bacteria. Indeed, quinolone prophylaxis has contributed significantly to the emergence of these latter organisms as the predominant pathogens in the neutropenic patient. Combining a quinolone with either benzylpenicillin or a macrolide has been proposed as a means of preventing streptococcal bacteraemia. Although this strategy has been used successfully in some trials, it was not protective in others and still allowed the development of resistance. Initial enthusiasm for the use of quinolones in this context has been further tempered by recent reports of the isolation of quinolone-resistant strains of *Esch. coli* from bacteraemic neutropenic patients who had been receiving one of these agents as prophylaxis. There is an immediate need, therefore, to reassess the benefits and risks of administering quinolones to prevent infection in this group of patients.

As empirical therapy of febrile episodes in neutropenic patients, ciprofloxacin or ofloxacin, in combination with another antibiotic (benzylpenicillin, an aminoglycoside, a glycopeptide or an extended-spectrum penicillin), has been shown in most trials to be at least as effective as a standard therapeutic regimen. On the other hand, the results of studies which have compared a quinolone as monotherapy with a standard regimen have been more conflicting. There have also been reports of superinfections with Gram-positive cocci (mainly streptococci) and of an outbreak of bacteraemia caused by ciprofloxacin-resistant coagulase-negative staphylococci when quinolones were administered alone. It is reasonable to conclude that quinolone monotherapy should not replace a standard β-lactam/aminoglycoside regimen unless the latter is contraindicated, in which case the quinolone should be combined with an agent which has greater activity against Gram-positive pathogens.

Meningitis

Fluoroquinolones penetrate into CSF in concentrations which are bactericidal against *H. influenzae*, *N. meningitidis* and AGNB, but the concentrations of these drugs, even following intravenous administration, are unlikely to exceed the MIC_{90} for *Str. pneumoniae*. Clinical experience to date has been largely confined to neurosurgical patients with Gram-negative bacillary meningitis, most of whom were cured with intravenous therapy.

There is no published evidence regarding the efficacy of quinolones in patients with infections caused by the organisms most commonly associated with community-acquired bacterial meningitis and they cannot be considered as first-line therapy for bacterial meningitis of unknown aetiology. They are also inappropriate for patients with CSF shunt infections in whom the predominant pathogens are coagulase-negative staphylococci and the degree of meningeal inflammation is usually minimal. However, they may be life-saving alternatives to standard agents in patients with infections caused by multiresistant strains of AGNB, including *Ps. aeruginosa*.

Ciprofloxacin, in a single dose or twice daily for 2 days, is highly effective (93–96%) at eradicating nasopharyngeal carriage of *N. meningitidis* and is, therefore, an appropriate alternative to rifampicin for this purpose and as prophylaxis in close contacts of patients with meningococcal disease (see p. 748).

Miscellaneous use

In patients receiving continuous ambulatory peritoneal dialysis (CAPD), the relative lack of efficacy of quinolones as treatment of episodes of peritonitis caused by Gram-positive cocci, particularly staphylococci, the collation of these drugs with co-administered oral bivalent and trivalent metal ions (frequently given to patients with end-stage renal disease) and the variable bioavailabilities of oral formulations combine to restrict the use of fluoroquinolones to the treatment of exit-site infections.

Fluoroquinolones are highly effective as therapy of malignant otitis externa (caused primarily by *Ps. aeruginosa*) and might be used empirically in place of standard antipseudomonal regimens. Topical preparations have also been used successfully to treat bacterial conjunctivitis and blepharitis.

Prophylaxis

Ciprofloxacin has been shown to be effective in preventing genito-urinary tract infections following transurethral prostatectomy and as prophylaxis in patients undergoing biliary tract, orthopaedic implant, cardiac and vascular surgery. Advantages of quinolones over alternative regimens are most apparent in prostatic and biliary surgery, particularly if these agents are administered by the oral route.

Quinolones have been shown to prevent bacterial infections in patients following liver transplantation, in those with acute hepatic failure and in cirrhotic patients with gastro-intestinal tract haemorrhage. When a quinolone (norfloxacin) was used as the only antibacterial agent or in place of an aminoglycoside for selective digestive tract decontamination in intensive care unit patients, the incidence of nosocomial infections was reduced. Nonetheless, there are justifiable concerns about the use of quinolones in this clinical setting.

Further information

Andriole V T (ed) 1988 The quinolones. Academic Press, London

Ball A P 1994 Editorial response: is resistant *Escherichia coli* bacteremia an inevitable outcome for neutropenic patients receiving a fluoroquinolone as prophylaxis. *Clinical Infectious Diseases* 20: 561–563

Brown E M 1992 The role of ciprofloxacin in hospitals. *Reviews in Contemporary Pharmacotherapy* 3: 153–165

Carratala J, Fernandez-Sevilla A, Tubau F, Callis M, Gudiol F 1995 Emergence of quinolone-resistant *Escherichia coli* bacteremia in neutropenic patients with cancer who have received prophylactic norfloxacin. *Clinical Infectious Diseases* 20: 557–560

Courvalin P 1990 Plasma-mediated 4-quinolone resistance; a real or apparent absence? *Antimicrobial Agents and Chemotherapy* 34: 681–684

Cruciani M, Bassetti D 1994 The fluoroquinolones as treatment for infections caused by Gram-positive bacteria. *Journal of Antimicrobial Chemotherapy* 33: 403–417

Dalhoff A, Doring G 1987 Action of quinolones on gene expression and bacterial membranes. *Antibiotics and Chemotherapy* 39: 209–214

Edlund C, Nord C E 1988 A review of the impact of 4-quinolones on the normal oropharyngeal and intestinal human microflora. *Infection* 16: 8–12

Fernandes P B 1988 Mode of action and in vitro and in vivo activities of fluoroquinolones. *Journal of Clinical Pharmacology* 28: 154–168

Fillastre J P, Leroy A, Moulin B, Dhib M, Borsa-Lebus F, Humbert G 1990 Pharmacokinetics of quinolones in renal insufficiency. *Journal of Antimicrobial Chemotherapy* 26 (suppl B): 51–60

Garcia-Rodriguez J A, Gomez Garcia A C 1993 In-vitro activities of quinolones against mycobacteria. *Journal of Antimicrobial Chemotherapy* 32: 797–808

Gruneberg R N 1994 Changes in urinary pathogens and their antibiotic sensitivities, 1971–1992. *Journal of Antimicrobial Chemotherapy* 33 (suppl A): 1–8

Harnett N, McLeod S, Au Yong Y, Hewitt C, Vearncombe M, Krishnan C 1995 Quinolone resistance in clinical strains of *Campylobacter jejuni* and *Campylobacter coli*. *Journal of Antimicrobial Chemotherapy* 36: 269–270

Hooper D C, Wolfson J S 1991 Fluoroquinolone antimicrobial agents. *New England Journal of Medicine* 324: 384–394

Janknegt R 1990 Drug interactions with quinolones. *Journal of Antimicrobial Chemotherapy* 26 (suppl D): 7–29

Lewin C S, Allen R, Amyes S G B 1990 Potential mechanisms of resistance to the modern fluorinated 4-quinolones. *Journal of Medical Microbiology* 31: 153–161

Leysen D C, Haemers A, Pattyn S R 1989 Mycobacteria and the new quinolones. *Antimicrobial Agents and Chemotherapy* 33: 1–5

Lode H, Höffken G, Boeckk M, Deppermann N, Borner K, Koeppe P 1990 Quinolone pharmacokinetics and metabolism. *Journal of Antimicrobial Chemotherapy* 26 (suppl B): 41–49

Maggioli F, Caprioli S, Suter F 1990 Risk/benefit analysis of quinolone use in children: the effect on diarthrodial joints. *Journal of Antimicrobial Chemotherapy* 26: 469–471

Nix D E, Schentag J J 1988 The quinolones: an overview and comparative appraisal of their pharmacokinetics and pharmacodynamics. *Journal of Clinical Pharmacology* 28: 169–178

Nord C E, Edlund C 1989 Clinical impact of newer quinolones: influence on normal microflora. *Journal of Chemotherapy* 1: 18–23

Paton J H, Reeves D S 1988 Fluoroquinolone antibiotics: microbiology, pharmacokinetics and clinical use. *Drugs* 36: 193–228

Paton J H, Reeves D S 1991 Clinical features and management of adverse effects of quinolone antibacterials. *Drug Safety* 6: 8–27

Phillips I 1987 Bacterial mutagenicity and the 4-quinolones. *Journal of Antimicrobial Chemotherapy* 20: 771–773

Smith J T 1985 The 4-quinolone antibacterials. *Symposium of the Society for General Microbiology* 38: 69–94

Stahlmann R 1990 Safety profile of the quinolones. *Journal of Antimicrobial Chemotherapy* 26 (suppl D): 31–44

Symposium 1988 International Symposium on New Quinolones. *Reviews of Infectious Diseases* 10 (suppl): S1–S262

Wijnands W J, Vree T B 1988 Interaction between the fluoroquinolones and the bronchodilator theophylline. *Journal of Antimicrobial Chemotherapy* 21 (suppl C): 109–114

Wiström J, Jertborn M, Ekwall E et al 1992 Empiric treatment of acute diarrheal disease with norfloxacin. A randomized, placebo-controlled study. *Annals of Internal Medicine* 117: 202–208

Wiström J, Norrby S R 1995 Fluoroquinolones and bacterial enteritis, when and for whom? *Journal of Antimicrobial Chemotherapy* 36: 23–39

Wolfson J S, Hooper D C (eds) 1989 Quinolone antimicrobial agents. American Society for Microbiology, Washington DC

4-Quinolones

ACROSOXACIN
Rosoxacin

A 4-quinolone.

Its antimicrobial spectrum and potency resemble those of other members of the group (Table 32.1), but it is particularly active against *N. gonorrhoeae*, including those strains which are β-lactamase producers. *C. trachomatis* is also susceptible and acrosoxacin is the most active of this group of quinolones against *Legionella pneumophila*.

A single oral dose of 300 mg produces a mean peak plasma concentration of 4–5 mg/l at about 2–4 h, with a plasma elimination half-life of approximately 6 h. Excretion in the urine is largely as the *N*-oxide metabolite and the glucuronides of this metabolite and acrosoxacin.

Side-effects are those common to the quinolones (p. 432), notably gastro-intestinal tract and CNS disturbances. About 50% of patients treated with single oral doses of 100–400 mg developed dizziness, drowsiness, altered visual perception and other CNS effects, none of which was clearly dose-related.

It is effective as single-dose treatment of patients with urethral and anorectal gonorrhoea, but coexistent *C. trachomatis* infection has not been eliminated from the majority of patients and postgonococcal urethritis has developed in up to a third. It may have a role as monotherapy of gonorrhoea caused by β-lactamase-producing strains (p. 818).

Preparations and dosage

Proprietary name: Eradacin.

Preparation: Capsules.

Dosage: 300 mg as a single dose.

Widely available.

Further information

Dobson R A, O'Connor J R, Poulin S A, Knudsin R B, Smith T F, Came P E 1980 In vitro antimicrobial activity of rosoxacin against *Neisseria gonorrhoeae*, *Chlamydia trachomatis* and *Ureaplasma urealyticum*. *Antimicrobial Agents and Chemotherapy* 18: 738–740

Handsfield H H, Judson F N, Holmes K K 1981 Treatment of uncomplicated gonorrhoea with rosoxacin. *Antimicrobial Agents and Chemotherapy* 20: 625–629

Park G B, Saneski J, Weng T, Edelson J 1982 Pharmacokinetics of rosoxacin in human volunteers. *Journal of Pharmaceutical Sciences* 71: 461–462

Pohlod D J, Saravolatz L D 1986 Activity of quinolones against Legionellaceae. *Journal of Antimicrobial Chemotherapy* 17: 540–541

Romanowski B, Austin T W, Pattison F L M et al 1984 Rosoxacin in the therapy of uncomplicated gonorrhoea. *Antimicrobial Agents and Chemotherapy* 25: 445–457

CINOXACIN

Antimicrobial activity

Cinoxacin is active against the majority of Enterobacteriaeceae, notably *Esch. coli*, *Proteus* spp. (both indole positive and negative) and *Klebsiella*, *Enterobacter*, *Citrobacter* and *Serratia* spp. *Ps. aeruginosa*, Gram-positive bacteria and anaerobes are resistant. Its activity against common pathogens is shown in Table 32.1.

Acquired resistance

Resistant mutants are relatively easily selected by serial passage in the presence of the drug and have emerged during courses of treatment.

Pharmacokinetics

It is relatively well absorbed when administered by mouth. A 500-mg dose produces mean peak plasma concentrations after 1–3 h of around 15 mg/l. Administration with food reduces the peak concentration by about a third, but the area under the curve (AUC) remains unchanged. Binding to plasma protein is 60–70% and the plasma elimination half-life is 1–1.5 h. Concentrations in prostatic and bladder tissues reach 60% and 80%, respectively, of the simultaneous serum concentrations.

Cinoxacin is almost entirely excreted in the urine, about 40–60% as unchanged drug and the rest as metabolites, most of which have no antimicrobial activity. Urinary concentrations of active drug in the first 2 h after administration of a dose are 100–500 mg/l. Elimination is reduced by probenecid and by renal impairment, the half-life rising to about 12 h in end-stage renal failure.

Toxicity and side-effects

The drug is generally well tolerated, adverse reactions which are common to the group (p. 427) being reported in 4–5% of patients; these are primarily gastro-intestinal tract disturbances, but rashes occur in up to 3% and CNS disturbances in less than 1%. Crystalluria and effects on the cartilage of weight-bearing joints, as observed in animal models, are the same as those produced by other members of the group. No embryopathic effects have been detected in experimental models. As with other quinolones, the numbers of AGNB in the faecal and vaginal flora are markedly depressed, but are not replaced by resistant strains.

Clinical use

The principal indication of cinoxacin in clinical practice is the treatment of patients with urinary tract infections. Its effects on the faecal and vaginal flora suggest that it may have a particular role as prophylaxis of recurrent infections, although the results of studies which have evaluated it in this clinical setting have been equivocal. As with other quinolones, it is not recommended for use in pregnant or lactating women or in children.

Preparations and dosage

Proprietary name: Cinobac.

Preparation: Capsules.

Dosage: 500 mg every 12 h; prophylaxis 500 mg/day.

Widely available.

Further information

Guay D R 1982 Cinoxacin (Cinobac, Eli Lilly and Co.) *Drug Intelligence and Clinical Pharmacy* 16: 916–921

Scavone J M, Gleckman R A, Fraser D G 1982 Cinoxacin: mechanism of action, spectrum of activity, pharmaco-kinetics, adverse reactions and therapeutic indications. *Pharmacotherapy* 2: 266–272

Sisca T S, Heel R C, Romakiewicz J A 1983 Cinoxacin. A review of its pharmacological properties and therapeutic efficacy in the treatment of urinary tract infections. *Drugs* 25: 544–569

NALIDIXIC ACID

A 4-quinolone.

Antimicrobial activity

Nalidixic acid is active in vitro against a wide range of Enterobacteriaceae, particularly *Esch. coli* and *Klebsiella,*

Enterobacter, Proteus (both indole positive and negative), *Citrobacter* and *Serratia* spp. Many strains which are resistant to multiple non-quinolone antibiotics are susceptible to this agent and most isolates are inhibited by concentrations of ≤8 mg/l. *Ps. aeruginosa*, Gram-positive bacteria and anaerobes are resistant. Nalidixic acid is also active against *H. influenzae* and *Neisseria* spp., including β-lactamase-producing strains. Its activity against common pathogenic organisms is shown in Table 32.1.

Nalidixic acid is bactericidal, although the MBCs for some strains are substantially in excess of the corresponding MICs. Synergy has been observed with both aminoglycosides and colistin against Enterobacteriaceae and with metronidazole against *B. fragilis*, while antagonism with nitrofurantoin has been demonstrated against *Proteus* spp.

Acquired resistance

Resistance of the form common to all quinolones (p. 423) develops readily following serial passage in the presence of nalidixic acid, although primary resistance amongst urinary pathogens is unusual. The development of resistance is observed more frequently with *Proteus, Klebsiella* and *Enterobacter* spp. than with *Esch. coli*. The frequency with which the emergence of resistance has been responsible for treatment failure has varied widely from one series to another, the factor contributing most significantly to this phenomenon being underdosage.

Pharmacokinetics

Nalidixic acid is readily absorbed from the gut, the mean peak plasma concentration in normal subjects following a 1-g dose being about 25 mg/l; however, the concentrations in individual subjects vary widely. In infants with acute shigellosis, absorption is much impaired by diarrhoea. Administration with an alkaline compound leads to higher plasma concentrations, partly as the result of enhanced dissolution (nalidixic acid is much more soluble at higher pH) and absorption and partly because of reduced tubular reabsorption. The plasma half-life is about 1.5 h. A high proportion of the drug is bound to plasma protein, from which it may displace other drugs. It is rapidly metabolized, principally to the hydroxy acid which is also microbiologically active.

Virtually all of a dose appears in the urine over 24 h, approximately 13% as the hydroxy acid and 4% as the dicarboxylic derivative and their glucuronides. Excretion is reduced when probenecid is administered concurrently. In the presence of renal impairment there is little accumulation of the active compound because it continues to be metabolized. However, elimination of metabolites is progressively delayed as renal function declines. About 4% of a dose appears in the faeces.

Toxicity and side-effects

Adverse reactions are generally those common to all quinolones (p. 427), i.e. gastro-intestinal tract and CNS disturbances and skin rashes, including eruptions related to photosensitivity. About half of the reported CNS reactions involve visual disturbances, hallucinations or disordered sensory perception. Severe excitatory states, including acute psychoses and convulsions, are usually observed in patients receiving high dosages. The drug should therefore be avoided in patients with psychiatric disorders or epilepsy.

About a quarter of skin reactions are attributable to phototoxicity and a further quarter are urticarial. Several cases of bullous eruptions have been reported with variable responses to phototesting. Acute intracranial hypertension has been observed in children, some of whom have also manifested cranial nerve palsies. Haemorrhage has occurred in patients who were also receiving warfarin, presumably due to displacement of the anticoagulant from its protein binding sites by the nalidixic acid. Haemolytic anaemia has been described several times in infants with or without glucose-6-phosphate dehydrogenase (G-6PD) deficiency; in adults, death has occurred from autoimmune haemolytic anaemia. Arthralgia and severe metabolic acidosis have been reported rarely.

Clinical use

Nalidixic acid has been used successfully as oral and, rarely, parenteral treatment of patients with urinary tract infections and has occasionally been instilled directly into the bladder. It has also been used as prophylaxis in patients undergoing transurethral surgery in order to cover the period of catheterization. Early claims of success in systemic diseases, notably brucellosis and enteric fever, have not been substantiated, but it has been effective in the treatment of patients with acute shigellosis.

Preparations and dosage

Proprietary names: Mictral, Negram, Uriben.

Preparations: Tablets, suspension.

Dosage: Adults, oral, 1 g every 6 h for 7 days; for chronic infections, 500 mg every 6 h. Children, >3 months, oral, 50 mg/kg per day in divided doses; reduced in prolonged therapy to 30 mg/kg per day.

Widely available.

Further information

Barbeau G, Belanger P-M 1982 Pharmacokinetics of nalidixic acid in old and young volunteers. *Journal of Clinical Pharmacology* 22: 490–496

Gleckman R, Alvarez S, Joubert D W, Matthews S J 1979 Drug therapy reviews: nalidixic acid. *American Journal of Hospital Pharmacy* 36: 1071–1076

Munshi M H, Sack D A, Haider K, Ahmed Z U, Rahaman M M, Morshed M G 1987 Plasmid-mediated resistance to nalidixic acid in *Shigella dysenteriae* type 1. *Lancet* ii: 419–421

Piddock L J, Diver J M, Wise R 1986 Cross-resistance of nalidixic acid resistant Enterobacteriaceae to new quinolones and other antibacterials. *European Journal of Clinical Microbiology* 5: 411–415

Schaad U B, Wedgwood-Krucko J 1987 Nalidixic acid in children: retrospective matched controlled study for cartilage toxicity. *Infection* 15: 165–168

OXOLINIC ACID

A 4-quinolone.

Antimicrobial activity

Oxolinic acid is active against many Enterobacteriaceae, notably *Esch. coli* and *Klebsiella*, *Proteus*, *Enterobacter*, *Citrobacter* and *Serratia* spp. It is also active against *Staph. aureus*, but other Gram-positive bacteria, *Ps. aeruginosa* and anaerobes are resistant. Its activity against common pathogenic organisms is shown in Table 32.1.

Acquired resistance

Bacteria which have been serially passaged in the presence of the drug readily acquire resistance which is common to other quinolones, although some wild-type strains resistant to nalidixic acid remain susceptible to oxolinic acid. In some series, the emergence of resistant strains has been a notable cause of treatment failure.

Pharmacokinetics

It is poorly and erratically absorbed when administered by mouth. In patients receiving 250 mg 4 times daily, mean plasma concentrations were shown to be 2–4 mg/l. In those receiving 750 mg twice daily, mean plasma concentrations were also very low on the first day (1.4 mg/l total and 0.7 mg/l free), but by the third day, the levels of free drug had risen to around 3.5 mg/l. When oxolinic acid was administered with food, the peak plasma concentration was delayed, although absorption was not impaired overall. Binding to plasma protein is about 80%.

Oxolinic acid undergoes complex biotransformation, and enterohepatic recycling may account for the increase in the plasma elimination half-life from 4 to 15 h over 7 days of treatment and for the 20% of a dose which can be recovered from the faeces.

About 50% of a dose appears in the urine in the first 24 h, partly in the form of at least eight metabolites, some of which are microbiologically active, and their glucuronides.

Toxicity and side-effects

Side-effects common to the 4-quinolones (p. 427) occur frequently. Of patients treated with a dosage regimen of 750 mg twice daily, about a quarter suffered nausea and vomiting or restlessness and insomnia.

Clinical use

Its only use is in the treatment of patients with lower urinary tract infections where its efficacy is undermined by irregular absorption and the frequency of side-effects.

Preparations and dosage

Dosage: Adults, oral, 750 mg every 12 h.
Widely available in continental Europe.

Further information

Gleckman R, Alvarez S, Joubert D W, Matthews S J 1979 Drug therapy reviews: oxolinic acid. *American Journal of Hospital Pharmacy* 36: 1077–1079

PIPEMIDIC ACID

A 4-quinolone.

Antimicrobial activity

The effects of substituting piperazine for the pyrrole group at position 7 in piromidic acid in increasing in vitro activity against Enterobacteriaceae and *Ps. aeruginosa* are shown in Table 32.1. Pipemidic acid exhibits no useful activity against Gram-positive bacteria or anaerobes.

Acquired resistance

Resistant mutants develop following serial passage in the presence of the drug and can emerge during courses of treatment. Most treatment failures in patients with urinary tract infections have been due to the emergence of resistant strains. Some strains resistant to other quinolones are more susceptible to pipemidic acid because of differential permeability to it. Susceptibility to pipemidic acid distinguishes *M. fortuitum* from *M. chelonei*.

Pharmacokinetics

Pipemidic acid is absorbed by mouth, 400- or 500-mg doses producing mean peak plasma concentrations after 1–2 h of 3–4 mg/l. Oral bioavailability exceeds 90%. Binding to plasma protein is 15–40% and the plasma elimination half-life is around 3.5 h.

With a regimen of 500 mg twice daily, a steady state plasma concentration of approximately 4.3 mg/l was reached. Pipemidic acid is rapidly metabolized, primarily to acetyl, formyl and oxo derivatives which exhibit 10–30% of the antimicrobial activity of the parent compound.

It is excreted in the urine, 50–85% of a dose appearing over the first 24 h, less than 2% as inactive metabolites. Non-renal clearance accounts for 10–40% of a dose in the young, rising to 40–70% in the elderly and thereby compensating for renal insufficiency. In elderly patients with measurable renal impairment, some delay in absorption has been observed, but the mean peak plasma concentration and the plasma elimination half-life were not significantly affected. No dosage adjustment is necessary in patients with mild renal insufficiency. Some of the drug is eliminated in the bile and a significant portion of a dose appears in the faeces.

Toxicity and side-effects

Untoward reactions are those common to quinolones in general (p. 427), i.e. nausea and vomiting; dizziness, weakness and grand mal seizures have been observed principally in the elderly. A number of reactions have been sufficiently severe to require discontinuation of therapy.

Clinical use

Its principal indication is the treatment of patients with urinary tract infections. In common with other quinolones, it markedly suppresses the multiplication of faecal Enterobacteriaceae and has been used, in combination with an antifungal agent, as selective decontamination of the gut in neutropenic patients.

Preparations and dosage

Dosage: Adults, oral, 400 mg twice daily.

Widely available in continental Europe.

Further information

Casal M J, Rodriguez F C 1981 Simple, new test for rapid differentiation of the *Mycobacterium fortuitum* complex. *Journal of Clinical Microbiology* 13: 989–990

Klinge E, Mannisto P T, Mantyla R, Mattila J, Hanninen U 1984 Single- and multiple-dose pharmacokinetics of pipemidic acid in normal human volunteers. *Antimicrobial Agents and Chemotherapy* 26: 69–73

Mannisto P, Solkinen A, Mantyla R et al 1984 Pharmacokinetics of pipemidic acid in healthy middle-aged volunteers and elderly patients with renal insufficiency. *Xenobiotica* 14: 339–347

Muytjens H L, van Veldhuizen G L, Welling G W, van der Ros-van de Repe J, Boerema H B J, van der Waaij D 1983 Selective decontamination of the digestive tract by pipemidic acid. *Antimicrobial Agents and Chemotherapy* 24: 902–904

Fluoroquinolones

CIPROFLOXACIN

A fluoropiperazinyl quinolone.

Antimicrobial activity

Overall, ciprofloxacin is the most potent of the currently available fluoroquinolones against Gram-negative bacteria (Table 32.2). It is particularly active against the majority of Enterobacteriaceae, including many strains resistant to unrelated agents, and against *Ps. aeruginosa* and *Acinetobacter* spp.; other non-fermenting AGNB are less susceptible. *H. influenzae*, *M. catarrhalis* and *Neisseria* spp., including β-lactamase-producing strains of *N. gonorrhoeae*, are also highly susceptible. Both methicillin-susceptible and -resistant strains of *Staph. aureus* and coagulase-negative staphylococci and *Str. pyogenes* are susceptible, while *Str. pneumoniae* and enterococci are less so. Ciprofloxacin has minimal activity against anaerobes, but useful activity against *M. tuberculosis* and other *Mycobacterium* spp. Intracellular pathogens such as *Chlamydia*, *Legionella* and *Mycoplasma* spp. are also susceptible.

Acquired resistance

Resistant mutants can be selected by passage in the presence of increasing concentrations of the drug and have emerged during courses of treatment of some patients, particularly those infected with *Ps. aeruginosa* or methicillin-resistant strains of *Staph. aureus* or coagulase-negative staphylococci. In such cases, there is complete cross-resistance with other fluoroquinolones.

The spread of resistant strains of *Staph. aureus* has been reported by several hospitals. In one, where ciprofloxacin replaced vancomycin as treatment of infections caused by methicillin-resistant strains, the prevalence of ciprofloxacin-resistant isolates increased from 10% to 80% in the course of one year. In another American institution, substantial numbers of new patients were found to be colonized by strains of *Staph. aureus* resistant to both ciprofloxacin and methicillin one year after the introduction of ciprofloxacin; less than a third of these patients had themselves received ciprofloxacin. In the UK, there has been an outbreak of bacteraemias caused by ciprofloxacin-resistant coagulase-negative staphylococci in a leukaemia unit; the outbreak occurred during a trial of ciprofloxacin as empirical treatment of febrile neutropenic patients.

Pharmacokinetics

Ciprofloxacin is absorbed by mouth, mean peak plasma concentrations increasing proportionately with dosages of between 50 mg and 1 g from around 0.3 to 5.9 mg/l 0.5–2 h after the dose. The plasma elimination half-life is 3–4 h. Some accumulation occurs with 500-mg oral doses or 200-mg i.v. doses twice daily and the plasma half-life has been reported to rise to about 6 h after a regimen of 250 mg twice daily for 6 days. Absorption is delayed but otherwise unaffected by food and, in common with other quinolones, is depressed by certain antacids; it is postulated that the 3-carbonyl and 4-oxo functional groups bind aluminium to form an unabsorbed complex. Each molecule of sucralfate (used to provide a protective mucosal barrier in the management of patients with peptic ulcers) contains 16 aluminium atoms which are released in the stomach. Its co-administration reduced the peak plasma concentrations of ciprofloxacin to undetectable levels in a number of subjects and the mean value from 2 to 0.2 mg/l. The AUC was reduced to 12% of the value obtained when ciprofloxacin was administered alone. Ferrous sulphate and multivitamin preparations containing zinc significantly reduce absorption which is also impaired in patients receiving cytotoxic chemotherapy for haematological malignancies. Calculated total bioavailability is 60–70%. Following i.v. infusion of a 200-mg dose over 15 min, the end-infusion concentration was around 3.5 mg/l. Binding to plasma protein is 20–40%. Ciprofloxacin is partly metabolized, some of the products of this process being microbiologically active.

Distribution

The drug is widely distributed in body water, concentrations in most tissues and in phagocytic cells approximating those in plasma. Concentrations in the CSF, even in the presence of meningitis, are about half the simultaneous plasma levels. In patients with hydrocephalus without meningeal inflammation who received 200 mg twice daily by i.v. infusion over 30 min, CSF concentrations reached 0.04–0.2 mg/l and did not significantly increase as the course of treatment proceeded. In the prostate, and particularly in the lung, concentrations can exceed those in plasma by many-fold.

Elimination

About 95% of a dose of ciprofloxacin can be recovered from the faeces and urine; about 40% of an oral and 75% of an i.v. dose appear in the urine over 24 h. Excretion is by both glomerular filtration and tubular secretion (60–70%) and is depressed by concurrently administered probenecid and by renal insufficiency. Other organic acids can compete for elimination, and administration with azlocillin results in reduced clearance and significantly elevated and prolonged plasma concentrations of ciprofloxacin, without any change in the pharmacokinetics of azlocillin. It is poorly removed by haemodialysis. Some is excreted in the bile, and enterohepatic recirculation evidently plays some part in prolonging the half-life, although most of the drug detected in the faeces is unabsorbed. Small quantities of four metabolites are present in the urine and faeces where concentrations of active agent after conventional dosages have been around 100–200 mg/l and 200–2000 mg/g, respectively.

Toxicity and side-effects

Significant untoward reactions are uncommon, those encountered being typical of the group (p. 427). Reactions severe enough to require withdrawal of treatment have occurred in less than 2% of patients. The commonest reactions, gastro-intestinal tract disturbances, have been seen in 5% of patients and rashes (rarely photosensitive) in about 1%. CNS disturbances typical of quinolones have been reported in 1–2% of patients. Potentiation of the action of theophylline and other drugs metabolized by microsomal

enzymes can occur. Crystalluria and transient arthralgia have been rarely reported. In volunteers, dosages of up to 750 mg produced no change in the numbers of faecal streptococci and anaerobes, but a marked decline $(2.5 \times \log_{10})$ in the numbers of Enterobacteriaceae which lasted 1 week. There were no changes in the MICs of the affected organisms and no overgrowth by resistant strains. As with other quinolones, ciprofloxacin is not recommended for use in children or in pregnant or lactating women.

Clinical use

Ciprofloxacin has been shown to be of benefit as treatment of patients with a wide range of infections. It is highly effective as therapy of urinary tract infections of all complexities, although for the time being it should be reserved for use against those pathogens which are resistant to standard agents. It shows promise as treatment of patients with prostatitis, but further studies are needed to confirm its efficacy in this clinical setting. A single dose of ciprofloxacin is effective against uncomplicated urogenital and rectal gonorrhoea, including those infections caused by β-lactamase-producing strains. However, it is inferior to conventional agents and some of the other fluoroquinolones in the treatment of genital tract infections caused by *C. trachomatis*.

Many studies have shown ciprofloxacin to be at least comparable to standard antibiotics as therapy of purulent bronchitis, bronchopneumonia, acute exacerbations of chronic obstructive airways disease, pneumonia (both community and hospital acquired) and bronchiectasis. However, it should be used only in patients who have failed to respond to conventional agents and should be avoided when it is suspected or confirmed that infections are caused by *Str. pneumoniae*, *M. pneumoniae* or *C. pneumoniae*. On the other hand, it has a definite therapeutic role in the management of pulmonary exacerbations in patients with cystic fibrosis, as an alternative to macrolides in patients with infections caused by *Legionella* spp. and as part of multidrug regimens in patients with infections caused by multiple drug resistant *M. tuberculosis* or MAC.

Ciprofloxacin has been used successfully to treat patients with a broad range of skin and soft-tissue infections and osteomyelitis caused by Gram-negative bacteria, but should not replace standard antibiotics where staphylococci and/or streptococci are the causative agents.

It is highly active against virtually all bacterial enteropathogens and is therefore widely considered to be the drug of choice for patients with enteric fever (including chronic carriage) or severe gastroenteritis; it has also been used effectively to treat patients with cholera and to eradicate salmonella carriage during institutional outbreaks.

Ciprofloxacin has been shown to be effective prophylaxis in neutropenic patients. However, it does not provide adequate cover against Gram-positive pathogens and concerns about its use in this setting have been justified by reports of the isolation of quinolone-resistant strains of *Esch. coli* from bacteraemic, neutropenic patients who had received quinolone prophylaxis. Evidence to date suggests that ciprofloxacin should not be substituted for standard regimens as empirical therapy of febrile neutropenic patients.

Other settings where ciprofloxacin has been shown to be effective include the eradication of nasopharyngeal carriage of *N. meningitidis*, the treatment of patients with malignant otitis externa or cat-scratch disease, the prevention of infection in patients undergoing biliary tract surgery and the treatment of infections of the biliary tract. A topical preparation of ciprofloxacin for use in the treatment of ocular infections is available, but is neither more effective nor safer than established topical agents and is more expensive; however, it may be indicated as treatment of superficial eye infections caused by pathogens which are resistant to conventional drugs or in patients who are unable to tolerate standard therapeutic agents.

Preparations and dosage

Proprietary name: Ciproxin.

Preparations: Tablets, injection, ophthalmic.

Dosage: Adults, oral, 250–750 mg twice daily; i.v. infusion, 200–400 mg twice daily. Children, where the benefits outweigh the risks, oral, 7.5–15 mg/kg per day in 2 divided doses; i.v., 5–10 mg/kg per day in 2 divided doses.

Widely available.

Further information

Barriere S L, Catlin D H, Orlando P L, Noe A, Frost R W 1990 Alteration to the pharmacokinetic disposition of ciprofloxacin by simultaneous administration of azlocillin. *Antimicrobial Agents and Chemotherapy* 34: 823–826

Bergan T 1989 Pharmacokinetics of ciprofloxacin with reference to other fluorinated quinolones. *Journal of Chemotherapy* 1: 10–17

Campoli-Richards D M, Monk J P, Price A, Benfield P, Todd F A, Ward A 1988 Ciprofloxacin. A review of its antibacterial activity, pharmacokinetic properties and therapeutic use. *Drugs* 35: 373–447

Garretts J C, Godley P J, Peterie J D, Gerlach E H, Yakshe C C 1990 Sucralfate significantly reduces ciprofloxacin concentrations in serum. *Antimicrobial Agents and Chemotherapy* 34: 931–933

Hawkey P M 1989 Where are we now with ciprofloxacin? *Journal of Antimicrobial Chemotherapy* 24: 477–480

Hirata C A I, Guay D R P, Awni W M, Stein D J, Peterson P K 1989 Steady-state pharmacokinetics of intravenous and oral ciprofloxacin in elderly patients. *Antimicrobial Agents and Chemotherapy* 33: 1927–1931

Jacobs F, Marchal M, de Francquen P, Kains J-P, Ganji D, Thys J-P 1990 Penetration of ciprofloxacin into human pleural fluid. *Antimicrobial Agents and Chemotherapy* 34: 934–936

Johnson E J, MacGowan A P, Potter M N et al 1990 Reduced absorption of oral ciprofloxacin after chemotherapy for haematological malignancy. *Journal of Antimicrobial Chemotherapy* 25: 837–842

Koestner J A 1989 Ciprofloxacin: a new fluoroquinolone. *American Journal of Medical Sciences* 297: 128–131

LeBel M 1988 Ciprofloxacin: chemistry, mechanism of action, resistance, antimicrobial spectrum, pharmacokinetics, clinical trials and adverse reactions. *Pharmacotherapy* 8: 3–33

Lettieri J T, Rogge M C, Kaiser K, Echols R M, Meller A N 1992 Pharmacokinetic profile of ciprofloxacin after single intravenous and oral doses. *Antimicrobial Agents and Chemotherapy* 36: 993–996

Nau R, Prange H W, Martell J, Sharifi S, Kolenda H, Bircher J 1990 Penetration of ciprofloxacin into the cerebrospinal fluid of patients with uninflamed meninges. *Journal of Antimicrobial Chemotherapy* 25: 956–973

Oppenheim B A, Hartley J W, Lee W, Burnie J P 1989 Outbreak of coagulase negative staphylococcus highly resistant to ciprofloxacin in a leukaemia unit. *British Medical Journal* 299: 294–297

Pecquet S, Ravoie S, Andremont A 1990 Faecal excretion of ciprofloxacin after a single oral dose and its effect on faecal bacteria in healthy volunteers. *Journal of Antimicrobial Chemotherapy* 26: 125–129

Polk R E, Healy D P, Sahai J, Orwal L, Racht E 1989 Effect of ferrous sulfate and multivitamins with zinc on absorption of ciprofloxacin in normal volunteers. *Antimicrobial Agents and Chemotherapy* 33: 1841–1844

Raviglione M C, Boyle J F, Mariuz P, Pablos-Mendez A, Cortes H, Merlo A 1990 Ciprofloxacin-resistant methicillin-resistant *Staphylococcus aureus* in an acute-care hospital. *Antimicrobial Agents and Chemotherapy* 34: 2050–2054

Sanders C C 1988 Ciprofloxacin: in vitro activity, mechanism of action, and resistance. *Reviews of Infectious Diseases* 10: 516–527

Smith D M, Eng R H K, Bais P, Fan-Havard P, Tecson-Tumang F 1990 Epidemiology of ciprofloxacin resistance among patients with methicillin-resistant *Staphylococcus aureus*. *Journal of Antimicrobial Chemotherapy* 26: 567–572

Symposium 1986 Ciprofloxacin: quinolones in practice. *Journal of Antimicrobial Chemotherapy* 18 (suppl D): 1–193

Symposium 1987 Ciprofloxacin: a major advance in quinolone therapy. *American Journal of Medicine* 82 (suppl 4A): 1–404

Symposium 1990 Ciprofloxacin – defining its role today. *Journal of Antimicrobial Chemotherapy* 26 (suppl F): 1–193

Waite N M, Edwards D J, Arnott W S, Warbasse L H 1989 Effect of ciprofloxacin on testosterone and cortisone concentrations in healthy males. *Antimicrobial Agents and Chemotherapy* 33: 1875–1877

isolates. Fourth International Symposium on New Quinolones, Abstract 31

Fuchs P C, Barry A L, Pfaller M A, Allen S D, Gerlach E H 1991 Multicenter evaluation of the in vitro activities of three new quinolones, sparfloxacin, CI-960, and PD-131,628 compared with the activity of ciprofloxacin against 5,252 clinical bacterial isolates. *Antimicrobial Agents and Chemotherapy* 35: 764–766

Yew W W, Piddock L J V, Li M S K, Lyon D, Chan C Y, Cheng A F B 1994 In-vitro activity of quinolones and macrolides against mycobacteria. *Journal of Antimicrobial Chemotherapy* 34: 343–351

CLINAFLOXACIN

Clinafloxacin is a naphthyridine derivative with a pyrrolidinyl substituent at position 7. It has excellent activity against members of the Enterobacteriaceae, *Neisseria* spp., *H. influenzae*, *M. catarrhalis*, *L. pneumophila*, *Acinetobacter* spp., *M. pneumoniae* and *M. hominis*. *Ps. aeruginosa* is only moderately susceptible. It is also one of the most active quinolones against Gram-positive bacteria, particularly staphylococci and streptococci (including *Str. pyogenes*, *Str. pneumoniae* and enterococci) and has moderate activity against some anaerobes. After sparfloxacin, it is the most active of the quinolones against *M. tuberculosis* (Table 32.2).

DIFLOXACIN

A difluoropiperazinyl quinolone.

Its spectrum and activity are typical of those of the group (Table 32.2). It is particularly notable for its activity against *N. gonorrhoeae* and *H. ducreyi*. It is claimed to be rapidly bactericidal against Grám-negative bacteria, but not against Gram-positive organisms. The desmethyl derivative is more active against some organisms.

In volunteers given single oral doses of 200, 400 or 600 mg, mean peak plasma concentrations approximated 2, 4 and 6 mg/l, respectively. The plasma elimination half-life is exceptionally long (25–30 h), presumably because the drug undergoes extensive tubular reabsorption. Very little metabolite is detectable in the plasma.

Less than 25% of a dose appears in the urine – 10% each of the unchanged drug and its glucuronide and the rest (2–4%) as desmethyl and *N*-oxide metabolites.

It is effective as single-dose therapy of patients with gonorrhoea.

Further information

Andrews J M, Cooper M A, Wise R 1992 The in vitro activity of PD131,628, the active component of the prodrug CI-990 (PD131,112). Fourth International Symposium on New Quinolones, Abstract 33

Barrett M S, Jones R M, Erwin M E, Johnson D M, Briggs B M 1991 Antimicrobial activity evaluations of two new quinolones, PD127391 (CI-960 and AM-1091) and PD131628. *Diagnostic Microbiology and Infectious Diseases* 14: 389–401

Felmingham D, Robbins M J, Ghosh G et al 1992 Comparative in vitro activity of PD131,628, the microbiologically active constituent of the prodrug CI-990 against clinical bacterial

Further information

Bansal M B, Thadepalli H 1987 Activity of difloxacin (A-56619) and A-56620 against clinical anaerobic bacteria in vitro. *Antimicrobial Agents and Chemotherapy* 31: 619–621

Fernandes P B, Chu D T W, Bower R R, Jarvis K P, Ramer N R, Shipkowitz N 1986 In vivo evaluation of A-56619 (Difloxacin) and A-56620: new aryl-fluoroquinolones. *Antimicrobial Agents and Chemotherapy* 29: 201–208

Granneman G R, Snyder K M, Shu V S 1986 Difloxacin metabolism and pharmacokinetics after single oral doses. *Antimicrobial Agents and Chemotherapy* 30: 689–693

ENOXACIN

A fluoropiperazinyl quinolone.

Antimicrobial activity

Enoxacin is active against a wide range of Entero-bacteriaceae, although *Serratia* and *Citrobacter* spp. are less susceptible. *Campylobacter* spp. are susceptible, *Ps. aeruginosa* less so and *Acinetobacter* spp. resistant. *Neisseria* spp., *M. catarrhalis* and *H. influenzae* are highly susceptible. *Staph. aureus* and coagulase-negative staphylococci are also susceptible, but streptococci, including enterococci, are only moderately susceptible. It has poor activity against *L. monocytogenes*, *Nocardia* spp. and *Mycobacterium* spp. Anaerobes and *Chlamydia* and *Ureaplasma* spp. are all moderately resistant. Enoxacin is active against some strains which are resistant to nalidixic acid.

Acquired resistance

Resistant mutants are selected following serial passage in the presence of the drug and have occasionally emerged during courses of treatment. There is cross-resistance with other quinolones, but not with unrelated agents. Enoxacin exerts effects on plasmids typical of quinolones.

Pharmacokinetics

Following an oral dose of 400 mg, mean peak plasma concentrations of 2–3 mg/l are achieved in 1–2 h. With a regimen of 400 mg twice daily for 14 days, mean peak plasma concentrations reach 3.5–4.5 mg/l, a steady state being achieved in 3–4 days. Absorption is not significantly affected by food, but ranitidine, sucralfate, some antacids and some mineral supplements may interfere with absorption. The plasma elimination half-life is 3–6 h. Plasma pharmacokinetics are essentially the same after an i.v. infusion of 400 mg given over 1 h.

It is widely distributed; concentrations close to, or exceeding by up to two-fold, those in plasma are found in saliva, sputum, prostatic fluid, bone and blister fluid. Very high concentrations (>100 mg/kg) have been detected in lung tissue after 400 mg twice daily for 5 days.

Some 40–60% of a dose is excreted unchanged in the urine with less than 10% as the 3-oxo metabolite which is 10–20 times less active microbiologically. In renal failure, the plasma elimination half-life rises to >20 h, with marked reduction in the elimination of the oxo metabolite. Haemodialysis removes insignificant amounts of both compounds. Some is excreted in bile, where concentrations of 4.5–25 mg/l have been found when the corresponding serum levels were 0.5–2 mg/l.

Toxicity and side-effects

Enoxacin is well tolerated, about 6% of patients experiencing mild and transient effects typical of the quinolones, i.e. gastro-intestinal tract disturbances, rashes, headaches and dizziness. Epileptiform and asthmatic attacks have occurred, but serious effects have been rare, except in patients also receiving theophylline, the quinolone causing significantly raised concentrations of this compound when they are administered concurrently.

Clinical use

Enoxacin has been shown to be effective in the treatment of patients with simple or complicated urinary tract infections.

In clinical trials involving patients with lower respiratory tract infections, including purulent bronchitis, acute exacerbations of chronic obstructive airways disease, community- and hospital-acquired pneumonia and bronchiectasis, the drug has produced clinical response rates which were at least equivalent to those produced by the comparator agents. However, bacteriological eradication rates for *Str. pneumoniae* were significantly lower than those for Gram-negative bacteria such as *H. influenzae*.

Although it has also been effective (even in a single dose) as therapy for patients with urogenital or anorectal gonorrhoea, it is inferior to other novel fluoroquinolones in these clinical settings. Enoxacin has also been used successfully to treat chancroid, but it has frequently failed to cure patients with infections caused by *C. trachomatis* or genital mycoplasmas.

While experience of treating skin and soft-tissue infections with enoxacin is limited, it has been shown to be effective as therapy of a wide range of infections caused by a variety of pathogens. It should not replace standard agents for use against staphylococci or streptococci, but might be of value as therapy of infections caused by Gram-negative bacteria.

> **Preparations and dosage**
> *Dosage:* Adults, oral, 400 mg twice daily.
> Available in the USA and continental Europe.

Further information

Henwood J M, Monk J P 1988 Enoxacin. A review of its antibacterial activity, pharmacokinetic properties and therapeutic use. *Drugs* 36: 32–66

Jaber L A, Bailey E M, Rybak M J 1989 Enoxacin: a new fluoroquinolone. *Clinical Pharmacy* 8: 97–107

Koup J R, Toothaker R D, Posvar E, Sedman A J, Colburn W A 1990 Theophylline dosage adjustment during enoxacin co-administration. *Antimicrobial Agents and Chemotherapy* 34: 803–807

Phillips I, Reeves D, Lewis D (eds) 1984. Enoxacin in antibiotic therapy: a look forward. *Journal of Antimicrobial Chemptherapy* 14: (suppl C): 1–94

Speller D, Wise R (eds) 1988 Enoxacin – a laboratory and clinical assessment. *Journal of Antimicrobial Chemotherapy* 21 (suppl B): 1–136

Van der Auwera P, Stolear J C, George B, Dudley M N 1990 Pharmacokinetics of enoxacin and its oxometabolite following intravenous administration in patients with different degrees of renal impairment. *Antimicrobial Agents and Chemotherapy* 34: 1491–1497

FLEROXACIN

A trifluorinated quinolone.

Antimicrobial activity

The spectrum and activity of fleroxacin are typical of those of potent fluoroquinolones in general. It exhibits a high degree of activity against Enterobacteriaceae, *Neisseria* spp. and *H. influenzae* (including β-lactamase-producing strains). It is active, albeit less so, against staphylococci (including some methicillin-resistant strains) and has only modest activity against streptococci. The susceptibility of *Ps. aeruginosa* is reduced, compared with other AGNB, and its activity against anaerobes is poor. The activity of fleroxacin against *C. trachomatis* is intermediate to that of other fluoroquinolones. *M. tuberculosis* and *M. kansasii* are both susceptible, while MAC strains are less so. Its activity against common pathogenic organisms is shown in Table 32.2.

Fleroxacin has been chemically linked to desacetyl cefotaxime, endowing the ester-linked molecule with activity characteristic of each of the constituent compounds; most noteworthy is the enhanced activity, compared with fleroxacin alone, against *Str. pneumoniae*.

Pharmacokinetics

Following oral doses of 100, 200 or 400 mg, mean peak plasma concentrations of 1.5, 3 and 6 mg/l, respectively, were obtained at 1–2 h. Absorption is not affected by food. Bioavailability is virtually complete and binding to plasma protein is around 30%. The plasma elimination half-life is around 10 h and there is a close correlation between dosage and AUC. Steady-state plasma concentrations in subjects receiving 200 or 400 mg twice daily are 2–4 and 4–9 mg/l, respectively. Accumulation occurs following multiple dosing of 800 mg or more over 10 days. Plasma concentrations of metabolites are low, but their elimination half-lives are longer. It is widely distributed in a large volume of distribution, with tissue or fluid/plasma ratios of 0.6 in saliva, 0.3–2 in prostate and 1.7 in seminal fluid; the volume of distribution of the metabolites is even greater.

Elimination is largely renal, with about 50% of a dose appearing in the urine as unchanged drug and about 5% as each of the principal (desmethyl and N-oxide) metabolites, giving urinary concentrations of the active compound of around 150–300 mg/l. The ratio of unchanged drug to metabolites does not change on repeated dosing. In moderate renal failure (CL_{CR} 30–10 ml/min), the dosage interval (normally 24 h) should be increased to 36 h and extended further to 48 h when the CL_{CR} is <10 ml/min. The pharmacokinetic behaviour of the drug in patients with biliary tract infections is similar to that in normal subjects; concentrations in bile obtained from T-tubes are 2–3 times those in plasma. About 3% of a 400-mg oral dose appears in the faeces, producing concentrations of 100–150 mg/g.

Toxicity and side-effects

It is generally well tolerated, untoward effects being those typical of the group (p. 427); gastro-intestinal tract and CNS disturbances (particularly insomnia and bad dreams) occur most frequently. The drug produces a marked reduction in the numbers of Enterobacteriaceae in the faeces.

Clinical use

Fleroxacin has produced high clinical and bacteriological cure rates in patients with either simple or complicated urinary tract infections. Uncomplicated gonococcal infections have been effectively eradicated with single doses of the drug and a once-daily regimen has produced results which have been comparable to those obtained with doxycycline in the treatment of patients with chlamydial genital tract infections. Single doses of fleroxacin have also been highly successful as therapy of chancroid.

Fleroxacin has been shown to be effective in patients with respiratory tract infections, including acute exacerbations of chronic obstructive airways disease, bronchitis and pneumonia. *H. influenzae* has been eradicated from sputum in almost all cases, but the rates for *Str. pneumoniae* have been much lower; in common with the majority of fluoroquinolones, its use should be avoided in patients with infections which are known or suspected to be caused by this latter pathogen.

Fleroxacin is effective therapy of patients with typhoid fever and even single doses have been used successfully to treat bacterial enteritis caused by a variety of pathogens. Similar clinical and bacteriological response rates have been achieved with fleroxacin and co-amoxiclav in patients with skin and soft-tissue infections, although the cure rates for infections caused by *Staph. aureus* have been lower. Only limited data are available, but fleroxacin has also been demonstrated to be effective therapy in patients with osteomyelitis and biliary tract infections.

Further information

DeLepeleire I, Van Hecken A, Verbesselt R, Tjandra-Maga T B, DeShepper P J 1988 Comparative oral pharmacokinetics of fleroxacin and pefloxacin. *Journal of Antimicrobial Chemotherapy* 22: 197–202

Hayton W L, Vishov V, Bacracheva N et al 1990 Pharmacokinetics and biliary concentrations of fleroxacin in cholecystectomised patients. *Antimicrobial Agents and Chemotherapy* 34: 2375–2380

Heim-Duthoy K 1990 Steady-state pharmacokinetics of fleroxacin in patients with skin and skin structure infections. *Antimicrobial Agents and Chemotherapy* 34: 922–923

Singlas E, Leroy A, Sultan E et al 1990 Disposition of fleroxacin, a new trifluoroquinolone, and its metabolites. Pharmacokinetics in renal failure and influence of haemodialysis. *Clinical Pharmacokinetics* 19: 67–79

Symposium 1988 Fleroxacin, a long acting fluoroquinolone with broad spectrum activity. *Journal of Antimicrobial Chemotherapy* 22 (suppl D): 1–230

Taburet A M, Devillers A, Thomare P et al 1990 Disposition of fleroxacin, a new trifluoroquinolone, and its metabolites. Pharmacokinetics in elderly patients. *Clinical Pharmacokinetics* 19: 80–88

FLUMEQUINE

A monofluoroquinolone.

Antimicrobial activity

It is active against a broad range of Enterobacteriaceae, notably *Esch. coli*, *Klebsiella* and *Enterobacter* spp. and *Pr. mirabilis*, including some strains which are resistant to nalidixic acid. Its activity against common pathogenic bacteria is shown in Table 32.2.

Acquired resistance

There is generally cross-resistance with nalidixic and oxolinic acids. Resistant strains have emerged during courses of treatment.

Pharmacokinetics

Following oral doses of 400, 800 or 1200 mg, mean peak plasma concentrations, obtained at about 2 h, are 13.5, 23.8 and 31.9 mg/l, respectively. On repeated dosing of 800 mg four times daily, the mean peak plasma concentration rises from 27 to 41 mg/l, but the plasma elimination half-life (around 7 h) remains the same. The principal metabolite, hydroxyflumequine, is much more rapidly eliminated.

Excretion is principally renal, about 60% of a dose appearing in the urine, mostly in the form of acid-hydrolysable conjugates. Urinary concentrations following an 800-mg dose are 10–35 mg/l, with a peak of 105 mg/l. Flumequine has no effect on the pharmacokinetics of theophylline.

Toxicity and side-effects

It is generally well tolerated, side-effects being those typical of quinolones (p. 427), i.e. mild gastro-intestinal tract disturbances, rashes, dizziness and confusion.

Clinical use

Flumequine is effective treatment of patients with urinary tract infections. While single-dose therapy of uncomplicated gonorrhoea has been unsuccessful, two- or three-dose regimens have been shown to be effective; however, the emergence of resistant strains has been noted.

Further information

Schuppan D, Harrison L I, Rohlfing S R et al 1985 Plasma and urine levels of flumequine and 7-hydroxyflumequine following single and multile oral dosing. *Journal of Antimicrobial Chemotherapy* 15: 337–343

LEVOFLOXACIN

A fluoropiperazinyl quinolone; the L isomer of ofloxacin.

Levofloxacin is the more active of the two optically active isomers and is generally twice as active as ofloxacin. It exhibits excellent activity against *Neisseria* spp., *H. influenzae* and *M. catarrhalis*, but only moderate activity against Enterobacteriaceae; *Ps. aeruginosa* and *Acinetobacter* spp. are even less susceptible. The drug also has only modest activity against Gram-positive bacteria (*Staph. aureus* being the most susceptible), *C. trachomatis* and *B. fragilis*. However, levofloxacin is one of the most active of the currently available quinolones against *M. tuberculosis*.

Following an oral dose of 200 mg, peak plasma concentrations are about 2.5 mg/l at 3 h, the plasma half-life being 3–4 h. After a 500-mg dose, the concentrations are 4–5 mg/l and the half-life is 7–8 h.

Further information

Child J, Andrews J, Boswell N, Brenwald N, Wise R 1995 The in-vitro activity of CP 99,219, a new naphthyridine antimicrobial agent: a comparison with fluoroquinolone agents. *Journal of Antimicrobial Chemotherapy* 35: 869–876

Chow A T, Wong F A, Rogge M C, Flor S C 1992 Pharmacokinetics of levofloxacin after 500 mg BID and 500 mg OD oral doses to two different groups of healthy volunteers. Fourth International Symposium on New Quinolones, Abstract 113

Yew W W, Piddock L J V, Li M S K, Lyon D, Chan C Y, Cheng A F B 1994 In-vitro activity of quinolones and macrolides against mycobacteria. *Journal of Antimicrobial Chemotherapy* 34: 343–351

LOMEFLOXACIN

A difluoropiperazinyl quinolone.

Antimicrobial activity

The spectrum and activity of lomefloxacin are typical of those of other members of the group (Table 32.2). It is particularly active against Enterobacteriaceae, *Neisseria* spp., *H. influenzae*, *M. catarrhalis* and *L. pneumophila*. Less susceptible are *Campylobacter* spp., *Ps. aeruginosa*, *Acinetobacter* and *Chlamydia* spp. Lomefloxacin has reduced activity against staphylococci and poor activity against streptococci (including *Str. pneumoniae* and enterococci), *L. monocytogenes*, anaerobes and *Mycobacterium* spp.

Pharmacokinetics

In volunteers given oral doses of between 100 and 800 mg, peak plasma concentrations were obtained in 1–1.5 h; the AUC was essentially proportional to the dosage and the mean plasma concentrations following 100-, 400- and 800-mg doses were around 1.1, 4.7 and 7.5 mg/l, respectively. The plasma elimination half-life was 7–8 h. Some accumulation occured in volunteers receiving 200 mg twice daily for 5 days, with a 20% increase in the AUC. Blister fluid contains around 3.5 mg/l 2.7 h after an oral dose of 400 mg. The drug is concentrated in various tissues.

Lomefloxacin is excreted principally by the kidneys and 50–70% of a dose, a small fraction as metabolites, appears in the urine over 24 h. In patients with impaired renal function given 400 mg orally, the plasma elimination half-life ranged from 8 to 44 h, depending on the degree of renal failure. Non-renal clearance was also impaired, but there was no significant change in other pharmacokinetic parameters. Mean urinary excretion of the drug and its glucuronide fell from 60% to 1% over 48 h. The daily dosage (normally 400 mg) should be reduced to 280 mg when the CL_{CR} falls below 30 ml/min. Haemodialysis has no effect on the plasma concentration. The effect of lomefloxacin on the plasma concentration of theophylline is clinically insignificant and no dosage adjustment is required.

Clinical use

Lomefloxacin is effective treatment of patients with urinary tract infections of varying degrees of complexity; in patients with simple urinary tract infections, equally high cure rates were achieved with 3- and 7-day regimens. The drug has also been very effective in a limited number of studies which have evaluated its efficacy in patients with uncomplicated gonorrhoea. However, its antichlamydial activity is not sufficient to justify its use as therapy of urogenital infections caused by this organism.

High clinical and bacteriological response rates have been recorded in patients with respiratory tract infections caused by *H. influenzae*, but the rates for infections caused by *Str. pneumoniae* have been significantly lower. Lomefloxacin has been shown to be as effective as tetracycline in the management of patients with severe cholera.

Further information

Blum R A, Schultz R W, Schentag J J 1990 Pharmacokinetics of lomefloxacin in renally compromised patients. *Antimicrobial Agents and Chemotherapy* 34: 2364–2368

Chin N-X, Novelli A, Neu H C 1988 In vitro activity of lomefloxacin (Sc-47111; NY-198) a difluoroquinolone 3-carboxylic acid, compared with those of other quinolones. *Antimicrobial Agents and Chemotherapy* 32: 656–662

Freeman C D, Nicolau D P, Belliveau P P, Nightingale C H 1993 Lomefloxacin clinical pharmacokinetics. *Clinical Pharmacokinetics* 25: 6–19

Gros J, Carbon C 1990 Pharmacokinetics of lomefloxacin in healthy volunteers: comparison of 400 milligrams once daily and 200 milligrams twice daily given orally for 5 days. *Antimicrobial Agents and Chemotherapy* 34: 150–152

Kumamoto Y, Henmi I, Tsunekawa T et al 1990 Epidemiological and therapeutic study on gonorrheal infection: a study on NY-198 (lomefloxacin) single administration therapy. *Acta Urologica Japonica* 36: 969–977

Kumamoto Y, Miyagishi T, Hirose T et al 1990 Epidemiological and therapeutic study on urethritis of male and cervicitis from viewpoint of STD: a study using NY-198. *Acta Urologica Japonica* 36: 979–987

Morrison P J, Mant G K, Norman G T, Robinson J, Kunka R L 1988 Pharmacokinetics and tolerance of lomefloxacin after sequentially increasing oral doses. *Antimicrobial Agents and Chemotherapy* 32: 1503–1507

Nix D E, Norman A, Schentag J J 1989 Effect of lomefloxacin on theophylline pharmacokinetics. *Antimicrobial Agents and Chemotherapy* 33: 1006–1008

Segreti J 1989 In vitro activities of lomefloxacin and temafloxacin against pathogens causing diarrhoea. *Antimicrobial Agents and Chemotherapy* 33: 1385–1387

Stone J W, Andrews J M, Ashby J P, Griggs D, Wise R 1988 Pharmacokinetics and tissue penetration of orally administered lomefloxacin. *Antimicrobial Agents and Chemotherapy* 32: 1508–1510

van der Auwera P, Grenier P, Glupczynski Y, Pierard D 1989 In vitro activity of lomefloxacin in comparison with pefloxacin and ofloxacin. *Journal of Antimicrobial Chemotherapy* 23: 209–219

NORFLOXACIN

A fluoropiperazinyl quinolone.

Antimicrobial activity

Norfloxacin is particularly active against a wide range of Enterobacteriaceae, including *Esch. coli*, *Klebsiella*, *Enterobacter*, *Proteus*, *Salmonella*, *Shigella*, *Citrobacter* and *Neisseria* spp., *H. influenzae* and *Campylobacter* spp. *Ps. aeruginosa* and *Acinetobacter*, *Serratia* and *Providencia* spp. are less susceptible (and often resistant).

While *Staph. aureus* is susceptible, norfloxacin is, in general, less active against Gram-positive bacteria, particularly pneumococci and enterococci; anaerobes are resistant. It has no useful activity against *Chlamydia*, *Mycoplasma* and *Mycobacterium* spp. Its activity against common pathogenic organisms is shown in Table 32.2.

Acquired resistance

Resistant mutants emerge readily on passage in the presence of the agent and have been the cause of treatment failures. The prevalence of resistance in wild-type strains of Enterobacteriaceae causing urinary tract infections is currently less than 5%. There is complete cross-resistance with other quinolones but none with unrelated agents.

Pharmacokinetics

Norfloxacin is absorbed by mouth, a 400-mg oral dose producing mean peak plasma concentrations at 1–2 h of around 1.4–1.6 mg/l. Doubling the dosage approximately doubles the peak plasma concentration. There is no significant accumulation with the recommended dosage of 400 mg twice daily. Food slightly delays but does not otherwise impair absorption. Bioavailability is around 70%. The plasma elimination half-life is 3–4 h. Six or more metabolites are produced, the majority of these being microbiologically inactive. It is widely distributed, but concentrations in tissues other than those of the urinary tract are low; levels in the prostate are around 2.5 mg/g.

Norfloxacin is excreted in the urine where 30% of a dose appears as unchanged drug and less than 10% as metabolites, producing peak concentrations of microbiologically active drug of around 100–400 mg/l. Urinary recovery is halved by probenecid, with little effect on the plasma concentration. The plasma elimination half-life increases with renal impairment, rising to around 8 h in the anuric patient. Some of the drug appears in the bile where concentrations 3- to 7-fold greater than the simultaneous plasma levels are achieved, but this is not a significant route of elimination and hepatic impairment is without effect. Very variable quantities, averaging 30% of a dose, appear in the faeces, producing concentrations of active agent of around 200–2000 mg/g.

Toxicity and side-effects

It is generally well tolerated, untoward reactions, interactions with other drugs and precautions in administration being those common to the fluoroquinolones (p. 427). Gastro-intestinal tract disturbances, which are generally mild, have been reported in 2–4% of patients. CNS disturbances have largely been limited to headache, drowsiness and dizziness.

Clinical use

The principal use of norfloxacin is in the treatment of simple or complicated urinary tract infections; it is also prescribed as prophylaxis in patients with recurrent infections. It has produced high cure rates in patients with prostatitis and, as a single dose, in patients with uncomplicated gonorrhoea. However, its activity against *C. trachomatis* is not sufficient to allow it to be used as therapy of patients with infections of the urogenital tract caused by this pathogen and, indeed, failure rates have been unacceptably high.

Norfloxacin has been used successfully to treat travellers' diarrhoea and gastroenteritis caused by *Salmonella*, *Shigella* and *Campylobacter* spp. It has also been used effectively to eradicate chronic *Salm. typhi* carriage and has been shown to be comparable to tetracycline in the management of patients with severe cholera. The high concentration of the drug in faeces has enabled it to be prescribed as selective decontamination of the digestive tract in neutropenic patients and to reduce the incidence of Gram-negative

infections, but not that of Gram-positive infections, in this patient population.

Preparations and dosage

Proprietary name: Utinor.

Preparations: Tablets, ophthalmic.

Dosage: Adults, oral, 400 mg twice daily for 7–10 days; uncomplicated lower urinary tract infections, 400 mg twice daily for 3 days; chronic relapsing urinary tract infections, 400 mg twice daily for 12 weeks, reduced to 400 mg/day if adequate suppression within first 4 weeks. Widely available.

Further information

Holmes B, Brogden R N, Richards D M 1985 Norfloxacin. A review of its antibacterial activity, pharmacokinetic properties and therapeutic use. *Drugs* 30: 482–513

Marble D A, Bosso J A 1986 Norfloxacin: a quinolone antibiotic. *Drug Intelligence and Clinical Pharmacy* 20: 261–266

Rowen R C, Michel D J, Thompson J C 1987 Norfloxacin: clinical pharmacology and clinical use. *Pharmacotherapy* 7: 92–110

Symposium 1987 Norfloxacin: a fluoroquinolone carboxylic acid antimicrobial agent. *American Journal of Medicine* 82 (suppl 6B): 1–92

Wolfson J S, Hooper D C 1988 Norfloxacin: a new targeted fluoroquinolone antimicrobial agent. *Annals of Internal Medicine* 198: 238–251

OFLOXACIN

A fluoropiperazinyl quinolone.

Antimicrobial activity

Ofloxacin exhibits potent activity against a wide range of Enterobacteriaceae, including strains resistant to nalidixic acid, as well as against *Aeromonas*, *Campylobacter*, *Vibrio* and *Neisseria* spp., *H. influenzae* and *M. catarrhalis.* Staphylococci are more susceptible than streptococci, including pneumococci and enterococci, against which activity is limited. Most anaerobes are either moderately or completely resistant. Ofloxacin is also active against the intracellular pathogens causing atypical pneumonias (*L. pneumophila*, *M. pneumoniae* and *C. pneumoniae*) and genital tract infections (*C. trachomatis*, *U. urealyticum* and *M. hominis*). *M. tuberculosis*, *M. fortuitum*, *M. kansasii* and *M. chelonei* are moderately susceptible, and MAC strains less so. The susceptibilities of common pathogens are summarized in Table 32.2.

Acquired resistance

Resistant mutants can be generated by a single passage in the presence of the agent: *Staph. aureus* and *Esch. coli* in the presence of 4–8 times the MIC with a frequency of around 10^{-10} and *Ps. aeruginosa* with a frequency of around 10^{-8} or more. There is complete cross-resistance with other quinolones, but not with unrelated agents.

Pharmacokinetics

Ofloxacin is rapidly absorbed when administered by mouth, a 400-mg dose producing a mean peak plasma concentration at 1–1.5 h of around 3–5 mg/l. There is no significant interference with absorption by magnesium–aluminium hydroxide or calcium carbonate compounds which normally impair quinolone absorption, providing administration is separated by at least 2 h. In patients receiving repeated 200-mg doses, the mean peak plasma concentration rises from 2.7 mg/l after the first dose to 3.4 mg/l after the seventh. Following i.v. infusion of 100 or 200 mg over 30 min, mean plasma concentrations 1 h after the end of the infusion are around 0.8 and 1.8 mg/l, respectively. The plasma elimination half-life is 5–7 h.

There is limited metabolism to the desmethyl and *N*-oxide derivatives, only about 20% of a dose being eliminated by non-renal routes. There is a very slight effect on cytochrome-P_{450}-related isoenzymes and no significant effect on the metabolism of theophylline in dosages of up to 800 mg.

Ofloxacin is widely distributed, achieving concentrations in many tissues, including lung and bronchial secretions, of 50% or more of the simultaneous plasma concentrations. In cantharides and suction blisters the peak concentrations exceed those in plasma, while the elimination half-life is similar. In patients with non-inflamed meninges, 200 mg administered orally or by i.v. infusion over 30 min produced CSF concentrations of around 0.4–1 mg/l at 2–4 h when the plasma concentration was 1.7–4 mg/l; a 400-mg i.v. infusion yielded a CSF concentration of 2 mg/l, which is adequate for some Gram-negative bacteria, but not for Gram-positive bacteria or *Ps. aeruginosa.*

The drug is eliminated principally by the renal route, about 60% and 80–90% of a dose appearing over 12 and 48 h, respectively. The plasma elimination half-life is prolonged in renal failure, reaching 30–50 h in anuria, and therefore necessitating a dosage reduction. The desmethyl metabolite accumulates in all patients and the *N*-oxide in 50%. Absorption and distribution are not affected by renal failure. Significant amounts of the drug appear in the faeces, producing very variable concentrations up to 100 mg/l.

Toxicity and side-effects

It is generally well tolerated, untoward reactions, which have been described in 2.5–7.5% of patients, being those common to the group, i.e. gastro-intestinal tract disturbances, rashes and insomnia. More dramatic CNS effects in some patients have included hallucinations, mostly visual, and psychotic reactions. In some patients, influenza-like symptoms have been described.

The presence of the drug in faeces results in rapid and virtually complete elimination of Enterobacteriaceae, with some increase in the numbers of streptococci, but no effect on the numbers of anaerobes. The faecal flora returns to normal 3–26 days after discontinuing treatment.

Clinical use

Ofloxacin has been shown in many studies to be effective therapy of both simple and complicated infections of the urinary tract. It achieves high concentrations in prostatic fluid and has produced a clinical cure rate of 85% in evaluable patients with prostatitis. The drug, even in a single dose, has been highly effective in the treatment of patients with uncomplicated urogenital and anorectal gonorrhoea. Three-day courses of ofloxacin have successfully treated patients with chancroid and 7-day courses have produced cure rates of up to 100% (comparable to those produced by doxycycline) when given to patients with genital chlamydial infections.

Ofloxacin has been effective therapy of a wide variety of respiratory tract infections, including bronchopneumonia, community- and hospital-acquired pneumonia, acute exacerbations of chronic obstructive airways disease and bronchiectasis. *H. influenzae*, *Mor. catarrhalis* and AGNB have been consistently eradicated from sputum, but persistence of *Str. pneumoniae* has been observed frequently. Therefore, despite the drug having produced high clinical cure rates in patients with pneumococcal pneumonia, it should probably not be used as initial therapy of this infection. On the other hand, it has been used successfully in patients with cystic fibrosis and, although it has been evaluated in only a small number of studies, patients with atypical pneumonias have also responded favourably. In clinical trials, ofloxacin, in combination with other agents, has eradicated MDR-TB from sputum and produced clinical cures in patients infected with these strains.

It has been demonstrated to be effective treatment of patients with enteric fever, including the chronic carrier state, and of those with gastroenteritis caused by enterotoxigenic *Esch. coli* and *Salmonella*, *Shigella* and *Campylobacter* spp. Administration of ofloxacin has been associated with high clinical and bacteriological cure rates in patients with skin and soft-tissue infections and bone and joint infections, particularly those caused by Gram-negative bacteria. The drug has also been effective therapy of infections caused by *Staph. aureus*, but it should not routinely replace standard antistaphylococcal agents in these clinical settings. When given to neutropenic patients as prophylaxis, ofloxacin has resulted in reductions in the incidence of bacteraemia caused by Gram-negative bacteria. However, it has not had the same impact on the incidence of infections caused by Gram-positive organisms and the use of quinolones in this context has been associated with septicaemic episodes caused by quinolone-resistant strains of Gram-negative bacteria. Ofloxacin has been used effectively in the treatment of patients with malignant otitis externa and a topical preparation is available for use in patients with ocular infections, although it should not routinely replace conventional agents which are equally effective and less expensive.

Guay D R P, Opsahl J A, McMahon F G, Vargas R, Matzke G R, Flor S 1992 Safety and pharmacokinetics of multiple doses of intravenous ofloxacin in healthy volunteers. *Antimicrobial Agents and Chemotherapy* 36: 308–312

Navarro A S, Lanao J M, Recio M M S et al 1990 Effect of renal impairment on distribution of ofloxacin. *Antimicrobial Agents and Chemotherapy* 34: 455–459

Neu H C, Chin N Y 1989 In vitro activity of S-ofloxacin. *Antimicrobial Agents and Chemotherapy* 33: 1105–1107

Pioget J C, Wolff M, Singlas E et al 1989 Diffusion of ofloxacin into cerebrospinal fluid of patients with purulent meningitis or ventriculitis. *Antimicrobial Agents and Chemotherapy* 33: 933–936

Symposium 1988 Focus on ofloxacin – a new 4-quinolone antimicrobial agent. *Journal of Antimicrobial Chemotherapy* 22 (suppl C): 1–175

Symposium 1990 Ofloxacin – developments in therapy. *Journal of Antimicrobial Chemotherapy* 26 (suppl D): 1–142

Warlich R, Korting H C, Schafer-Korting M, Mutschler E 1989 Multiple dose pharmacokinetics of ofloxacin in serum, saliva and skin blister fluid of healthy volunteers. *Antimicrobial Agents and Chemotherapy* 34: 78–81

Preparations and dosage

Proprietary name: Tarivid.

Preparations: Tablets, injection, ophthalmic.

Dosage: Adults, oral, 200–400 mg/day, increased to 400 mg twice daily in severe infections; i.v., 200–400 mg once or twice a day depending on severity of infection. Widely available.

Further information

Bitar N, Claes R, Van der Auwera P 1989 Concentration of ofloxacin in serum and cerebrospinal fluid of patients without meningitis receiving the drug intravenously and orally. *Antimicrobial Agents and Chemotherapy* 33: 1686–1690

Farinotti R, Trouvin J H, Bocquet V, Vermerie N, Carbon C 1988 Pharmacokinetics of ofloxacin after single and multiple intravenous infusions in healthy subjects. *Antimicrobial Agents and Chemotherapy* 22: 1590–1592

Flors S, Guay D R P, Opsahl J A, Tack K, Matzke G R 1990 Effects of magnesium-aluminium hydroxide and calcium carbonate antacids on bioavailability of ofloxacin. *Antimicrobial Agents and Chemotherapy* 34: 2436–2438

PEFLOXACIN

A fluoropiperazinyl quinolone.

Antimicrobial activity

Pefloxacin is highly active against a wide range of Enterobacteriaceae (Table 32.2), as well as *Aeromonas*, *Legionella*, *Vibrio* and *Neisseria* spp., *H. influenzae*, *M. catarrhalis* and *H. ducreyi*. *Campylobacter* and *Acinetobacter* spp. and *Ps. aeruginosa* are only moderately susceptible, and other *Pseudomonas* spp. vary in their susceptibilities.

Staphylococci, including multiresistant strains, are susceptible; streptococci, including pneumococci and enterococci, less so. It has poor activity against *Mycobacterium*, *Chlamydia* and *Mycoplasma* spp. and *U. urealyticum*. *L. monocytogenes*, *Nocardia* spp. and anaerobes are resistant.

Pharmacokinetics

Pefloxacin is absorbed when administered by mouth, mean peak plasma concentrations 1–1.5 h after a 400-mg dose being around 4.5–6 mg/l. Binding to plasma protein is 20–30%. The plasma elimination half-life is 8.5–13 h, rising to 15 h after multiple dosing when the steady-state concentration is achieved in less than 48 h. Bioavailability is virtually complete. It is widely distributed, concentrations in bone, brain, blister fluid, CSF, saliva, sputum and prostate all approximating, and in some cases exceeding, the simultaneous plasma concentration. It is extensively metabolized to the desmethyl and N-oxide derivatives. Some 60–70% of a dose, only about 10% of which is unchanged, appears in the urine; 25% of a dose appears in the faeces, a small part contributed by excretion in the bile.

In keeping with its handling, the plasma elimination half-life increases with hepatic impairment, but is virtually unaffected by renal failure. In patients on CAPD given 800 mg followed by 400 mg twice daily for 10–12 days, there was no significant accumulation of pefloxacin or its metabolite, norfloxacin, but concentrations of pefloxacin N-oxide rose continuously in plasma and dialysate; all concentrations fell rapidly when treatment was discontinued.

Toxicity and side-effects

It is generally well tolerated, untoward reactions being those common to the group (p. 427). Most of these (50% or more) are gastro-intestinal tract disturbances, although some typical CNS reactions have been encountered. Skin eruptions (some photosensitive) occur and rashes appeared in about one-third of a group of patients who were given long-term therapy.

Clinical use

Pefloxacin (even as a single dose) has been shown to be highly effective as therapy of patients with simple or complicated urinary tract infections; the cure rates in patients with prostatitis have also been at least comparable to those obtained with conventional agents. Uncomplicated gonococcal infections have responded well to this quinolone, but its activity against *C. trachomatis* is not sufficient to enable it to be used as therapy of genital tract infections caused by this pathogen.

The drug has produced high clinical response rates in patients with a variety of respiratory tract infections, including acute bronchitis, acute exacerbations of chronic obstructive airways disease and pneumonia (both hospital and community acquired). While Gram-negative pathogens (*H. influenzae*, *M. catarrhalis* and AGNB) have been consistently eradicated from sputum, lower bacteriological cure rates have been achieved in patients with infections caused by *Str. pneumoniae* and, in common with most other fluoroquinolones, there remain concerns about the reliability of pefloxacin as therapy of severe pneumococcal infections.

The drug has been used effectively to treat infections caused by most bacterial enteric pathogens, including *Salm. typhi*. Pefloxacin has produced cure rates equivalent to those achieved with comparator agents in patients with skin and soft-tissue and bone and joint infections. However, the incidence of treatment failure associated with infections caused by Gram-negative organisms has been lower than that associated with infections caused by Gram-positive organisms, especially *Staph. aureus*, some strains of this pathogen becoming resistant during courses of therapy. The drug has also been used effectively as therapy of malignant otitis externa and meningitis caused by Gram-negative bacteria, to prevent infections in patients undergoing biliary tract surgery and in the treatment of patients with infections of the biliary tract. While pefloxacin has been shown to prevent infections caused by Gram-negative bacteria in neutropenic patients, prophylaxis with this agent has reduced the incidence of infections caused by Gram-positive organisms only when it was combined with penicillin.

Preparations and dosage

Dosage: Adults, oral, i.v., 400 mg twice daily.
Available in continental Europe.

Further information

Gonzalez J P, Henwood J M 1989 Pefloxacin: a review of its antibacterial activity, pharmacokinetic properties and therapeutic use. *Drugs* 37: 628–668

Jones R N 1989 Antimicrobial activity and interaction of pefloxacin and its principal metabolites. Collaborative Antimicrobial Susceptibility Testing Group. *European Journal of Clinical Microbiology and Infectious Diseases* 8: 551–556

Rose T F, Bremner D A, Collins J et al 1990 Plasma and dialysate levels of pefloxacin and its metabolites in CAPD patients with peritonitis. *Journal of Antimicrobial Chemotherapy* 25: 657–664

Symposium 1986 Pefloxacin – a laboratory and clinical evaluation of a new quinolone. *Journal of Antimicrobial Chemotherapy* 17 (suppl B): 1–115

Symposium 1990 Pefloxacin in clinical practice. *Journal of Antimicrobial Chemotherapy* 26 (suppl B): 1–229

RUFLOXACIN

A fluoropiperazinyl quinolone.

Antimicrobial activity

Rufloxacin has only moderate to poor activity against the majority of Enterobacteriaceae and some genera (*Klebsiella, Enterobacter, Serratia*) are virtually resistant. *H. influenzae, Neisseria* spp. and *M. catarrhalis* are susceptible, but the drug has only modest activity against *Ps. aeruginosa, Acinetobacter* spp., staphylococci and *Chlamydia* spp. Streptococci (including β-haemolytic species, enterococci and pneumococci) and anaerobes are resistant.

Pharmacokinetics

Rufloxacin is rapidly and well absorbed after oral administration, 400-mg doses giving maximum concentrations at 2–4 h of 3.5–4.5 mg/l. The plasma half-life is very long (30–45 h) and, not surprisingly, the total (2.7 l/h) and renal (1.0 l/h) clearances are low. In common with other fluoroquinolones, the volume of distribution of rufloxacin (100 l) greatly exceeds the body water volume. It is widely distributed in tissues where it is found in therapeutic concentrations. In bronchial mucosa, alveolar macrophages and lung epithelial lining fluid, concentrations exceed, greatly in some instances, those in the plasma, as do concentrations in prostatic tissue and secretions.

Rufloxacin undergoes extensive metabolism to the active *N*-desmethyl metabolite, the plasma concentrations of which exceed by about two-fold those of the parent drug. In 72 h about 27% of a dose is recovered in the urine and 1% in the bile; biliary concentrations are sufficiently high to suggest utility in treating biliary infections. Urinary concentrations (30–50 mg/l) comfortably exceed the MICs of susceptible pathogens, and concentrations of about 20 mg/l can still be found 3 days after dosing.

The renal clearance of rufloxacin diminishes with falling renal function, but the plasma half-life does not increase greatly, presumably because of the drug's substantial metabolism. It has been suggested that the dosage interval should be doubled to 48 h in patients with creatinine clearances of <30 ml/min per 1.73 m^2.

Clinical use

There are relatively few published data regarding clinical experience with rufloxacin. In a limited number of trials, the drug has been shown to be effective treatment of both simple and complicated urinary tract infections and has produced high clinical and bacteriological cure rates in patients with prostatitis. Its in vitro activity and pharmacokinetic properties suggest that it might be useful as therapy of bacterial gastroenteritis and of genital tract infections caused by *N. gonorrhoeae*. Although rufloxacin is active against *H. influenzae* and *M. catarrhalis* and has been shown to be effective treatment in patients with lower respiratory tract infections (including bronchopneumonia, acute exacerbations of chronic obstructive airways disease and pneumonia), its very poor activity against *Str. pneumoniae* precludes its use in patients with severe pneumococcal respiratory tract infections.

Further information

Boerema J B J, Bischoff W, Focht J, Naber K G 1991 An open multicentre study on the efficacy and safety of rufloxacin in patients with chronic bacterial prostatitis. *Journal of Antimicrobial Chemotherapy* 28: 587–597

Dirksen M, Focht J, Boerema J 1991 Rufloxacin once daily in acute exacerbations of chronic bronchitis. *Infection* 19: 297–300

Imbimbo B P, Broccali G P, Cesana M, Crema F, Attardo-Parrinello G 1991 Inter- and intrasubject variabilities in the pharmacokinetics of rufloxacin after single oral administration to healthy volunteers. *Antimicrobial Agents and Chemotherapy* 35: 390–393

Mattina R, Bonfiglio G, Cocuzza C E, Gulisano G, Cesana M, Imbimbo B P 1991 Pharmacokinetics of rufloxacin in healthy volunteers after repeated oral doses. *Chemotherapy* 37: 389–397

Mattina R, Cocuzza C E, Cesana M, Bonfiglio G 1991 In vitro activity of a new quinolone, rufloxacin, against nosocomial isolates. *Chemotherapy* 37: 260–269

Wise R, Andrews J M, Matthews R, Wostenholme M 1992 The in-vitro activity of two new quinolones: rufloxacin and MF 961. *Journal of Antimicrobial Chemotherapy* 29: 649–660

SPARFLOXACIN

A dimethylpiperazinyl fluoroquinolone.

Antimicrobial activity

Sparfloxacin is, overall, the most active of the currently

available fluoroquinolones. It is highly active (and comparable to ciprofloxacin) against Enterobacteriaceae, *H. influenzae*, *Neisseria* spp., *M. catarrhalis*, *Acinetobacter* spp., *Campylobacter* spp., *Legionella* spp. and *C. trachomatis*; *Ps. aeruginosa* is less susceptible. Sparfloxacin is the most active quinolone against Gram-positive bacteria, with moderate to excellent activity against staphylococci (both methicillin-resistant and -susceptible strains) and streptococci (including pneumococci and enterococci). The genital mycoplasmas, *M. hominis* and *U. urealyticum*, are susceptible and sparfloxacin is the most active fluoro-quinolone against *Mycobacterium* spp., including MAC strains. It is also moderately active against some anaerobes (including the *B. fragilis* group); *L. monocytogenes* is resistant. Its activity against common pathogenic bacteria is shown in Table 32.2.

Pharmacokinetics

Following a 400-mg oral dose, plasma concentrations peak at 1–1.5 mg/l at 4–5 h; absorption is decreased in the presence of antacids due to the formation of chelates with metallic ions. The low plasma concentrations are presumably a reflection of the very large apparent volume of distribution (>300 l). The plasma elimination half-life is 15–20 h, with a total clearance of 10–15 l/h, of which only about 10% is renal. Not surprisingly, the plasma half-life increases only modestly in renal failure to 30–40 h. In the urine, only 5–10% of a dose is excreted unchanged, with about 30% appearing as the glucuronide. In the faeces, about 50–60% of the dose appears as unchanged drug, as a result of unabsorption or, perhaps, excretion into the bowel, with biliary excretion, mainly as the glucuronide, accounting for 10–20% of a dose.

Sparfloxacin is concentrated in many tissues, in some greatly so, and tissue concentrations generally exceed those in plasma. In the lungs, concentrations of the drug exceed the MICs for the bacterial pathogens normally implicated in respiratory tract infections. The drug accumulates rapidly in macrophages, polymorphonuclear cells and fibroblasts. CSF penetration is limited, with CSF concentrations <0.1 mg/l after a single 200-mg oral dose.

Toxicity and side-effects

The adverse events associated with the administration of sparfloxacin have been those common to fluoroquinolones in general (p. 427), in particular, gastro-intestinal tract disturbances, CNS effects (mainly headache and insomnia) and rashes. Photosensitivity reactions have been observed in approximately 1% of patients. Sparfloxacin does not potentiate the toxicity of theophylline, but its use is contraindicated during pregnancy and lactation.

Clinical use

The relatively few published clinical trials to date make it difficult to decide whether the therapeutic efficacy of sparfloxacin matches its excellent in vitro activity. It has been shown to be effective in the treatment of gonococcal and chlamydial genital tract infections and has produced high clinical and bacteriological cure rates in patients with bronchopneumonia, acute exacerbations of chronic obstructive airways disease and community-acquired pneumonia, including those infections due to *Str. pneumoniae* and atypical pathogens.

Further information

Barry A L, Fuchs P C 1991 In vitro activities of sparfloxacin, tosufloxacin, ciprofloxacin and fleroxacin. *Antimicrobial Agents and Chemotherapy* 35: 955–960

Canton N, Peman J, Jimenez M T, Ramon M S, Gobernado M 1992 In vitro activity of sparfloxacin compared with those of five other quinolones. *Antimicrobial Agents and Chemotherapy* 36: 558–565

Chaudhry A Z, Knapp C C, Sierra-Madero J, Washington J A 1990 Antistaphylococcal activities of sparfloxacin (CI-978; AT-4140), ofloxacin, and ciprofloxacin. *Antimicrobial Agents and Chemotherapy* 34: 1843–1845

Cooper M A, Andrews J M, Ashby J P, Matthews R S, Wise R 1990 In-vitro activity of sparfloxacin, a new quinolone antimicrobial agent. *Journal of Antimicrobial Chemotherapy* 26: 667–676

Hara K, Kobayashi H, Tanimota H, Matsumoto K, Oizumi K 1991 A multicenter double blind comparative study of sparfloxacin and ofloxacin in the treatment of chronic respiratory tract infections. In: Program and abstracts of the thirty-first interscience conference on antimicrobial agents and chemotherapy, Chicago, IL, 1991. American Society for Microbiology, Washington, DC, Abstract 878, p 245

Kenny G E, Bien P A, Cartwright F D 1990 Susceptibilities of genital mycoplasmas to sparfloxacin compared to ofloxacin and tetracycline. In: Programme and abstracts of the third international symposium on new quinolones, Vancouver, Canada

Nakata K, Maeda H, Fujii A, Arakawa S, Umeza K, Kamidono S 1992 In vitro and in vivo activities of sparfloxacin, other quinolones, and tetracyclines against *Chlamydia trachomatis*. *Antimicrobial Agents and Chemotherapy* 36: 188–190

Rastogi N, Goh K S 1991 In vitro activity of the new difluorinated quinolone sparfloxacin (AT-4140) against *Mycobacterium tuberculosis* compared with activities of ofloxacin and ciprofloxacin. *Antimicrobial Agents and Chemotherapy* 35: 1933–1936

Rolston K V I, Nguyen H, Messer M, Le Blanc B, Ho D H, Bodey G P 1990 In vitro activity of sparfloxacin (CI-978; AT-4140) against clinical isolates from cancer patients. *Antimicrobial Agents and Chemotherapy* 34: 2263–2266

Shimada J, Nogita T, Ishibashi Y 1993 Clinical pharmacokinetics of sparfloxacin. *Clinical Pharmacokinetics* 25: 358–369

Soejima R, Shimada K, Matsumoto F, Miki F, Saito A 1991 A multicenter double blind comparative study of sparfloxacin and ofloxacin in the treatment of bacterial pneumonia. In: Program and abstracts of the thirty-first interscience conference on antimicrobial agents and chemotherapy, Chicago, IL, 1991. American Society for Microbiology, Washington, DC, Abstract 877, p 245

TOSUFLOXACIN

Tosufloxacin is a naphthyridine derivative with a pyrrolidinyl substituent at position 7. It is highly active against Enterobacteriaceae, *Neisseria* spp., *H. influenzae*, *M. catarrhalis*, *L. pneumophila* and *Campylobacter* spp. It is only moderately active against *Ps. aeruginosa*, but is one of the most active quinolones to date against *Acinetobacter* spp. Tosufloxacin exhibits good activity against Gram-positive bacteria, particularly staphylococci (both methicillin-susceptible and -resistant strains) and streptococci (including *Str. pyogenes* and *Str. pneumoniae*). Enterococci are less susceptible, but, unlike many of the new quinolones, the drug is moderately active against *L. monocytogenes*. *C. trachomatis* is also moderately susceptible. It is active against some anaerobes, including the *B. fragilis* group. Activity against *Mycobacterium* spp. is limited (Table 32.2).

Tosufloxacin is poorly absorbed when administered by the non-oral route. Following an oral dose of 300 mg, a mean peak plasma concentration of 1 mg/l was found in a group of volunteers. The plasma half-life was 6–7 h. Around 30–35% of the dose was recovered in the urine. The concentration in prostatic tissue was similar to that seen in plasma.

Clinical experience with tosufloxacin is limited, but high clinical and bacteriological cure rates have been obtained in patients with skin and soft-tissue infections.

Further information

Arguedas A G, Akaniro J C, Stutman H R, Marks M I 1990 In vitro activity of tosufloxacin, a new quinolone, against respiratory pathogens derived from cystic fibrosis sputum. *Antimicrobial Agents and Chemotherapy* 34: 2223–2227

Barry A L, Fuchs P C 1991 In vitro activities of sparfloxacin, tosufloxacin, ciprofloxacin and fleroxacin. *Antimicrobial Agents and Chemotherapy* 35: 955–960

Barry A L, Jones R N 1989 In vitro activities of temafloxacin, tosufloxacin (A-61827) and five other fluoroquinolone agents. *Journal of Antimicrobial Chemotherapy* 23: 527–535

Bryan J P, Waters C, Sheffield J, Krieg R E, Perine P, Wagner K 1989 In vitro activities of tosufloxacin, temafloxacin and A-56620 against pathogens of diarrhoea. *Antimicrobial Agents and Chemotherapy* 34: 368–370

Kinzig M, Sörgel F, Shah A, Greene D, Faulkner R, Tonelli A et al 1991 The pharmacokinetics of tosufloxacin in man. In: Program and abstracts of the thirty-first interscience conference on antimicrobial agents and chemotherapy, Chicago, IL, 1991. American Society for Microbiology, Washington, DC, Abstract 595, p 198

Rifamycins

F. Parenti   G. Lancini

Introduction

The rifamycins are a family of antibiotics produced by a strain of a species originally denoted as Streptomyces mediterranei, later reclassified as Nocardia mediterranea and, more recently as Amycolatopsis mediterranei. All the therapeutically useful rifamycins are semi-synthetic derivatives of rifamycin B, a fermentation product poorly active but easily produced and readily converted chemically into rifamycin S from which the majority of active derivatives are prepared. The general structure of rifamycins is:

Natural products, like rifamycins, which are characterized by an aromatic ring spanned by an aliphatic bridge (ansa) are called 'ansamycins'. To this class belong the streptovaricins and the tolypomycins, chemically and biologically similar to rifamycins, and geldanamycin and the maytansines that have quite different, antiblastic, biological activities. Among the vast number of rifamycin derivatives investigated, rifampicin is by far the most important and most widely used. Rifamycin SV (also produced naturally by some strains of A. mediterranei) is available in several countries, whereas rifaximin and rifamide are used in a few

countries only. Rifabutin has been recently approved for clinical use in the USA, and rifapentine is still under clinical development.

Interest in these antibiotics is centred on their potent activity against pathogenic Gram-positive cocci and mycobacteria. They were the first substances encountered with MICs below 0.01 mg/l – described in earlier editions of this book as 'almost incredibly low'. Neisseria are susceptible, as are some other Gram-negative organisms, but the MICs for enterobacteria are, at best, several milligrams per litre.

Knowledge of the general properties of the group is largely based on extensive study and use of rifampicin but, insofar as they have been investigated, the main features are exhibited also by the other congeners: action through inactivation of bacterial DNA-dependent RNA polymerase; bactericidal effect; relatively high frequency of resistant mutants; stimulation of hepatic metabolism and significant biliary excretion. Rifampicin was reported to exert a certain degree of activity against some eukaryotic organisms, such as fungi (in combination with amphotericin B), Leishmania spp., and Plasmodium falciparum, but clinical efficacy against these organisms has not been sufficiently proven. Rifampicin inhibits in vitro vaccinia viruses, an activity originally interpreted as due to inhibition of viral RNA polymerase, but later shown to be due to interference with capsid assembly. Several other rifamycins have been studied for their ability to inhibit various polymerizing enzymes, such as eukaryotic DNA and RNA polymerases and viral reverse transcriptase, but without any practical success. Several rifamycins have been shown to exert some immuno-suppressive effect in animals, but again without clinical significance.

Rifamycin SV and rifamide were originally released for the treatment of infections with susceptible Gram-positive organisms and infections of the biliary tract, but the principal use of rifampicin and the recently introduced rifabutin has been in the treatment of mycobacterial infections. Rifampicin proved so important in the treatment of tuberculosis, where its potent action allowed the introduction of short-course therapy, that in many countries its use was restricted to that indication, for fear that more widespread use would encourage the emergence of resistant Mycobacterium tuberculosis. Those fears have proven to be exaggerated (the frequency of resistant mutants in sensitive bacterial populations is high, but resistance is not transferable) and, increasingly, interest has been refocused on what was originally anticipated to be an important use: treatment of severe Gram-positive infections. To prevent emergence of resistance co-administration of another effective agent is required.

Rifaximin, like rifamide and rifamycin SV is poorly absorbed from the gut, and is used in the treatment of a variety of gastro-intestinal infections.

RIFABUTIN
Rifabutine; ansamycin; LM-427

A semi-synthetic spiropiperidyl derivative of rifamycin S.

It exhibits good activity against most mycobacteria, including the *Mycobacterium avium/intracellulare* complex (MIC 0.01–2 mg/l) and some strains of *M. tuberculosis* and *Mycobacterium leprae* resistant to rifampicin. Campylobacter is inhibited by 0.25–1 mg/l. It appears that the frequency of resistance in several bacterial species, including *Staphylococcus aureus* and *Chlamydia trachomatis* is somewhat lower with rifabutin than with some other rifamycins.

It has been reported to inhibit the replication of human immunodeficiency virus I (HIV I) in concentrations (10 mg/l) that are not toxic to lymphoid cells, but no efficacy on HIV infections has been demonstrated.

Oral absorption is rapid but incomplete, oral bioavailability being only 12–20% with considerable interpatient variation. Binding to plasma protein is about 70%. It is widely distributed in a large volume, producing tissue levels 5–10 times the simultaneous plasma concentration. The plasma elimination half-life is very long (around 16 h). It exhibits hepatic-enzyme-inducing properties and the area under the curve (AUC) declines as treatment continues. It is mainly metabolized to the desacetyl derivative, although several other oxidation products have been detected in urine, where some 10% of the dose is eliminated. About 30–50% of the dose can be recovered from the faeces.

Rifabutin has been proven of value in preventing or delaying mycobacterial infections in immunocompromised patients. It has been approved in the USA and in Italy for the prevention of *M. avium/intracellulare* infections in acquired immune deficiency syndrome (AIDS) patients.

Preparations and dosage

Proprietary name: Mycobutin.

Preparation: Capsules.

Dosage: Adults, oral, prophylaxis of *M. avium* complex infections in immunocompromised patients with low CD4 count, 300 mg/day as a single dose. Treatment of non-tuberculous mycobacterial disease, in combination with other drugs, 450–600 mg/day as a single dose for up to 6 months after cultures negative. Treatment of pulmonary tuberculosis, in combination with other drugs, 150–450 mg/day as a single dose for at least 6 months.

Available in the UK and the USA.

Further information

Cocchiara G, Strolin-Benedetti M, Vicario G P et al 1989 Urinary metabolites of rifabutin, a new antimycobacterial agent in human volunteers. *Xenobiotica* 19: 769–780

Klemens S P, Grossi M A, Cynamon M H 1994 Comparative in vivo activities of rifabutin and rifapentine against *Mycobacterium avium* complex. *Antimicrobial Agents and Chemotherapy* 38: 243–237

Masur H 1993 Recommendations on prophylaxis and therapy for disseminated *Mycobacterium avis* complex disease in patients infected with the human immunodeficiency virus. *New England Journal of Medicine* 329: 898–904

Nightingale S D, Cameron D W, Gordin F M et al 1993 Two controlled trials of rifabutin prophylaxis against *Mycobacterium avis* complex infection in AIDS. *New England Journal of Medicine* 329: 828–833

O'Brien R J, Lyle M A, Snider D E Jr 1987 Rifabutin (Ansamycin LM 427): a new rifamycin S derivative for the treatment of mycobacterial diseases. *Reviews of Infectious Diseases* 9: 519–530

Skinner M H, Hsieh M, Torseth J et al 1989 Pharmacokinetics of rifabutin. *Antimicrobial Agents and Chemotherapy* 33: 1237–1241

RIFAMPICIN
Rifampin

A semi-synthetic derivative of rifamycin SV.

Antimicrobial activity

Rifampicin exibits in vitro various degrees of antimicrobial activity against a large spectrum of microorganisms, including (Table 33.1) Gram-positive cocci and bacilli, Gram-negative cocci and bacilli, Mycobacterium spp., Chlamydia spp., some eukariotic parasites and some viruses.

Potent activity (minimum inhibitory concentration (MIC) <0.025–0.5 mg/l) is exerted against both coagulase-positive and -negative staphylococci, including methicillin-resistant strains, and streptococci including penicillin-resistant *Streptococcus pneumoniae*. Group B streptococci are somewhat sensitive and enterococci are substantially less sensitive. Gram-positive bacilli including *Bacillus* spp., *Clostridium difficile*, Corynebacterium spp. and *Leisteria monocytogenes* are highly susceptible (MIC 0.025–0.5 mg/ml). The pathogenic nesseria and *Moraxella* spp. are also highly susceptible to rifampicin.

Table 33.1 *Activity of rifampicin against common pathogenic bacteria: MIC (mg/l)*

Staph. aureus	0.008 – 0.06
Strep. pyogenes	0.03 – 0.1
Strep. pneumoniae	0.06 – 4
Ent. faecalis	1 – 4
M. tuberculosis	0.1 – 1
N. gonorrheae	0.06 – 0.5
N. meningitidis	0.01 – 0.5
H. influenzae	0.5 – 1
Esch. coli	8 – 16
Klebsiella	16 – 32
Pr. mirabilis	4 – 8
Proteus indole +	8 – 32
Enterobacter	8 – 64
Salmonella	8 – 16
Shigella	16 – 64
Ser. marcescens	32 – 64
Citrobacter	32
Ps. aeruginosa	32 – 64

The enteric Gram-negative bacteria are generally less sensitive to rifampicin (MIC 1–32 mg/ml), except *Bacteroides fragilis* which is highly susceptible. Among other Gram-negative bacilli, *Haemophilus influenzae* and *Haemophilus ducreyi, Flavobacterium meningosepticum* and Legionella spp. are highly susceptible (MIC <0.025–2 mg/l). *Chlamydia trachomatis* and *C. psittaci* are inhibited by low concentrations (0.025–0.5 mg/ml).

M. tuberculosis, Mycobacterium kansasi and *Mycobacterium marinum* are all susceptible, the majority of strains being inhibited by <0.01–0.1 mg/l, but *Mycobacterium fortuitum* members of the *M. avium* complex are resistant. *M. leprae* is highly sensitive to rifampicin. It is active against some eukaryotic parasites through unknown mechanisms, although inhibition of the prokaryote-like polymerase of kinetoplasts or mitochondria has been postulated. Maturation of *Plasmodium falciparum* is inhibited by 2–10 mg/l; at higher concentrations *Leishmania* spp. are also inhibited.

High concentrations of rifampicin inhibit growth of a variety of poxviruses, by interference with viral-particle maturation; viral reverse transcriptase is insensitive to rifampicin.

Combined activity

Because of the relative ease with which resistant mutants emerge, it appears advisable to use rifampicin in combination with other unrelated antibiotics. Consequently, considerable attention has been paid to its interaction with other agents. The general experience has been that combinations with β-lactams or glycopeptides (vancomycin and teicoplanin) are antagonistic or indifferent, but synergy has been found with some penicillins against some strains of *Staph. aureus* and the combination has proved effective in some cases in vivo. It antagonizes the bactericidal effect of ciprofloxacin against *Staph. aureus*. Rifampicin is synergic in vitro with aminoglycosides against *Esch. coli* and with polymyxin B against multiresistant *Serratia marcescens*. Synergy with trimethoprim against enterobacteria, strepto-cocci and staphylococci has been reported by several authors, but others have found indifference, or sometimes antagonism, and there appears to be substantial individual strain variation. Synergy against some strains of *Staph. aureus* has also been demonstrated with erythromycin, clindamycin and other antistaphylococcal agents.

In vitro activity against *Myc. tuberculosis* is increased in the presence of streptomycin and isoniazid but not ethambutol. Rifampicin acts synergically with amphotericin B against *Candida albicans* and against the mycelial, but not the spherule-endospore phase of *Coccidium immitis*. However, combined therapy was no more effective against murine coccidiomycosis than was amphotericin alone.

All together the principal value of the addition of a second unrelated agent appears to be the suppression of emergence of resistant mutants.

Acquired resistance

Most large bacterial populations contain resistant mutants which readily emerge in the presence of the drug and can emerge during treatment. The mutation rate to resistance in *Staph. aureus, Str. pyogenes, Str. pneumoniae, Esch. coli* and *Proteus mirabilis* is about 10^{-7} and that to *M. tuberculosis* and *M. marinum* around 10^{-9} to 10^{-10}. Primary resistance of *M. tuberculosis* remained constantly low for many years, but is now somewhat increasing.

Resistance is of the one-step type, and several classes of mutants exhibiting resistance to different concentrations of the antibiotic can be selected by treatment of a large population with a relatively low concentration of the drug. Some of these mutants may be susceptible to other rifamycin derivatives. Resistance is not due to enzymic destruction and is not transferable. It is due to a change in a single amino acid of the β subunit of DNA-dependent RNA polymerase. The mutant enzyme no longer forms a stable complex with rifampicin. There is no cross-resistance with any other class of antibiotics presently in clinical use. The susceptible strains of the gastro-intestinal flora become rapidly resistant during rifampicin treatment without alteration in the flora composition, and revert to susceptibility within a few weeks upon treatment cessation.

Pharmacokinetics

Rifampicin is virtually completely absorbed when administered orally, but a high degree of variability has been found among different pharmaceutical preparations. Substantial differences in blood levels have been reported comparing capsules or tablets from different manufacturers. Peak plasma levels differ noticeably between individuals, and food also affects absorption, the peak plasma levels being delayed and about 2 mg/l lower after a meal. Although the AUC and the length of time for which effective antibacterial levels are maintained are little affected, it is preferable that patients do not take the drug with or after meals.

Plasma levels and elimination half-lives increase more than proportionally with the dose: whilst a 300 mg dose can give average peak serum levels of 4 mg/l with an elimination half-life of 2.5 h, 600 mg gives peaks of 10 mg/l and an elimination half-life of 3 h. Elimination half-life may be as long as 5 h with a 900 mg dose. The reason for this phenomenon is that rifampicin is mainly excreted and metabolized through the liver (see below), and there is a limit to the rate at which the liver can deliver the drug to the bile. Binding to plasma protein is about 80%, but the drug's lipid solubility facilitates its distribution. Intravenous administration produces AUCs and elimination half-lives similar to those obtained after oral doses.

It is metabolized principally to its desacetyl derivative, which is also antimicrobially active, and this process is accelerated by its stimulatory effect on hepatic microsomal enzymes. As a consequence, hepatic clearance increases on continuous administration and, especially with high doses, the serum half-life becomes shorter after a few days of treatment. It is widely distributed in the internal organs, bones, and fluids, including tears, saliva, ascitic fluid, and abscesses. It penetrates into cells, and is active against intracellular bacteria. Low concentrations are found in the cerebrospinal fluid (CSF), but these are substantially higher when the meninges are inflamed. Concentrations around 60% of the simultaneous plasma value were found in the heart valves of patients receiving a 600 mg dose before surgery.

Elimination is principally by secretion into the bile, a process that is dose dependent, being efficient at low dosage but limited at high dosage. As a result, the dose determines the proportion excreted via the bile or passing the liver to be excreted in the urine. The desacetyl compound is mainly found in the bile where the parent compound accounts for only 15% of the total. Plasma levels are increased by hepatic insufficiency, biliary obstruction and by probenecid which depresses hepatic uptake. The drug escaping biliary excretion appears in the urine, to which it imparts an orange-red colour, the parent compound and the desacetyl metabolites being present in about equal proportions. The plasma concentrations and half-life are not significantly affected by renal failure. The drug is not removed by haemodialysis.

Toxicity and side-effects

Rifampicin appears relatively non-toxic, even when administered for a long period as in the treatment of tuberculosis. However several unwanted effects, including pink staining of soft contact lenses, have been associated with its use. Adverse reactions have been divided into those associated with daily or intermittent administration, and those found only with intermittent therapy.

The former group includes: skin reactions, mostly flushing with or without rash, and often transient even when therapy is continued; gastro-intestinal disturbances, usually mild and most common in the early weeks of treatment; and disturbance of hepatic function. Transient abnormalities of liver function, especially a rise in serum transaminases and, less commonly, a raised bilirubin level, are common during rifampicin treatment, and clinical hepatitis, usually of mild degree, also occurs. Hepatitis was commonly recorded in some early studies, but the incidence in short-course regimens appears to be low. Earlier suggestions that hepatic damage was more common in rapid acetylators, and when given in combination with isoniazid, were not borne out by subsequent studies.

Thrombocytopenia, associated with complement-fixing serum antibodies, is an uncommon adverse reaction. The platelet count falls within a few hours, returning to normal within a day or two. Rifampicin administration should be discontinued at once. Thrombocytopenia is more common with intermittent schemes, but is also encountered in patients receiving daily treatment. Other adverse effects are confined to patients receiving intermittent therapy. The most important is the 'flu' syndrome, with fever, chills and malaise usually developing after 3–6 months of treatment. Its incidence is less with frequent than infrequent dosage, less with lower than higher doses, and less when intermittent therapy is preceded by an initial phase of daily treatment. It was not, however, prevented by a daily supplement of 25 mg in an intermittent regimen. Circulating immunoglobulin M (IgM) antibodies to rifampicin are found in serum, and the 'flu' syndrome may be caused by resulting complement activation.

Other rare syndromes associated with intermittent administration are acute renal failure, sometimes associated with acute haemolysis. Shortness of breath, wheezing and fall of blood pressure have occasionally been recorded.

In addition to these unwanted effects, the drug is a potent inducer of hepatic P_{450} microsomal enzymes, and this leads not only to more rapid elimination of rifampicin itself, but also to that of other agents handled by the same process. The effect is selective and it is not possible to predict which drugs may be affected. The most important are warfarin, the anticoagulant effect of which is thereby diminished, and oral contraceptives, with possible breakthrough bleeding and unwanted pregnancy. Addisonian crises have been described, and adjustments to steroid dosage in patients with Addison's disease may be necessary. Plasma concentrations of a number of other drugs may be affected, including digoxin, quinidine, methadone, hypoglycaemic agents and barbiturates, with corresponding pharmacological effects.

There is considerable evidence that rifampicin has immunosuppressive properties, demonstrable in a number of experimental systems, but no effect in man resulting from these properties has been demonstrated.

Clinical use

Treatment failure from emergence of resistant mutants is likely to occur if rifampicin is used alone in severe or chronic infections; therefore it must be combined with an unrelated drug to which the infecting organism is susceptible.

The most important use of rifampicin is in the treatment of tuberculosis, which is discussed in Chapter 59 where rifampicin's use in leprosy is also considered.

Because of its outstanding importance in the treatment of tuberculosis, the view has been taken that it should be reserved solely for this purpose, because of the danger that widespread use could lead to the emergence of resistant organisms in patients with unsuspected tuberculosis. This fear was exaggerated (several weeks of treatment are required for selection of resistant bacilli in tuberculosis patients treated with rifampicin alone) and the drug has re-emerged as an important agent for the treatment of severe infections due to a number of susceptible organisms. Its use has been proposed, in combination with a glycopeptide (teicoplanin or vancomycin), for the treatment of highly penicillin-resistant pneumococci, for pneumococcal or staphylococcal meningitis, *Staph. aureus* endocarditis (p. 704), severe staphylococcal sepsis (p. 586) and osteomyelitis (p. 762).

It is used for elimination of nasopharyngeal carriage of *Neisseria meningitidis* (p. 747) and of *H. influenzae* (p. 749); in both cases the emergence of resistant strains has been noted. Treatment for 5 days produced highly significant reduction in the nasal carriage of *Staph. aureus*, without emergence of resistance.

The combination with trimethoprim has been recommended in infections of the urinary tract and was shown to be effective against *H. ducreyi. Neisseria gonorrhoeae* infections have been successfully treated with combinations of erythromycin and rifampicin. Data from human studies suggest that *Cl. difficile* colitis can be successfully treated with rifampicin plus vancomycin. Reference is also made to its use in legionellosis (p. 687), meningitis (pp. 748, 750) and brucellosis (p. 883). In combination with primaquine it may be useful in the treatment of malaria.

Preparations and dosage

Proprietary names: Rifadin, Rimactane. In combination with Isoniazid: Rifinah, Rimactazid. In combination with Isoniazid and with Pyrazinamide: Rifater.

Preparations: Capsules, syrup, i.v. infusion.

Dosage: Oral, adults, 450–600 mg/day as a single dose, base on approx. 10 mg/kg daily. Children up to 20 mg/kg daily, as a single dose, to a maximum of 600 mg as a single dose. Premature and newborn infants, 10 mg/kg once daily; treat only in cases of emergency and with extreme caution since their liver enzyme system may not be fully developed.

I.v. infusion, adults, 450–600 mg/day as a single dose, based on approx. 10 mg/kg daily. Lower doses are recommended for small or frail patients. Children, 20 mg/kg daily, with a maximum daily dose of 600 mg. Premature and newborn infants, 10 mg/kg daily with caution, as for oral dose.

Chemoprophylaxis of meningococcal meningitis: oral, adults, 600 mg every 12 h (twice daily) for 2 days; children 1–12 years, 10 mg/kg every 12 h for 2 days; infants up to 1 year, 5 mg/kg every 12 h for 2 days.

Widely available.

Further information

Ball P, Williams T 1989 Attitudes to use of rifampicin in non-tuberculous infections. *Journal of Antimicrobial Chemotherapy* 24: 824–826

Buniva G, Pagani V, Carozzi A 1983 Bioavailability of rifampicin capsules. *International Journal of Clinical Pharmacology, Therapy and Toxicology* 21: 404–409

Cartwright K A V, Begg N T, Rudd P 1994 Use of vaccines and antibiotic prophylaxis in contacts and cases of *Haemophilus influenzae* type B (Hib) disease. *Communicable Disease Report Reviews* 4: R16–R17

Cohn J R, Fye D L, Sills J M, Francos G C 1985 Rifampicin-induced renal failure. *Tubercle* 66: 289–293

Konrad P, Stenberg P 1988 Rifampicin quinone is an immunosuppressant, but not rifampicin itself. *Clinical Immunology and Immunopathology* 46: 162–166

Morris A B, Brown R B, Sands M 1993 Use of rifampin in nonstaphylococcal, non-mycobacterial disease. *Antimicrobial Agents and Chemotherapy* 37: 1–7

Pukrittayakamee S, Viravan C, Charoenlarp P, Yeamput C, Wilson R J M, White N J 1994 Antimalarial effects of rifampin in *Plasmodium vivax* malaria. *Antimicrobial Agents and Chemotherapy* 38: 511–514

Venkatesan K 1992 Pharmacokinetic drug interactions with rifampicin. *Clinical Pharmacokinetics* 22: 47–65

poor results were obtained in tuberculosis, because of insufficient distribution to the tissues. There is anecdotal evidence of the efficacy of topical applications of rifamycin SV in curing wounds, particularly bedsores. The introduction in the UK of an injectable form of rifampicin superseded the use of rifamide which was withdrawn from the UK market.

Preparations and dosage

Proprietary names: Chibro-Rifamycin, Otofa, Rifocine.
Preparations: Parenteral injection, i.m., i.v., topical.
Dosage: I.m., 250 mg three times daily i.v. infusion (slow), up to 750 mg every 12 h.
Available in Italy, Switzerland, Germany.

Further information

Bergamini G, Fowst G 1965 Rifamycin SV. A review. *Arzneimittel Forschung* 15: 951–1002

Khan G A, Scott A G 1967 The place of rifamycin B diethylamide in the treatment of cholangitis complicating biliary obstructions. *British Journal of Pharmacology and Chemotherapy* 31: 506–512

Pallanza R, Füresz S, Timbal M T, Carniti G 1965 In vitro bacteriological studies on rifamycin B diethylamide (rifamide). *Arzneimittel Forschung* 15: 800–802

RIFAMYCIN SV AND RIFAMIDE

Rifamycin SV, the simplest rifamycin in clinical use, is obtained by elimination of a glycolic moiety from rifamycin B. Rifamide is the diethyl amide of rifamycin B.

These two products share very similar biological properties and have been marketed as alternatives to one another in several countries. They exhibit high activity against Gram-positive organisms and *M. tuberculosis* typical of the group. MICs for Gram-negative bacilli are of the order of 20–50 mg/l. Both drugs are poorly absorbed orally, but have some clinical usefulness because, in contrast to rifampicin, they can easily be administered as the sodium salt by intramuscular (i.m.) injection. A dose of 250 mg i.m. of rifamycin SV produces mean plasma levels of about 2 mg/l and a dose of 150 mg of rifamide gives around 1 mg/l. In both cases elimination is through the bile, with serum half-lives of about 2 h.

Because of the high concentrations reached in the bile, both drugs have been used successfully to treat infections of the biliary tract, even when due to Gram-negative bacilli. Efficacy has been shown in staphyloccal infections, whereas

RIFAPENTINE

An analogue of rifampicin in which a cyclopentyl group is substituted for a methyl group on the piperazine ring.

Rifapentine shows potent activity typical of the group against staphylococci and streptococci (MIC 0.01–0.5 mg/l), *Listeria monocytogenes* and *Brucella* spp., less against *Enterococcus faecalis* (MIC 1–4 mg/l). It is active against Mycobacteria, including the *M. avium* complex (MIC <0.06–0.5 mg/l). *Bacteroides* spp. are inhibited by 0.5–2 mg/l. Gram-negative cocci are susceptible, and some Gram-negative bacilli are inhibited by 4–32 mg/l, including *Esch. coli* and some *Pseudomonas* spp., but most are resistant. Indifference was the predominant response when combined with a variety of antistaphylococcal agents.

A dose of 600 mg produced mean peak plasma concentrations around 17 mg/l. The concentrations were around 21 mg/l when the same dose was administered after a meal. Elimination is mainly through the liver, and the terminal half-life in serum is about 12 h. An average of 9% of the administered dose is recovered in the urine. There is evidence that the drug is a potent inducer of liver oxidases in man. Rifapentine penetrates into cells, achieving concentrations several times higher than those of rifampicin under the same conditions. Experiments with animal models indicate the potential usefulness of rifapentine in the prevention and cure of mycobacterial infections. A dose of 20 mg/kg was shown effective in reducing substantially the number of infecting cells in the beige mouse model of disseminated *M. avium* infection.

Further information

Dickinson J M, Mitchinson D A 1987 In vitro properties of rifapentine (MDL 473) relevant to its use in intermittent chemotherapy of tuberculosis. *Tubercle* 68: 113–118

Fattorini L, Hu C Q, Jin S H et al 1992 Activity of antimicrobial agents against *Mycobacterium avium–intracellulare* complex (MAC) strains isolated in Italy from AIDS patients. *Zentralblatt Bakteriologie* 276: 512–520

Heifets L B, Lindholm-Levy P, Flory M 1990 Bactericidal activity in vitro of various rifamycins against *Mycobacterium avium* and *Mycobacterium tuberculosis. American Review of Respiratory Diseases* 141: 626–630

Ji B, Truffot-Pernot C, Lacroix C et al 1993 Effectiveness of rifampin, rifabutin and rifapentine for preventive therapy of tuberculosis in mice. *American Review of Respiratory Disease* 148: 1541–1546

Klemens S P, Cynamon M H 1992 Activity of rifapentine against *Mycobacterium avium* infection in beige mice. *Journal of Antimicrobial Chemotherapy* 29: 555–561

RIFAXIMIN

A semi-synthetic derivative of rifamycin S.

Antimicrobial activity

Its activity and range resemble those of the group. It is poorly absorbed from the gastro-intestinal tract, where the high concentrations are effective against a variety of gastro-intestinal pathogens. It is used in the treatment of gastro-intestinal infections. It has been also proposed for the treatment of chronic hepatic encephalopathy and for topical treatment of bacterial vaginitis.

Preparations and dosage

Proprietary names: Normix, Rifacol.
Dosage: Adults, 10–15 mg/kg per day.
Available in Italy.

Further information

Corazza G R, Ventrucci M, Strocchi A et al 1988 Treatment of small intestine bacterial overgrowth with rifaximin, a non-absorbable rifamycin. *Journal of International Medical Research* 16: 312–316

Festi D, Mazzella G, Orsini M et al 1993 Rifaximin in the treatment of chronic hepatic encephalopathy; results of a multicenter study of efficacy and safety. *Current Therapeutic Research: Clinical and Experimental* 54: 598–609

Ripa S, Mignini F, Prenna M, Falcioni E 1987 In vitro antibacterial activity of rifaximin against *Clostridium difficile, Campylobacter jejeuni* and *Yersinia* spp. *Drugs under Experimental and Clinical Research* 13: 483–488

34

Sulphonamides

D. T. D. Hughes

Introduction

The discovery and early history of the sulphonamides are described in Chapter 1. All compounds of this group are derived from sulphanilamide:

$$H_2N \text{—} \bigcirc \text{—} SO_2NH_2$$

Sulphonamides act as competitive antagonists of p-aminobenzoic acid (PABA) and thus as inhibitors of folic acid synthesis, since PABA is an integral component of the structure of folic acid.

Many compounds have been developed since their introduction. Advances have included increased antibacterial potency, decreased toxicity, and the introduction of sulphonamides with special properties such as high solubility, low solubility and prolonged duration of action. Combinations of sulphonamides with trimethoprim and pyrimethamine are widely used for certain purposes (see Ch. 21).

GENERAL PROPERTIES

Antibacterial activity

Sulphonamides exhibit broad-spectrum activity. Group A streptococci and pneumococci are highly susceptible; staphylococci and *Clostridium perfringens* moderately so, other clostridia are more resistant; and *Enterococcus faecalis* is resistant. Neisseriae are highly susceptible and many enterobacteria, *Haemophilus influenzae* and *Bordetella pertussis* are susceptible. Other organisms commonly susceptible include *Yersinia pestis*, *Actinomyces* spp., *Nocardia* spp., *Bacillus anthracis*, *Corynebacterium diphtheriae*, *Legionella pneumophila*, *Brucella* spp. and several important causes of sexually transmitted diseases (*Chlamydia trachomatis*, *Haemophilus ducreyi* and *Calymmatobacterium granulomatis*). *Pseudomonas aeruginosa* is usually resistant. *Leptospira*, *Treponema* and *Borrelia* spp. are resistant, as are rickettsiae, *Coxiella burnetii* and mycoplasmas. Mycobacteria are resistant, except for modest activity of some long-acting compounds against *Mycobacterium leprae*. The related sulphone, dapsone, exhibits good activity against *M. leprae* (see p. 846) and *p*-aminosalcylic acid, which is structurally similar, was formerly widely used in tuberculosis. In combination with other agents which inhibit folic acid synthesis, sulphonamides show activity against plasmodia and *Toxoplasma gondii*.

In vitro tests are markedly influenced by the composition of the culture medium and the size of the inoculum. Sulphacetamide and sulphadimidine show comparatively low activity. The most active among the shorter acting drugs are sulphadiazine, sulphafurazole and sulphamethoxazole, the sulphonamide combined with trimethoprim in co-trimoxazole (p. 353).

Acquired bacterial resistance

There is complete cross-resistance among sulphonamides. Sulphonamide resistance occurred early and rapidly in gonococci but, with widespread use of penicillin in treatment, they reverted to sulphonamide susceptibility in many, but not all, areas. Resistance is now widespread among meningococci. In the UK, about 15% of strains are resistant. Resistant strains of *Streptococcus pyogenes* (now uncommon) and of pneumococci also appeared early. Resistance in all enterobacteria is now common, and in shigella almost invariable. Resistance is found in 25–40% of strains of *Escherichia coli* and other enterobacteria infecting the urinary tract. Sulphonamides act synergically with polymyxin and with some diaminopyrimidines, notably trimethoprim (co-trimoxazole, co-trimazine, co-trifamole) and pyrimethamine (Fansidar) (see Ch. 21).

Pharmacokinetics

Most sulphonamides are well absorbed after oral administration, reaching a peak concentration in the blood after 2–4 h, which after a dose of 2 g is of the order of 100 mg/l. After absorption, the behaviour of the individual compounds varies widely depending on their degree of plasma binding and their rates of conjugation. The main metabolic pathway is conjugation by acetylation in the liver, although glucuronidation and oxidation also occur. Sulphonamide acetylation shows a bimodal distribution in the population, rapid and slow inactivators corresponding with rapid and slow inactivators of isoniazid. The conjugates are inactive antibacterially and the low solubility of the acetyl conjugates of some of the earlier compounds may give rise to renal toxicity.

A proportion, varying considerably with different compounds, is contained in the red cells, some is free in the plasma and some is bound to plasma albumin. Sulphanilamide is present mainly in its free diffusible form and, of the compounds still in use, sulphadiazine is the least (about 20%) and the long-acting sulphonamides generally the most (75–90%) protein bound. The degree of binding depends on the serum albumin concentration and on the total drug concentration in the blood, the proportion of protein-bound drug decreasing as the total drug concentration rises.

Sulphonamides can be displaced from their protein binding sites by a variety of compounds, the most important clinically being oral anticoagulant drugs. Simultaneous administration of these compounds with sulphonamides potentiates the anticoagulant effect and produces higher concentrations of diffusible sulphonamide. Competition for plasma albumin binding sites causes sulphonamide to displace albumin-bound bilirubin.

Sulphonamides are distributed throughout the body tissues. Protein-bound drug is distributed as protein, so that drug is present in the unbound and antibacterially active form in tissues of low protein content. Access to the cerebrospinal fluid (CSF) is normally limited to the unbound drug, but with increasing capillary permeability and the passage of protein into the CSF in inflammation, protein-bound sulphonamide enters and the total concentration of sulphonamide in the CSF rises. The concentration of short-acting sulphonamides in CSF varies between 30% and 80% of the corresponding plasma concentration. Sulphonamides also enter other body fluids, including the eye. Sulphonamides pass readily through the placenta into the

fetal circulation and may circulate in the fetus for several days or even weeks. They also reach the infant via the breast milk.

Sulphonamides are excreted mainly in the urine, the free drug and its conjugates being frequently excreted at different rates and by different mechanisms. As a result, the peak plasma concentrations of free drug and conjugate may occur at different times and the proportion of free drug to conjugate may be very different in the plasma and urine.

Sulphonamides are partly filtered through the glomeruli and partly secreted by the tubules, where some of the excreted drug is reabsorbed. The extent of these processes differs among the sulphonamides and may differ markedly for the free drug and its conjugates. As a result, the plasma clearance values vary from 10 to >200 ml/min. Substances with high clearances like sulphafurazole are rapidly eliminated from the plasma and achieve high concentrations in the urine. Substances with low clearances are slowly excreted, plasma levels are maintained for long periods, and low concentrations appear in the urine. If renal function is impaired, excretion may be delayed still further and therapeutic levels may persist for considerably longer; if the drugs are given repeatedly, high and possibly toxic levels may develop. Highly protein-bound compounds are in general long-acting, but correspondence between the two properties is far from exact because of differences in the degree of tubular reabsorption, which may be a major factor in maintaining the plasma level.

Less than 1% of the dose of the older sulphonamides is excreted in the bile, but the proportion is greater (2.4–6.3%) for the long-acting compounds.

Toxicity and side-effects

Cyanosis and renal blockage from crystalluria caused by earlier compounds are now rare. Side-effects from the more recent compounds, given with proper attention to dosage, are relatively uncommon, but some are serious. Crystals of less soluble compounds, such as sulphathiazole, sulphadiazine and sulphamerazine or of less soluble conjugates may deposit in the urine and block either the renal tubules or the upper orifice of the ureter. Haematuria is a common early sign. However, renal damage during sulphonamide therapy is often due to a hypersensitivity reaction, rather than to tubular blockage, with changes of tubular necrosis or vasculitis. Renal failure has been recorded in several patients after treatment with sulphamethoxazole, as a component of co-trimoxazole. The risk is diminished by giving alkali and copious fluid and by the use of triple sulphonamide mixtures.

Hypersensitivity reactions usually occur as moderate fever with a rash on about the 9th day of a course of treatment. Repetition after an interval elicits the reaction immediately. Rashes are commonly erythematous, maculopapular or urticarial, and recur if the drug is given again. Well-documented but uncommon is a severe serum-sickness-like reaction with fever, urticarial rash, polyarthropathy and eosinophilia. Eosinophilia may occur without other allergic manifestations.

Stevens–Johnson syndrome is rare, but often serious and sometimes fatal. The relative risks of different sulphonamides in the aetiology of this syndrome cannot be known accurately, but there are many reports of this complication following the use of long-acting sulphonamides. Among 116 cases, 79 were under the age of 15 years and there were 20 deaths. Of the 37 adults, 9 died. The time of onset varied from 2 to 24 days, sometimes as long as 6 weeks after discontinuing the drug. It was estimated that there has been 1 or 2 cases per 10 million doses distributed. Toxic epidermal necrolysis (Lyell's syndrome) has also been recorded after administration of long-acting sulphonamides.

Drug fever without other features may also occur. A special problem of hypersensitivity to the sulphonamide component of co-trimoxazole is its frequency in the treatment of acquired immune deficiency syndrome (AIDS). Sulphonamides are among the compounds reported to provoke systemic lupus erythematosus (LE). The earlier compounds were alleged to be implicated in polyarteritis nodosa. Myocarditis has also been reported a few times. A very intractable type of sensitization may result from local applications manifested at first by a local dermatitis, later by extension to other areas and sometimes by fever, and persistence of the reaction long after the treatment has been stopped.

In patients with inherited glucose-6-phosphate dehydrogenase deficiency, treatment with sulphonamides may cause denatured haemoglobin to accumulate in the red cells in the form of Heinz bodies, and intravascular haemolysis and haemoglobinuria to occur. Haemolysis may also occur as part of a generalized sensitivity reaction, or as a single manifestation not related to glucose-6-phosphate dehydrogenase deficiency. Another effect of sulphonamides on the bone marrow is a depression of leucopoiesis, rarely proceeding to agranulocytosis. Later sulphonamides seem less liable to have this effect than the earlier ones. Aplastic anaemia and thrombocytopenia occur rarely.

Megaloblastic anaemia has been reported, as also has bone marrow necrosis, a rare haematological finding, following the use of sulphasalazine. Methaemoglobinaemia was apparently fairly common after administration of sulphapyridine, but is rarely seen with the compounds in current use.

Liver injury is rare but well documented. Reversible chronic active hepatitis, with LE cells and positive tests for antinuclear factor in which a provocation test caused immediate deterioration of liver function tests has been described. Evidence of hepatotoxicity usually develops within days or weeks of drug administration, but one patient has been reported who developed this complication after 15 years of treatment with sulphasalazine for ulcerative colitis.

Interference with bilirubin transport in the fetus by sulphonamide administered to the mother may increase the free plasma bilirubin level and result in kernicterus. Respiratory disease in the form of a fibrosing alveolitis has been noted a few times after sulphasalazine. The changes develop only after several months of drug administration, may progress to severe disability and even death if the association is unrecognized, but tend to abate if the drug is discontinued.

In a retrospective study, no evidence was found of embryopathy in man. Benign intracranial hypertension has been reported in children receiving sulphamethoxazole.

Interactions

Many interactions between sulphonamides and other drugs arise as a result of competition for plasma albumin binding sites. Those of greatest potential clinical importance are increases in the actions of oral anticoagulants and phenylthiourea (but not biguanide) oral hypoglycaemic agents and increased toxicity of methotrexate. Simultaneous administration of indomethacin or salicylates may increase the peak plasma concentration and decrease the plasma half-life of sulphonamides. The action of phenytoin is enhanced by some sulphonamides (sulphadiazine and sulphamethizole). A serious interaction between cyclosporin A and sulphadimidine in transplant recipients, leading to diminution of levels of the former drug, has been reported.

Clinical use

Absolute indications for their use are very few and have been restricted by the emergence of acquired resistance in many previously susceptible organisms. Their principal value, alone or in combination with trimethoprim, has been for the treatment of urinary tract infection (Ch. 56). Their use in the treatment of respiratory infections is now confined to a few special problems, notably nocardiasis (and also for cerebral nocardiasis) and, in combination with trimethoprim, in the prevention and treatment of *Pneumocystis carinii* pneumonia. Some success has been claimed in the prevention of recurrent otitis media in childhood. The value of sulphonamides in meningococcal infection and in bacterial gut infection is now greatly reduced by bacterial resistance. Poorly absorbed compounds were formerly used as chemoprophylactic agents in abdominal surgery. Sulphonamides are sometimes used for trachoma, for sexually transmitted chlamydial infections and for chancroid. Combined preparations with pyrimethamine are used in the treatment of drug resistant malaria and for toxoplasmosis (Chs 63 and 62).

Toxicity may become manifest when sulphonamides are administered for prolonged periods, as in the use of sulphamethoxazole (as co-trimoxazole) for the control of chronic urinary tract infection and of sulphasalazine for ulcerative colitis or Crohn's disease.

Further information

Editorial 1986 Hypersensitivity and sulphonamides: a clue? *Lancet* ii: 958–959

Foltzer M A, Reese R E 1987 Trimethoprim–sulpha-methoxazole and other sulphonamides. *Medical Clinics of North America* 71: 1177–1194

Vree T B, Hekster Y A 1985 Renal excretion of sulphonamide. *Antibiotics and Chemotherapy* 34: 66–120

Vree T B, Hekster Y A 1987 Clinical pharmacokinetics of sulphonamides and their metabolites. *Antibiotics and Chemotherapy* 37: 1–208

Classification of sulphonamides

The range of compounds available differs from country to country, and we discuss mainly those available in the UK and the USA. Of the older compounds, sulphanilamide, sulphapyridine (but see under sulphasalazine), sulpha-merazine and sulphacetamide (except for local use as eye drops) have now been discarded because of low activity, high toxicity or both. Parenteral preparations of some are available, usually sodium salts which are strongly alkaline and can only be given intravenously or, in the case of sodium sulphadimidine, by deep intramuscular injection. The compounds available may be classified according to their elimination rates and other features into the following groups: general use; high solubility; low solubility; medium- and long-acting; and special purposes.

Sulphonamides for general use

SULPHATHIAZOLE
2-Sulphanilamidothiazole

Although highly active in comparison with other sulphonamides, its use has declined because of a high incidence of side-effects. It is one of the constituents of triple sulphonamide mixtures, of which local preparations are still available.

Preparations

Tablets, 0.5 g (for cream see under Triple sulphonamides, p. 464).
Widely available in multi-ingredient preparations.

SULPHADIAZINE
2-Sulphanilamidopyrimidine

It is a compound of high potency. Adequate blood concentrations are easily achieved and maintained, and protein binding is low (of the order of 20%). It penetrates well into the CSF and for this reason was often the sulphonamide of choice in meningitis, before drug resistance rendered this group ineffective. Its low solubility in urine led to its general replacement by other components, but it remains one of the few sulphonamides available for intravenous injection on the rare occasion when indicated; the solution is highly alkaline and should not be given by any other route.

Preparations and dosage

Preparations: 4 ml ampoules, each containing 1 g for i.v. injection.
Dosage: Adult, 1–1.5 g, 4-hourly for 2 days, then oral. Available in the UK, the USA, Canada, Belgium and Australia. Widely available in multi-ingredient preparations.

SULPHADIMIDINE
2-Sulphanilamido-4,6-methylpyrimidine

It is well absorbed and excreted moderately slowly. Both the drug and its acetyl derivative are highly soluble and toxic effects and sensitivity reactions are rare. Its disadvantages are its relatively low potency and high degree of protein binding (80–90%). Plasma half-life varies from 1.5 to 5.5 h.

Preparations and dosage

Preparations: Tablets, injection.
Dosage: Adults, oral, 2 g initially, then 0.5–1 g every 6–8 h; i.m., i.v., 3 g initially, then 1.5 g every 6 h.
Widely available in multi-ingredient preparations, limited availability in tablet and injectable forms. No longer available in the UK.

TRIPLE SULPHONAMIDES

The mixture originally advocated contained 37% of each of sulphadiazine and sulphathiazole and 26% of sulphamerazine. The main advantage of the mixture is that each drug retains its individual solubility in the urine, and since the dose of each is small so is the risk of renal blockage; indeed, if adequate fluids and alkali are given, it may well be negligible. Other advantages claimed were a reduced risk of sensitization reactions and the maintenance of a steadier blood level.

Several modifications of the original mixture (Sulphatriad) were later introduced, and one of them is still available for local use as an intravaginal cream. For systemic use, they have generally been replaced by other compounds.

Preparations

Proprietary name: Sultrin. Triple sulpha cream containing sulphathiazole 3.42% sulphacetamide 2.86% and sulphabenzamide 3.7% w/v.

Highly soluble compounds

These sulphonamides are highly soluble, even in acid urine. They attain high concentrations in urine and have been used mainly in the treatment of urinary infections.

SULPHAFURAZOLE
3,4-Dimethyl-5-sulphanilamidoisoxazole; sulfisoxazole

The plasma half-life is 6 h and the protein binding is 90%. If given in sufficiently frequent doses to compensate for its rapid excretion, sulphafurazole can be used for treating infection elsewhere as well as in the urinary tract. Improvement occurs in children with chronic granulomatous disease too great to be attributed to the direct antibacterial effect of the drug, and has been explained by its apparent ability to enhance the bactericidal activity of leucocytes from patients with this disorder. It has also been used, in combination with pyrimethamine, as an antimalarial agent.

Preparations and dosage

Preparations: Tablets, suspension, ophthalmic preparations.
Dosage: Adults, oral, 2–4 g initially, then 4–8 g/day in divided doses every 4–6 h.
Limited availability; not available in the UK.

Further information

Pang L W, Limsomwong N, Singharaj P, Canfield C J 1989 Malaria prophylaxis with proguanil and sulfisoxazole in children living in a malaria endemic area. *Bulletin of the World Health Organization* 67: 51–58

SULPHAMETHIZOLE
2-Sulphanilamido-5-methyl-1,3,4-thiodiazole

The plasma half-life is 2.5 h and protein binding 85%. Its rapid rate of excretion makes it unsuitable for use in systemic infection. About 60% is excreted in the urine within 5 h.

Preparations and dosage

Proprietary name: Urolucosil.
Preparation: Tablets.
Dosage: Adult, oral, 1.5–4 g/day in 3–4 divided doses.
Widely available; not available in the UK.

SULPHASOMIDINE
6-Sulphanilamido-2,4-dimethylpyrimidine

A short-acting sulphonamide with a plasma half-life of 6–8 h. Protein binding is about 90%.

Preparations and dosage

Proprietary name: Elkosin.
Preparations: Tablets, topical preparations.
Available in some European countries, Mexico, Japan and South Africa.

Compounds of low solubility

PHTHALYLSULPHATHIAZOLE
2-(*p*-Pthalylsulphanilamido)thiazole; sulfathalidine

It is very little absorbed and owes its activity to the slow liberation of sulphathiazole in the bowel. It was formerly used in the treatment of shigellosis (but resistance to sulphonamides is now widespread) and in bowel preparation before surgery.

Preparations and dosage

Proprietary name: Thalazole.
Dosage: 5 g/day or more in divided doses for shigellosis; 12 g/day in divided doses for bowel preparation.
Widely available in multi-ingredient preparations; limited availability as a single preparation; not available in the UK.

SUCCINYLSULPHATHIAZOLE
2-(*p*-Succinylsulphanilamido)thiazole; sulfasuxidine

Like phthalylsulphathiazole, this compound is hydrolysed to sulphathiazole in the large intestine, and little is absorbed.

Preparations
Very limited availability in multi-ingredient preparations; not available in the UK.

SULPHAGUANIDINE
1-Sulphanilylguanidine

It is less potent and better absorbed than succinylsulphathiazole. There is variable absorption from the gastrointestinal tract, with blood concentrations of 15–40 mg/l after single doses of 1–7 g. Excretion in the urine is rapid.

Preparations
Available in multi-ingredient preparations; not available in the UK.

CALCIUM SULPHALOXATE

Absorption is low, about 5%.

Preparations
Preparation: Tablets.
Very limited availability in continental Europe.

Medium- and long-acting compounds

SULPHAMETHOXAZOLE
5-Methyl-3-sulphanilamidoisoxazole

This is the sulphonamide component of co-trimoxazole, and is a 'medium' long-acting compound, with a plasma half-life of 12 h, requiring twice-daily dosage.

It has a moderate degree of binding to plasma protein (65%). Penetration of extravascular sites, including the CSF, is good, and high concentrations are achieved in urine.

Unwanted effects are in general those common to sulphonamides. In addition to the more serious syndromes described on p. 462, minor gastro-intestinal effects, nausea,

vomiting and diarrhoea are common. Patients with AIDS treated with co-trimoxazole for pneumocystis pneumonia have shown a special propensity to develop hypersensitivity reactions and other unwanted effects. A severe rash occurs in 10–15% of patients, and leucopenia, thrombocytopenia and raised liver enzymes are also common. Sulphamethoxazole may sometimes precipitate haemolysis in patients with glucose-6-phosphate dehydrogenase deficiency.

Clinical uses

In combination with trimethoprim (p. 354), sulphamethoxazole is used extensively throughout the world, principally for urinary tract and respiratory tract infections, including otitis media and sinusitis. Other uses are for typhoid and paratyphoid and for shigellosis and cholera, provided that the organisms responsible are not resistant to the combination. It is used in combination therapy for brucellosis and, when appropriate, for some generalized septicaemias and selected cases of meningitis. It is often appropriately used in bacterial prostatitis and sometimes in gonorrhoea.

Apart from these infections, benefit has been described from its use in Wegener's granulomatosis.

Preparations
Very limited availability as a single agent; available in combination with trimethoprim (p. 354).

Further information

Bowden F J, Harman P J, Lucas C R 1986 Serum trimethoprim and sulphamethoxazole levels in AIDS. *Lancet* i: 853

Lode H, Marget W 1987 Benefits and risks of co-trimoxazole therapy. *Infection* 15 (suppl 5): S222–S266

Siber G R, Gorham C C, Ericson J F, Smith A L 1982 Pharmacokinetics of intravenous trimethoprim–sulphamethoxazole in children and adults with normal and impaired renal function. *Reviews of Infectious Diseases* 4: 566–578

Wormser G P, Keusch G T, Heel R C 1982 Co-trimoxazole (trimethoprim–sulfamethoxazole). An updated review of its antibacterial activity and clinical efficiency. *Drugs* 24: 459–518

SULPHAMETHOXYPYRIDAZINE
3-Sulphanilamido-6-methoxypyridazine

A long-acting compound, with a half-life of 38 h and a high degree of protein binding (96%). It is rapidly absorbed, with a peak plasma concentration at 5 h, and slowly excreted, being detectable up to 7 days after the last dose. Daily dosage of 500 mg maintains adequate levels. It use has been largely discontinued because of frequent adverse effects, but there are reports of benefit in dermatitis herpetiformis. It has been used in combination with trimethoprim.

Preparations

Preparation: Tablets.

Very limited availability in Continental Europe.

SULPHADIMETHOXINE
2,4-Dimethoxy-6-sulphanilamido-1,3-diazine

Properties are similar to those of sulphamethoxypyridazine: rapid absorption, a long half-life (38–40 h), and a high degree of protein binding (98%). Renal clearance is very slow, and daily dosage maintains adequate plasma levels.

Other sulphonamides with a similar pharmacokinetic profile to that of sulphamethoxypyridazine and sulphadimethoxine, and similarly permitting once-daily dosage, are: sulphaphenazole (3-sulphanilamido-2-phenylpyrazole, Orisulf) and sulphamethoxydiazine (2-sulphanilamido-5-methoxypyrimidine, Durenate). Neither of these drugs is now in general use.

Preparations and dosage

Proprietary name: Madribon.

Preparation: Tablets.

Dosage: 1–2 g followed by 0.5–1.0 g/day.

Fairly widely available in Europe, Japan, South America and South Africa.

SULFADOXINE
4-Sulphanilamido-5,6-dimethoxypyrimidine

An ultra-long-acting sulphonamide, with a half-life of about 100–120 h and requiring only weekly administration. It is highly protein bound (93%). Its acetyl metabolite has a similarly long half-life. No longer prescribed alone, it is used in combination with pyrimethamine as the antimalarial agent, Fansidar (p. 349). It is effective in the prophylaxis and treatment of malaria resistant to chloroquine. Its role for prophylaxis has, however, greatly diminished after many reports of Stevens–Johnson syndrome following its use. Some malaria strains are now resistant to the combination.

Preparations and dosage

Proprietary names: Fansidar, Fanasil, in combination with pyrimethamine.

Preparations: Tablets containing 500 mg sulfadoxine and 25 mg pyrimethamine.

Dosage: Adults, Fansidar prophylaxis 1 tablet weekly; treatment 2–3 tablets as a single dose. Children, Fansidar prophylaxis: 9–14 years, $^3/_4$ tablet; 4–8 years, $^1/_2$ tablet; under 4 years, $^1/_4$ tablet. Treatment: 10–14 years, 2 tablets; 7–9 years, 1$^1/_2$ tablet; 4–6 years 1 tablet; under 4 years $^1/_2$ tablet.

Very limited availability as a single agent; widely available in combination with pyrimethamine as Fansidar.

Further information

Hellgren U, Rombo L, Berg B, Carlson J, Wilholm B-E 1987 Adverse reactions to sulfadoxine–pyrimethamine in Swedish travellers. Implications for prophylaxis. *British Medical Journal* 295: 365–366

Selby C D, Ladusans E J, Smith P G 1985 Fatal multisystem toxicity associated with prophylaxis with pyrimethamine and sulfadoxine (Fansidar). *British Medical Journal* 290: 113–114

SULFAMETOPYRAZINE
2-Sulphanilamido-3-methoxypyrazine

A very long-acting compound of which adequate blood levels can be maintained by giving a dose of 2 g once-weekly. The plasma half-life is 60 h and protein binding 60–80%.

It has been successfully used in the single-dose treatment of urinary tract infection.

Preparations and dosage

Proprietary name: Kelfizine W.

Preparation: Tablets.

Dosage: Adults, oral, 2 g once-weekly.

Limited availability; available in the UK.

Sulphonamides for special purposes

SULPHASALAZINE

One of the earliest and most successful sulphonamides to be developed was sulphapyridine (2-sulphanilamidopyridine) which fell into disuse because of unwanted effects such as crystalluria. Later, a number of salicylazosulphonamides, developed because of their increased water solubility, showed anti-inflammatory properties, and one of them, salicylazosulphapyridine, has come into general use for ulcerative colitis under the name of sulphasalazine or Salazopyrine.

The intact compound is absorbed from the upper gastro-intestinal tract, appearing in the blood in 1–2 h, but cleavage of the azo bond is brought about by colonic bacteria and sulphapyridine is found in the blood 3–6 h after administration. The other breakdown product, 5-aminosalicylic acid (mesalazine), is partly excreted in the faeces, but its acetyl derivative appears in faeces and urine.

Antibacterial, anti-inflammatory and immune suppressing effects have all been claimed as the mode of action of sulphasalazine. It has been shown to correct the abnormal sodium and water fluxes across diseased bowel mucosa, and it has been postulated that the action of 5-aminosalicylic acid in inhibiting prostaglandin is responsible for the beneficial effect, the sulphapyridine component acting merely as a carrier enabling the active component to reach the colon. Although disputed, this is supported by the finding that retention enemas of sulphasalazine or 5-aminosalicylic acid, but not of sulphapyridine, caused substantial improvement and that, in order to be effective, metabolites of sulphasalazine must reach the lumen of the diseased distal colon. In a controlled trial, remission rates of 86% followed the administration of 5-aminosalicylic acid suppositories, 79% oral sulphasalazine and 14% oral sulphapyridine.

Unwanted reactions are generally uncommon, but the sulphonamide moiety is sulphapyridine, the earliest of the compounds in general use and one associated with a number of ill-effects. Unwanted effects common to other sulphonamides are shared by sulphasalazine and are described on p. 461. Some unwanted effects are related to high dosage of more than 4 g/day, and can be related to high serum concentration of sulphapyridine itself. The concentrations of other metabolites are not related to toxicity. Many patients with unwanted effects are slow inactivators and their mean serum concentration of sulphapyridine is higher (54 mg/l) than that of the fast inactivators (32 mg/l).

Fibrosing alveolitis has been noted a few times after sulphasalazine. The changes develop only after several months of drug administration, may progress to severe disability and even death if the association is not recognized, but tend to abate if the drug is discontinued.

Another rare complication of sulphasalazine administration is an acquired deficiency of immunoglobulin A (IgA). Sulphasalazine also causes reversible infertility in men. Sperm counts recover 2 months after the drug is discontinued.

Patients receiving sulphasalazine may develop a yellow-orange tinge in the skin and the urine may be similarly discoloured. Extended-use soft contact lenses may also become discoloured.

It is effective in the management and prevention of relapse of acute attacks of ulcerative colitis and is also of benefit in some patients with Crohn's disease, especially those with ileocolonic or colonic disease. This success has led to the extensive use of this agent, often for extremely prolonged periods of time. In such patients receiving the drug uneventfully for a long time unusual reactions may easily be overlooked, especially since very severe multisystem illness is sometimes encountered.

Preparations and dosage

Proprietary name: Salazopyrin.

Preparations: Tablets, enema, suppositories, suspension.

Dosage: Adults, oral, acute attack 1–2 g, 4 times daily until remission occurs, reducing to a maintenance dose of 500 mg, 4 times daily. Children over 2 years, acute attack, 40–60 mg/kg daily reducing to 20–30 mg/kg maintenance dose.

Widely available.

Further information

Azad Khan A K, Piris J, Truelove S C 1977 An experiment to determine the active moiety of sulphasalazine. *Lancet* ii: 892–895

Delamere J P, Farr M, Grindulis K A 1983 Sulphasalazine induced selective IgA deficiency in rheumatoid arthritis. *British Medical Journal* 286: 1547–1548

Levi A J, Fisher A M, Hughes L, Hendry W F 1979 Male infertility due to sulphasalazine. *Lancet* ii: 276–278

Peppercorn M A 1984 Sulphasalazine – pharmacology, clinical use, toxicity and related new drug development. *Annals of Internal Medicine* 101: 377–386

SILVER SULPHADIAZINE CREAM

This preparation has been widely used in the local treatment of burns. In addition to the usual antibacterial range of the sulphonamides, it is active against *Ps. aeruginosa* and against a number of dermatophytic fungi. Its value has often been limited by the emergence of sulphonamide-resistant enterobacteria during its use, although susceptibility can be re-established after its use is discontinued.

Preparations

Proprietary name: Flamazine.

Preparation: Topical cream containing 1% w/w silver sulphadiazine.

Widely available.

MAFENIDE
p-Aminomethylbenzene sulphonamide; mafanil; sulphamylar; sulfamylon

It was formerly used extensively in burns, especially for its action in suppressing *Ps. aeruginosa*. It is rapidly absorbed through burned skin and is unusual in that it is not neutralized by *p*-aminobenzoic acid or by tissue exudates.

Disadvantages of its use were local pain and burning, a variety of allergic reactions including erythema multiforme and its capacity to inhibit carbonic anhydrase, necessitating careful observation to detect the development of metabolic acidosis. Its metabolite, *p*-carboxybenzene sulphonamide, also inhibits carbonic anhydrase but has no antibacterial activity.

Tetracyclines

R. G. Finch

Introduction

A group of natural products derived from Streptomyces *spp. and their semi-synthetic derivatives based on a hydronaphthacene nucleus containing four fused rings:*

The natural products include chlortetracycline, oxytetracycline, tetracycline and demeclocycline (demethylchlortetracycline). Semi-synthetic derivatives include methacycline, doxycycline, minocycline, clomocycline, lymecycline, rolitetracycline and the new investigational class of glycylcyclines. Closely related compounds include β-chelocardin, which lacks the $N(CH_2)_3$ group at position 4 and the thiacyclines which have sulphur in place of carbon at position 6.

Antimicrobial activity

Tetracyclines exhibit broad-spectrum activity which includes bacteria and protozoa. They are active against many common Gram-positive and Gram-negative bacteria, chlamydiae, mycoplasmas, rickettsiae, coxiellae, spirochaetes and some mycobacteria. They are generally inactive against fungi, although minocycline shows some activity against *Candida albicans*. They show useful activity against *Entamoeba histolytica* and plasmodia. In general, they are more active against Gram-positive than against Gram-negative bacteria. The hydrophilic congeners (e.g. tetracycline) are generally less active than the lipophilic congeners (e.g. minocycline and doxycycline). *Staphylo-*

coccus aureus, including β-lactamase-producing strains, is susceptible, while coagulase-negative staphylococci are less predictably so. Most streptococci are susceptible, except *Streptococcus agalactiae* and enterococci. Other susceptible Gram-positive bacilli include *Actinomyces israelii*, *Arachnia propionica*, *Listeria monocytogenes*, most clostridia and *Bacillus anthracis*. Nocardia are much less susceptible, minocycline demonstrating the greatest activity.

Neisseriae and *Moraxella* (*Branhamella*) *catarrhalis*, including β-lactamase-producing strains, are susceptible, although resistant strains of *Neisseria gonorrhoeae* are ubiquitous and those of *Neisseria meningitidis* no longer uncommon. *Haemophilus influenzae* is susceptible, with doxycycline the most active agent, as are legionellae, brucellae and *Francisella tularensis*. Enterobacteria are generally susceptible, minocycline again being the most active compound. None of the tetracyclines has useful activity against *Proteus* spp., *Pseudomonas aeruginosa* or *Providencia* spp., but *Burkholderia* (*Pseudomonas*) *pseudomallei* and *Stenotrophomonas* (*Xanthomonas*) *maltophilia* are usually susceptible. Salmonellae and shigellae are susceptible, although resistant strains are now widespread, as are vibrios, *Campylobacter* spp., *Helicobacter pylori*, *Plesiomonas shigelloides* and *Aeromonas hydrophila*. Most anaerobic bacteria are susceptible, doxycycline and minocycline being most active, but wild strains of bacteroides are now commonly resistant.

Rickettsiae are more susceptible to doxycycline, minocycline and tetracycline than to other tetracyclines. Doxycycline and minocycline are often more active against common anaerobic bacteria in comparison with tetracycline and oxytetracycline. Approximately 90% of isolates are inhibited by 4 mg/l, with the exception of *Prevotella* (*Bacteroides*) *bivius* which appears more resistant. In the case of clostridia, doxycycline is more active than tetracycline; 96% of *Clostridium perfringens* are inhibited by 2 mg/l. Their activity is essentially bacteriostatic.

The glycylcyclines currently under investigation include 9-aminominocycline and 9-amino-6-demethyl-6-deoxytetracycline. They have good activity against tetracycline-resistant strains caused by *tet(A), tet(B), tet(C), tet(D)* and *tet(K)* determinants. They are as active against tetracycline-resistant bacteria as against those which are susceptible. For example, an MIC$_{90}$ of <0.5 mg/l for multiply-resistant *Staph. aureus* (MRSA) and vancomycin-resistant enterococci and an MIC$_{90}$ of <0.5 mg/l for penicillin-resistant pneumococci. Clinical studies are awaited with interest.

Acquired resistance

Resistance (see also Ch. 3) has emerged gradually in an ever-increasing number of species, but it has tended to fluctuate both temporally and geographically. Fortunately, resistance has not yet become a problem in those few diseases for which tetracycline is the drug of choice.

Resistance is primarily transferable and plasmid mediated, and hence is frequently associated with multiple drug resistance. There are three mechanisms of resistance to the tetracyclines. Firstly, there is inhibition of cell membrane transportation, which decreases antibiotic entry and facilitates drug efflux. The efficacy of this mechanism differs between the various tetracyclines and explains why certain resistant strains remain susceptible to minocycline. Ribosomal protection resulting from formation of a cytoplasmic protein is a second mechanism, while chemical modification requiring NADPH and oxygen is a third less common cause of resistance. Resistance is now common among the enterobacteria, staphylococci, streptococci, neisseriae and bacteroides.

Resistance in group A haemolytic streptococci was first noted in 1952 and by 1975 had risen to 36%, but in 1990 had fallen to 6.1% in the UK, although there are wide international differences which reflect the variation in usage of these agents. Likewise, viridans streptococci are commonly resistant to tetracyclines. Resistance is even more common in group B streptococci, in which it is plasmid-mediated. Tetracycline-resistant pneumococci were first reported in 1962 from Australia; resistance rates world-wide have since varied from 3 to 23%, with multiple drug resistance becoming common.

Staph. aureus is commonly, and coagulase-negative staphylococci still more commonly resistant, such strains frequently exhibiting multiple resistance. Doxycycline is active against some tetracycline resistant *Staph. aureus*, including multiply-resistant strains. Occasional β-haemolytic streptococci and pneumococci may be susceptible to minocycline when resistant to other tetracyclines.

Resistance is especially common among Gram-negative bacteria. Enterobacteria commonly show high levels of plasmid-mediated resistance, particularly in hospital-associated isolates. *Enterobacter, Shigella* and *Salmonella*

spp., especially in developing countries, are frequently multiply resistant. Some tetracycline-resistant enterobacteria are susceptible to minocycline. Resistance is not seen to the same extent in *Vibrio cholerae*. Resistant *N. gonorrhoeae* carrying the Tet M determinant on a 25.2 MDa plasmid have been identified on both sides of the Atlantic. Tetracycline-resistant strains of gonococci are now common and are often resistant to more than one agent, including penicillin and spectinomycin. Plasmid-mediated resistance to tetracycline among *N. meningitidis* is also increasing.

A recent (1992) UK survey found 1.4% of *H. influenzae* strains to be resistant. Higher figures, including multiresistant isolates, have been reported from Hong Kong, Spain and Australia. *Haemophilus ducreyii* resistant to the tetracyclines and β-lactams have also been reported.

Clostridia other than *Clostridium tetani* are notable for their frequent resistance. *Bacteroides fragilis* resistance ranges from <5% to >60% according to geographic area.

Pharmacokinetics

Tetracyclines are usually administered by mouth. Tetracycline, oxytetracycline, lymecycline, rolitetracycline, doxycycline and minocycline have all been prepared in forms suitable for injection. Absorption occurs largely in the proximal small bowel, where the proportion of absorbed drug may be diminished by the simultaneous presence of food, milk or divalent cations, especially calcium with which the tetracyclines form non-absorbable chelates. Concomitant administration of iron reduces peak serum concentrations of several tetracyclines, including doxycycline. Cimetidine and presumably other H$_2$ antagonists also impair absorption of the tetracyclines by interfering with their dissolution, which is pH dependent.

The problems of absorption of the earlier compounds have been mitigated to a variable extent in the later tetracyclines. Improved absorption is claimed for lymecycline, demeclocycline, clomocycline and methacycline, but is best established for doxycycline and minocycline, which may be administered with food and for which the proportion of administered dose absorbed is more than 90%.

Peak plasma concentrations are produced 1–3 h after ingestion. The pharmacokinetics of some of the tetracyclines are summarized in Table 35.1. The plasma concentration curve for tetracyclines is plateau shaped, having a small rise and a still slower fall. Factors contributing to this are continued absorption, biliary recirculation and protein binding, estimated to be 20–35% for oxytetracycline and somewhat higher for tetracycline. Demeclocycline, doxycycline and minocycline are all highly protein bound (80–90%). Blood levels achieved after normal oral dosage are of the order of 1.5–4.0 mg/l, with a small cumulative increase with time. Most of the compounds must be given four times daily to maintain therapeutic concentrations in the blood,

Table 35.1   *Selected pharmacokinetic characteristics of some tetracyclines*

Drug	Dose (mg)	C_{max} (mg/l)	$t_{1/2}$ (h)	Recovery from urine (%)	Protein binding (%)
Tetracycline	500	3.5	8	60	24–65
Chlortetracycline	500	2.5	6	18	47
Oxytetracycline	500	1.5	9	20	20–35
Demeclocycline	300	2.0	12	39	90
Methacycline	300	1.5	14	60	80–95
Doxycycline	200	2.5	18	42	90
Minocycline	200	2.5	16	6	75

but the plateau curves of demeclocycline, minocycline and doxycycline enable the first two to be administered twice daily and doxycycline once daily. The serum half-life of tetracycline is 8 h, compared with 16 h for minocycline and 18 h for doxycycline.

Tetracyclines generally penetrate moderately well into body fluids and tissues. This is reflected in their large volumes of distribution, which exceed 100 l except for methacycline (25 l) and doxycycline and minocycline (approximately 50 l). Tissue concentrations are generally related to lipid solubility, which is in the order: minocycline > doxycycline > older tetracyclines. Concentrations of tetracycline in the cerebrospinal fluid (CSF) are about 10–25% of those in the blood. Concentrations achieved in breast milk and in fetal blood are also high, but tetracycline in milk may not be important because it is chelated by calcium and is not absorbed by the infant gut. A unique feature of their behaviour is deposition and persistence in areas where bone and teeth are being laid down.

Tetracyclines are also found in substantial concentrations in the eye.

The mean sputum level, about 20% of that in serum, is high enough to inhibit all (tetracycline susceptible) pneumococci and most strains of *H. influenzae*, the penetration of tetracycline and minocycline being superior to that of doxycycline.

The main excretory route is the kidney, but tetracyclines are also eliminated to a greater or lesser extent in the faeces. Faecal excretion occurs even after parenteral administration as a result of passage of the drug into the bile. The concentrations obtained in bile are 5–25 times those in the blood, doxycycline attaining especially high levels. These concentrations are lowered in the presence of biliary obstruction. The proportion of administered dose found in the urine is, for most tetracyclines, in the range 20–60%, but is less in the case of chlortetracycline and

doxycycline and least for minocycline. Glomerular filtration is the main determinant of renal excretion, with the exception of doxycycline. They are removed slowly by haemodialysis and minimally by peritoneal dialysis.

Toxicity and side-effects

The most important adverse effects of the tetracyclines relate to gastro-intestinal intolerance, which is dose dependent. Allergic reactions are uncommon. Photosensitivity is a class phenomenon and is most marked for demeclocycline. Deposition in developing bones and teeth precludes their use in young children and during late pregnancy. The majority of compounds show anti-anabolic effects and accumulate in renal failure, with the notable exception of doxycycline. Intravenous administration of tetracycline during pregnancy has been complicated by acute fatty liver. Benign intracranial hypertension is another uncommon adverse effect.

Gastro-intestinal disturbances are much more common when larger doses (2 g or more) are given. Nausea and vomiting are presumed to be due to a direct irritant effect of the drug on the gastric mucosa, but diarrhoea is believed to be the result of disturbance of the normal flora. The frequency and nature of superinfection with resistant organisms depends much on local ecology. Pseudomembranous colitis has been associated with tetracyclines, but they do not appear to be a particularly common precursor of that complication. Other organisms which often become dominant in the faecal flora after administration of tetracyclines are *Candida, Proteus* or *Pseudomonas* spp. Some serious consequences of superinfection are well documented, including *Staph. aureus* enterocolitis, which was much more common in hospital when the tetracyclines were more widely prescribed.

Glossitis and pruritus ani, vulvitis and vaginitis are well recognized; less common side-effects include oesophageal ulceration and acute pancreatitis.

Another result of the antibacterial activity of tetracycline is that complex changes occur in the surface lipids of the skin, notably a decrease in fatty acids and reciprocal increase in triglycerides, probably caused by inhibition of extracellular bacterial lipase production by *Propionibacterium acnes*.

In patients with impaired renal function, treatment with tetracyclines may lead to biochemical deterioration and even to irreversible renal failure. The changes are proportional to the degree of renal impairment and to the dose and duration of tetracycline administration. The maximal effects are often reached some days after the course of tetracycline has finished. An exception to this is doxycycline, for which an alternative path of elimination exists.

Tetracyclines are deposited in teeth and bone during the early stages of calcification. This may occur in utero if the mother is treated after the fifth month, when calcification of the deciduous teeth begins, or be produced by treatment of the child after birth. For the effect to be visible as yellow staining a certain total dose must be exceeded. Different tetracyclines produce different degrees and shades of pigmentation—and varying degrees of hypoplasia may accompany it. The main objection to this change is cosmetic, and this applies particularly to the second dentition. The permanent incisors begin to be formed 6 months after birth, the canines and premolars after 2 years and the molars after 3–4 years. Tetracycline treatment is therefore to be avoided in early childhood up to the age of 8 years, except for imperative indications or unless a short course will suffice. Doxycycline, which binds less with calcium than other tetracyclines, is said to cause dental changes less frequently. Direct ill-effects on teeth are compounded by the use in children of liquid preparations containing sucrose, which have been shown to be associated with a much increased risk of dental caries. Paediatric formulations of tetracyclines have been discontinued in Australia and the UK, although dispersible formulations of some tablet forms are available for use in adults and older children.

A number of deaths have been reported in pregnant women given tetracycline in large intravenous doses (>1.0 g/day) usually for the treatment of pyelonephritis. The main lesion found at autopsy was diffuse fatty degeneration of the liver, which may also involve the pancreas, kidneys and brain. In contrast, mild derangements of liver enzyme function are not uncommon with the tetracyclines, as with many other antibiotics, although tetracycline and oxytetracycline have a lower incidence in comparison with other tetracyclines.

A number of infants treated with tetracyclines have developed bulging of the anterior fontanelle; benign intracranial hypertension has also been described in older children and even in adults, with headache, photophobia and papilloedema. Symptoms disappear quickly after the drug is stopped, but papilloedema may persist in some patients for many months or reappear when tetracycline is given again. The mechanism is unknown.

Hypersensitivity rashes, including exfoliation, occasionally occur, but skin reactions after tetracyclines are more often manifestations of photosensitivity. This reaction is especially associated with demeclocycline but may occur after any tetracycline, although it is said to be less common with doxycycline and minocycline. Fixed drug eruptions, onycholysis and nail and thyroid pigmentation have also been reported. Angioedema and anaphylaxis are rare adverse effects. Hypersensitivity reactions to one tetracycline generally infer cross-hypersensitivity to the other agents. Reported inhibitory effects on several human polymorphonuclear leucocyte and lymphocyte functions in vitro have yet to be shown to have any therapeutic significance.

Drug interactions with the tetracyclines include the complexes with divalent and trivalent cations together with chelation by iron-containing preparations. The anticonvulsants carbamazepine, phenytoin and barbiturates decrease the half-life of doxycycline through enzyme induction. The anaesthetic methoxyflurane has been reported to cause nephrotoxicity when co-administered with tetracyclines. The efficiency of the oral contraceptive pill is reduced with the co-administration of tetracyclines, as with many other broad-spectrum antibiotics.

Clinical use

Despite their wide range of activity, the clinical use of tetracyclines has significantly declined with the increase of drug resistance among common bacterial pathogens and the availability of more active and better tolerated agents. They remain popular in developing countries, largely on account of their relative cheapness. They continue to be the drugs of choice for the treatment of infections due to chlamydiae (pp. 687, 820), mycoplasmas and rickettsiae (p. 889), although alternatives exist. They may provide adjunctive care in the management of cholera (p. 711), where they both abbreviate the duration of the illness and speed up the elimination of *V. cholerae* from the bowel, and parasitic diseases such as amoebiasis. Their activity against malaria has unexpectedly become important with the rapid spread of resistance to first-line drugs. They have recently received widespread use as part of a multidrug regimen for the management of *Helicobacter pylori* associated gastritis and peptic ulcer disease.

They also provide alternative therapy for a range of diseases where there is intolerance to first-line agents, such as syphilis, Lyme disease (p. 888), leptospirosis (p. 887), actinomycosis (p. 739) and anthrax (p. 737). Much of their prescription is for infections of the respiratory tract, but variable susceptibility of haemolytic streptococci and pneumococci has led to a reduction in such use, including that for infective exacerbations of chronic bronchitis (p. 691). They remain active against *Chlamydia* spp., *Coxiella burnetii* (p. 687) and *Mycoplasma pneumoniae*, and therefore provide a valuable alternative to erythromycin in the treatment of atypical pneumonias due to those organisms. Resistance among haemolytic streptococci has limited their value in skin sepsis such as impetigo and erysipelas, but they continue to play a valuable role in the long-term management of acne (p. 740). They have also found some use in the treatment of rosacea.

They continue to be recommended for a variety of sexually transmitted diseases. In particular, their activity against chlamydiae has made them agents of choice for the treatment of infections such as nongonococcal urethritis and cervicitis and lymphogranuloma venereum (p. 824). They offer alternative treatment for syphilis and gonorrhoea, although other agents are preferred and the increasing incidence of tetracycline-resistant *N. gonorrhoeae* is of concern, particularly since this is frequently linked to resistance to other antibiotics (Ch. 3). Tetracyclines also continue to be popular in the treatment of pelvic inflammatory disease (p. 821) owing to their broad spectrum of activity against sexually transmitted pathogens and anaerobic bacteria which predominate in these infections. Tetracycline is the drug of choice for granuloma inguinale, but increasing resistance among *H. ducreyi* has limited its use in chancroid (p. 824).

Their value in anaerobic infections is now limited by widespread drug resistance, but actinomycosis can still be treated effectively, as can its aerobic counterpart, nocardiosis.

Resistance has substantially limited their value in treating infections due to *Shigella* and *Salmonella* spp. They are also useful in other gastro-intestinal diseases such as Whipple's disease (p. 714), tropical sprue and the blind loop syndrome. Doxycycline has proved effective in the prevention and treatment of travellers' diarrhoea.

They continue to prove of value in tularaemia (p. 884) and the rickettsial infections such as the various types of typhus, rickettsialpox and Rocky Mountain spotted fever (p. 889). Borreliosis in the form of relapsing fever responds to single dose treatment with tetracycline (p. 889) or doxycycline which provide the treatment of choice. Melioidosis is now less commonly treated with tetracyclines. Trachoma has been managed with topical tetracycline ointment, although oral treatment with doxycycline has proved most effective. The spirochaetal infections, yaws and relapsing fever, respond successfully as does acute Lyme borreliosis, although the late manifestations are less satisfactorily managed. Brucellosis in its acute form responds to tetracycline (p. 883), although a combination of doxycycline and another agent such as streptomycin or rifampicin is preferred, especially when treating more prolonged infections.

Selected mycobacterial diseases such as *Mycobacterium marinum* infection also respond. Doxycycline contributes useful activity to a multidrug regimen against infection with *M. fortuitum* and *M. chelonei*.

Further information

Acar J F, Goldstein F W, Kitzis M D, Eyquem M T 1981 Resistance pattern of anaerobic bacteria isolated in a general hospital during a two-year period. *Journal of Antimicrobial Chemotherapy* 8 (suppl D): 9–16

Backmann A, Danielsson D, Olcen P 1993 Plasmid carriage and antibiotic susceptibility of *Neisseria meningitidis* strains isolated in Sweden 1981–1990. *European Journal of Clinical Microbiology and Infectious Diseases* 12: 683–689

Chopra I, Hawkey P M, Hinton M 1992 Tetracyclines, molecular and clinical aspects. *Journal of Antimicrobial Chemotherapy* 29: 245–277

Collignon P J, Bell J M, MacInnes S J, Gilbert G L, Tookey M, Australian Group for Antimicrobial Resistance 1992 A national collaborative study of resistance to antimicrobial agents in *Haemophilus influenzae* in Australian hospitals. *Journal of Antimicrobial Chemotherapy* 30: 153–164

Fekete T, Woodwell J, Cundy K R 1991 Susceptibility of *Neisseria gonorrhoeae* to cefpodoxime: determination of MICs and disk diffusion zone diameters. *Antimicrobial Agents and Chemotherapy* 35: 497–499

Pedrazzoli J, Magalhaes A F, Ferraz J G, Trevisan M, De Nucci G 1994 Triple therapy with sucralfate is not effective in eradicating *Helicobacter pylori* and does not reduce duodenal ulcer relapse rates. *American Journal of Gastroenterology* 89: 1501–1504

Potgieter E, Carmichael M, Koornof H J, Chalkley L J 1992 In vitro antimicrobial susceptibility of viridans streptococci isolated from blood cultures. *European Journal of Clinical Microbiology and Infectious Diseases* 11: 543–546

Schwarz S, Cardoso M, Wegener H C 1992 Nucleotide sequence and phylogeny of the *tet(L)* tetracycline resistance determinant encoded by plasmid pSTE1 from *Staphylococcus hyicus*. *Antimicrobial Agents and Chemotherapy* 36: 580–588

Speer B S, Shoemaker N B, Salyers A A 1992 Bacterial resistance to tetracycline: mechanisms, transfer, and clinical significance. *Clinical Microbiology Reviews* 5: 387–399

Tally P P, Cuchural G J, Jacobus N V et al 1985 Nationwide study of the susceptibility of the *Bacteroides fragilis* in the United States. *Antimicrobial Agents and Chemotherapy* 28: 675–677

Testa R T, Petersen P J, Jacobus N V, Sum P E, Lee V J, Tally F P 1993 In vitro and in vivo antibacterial activities of the glycylcyclines, a new class of semisynthetic tetracyclines. *Antimicrobial Agents and Chemotherapy* 37: 2270–2277

Welsh L E, Gaydos C A, Quinn T C 1992 In vitro evaluation of activities of azithromycin, erythromycin and tetracycline against *Chlamydia trachomatis* and *Chlamydia pneumoniae*. *Antimicrobial Agents and Chemotherapy* 36: 291–294

Winstanley T G, Wilcox M H, Spencer R C 1991 Combined resistance to erythromycin and tetracycline in streptococci. *Journal of Antimicrobial Chemotherapy* 28: 154–156

Wright A L, Colver G B 1988 Tetracyclines – how safe are they? *Clinical and Experimental Dermatology* 13: 57–61

CHLORTETRACYCLINE

A fermentation product of certain strains of *Streptomyces aureofaciens.*

Antimicrobial activity

Its activity is slightly less than that of tetracycline against many bacteria, with the exception of Gram-positive organisms. Its spectrum and resistance patterns are typical of the group. Its activity against common pathogenic bacteria is shown in Table 35.2.

Pharmacokinetics

Chlortetracycline is relatively poorly absorbed compared with other tetracyclines. The half-life ranges from 2.3 to 5.6 h. It is 47–65% protein bound. It undergoes rapid metabolism and is largely eliminated by biliary excretion, with only a small proportion eliminated via the kidney.

Despite this, it is not recommended for patients in renal failure, since accumulation occurs as a consequence of the half-life increase to approximately 7–11 h.

Toxicity and side-effects

Side-effects are typical of the group (p. 471). There are no particular issues of note, although contact hypersensitivity has been reported with topical application to abraded skin and varicose ulcers.

Clinical use

Its uses are those common to the group (p. 472). It has no particular advantages. It has been widely used in animal husbandry as a growth promoter.

It has been used topically in the management of recurrent aphthous ulcers of the mouth, but experience is limited and the mechanism of action is unknown.

Preparations and dosage

Proprietary name: Aureomycin.

Preparations: Topical, ophthalmic, capsules.

Dosage: Adults, oral, 250–500 mg, four times daily.

Widely available; oral preparation not available in the UK.

Table 35.2 *Activity of tetracyclines against common pathogenic bacteria: MIC (mg/l)*

	Chlortetra-cycline	Demeclo-cycline	Doxy-cycline	Metha-cycline	Mino-cycline	Oxytetra-cycline	Tetra-cycline
Staph. aureus	0.5–4	1–4	0.5–2	0.5–2	0.5–1	2–8	2–4
Str. pyogenes	0.1–1	0.25–1	0.1–1	0.1–0.5	0.1–0.5	0.25–1	0.25–1
Str. pneumoniae	0.1–1	0.1–0.55	0.1–0.25	0.06–0.1	0.06–0.25	0.1–0.25	0.25–1
Ent. faecalis	4–128	2–128	2–64	4–R	2–128	8–128	8–R
N. gonorrhoeae	0.25–0.5	0.5–1	0.1–0.5	0.1–0.5	0.25–0.5	1–2	0.5–1
N. meningitidis			1–2		1–2		0.5–1
H. influenzae	1–2	2–4	1–2	1–2	1–4	4–16	0.25–4
Esch. coli	8–16	4–16	2–16	4–16	4–8	2–16	2–16
K. pneumoniae	8–128	8–128	8–64	8–128	4–32	16–128	4–64
Pr. mirabilis	128–R	32–64	64–R	64–R	64–R	128–R	32–R
Pr. vulgaris/Providencia spp.							4–R
Enterobacter spp.	8–R	8–R	16–R	8–R	8–R	8–R	4–R
Salmonella spp.							1–2
Shigella spp.			4–128		2–128		1–2
Ser. marcescens	128–R	128–R	64	R	32	R	16–4
Ps. aeruginosa	64–R	32–128	32–128	64–128	128–256	64–128	32–R
B. fragilis			0.1–8		0.1–16	0.5–64	0.5–2

R, resistant.

CLOMOCYCLINE

Semi-synthetic hydroxymethyl chlortetracycline; supplied as the sodium salt.

Its activity and spectrum are typical of the group of which, with chlortetracycline, it is the most active, especially against staphylococci and pneumococci.

It is highly water soluble and is, therefore, readily absorbed from the gastro-intestinal tract, especially in the presence of food. Peak plasma concentrations of 2–5 mg/l are achieved at approximately 3 h. The plasma elimination half-life is about 6 h. Approximately 30% of the dose is excreted unchanged in the urine.

Its adverse effects and clinical uses are those common to the group, although its improved absorption is associated with relatively few gastro-intestinal side-effects.

It formerly found some use in the treatment of dermatological conditions, and its improved gastro-intestinal tolerance led to its use in the treatment of acne.

> **Preparations**
> No longer marketed.

DEMECLOCYCLINE

A fermentation product of a mutant strain of *Streptomyces aureofaciens*. It differs from chlortetracycline in lacking the methyl group at position 6.

Antimicrobial activity

Its activity and spectrum are typical of the group (p. 469). Its activity is comparable with that of tetracycline, although occasional strains are more susceptible, including viridans streptococci, *N. gonorrhoeae* and *H. influenzae*. It is the most active tetracycline against *Brucella* spp. Its activity against common pathogenic bacteria is shown in Table 35.2. It shares resistance mechanisms and prevalence with the rest of the group.

Pharmacokinetics

It is promptly yet incompletely absorbed by mouth, giving mean peak plasma levels after a single dose at 3–6 h which are slightly higher than those produced by oxytetracycline and chlortetracycline, but less than those achieved by tetracycline. However, with repeat dosing, steady-state concentrations exceed those for tetracycline. Simultaneous administration of antacids markedly depresses blood levels. The volume of distribution is about 1–7 l/kg. The plasma elimination half-life is approximately 12 h. It is 40–90% protein bound.

It is widely distributed, achieving concentrations in pleural exudates similar to those of blood. CSF penetration is poor, especially in the absence of inflammation. Biliary concentrations are 20–30 times higher than those of plasma, and 40–50% of the drug can be recovered from faeces. The other route of elimination is via glomerular filtration without reabsorption and accumulation occurs in renal failure.

Toxicity and side-effects

Untoward reactions, notably gastro-intestinal intolerance, are generally those typical of the group (p. 471) and occur to a similar degree to tetracycline. Occasional patients develop transient steatorrhoea.

Of particular note is the occurrence of nephrogenic diabetes insipidus. This effect is dose dependent and occurs with daily doses in excess of 1200 mg. The polyuria which develops is vasopressin resistant. The drug inhibits activation of adenylate cyclase and protein kinase which are both important in the interaction of antidiuretic hormone (ADH) with receptors within the renal tubule, thus decreasing the effect of ADH on the kidney. As a result, it has found a place in the treatment of inappropriate ADH secretion.

Renal failure may occur, particularly if prescribed for those with advanced liver cirrhosis. The mechanism is uncertain but may in part be related to the antianabolic effect of the tetracyclines as well as a direct toxic effect.

Photosensitivity may be severe and accompanied by vesiculation, oedema and onycholysis. It is largely restricted to exposed skin and therefore it has been suggested that patients should avoid prolonged exposure to sunlight.

Clinical use

Its uses are those common to the group (p. 472) and it has not found any specific therapeutic niches. However, it has been extensively used in the management of the syndrome of inappropriate ADH secretion in a dose of at least 1200 mg/day; therapeutic response may take several days, but has been shown to be superior to that of lithium. It has also found occasional use in patients with water retention as a result of congestive cardiac failure and in those with alcoholic cirrhosis and water and electrolyte retention.

Further information

de Troyer A 1977 Demeclocycline treatment for syndrome of inappropriate antidiuretic hormone secretion. *Journal of the American Medical Association* 237: 2723–2726

Geheb M, Cox M 1980 Renal effects of demeclocycline. *Journal of the American Medical Association* 243: 2519–2520

Miller P D, Linas S L, Schrier R W 1980 Plasma demeclocycline levels and nephrotoxicity. Correlation in hyponatremic cirrhotic patients. *Journal of the American Medical Association* 243: 2513–2515

DOXYCYCLINE

Semi-synthetic 6-deoxy-5β-hydroxytetracycline supplied as the hydrochloride.

Antimicrobial activity

Its activity and spectrum are typical of the group (Table 35.2).

It is active against a proportion of tetracycline-resistant *Staph. aureus*. It is more active than other tetracyclines against *Streptococcus pyogenes*, enterococci and *Nocardia* spp.

M. catarrhalis, regardless of β-lactamase production, is inhibited by 0.5 mg/l. *Legionella pneumophila* is susceptible. The majority of strains of *Ureaplasma urealyticum* are inhibited by 0.5 mg/l.

Acquired resistance

It shares the resistance mechanisms and generally the prevalence common to the group (p. 470), but it has been suggested that it may be associated with less increase in resistance among faecal *Esch. coli* during treatment.

Pharmacokinetics

It is rapidly absorbed from the upper gastro-intestinal tract, where 80–95% of the drug is taken up. Following a single oral 100–200 mg dose, mean peak plasma concentrations range from 1.7 to 5.7 mg/l and occur 2–3.5 h after administration. Absorption appears to be linearly related to the administered dose. Food, especially dairy products, reduces peak serum concentrations by 20%. Alcohol also delays absorption. As with other tetracyclines, divalent and trivalent cations, as in antacids and ferrous sulphate, form chelates which reduce absorption. The volume of distribution at steady state varies between 50 and 135 l. Protein binding ranges from 80 to 90%: the highest degree of binding among the tetracyclines.

The greater lipophilicity of doxycycline is responsible for its widespread tissue distribution where concentrations are approximately twice those in plasma – in liver, biliary system, kidneys and the digestive tract. The volume of distribution is 0.9–1.18 l/kg. Within the respiratory tract, doxycycline achieves concentrations of 2.3–6.7 mg/kg in tonsils and 2.3–7.5 mg/kg in maxillary sinus mucosa. In bronchial secretions, approximately 20% of plasma concentrations is achieved, increasing to about 25–35% in the presence of pleurisy. Gallbladder concentrations are approximately 75%, and those of plasma and prostate concentrations are 60–100%. It penetrates well into the aqueous humour. CSF concentrations range from 11 to 56% of plasma levels and are not affected by inflammation. In the elderly, tissue concentrations are 50–100% higher than in young adults. The half-life remains unaltered and one explanation is reduced faecal elimination.

Doxycycline is largely excreted unchanged. Approximately 35% is eliminated through the kidneys and the remainder through the digestive tract. Renal clearance ranges from 1.8 to 2.1 l/h, and is largely via glomerular filtration, with approximately 70% tubular reabsorption. Alkalinization enhances renal clearance. Faecal elimination partly reflects biliary excretion but also includes diffusion across the intestinal wall. Provided the drug is not chelated, reabsorption occurs with enterohepatic recycling. The elimination half-life is long (15–25 h).

The half-life and area under the curve (AUC) are little altered in renal insufficiency, with no evidence of accumulation after repeat dosing, even in anuric patients, evidently as a result of increased clearance through the liver or gastro-intestinal tract, since biliary and faecal concentrations increase in renal failure. Although the plasma elimination half-life is unchanged, the drug appears to accumulate in tissues with increasing renal failure, and it has been suggested that less drug is bound to plasma protein and red cells through competition with other metabolites, which in turn increases hepatic elimination. Neither haemodialysis nor peritoneal dialysis modify doxycycline pharmacokinetics. Clearance is decreased by approximately half in patients with type IIa and type IV hyperlipidaemia.

The plasma elimination half-life is shortened by a variety of antiepileptic agents including phenytoin, barbiturates and carbamazepine, presumably as a result of liver enzyme induction, although there is also evidence for some interference with the protein binding of doxycycline.

Toxicity and side-effects

Untoward reactions are generally those typical of the group (p. 471) but gastro-intestinal side-effects are less common than with other tetracyclines, as a result of the lower total dosage and the ability to administer the drug with meals. As with other tetracyclines, oesophageal ulceration as a result of capsule impaction has been reported. Dental and bone deposition appear to be less common with doxycycline than other tetracycline derivatives. Other adverse phenomena include occasional vestibular toxicity.

Hypersensitivity reactions include photosensitivity and eosinophilia, but rarely anaphylaxis. In common with demeclocycline and chlortetracycline it may be a more powerful sensitizer than other tetracyclines. It is contraindicated in patients with acute porphyria, since it has been demonstrated to be porphyrinogenic in animals.

Clinical use

Its uses are generally those common to the group (p. 472), but advantage has been taken of its once-daily administration and safety in renal insufficiency.

It has been most widely used for the treatment of respiratory infections but shares in increasing tetracycline resistance among pneumococci and *H. influenzae* (p. 36). It provides a valuable alternative to erythromycin, with or without rifampicin, in legionnaires' disease (p. 686).

Louse-borne typhus is cured with a single adult dose of 100–200 mg; scrub typhus responds promptly, even to a single dose (p. 889). Mediterranean spotted fever has responded, and it has been used prophylactically in some rickettsial infections and in leptospirosis (p. 887).

It has proved an effective alternative to benzylpenicillin in leptospirosis and tick-borne relapsing fever (p. 889), and cutaneous anthrax. It is currently recommended for the treatment of acute brucellosis, either alone or in combination with other agents (p. 883). Other uses include adult chlamydial ophthalmia and for the treatment of infection with *Norcardia brasiliensis*.

It is as effective as other tetracyclines in the treatment of genital infections, but is subject to the same limitations resulting from increased resistance. It is recommended by the Centers for Disease Control for the initial treatment of pelvic inflammatory disease (p. 821) in a regimen combined with cefoxitin. Its efficacy in genital tract infections has led to its use in the treatment of infertility; 4 weeks' treatment has been associated with an increase in successful pregnancies compared with controls within a 3-year follow-up period. Reference is also made to its use in Q fever and gut infections (pp. 687, 709).

Further information

Bocker R, Muhlberg W, Platt D et al 1986 Serum level, half-life and apparent volume of distribution of doxycycline in geriatric patients. *European Journal of Clinical Pharmacology* 30: 105–108

Carta F, Zanetti S, Pinna A, Sotgiu M, Fadda G 1994 The treatment and follow-up of adult chlamydial ophthalmia. *British Journal of Ophthalmology* 78: 206–208

Centers for Disease Control & Prevention 1993 Sexually transmitted diseases treatment guidelines. *Mortality & Morbidity Weekly Report* 42: 75–81

Cunha B A, Sibley C M, Ristuccia A M 1982 Review. Doxycycline. *Therapeutic Drug Monitoring* 11: 5–135

Forsgren A, Walder M 1982 *Haemophilus influenzae*, pneumococci, group A streptococci and *Staphylococcus aureus*: sensitivity of outpatient strains to commonly prescribed antibiotics. *Scandinavian Journal of Infectious Diseases* 14: 39–43

Houin G, Brunner F, Nebout Th et al 1983 The effects of chronic renal insufficiency on the pharmacokinetics of doxycycline in man. *British Journal of Clinical Pharmacology* 16: 245–252

Robbins M, Marais R, Felmingham D, Ridgway G L 1987 The in-vitro activity of doxycycline and minocycline against anaerobic bacteria. *Journal of Antimicrobial Chemotherapy* 20: 379–382

Whelton A, Blanco L J, Carter G G 1980 Therapeutic implication of doxycycline and cephalothin concentrations in the female genital tract. *Obstetrics and Gynecology* 55: 28–32

Wisseman C L, Ordonez S V 1986 Actions of antibiotics on *Rickettsia rickettsii. Journal of Infectious Diseases* 153: 626–628

Wojcicki J, Kalinowski W, Gawronska-Szlarz B 1985 Comparative pharmacokinetics of doxycycline and oxytetracycline in patients with hyperlipidemia. *Arzneimittelforschung* 35: 991–993

LYMECYCLINE

Tetracycline-L-methylene lysine, a water-soluble combination of tetracycline, lysine and formaldehyde.

Its antimicrobial activity is that of the tetracycline content. It is lipophilic and rapidly absorbed from the gastro-intestinal tract and widely distributed. In maxillary sinus tissue concentrations around 1 mg/kg have been found some 3 h after administration of a conventional dose. Its C_{max} is 2 h and half-life is 7–14 h. Approximately 30% of an orally administered dose is excreted as active drug in the urine, where it achieves concentrations of 300 mg/l.

Its untoward effects and clinical uses are those of tetracycline (p. 482), although it is said to be better tolerated.

Preparations and dosage

Proprietary name: Tetralysal 300.

Preparation: Capsules.

Dosage: Adults, oral, 408 mg every 12 h.

Available in the UK and continental Europe.

Further information

Bergholm A M 1987 Studies of the penetration of lymecycline into paranasal sinus in man. *Acta Oto-Rhino-Laryngologia Belgica* 37: 649–653

Forsberg G S, Hermansson J 1984 Comparative bioavailability of tetracycline and lymecycline. *British Journal of Pharmacology* 18: 529–533

METHACYCLINE

Semi-synthetic methylene oxytetracycline supplied as the hydrochloride.

Its activity and spectrum are typical of the group (p. 469). Its activity against common pathogenic bacteria is shown in Table 35.2.

It is absorbed by mouth, mean peak plasma concentrations around 2–6 mg/l being found about 4 h after a 300 mg dose. Food or milk reduces uptake by half. Protein binding is 80–90%. The plasma elimination half-life varies between 7 and 15 h and increases to 44 h in those with severe renal impairment.

It is widely distributed, producing lung concentrations similar to, or greater than, the simultaneous plasma concentration. About a third is excreted in the urine.

Untoward reactions are generally those common to the group (p. 471), although gastro-intestinal intolerance is reported to be less frequent than with other tetracyclines, largely because of the lower dosages used. There are no unique adverse drug reactions, although skin and conjunctival pigmentation have been reported.

Its clinical uses are those common to the group (p. 472).

Preparations and dosage

Dosage: Adults, oral, 600 mg/day in 2–4 divided doses.

Widely available in continental Europe.

Further information

Wright A L, Colver G B 1988 Tetracyclines – how safe are they? *Clinical and Experimental Dermatology* 13: 57–61

MINOCYCLINE

Semi-synthetic 6-demethyl-6-deoxy-7-dimethylamino tetracycline supplied as the hydrochloride.

Antimicrobial activity

It exhibits the broad-spectrum activity typical of the group, but it is more active than other tetracyclines against *Staph. aureus*, including tetracycline-resistant strains. It is also the most active tetracycline against β-haemolytic streptococci and is active against tetracycline-resistant pneumococci.

It is also active against a number of enterobacteria resistant to other tetracyclines, possibly as a result of differences in cell wall transportation. Some strains of *H. influenzae* resistant to other tetracyclines are also susceptible. *Sten. maltophilia* is susceptible, as are most strains of *Acinetobacter* spp. and *L. pneumophila.*

It is notable for its activity against *Bacteroides* and *Fusobacterium* spp., and is more active than other tetracyclines against *C. trachomatis*, brucellae and nocardiae. It inhibits *M. tuberculosis*, *M. bovis*, *M. kansasii* and *M. intracellulare* at 5–6 mg/l. *Cand. albicans* and *Cand. tropicalis* are also slightly susceptible.

Acquired resistance

It shares in general the resistance mechanisms and prevalence common to the group (p. 470), but is active against some strains resistant to earlier tetracyclines.

Clinical failure in the treatment of non-gonococcal urethritis caused by minocycline-resistant *U. urealyticum* has been reported from Brazil, where approximately one-third of isolates are resistant in vitro.

Pharmacokinetics

Following oral administration, 95–100% is absorbed from the stomach and upper small bowel. Peak plasma concentrations at approximately 2 h are 2–4 mg/l after 150 and 300 mg, respectively. The volume of distribution varies between 80 and 115 l. Food does not significantly affect absorption, which is depressed by co-administration with milk. It is chelated by heavy metals and suffers the effects of antacids and ferrous sulphate common to tetracyclines. Following intravenous infusion of 200 mg, the mean plasma concentration at 1 h was 3.5 mg/l. On a regimen of 100 mg 12-hourly, steady-state concentrations ranged between 2.3 and 3.5 mg/l. The plasma elimination half-life is 12–24 h and protein binding ranged from 75 to 85%.

Its high lipophilicity provides wide distribution and tissue concentrations which often exceed those of the plasma. The tissue:plasma ratio in maxillary sinus and tonsillar tissue is 1.6; that in lung is 3–4. Sputum concentrations may reach 37–60% of simultaneous plasma levels. In bile, liver and gallbladder the ratios are 38, 12 and 6.5, respectively.

Prostatic and seminal fluid concentrations range from 40 to 100% of those of serum. CSF penetration is poor, especially in the non-inflamed state. Concentrations in tears and saliva are high, and may explain its beneficial effect in the treatment of meningococcal carriage.

Only 4–9% of orally or parenterally administered drug is excreted in the urine, and in renal failure elimination is little affected. Neither haemodialysis nor peritoneal dialysis affect drug elimination. Faecal excretion is relatively low and evidence for enterohepatic recirculation remains uncertain. Biotransformation to three microbiologically inactive metabolites occurs in the liver; the most abundant is 9-hydroxyminocycline. Despite high hepatic excretion, dose accumulation does not occur in liver disease, such as cirrhosis. Type IIa and type IV hyperlipidaemic patients show a decreased minocycline clearance of 50%, suggesting that dose modification may be necessary.

Toxicity and side-effects

It shares the untoward reactions common to the group (p. 471), with gastro-intestinal side-effects being the most common adverse effect and more prevalent in females. Diarrhoea is less common than with other tetracyclines, presumably as a result of its lower faecal concentrations. Other side-effects include hypersensitivity reactions, including rashes and interstitial nephritis and pulmonary eosinophilia.

Staining of the permanent dentition is common to all tetracyclines; a side-effect which appears to be unique to minocycline is that of tissue discoloration and skin pigmentation. Tissues which have become pigmented include the skin, skull and other bones and the thyroid gland which at autopsy appears blackened. The pigmentation tends to resolve slowly with discontinuation of the drug and is more related to the length of therapy. Three types of pigmentation have been identified: a brown macular discoloration ('muddy skin syndrome'), which occurs in sun-exposed parts and is histologically associated with melanin deposition; blue-black macular pigmentation occurring within inflamed areas and scars associated with haemosiderin deposition; and circumscribed macular blue-grey pigmented areas occurring in normal skin, sun-exposed and unexposed, which appears to be linked to a breakdown product of minocycline.

Central nervous system toxicity has been prominent, notably benign intracranial hypertension which resolves on discontinuation of the drug and, more commonly, dizziness, ataxia, vertigo, tinnitus, nausea and vomiting, which appear to be more frequent in women. These primarily vestibular side-effects have ranged in frequency from 4.5 to 86%. They partly coincide with plasma concentration peaks, but their exact pathogenesis has yet to be determined.

Clinical use

Its uses are those common to the group (p. 472) and there appear to be few situations in which minocycline has a unique therapeutic advantage. Its use has been tempered by the high incidence of vestibular side-effects. It has been promoted for the chemoprophylaxis of meningococcal infection (p. 748). Resistance does not appear to emerge with such short-term use.

Although used in the long-term management of acne, the potential for skin pigmentation must be considered. Because of its high tissue concentrations, it may occasionally provide a useful alternative to other agents for the treatment of chronic prostatitis. Reference is also made to its use in chlamydial infections (p. 773).

Preparations and dosage

Proprietary name: Minocin MR.

Preparations: Tablets, capsules.

Dosage: Adults, oral, 100 mg twice daily; acne, 100 mg/day as a single or two divided doses.

Widely available.

Further information

Basler R S W 1985 Minocycline-related hyperpigmentation. *Archives of Dermatology* 121: 606–608

Dykhuizen R S, Zaidi A M, Godden D J, Jegarajah S, Legge J S 1995 Minocycline and pulmonary eosinophilia. *British Medical Journal* 310: 1520–1521

Freeman C D, Nightingale C H, Quintiliani R 1994 Minocycline: old and new therapeutic uses. *International Journal of Antimicrobial Agents* 4: 325–335

Jonar A, Cunha B A 1982 Minocycline. *Therapeutic Drug Monitoring* 4: 137–145

Magalhaes M, Veras A 1984 Minocycline resistance among clinical isolates of *Ureaplasma urealyticum*. *Journal of Infectious Diseases* 149: 117

Nelis H J C F, De Leenheer A P 1982 Metabolism of minocycline in humans. *Drug Metabolism and Disposition* 10: 142–146

Noble J G, Christmas T J, Chapple C et al 1989 The black thyroid: an unusual finding during neck exploration. *Postgraduate Medical Journal* 64: 34–35

Okada N, Moriya K, Nishida K et al 1989 Skin pigmentation associated with minocycline therapy. *British Journal of Dermatology* 121: 247–257

Pearson M G, Littlewoods S M, Bowden A N 1981 Tetracycline and benign intracranial hypertension. *British Medical Journal* 282: 568–569

Poliak S C, D'Giovanna J J, Gross E G et al 1985 Minocycline-associated tooth discoloration in young adults. *Journal of the American Medical Association* 254: 2930–2932

Ridgway H A, Sonnex T S, Kennedy C T et al 1982 Hyperpigmentation associated with oral minocycline. *British Journal of Dermatology* 107: 95–102

Saivin S, Houin G 1988 Clinical pharmacokinetics of doxycycline and minocycline. *Clinical Pharmacokinetics* 15: 355–366

Simon C 1981 Penetration of various antibiotics into sputum. In: Van Furth R (ed) Developments in antibiotic treatment of respiratory infections. Martinus Njhoff, The Hague, p 86–97

Tsukamura M 1980 In vitro antimycobacterial activity of minocycline. *Tubercule* 61: 37–38

Wilkinson S P, Stewart W K, Spiers E M, Pears J 1989 Protracted systemic illness and interstitial nephritis due to minocycline. *Postgraduate Medical Journal* 65: 53–56

Yoshida S, Mizuguchi V, Ohta H et al 1985 Effect of tetracyclines on experimental *Legionella pneumophila* infection in guinea-pigs. *Journal of Antimicrobial Chemotherapy* 16: 199–204

OXYTETRACYCLINE

A fermentation product of certain strains of *Streptomyces rimosus*.

Antimicrobial activity

Its spectrum and activity are typical of the group (p. 469). It is generally slightly less active than other tetracyclines against most common pathogenic bacteria (Table 35.2). It shares resistance mechanisms and patterns with the rest of the group (p. 470).

Pharmacokinetics

It is moderately well absorbed from the upper gastro-intestinal tract, producing serum concentrations around 3–4 mg/l after a dose of 500 mg, 6-hourly. The plasma elimination half-life is about 9 h. Food decreases plasma levels by approximately 50%. The drug is 20–35% protein bound. Although widely distributed in the tissues, it achieves lower concentrations than related agents such as minocycline. Sputum concentrations of 1 mg/l have been recorded on a daily dosage of 2 g. Approximately 60% is excreted in the urine and the half-life is prolonged in renal insufficiency.

Toxicity and side-effects

Gastro-intestinal intolerance is responsible for the majority of side-effects, and tends to be more severe than with other tetracyclines. Oesophageal irritation may result from the local effects of the swallowed drug. Potentially serious adverse reactions have included neuromuscular paralysis following intravenous administration to patients with myasthenia gravis. Thrombocytopenic purpura and lupus erythematosus syndrome have been reported, although responsibility of the drug for the latter remains uncertain. Apart from the effect on nitrogen balance common to many tetracyclines, a metabolic effect on glucose homeostasis has been noted in insulin dependent diabetes mellitus. Allergic contact sensitivity reactions have also been reported.

Clinical use

Its uses are those common to the group (p. 472). Oxytetracycline offers no unique therapeutic advantages, although it is one of the cheaper preparations.

Preparations and dosage

Proprietary name: Terramycin.
Preparations: Tablets, capsules.
Dosage: Adults, oral, 250–500 mg every 6 h.
Widely available.

Further information

Snaveley S R, Hodges G R 1984 The neurotoxicity of antibacterial agents. *Annals of Internal Medicine* 101: 92–104

Wright A L, Colver G B 1988 Tetracyclines – how safe are they? *Clinical and Experimental Dermatology* 13: 57–61

ROLITETRACYCLINE

Semi-synthetic pyrrolidinomethyltetracycline supplied as the nitrate sesquihydrate.

Its antimicrobial activity and spectrum are typical of the group (p. 469).

It is not absorbed from the gastro-intestinal tract. It is highly soluble and therefore can be administered parenterally. Peak plasma concentration of 4–6 mg/l occur at 0.5–1 h after 350 mg i.v. The plasma elimination half-life is 5–8 h. About 50% of the dose is excreted in the urine producing high concentrations.

Intravenous administration is occasionally accompanied by abnormal taste, shivering and rigors, hot flushes, facial reddening, dizziness and, rarely, circulatory collapse. Symptoms of myasthenia gravis have occasionally been exacerbated. Its clinical uses are those common to the group (p. 472).

Preparations and dosage

Preparation: Injection.
Dosage: Adults, i.m., 350 mg/day; i.v., 275 mg/day.
Limited availability in continental Europe.

TETRACYCLINE

Fermentation product of certain *Streptomyces aureofaciens*, also produced from chlortetracycline.

Antimicrobial activity

Its activity against common pathogenic bacteria, which is typical of the group, is shown in Table 35.2. It is also active against *V. cholerae, Aer. hydrophila* and *Ples. shigelloides*.

Acquired resistance

Tetracycline shares in resistance to the group, which has proved a major limiting factor in their continuing use against many common pathogens. Among Gram-positive pathogens, tetracycline resistance has been particularly marked among staphylococci. Streptococci also vary widely in their susceptibility, with resistance rates in group B streptococci more than 85% and in pneumococci ranging from 10% up to 65%.

Reported resistance rates for clostridia are: *Cl. perfringens* 19–54%, *Cl. ramosum* 56% and *Cl. difficile* 16%. No resistance was noted among *Cl. septicum* or *Cl. tetani*. Resistant strains have also been reported in: *Peptococcus, Peptostreptococcus, Eubacterium* and *Actinomyces* spp.

Tetracycline resistance among Gram-negative enteric pathogens is particularly widespread; resistance has steadily increased in shigella, salmonellae and *V. cholerae*, including the El Tor biotype.

Resistant *N. gonorrhoeae* are now widespread, with no distinction between β-lactamase-positive and -negative strains and rates of 20–47% have been recorded. High-level resistance (MIC 26–32 mg/l) has been increasingly noted in the USA, although such strains usually remain susceptible to penicillin.

Resistance is rare in *M. catarrhalis* and relatively uncommon in *H. influenzae* (UK, 1.4% in 1992). Resistance is common among *Haemophilus* species isolated from patients with chronic bronchitis and may occur during treatment. The highest resistance rates have been reported from Hong Kong (23%).

Anaerobic Gram-negative bacilli, including *Bacteroides* spp., have also become less commonly susceptible, with resistance noted in 6% of strains in the UK and two-thirds of strains in the USA and France. Among other pathogens, resistance has been noted in 7% of isolates of *U. urealyticum* from the USA and one-third of isolates from Brazil. Resistance in *Mycoplasma hominis* has been noted occasionally.

Pharmacokinetics

Steady-state plasma concentrations of 4–5 mg/l occur after oral doses of 500 mg, 6-hourly. The C_{max} after a single dose is 2–4 mg/l. The plasma elimination half-life after oral administration is approximately 8.5 h and the volume of distribution approximately 1.3 l/kg. When taken with food, absorption is reduced by approximately 50%. Females appear to produce higher concentrations than males. Divalent and trivalent cations such as calcium and aluminium present in antacids and milk interfere with absorption through chelation, as does ferrous sulphate. H_2 antagonists, by raising gastric pH, also interfere with absorption through impaired drug dissolution. Despite the effect of gastric pH, oral absorption has not been shown to be affected in elderly patients with achlorhydria.

The drug is protein bound to about 24–65%, which is reduced in states of malnutrition.

It is widely distributed in the body tissues; in particular, it penetrates well into the prostate, uterus, ovary and bladder, and also appears to be preferentially taken up by the gastro-intestinal tract. It is also detectable within reticulo-endothelial cells of the liver, spleen and bone marrow.

It is also bound to bone, dentine and tooth enamel of unerupted teeth. Sputum concentrations of 0.4–2.6 mg/l have been detected after 250 mg oral dosage, three times daily. Maxillary sinus secretions and bronchial mucosal tissue have been noted to have concentrations comparable to those of serum.

Following 500 mg i.v. concentrations up to 7 mg/l have been found in the aqueous humour. CSF penetration is poor but increases with meningeal inflammation. Tetracycline crosses the placenta readily to enter the fetal circulation, where it achieves 25–75% of the maternal plasma concentration. It is also present in breast milk.

It is largely eliminated unchanged by glomerular filtration, with more than 50% excreted within 24 h after oral administration. This rises to approximately 70% following parenteral administration. Urinary concentrations of 300 mg/l occur within the first 2 h and persist for up to 12 h. Urinary excretion is enhanced in alkaline urine. Renal clearance is reduced in severe protein calorie malnutrition, possibly through reduced glomerular filtration. It accumulates in the presence of renal failure and is only slowly removed by haemodialysis and minimally by peritoneal dialysis.

The bile is an important route of excretion accounting for approximately one-third. Biliary concentrations may be 10–25 times those found in serum. Impaired hepatic function or biliary obstruction reduces this route of excretion with a consequent increase in blood levels.

Toxicity and side-effects

The gastro-intestinal side-effects which are the most frequent cause of intolerance to tetracycline are common to the group (p. 471). Metallic taste and glossitis are less burdensome than diarrhoea. Tetracycline has also been responsible for antibiotic-associated enterocolitis caused by *Cl. difficile* toxin and staphylococcal enterocolitis. Steatorrhoea and acute pancreatitis have been described. Irritation and ulceration of the oesophagus has occurred with local impaction of the drug.

Cand. albicans overgrowth is common and may result in symptomatic oral or vaginal candidiasis and occasionally candida diarrhoea.

Hypersensitivity reactions include contact dermatitis, urticaria, facial oedema and asthma. Anaphylaxis is rare. A lupus syndrome has been reported but its cause is uncertain. Photosensitivity can be severe and cause vesiculation, desquamation and onycholysis. The Jarisch–Herxheimer reaction has been observed when tetracycline has been used to treat syphilis, louse-borne relapsing fever, leptospirosis, brucellosis and tularaemia. Tetracycline deposition in deciduous teeth (p. 114) is of continuing concern, and although a survey in 1988 reported a reduction, it remains necessary to emphasize that tetracyclines are contra-indicated in children under 8 years of age and in pregnancy, not only because of the effect on teeth but also because tetracycline is deposited in bone and may temporarily inhibit growth. Between 3 and 44% of administered tetracycline is incorporated in the inorganic phase of bone, which may become visibly discolored and fluoresce. Concentrations as high as 290 mg/g have been recorded in bone in those on long-term tetracycline treatment for acne.

Tetracycline-induced nephrotoxicity can take several forms. Existing renal insufficiency may be aggravated and is probably related to the anti-anabolic effect of this class of drugs; interference with protein synthesis places an additional burden on the kidney from amino acid metabolism.

Acute renal failure may occur and can be aggravated by drug-induced diarrhoea. Dehydration and salt loss from diuretic therapy may aggravate nephrotoxicity. Methoxyflurane and tetracycline in combination may be synergically nephrotoxic.

Acute fatty liver is an uncommon but serious adverse reaction which may be complicated by renal insufficiency and electrolyte abnormalities. This is most likely to occur with high dose intravenous administration, especially during pregnancy.

Haematological toxicity is uncommon. Leucopenia, thrombocytopenia and haemolytic anaemia have been reported. Altered coagulation may also occur with high intravenous dosage. Phagocyte function may theoretically be impaired as a result of the increased excretion of vitamin C during tetracycline administration.

Neurological toxicity is uncommon but includes benign intracranial hypertension. In infancy it has been described as the 'bulging fontanelle syndrome' and in adults as 'pseudotumour cerebri'. The CSF pressure is raised but the fluid is otherwise normal; the syndrome is reversible on stopping the drug.

Other toxicities include interference with neuromuscular function; a transient myopathy has complicated long-term use of oral tetracycline for the treatment of acne, while intravenous administration has caused increased muscle weakness in those with myasthenia gravis and has also potentiated curare-induced neuromuscular blockade.

A variety of metabolic effects have been recorded. These include: precipitation of lactic acidosis in diabetic patients receiving phenformin; a reduction in vitamins B_{12} and B_6 and pantothenic acid with long-term therapy; interference with laboratory tests of urinary catecholamines and urinary tests for glucose (Clinitest and Benedict's); and elevation of serum lithium concentrations. In addition, warfarin is potentiated and failures of oral contraceptives also occur, justifying advice concerning the simultaneous use of a barrier contraceptive method in women of childbearing potential.

Clinical use

Respiratory infections continue as the commonest indication world-wide for the use of tetracyclines (Ch. 48). It is the drug of choice for the treatment of psittacosis. Acute Q fever, although self-limiting, on occasion justifies treatment with tetracycline which is the drug of choice for more severe infections. In the case of chronic Q fever infection, long-term treatment is necessary; its place in endocarditis is discussed on page 890. Tetracycline has been widely used in high dose for prolonged periods for melioidosis with some benefit, although other agents are now preferred.

Gastro-intestinal infections against which tetracyclines may prove of value include cholera and severe shigellosis (p. 711) and travellers' diarrhoea caused by enterotoxigenic *Esch. coli* shows modest benefit. Tetracycline has been extensively studied in recent years as part of a multidrug regimens in the management of *H. pylori* gastritis and peptic ulcer disease. Regimens have included tetracycline, amoxycillin and clarithromycin in combination with an H_2 antagonist, omeprazole or bismuth preparations.

Sexually transmitted diseases are still an important target for tetracycline use. They include gonorrhoea, chancroid, granuloma inguinale and lymphogranuloma venereum, and infection with *U. urealyticum* and *Chlamydia trachomatis*, but in some of these infections, resistance is a problem (Ch. 58). Prolonged tetracycline treatment may be used in those allergic to penicillin, and it is effective in a number of other spirochaetoses. Rickettsial infections, such as murine typhus, Scrub typhus, Boutonneuse fever, rickettsialpox and Rocky Mountain spotted fever are effectively treated with a short course, although the latter may require more prolonged treatment (p. 889).

Topical application has been used to prevent ophthalmia neonatorum caused by gonococci or chlamydiae. Trachoma responds to topical application, although oral administration is preferred.

It is of some benefit in a variety of parasitic diseases, including acute amoebic dysentery, possibly toxoplasmosis, balantidiasis, and chloroquine-resistant malaria.

Acne and rosacea have been widely treated with tetracyclines (p. 740), and it is effective in actinomycosis (p. 739), cutaneous anthrax (p. 737) and *M. marinum* infections.

Other infections that have been successfully treated include plague and tularaemia (p. 884), tropical sprue and Whipple's disease. The sclerosing properties of tetracycline have been exploited in various body sites for the management of recurrent pneumothorax, malignant pleural effusions, pericardial effusions, hydroceles and also thyroid cysts.

Further information

Boer de W A, Driessen W M, Potters V P, Tytgat G N 1994 Randomized study comparing 1 with 2 weeks of quadruple therapy for eradicating *Helicobacter pylori*. *American Journal of Gastroenterology* 89: 1993–1997

Bourbeau P, Campos J M 1982 Current antibiotic susceptibility of group A β-hemolytic streptococci. *Journal of Infectious Diseases* 145: 916

Brown B A, Wallace R J, Flanagan C W et al 1989 Tetracycline and erythromycin resistance among clinical isolates of *Branhamella catarrhalis*. *Antimicrobial Agents and Chemotherapy* 33: 1631–1633

Enderlin G, Morales L, Jacobs R F, Cross J T 1994 Streptomycin and alternative agents for the treatment of tularemia: review of the literature. *Clinical Infectious Diseases* 19: 42–47

Feurle G E, Marth T 1994 An evaluation of antimicrobial treatment for Whipple's disease. Tetracycline versus trimethoprim–sulfamethoxazole. *Digestive Diseases and Sciences* 39: 1642–1648

Forsgren A, Walder M 1982 *Haemophilus influenzae*, pneumococci, group A streptococci and *Staphylococcus aureus*: sensitivity of outpatient strains to commonly prescribed antibiotics. *Scandinavian Journal of Infectious Diseases* 14: 39–43

Gebbia N, Mannino R, Di Dino A et al 1994 Intracavitary treatment of malignant pleural and peritoneal effusions in cancer patients. *Anticancer Research* 14 (2B): 739–745

Gross R J, Threlfall E J, Ward L R, Rowe B 1987 Drug resistance in *Shigella dysenteriae, S. flexneri* and *S. boydii* in England and Wales: increasing incidence of resistance to trimethoprim. *British Medical Journal* 288: 784–786

Islam M R 1987 Single dose tetracycline in cholera. *Gut* 28: 1029–1032

Khan M V 1982 Efficacy of short course antibiotic prophylaxis in controlling cholera in contacts during epidemic. *Journal of Tropical Medicine and Hygiene* 85: 27–29

Kinirons M J 1983 Reduction in evidence in children's teeth of use of tetracyclines. *British Medical Journal* 287: 1515

Labenz J, Ruhl G H, Bertrams J, Borsch G 1994 Effective treatment after failure of omeprazole plus amoxycillin to eradicate *Helicobacter pylori* infection in peptic ulcer disease. *Alimentary Pharmacology and Therapeutics* 8: 323–327

Linares J, Garau J, Dominguez C, Perez J L 1983 Antibiotic resistance and serotypes of *Streptococcus pneumoniae* from patients with community acquired pneumococcal disease. *Antimicrobial Agents and Chemotherapy* 23: 545–547

Ling J, Chau P Y, Leung Y K et al 1983 Antibiotic susceptibility of pneumococci and *Haemophilus influenzae* isolated from patients with acute exacerbations of chronic bronchitis: prevalence of tetracycline-resistant strains in Hong Kong. *Journal of Infection* 6: 33–37

Looareesuwan S, Vanijanota S, Viravan C et al 1994 Randomised trial of mefloquine-tetracycline and quinine-tetracycline for acute uncomplicated falciparum malaria. *Acta Tropica* 57: 47–53

Murphy A A, Zacur H A, Charache P, Burkman R T 1991 The effect of tetracycline on levels of oral contraceptives. *American Journal of Obstetrics and Gynecology* 164: 28–33

Nicolau D P, Mengedoht D E, Kline J J 1991 Tetracycline-induced pancreatitis. *American Journal of Gastroenterology* 86: 1669–1671

Oklund S A, Prolo D J, Gutierrez R V 1981 The significance of yellow bone. Evidence for tetracycline in adult human bone. *Journal of the American Medical Association* 246: 761–763

Powell M, Fah S, Seymour A, Yuan M, Williams J D 1992 Antimicrobial resistance in *Haemophilus influenzae* from England and Scotland in 1991. *Journal of Antimicrobial Chemotherapy* 29: 547–554

Pierog S H, Al-Salimi F L, Cinotti D 1986 Pseudotumor cerebri – a complication of tetracycline treatment of acne. *Journal of Adolescent Health Care* 7: 139–140

Rajatanavin R, Chailurkit L, Chiemchanya S 1994 The efficacy of percutaneous tetracycline instillation for sclerosis of recurrent thyroid cysts: a multivariate analysis. *Journal of Endocrinological Investigation* 17: 123–125

Sankari B R, Boullier J A, Garvin P J, Parra R O 1992 Sclerotherapy with tetracycline for hydroceles in renal transplant patients. *Journal of Urology* 148: 1188–1189

Shepherd F A, Morgan C, Evans W K et al 1987 Medical management of malignant pericardial effusion by tetracycline sclerosis. *American Journal of Cardiology* 60: 1161–1166

Sinclair D, Phillips C 1982 Transient myopathy apparently due to tetracycline. *New England Journal of Medicine* 307: 821–822

Stephenson L W 1985 Treatment of pneumothorax with intrapleural tetracycline. *Chest* 88: 803–804

Stimson J B, Hale J, Bowie W R, Holmes K K 1981 Tetracycline-resistant *Ureaplasma urealyticum*: a cause of persistent nongonococcal urethritis. *Annals of Internal Medicine* 94: 192–914

Thomas E 1980 Towards better antimicrobial treatment of sexually transmitted diseases. *Journal of Antimicrobial Chemotherapy* 6: 570–573

36

Antifungal agents

D. W. Warnock

Introduction

Effective drugs are now available for a wide range of fungal infections, covering most of the major pathogens and providing a choice for many conditions. In the more common superficial infections it is now possible to cure most patients with topical treatment, and the details of administration are often more important than the choice of agent. There is less satisfactory provision for systemic fungal infections, and there are still conditions for which there is no effective treatment.

There are three main families of antifungal agents: the allylamines, the azoles and the polyenes. In addition, there is a miscellaneous group of drugs that includes flucytosine, griseofulvin, amorolfine and various other agents that are used for topical treatment. New groups of compounds and new ways of using the older agents, such as liposomal formulations, are under constant development and review. Resistance, although not a major problem, has now been recorded with some azole antifungals, as well as with flucytosine, usually in situations where the drugs have been given for long periods of time in the face of persistent infection.

Further information

British Society for Antimicrobial Chemotherapy Working Party 1991 Laboratory monitoring of antifungal chemotherapy. *Lancet* 337: 1577–1580

Fernandes P B (ed) 1992 New approaches for antifungal drugs. Birkhauser, Boston

Fromtling R A (ed) 1987 Recent trends in the discovery, development and evaluation of antifungal agents. Prous, Barcelona

Georgopapadakov N H, Walsh T J 1996 Antifungal agents: chemotherapeutic targets and immunologic strategies. *Antimicrobial Agents and Chemotherapy* 40: 279–291

Kerridge D 1986 Mode of action of clinically important antifungal drugs. *Advances in Microbial Physiology* 27: 1–72

Rex J H, Pfaller M A, Rinaldi M G, Polak A, Galgiani J N 1993 Antifungal susceptibility testing. *Clinical Microbiology Reviews* 6: 367–381

Ryley J F (ed) 1990 Chemotherapy of fungal diseases. Springer, Berlin

Vanden Bossche H, Marichal P, Odds F C 1994 Molecular mechanisms of drug resistance in fungi. *Trends in Microbiology* 2: 393–400

Allylamines

This group of synthetic agents contains compounds that are effective in the topical and oral treatment of dermato-phytoses and superficial forms of candidosis. Like the azoles, the allylamines inhibit fungal ergosterol biosynthesis, but act through inhibition of the non-cytochrome-P450-mediated enzyme, squalene epoxidase. Two drugs, naftifine and terbinafine, have entered clinical use.

Naftifine is useful for the topical treatment of dermato-phytoses, including tinea corporis and tinea cruris, but is less effective in the treatment of cutaneous candidiasis. It has been licensed for use as a 1% cream in some countries, including the USA.

Further information

Ryder N S 1987 Mechanism of action of the allylamine antimycotics. In: Fromtling R A (ed) Recent trends in the discovery, development and evaluation of antifungal agents. Prous, Barcelona, p 451–459

TERBINAFINE

A synthetic allylamine.

Antimicrobial activity

Terbinafine is active against a range of superficial fungal pathogens, including the aetiological agents of the dermatophytoses and pityriasis versicolor. It has a fungistatic effect on *Candida albicans*, but is fungicidal for some other *Candida* species, including *Candida parapsilosis*. It has also been shown to be effective in vitro against a number of dimorphic fungi, including *Blastomyces dermatitidis*, *Histoplasma capsulatum* and *Sporothrix schenckii*. It has been used successfully in patients with cutaneous sporotrichosis.

Acquired resistance

This has not been reported.

Pharmacokinetics

It is well absorbed (>70%) after oral administration, blood concentrations of the drug increasing in proportion to dosage. Peak plasma concentrations of about 1 mg/l are achieved within 2 h of a 250 mg dose. Plasma protein binding is >95%. Terbinafine is a lipophilic compound and this results in its accumulation in adipose tissue. It reaches the stratum corneum as a result of diffusion through the dermis and epidermis, and secretion in sebum. Diffusion from the nail bed is the major factor in its rapid penetration of nails. Terbinafine is metabolized by the liver and the inactive metabolites are excreted in the urine. The elimination half-life is about 17 h, but this is prolonged in patients with hepatic or renal impairment.

Terbinafine does not affect the clearance of drugs, such as cyclosporin, that undergo cytochrome-P_{450}-mediated hepatic metabolism. However, blood concentrations of terbinafine are reduced following concomitant administration with drugs, such as rifampicin, which induce cytochrome-P_{450}-mediated metabolism. Levels are increased if terbinafine is given with drugs, such as cimetidine, which inhibit hepatic metabolism.

Toxicity and side-effects

It has no effect on mammalian cholesterol synthesis. It is generally well tolerated apart from some gastro-intestinal disturbance, impairment of taste and occasional allergic skin reactions. There have been a few anecdotal reports of hepatotoxic reactions (including one death) and it is not recommended in patients with severe renal or hepatic impairment.

Clinical use

Oral terbinafine is an effective treatment for dermatophytoses of the skin and nails for which topical treatment is considered inappropriate or has failed. Clinical trials suggest it is more effective than griseofulvin, ketoconazole or itraconazole for treatment of skin or nail infections. It does not appear to be particularly effective in superficial candidosis.

Preparations and dosage

Proprietary name: Lamisil.

Preparations: Tablets, cream.

Dosage: Adults, oral, 250 mg/day for 2–6 weeks in tinea pedis, 2–4 weeks in tinea cruris, 4 weeks in tinea corporis, 6 weeks to 3 months or longer in nail infections.

Available in the UK.

Further information

Goodfield M J D, Rowell N R, Forster R A, Evans E G V, Raven A 1989 Treatment of dermatophyte infections of the finger or toe nails with terbinafine (SF86-327, Lamisil), an orally active fungicidal agent. *British Journal of Dermatology* 121: 359–366

Jensen J C 1989 Clinical pharmacokinetics of terbinafine (Lamisil). *Clinical and Experimental Dermatology* 14: 110–113

De Keyser P, De Backer M, Massart D L, Westelinck K J 1994 Two-week oral treatment of tinea pedis, comparing terbinafine (250 mg/day) with itraconazole (100 mg/day): a double-blind, multicentre study. *British Journal of Dermatology* 130 (suppl 43): 22–25

Azoles

This large group of synthetic agents, which includes drugs used in bacterial and parasitic infections (5-nitroimidazoles, benzimidazoles), contains many compounds that are effective in the topical treatment of dermatophytoses and superficial forms of candidosis; a few are suitable for systemic administration.

Members of this group have in common an imidazole or triazole ring with *N*-carbon substitution. Azoles damage the fungal cell membrane by blocking the cytochrome-P450-mediated 14α-demethylation step in the biosynthesis of ergosterol, the principal sterol in the membrane of susceptible fungal cells. The consequent depletion of ergosterol and accumulation of methylated sterols leads to alterations in a number of membrane-associated functions. At high concentrations, some azoles can exert fungicidal effects by directly damaging cell membranes, causing leakage of cellular constituents and other effects.

In addition to the systemic agents (fluconazole, itraconazole, ketoconazole, miconazole), numerous imidazoles are presently available for topical use. They include:

- **Bifonazole** Used for the topical treatment of dermatophytoses and pityriasis versicolor.
- **Clotrimazole** Used for the topical treatment of dermatophytoses, and oral, cutaneous and genital candidosis.
- **Econazole nitrate** Used for the topical treatment of dermatophytoses and cutaneous and genital candidosis.
- **Isoconazole nitrate** Used for the topical treatment of vaginal candidosis.
- **Sulconazole nitrate** Used for the topical treatment of dermatophytoses and cutaneous candidosis.
- **Tioconazole** Used for the topical treatment of dermatophytoses (including nail infections) and, in some countries, for cutaneous and vaginal candidosis.

Preparations and dosages

Bifonazole

Preparation: Topical.

Available in continental Europe.

Clotrimazole

Proprietary name: Canesten.

Preparations: Vaginal cream, vaginal tablets, topical.

Dosage: Adults, vaginal tablets, 200 mg/day for 3 days, or 100 mg/day for 6 consecutive days. For fungal skin infections dosage and duration of treatment varies according to condition.

Widely available.

Econazole nitrate

Proprietary names: Ecostatin, Gyno-Pevaryl.

Preparations: Pessaries, topical.

Dosage: Adults, pessaries, 150 mg/day for 3 consecutive days. For fungal skin infections dosage and duration of treatment varies according to condition.

Widely available.

Isoconazole

Proprietary name: Travogyn.

Preparation: Vaginal tablets.

Dosage: Adult, 600 mg as a single dose.

Widely available.

Sulconazole nitrate

Proprietary name: Exelderm.

Preparation: Topical.

Dosage: For fungal skin infections dosage and duration of treatment varies according to the condition being treated.

Available in the UK.

Tioconazole

Proprietary name: Trosyl.

Preparation: Nail solution, cream.

Dosage: For fungal skin and nail infections dosage and duration of treatment varies according to the condition being treated.

Widely available.

Further information

Como J A, Dismukes W E 1994 Oral azole drugs as systemic antifungal therapy. *New England Journal of Medicine* 330: 263–272

Fromtling R A 1988 Overview of medically important antifungal azole derivatives. *Clinical Microbiology Reviews* 1: 187–217

Odds F C 1993 Resistance of yeasts to azole-derivative antifungals. *Journal of Antimicrobial Chemotherapy* 31: 463–471

FLUCONAZOLE

A synthetic bis(triazole).

Antimicrobial activity

Fluconazole has a broad-spectrum of activity, including *Blast. dermatitidis, Coccidioides immitis, Cryptococcus neoformans*, *Hist. capsulatum* and *Paracoccidioides brasiliensis*. It is active in dermatophytosis, but appears to be ineffective in aspergillosis. It is active against *Candida albicans*, *Cand. parapsilosis* and *Cand. tropicalis*, but most strains of *Cand. krusei* and *Torulopsis glabrata* (now reclassified as *Cand. glabrata*) appear to be insensitive.

Acquired resistance

An increasing number of resistant strains of *Cand. albicans* are now being isolated from acquired immune deficiency syndrome (AIDS) patients given long-term fluconazole treatment for oral or oesophageal candidosis. There are a few reports of fluconazole-resistant strains of· *Cryp. neoformans* recovered from AIDS patients with relapsed meningitis. Some, but not all, *Cand. albicans* strains resistant to fluconazole are cross-resistant to other azoles.

Pharmacokinetics

Oral administration leads to rapid and almost complete absorption of the drug, blood concentrations increasing in proportion to dosage. Two hours after a single 50 mg oral dose, maximal serum concentrations in the region of 1.0 mg/l can be anticipated, but after repeated dosing this increases to about 2.0–3.0 mg/l. Administration of the drug with food does not affect absorption. Unlike other azole antifungals, the protein binding of fluconazole is about 12%, resulting in high levels of circulating unbound drug. Concentrations of fluconazole in the cerebrospinal fluid (CSF) are between 50 and 60% of the simultaneous serum concentration in normal individuals and even higher in patients with meningitis. More than 90% of a given dose of fluconazole is eliminated in the urine: about 80% as unchanged drug and 10% as metabolites. The drug is cleared through glomerular filtration, but there is significant tubular reabsorption. The serum half-life of fluconazole is 25–30 h, but this is prolonged in renal failure, necessitating adjustment of the dosage regimen. Fluconazole can enhance the anticoagulant effect of warfarin and the hypoglycaemic effects of drugs, such as chlorpropamide, glipizide and tolbutamide.

Toxicity and side-effects

It does not affect human steroid metabolism. Minor side-effects, such as nausea, headache and abdominal discomfort, have been seen in a few patients, as have transient asymptomatic transaminase elevations.

Clinical use

For patients with mucosal candidosis, fluconazole appears to be as effective as or better than other drugs: duration of treatment is shorter and there are fewer relapses. The results of a recent randomized trial suggest that fluconazole, at a dosage of 400 mg, is as effective as amphotericin B in treating candidaemia in patients without neutropenia. Fluconazole is an effective initial treatment for cryptococcal meningitis in patients with AIDS, but because of faster sterilization of the CSF and fewer deaths, amphotericin B is the better choice for induction. However, long-term maintenance treatment with fluconazole to prevent relapse in this population has proved to be better, and also better tolerated than amphotericin B. Fluconazole has also proved to be a useful prophylactic treatment against candidosis in patients at risk of neutropenia. However, it is ineffective in aspergillosis.

Preparations and dosage

Proprietary name: Diflucan.

Preparations: Capsules, suspension, i.v. infusion

Dosage: Adults, oral, vaginal candidiasis, 150 mg as a single dose; oropharyngeal candidiasis, 50 mg/day for 7–14 days; atrophic candidiasis, 50 mg/day for 14 days; oesophageal and mucocutaneous candidiasis, and candiduria, 50 mg/day for 14–30 days. Tinea pedis, corporis, cruris, pityriasis versicolor, 50 mg/day for 2–4 weeks. Systemic candidiasis, cryptococcal meningitis and other forms of cryptococcosis, oral or i.v. infusion, 400 mg initially, then 200 mg/day; treatment is continued according to response. For the prevention or relapse of cryptococcal meningitis in AIDS patients, 100–200 mg/day, indefinitely. Prevention of fungal infections in immunocompromised patients following radiotherapy or cytotoxic chemotherapy, 50–400 mg/day.

Children >1 year, oral, i.v. infusion, superficial candidal infections, 1–2 mg/kg daily; systemic candidiasis and cryptococcal infections, 3–6 mg/kg daily.

Widely available.

Further information

Brammer K W, Tarbit M H 1987 A review of the pharmacokinetics of fluconazole (UK-49,858) in laboratory animals and man. In: Fromtling R A (ed) Recent trends in the discovery, development and evaluation of antifungal agents. Prous, Barcelona, p 144–149

Goodman J L, Winston D J, Greenfield R A et al 1992 A controlled trial of fluconazole to prevent fungal infections in patients undergoing bone marrow transplantation. *New England Journal of Medicine* 326: 845–851

Laine L, Dretler R H, Conteas C N et al 1992 Fluconazole compared with ketoconazole for the treatment of candida esophagitis in AIDS. *Annals of Internal Medicine* 117: 655–660

Powderly W G, Saag M S, Cloud G A et al 1992 A controlled trial of fluconazole or amphotericin B to prevent relapse of cryptococcal meningitis in patients with the acquired immunodeficiency syndrome. *New England Journal of Medicine* 326: 793–798

Rex J H, Bennett J E, Sugar A M et al 1994 A randomized trial comparing fluconazole with amphotericin B for the treatment of candidemia in patients without neutropenia. *New England Journal of Medicine* 331: 1325–1330

Rex J H, Rinaldi M G, Pfaller M A 1995 Resistance of Candida species to fluconazole. *Antimicrobial Agents and Chemotherapy* 39: 1–8

Saag M S, Powderly W G, Cloud G A, Robinson P, Grieco M H, Sharkey P K 1992 Comparison of amphotericin B with fluconazole in the treatment of acute AIDS-associated cryptococcal meningitis. *New England Journal of Medicine* 326: 83–89

ITRACONAZOLE

A synthetic dioxolane triazole.

Antimicrobial activity

Itraconazole has a wide spectrum of activity including *Aspergillus* spp., *Blast. dermatitidis*, *Candida* spp., *Cocc. immitis*, *Cryp. neoformans*, *Hist. capsulatum*, *Malassezia furfur*, *Paracocc. brasiliensis*, *Spor. schenckii* and the dermatophytes.

Acquired resistance

This is still rare, but ketoconazole- and some fluconazole-resistant *Cand. albicans* have been found to be cross-resistant to itraconazole.

Pharmacokinetics

It is a lipophilic compound. Absorption from the gastrointestinal tract is incomplete (55%), but is improved if the drug is given with food. Oral administration of a single 100 mg dose will produce maximal serum concentrations in the region of 0.1–0.2 mg/l about 2–4 h later. Much higher concentrations are obtained with repeated dosing, but there is much variation among individuals. Itraconazole is >99% protein bound in serum and levels in body fluids, such as the CSF, are negligible. In contrast, itraconazole concentrations in tissues such as lung, liver and bone are 2–3 times higher than in serum, and concentrations in the genital tract are 3–10 times higher. High concentrations are also found in the stratum corneum, as a result of drug secretion in sebum. It is degraded by the liver into a large number of metabolites, most of which are inactive, and these are excreted with the bile. It is not excreted as unchanged drug in the urine. The serum half-life is of the order of 20–30 h, increasing to 40 h after repeated dosing. No adjustment of dosage is required in hepatic or renal failure.

Absorption of itraconazole is reduced if it is given together with compounds that reduce gastric acid secretion. Much reduced blood levels have also been noted during concomitant administration with rifampicin. Like rifampicin, phenytoin undergoes cytochrome-P_{450}-mediated hepatic metabolism and its concomitant administration with itraconazole can alter the clearance of one or both drugs. Itraconazole should not be taken with H_1-receptor antagonists, such as terfenadine or astemizole, because of the potential for cardiac ventricular dysrhythmias. Itraconazole can augment the anticoagulant effect of warfarin and the hypoglycaemic effect of drugs such as chlorpropamide, glipizide and tolbutamide.

Toxicity and side-effects

Unlike ketoconazole, it does not affect human steroid metabolism. Minor side-effects, such as nausea, headache and abdominal discomfort, have been seen in a few patients, as have transient asymptomatic transaminase elevations.

There have been a few reports of reversible idiosyncratic hepatitis in patients treated with itraconazole. Hypokalaemia has also occasionally been reported.

Clinical use

It is effective in various superficial mycoses, including the dermatophytoses, pityriasis versicolor and oral and vaginal forms of candidosis. It is also effective in patients with subcutaneous mycoses, such as sporotrichosis. It has become the drug of choice for non-meningeal, non-life-threatening forms of blastomycosis and histoplasmosis and may be an effective alternative to amphotericin B for invasive aspergillosis. Itraconazole has also proved to be a useful prophylactic treatment against aspergillosis and candidosis in patients at risk of neutropenia. However, it has not been adequately evaluated as an oral treatment for systemic candidosis.

Preparations and dosage

Proprietary name: Sporanox.

Preparations: Capsules, oral solution.

Dosage: Adults, oral, oropharyngeal candidiasis, 100 mg/day (200 mg/day in AIDS or neutropenia) for 15 days. Vulvovaginal candidiasis, 200 mg twice daily for 1 day. Pityriasis versicolor, 200 mg daily for 7 days; tinea corporis, tinea cruris, 100 mg/day for 15 days; tinea pedis, tinea manuum, 100 mg/day for 30 days. Onychomycosis, 200 mg once daily for 3 months.

Widely available.

Further information

Denning D W, Tucker R M, Hanson L H, Hamilton J R, Stevens D A 1989 Itraconazole therapy for cryptococcal meningitis and cryptococcosis. *Archives of Internal Medicine* 149: 2301–2308

Denning D W, Lee J Y, Hostetler J S et al 1994 NIAID mycoses study group multicenter trial of oral itraconazole therapy for invasive aspergillosis. *American Journal of Medicine* 97: 135–144

Dismukes W E, Bradsher R W, Cloud G C et al 1992 Itraconazole therapy for blastomycosis and histoplasmosis. *American Journal of Medicine* 93: 489–497

Hay R J, Dupont B, Graybill J R 1987 First international symposium on itraconazole. *Reviews of Infectious Diseases* 9 (suppl 1)

Heykants J, Van Peer A, Van de Velde V et al 1989 The clinical pharmacokinetics of itraconazole: an overview. In: Fromtling R A (ed) Recent trends in the discovery, development and evaluation of antifungal agents. Prous, Barcelona, p 223–249

Sharkey P K, Graybill J R, Rinaldi M G et al 1990 Itraconazole treatment of phaeohyphomycosis. *Journal of the American Academy of Dermatology* 23: 577–586

Sharkey-Mathis P K, Kauffman C A, Graybill J R et al 1993 Treatment of sporotrichosis with itraconazole. *American Journal of Medicine* 95: 279–285

KETOCONAZOLE

A synthetic dioxolane imidazole.

Antimicrobial activity

Ketoconazole has a wide spectrum of activity, including *Blast. dermatitidis*, *Candida* spp., *Cocc. immitis*, *Cryp. neoformans*, *Hist. capsulatum* and *Paracocc. brasiliensis*. It is active in dermatophytosis and pityriasis versicolor, but ineffective in aspergillosis and mucormycosis.

Acquired resistance

This is rare, but occasional instances have been documented in patients treated for chronic mucocutaneous candidosis and AIDS patients with oropharyngeal or oesophageal candidosis. Some fluconazole-resistant *Cand. albicans* have been found to be cross-resistant to ketoconazole.

Pharmacokinetics

It is well absorbed after oral administration, peak serum concentrations being reached 2–4 h later. Absorption is favoured by an acid pH. Food delays absorption, but does not significantly reduce the peak serum concentration. Two hours after a 400 mg dose serum concentrations in the region of 5–6 mg/l can be expected, but there is much variation among individuals. Much higher concentrations can be obtained with doses of 600–1000 mg. Penetration into CSF is generally poor and unreliable, although effective concentrations have been recorded with high doses in some cases of active meningitis. Ketoconazole is metabolized by the liver, and the metabolites are excreted in the bile. Less than 1% of an oral dose is excreted unchanged in the urine. The half-life appears to be dose dependent. There is an initial half-life of 1–4 h, and an elimination half-life ranging from 6 to 10 h.

Absorption of ketoconazole is reduced if it is given together with compounds that reduce gastric acid secretion. Much reduced blood levels have also been noted during concomitant administration with rifampicin. Ketoconazole should not be taken with H_1-receptor antagonists, such as terfenadine or astemizole, because of the potential for cardiac ventricular dysrhythmias. Ketoconazole prolongs the half-life of cyclosporin in organ-transplant recipients, at times raising blood concentrations of that drug to toxic levels. It can augment the anticoagulant effect of warfarin.

Toxicity and side-effects

Transient transaminase elevations develop in 5–10% of patients on oral ketoconazole. Treatment should be discontinued if these persist, if the abnormalities increase, or if symptoms associated with hepatic dysfunction appear. The serious hepatotoxic side-effects of ketoconazole are idiosyncratic and rare, occurring in between 1 in 10 000 and 1 in 15 000 patients treated for longer than 2 weeks. In most cases, hepatic damage is reversible when the drug is discontinued. Liver function tests should be performed at monthly intervals and treatment discontinued in patients with elevated total serum bilirubin or progressively increasing transaminase levels. High doses of ketoconazole (>800 mg/day) inhibit human steroid synthesis. Clinical manifestations of interference with testosterone synthesis may occur, including painful gynaecomastia, loss of libido and, sometimes, loss of hair.

Clinical use

Until the introduction of itraconazole and fluconazole, ketoconazole was regarded as the drug of choice in chronic mucocutaneous candidosis and an effective alternative for non-meningeal, non-life-threatening forms of blastomycosis, coccidioidomycosis, histoplasmosis and paracoccidioidomycosis. However, prolonged administration of high doses was often required and later relapse was a common problem. It has not been adequately evaluated in systemic candidosis or cryptococcosis and it is ineffective in aspergillosis. It is less effective in dermatophytoses and vaginal candidosis than are itraconazole or fluconazole, and because of the possible effects on the liver and on steroid metabolism, it should not be used as first-line treatment for cutaneous or vaginal infections.

Topical formulations have produced excellent results in seborrhoeic dermatitis.

Preparations and dosage

Proprietary name: Nizoral.

Preparations: Tablets, suspension, topical cream, shampoo.

Dosage: Adult, oral, 200 mg/day for 14 days; if inadequate response after 14 days, continue until at least 1 week after symptoms have cleared and cultures become negative; maximum dose 400 mg/day. Children, oral, 3 mg/kg daily.

Widely available.

Further information

Daneshmend T K, Warnock D W 1988 Clinical pharmacokinetics of ketoconazole. *Clinical Pharmacokinetics* 14: 13–34

Lake-Bakkar G, Scheuer P J, Sherlock S 1987 Hepatic reactions associated with ketoconazole in the United Kingdom. *British Medical Journal* 294: 419–422

National Institutes of Allergy and Infectious Disease Mycoses Study Group 1985 Treatment of blastomycosis and histoplasmosis with ketoconazole. *Annals of Internal Medicine* 103: 861–872

Smith K J, Warnock D W, Kennedy C T C et al 1986 Azole resistance in *Candida albicans. Journal of Medical and Veterinary Mycology* 24: 133–144

Sobel J D 1986 Recurrent vulvovaginal candidiasis: a prospective study of the efficacy of maintenance ketoconazole therapy. *New England Journal of Medicine* 315: 1455–1458

Sugar A M, Alsip S G, Galgiani J N et al 1987 Pharmacology and toxicity of high-dose ketoconazole. *Antimicrobial Agents and Chemotherapy* 31: 1874–1878

MICONAZOLE

A synthetic phenethyl imidazole.

Antimicrobial activity

It has a wide spectrum of activity including *Aspergillus* spp., *Candida* spp., *Cocc. immitis*, *Cryp. neoformans*, *Hist. capsulatum*, *Paracocc. brasiliensis* and *Scedosporium apiospermum* (*Pseudallescheria boydii*). It is also active against dermatophytes.

Acquired resistance

This is rare, but *Cand. albicans* resistant to other azoles has been found to be cross-resistant to miconazole.

Pharmacokinetics

There is little absorption from the gut, and for treatment of systemic infections miconazole is prepared in Cremophor EL (an emulsifying agent) for intravenous use. Parenteral administration of a single 1000 mg dose will produce maximal serum concentrations as high as 7.5 mg/l. There is rapid decline, with an initial serum half-life of 20–30 min and an elimination half-life of about 20 h. There is good penetration into some tissues, such as the eyes and joints, but generally poor penetration into the CSF. Miconazole is eliminated by hepatic metabolism with excretion of inactive metabolites in the bile. Less than 1% of a given dose is excreted unchanged in the urine.

Miconazole intravenous solution may augment the anticoagulant effect of warfarin. It can potentiate the effect of hypoglycaemic drugs.

Toxicity and side-effects

Particularly in the high dosage regimens used in the USA, reactions including phlebitis, severe and intractable pruritus, gastro-intestinal upsets, fever and rashes have required termination of treatment in some patients. Cardiac dysrhythmias have also been described, but can be avoided by slow infusion over an hour or more.

Clinical use

Early reports suggested that miconazole might be effective in coccidioidomycosis, paracoccidioidomycosis and opportunistic mycoses such as systemic candidosis and cryptococcosis, but, more recently, advancing disease has been seen in the presence of 'effective' concentrations and relapse after cessation of even long courses has been common. Intravenous administration is effective in *Sced. apiospermum* (*Pseud. boydii*) infection and in such localized conditions as oesophageal candidosis, but in systemic mycoses it is now rarely used. Intrathecal miconazole has been used in doses up to 20 mg in central nervous system (CNS) infection.

Preparations and dosage

Proprietary names: Daktarin, Gyno-Daktarin, Femeron.

Preparations: Tablets, oral gel, i.v. infusion, cream, pessary, intravaginal cream.

Dosage: Adults, oral, 250 mg every 6 h for 10 days, or for up to 2 days after symptoms have cleared. Children >6 years, oral gel, 125 mg, 4 times daily; 2–6 years, 125 mg twice daily; infants <2 years, 62.5 mg twice daily. Adults, i.v. infusion, 600 mg every 8 h; children 15 mg/kg every 8 h up to 40 mg/kg daily.

Widely available.

Further information

Bennett J E, Remington J S 1981 Miconazole in cryptococcosis and systemic candidiasis: a word of caution. *Annals of Internal Medicine* 94: 708–709

Lutwick L I, Rytel M W, Yanez J P, Galgiani J N, Stevens D A 1979 Deep infections from *Petriellidium boydii* treated with miconazole. *Journal of the American Medical Association* 241: 272–273

Stevens D A 1977 Miconazole in the treatment of systemic fungal infections. *American Review of Respiratory Disease* 116: 801–806

Stevens D A 1983 Miconazole in the treatment of coccidioidomycosis. *Drugs* 26: 347–354

Polyenes

Around 100 polyene antibiotics have been described, but few have been developed for clinical use. They have large amphipathic molecules: closed macrolide rings with a variable number of hydroxyl groups along the hydrophilic side, and along the hydrophobic side a variable number of conjugated double bonds to which they owe the name 'polyene'; e.g. tetraene (four double bonds), heptaene (seven double bonds). They bind to sterols in eukaryotic cell membranes, causing impairment of barrier function, leakage of cell constituents, metabolic disruption and cell death. At low concentrations leakage of cell constituents is restricted to small molecules or ions such as sodium and potassium and is still reversible. At higher concentrations, larger molecules are transported through the membrane, producing irreversible loss of cell constituents. The most useful polyenes are those which bind to ergosterol, the principal sterol in the membrane of susceptible fungal cells, but even these compounds often bind to host cell membranes as well, and are toxic to both fungal and mammalian cells.

The most important member of the group is amphotericin B, a heptaene which is administered parenterally for the treatment of systemic fungal infections. Other clinically useful polyenes, which in general resemble amphotericin B in antifungal action and spectrum of activity, but are mostly used only topically, are:

- **Candicidin** (heptaene) A product of *Streptomyces griseus*. Used for the topical treatment of vaginal candidosis.
- **Mepartricin**; methyl partricin (heptaene) A product of *Streptomyces aureofaciens* used for intravenous treatment of deep candidosis and for the topical treatment of vaginal candidosis. It offers no conspicuous advantages over amphotericin B as a systemic antifungal.
- **Natamycin**; pimaricin (tetraene) A product of *Streptomyces chatanoogensis* or *Streptomyces natalensis* used for the topical treatment of ophthalmic and bronchopulmonary infections and vaginal candidosis.
- **Nystatin** (tetraene) A product of *Streptomyces albulus* or *Streptomyces noursei* used for the topical treatment of oral, oesophageal, gastro-intestinal and genital candidosis, and gastro-intestinal prophylaxis.
- **Pecilocin**; variotin (tetraene) A product of *Paecilomyces variotii* used for the topical treatment of dermatophytoses.
- **Trichomycin** (heptaene) A product of *Streptomyces hachijoensis* or *Streptomyces abikoensis* used for the topical treatment of vaginal candidosis.

Preparations and dosages

Candicidin

Preparation: Vaginal tablet.

Dosage: 3 mg, twice daily for 2 weeks.

Not available in the UK.

Mepartricin

Preparations: Tablets, vaginal preparations.

Not available in the UK.

Natamycin

Preparations: Oral suspension, cream, vaginal preparations.

Dosage: Vaginal pessary, 25 mg/day for 20 days.

Not available in the UK.

Nystatin

Proprietary name: Nystan.

Preparations: Tablets, pastilles, suspension, vaginal and topical preparations.

Dosage: Adults, oral, 500 000 units every 6 h, doubled in severe infections. Prophylaxis: adults, 1 million units daily; children, 100 000 units 4 times daily; neonates, 100 000

units daily as a single dose. Vaginal pessaries, 1–2 at night for at least 14 nights.

Widely available.

Trichomycin

Topical.

Not available in the UK.

Further information

Medoff G, Kobayashi G A 1980 The polyenes. In: Speller D C E (ed) Antifungal chemotherapy. Wiley, Chichester, ch 1, p 3–33

Sugar A M 1986 The polyene macrolide antifungal drugs. In: Peterson P K, Verhoef J (eds) The antimicrobial agents annual. Elsevier, Amsterdam, vol 1, p 229–244

AMPHOTERICIN B

A fermentation product of *Streptomyces nodosus*.

The traditional micellar suspension formulation of this drug is often associated with serious toxic side-effects, in particular renal damage, and this has stimulated efforts to develop chemical modifications and new formulations. Most of the chemical modifications that have been devised have been less toxic, but also less active than amphotericin B. None has achieved clinical importance. Three lipid-associated formulations have been licensed for use in a number of countries: liposomal amphotericin B (AmBisome), in which the drug is encapsulated in phospholipid-containing liposomes; amphotericin B colloidal dispersion (Amphocil), in which the drug is packaged into small lipid discs containing cholesterol sulphate; and amphotericin B lipid complex (Abelcet), in which the drug is complexed with phospholipids to produce ribbon-like structures. These formulations appear to be less toxic than the micellar suspension because of their altered pharmacological distribution. They permit higher doses of amphotericin B to be administered and encouraging results have been reported in patients with serious fungal infection.

Antimicrobial activity

It has a wide spectrum of antifungal activity, including most fungi that cause disease in humans: *Aspergillus fumigatus*, *Blast. dermatitidis*, *Candida* spp., *Cocc. immitis*, *Cryp. neoformans*, *Hist. capsulatum*, *Paracocc. brasiliensis* and *Spor. schenckii*. dermatophytes, *Fusarium* spp. and some other *Aspergillus* spp. may be less sensitive, while *Sced. apiospermum* (*Pseud. boydii*), *Trichosporon beigelii* and some fungi that cause mucormycosis are resistant.

Apart from fungi it exhibits useful activity against *Prototheca* spp., and some protozoa, including *Leishmania* spp., and the genera *Naegleria* and *Hartmanella* (p. 754).

Acquired resistance

This is a rare problem. Resistant strains of *Cand. tropicalis*, *Cand. lusitaniae*, *Cand. krusei* and *Cand. guilliermondii* with alterations in the cell membrane including reduced amounts of ergosterol, have occasionally been isolated after prolonged treatment, particularly of infections in partially protected sites, such as the vegetations of endocarditis. Significant resistance in yeasts, including *Cand. albicans* and *Cand.* (*Torulops*) *glabrata*, has also been reported in isolates from cancer patients with prolonged neutropenia. In some cases resistant strains have caused disseminated infection. There are a few reports of amphotericin-resistant strains of *Cryp. neoformans* recovered from AIDS patients with relapsed meningitis.

Pharmacokinetics

It is poorly absorbed following oral administration. Less than 10% of a parenteral dose of the conventional micellar suspension formulation of amphotericin B remains in the blood 12 h after administration, and >90% of this is protein bound. The remainder is thought to bind to tissue cell membranes, the highest concentrations being found in the liver (up to 40% of the dose). Levels in the CSF are less than 5% of the simultaneous blood concentration. Administration of lipid-associated formulations of amphotericin B results in lower renal concentrations of the drug and its nephrotoxic side-effects are much reduced. Hepatic or renal failure does not influence serum concentrations.

The conventional micellar suspension formulation has a second-phase elimination half-life of about 24–48 h and a third-phase half-life of about 2 weeks. About 2–5% of a given dose appears in the urine within 24 h, but the fate of the rest is unknown. No metabolites have been identified.

Amphotericin B can add to the nephrotoxic effects of other drugs, such as aminoglycoside antibiotics and certain antineoplastic agents. It can also augment corticosteroid-induced potassium loss.

Toxicity and side-effects

The immediate side-effects of amphotericin B micellar suspension include fever, rigors, headache, backache, vomiting and thrombophlebitis. These unpleasant reactions differ from patient to patient, but are most common during the first week of treatment and often diminish thereafter. Infusion-related reactions are uncommon in patients receiving liposomal amphotericin B, but fever, rigors and hypotension have developed in up to 40% of patients given amphotericin B colloidal dispersion.

In the longer term, the most serious toxic effect of the conventional micellar suspension formulation is renal tubular damage. This is almost invariable with effective courses, and to some extent irreversible. Hypokalaemia (treated with oral potassium supplements) and mild anaemia (unresponsive to iron, and not usually requiring transfusion) are also common. Renal function should be measured at regular intervals and the treatment interrupted or the dosage modified if the serum creatinine concentration exceeds 250 mol/l. Intravenous sodium supplementation may help to prevent amphotericin-induced renal damage. Patients who have developed renal impairment while receiving the conventional formulation of amphotericin B have improved or stabilized when lipid-associated amphotericin B was substituted, even when the dose was increased.

Clinical use

Amphotericin B is still the drug of choice in most systemic fungal infections seen in Europe, giving the best chance of cure in disseminated candidosis, cryptococcosis and aspergillosis and the only hope of success in mucormycosis. It may advantageously be combined with flucytosine in cryptococcosis, and this combination is often used in systemic candidosis. Other uses of combinations of flucytosine or other drugs with amphotericin B are more controversial. The results of small open trials with the lipid-associated formulations of amphotericin B in aspergillosis, systemic candidosis and cryptococcosis have been encouraging, but proof of their effectiveness will only come from larger randomized trials. In the meantime it is reasonable to use a lipid-associated formulation in a patient with an invasive fungal infection who has failed to respond to conventional amphotericin B or in whom the conventional formulation is contraindicated because of renal impairment.

For the micellar suspension formulation, a 'test' dose of 1 mg in 50–100 ml 5% dextrose is given over 1–2 h (0.5 mg in children weighing <30 kg), with general clinical observation and monitoring of temperature, pulse and blood pressure. If this is well tolerated there can be progression to larger doses. In patients who are not immunocompromised or seriously ill, optimal dosage can be achieved gradually with daily augmentation of the dose over 5–7 days. In other circumstances the dosage is increased more rapidly, as the patient's tolerance of the drug allows. Rapid augmentation of the dose carries the risk of acute renal failure, but immunocompromised patients generally tolerate these regimens well. Appropriate regimens for adults are shown in Table 36.2. The patient's renal function should be monitored frequently and the treatment interrupted or the dosage temporarily modified if the plasma urea exceeds 15 mmol/l or the plasma creatinine exceeds 250 mol/l. Plasma potassium concentrations and haemoglobin should also be followed. Laboratory determination of sensitivity of isolates is not usually advantageous unless there is an unusual fungal species of variable sensitivity or a failure of treatment with reisolation of the causative organism. Likewise, assay of serum concentration is not usually thought to be helpful.

When optimal dosage has been reached, and the patient's condition is stable, it is possible to change to alternate daily or even thrice weekly infusions, as the drug persists for long periods. The duration of therapy depends upon the infection and the underlying illness of the patient. Oesophageal candidosis may respond in days; 2–3 weeks may be required for candidaemia; and 6–10 weeks may be necessary for aspergillosis and cryptococcosis.

The optimal dosage and duration of use of the lipid-associated formulations has not been established. Doses of up to 6 mg/kg of liposomal amphotericin B have been well tolerated. It appears that gradual escalation of drug dose is not required. However, it is recommended that treatment with lipid-associated amphotericin B is started at a dosage of 1 mg/kg, with a stepwise increase in dose in 1 mg/kg increments as required.

The recommended adult and paediatric dose of amphotericin B lipid complex for deep-seated fungal infections is 5 mg/kg, given as a single infusion at a rate of 2.5 mg/kg per hour. It is always advisable to precede larger doses with a 1 mg test dose.

The conventional intravenous preparation of amphotericin is useful for local treatment of yeast infections of the bladder (50 mg/l in sterile water, by continuous irrigation, or by intermittent instillation of 200–300 ml three to four times daily for 5–7 days). Intrathecal use (0.1–0.5 mg, with 10–20 mg hydrocortisone, well diluted in CSF, 2–3 times weekly) is reserved for patients with CNS infections that fail to respond to parenteral treatment, or in whom full parenteral dosage cannot be given because of renal failure. This use is laborious and liable to be complicated by headache, vomiting and arachnoiditis. Amphotericin B has also been administered by instillation into cavities and injection into joints.

Table 36.2 *Regimens (adults) for administration of intravenous amphotericin B, to achieve effective dosage rapidly*

Time infusion started (h)	Duration of infusion (h)	Amphotericin B dosage (mg)	Volume of infusion (ml)
Rapid regimen			
0	2	1	50
2	5	9	450
12	6	10	500
24	6	20	500
48	6	30	1000
(Then every 24 h, with increments of 10 mg until optimal dosage is reached)			
Very rapid regimen (for grave infection in the compromised patient)			
0	2	1	100
4	6	24	900
16	6	25	1000
Then at 24-h intervals	6	Optimal dosage*	1000
(Satisfactory tolerance of each infusion is necessary for proceeding to next increment; see text)			

* Optimal dosage: usually 0.5–0.6 mg/kg per day; not to exceed 50 mg/day (see text).

Preparations and dosage

Proprietary names: Fungilin, Fungizone, AmBisome, Amphocil, Abelcet.

Preparations: Tablets, lozenges, suspension, i.v. infusion, lipid formulation.

Dosage: Adults, oral, 100–200 mg, 4 times daily. Lozenges, 1–2, 4 times daily. Infants and children, 1 ml of suspension 4 times daily. I.v. infusion, adults and children, 0.25 mg/kg daily gradually increasing to 1 mg/kg daily. In severely ill patients the dose can be increased to 1.5 mg/kg daily. Lipid formulations, adults and children, i.v. infusion 1–5 mg/kg daily as a single dose, daily.

Widely available.

Further information

Gallis H A, Drew R H, Packard W W 1990 Amphotericin B: 30 years of clinical experience. *Reviews of Infectious Diseases* 12: 308–329

Graybill J R 1996 Lipid formulations for amphotericin B: does the emperor need new clothes? *Annals of Internal Medicine* 124: 921–923

Hay R J 1994 Liposomal amphotericin B, AmBisome. *Journal of Infection* 28 (suppl 1): 35–43

Janknegt R, de Marie S, Bakker-Woudenberg I A, Crommelin D 1992 Liposomal and lipid formulations of amphotericin B: clinical pharmacokinetics. *Clinical Pharmacokinetics* 23: 279–291

Khoo S H, Bond J, Denning D W 1994 Administering amphotericin B – a practical approach. *Journal of Antimicrobial Chemotherapy* 33: 203–213

Medoff G 1987 Controversial areas in antifungal chemotherapy: short-course and combination therapy with amphotericin B. *Reviews of Infectious Diseases* 9: 403–407

Meyer R D 1992 Current role of therapy with amphotericin B. *Clinical Infectious Diseases* 14 (suppl 1): S154–S160

Walsh T J, Lee J, Lecciones J et al 1991 Empiric therapy with amphotericin B in febrile granulocytopenic patients. *Reviews of Infectious Diseases* 13: 496–503

Other systemic agents

FLUCYTOSINE, 5-FLUOROCYTOSINE

A synthetic fluorinated pyrimidine.

Antimicrobial activity

Flucytosine has a restricted spectrum of activity including *Candida* spp., *Cryp. neoformans* and some fungi causing chromoblastomycosis. It is transported across the membrane of susceptible fungal cells by the action of cytosine permease and then deaminated to 5-fluorouracil, which is incorporated into RNA in place of uracil, with resulting abnormalities of protein synthesis. In addition, it blocks thymidylate synthetase causing inhibition of fungal DNA synthesis.

Acquired resistance

The usefulness of flucytosine is further limited by the pretreatment occurrence of resistant strains (about 10% of *Cand. albicans* isolates, and more in some centres), and the development of resistance during treatment. The most common cause of resistance appears to be loss of the enzyme uridine monophosphate pyrophosphorylase.

Pharmacokinetics

Oral administration of flucytosine leads to rapid and almost complete absorption of the drug. A dose of 25 mg/kg given at 6-h intervals will give a peak serum concentration at 1–2 h of 70–80 mg/l. Absorption is slower in persons with impaired renal function, but peak concentrations are higher. The protein binding of flucytosine is low (about 12%), resulting in high levels of circulating unbound drug. Levels in the CSF are around 75% of the simultaneous serum concentration. More than 90% of a dose of flucytosine is excreted in the urine in unchanged form. The serum half-life is 3–6 h, but is much longer in renal failure, necessitating modification of the dosage regimen.

The nephrotoxic effects of amphotericin B can result in elevated blood concentrations of flucytosine, and levels of the latter drug should be monitored when these compounds are administered together.

Toxicity and side-effects

Nausea, vomiting and diarrhoea are the commonest side-effects. Thrombocytopenia and leucopenia can occur if excessive blood concentrations of flucytosine (more than 100 mg/l) are maintained. The effect is usually reversible if treatment is discontinued. Elevated transaminase levels develop in some patients, but usually return to normal after the drug is stopped. Liver necrosis leading or contributing to death has been reported in occasional patients.

Clinical use

Flucytosine as a single drug (100–150 mg/kg daily in four divided doses) is indicated only in lower urinary tract candidosis and possibly in chromoblastomycosis caused by susceptible fungi. Its principal use is in combination with amphotericin B in the treatment of cryptococcosis, systemic candidosis and fungal endocarditis. It has been suggested that the combination may also be beneficial in severe or unresponsive aspergillosis. The lower dose of amphotericin (0.3–0.5 mg/kg daily) is advantageous, but monitoring of flucytosine concentrations is essential. Indeed, assay of serum concentrations is desirable in all patients, and mandatory in those with renal impairment in whom the dosage must be modified (Table 36.1).

Table 36.1 *Regimens for administration of flucytosine in renal failure**

Creatinine clearance (ml/min)	Individual dosage (mg/kg)	Dosage interval (h)
>40	(25–) 37.5	6
40–20	(25–) 37.5	12
20–10	(25–) 37.5	24
<10		>24†

* Renal function is considered to be normal when creatinine clearance is greater than 40–50 ml/min or the concentration of creatinine in serum is less than 180 mmol/l; concentration of creatinine in serum is not reliable unless renal function is stable.
† Dosage interval must be based on serum drug concentration measurement at frequent intervals. Maximum serum concentration should not exceed 80 mg/l.

Preparations and dosage

Proprietary name: Alcobon.

Preparations: Tablets, i.v. infusion.

Dosage: Adults, oral, i.v., 200 mg/kg daily in 4 divided doses. For extremely sensitive organisms, 100–150 mg/kg daily may be sufficient.

Widely available.

Further information

Scholer H J 1980 Flucytosine. In: Speller D C E (ed) Antifungal chemotherapy. Wiley, Chichester, ch 2, p 35–106

Scholer H J, Polak A 1984 Resistance to systemic antifungal agents. In: Bryan L E (ed) Antimicrobial drug resistance. Academic Press, Orlando, p 393–460

Wise G J, Kozinn P J, Goldberg P 1982 Flucytosine in the management of genitourinary candidiasis: 5 years of experience. *Journal of Urology* 124: 70–72

Working Group of the British Society for Mycopathology 1984 Laboratory methods for flucytosine (5-fluorocytosine). *Journal of Antimicrobial Chemotherapy* 14: 1–8

GRISEOFULVIN

A fermentation product of various species of *Penicillium*, including *Penicillium griseofulvum*.

Antimicrobial activity

It has a limited spectrum of activity and its clinical use is restricted to the dermatophytoses. Griseofulvin binds to microtubular proteins and inhibits fungal cell mitosis. It also acts as an inhibitor of nucleic acid biosynthesis.

Acquired resistance

This has seldom been reported.

Pharmacokinetics

Absorption of griseofulvin from the gastro-intestinal tract is dependent on drug formulation. Administration with a high-fat meal will increase the rate and extent of absorption, but individuals tend to achieve consistently high or low blood concentrations. It appears in the stratum corneum within 4–8 h, as a result of secretion in perspiration. However, levels begin to fall soon after the drug is discontinued, and within 48–72 h it can no longer be detected. Griseofulvin is metabolized in the liver, the metabolites then being excreted in the urine. The drug has an elimination half-life of 9–21 h. Griseofulvin can diminish the anticoagulant effect of warfarin. Its absorption is reduced in persons receiving concomitant treatment with phenobarbitone.

Toxicity and side-effects

Up to 15% of patients treated with griseofulvin develop adverse reactions. These include headache, nausea and abdominal discomfort. Occasional patients develop urticarial reactions or erythematous rashes. The drug should not be used in persons with liver disease.

Clinical use

It is indicated for moderate to severe dermatophytoses of the skin, scalp hair or nails where topical treatment is considered inappropriate or has failed. It is important to adjust the dose to the weight of the patient, most of whom require treatment for 4 weeks or more. Long courses (usually 4–8 months) and high doses may be needed for nail infections.

Preparations and dosage

Proprietary names: Grisovin, Fulcin.

Preparations: Tablets, suspension.

Dosage: Adults, oral, 500 mg/day as a single or divided dose. In severe infections the dose may be doubled, reducing when response occurs. Children, 10 mg/kg daily in divided doses, or as a single dose.

Widely available.

Further information

Davies R R 1980 Griseofulvin. In: Speller D C E (ed) Antifungal chemotherapy. Wiley, Chichester, ch 4, p 149–182

Roberts S O B 1980 Treatment of superficial and sub-cutaneous mycoses. In: Speller D C E (ed) Antifungal chemotherapy. Wiley, Chichester, ch 7, p 225–283

Other topical agents

AMOROLFINE

This synthetic phenylmorpholine derivative is an ergosterol biosynthesis inhibitor. It is active against the dermatophytes and some moulds that cause onychomycosis.

Preparations and dosage

Proprietary name: Loceryl.

Preparation: Nail lacquer.

Dosage: Applied once or twice weekly.

Widely available.

Further information

Hay R J (ed) 1992 Amorolfine: an innovation in antimycotic therapy. *Clinical and Experimental Dermatology* 17 (suppl 1)

MISCELLANEOUS DRUGS

There is also a large and miscellaneous group of topical antifungal agents, such as tolnaftate, cicloprixolamine and haloprogin, all of which are effective treatments for superficial mycoses.

- **Tolnaftate** A thiocarbamate used in tinea pedis, although it is less effective than azole antifungals. It is ineffective in candidosis.
- **Ciclopiroxolamine** A 1% cream is effective in cutaneous candidioasis, pityriasis versicolor, tinea pedis and tinea cruris. It is ineffective in nail infections.
- **Haloprogin** A halogenated phenolic which is effective in pityriasis versicolor and the dermatophytoses.

37

Antimycobacterial agents

J. Grange

Introduction

The mycobacteria causing human disease, and therefore requiring treatment by antibacterial agents, are divisible into three groups: the tuberculosis complex (Mycobacterium tuberculosis, Mycobacterium bovis and Mycobacterium africanum), the leprosy bacillus (Mycobacterium leprae) and various environmental saprophytes that occasionally cause human disease. Patients with acquired immune deficiency syndrome (AIDS) are particularly likely to develop disease due to the latter species, notably the Mycobacterium avium complex (MAC).

Antimycobacterial agents include natural and semi-synthetic antibiotics and synthetic agents. Some agents are active against a wide range of bacteria, but their use is mostly restricted to the treatment of mycobacterial disease and some are active only against mycobacteria. In recent years, the occurrence of multidrug resistant tuberculosis has led to the increasing use of agents principally used for other infections. These include macrolides, quinolones and minocycline. The two rapidly growing mycobacteria that cause disease in man, Mycobacterium chelonae and Mycobacterium fortuitum, are resistant to the standard antituberculosis agents, but are often susceptible to agents used for other purposes, including macrolides, quinolones, sulphonamides, trimethoprim, cephalosporins, gentamicin and amikacin.

The rifamycins are among the most important of the antimycobacterial agents. Rifampicin is included in drug regimens for the treatment of tuberculosis and leprosy and rifabutin is effective against MAC infection in AIDS patients. The aminoglycoside streptomycin is used in some anti-tuberculosis regimens, particularly when resistance to other agents is suspected or known. Other aminoglycosides,

notably amikacin, are sometimes used in the treatment of disease due to environmental mycobacteria, particularly AIDS-related MAC infection.

Synthetic agents, which for practical purposes are only active against mycobacteria, are chemically diverse and were principally found as a result of extensive screening of compounds for activity against M. tuberculosis. Isoniazid and pyrazinamide are principal components of modern short-course antituberculosis regimens. Ethambutol is often included in short-course antituberculosis regimens, especially when resistance to one of the other drugs is suspected or intermittent therapy (twice- or thrice-weekly doses) is used. p-aminosalicylic acid, a key component of antituberculosis regimens in the pre-rifampicin era, is now rarely used except for multidrug resistant tuberculosis. Thiacetazone is still used in some countries on account of its cheapness, although it is of poor efficacy and toxic side-effects, especially rashes and the more serious exfoliative dermatitis, are common. Ethionamide and the closely related prothionamide are used for treating drug-resistant tuber-culosis and leprosy. Dapsone is the key drug in the treatment of leprosy, although it is now used together with rifampicin and clofazimine. The latter drug is also used, principally with rifabutin and the newer macrolides, for the treatment of AIDS-related MAC infection.

Antimicrobial activity

The action of antimycobacterial agents in vivo depends on the population dynamics of the mycobacteria within the lesions. In the case of tuberculosis, some bacilli replicate freely in the walls of well-oxygenated cavities, some replicate more slowly in acidic and anoxic tissue and within macrophages and a few are in a near-dormant 'persister' state. Isoniazid exerts a powerful and rapid bactericidal activity against the freely replicating bacilli, but has little or no effect against the near-dormant bacilli. The latter are killed by rifampicin, while the slowly replicating bacilli in acidic environments are killed by pyrazinamide, which is only active at low pH. Thus a distinction is drawn between agents that are bactericidal in vitro and those that actually 'sterilize' lesions in vivo. Accordingly, modern short-course antituberculosis regimens commence with an intensive phase of isoniazid, rifampicin and pyrazinamide during which all except a few persisters are killed, and a continuation phase of rifampicin which kills persisters during shorter bursts of metabolic activity. A second drug, usually isoniazid, is included in the continuation phase to kill any rifampicin-resistant mutants that commence replication. Ethambutol and streptomycin, included in some short-course regimens, add little if the organisms are fully susceptible.

In both tuberculosis and leprosy, the great majority of bacilli are killed during the first few weeks of therapy; prolonged therapy, with its associated problems of cost, compliance and the need for supervision, is required to kill a few remaining metabolically inactive persisters and thus prevent relapse. Accordingly, attempts have been made to stimulate the immune system to destroy these residual bacilli and success has been obtained by the use of a heat-killed injectable suspension of a rapidly growing mycobacterium, *Mycobacterium vaccae*, as an adjunct to chemotherapy in both drug-susceptible and drug-resistant tuberculosis.

In the absence of acquired drug resistance, strains of *M. tuberculosis* and related members of the tuberculosis complex are remarkably constant in their susceptibility to the antituberculosis drugs. All strains of *M. bovis* and some strains of *M. africanum* are, however, naturally resistant to pyrazinamide. Environmental mycobacteria are often resistant to antituberculosis agents in vitro, although in patients with disease due to the slowly growing species (*Mycobacterium kansasii*, *Mycobacterium xenopi*, *Mycobacterium avium/Mycobacterium intracellulare* and *Mycobacterium malmoense*) good clinical responses to regimens containing rifampicin, ethambutol and isoniazid often occur. The rapidly growing pathogens *M. chelonae* and *M. fortuitum*, are resistant to the antituberculosis drugs but susceptible to a range of other agents.

Acquired resistance

Mutation to drug resistance occurs at a low but constant rate in all mycobacterial populations and such mutants are readily selected if the patient is treated with a single drug. Successful therapy thus requires the use of at least two drugs to which the strain is susceptible. An exception is the use of a single drug, usually isoniazid, to prevent the emergence of active tuberculosis in infected but healthy persons who are assumed to have very small numbers of bacilli in their tissues. Emergence of drug resistance is very uncommon in patients receiving a full course of modern short-course chemotherapy based on drugs of known quality.

Unfortunately, poor prescribing habits, unavailability of drugs, inadvertent use of time-expired or even counterfeit drugs, poor supervision of therapy and unregulated 'over-the-counter' sales of drugs has led to the emergence of single- or multiple-drug-resistant tubercle bacilli in many countries. Resistance may develop in an inadequately treated patient (acquired or secondary resistance) or a person may become infected with a resistant strain (initial or primary resistance). Likewise, primary and acquired drug resistance is encountered in leprosy and the World Health Organization (WHO) has therefore advised that all cases of leprosy should be treated by combination therapy.

The WHO recommends that surveys of primary drug resistance should be undertaken as these give a good measure of the efficiency of control programmes. The extent to which such surveys have been, and are being, carried out varies considerably from country to country. Whereas in developed nations drug susceptibility tests are carried out on most clinical isolates of *M. tuberculosis*, such testing is often only carried out sporadically, and perhaps on unrepresentative isolates, in many developing countries. Figure 37.1 shows the range of reported incidences of initial drug resistance from countries in the WHO regions in the years 1988–1992.

Trends in drug resistance also vary from region to region. In the USA, the incidence of initial resistance to isoniazid rose fairly steadily from less than 2% in 1961–1968 to 9% in 1991. Rifampicin and multidrug (rifampicin and isoniazid) resistance rose from less than 1% in 1982–1986 to almost 4% in 1991. There is also considerable regional variation; in New York, where about 40% of tuberculosis patients were human immunodeficiency virus (HIV) positive, 19% of isolates were multidrug resistant in 1991. It is important to note that HIV per se does not cause drug resistance, but facilitates its more rapid dissemination in the community. In the UK and Zaire, the prevalence of drug resistance is no greater in HIV-positive patients than in those who are HIV negative.

Within a country, ethnic differences are observed, with higher incidences of drug resistance in populations originating in regions where such resistance is prevalent. Table 37.1 shows the percentages of drug-resistant strains according to ethnic origin in south-east England.

Well-organized tuberculosis-control programmes can reduce the incidence of both initial and acquired drug resistance. In south Korea the incidence of initial resistance to any single drug dropped from 30.6% in 1980 to 15% in 1990, and in Algeria there was a drop from 15% to 6.3% between 1981 and 1985.

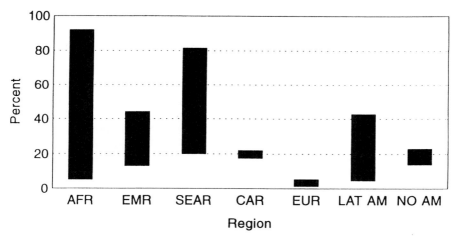

Fig. 37.1 *Range of initial tuberculosis drug resistance data, WHO world regions 1988–1992. AFR, Africa; EMR, Eastern Mediterranean; SEAR, South-East Asia; CAR, Caribbean; EUR, European; LAT AM, Latin America; NO AM, North America. Reproduced by permission of the WHO Tuberculosis Unit.*

Table 37.1 *Drug resistant* M. tuberculosis *isolated in south-east England, 1984–1991, according to the ethnic origin of the patient*

Resistance*	European (n = 4594)		Indian subcontinent (n = 4099)		Other (n = 625)	
	No.	%	No.	%	No.	%
Single drug						
INH	60	1.3	119	2.9	16	2.56
SM	30	0.65	72	1.76	21	3.36
PZA	15	0.33	12	0.29	2	0.32
RIF	3	<0.1	5	0.12	1	0.16
EMB	1	<0.1	–		–	
Two drugs						
INH + SM	16	0.35	83	2.02	22	3.52
INH + RIF	4	<0.1	4	<0.1	4	0.64
Other	1	<0.1	7	0.17	–	–
Three drugs	1	<0.1	28	0.68	1	0.16
Four drugs	1	<0.1	14	0.34	5	0.8
Five drugs	1	<0.1	3	<0.1	1	0.16
Six drugs	–	–	1	<0.1	–	–
Total	133	2.9	348	8.5	73†	11.7

* EMB, ethambutol; INH, isoniazid; PZA, pyrazinamide; RIF, rifampicin; SM, streptomycin.
† 35, Africa; 31, Far East; 7, other.

Pharmacokinetics

With the exception of streptomycin (and other aminoglycosides) and the peptides, all the antimycobacterial agents currently in use are absorbed adequately when given orally. They are distributed to all tissues and organs and adequate amounts of the first-line antituberculosis agents cross the blood–brain barrier. Thus, in principle, standard regimens and doses are suitable for treatment of all forms of tuberculosis, although many clinicians prescribe more prolonged courses of therapy for extrapulmonary tuberculosis, particularly tuberculous meningitis. Rifampicin, isoniazid, pyrazinamide, ethionamide and prothionamide are either eliminated in the bile or metabolized, and may therefore be given in standard doses to patients with impaired renal function. Ethambutol is eliminated predominantly by the kidney, and streptomycin and other aminoglycosides are excreted entirely by the kidney: these drugs should be avoided, if possible, in patients with impaired renal function.

Small amounts of isoniazid and even smaller amounts of the other antituberculosis drugs enter the milk, so breast feeding is not contraindicated.

Toxicity and side-effects

Unwanted side-effects occur with all antituberculosis agents, but those caused by the first-line drugs (rifampicin, isoniazid, pyrazinamide) are less frequent and severe than those due to the older agents (streptomycin, *p*-aminosalicylic acid, thiacetazone). Side-effects are particularly likely to occur in HIV-positive patients who should never be given thiacetazone as fatal exfoliative dermatitis may occur. Specific toxicities are discussed under the individual drugs. Transient and clinically insignificant rise in serum hepatic enzyme levels commonly occurs during the first few weeks of therapy and, unless the patient is known to have liver disease, routine assay of these enzymes is unnecessary.

Clinically evident hepatitis occurs in about 1% of patients and the incidence increases with age. It usually resolves rapidly when therapy is stopped. In most cases therapy with the same drugs can be continued. More generalized reactions, with rashes, influenza-like symptoms and, sometimes, lymphadenopathy and hepatic enlargement with or without jaundice may occur in the first 2 months of therapy. Therapy must be stopped, the responsible drug identified by giving small challenge doses sequentially, and treatment resumed with omission of that drug.

Interactions between the antimycobacterial drugs themselves have been described: pyrazinamide and ethionamide may increase serum concentrations of isoniazid, while pyrazinamide may decrease that of rifampicin, but these effects are of no known clinical significance. More significant interactions occur between the antimycobacterial agents and drugs used for other purposes. Most recorded drug interactions involve rifampicin (p. 106) and quinolones (p. 104) but some interactions with isoniazid have been described, especially in slow acetylators (p. 509). In particular, isoniazid increases the plasma concentrations of the antiepileptics phenytoin and carbamazepine, sometimes enough to cause toxicity. It enhances the defluorination of the anaesthetic enfluorane. The bioavailability of both isoniazid and ethambutol is reduced by aluminium hydroxide.

Clinical use

There are four principal clinical uses for the antimyco-bacterial drugs: tuberculosis, leprosy, other mycobacterial infections in HIV-negative persons (Ch. 59) and such infections in HIV-positive persons (p. 668). Definite recommendations for the first two uses have been made by the WHO and these regimens are also used for treating human tuberculosis due to *M. bovis* and for the rare cases of disseminated disease due to the vaccine strain Bacille Calmette–Guerin (BCG), although both are naturally resistant to pyrazinamide.

Opinions differ as to the most suitable regimens for other mycobacterial infections. While standard regimens have been proposed, drug susceptibilities vary from species to species, and from strain to strain, so that some workers advocate individualized therapy.

The British and American Thoracic Societies recommend an 18-month course of rifampicin, ethambutol and isoniazid for treatment of pulmonary disease due to MAC, *M. kansasii, M. xenopi* and *M. malmoense.* The need for isoniazid has been questioned, but ethambutol is a key component and must be given throughout. A nine month course appears adequate for *M. kansasii.* These recommendations are likely to be revised when the results of trials involving quinolones and macrolides are available.

HIV-related disease, which is usually caused by MAC, was treated with regimens containing rifabutin, clofazimine and ethambutol. The US Task Force on MAC now recommends that all patients should receive clarithromycin or azithromycin with companion drugs selected on the basis of in vitro susceptibility tests.

No controlled clinical trials on the therapy of disease due to the rapidly growing mycobacteria *M. chelonae* and *M. fortuitum* have been carried out. Therapy is therefore empirical, but may be assisted by in vitro susceptibility testing. Limited infections such as postinjection abscesses respond to trimethoprim with sulphamethoxazole together with erythromycin. More serious infections have responded to cefoxitin with amikacin. The outcome of therapy is, however, very unpredictable.

Formulations

Compliance with antituberculosis therapy is aided by use of combination drug preparations and calendar blister-packs. Examples of combination preparations are rifampicin + isoniazid (Rifinah, Rimactizid), isoniazid with ethambutol (Mynah), rifampicin + isoniazid + pyrazinamide (Rifater), and dapsone + prothionamide + isoniazid (Isoprodian). It is essential that combination drugs be obtained from reputable manufacturers as the bioavailability of the component drugs may be seriously affected by the manufacturing process. Blister-packs are available for treatment of paucibacillary and multibacillary leprosy (PB-Combi, MB-Combi).

Further information

Acocella G 1990 The use of fixed-dose combinations in antituberculosis chemotherapy. Rationale for their application in daily, intermittent and pediatric regimens. *Bulletin of the International Union Against Tuberculosis and Lung Disease* 65 (2–3): 77–83

Baker R J 1990 The need for new drugs in the treatment and control of leprosy. *International Journal of Leprosy* 58: 78–97

Bartmann K (ed) 1988 Antituberculosis drugs. In: Handbook of experimental pharmacology, vol 84. Springer, Berlin

Bartmann K 1991 Clinical evaluation of the efficacy of antituberculosis chemotherapy. A review of the methods. *Zeitung der Erkrankungen Atmungsorgane* 177: 6–19

Centres for Disease Control and Prevention 1993 Initial therapy for tuberculosis in the era of multidrug resistance. Recommendations of the Advisory Council for the Elimination of Tuberculosis. *Journal of the American Medical Association* 270: 694–698

Ellard G A, Humphries M J, Allen B W 1993 Cerebrospinal fluid drug concentrations and the treatment of tuberculous meningitis. *American Review of Respiratory Disease* 148: 650–655

Fox W 1990 Drug combinations and the bioavailability of rifampicin. *Tubercule* 71: 241–245

Grange J M, Winstanley P A, Davies P D O 1994 Clinically significant drug interactions with antituberculosis agents. *Drug Safety* 11: 242–251

Grosset J H 1992 Treatment of tuberculosis in HIV infection. *Tubercle and Lung Disease* 73: 378–383

Grosset J H 1994 Progress in the chemotherapy of leprosy *International Journal of Leprosy* 62: 268–277

Heifets L B (ed) 1991 Drug susceptibility in the chemotherapy of mycobacterial infections. CRC Press, Boca Raton, FL

Heifets L B 1994 Antimycobacterial drugs. *Seminars in Respiratory Infections* 9: 84–103

Hopewell P 1992 Evaluation of new anti-infective drugs for the treatment and prevention of tuberculosis. *Clinical Infectious Diseases* 15 (suppl 1): S282–S295

Iseman M D 1993 Treatment of multidrug resistant tuberculosis. *New England Journal of Medicine* 329: 784–791

Israel H L 1993 Chemoprophylaxis for tuberculosis. *Respiratory Medicine* 87: 81–83

Mitchison D A 1985 The action of antituberculosis drugs in short course chemotherapy. *Tubercle* 66: 219–225

Mitchison D A 1992 The Garrod lecture. Understanding the chemotherapy of tuberculosis in current problems. *Journal of Antimicrobial Chemotherapy* 29: 477–493

Stanford J L, Stanford C A, Rook G A W, Grange J M 1994 Immunotherapy for tuberculosis. Investigative and practical aspects. *Clinical Immunotherapeutics* 1: 430–440

Winstanley P A 1994 The clinical pharmacology of anti-tuberculosis drugs. In: Davies P D O (ed) Clinical tuberculosis. Chapman & Hall, London, p 129–140

World Health Organization 1991 WHO model prescribing information. Drugs used in mycobacterial diseases. WHO, Geneva

AMINOSALICYLIC ACID
p-Aminosalicylic acid; PAS

Antimicrobial activity

Originally thought to be a competitive inhibitor of *p*-aminobenzoic acid in the folic acid synthetic pathway, it is now more likely that it interferes with the salicylate-dependent biosynthesis of iron-chelating lipids termed 'mycobactins'. Inhibitory concentrations for *M. tuberculosis* are reported to be 0.5–10 mg/l, depending on the medium used and the inoculum size. Other mycobacterial species are resistant to 8 mg/l. Its activity is bacteriostatic.

Acquired resistance

Resistance is very uncommon as the drug is rarely used.

Pharmacokinetics

It is readily absorbed from the intestine; a dose of 4 g gives a peak plasma concentration of 70–80 mg/l at 1–2 h (many publications erroneously cite concentrations of 7–8 mg/l). The plasma elimination half-life is 0.75–1.0 h. It is rapidly acetylated in the liver and about 80% is excreted in the urine, mostly in the acetylated form.

Toxicity and side-effects

Adverse effects, leading to problems of compliance, occur in 10–30% of patients. Gastro-intestinal effects, including abdominal pain, nausea and diarrhoea are very common. It interferes with iodine metabolism in the thyroid, and prolonged therapy may lead to goitre, and less frequently to myxoedema, which respond to thyroxine therapy. Allergic skin reactions are common. Other less common reactions include blood dyscrasias, crystalluria, a syndrome resembling infectious mononucleosis and, rarely, Löeffler's syndrome and encephalitis.

Clinical use

It was virtually abandoned following the introduction of modern short-course antituberculosis regimens, but is now occasionally included in regimens for the treatment of multidrug-resistant tuberculosis.

Preparations and dosage

Dosage: Adults and children, oral, 150–300 mg/kg per day in 2 divided doses.
Limited availability; not available in the UK.

Further information

Held H, Fried F 1977 Elimination of para-aminosalicylic acid in patients with liver disease and renal insufficiency. *Chemotherapy* 23: 405–415

Lehmann J 1969 The role of metabolism of *p*-aminosalicylic acid (PAS) in the treatment of tuberculosis. *Scandinavian Journal of Respiratory Diseases* 50: 169–185

Trnka L, Mison P 1988 *p*-Aminosalicylic acid (PAS). In: Bartmann K (ed) Antituberculosis drugs (Handbook of experimental pharmacology, vol 84). Springer, Berlin, p 191–197

CAPREOMYCIN

A mixture of four cyclic polypeptides, CM IA, CM IB, CM IIA and CM IIB, produced by *Streptomyces capreolus*. It is supplied as a water-soluble sulphate and at least 90% consists of capreomycin IA and IB.

Antimicrobial activity

There is little direct information on its mode of action, but as it is structurally similar to viomycin, and shows cross-resistance, it is likely that the two agents act similarly (p. 512).

It inhibits *M. tuberculosis*, including strains resistant to most other antituberculosis agents, at a minimum inhibitory concentration (MIC) of 1.25–2.5 mg/l in liquid media. MICs are higher (8–16 mg/l) on egg media owing to protein binding. It has not been adequately determined whether it is bacteriostatic or bactericidal.

Acquired resistance

Resistant strains are cross-resistant with viomycin and partly cross-resistant with aminoglycosides.

Pharmacokinetics

It is not absorbed from the intestine. Intramuscular injection of 1 g gives peak serum concentrations of 30–50 mg/l. It is mostly excreted unchanged in the urine. No metabolites have been described.

Toxicity and side-effects

Pain, induration and excessive bleeding may occur at the injection site. It is ototoxic, affecting both cochlear and vestibular functions, and nephrotoxic, causing loss of K^+, Ca^{2+} and Mg^{2+}, leading to neuromuscular blockade. These toxic effects are uncommon if the drug is given two or three times weekly.

Clinical use

It is very rarely used for the treatment of tuberculosis, except in occasional cases of multidrug resistance. It has no established place in the therapy of other mycobacterial infections. Auditory and vestibular functions and serum K^+ should be monitored before and regularly during therapy.

Preparations and dosage

Proprietary name: Capastat.

Preparation: Injection.

Dosage: Adults, deep i.m. injection, 1 g/day (with a maximum of 20 mg/kg) for 2–4 months, then 1 g 2–3 times a week for the remainder of the therapy.

Limited availability, including the UK and the USA.

Further information

Black H R, Griffith R S, Peabody A M 1966 Absorption, excretion and metabolism of capreomycin in normal and diseased states. *Annals of the New York Academy of Science* 135: 974–982

Heifets L, Lindholm-Levy P 1989 Comparison of bactericidal activities of streptomycin, amikacin, kanamycin and capreomycin against *Mycobacterium avium* and *Mycobacterium tuberculosis*. *Antimicrobial Agents and Chemotherapy* 33: 1298–1301

Lehmann C R, Garrett L E, Winn R E et al 1988 Capreomycin kinetics in renal impairment and clearance by hemodialysis. *American Review of Respiratory Disease* 138: 1312–1313

Otten H 1988 Capreomycin. In Bartmann K (ed) Antituberculosis drugs (Handbook of experimental pharmacology, vol 84). Springer, Berlin, p 191–197

CLOFAZIMINE

One of a number of substituted iminophenazines originally produced as potential antituberculosis agents. It stimulates various phagocyte functions including release of free oxygen radicals, but it is not clear whether this is its sole mode of action. There is some evidence that it resembles rifampicin in interfering with RNA polymerase activity. It also has anti-inflammatory properties, probably due to its ability to stimulate prostaglandin E_2 synthesis and release.

Antimicrobial activity

It is active against several species of mycobacteria and some species of *Actinomyces* and *Nocardia*. In vitro MICs (mg/l) are: *M. tuberculosis*, 0.5; *M. scrofulaceum*, 0.5; *M. leprae*, 0.1–1; *M. avium/intracellulare*, 1–2; *M. chelonae*, 0.2–4; and *M. fortuitum*, 0.5–8 mg/l. These MICs have limited clinical relevance as clofazimine shows marked differences in accumulation in various tissues. It is weakly bactericidal; activity against *M. leprae* is only demonstrable in humans after 50 days of therapy; clofazimine-resistance, though reported, is rare.

Pharmacokinetics

It is well absorbed by the intestine and is taken up by adipose tissue and cells of the macrophage/monocyte series, including those in the wall of the small intestine. It has a very long half-life (70 days) and is eliminated in the urine and faeces.

Toxicity and side-effects

It is usually well tolerated, but some patients develop nausea, abdominal pain and diarrhoea, relieved to some extent by taking the drug with a meal or glass of milk. Dose-related, reversible, skin discolouration is very common and is unacceptable to some patients. Discolouration of the hair, cornea, urine, sweat and tears also occurs. Infants born to mothers receiving clofazimine are reversibly pigmented at birth.

Oedema of the wall of the small intestine leading to subacute obstruction is a rare but serious complication of prolonged, high-dose therapy for leprosy reactions. Deposition of clofazimine in lymph nodes may interfere with lymphatic drainage, occasionally manifesting as oedema of the feet.

Clinical use

Its principal use is in the treatment of multibacillary leprosy, in conjunction with dapsone and rifampicin. Being anti-inflammatory, it is also used to treat leprosy reactions, particularly type 2 reactions (erythema nodosum leprosum). It is included in some multidrug regimens for treatment of disseminated AIDS-related MAC infection. It has been suggested as a drug for treatment of multidrug resistant

tuberculosis, although its efficacy is unproven. It has been used to treat *Mycobacterium ulcerans* infection (Buruli ulcer) but with limited responses.

Preparations and dosage

Proprietary name: Lamprene.

Preparation: Capsules.

Dosage: Multibacillary forms of leprosy: adults, oral, 300 mg once a month, supervised, and 50 mg/day self-administered. Erythema nodosum leprosum: 300 mg once a day for no longer than 3 months.

Limited availability.

Further information

Anderson R, Zeis B M, Anderson I F 1988 Clofazimine-mediated enhancement of reactive oxidant production by human phagocytes as a possible therapeutic mechanism. *Dermatologia* 176: 234–242

Grange J M 1991 Detection of drug resistance in *Mycobacterium leprae* and the design of treatment regimens for leprosy. In: Heifets L (ed) Drug susceptibility in the chemotherapy of mycobacterial infections. CRC Press, Boca Raton, FL, p 161–177

Jamet P, Traore I, Husser J A, Ji B 1992 Short-term trial of clofazimine in previously untreated lepromatous leprosy. *International Journal of Leprosy* 60: 542–548

Levy L 1986 Clofazimine-resistant *M. leprae*. *International Journal of Leprosy* 54: 137–140

Moore U J 1983 A review of the side effects experienced by patients taking clofazimine. *Leprosy Review* 54: 327–335

Oommen S T, Natu M V, Mahajan M K, Kadyan R S 1994 Lymphangiographic evaluation of patients with clinical lepromatous leprosy on clofazimine. *International Journal of Leprosy* 62: 32–36

Schaad-Lanyi Z, Dieterle W, Dubois J P, Theobold W, Vischer W 1987 Pharmacokinetics of clofazimine in healthy volunteers. *International Journal of Leprosy* 55: 9–15

Venkatesan K, Mathur A, Girdhar B K, Bharadwaj V P 1986 The effect of clofazimine on the pharmacokinetics of rifampicin and dapsone in leprosy. *Journal of Antimicrobial Chemotherapy* 18: 715–718

Zeis B M, Anderson R 1986 Clofazimine-mediated stimulation of prostaglandin synthesis and free oxygen radical production as novel mechanisms of drug-induced immunosuppression. *International Journal of Immunopharmacology* 8: 731–739

DAPSONE
Diaminodiphenyl sulphone (DDS)

Antimicrobial activity

It is active against many bacteria and some protozoa. In many susceptible bacteria, including some mycobacteria, it inhibits folic acid synthesis, but this does not appear to be the mode of action in *M. leprae*. Fully susceptible strains of *M. leprae* are inhibited by 0.003 mg/l.

Acquired resistance

Resistance to high levels is acquired by several sequential mutations. As a result of prolonged use of dapsone monotherapy, acquired resistance emerged in patients with multibacillary leprosy in many countries. Initial resistance also occurs in patients with both paucibacillary and multibacillary leprosy. Thus, leprosy should always be treated with multidrug regimens.

Pharmacokinetics

It is slowly but almost completely absorbed from the intestine. It is widely distributed in the tissues but is selectively retained in skin, muscle, kidneys and liver. Peak plasma levels of about 2 mg/l occur 3–6 h after a dose of 100 mg. It is metabolized by *N*-oxidation and also by acetylation which is subject to the same genetic polymorphism seen with isoniazid (p. 509). Thus the elimination half-life varies considerably (18–45 h), but on standard therapy the trough levels are always well in excess of the inhibitory concentrations.

It is mostly excreted in the urine: in the unchanged form (20%), as *N*-oxidation products (30%) and as other metabolites.

Toxicity and side-effects

Although usually well tolerated at standard doses, gastro-intestinal upsets, anorexia, headaches, dizziness and insomnia may occur. Less frequent reactions include skin rashes and photosensitivity, peripheral neuropathy, psychoses, hepatitis, nephrotic syndrome and generalized lymphadenopathy.

The term 'dapsone syndrome' is applied to a skin rash and fever, occurring 2–8 weeks after starting therapy and sometimes accompanied by lymphadenopathy, hepatomegaly, jaundice and/or mononucleosis.

Blood disorders include anaemia, methaemoglobinaemia, haemolysis, notably in patients with glucose-6-phosphate dehydrogenase deficiency, mononucleosis and, rarely, agranulocytosis. Severe anaemia should be treated before patients receive dapsone.

There is some evidence that the incidence of adverse reactions declined in the 1960s but reappeared around 1982, the time when multidrug therapy was introduced, and may represent an unexplained drug interaction with rifampicin.

Clinical use

It is a principal component of multidrug regimens for all forms of leprosy and is used in combination with pyrimethamine (maloprim), in the prophylaxis of malaria and in combination therapy of chloroquine-resistant malaria. It is used in the prophylaxis of toxoplasmosis and, in combination with trimethoprim, for the prophylaxis and therapy of *Pneumocystis carinii* pneumonia (p. 669). There is experimental evidence of efficacy in treatment of MAC infections. It is also used in the treatment of dermatitis herpetiformis and related skin disorders.

Preparations and dosage

Preparations: Tablets. Also available as a combination tablet with prothionamide and isoniazid (Isoprodian).

Dosage: Paucibacillary leprosy (in combination with rifampicin): Adults 100 mg/day, children 1–2 mg/kg daily, for at least 6 months. Multibacillary leprosy (in combination with rifampicin and clofazimine) adults 100 mg/day, children 1–2 mg/kg daily, for at least 2 years. Limited availability; available in the UK.

Further information

Ahrens E M, Meckler R J, Callen J P 1986 Dapsone-induced peripheral neuropathy. *International Journal of Dermatology* 25: 314–316

Byrd S R, Gelber R H 1991 Effect of dapsone on haemoglobin concentration in patients with leprosy. *Leprosy Review* 62: 171–178

Daneshmend T K 1984 The neurotoxicity of dapsone. *Adverse Drug Reactions and Acute Poisoning Reviews* 3: 43–58

Johnson D A, Cattau E L, Kuritsky J N, Zimmerman H J 1986 Liver involvement in the sulphone syndrome. *Archives of Internal Medicine* 146: 875–877

Kromann N P, Vilhelmsen R, Stahl D 1982 The dapsone syndrome. *Archives of Dermatology* 118: 531–532

Rai P P, Aschhoff M, Lilly L, Balakrishnan S 1988 Influence of acetylator phenotype of the leprosy patient on the emergence of dapsone resistant leprosy. *Indian Journal of Leprosy* 60: 400–406

Rastogi N, Goh K S, Labrousse V 1993 Activity of subinhibitory concentrations of dapsone alone and in combination with cell wall inhibitors against *Mycobacterium avium* complex organisms. *European Journal of Clinical Microbiology* 12: 954–958

Richardus J H, Smith T C 1989 Increased incidence in leprosy of hypersensitivity reactions to dapsone after introduction of multidrug therapy. *Leprosy Review* 60: 267–273

Smith W C S 1988 Are hypersensitivity reactions to dapsone becoming more frequent? *Leprosy Review* 59: 53–58

Wozel G, Barth J 1988 Current aspects of the modes of action of dapsone. *International Journal of Dermatology* 27: 547–552

Zuidema J, Hilbers-Modderman E S, Merkus F W 1986 Clinical pharmacokinetics of dapsone. *Clinical Pharmacokinetics* 11: 299–315

ETHAMBUTOL
Hydroxymethylpropylethylene diamine

$$\begin{array}{ccc}
CH_2OH & & C_2H_5 \\
| & & | \\
HC-NH-CH_2-CH_2-NH-CH \\
| & & | \\
C_2H_5 & & CH_2OH
\end{array}$$

Antimicrobial activity

It inhibits the biosynthesis of arabinogalactan, a cell-wall polysaccharide to which mycolic acids are attached by an ester bond. Thus it indirectly inhibits incorporation of mycolic acids into the cell wall. It is active against several species of mycobacteria and nocardia. MICs (mg/l) on solid media are: *M. tuberculosis*, 0.5–2; *M. kansasii*, 1–4; other slowly growing mycobacteria, 2–8; rapidly growing pathogens, 2–16; and Nocardia spp., 8–32. Resistance is uncommon.

Pharmacokinetics

About 80% of a dose is absorbed from the gastro-intestinal tract. Absorption is impeded by aluminium hydroxide and alcohol. A dose of 25 mg/kg gives peak plasma concentrations of 2.6–5 mg/l at 2 h after ingestion. It is concentrated in the phagolysosomes of alveolar macrophages. It does not enter the cerebrospinal fluid (CSF) in health but CSF levels of 25–40% of the plasma concentration occur in patients with tuberculous meningitis.

Various metabolites are produced, including dialdehyde, dicarboxylic acid and glucuronide derivatives. About 90% is excreted in the urine, mostly unchanged but 10–15% is excreted as metabolites.

Toxicity and side-effects

The most important side-effect is optic neuritis, which may be irreversible if treatment is not discontinued. This complication is rare if the higher dose (25 mg/kg) is not given for more than 2 months. National codes of practice for prevention of ocular toxicity should be adhered to; in particular, patients should be advised to stop therapy and seek medical advice if they notice any change in visual acuity, peripheral vision or colour perception, and the drug should not be given to young children and others unable to comply with this advice.

Other side-effects include peripheral neuritis, arthralgia, hyperuricaemia, rashes and, rarely, thrombocytopenia and jaundice.

Clinical use

Often used as an additional agent in short-course therapy when resistance to one or more of the first-line drugs is suspected or known or when intermittent therapy (twice- or thrice-weekly dosage) is used. It is used with rifampicin and isoniazid to treat disease due to slowly growing mycobacteria including *M. kansasii, M. xenopi, M. malmoense, M. avium/M. intracellulare*. It is included in several multidrug regimens for treatment of AIDS-associated disseminated *M. avium/M. intracellulare* infection.

Preparations and dosage

Proprietary names: Myambutol, Mynah (with isoniazid).

Preparations: Tablets (and syrup on special request). Also available as combination tablets with isoniazid.

Dosage: Adults and children, 15–25 mg/kg daily for 2 months. If more prolonged therapy is indicated, the daily dose should not exceed 15 mg/kg; retreatment 25 mg/kg daily in first 60 days.

Further information

Citron K M 1986 Ocular toxicity from ethambutol. *Thorax* 41: 737–739

Hoffner S E, Kallenius G, Beezer A E, Svenson S B 1989 Studies on the mechanisms of the synergistic effects of ethambutol and other antibacterial drugs on *Mycobacterium avium* complex. *Acta Leprologica* 7 (suppl 1): 195–199

Khanna B K, Gupta V P, Singh V P 1984 Ethambutol-induced hyperuricaemia. *Tubercle* 65: 215–217

Prasad R, Mukerji P K 1989 Ethambutol-induced thrombocytopenia. *Tubercle* 70: 211–212

Sarren M, Khuller G K 1990 Cell wall and membrane changes associated with ethambutol resistance in *Mycobacterium tuberculosis* H37Rv. *Antimicrobial Agents and Chemotherapy* 34: 1773–1776

Takayama K, Kilburn J O 1989 Inhibition of synthesis of arabinogalactan in *Mycobacterium smegmatis*. *Antimicrobial Agents and Chemotherapy* 33: 1493–1499

ETHIONAMIDE
Ethylthioisonicotinamide

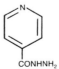

Antimicrobial activity

In common with isoniazid, to which it is structurally related, it is an inhibitor of mycolic acid synthesis. The MIC for *M. tuberculosis* on solid egg media is 8–16 mg/l. The MICs for other slowly growing mycobacteria (including *M. avium/ M. intracellulare*, *M. kansasii* and *M. malmoense*) are similar. Resistant strains show cross-resistance to prothionamide and thiacetazone, but not, despite the chemical similarity, isoniazid.

Pharmacokinetics

The uncoated drug is well absorbed from the intestine but not well tolerated. A dose of 250 mg produces peak serum levels of 1.8 mg/ml after 2–3 h. Enteric coated tablets, though better tolerated, produce serum levels about half those found after ingestion of uncoated drug. It is degraded to up to seven metabolites, including a biologically active sulphoxide and various inert compounds including nicotinic acid. Less than 1% is excreted unchanged in the urine and about 1.2% is excreted as the sulphoxide metabolite.

Toxicity and side-effects

Its principal side-effect is gastric irritation, which is commoner in adults and females. This effect is reduced by commencing with a low dose and gradually increasing to the full dose, by the use of antacids and by taking the drug at bedtime. Hypersensitivity reactions and hepatitis also occur. Rare effects include hypothyroidism, impotence, menstrual irregularities, gynaecomastia, alopecia, convulsions, deafness diplopia, peripheral neuropathy and mental disturbances.

Clinical use

Its side effects, notably gastric intolerance, limit its use to treatment of multidrug-resistant tuberculosis. It has also been used, with rifampicin and either dapsone or clofazimine, in short-course (13 week) regimens for multibacillary leprosy, but long-term follow-up results are required before it can be recommended for general use.

Preparations and dosage

Proprietary name: Trecator.

Preparation: Tablets.

Dosage: Adult, 750 mg, divided dose, with meals. Children, 15 mg/kg to maximum of 750 mg, divided dose, with meals.

Limited availability. Available in the USA and Spain. No longer available in the UK.

Further information

Donald P R, Seifart H I 1989 Cerebrospinal fluid concentrations of ethionamide in children with tuberculous meningitis. *Journal of Pediatrics* 115: 483–486

Jenner P J, Ellard G A, Gruer P J K, Aber V R 1984 Plasma levels and urinary excretion of ethionamide and prothionamide in man. *Journal of Antimicrobial Chemotherapy* 13: 267–277

Pattyn S R, Groenen G, Janssens L, Kuykens L, Mputu L B 1992 Treatment of multibacillary leprosy with a regimen of 13 weeks duration. *Leprosy Review* 63: 41–46

ISONIAZID
Isonicotinic acid hydrazide

Antimicrobial activity

Despite numerous studies and many theories, its mode of action is poorly understood, although it appears to inhibit mycolic acid synthesis. Susceptibility depends on the presence of a catalase–peroxidase enzyme.

It is highly bactericidal against actively replicating *M. tuberculosis* with MICs of 0.01–0.2 mg/l. Other mycobacteria are resistant, except for some strains of *M. xenopi* which are susceptible to 0.2 mg/l and a minority of strains of *M. kansasii* which are susceptible to 1 mg/l.

Acquired resistance

Some resistant strains have mutations in a gene (*inhA*) of unknown function, but resistance may also result from mutations in other, as yet undetermined, genes.

World-wide, isoniazid resistance is one of the two most frequently encountered forms of drug resistance in *M. tuberculosis*; the other being streptomycin resistance. Almost all multidrug-resistant strains are resistant to isoniazid (see p. 500).

Pharmacokinetics

It is readily absorbed from the gastro-intestinal tract. Absorption is impaired by aluminium hydroxide. Peak serum concentrations of 3–5 mg/l occur 1–2 h after a 300 mg dose. It is extensively metabolized to a variety of pharmacologically inactive derivatives, predominantly by acetylation. As a result of genetic polymorphism, patients are divisible into rapid and slow acetylators. About 50% of Caucasians and Blacks, but 80–90% of Chinese and Japanese, are rapid acetylators. The elimination half-lives in slow and rapid acetylators are 2–4 and 0.5–1.5 h, respectively. Acetylation status does not affect the efficacy of daily-administered therapy. The rate of acetylation is reduced in chronic renal failure.

Drug interactions may be more pronounced in slow acetylators. When given to patients stabilized on phenytoin or carbamazepine, it causes plasma levels of these antiepileptic drugs to rise and, notably in slow acetylators, may cause toxicity. Antiepileptic therapy thus requires monitoring and adjustment of dosage as necessary. Prednisolone reduces isoniazid levels in both slow and rapid acetylators, but the mechanism is unclear.

Toxicity and side-effects

Toxic effects are unusual on recommended doses and are more frequent in slow acetylators. Many side-effects are neurological, including restlessness, insomnia, muscle twitching and difficulty in starting micturition. More serious but less common neurological side-effects include peripheral neuropathy, optic neuritis, encephalopathy and a range of psychiatric disorders, including anxiety, depression and paranoia. Neurotoxicity is usually preventable by giving pyridoxine (vitamin B_6) 10 mg/day. Pyridoxine should not be given to patients with liver disease, pregnant women, alcoholics, renal dialysis patients, HIV-positive patients, the malnourished and the elderly.

Encephalopathy, which has been reported in patients on renal dialysis, may not be prevented by, or respond to, pyridoxine, but usually resolves on withdrawal of isoniazid.

Isoniazid-related hepatitis occurs in about 1% of patients receiving standard short-course chemotherapy. The incidence is unaffected by acetylator status. It is more common in those aged over 35 years and isoniazid prophylaxis should be used with care in older people.

Other less common side-effects include arthralgia, a 'flu'-like syndrome, hypersensitivity reactions with fever, rashes and, sometimes, eosinophilia, sideroblastic anaemia, pellagra, which responds to treatment with nicotinic acid, and haemolysis in patients with glucose-6-phosphatase deficiency. It exacerbates acute porphyria and it induces antinuclear antibodies, but overt systemic lupus erythematosus is rare.

Clinical use

It is a component of all WHO-recommended antituberculosis regimens during both the intensive and continuation phases. It is used as monotherapy to prevent primary tuberculosis in close contacts and reactivation disease in infected but healthy persons. Such monotherapy is usually given for 6–12 months, but HIV-positive patients may require preventive therapy for the rest of their lives.

Preparations and dosage

Proprietary name: Rimifon.

Preparations: Tablets, elixir, injection.

Dosage: Unsupervised: adults, oral, 300 mg/day; children, 10 mg/kg daily with a maximum dose of 300 mg/day. Adults, i.m., i.v., 200–300 mg as a single daily dose. Children, 10–20 mg/kg daily with a maximum of 300 mg/day. Neonates, 3–5 mg/kg daily, with a maximum of 10 mg/kg daily.

Widely available.

Further information

Cheung W C, Lo C Y, Lo W K, Ip M, Cheng I K P 1993 Isoniazid induced encephalopathy in dialysis patients. *Tubercle and Lung Disease* 74: 136–139

Ellard G A 1984 The potential clinical significance of the isoniazid acetylator phenotype in the treatment of pulmonary tuberculosis. *Tubercle* 65: 211–217

Grosset J 1990/1991 New experimental regimens for preventive therapy of tuberculosis. *Bulletin of the International Union Against Tuberculosis and Lung Disease* 66 (suppl 1990/1991): 15–16

Holdiness M R 1987 Neurological manifestations and toxicities of the antituberculosis drugs. *Medical Toxicology* 2: 33–51

Hutchings A D, Monie R D, Spragg B P, Routledge P A 1988 Saliva and plasma concentrations of isoniazid and acetylisoniazid in man. *British Journal of Clinical Pharmacology* 25: 585–589

Israel H L 1993 Chemoprophylaxis for tuberculosis. *Respiratory Medicine* 87: 81–83

Israel H L, Gottlieb J E, Maddrey W C 1992 Perspective: preventive isoniazid therapy and the liver. *Chest* 101: 1298–1301

Motion S, Humphries M J, Gabriel M 1989 Severe 'flu'-like symptoms due to isoniazid – a report of three cases. *Tubercle* 70: 57–60

Orlowski J P, Paganini E P, Pippenger C E 1988 Treatment of a potentially lethal dose isoniazid ingestion. *Annals of Emergency Medicine* 17: 73–76

Snider D E, Tabas G J 1992 Isoniazid associated hepatitis deaths: a review of available information. *American Review of Respiratory Disease* 145: 494–497

Statement: International Union Against Tuberculosis and Lung Disease/World Health Organization 1994 Tuberculosis preventive therapy in HIV-infected individuals. *Tubercle and Lung Disease* 75: 96–98

Tsukamura M 1990 In vitro bacteriostatic and bactericidal activity of isoniazid on the *Mycobacterium avium–Mycobacterium intracellulare* complex. *Tubercle* 71: 199–204

Weber W W 1986 The molecular basis of hereditary acetylation polymorphism. *Drug Metabolism and Disposition* 14: 377–381

Zhang Y, Young D B 1993 Molecular mechanisms of isoniazid: a drug at the front line of tuberculosis control. *Trends in Microbiology* 1: 109–113

PROTHIONAMIDE
Propylthioisonicotinamide

A very similar drug to ethionamide but said to be better tolerated. The antibacterial activity and pharmacokinetics of the two drugs are almost identical. It is seldom used in tuberculosis. It is used in combination with rifampicin and also with dapsone and isoniazid (Isoprodian) for treatment of leprosy patients who find clofazimine skin pigmentation unacceptable. As gastric irritation often leads to non-compliance, supervised therapy is recommended. If given simultaneously with isoniazid, the blood level of prothionamide may be raised, resulting in more side-effects unless the dosage is adjusted.

Preparations and dosage

Proprietary names: Peteha. Also available as a combination tablet with dapsone and isoniazid (Isoprodian).
Dosage: Adults, 750 mg, divided dose, with meals.
Children, 15 mg/kg to maximum of 750 mg, divided dose, with meals.
Very limited availability; not available in the UK.

Further information (see also ethionamide p. 508)

Ellard G A, Kiran K U, Stanley J N A 1988 Long-term prothionamide compliance: a study carried out in India using a combined formulation containing prothionamide, dapsone and isoniazid. *Leprosy Review* 59: 163–175

Kleeberg H H 1987 Pulmonary tuberculosis treated with isoprodian and rifampicin or pyrazinamide. *Chemotherapy* 33: 219–228

Van Brakel W H, Drever W 1993 Side effects of isoprodian compared with WHO-MDT in rural Nepal. *Leprosy Review* 64: 276–280

PYRAZINAMIDE
Pyrazinoic acid amide

Antimicrobial activity

Its mode of action is the least understood of all the antituberculosis drugs. Its activity against *M. tuberculosis* is highly pH dependent. At pH 5.6 the MIC is 8–16 mg/l, but it is almost inactive at neutral pH. Other mycobacterial species, including *M. bovis*, are resistant. Its activity requires its conversion to pyrazinoic acid by mycobacterial pyrazinamidase, which is present in *M. tuberculosis* but not *M. bovis*. It is principally active against intracellular bacilli and those in acidic, anoxic inflammatory lesions.

Acquired resistance

Resistant mutants are not cross-resistant to other antimycobacterial agents. Susceptibility testing is technically demanding as it requires very careful control of the pH of the medium. Resistant mutants lose pyrazinamidase activity, so tests for this activity offer an alternative to conventional susceptibility testing. Drug resistance is uncommon.

Pharmacokinetics

It is only given orally and is completely absorbed from the gastro-intestinal tract. It readily crosses the blood–brain barrier. Peak serum concentrations 2 h after a dose of 20–22 mg/kg are 10–50 mg/l. About 50% is bound to plasma protein. The plasma half-life is about 10 h. CSF levels are similar to plasma levels. It is metabolized to pyrazinoic acid in the liver and oxidized to inactive metabolites which are excreted in the urine.

Toxicity and side-effects

It is usually well tolerated. Moderate elevations of serum transaminases occur early in treatment. Severe hepato-toxicity is uncommon with standard dosage, except in patients with pre-existing liver disease.

Its principal metabolite, pyrazinoic acid, inhibits renal excretion of uric acid, occasionally causing gout requiring treatment with allopurinol. An unrelated arthralgia, notably of the shoulders and responsive to analgesics, also occurs.

Other side-effects include anorexia, nausea, mild flushing of the skin and photosensitization.

Clinical use

It is a component of modern short-course antituberculosis regimens as it has a key role in sterilizing acidic, inflammatory tissues and killing intracellular bacilli. In most regimens it is only used during the early, intensive, phase of therapy as it has little activity against near dormant persisting bacilli.

Preparations and dosage

Proprietary name: Zinamide.

Preparation: Tablets.

Dosage: Adult, oral, 2 g/day (over 50 kg), 1.5 g/day (under 50 kg); children, 35 mg/kg daily, in three to four divided doses.

Widely available.

Further information

Butler W R, Kilburn J O 1983 Susceptibility of *Mycobacterium tuberculosis* to pyrazinamide and its relationship to pyrazinamidase activity. *Antimicrobial Agents and Chemotherapy* 24: 600–601

Crowle A J, Sbarbaro J A, May M H 1986 Inhibition by pyrazinamide of tubercle bacilli within cultured human macrophages. *American Review of Respiratory Disease* 134: 1052–1055

Donald P R, Seifart H 1988 Cerebrospinal pyrazinamide concentrations in children with tuberculous meningitis. *Pediatric Infectious Diseases Journal* 7: 469–471

Jain A, Mehta V L, Kulshrestha S 1993 Effect of pyrazinamide on rifampicin kinetics in patients with tuberculosis. *Tubercle and Lung Disease* 74: 87–90

Lacroix C, Hoang T P, Nouveau J et al 1989 Pharmacokinetics of pyrazinamide and its metabolites in healthy subjects. *European Journal of Clinical Pharmacology* 36: 395–400

Stamatakis G, Montes C, Trouvin J H et al 1988 Pyrazinamide and pyrazinoic acid pharmacokinetics in patients with chronic renal failure. *Clinical Nephrology* 30: 230–234

Trivedi S S, Desai S G 1987 Pyrazinamidase activity of *Mycobacterium tuberculosis* – a test of sensitivity to pyrazinamide. *Tubercle* 68: 221–224

THIACETAZONE
Acetylaminobenzaldehyde thiosemicarbazone

$$CH_3COHN - \!\!\bigcirc\!\!- CH = N_2HCSNH_2$$

Antimicrobial activity

It inhibits mycolic acid synthesis by a poorly understood mechanism. *M. tuberculosis* is inhibited by 0.5–1 mg/l in Dubos Tween–albumin liquid media, but in vitro MICs vary considerably according to the medium used and bear little relation to in vivo efficacy.

Resistance

Many strains of *M. tuberculosis* isolated in East Africa, India and Hong Kong are naturally more resistant than strains from Europe. Acquired resistance, as a result of the use of monotherapy, is prevalent in the developing countries. Resistance develops rapidly in *M. leprae*.

Pharmacokinetics

It is rapidly absorbed from the intestine and does not bind to serum proteins. Peak plasma concentrations of 1–4 mg/l occur 2–4 h after a 100 mg dose. The plasma elimination half-life is 8–12 h. About 20% is eliminated in the urine: the fate of the remainder is unknown.

Toxicity and side-effects

Rashes are common, occurring in 2–4% of patients in Africa but much more frequently in those of Chinese ethnic origin. More severe skin reactions, exfoliative dermatitis and

Stevens–Johnson syndrome occur in less than 0.5% of patients, but there is a 10-fold increase of these reactions in HIV-positive patients, proving fatal in up to 3% of such patients.

Other common side-effects include gastro-intestinal reactions, vertigo and conjunctivitis. Less common reactions include hepatitis, erythema multiforme, haemolytic anaemia and, rarely, agranulocytosis. Prolonged therapy may rarely lead to hypertrichosis, gynaecomastia and osteoporosis.

Clinical use

It has the single virtue of low cost and has thus been used extensively, usually in combination with isoniazid. Owing to its low efficacy and frequent serious side-effects, it should be avoided whenever possible and never knowingly be given to an HIV-positive person. It has been evaluated in leprosy but abandoned because of the high incidence of side-effects and rapid emergence of drug resistance.

Preparations and dosage

Preparation: Tablets.

Dosage: Adults, oral, 150 mg/day. Children, 4 mg/kg to maximum of 150 mg/day.

Limited availability in the USA and Europe, including in the UK.

Further information

Heifets L B, Lindholm-Levy P J, Flory M 1990 Thiacetazone in vitro activity against *Mycobacterium avium* and *M. tuberculosis*. *Tubercle* 71: 287–292

Jenner P J, Ellard G A, Swat O B 1984 A study of thiacetazone blood levels and urinary excretion in man using high performance liquid chromatography. *Leprosy Review* 55: 121–128

World Health Organization 1992 Severe hypersensitivity reactions among HIV-seropositive patients with tuberculosis treated with thiacetazone. *Weekly Epidemiological Record* 67: 1–3

VIOMYCIN

A cyclic peptide, closely related to capreomycin, produced by several species of *Streptomyces*. It is supplied as the sulphate.

In common with the aminoglycosides, it inhibits protein synthesis by interfering with ribosomal function. It inhibits *M. tuberculosis* at concentrations of 2–12 mg/l. Although data are limited, other mycobacteria appear less susceptible. Resistance rapidly develops, with complete cross-resistance with capreomycin and one-way cross-resistance with streptomycin and kanamycin: strains resistant to streptomycin and kanamycin are usually susceptible to viomycin. It shows synergy with isoniazid against *M. tuberculosis*.

Low-level resistance, and cross-resistance with capreomycin, results from mutations in genes coding for the 50S (*vicA*) or 30S (*vicB*) ribosomal subunits. High-level resistance results from mutations in the v*icA* and *str* (streptomycin resistance) genes or in the *vicB* and both the *str* and *nek* (neomycin and kanamycin) genes. Thus cross-resistance with these aminoglycosides occurs.

It is not absorbed from the intestine. A dose of 1 g i.m. produces peak plasma concentrations of around 42 mg/l at 2 h after injection. It is distributed in the extracellular space, does not pass the blood–brain barrier readily and is mostly excreted unchanged in the urine.

Side-effects include ototoxicity, leading to deafness and giddiness, and nephrotoxicity. The incidence of these effects is greatly reduced by giving the drug on only 2 or 3 days each week.

It is now very rarely used and is of limited availability.

Further information

Hobby G L, Lenert T F, Donikian M, Pikula D 1951 The activity of viomycin against *Mycobacterium tuberculosis* and other microorganisms in vitro and in vivo. *American Review of Tuberculosis* 63: 17–24

McClatchy J K, Kanes W, Davidson P T, Moulding T S 1977 Cross resistance in *M. tuberculosis* to kanamycin, capreomycin and viomycin. *Tubercle* 58: 29–34

38

Anthelmintics

D. A. Denham

The helminths, or parasitic worms, comprise the nematodes (roundworms), trematodes (flukes) and cestodes (tapeworms). Most anthelmintics are more than 20 years old and few companies are searching for new ones for use in human medicine. Virtually every anthelmintic used against human nematode infections was developed for use in the veterinary field, where sheep, cattle, pigs and horses are hosts for large numbers of gastro-intestinal parasites. Commercial competition and the rapid development of drug resistance has meant that there has been a steady supply of new compounds for the veterinarian, although these have often been close relatives of previously available compounds. Antischistosome agents have usually been developed for use in humans, and because tapeworms and flukes are related some compounds are effective against both types of worm.

Despite the fact that most anthelmintics have been around for many years, satisfactory results can be achieved for nearly all helminth infections. The side-effects usually include gastro-intestinal upsets, but these are as likely to be related to the worm burden as to the drug. As extra-intestinal helminths are often present in large numbers their disintegration after chemotherapy must release much toxic material and this accounts for most of the side-effects after treatment.

The biggest problem still remaining to be solved is the treatment of *Echinococcus* infections. The only drugs showing anthelmintic effects with these parasites are the benzimidazole carbamates, but most of the huge amount of drug used in treatment of these patients is wasted as it is not absorbed from the gut. These compounds cannot be injected as they cause painful sterile abscesses.

Another problem is the treatment of disseminated strongyloidiasis. This condition occurs when patients with a latent infection are immunosuppressed. The *Strongyloides* multiply until the host is overwhelmed with worms in all tissues. The only cure is thiabendazole, but the drug has

such unpleasant side-effects that its use in patients who are already sick is a problem.

Although drug resistance is common in the veterinary field it has not been a problem in human medicine. This is because anthelmintics are very widely used in the veterinary world but much less so in human medicine due to the poverty of most of the people who are infected. With increasing wealth in tropical countries where these infections occur, anthelmintics are being used much more widely and there must be a fear that drug resistance will develop.

Further information

Campbell W C, Rew R S 1986 Chemotherapy of parasitic diseases. Plenum Press, New York

James D M, Gilles H M 1985 Human antiparasitic drugs. Pharmacology and usage. Wiley, Chichester

World Health Organization 1990 WHO model prescribing information. Drugs used in parasitic diseases, WHO, Geneva

Benzimidazoles and benzimidazole carbamates

Synthetic compounds with a broad-spectrum of anthelmintic activity, particularly against intestinal nematodes. They are widely used in veterinary medicine. The first compound of this type to be marketed for human use, thiabendazole, has been largely superseded by the benzimidazole carbamates, especially mebendazole and, more recently, albendazole.

Acquired resistance

There are no published records of any human nematode developing resistance to benzimidazole derivatives. However, one patient with persistent and recurring *Enterobius vermicularis* infection failed to respond to a 5-day course of mebendazole and was subsequently cured with albendazole. Since mebendazole is now available without prescription in the UK and elsewhere, there is a risk that resistance may develop in patients who do not complete the full course of treatment and such resistance may extend to related benzimidazoles. Experience in the veterinary world shows that if resistance to one benzimidazole carbamate occurs the parasite very rapidly becomes resistant to any new congener.

Further information

Various authors 1990 Benzimidazole anthelmintics. *Parasitology Today* 6: 106–136

ALBENDAZOLE

A benzimidazole carbamate

Anthelmintic activity

It has a wide spectrum of activity against intestinal nematodes, including *Ascaris lumbricoides,* hookworm and *Ent. vermicularis* (threadworm). It has useful, but lesser activity against *Trichuris trichiura* (whipworm) and *Strongyloides stercoralis* (Table 38.1). Albendazole also exhibits some activity against the larval stages of *Echinococcus granulosus* and *Echinococcus multilocularis*. It has been successfully used in infections with the protozoon

Giardia lamblia and is under trial in microsporidiosis (pp. 671, 916).

Pharmacokinetics

Albendazole is rather better absorbed after oral absorption than the other benzimidazole carbamates. It is extensively metabolized to albendazole sulphoxide, producing concentrations of the metabolite of about 0.25 mg/l at 2–3 h after a 400 mg oral dose. The half-life is about 8 h and the major route of excretion is via the bile.

Toxicity and side-effects

Various intestinal and other upsets have been reported, but equal numbers were reported by patients who were given a placebo in double-blind trials.

Clinical use

It is administered as a single oral dose for most intestinal worm infections. Mild *Trichuris* infections are cured by this regimen, but heavy infections respond better to 3 days' treatment, which should be repeated after 3 or 4 weeks. *Trichuris* infections specifically suppress the immune responses and the degree of suppression may be related to worm burden. Removal of the majority of the *Trichuris* with the first course of the treatment probably allows the immune response to improve so that it can act together with the drug in the follow-up treatment.

The drug has been used as an adjunct, or alternative, to surgery in hydatid disease. If used in high dosage and for very long periods against the hydatid cysts caused by *Ech. granulosus* and *Ech. multilocularis*, it induces remission in some cases. However, it does not kill *Ech. multilocularis* and if treatment is ceased the cysts start to grow again. Albendazole has been recommended for the treatment of

Table 38.1 *Activity of the commonly available anthelmintics against intestinal nematodes*

Agent	Ent. vermicularis	Trich. trichuris	Asc. lumbricoides	Hookworms	S. stercoralis
Piperazine	++	–	+++	–	–
Levamizole	++	+	+++	+++	?
Pyrantel	+++	–	+++	++	?
Oxantel	++	+++	–	++	?
Mebendazole	+++	++	+++	+++	++
Albendazole	+++	++	+++	+++	++
Ivermectin	+	+	+++	+	+++
Pyrvinium	+++	–	–	–	–

+++, Highly effective; ++, moderately effective; +, poorly effective; –, no useful activity; ?, no information.

cerebral cysticercosis, especially as it is much cheaper than praziquantel. It is reportedly more effective than mebendazole against the larvae of *Trichinella spiralis*. It is effective against *Fasciola hepatica* in cattle and may be useful in zoonotic human infections.

Preparations and dosage

Proprietary name: Eskazole.

Preparation: Tablets.

Dosage: Oral, adults (over 60 kg), *Ech. granulosus*, medical treatment 800 mg/day in divided doses for 28 days followed by 14 tablet-free days; up to 3 cycles of treatment may be given. Surgical treatment: pre-surgery, 800 mg/day in divided doses for 28 days followed by 14 drug-free days, repeat the cycle once prior to surgery; per- and post-surgery, two 28-day cycles separated by 14 days. In addition, where cysts are found to be viable after presurgical treatment, a full two-course cycle should be given.

Ech. multilocularis, 800 mg/day in divided doses.

Available in the UK and elsewhere.

Further information

Firth M (ed) 1983 Albendazole in helminthiasis. *Royal Society of Medicine, International Congress and Symposium Series,* Number 57. Royal Society of Medicine, London

Teggi A, Lastilla M G, De Rosa F 1993 Therapy of hydatid disease with mebendazole and albendazole. *Antimicrobial Agents and Chemotherapy* 37: 1679–1684

FLUBENDAZOLE

A benzimidazole carbamate that is chemically very closely related to mebendazole. It was initially developed as a replacement therapy for pigs infected with *Ascaris suum* because they react badly to mebendazole. It is used in some countries in place of mebendazole for the treatment of *Ascaris* infection. It is even less well absorbed after oral administration than mebendazole.

MEBENDAZOLE

A benzimidazole carbamate with a wide spectrum of activity against intestinal nematodes.

Anthelmintic activity

It is active against hookworms, threadworms, and ascaris, but less so against whipworm and *S. stercoralis* (Table 38.1).

Pharmacokinetics

Oral absorption is poor. Plasma concentrations achieved after a single oral dose are extremely low in fasting subjects, but rise substantially if the dose is taken with a fatty meal. About 90% of the drug is retained in the intestinal tract and passed in the faeces. The remainder is metabolized and passed in the urine.

Toxicity and side-effects

Diarrhoea and gastro-intestinal discomfort may occur, but adverse reactions are generally mild.

Clinical use

Its main use is in infections with *Asc. lumbricoides, Ent. vermicularis* and hookworm. It has partial activity against *Trichuris*. It is also used to kill the encysted larvae of *Trich. spiralis*. It has been used with variable success in hydatid disease.

Preparations and dosage

Proprietary name: Vermox.

Preparations: Tablets, suspension.

Dosage: Adults and children >2 years, threadworms, 100 mg as a single dose; if re-infection occurs a second dose may be needed after 2–3 weeks. Ascaris and hookworm, 100 mg twice daily for 3 days. Not recommended for children <2 years of age.

Widely available.

Further information

Raush R L, Wilson J F, McMahon B J, O'Gorman M A 1986 Consequences of continuous mebendazole therapy in alveolar hydatid disease – with a summary of a ten-year clinical trial. *Annals of Tropical Medicine and Parasitology* 80: 403–419

THIABENDAZOLE

A synthetic benzimidazole derivative first patented in 1961.

Anthelmintic activity

It is active against many intestinal nematodes, including *Asc. lumbricoides*, threadworm, hookworm, whipworm and *Trichostrongylus* spp. It is active against larvae and developing ova, and consequently is effective in infection with *S. stercoralis, Trich. spiralis,* and cutaneous larva migrans caused by animal hookworms.

Pharmacokinetics

It is well absorbed from the small intestine. Peak plasma levels around 5 mg/l are reached about 1 h after a single oral dose of 15 mg/kg. It is extensively metabolized in the liver to the 5-hydroxy derivative, which is inactive. About 90% is excreted in the urine, chiefly as glucuronide conjugates; the remainder is passed in the faeces within 24 h.

Toxicity and side-effects

Thiabendazole causes a wide range of very unpleasant side-effects, including nausea and other gastro-intestinal upsets, fever and neurological effects.

Clinical use

Despite its numerous side-effects, thiabendazole was widely used in the tropics as a general antinematode agent, but it has been largely replaced by the less toxic benzimidazole carbamates. It is still the drug of choice for disseminated strongyloidiasis, which is invariably fatal without chemotherapy. Emulsified in handcreams or Vaseline it has very good activity when applied topically to the cutaneous larva migrans lesions caused by animal hookworms.

Preparations and dosage

Proprietary names: Mintezol, Triasox.

Preparation: Tablets.

Dosage: Oral: <60 kg bodyweight, 25 mg/kg every 12 h; >60 kg body weight, 1.5 g twice daily; duration of therapy depends in the infection.

Strongyloidiasis: 2 doses a day on 2 successive days.

Cutaneous larva migrans: 2 doses a day on two successive days, and repeat if active lesions are still present 2 days after completion of therapy.

Visceral larva migrans: 2 doses a day on 7 successive days.

Widely available.

Miscellaneous anthelmintic agents

BEPHENIUM

A quaternary ammonium compound formulated as the hydroxynaphthoate. It is effective as a single 5 g dose against several nematodes, including *Asc. lumbricoides* and *Ancylostoma duodenale*, but not *Necator americanus*. It is extremely bitter and may induce vomiting. Bephenium has been largely superseded by other drugs and no longer

features in the World Health Organization (WHO) model prescribing information on drugs for use in parasitic diseases.

DIETHYLCARBAMAZINE

A synthetic carbamyl derivative of piperazine, first described in 1947.

Anthelmintic activity

Its useful activity is restricted to filarial worms. It is adulticidal and microfilaricidal against *Loa loa*. Against *Wuchereria bancrofti* and *Brugia malayi* it is predominantly microfilaricidal, but slowly kills adult worms. It kills microfilariae, but not adults of *Onchocerca volvulus*.

Pharmacokinetics

Like piperazine to which it is related, it is rapidly and completely absorbed, achieving a peak plasma concentration of about 0.1 mg/l at 1–2 h after a 50 mg oral dose. The plasma half-life is about 9–12 h. The apparent volume of distribution in adults is 200–240 l. About half the dose is excreted unchanged in the urine; the rest is metabolized and eliminated by renal and extrarenal routes.

Toxicity and side-effects

In uninfected people diethylcarbamazine has virtually no side-effects, but in people with various forms of filariasis it has unpleasant effects due to the death of, often, millions of blood or skin dwelling microfilariae. In onchocerciasis the severe skin reactions that occur in treated patients have been name 'Mazzotti reactions'. These reactions have been deliberately used as a diagnostic procedure but this is now regarded as unethical. In patients with *L. loa* who harbour very large numbers of microfilariae in their blood, neurological problems may be very severe. Cardiological damage has also been reported. In patients with *W. bancrofti* and *B. malayi* high fever occurs in the first few days after treatment

Clinical use

It is used for the treatment of filariasis. Dosage is gradually increased to avoid a severe side-reaction. A full schedule of 12 doses of 6 mg/kg is necessary to kill adult worms of *W. bancrofti* and *B. malayi*. Its use reverses the early signs of lymphoedema caused by lymphatic filarial worms. Diethylcarbamazine has also been used in visceral larva migrans caused by *Toxocara canis*, but experience is limited and there is little evidence of its efficacy.

Further information

Mackenzie C D, Kron M A 1985 Diethylcarbamazine: a review of its action in onchocerciasis, lymphatic filariasis and inflammation. *Tropical Diseases Bulletin* 82: R1–R37

Maizels R M, Denham D A 1993 Diethylcarbamazine (DEC): immunopharmacological interactions of an anti-filarial drug. *Parasitology* 105: S49–S60

IVERMECTIN

A mixture of two closely related semi-synthetic derivatives of avermectins, a complex of macrocyclic lactone antibiotics produced by *Streptomyces avermitilis*.

Anthelmintic activity

Ivermectin has quite broad-spectrum anthelmintic activity and has been widely used in the veterinary field, where use is also made of its effect on ectoparasites. In human medicine its widespread use is limited to the treatment of onchocerciasis, although it is also active against other filarial worms and against some intestinal nematodes, notably *S. stercoralis* and *Asc. lumbricoides* (Table 38.1). The effect against filarial worms is chiefly directed against the larva forms (microfilariae).

Pharmacokinetics

It is well absorbed from the gut and is rapidly metabolized. Peak values (about 30 μg/l after a dose of 12 mg) are achieved within 4 h. The half-life is about 12 h, but metabolites are excreted in the urine for about 2 weeks. It has a volume of distribution of 46.9 l and plasma protein binding of 93%. Highest concentrations occur in the liver and fat. Extremely small amounts are found in the brain.

Toxicity and side-effects

In the treatment of onchocerciasis, mild Mazzoti-type reactions occur, with occasional neurological problems. If the patient is harbouring *Ascaris*, the worms will be passed in the faeces. Head lice will also be killed, but this is very much welcomed by the treated patients. Although it is highly effective against *L. loa*, care must be taken to avoid treating patients with high microfilarial counts: there is one report of a patient with a concomitant *L. loa* infection who died when treated for onchocerciasis.

Clinical use

It is widely used in west Africa for the treatment of onchocerciasis in areas where vector control is difficult. Many of these patients are also infected with *Ascaris* and the hookworm, *Anc. duodenale*, and treatment inadvertently reduces the worm burden due to these parasites. Annual or six-monthly treatments may have macrofilaricidal effects. Higher doses than those presently used are also being evaluated after the demonstration that high levels kill *Onchocerca gibsoni* adults in cattle.

It has been used in many trials against lymphatic filariae. It is potently microfilaricidal but probably has no lethal effects on adult worms. Trials are underway to test its effects on clinical disease. There is also some interest in its possible use in scabies.

Further information

Campbell W C (ed) 1989 Ivermectin and abamectin, Springer, New York

Chodakewitz J 1995 Ivermectin and lymphatic filariasis: a clinical update. *Parasitology Today* 11: 233–235

Ottesen E A, Campbell W C 1994 Ivermectin in human medicine. *Journal of Antimicrobial Chemotherapy* 32: 195–203

Ottesen E A, Vijayasekaran V, Kumaraswami V et al 1990 A controlled trial of ivermectin and diethylcarbamazine in lymphatic filariasis. *New England Journal of Medicine* 322: 1113–1117

LEVAMISOLE

The laevorotatory isomer of tetramisole. The dextrorotatory isomer has no anthelmintic activity.

Anthelmintic activity

Its principal activity is against *Asc. lumbricoides* and hookworms. Worms are paralysed and passed out in the faeces within a few hours.

Pharmacokinetics

Levamisole is rapidly absorbed from the gut with peak plasma levels reached in about 2 h. It is extensively metabolized in the liver and is excreted, chiefly in the urine, with a half-life of about 4 h.

Toxicity and side-effects

Nausea, gastro-intestinal upsets and very mild neurological problems have been reported.

Clinical use

Levamisole is useful for the treatment of *Ascaris* and the hookworms. It has also been used in rheumatoid arthritis and some other conditions that are said to respond to its immunomodulatory activity.

Preparations and dosage

Preparation: Tablets.

Dosage: Adults, oral, 120–150 mg as a single dose.

Not available in the UK; available in France.

METRIPHONATE

An organophosphate compound. It is a pro-drug of the active form, dichlorvos.

Anthelmintic activity

Its use is restricted to infection with *Schistosoma haematobium*. It has little activity against other schistosomes (Table 38.2). Although it exhibits activity against several other helminths it is not used for their treatment.

Pharmacokinetics

Metrifonate is rapidly absorbed after oral administration, achieving a peak concentration in plasma within 1 h. It undergoes chemical transformation to dichlorvos, which is

Table 38.2 *Activity of commonly used antischistosome agents*

Agent	Schist. mansoni	Schist. haematobium	Schist. japonicum
Praziquantel	+++	+++	+++
Metriphonate	–	+++	–
Oxamniquine	++	+++	+++

+++, Highly effective; ++, moderately effective; –, no useful activity.

the active molecule. Dichlorvos is extensively metabolized and excreted mainly in the urine.

Toxicity and side-effects

Various side-effects such as abdominal pain, gastro-intestinal upsets and vertigo occur in many patients. As the worms release their hold of the veins in the bladder they pass through the blood system to the lungs where they disintegrate and this may cause some of the side-effects. Cholinesterase levels in the blood and on erythrocytes are depressed, but the significance of this is doubtful.

Clinical use

Because it is so cheap it has been used in mass chemotherapy control programmes for urinary schistosomiasis.

Preparations and dosage

Proprietary name: Bilarcil.

Preparation: Tablets.

Dosage: Adults, oral, *Schist. haematobium*: three doses of 7.5–10 mg/kg may be given at intervals of 2 weeks; single doses of 10 mg/kg at intervals of 3, 6 or 12 months have also been used.

Not available in the UK; limited availability in continental Europe.

NICLOSAMIDE

A chlorinated nitrosalylanilide.

Anthelmintic activity

Niclosamide is active against intestinal tapeworms, including *Taenia saginata, Taenia solium, Diphyllobothrium latum* and *Hymenolepis nana*.

Pharmacokinetics

Niclosamide is poorly absorbed from the gut and is passed in the faeces staining them yellow.

Toxicity and side-effects

Very few have been reported.

Clinical use

It is used exclusively for infections with adult *T. solium, T. saginata, D. latum* and *H. nana*. Since it is not absorbed from the intestine, it is not effective against larval stages of tapeworms.

Preparations and dosage

Proprietary name: Yomesan.
Preparation: Tablets.
Dosage:

Infection	Age range	Dose	Comment
T. solium	Adults and children >6 years	2 g	Take as a single dose after a light breakfast. Administer a purge 2 h later.
	Children 2–6 years	1 g	
	Children <2 years	500 mg	
T. saginata	As above	As above	As above but the dose may be divided, half being taken after breakfast and the remainder 1 h later. An aperient should be administered 2 h later.
D. latum	As above	As above	As above
H. nana	As above	As above	As above

Widely available.

OXAMNIQUINE

A synthetic quinolinemethanol derivative.

Anthelmintic activity

It is effective against *Schist. mansoni* but some geographical strains, particularly those in Egypt and southern Africa are partially resistant. Activity against *Schist. haematobium* and *Schist. japonicum* is unreliable.

Pharmacokinetics

It is rapidly absorbed after oral administration, achieving a peak concentration in plasma after 1–1.5 h. It is extensively metabolized to biologically inactive 6-carboxy and 2-carboxylic acid derivatives which are excreted in the urine, mostly within 12 h.

Toxicity and side-effects

Dizziness and sleepiness occur frequently. Other side-effects are probably due to the death and disintegration of the worms in the liver.

Clinical use

It is exclusively used in the treatment of infection with *Schist. mansoni.*

Preparations and dosage

Dosage: Adults, oral, *Schist. mansoni* infections only, total doses range from 15 mg/kg given as a single dose to 60 mg/kg given over 2–3 days.
Not available in the UK; limited availability in continental Europe.

PIPERAZINE

A synthetic antinematode agent widely available without prescription in many countries under numerous trade names. It is available as the adipate, citrate, edentate calcium and tartrate salts.

Anthelmintic activity

Its useful activity is restricted to *Ent. vermicularis* and *Asc. lumbricoides* (Table 38.1).

Pharmacokinetics

Its activity against intestinal worms requires that a substantial amount remains in the gut. However, after oral administration a variable amount is rapidly absorbed from the small intestine and subsequently excreted in the urine. Its half-life is very variable.

Toxicity and side-effects

Some people develop hypersensitivity requiring cessation of treatment. Transient neurological symptoms may occur.

Clinical use

It is very effective as a single dose against *Asc. lumbricoides*, but treatment for seven consecutive days is necessary in threadworm infection. It is of little or no use for other nematodes.

Preparations and dosage

Proprietary names: Pripsen (oral powder), Antepar, Helmezine.
Preparations: Elixir (as citrate), oral powder (as phosphate, also contains sennosides).
Dosage: Piperazine citrate, threadworms, oral: adult, 2.25 g/day for 7 days; children <2 years, 45–75 mg/kg daily for 7 days (on doctor's advice only); children 2–3 years 750 mg/day for 7 days; children 4–6 years, 1.125 g/day for 7 days; children 7–12 years, 1.5 g/day for 7 days. Repeat course after 1 week if necessary.

Piperazine citrate, roundworms, oral: adult, 4.5 g as a single dose; children <1 year, 120 mg/kg as a single dose (on doctor's advice only); children 1–3 years, 1.5 g as a single dose; children 4–5 years, 2.25 g as a single dose; children 6–8 years, 3 g as a single dose; children 9–12 years, 3.75 g as a single dose. Repeat doses after 2 weeks.

Piperazine phosphate, threadworms, oral: adults and children >6 years, 1 sachet (15.3 mg); infants 3 months to 1 year, one-third of a sachet; children 1-6 years, two-thirds of a sachet. Repeat doses after 14 days.

Piperazine phosphate, roundworms: first dose as for threadworms; repeat at monthly intervals for up to 3 months if reinfection risk.

Widely available.

PRAZIQUANTEL

A pyrazinoquinoline. It is one of the very few anthelmintics developed specifically for use in people rather than domestic animals.

Anthelmintic activity

It is active against a wide range of cestodes and trematodes (including the intestinal tapeworms and their larval forms) and all species of human schistosomes (Table 38.2). Praziquantel is also effective against the intestinal flukes *Fasciolopsis buski*, *Metagonimus yokogawi* and *Heterophyes heterophyes*; against *Opisthorchis* spp. in the bile ducts; and against *Paragonimus westermanni* in the lungs. It has little or no activity against zoonotic *Fasciola hepatica* infections.

Pharmacokinetics

It is rapidly absorbed when given orally, but it undergoes extensive presystemic metabolism and the concentration of unchanged drug in plasma is low. Peak concentrations are achieved after 1–2 h. The major metabolite, a 4-hydroxy derivative, retains some antiparasitic activity. About 80% of the oral dose is excreted in the urine in 24 h. The half-life of praziquantel plus its metabolites is 4–6 h. A higher peak plasma concentration is achieved in infected people, but other pharmacokinetic values are unchanged.

Toxicity and side-effects

Very few side-effects have been reported. In the treatment of cerebral cysticercosis the death of cysts in the brain may cause local inflammation and oedema, but this usually subsides quickly. Adverse events seen in the treatment of schistosomiasis, including abdominal pain, nausea and mild neurological effects, are almost certainly due to the death and disintegration of the large adult worms.

Clinical use

It is the drug of choice for the treatment of all forms of human schistosomiasis, and most other trematode infections, but *Fasciola hepatica* is usually refractory to treatment. It is also effective in cerebral cysticercosis due to the larval form of *T. solium*, although treatment may need to be prolonged. For most other cestode and trematode infections a single dose is usually effective.

Preparations and dosage

Proprietary name: Biltricide.

Preparation: Tablets.

Dosage: Adults, oral, schistosomiasis, 20 mg/kg in 3 divided doses 4–6 h apart on one day.

Not available in the UK, available in continental Europe.

Further information

Davis A 1993 Antischistosomal drugs and clinical practice. In: Jordan P, Webbe G, Sturrock R F (eds) Human schistosomiasis. CAB International, Wallingford, p 367–404

Kumar V, Gryseels B 1994 Use of praziquantel against schistosomiasis: a review of current status. *International Journal of Antimicrobial Agents* 4: 313–321

OXANTEL

A tetrahydropyrimidine formulated as the embonate (pamaote).

Anthelmintic activity

It has a very limited spectrum of activity with extremely good activity against *Trichuris trichiura*, but virtually no activity against other intestinal nematodes.

Pharmacokinetics

Very little is absorbed from the intestine, most being passed unchanged in the faeces. The portion that is absorbed is metabolized and excreted in the urine.

Toxicity and side-effects

Nausea, vomiting and other gastro-intestinal symptoms may occur.

Clinical use

It is used exclusively for whipworm infections. Because the spectrum is essentially the mirror image of the activity of pyrantel these drugs have been used in combination, especially in areas where *Trichuris* is a problem.

PYRANTEL

A tetrahydropyrimidine. Like oxantel it is formulated as the embonate (pamoate).

Anthelmintic activity

It is highly active against *Asc. lumbricoides*, *Ent. vermicularis* and *Anc. duodenale*, but less so against *N. americanus* (Table 38.1). It is also active against *Trichostrongylus* spp., but has no action on whipworm, *Trichuris trichiura*.

Pharmacokinetics

Very little pyrantel is absorbed from the intestine, most being passed unchanged in the faeces. The portion that is absorbed is metabolized and excreted in the urine.

Toxicity and side-effects

It should not be used at the same time as piperazine as their modes of action are antagonistic. Gastro-intestinal upsets and, rarely, very mild neurological symptoms occur.

Clinical use

It is used as a single dose of 10 mg/kg for most worm infections. Higher and more prolonged doses (20 mg/kg daily for 2 days, or 10 mg/kg daily for 3 days) may be necessary in hookworm infection caused by *N. americanus*. It is often used in combination with oxantel if concurrent whipworm infections is likely.

Preparations and dosage

Proprietary name: Combantrin.

Preparation: Tablets.

Dosage: Adults and children >6 months: *Asc. lumbricoides* alone, single dose of 5 mg/kg; mixed infections involving *Asc. lumbricoides*, single dose of 10 mg/kg; more severe infections of *N. americanus*, 20 mg/kg as a single dose on each of 2 consecutive days, or 10 mg/kg as a single dose on each of 3 consecutive days.

Widely available.

PYRVINIUM

A cyanine dye formulated as the almost insoluble pamoate. It is not absorbed from the gut and was formerly used for the treatment of *Ent. vermicularis* infection. It is a very bright red colour and stains the faeces red. Occasional nausea and vomiting occur. Depression of haematopoiesis has been reported, which is strange for a drug that is not absorbed from the gut. Because it is completely unrelated to the benzimidazole carbamates it may be useful as a cover if drug resistance to them is developed by *Enterobius*.

SURAMIN

A colourless derivative of the dye trypan blue, developed in Germany in the early 1920s for the treatment of African trypanosomiasis (p. 522). Its useful anthelmintic activity is restricted to *O. volvulus* and it has been used to achieve a radical cure of onchocerciasis by killing the adult worms. However, it is an extremely toxic drug and use has become increasingly uncommon since ivermectin became available. Pharmacokinetics, toxicity and side-effects are described in Chapter 39.

Other anthelmintic agents

Potassium antimony tartrate (tartar emetic), sodium antimony tartrate, the thioxanthone, hycanthone, and the 5-nitrothiazole, niridazole, were formerly used in the treatment of schistosomiasis, but have been largely superseded by less toxic compounds. Niridazole has also been used in Guinea worm (*Dracunculus medinensis*) infection, but no drug interrupts transmission and metronidazole (p. 407) or benzimidazole carbamates are much safer and as useful in providing symptomatic relief.

The chlorinated hydrocarbon, tetrachloroethylene has been used since the 1920s in the treatment of hookworm infection. It is more effective in eliminating *N. americanus* than *Anc. duodenale* and has no useful effect against other intestinal worms. It has now been replaced by safer and more effective agents.

Antiprotozoal agents

S. L. Croft

Introduction

The treatment and prophylaxis of many protozoal diseases, such as malaria which causes up to 250 million infections and 2 million deaths per annum, is inadequate. Malaria chemotherapy has been undermined by the development of resistance to pyrimethamine and chloroquine (Ch. 62). Treatment of African trypanosomiasis (sleeping sickness), leishmaniasis and South American trypanosomiasis (Chagas' disease), caused by closely related flagellate parasites, still depends upon arsenicals and antimonials or toxic nitro-heterocyclic compounds. During the past 15 years opportunistic protozoa, some previously unknown in humans, have emerged as important pathogens in immunocompromised patients. No drugs have so far proved effective against cryptosporidiosis, and those for toxoplasmosis and microsporidiosis are limited.

Protozoa are unicellular, eukaryotic cells with an enormous diversity in morphology, life cycles, genomic and biochemical characteristics. This diversity is reflected in their very different sensitivity to antiprotozoal drugs.

Several antiprotozoal agents developed in the 1920s and 1930s, for example suramin, mepacrine, primaquine, chloroquine and sodium stibogluconate, are still widely used. Identification of new drugs has been hampered, in part, by lack of suitable in vitro and in vivo models, for example suitable in vitro models for Plasmodium falciparum and Trypanosoma brucei were not discovered until the 1970s. Development of novel antiprotozoal drugs has also been hampered by unprofitability. Hence antibacterial, antifungal and anticancer drugs have frequently been turned to in a search for concordant activity.

Further information

Berman J D, Fleckenstein L 1991 Pharmacokinetic justification of antiprotozoal chemotherapy. Clinical Pharmacokinetics 21: 479–493

Coombs G, North M (eds) 1991 Biochemical protozoology. Taylor & Francis, London

Croft S L 1994 A rationale for antiparasite drug discovery. Parasitology Today 10: 385–386

Das S S, Simpson A J H 1993 Therapy of protozoan infections in patients with impaired immunity. Current Opinion in Infectious Diseases 6: 784–793

Schuster B G, Milhous W K 1993 Reduced resources applied to antimalarial drug development. Parasitology Today 9: 167–168

Organometals

The use of both arsenic and antimony in the treatment of infectious diseases originates from traditional treatments: Fowler's solution, containing potassium arsenite, and tartar emetic (antimony potassium tartrate). Arsenical compounds were used for the treatment of African sleeping sickness and antimonial compounds for the treatment of leishmaniasis before 1920. The compounds presently used are considerably less toxic than their predecessors; they were developed in the 1930s (sodium stibogluconate) and 1940s (melarsoprol, meglumine antimonate). Tryparsamide was formerly used in sleeping sickness, but it is highly toxic and there is intrinsic resistance. A water-soluble compound, trimelarsen (Mel W) has also been used, but it is less effective and more toxic than melarsoprol.

MELARSOPROL

A derivative of trivalent melarsen oxide and dimercaprol (BAL), possessing a melaminyl moiety.

Antimicrobial activity

It is highly and rapidly active against *T. brucei gambiense* and *T. brucei rhodesiense* in vitro at submicromolar concentrations and in vivo at single doses of 1–3 mg/kg. It has much lower activity against the animal trypanosomes *Trypanosoma congolense* and *Trypanosoma vivax*. Combinations of melarsoprol with eflornithine and nitroimidazoles are highly active against central nervous system (CNS) infection with *T. brucei* in rodents. Melarsoprol inhibits phosphofructokinase and interacts with trypanothione, which substitutes for glutathione in trypanosomatids. Melarsoprol forms an adduct with trypanothione which inhibits trypanothione reductase and lowers levels of this homeostatic thiol in the trypanosome.

Acquired resistance

Although 3–11% of patients with *T. b. gambiense* and *T. b. rhodesiense* infections relapse, this figure has remained constant for 40 years. Patients with *T. b. rhodesiense* normally respond to a second course of the drug, but patients with *T. b. gambiense* do not. Resistance is due to reduced uptake of the drug by trypanosomes. Resistant trypomastigotes lack an adenine/adenosine transporter that is also responsible for melarsoprol transport. Melarsoprol is active against trypanosomes resistant to tryparsamide.

Pharmacokinetics

Pharmacokinetic data is limited. Serum levels of 2–4 mg/l at 24 h after administration of 3.6 mg/kg, falling to 0.1 mg/l at 120 h after the 4th daily injection, have been reported. Elimination was biphasic with a half-life of 35 h and a volume of distribution of 100 l. Levels of melarsoprol in the cerebrospinal fluid (CSF) reached around 300 μg/l, about 50 times lower than serum levels.

Toxicity and side-effects

It is supplied in 3.6% propylene glycol, which can cause tissue trauma and long-term damage to veins. Reactions due to melarsoprol include fever on first administration, abdominal colic pain, dermatitis and arthralgia. Polyneuropathy has been reported in about 10% of patients. Reactive arsenical encephalopathy is a serious side-effect which occurs in around 10% of those treated, with death in 1–3% of cases. The frequency of encephalopathy increases with a rise in the white cell count or the presence of trypanosomes in the CSF. The causes of the immunological responses involved in the encephalopathy and the possible existence of two forms (reactive and haemorrhagic) are subjects of debate. Concomitant administration of prednisolone has reduced the frequency of reactive encephalopathy in late stage *T. b. gambiense* infection.

Clinical use

It is used in late-stage sleeping sickness caused by both *T. b. gambiense* and *T. b. rhodesiense*. It is not recommended for early-stage disease in which alternatives with less serious side-effects are available.

Preparations and dosage

Proprietary name: Arsobal.

Preparation: Injection.

Dosage: Adults, i.v., 3.6 mg/kg daily for 3–4 days and repeat 2–3 times with an interval of at least 7 days between courses.

Available in South Africa.

Further information

Bacchi C 1993 Resistance to clinical drugs in African trypanosomes. *Parasitology Today* 9: 190–193

Berger B J, Fairlamb A H 1994 High-performance liquid chromatographic method for the separation and quantitative estimation of anti-parasitic melaminophenyl arsenical compounds. *Transactions of the Royal Society of Tropical Medicine and Hygiene* 88: 357–359

Burri C, Baltz T, Giroud C, Doua F, Welker H A, Brun R 1993 Pharmacokinetic properties of the trypanocidal drug melarsoprol. *Chemotherapy* 39: 225–234

Jennings F 1993 Combination therapy of CNS trypanosomiasis. *Acta Tropica* 54: 205–213

Pepin J, Milord F 1994 The treatment of human African trypanosomiasis. *Advances in Parasitology* 33: 1–47

SODIUM STIBOGLUCONATE

Sodium antimony gluconate, antimony(V) gluconic acid. A pentavalent antimonial derivative of unknown chemical composition, probably a complex mixture polymeric forms. There is batch-to-batch variation and solutions may contain 32–34% antimony(V) (Sb(V)). The structural formula normally given is based upon that of tartar emetic.

$$
\begin{array}{lcccr}
CH_2OH & & & HOH_2C \\
| & & & | \\
CHOH & & & HOHC \\
| & & & | \\
CHO & OH & O^- & OHC \\
| & & & | \\
CHO \rightarrow Sb & \!\!-O-\!\! & Sb \leftarrow OHC & 3Na^+ \\
| & & & | \\
CHO & & & OHC \\
| & & & | \\
COO & & & OOC
\end{array}
$$

Antimicrobial activity

It has low activity against the extracellular promastigotes of *Leishmania* spp. in vitro, but is active against amastigotes in macrophages. It is more active against visceral than cutaneous leishmaniasis in animal models. Although several mechanisms of action have been proposed, no satisfactory explanation is yet available. Sodium stibogluconate cures CNS infections with *T. brucei* in rodents.

Acquired resistance

Increasing unresponsiveness and relapse in India and Kenya over the past 30 years is assumed to be due to increasing resistance. Resistance is also reported in patients with mucosal leishmaniasis caused by *Leishmania braziliensis*. Relapse is common in patients with visceral leishmaniasis who are immunodepressed, for example by human immunodeficiency virus (HIV) infection, but this is due to the immune dependence of drug activity and not acquired resistance.

Pharmacokinetics

It is rapidly excreted into urine with a half-life of about 2 h; 60–80% of the dose appears in the urine within 6 h of parenteral administration. Peak concentrations of about 12–15 mg Sb/l are achieved in serum 1 h after a dose of 10 mg Sb(V)/kg. There is a slow accumulation in the central compartment, and tissue concentrations reach a maximum after several days. In contrast to trivalent derivatives, pentavalent antimonials are not accumulated by erythrocytes, but there is evidence of protein binding. Antimony is detected in the skin for at least 5 days after treatment. Some of the dose of Sb(V) is converted to Sb(III) possibly by the liver. In a study on structurally related meglumine antimonate (see below) the pharmacokinetics of Sb(V) and Sb(III) were similar as measured by serum and urine levels.

Toxicity and side-effects

The toxic effects are limited by the rapid excretion, but cumulative toxicity increases in proportion to dose. Myalgia, arthralgia, anorexia and electrocardiographic changes have been reported as side-effects of high-dose regimens. Hepatocellular damage, hepatic and renal functional impairment and pancreatitis have also been reported. The changes are reversible on discontinuation of treatment.

Clinical use

Pentavalent antimonials are used exclusively in leishmaniasis. In visceral leishmaniasis relapse rates of 10% are common. Cutaneous leishmaniasis responds unpredictably, but mucocutaneous disease is usually unresponsive. Intralesional administration is practised in some countries for simple cutaneous lesions. Sodium stibogluconate has been used in combination with allopurinol for the treatment of visceral leishmaniasis and with paromomycin (aminosidine) for the treatment of both visceral and cutaneous forms of the disease which did not respond to the antimonial drugs alone.

Preparations and dosage

Proprietary name: Pentostam.

Preparation: Injection.

Dosage: Adults, i.m., i.v., 20 mg/kg per day with a maximum of 850 mg for at least 20 days; the dose varies with different geographical regions.

Limited availability; not available in the USA.

Further information

Bryceson A 1987 Therapy in man. In: Peters W, Killick-Kendrick R (eds) The leishmaniases. Academic Press, London, vol II, p 847–907

Chulay J D, Fleckenstein L, Smith D H 1988 Pharmacokinetics of antimony during treatment of visceral leishmaniasis with sodium stibogluconate or meglumine antimoniate. *Transactions of the Royal Society of Tropical Medicine and Hygiene* 82: 69–72

Herwaldt B L, Berman J D 1992 Recommendations for treating leishmaniasis with sodium stibogluconate (Pentostam) and review of pertinent clinical studies. *American Journal of Tropical Medicine and Hygiene* 46: 296–306

Navin T R, Arana B A, Arana F E, Berman J, Chajon J F 1992 Placebo-controlled clinical trial of sodium stibogluconate (Pentostam) versus ketoconazole for treating cutaneous leishmaniasis in Guatemala. *Journal of Infectious Diseases* 165: 528–534

Olliaro P L, Bryceson A D M 1993 Practical progress and new drugs for changing patterns of leishmaniasis. *Parasitology Today* 9: 323–328

World Health Organization 1990 Control of the leishmaniases. Technical report series 793. WHO, Geneva

MEGLUMINE ANTIMONATE

N-Methylglucamine   antimoniate,   methylaminoglucitol antimoniate

The Sb(V) content varies around 28% between batches.

Its activity, pharmacology and toxicology are similar to that of sodium stibogluconate; both are recommended for the treatment of visceral and cutaneous leishmaniasis and are essentially interchangeable. The predominant use of sodium stibogluconate in the Middle East and Africa and meglumine antimonate in South America is due to history and marketing policies. Studies in Central and South America have indicated that meglumine antimonate plus interferon-γ is effective in the treatment of visceral and cutaneous leishmaniasis cases unresponsive to antimony alone.

Preparations and dosage

Proprietary name: Glucantime.

Preparation: Injection.

Limited availability, not available in the UK.

Quinolines

Quinoline-containing drugs have been the mainstay of antimalarial chemotherapy since the 17th century in the form of *Cinchona* bark, which contains quinine and related alkaloids. Synthetic quinolines were developed in the 1920s and 1930s. The most important of these, the 4-aminoquinoline chloroquine, has succumbed to global resistance in *P. falciparum*. This has brought quinine and quinidine back into use for the therapy of severe malaria and prompted the search for new derivatives which led to mefloquine. Amodiaquine is active against chloroquine resistant strains of *P. falciparum*, but is not recommended for prophylaxis and is not often used in treatment because of the high rate of adverse effects (1 in 2000). Two bis(quinolines), piperaquine and hydroxypiperaquine, have been used in the treatment of drug resistant malaria in China. 8-Aminoquinolines are used for the radical cure of benign tertian malaria, but some investigational derivatives may have wider uses.

Further information

Foote S J, Cowman A F 1994 The mode of action and the mechanism of resistance to antimalarial drugs. *Acta Tropica* 56: 157–171

Kozarsky P E, Lobel H O 1994 Antimalarial agents: are we running out of options? *Current Opinions in Infectious Diseases* 7: 701–707

CHLOROQUINE

A synthetic 4-aminoquinoline.

Antimicrobial activity

It acts against the early erythrocytic stages of all four species of *Plasmodium* that cause human malaria. It is also active against the gametocytes of *Plasmodium vivax*, *Plasmodium ovale* and *Plasmodium malariae*, but not against the hepatic stages or mature erythrocytic schizonts and merozoites. The mechanism of action is related to the inhibition of degradation of haemoglobin in the parasite's food vacuole. Hypotheses to explain the selective toxicity of chloroquine include: (a) formation of a toxic haem–chloroquine complex; (b) inhibition of haemoglobin degradation through alteration of pH following accumulation in the food vacuole; and (c) inhibition of haemoglobin degradation through inhibition of haem polymerase, an enzyme which converts toxic haem into non-toxic haemozoin crystals. The 300-fold accumulation of chloroquine by infected erythrocytes is important to all these proposed mechanisms.

Acquired resistance

Resistance of *P. falciparum* was first reported in South America and South-East Asia in 1959 and has since spread to Africa and become a major problem in the control of malaria. The mechanism appears to be either decreased uptake of drug by the parasite or increased efflux from the parasite, or both. Verapamil and desipramine reverse chloroquine resistance in experimental models, but human trials have been disappointing. Chloroquine-resistant *P. vivax* has been reported in South America and South-East Asia.

Pharmacokinetics

Bioavailablity is 80–90% after oral administration. In the blood there is a large uptake by cells and 50–70% binding to plasma proteins. Peak plasma concentrations of 0.25 mg/l are achieved 1–6 h after doses of 300 mg. There is a large volume of distribution (200 l/kg) with extensive tissue binding and a high affinity for melanin-containing tissues. Chloroquine is extensively metabolized to a monodesethyl derivative which is biologically active and forms about 20% of the plasma level of the drug. The mean elimination half-life is approximately 9 days, resulting from a multi-component elimination with an initial phase (3–6 days), slow phase (12–14 days) and terminal phase (40 days). Renal clearance is about 50% of the dose.

Toxicity and side-effects

Minor side-effects such as dizziness, headache, rashes, nausea and diarrhoea are frequently reported. Pruritis occurs in up to 20% of Africans taking chloroquine. Long-term treatments can induce CNS effects and cumulative dosing over many years may cause retinopathy. Rarely, photosensitization, tinnitus and deafness have occurred.

Clinical use

It is used widely in the prophylaxis and treatment of all types of malaria, but activity against *P. falciparum* is seriously limited by the spread of resistance. Chloroquine is also used in an alternative treatment for hepatic amoebiasis in sequential combination with dehydroemetine.

Preparations and dosage

Proprietary names: Avloclor, Nivaquine.
Preparations: Tablets, syrup, injection.

Dosage: Treatment of benign malarias: adult, oral, 600 mg chloroquine base as initial dose then a single dose of 300 mg after 6–8 h, then a single dose of 300 mg/day for 2 days; children, oral, initial dose of 10 mg/kg of chloroquine base then a single dose of 5 mg/kg after 8 h, then a single dose of 5 mg/kg daily for 2 days.
Malaria prophylaxis: consult specialist guidelines.
Widely available.

Further information

Bradley D J, Warhurst D C 1995 Malaria prophylaxis: for travellers from Britain. *British Medical Journal* 310: 709–714

Dorn A, Stoffel R, Matile H, Bubendorf A, Ridley R G 1995 Malarial haemozoin/β-haematin supports haem polymerization in the absence of protein. *Nature* 374: 269–271

Murphy G, Basri H, Purnomo et al 1993 Vivax malaria resistant to treatment and prophylaxis with chloroquine. *Lancet* 341: 96–100

Slater A F G 1993 Chloroquine: mechanism of drug action and resistance in *Plasmodium falciparum*. *Pharmacology and Therapeutics* 57: 203–235

Wernsdorfer W H, Payne D 1991 The dynamics of drug resistance in *Plasmodium falciparum*. *Pharmacology and Therapeutics* 50: 95–121

White N J 1992 Antimalarial pharmacokinetics and treatment regimens. *British Journal of Clinical Pharmacology* 34: 1–10

World Health Organization 1990 Practical chemotherapy of malaria. Technical report series 805. WHO, Geneva

IODOQUINOL

Di-iodohydroxyquinoline, an 8-hydroxyquinoline derivative.

Antimicrobial activity

It has direct, but feeble activity against *Entamoeba histolytica* in vitro and in vivo. The mechanism of action is unknown.

Pharmacokinetics

Halogenated hydroxyquinolines are slowly and incompletely absorbed with <10% of an oral dose reaching the circulation. Absorbed drug is metabolized to sulphate or glucuronide conjugates and excreted.

Toxicity and side-effects

Side-effects are normally mild, including nausea, diarrhoea, rashes and cramps. Other halogenated hydroxyquinolines have been shown to cause subacute myelo-optic neuropathy from prolonged dosage and are banned in some countries.

Clinical use

It is used for the treatment of asymptomatic or mild intestinal amoebiasis and with nitroimidazoles or dehydro-emetine for severe cases.

Preparations and dosage

Preparation: Tablets.

Dosage: Adults, oral, 500 mg three times daily for 10 days. Children, oral, 20 mg/kg daily in divided doses for 10 days.

Not available in the UK.

MEFLOQUINE

A synthetic 4-quinolinemethanol.

Antimicrobial activity

It has rapid dose-related activity against erythrocytic stages of *Plasmodium* spp. with in vitro activity at 10–40 nM. It is effective against strains of *P. falciparum* that are resistant to chloroquine, sulphonamides and pyrimethamine. The C-11 (hydroxy) enantiomers have equal antimalarial activity. The mechanism of action is unclear, but it disrupts the parasites' digestive process, probably by binding to haematin or by the inhibition of haem polymerase, and intercalates into lipid bilayers with a high affinity for the erythrocyte membrane.

Acquired resistance

Resistance to mefloquine in *P. falciparum* has been increasing in South-East Asia; high-grade resistance occurs in 15% of patients and low-grade resistance in about 50%. There is cross-resistance with quinine and halofantrine, and an inverse relationship with chloroquine resistance has been reported. Resistant strains of *P. falciparum* appeared in Africa before the drug was used in that continent, perhaps because of quinine abuse or intrinsic resistance. The mechanism of resistance is unknown.

Pharmacokinetics

It is 70–80% absorbed after an oral dose of 1 g with peak plasma levels of 1 mg/l achieved in 2–12 h. The mean plasma elimination half-life is 20 days with <10% excreted in urine. Mefloquine is 98% plasma protein bound and is concentrated 2- to 5-fold in erythrocytes. The major metabolites do not have antimalarial activity. Pregnant women require larger doses than non-pregnant women to achieve comparable blood levels.

Toxicity and side-effects

At prophylactic doses risks of serious toxicity are about 1 in 10 000, similar to chloroquine. Doses used in therapy are more commonly associated with nausea, dizziness, fatigue, mental confusion and sleep loss. Psychosis, encephalopathy and convulsions are seen in about 1 in 1200 to 1 in 1700 patients.

Clinical use

It is a recommended antimalarial prophylactic for periods of less than 3 months in areas of chloroquine resistance. It is also an alternative to quinine and halofantrine in the treatment of uncomplicated multidrug-resistant malaria (p. 899). The combination with sulphadoxine–pyrimethamine is no longer favoured. A combination of mefloquine with artesunate has proved to be effective in Thailand.

Preparations and dosage

Proprietary names: Lariam, Mephaquine.

Preparation: Tablets.

Dosage: Malaria prophylaxis, see specialist guidelines.

Widely available.

Further information

Lobel H O, Miani M, Eng T et al 1993 Long term prophylaxis with weekly mefloquine. *Lancet* 341: 848–851

Pennie R A, Koren G, Crevoisier C 1993 Steady state pharmacokinetics of mefloquine in long-term travellers. *Transactions of the Royal Society of Tropical Medicine and Hygiene* 87: 459–462

Rojas-Rivero L, Gay F, Bustos M D et al 1992 Mefloquine–halofantrine cross-resistance in *Plasmodium falciparum* induced by intermittent mefloquine pressure. *American Journal of Tropical Medicine and Hygiene* 47: 372–377

Steffen R, Fuchs E, Schildknecht J, Naef U 1993 Mefloquine compared with other malaria chemoprophylactic regimens in tourists visiting East Africa. *Lancet* 341: 1299–1303

Ter Kuile F, Nosten F, Thieren M et al 1992 High dose mefloquine in the treatment of multidrug resistant falciparum malaria. *Journal of Infectious Diseases* 166: 1393–1400

White N J 1994 Mefloquine in the prophylaxis and treatment of falciparum malaria. *British Medical Journal* 308: 286–287

Wilson C M, Volkman S K, Thaithong S et al 1993 Amplification of *pfmdr 1* associated with mefloquine and halofantrine resistance in *Plasmodium falciparum* from Thailand. *Molecular and Biochemical Parasitology* 57: 151–160

PRIMAQUINE

A synthetic 8-aminoquinoline.

Antimicrobial activity

It is highly active against the hepatic stages of the malaria life cycle, including the latent hypnozoite stage of *P. vivax*. It has poor activity against erythrocytic stages of malaria parasites, but kills gametocytes. The isomers have similar antiplasmodial activity but differ in toxicity. In experimental models primaquine has activity against intracellular *Leishmania* and *Trypanosoma cruzi*. It has an effect on mitochondrial function, but the principal mechanism of action results from the formation of hydroxylated metabolites which are oxidized, forming toxic hydrogen peroxide and quinone–imine derivatives.

Acquired resistance

Failure rates of up to 35% have been reported in South-East Asia in patients treated with a standard course of primaquine for *P. vivax* infections.

Pharmacokinetics

Bioavailability estimates of 100% and 74% have been reported after oral administration. Peak plasma concentrations of 0.2 mg/l are achieved in 2–3 h after a 45 mg oral dose. There is extensive tissue distribution and a volume of distribution of only 2 l/kg. The elimination half-life is 4–10 h with urine containing <4% of the original dose. About 60% of the dose is metabolized to carboxyprimaquine which can reach levels 50-fold that of the parent drug; this metabolite has a half-life of 16 h, a low tissue distribution and is detectable at 120 h. Methoxy and hydroxy metabolites are also detectable.

Toxicity and side-effects

At standard doses there are mild side-effects, including abdominal cramps, anaemia, leucocytosis and methaemoglobinaemia. Patients with glucose-6-phosphate dehydrogenase deficiency, which occurs most frequently in Africans, are prone to intravascular haemolysis resulting from the oxidant stress induced by the drug.

Clinical use

It is principally used for radical cure of malaria caused by *P. vivax* or *P. ovale* (p. 898). Because of its gametocytocidal properties it has been used rarely in a single dose to prevent the spread of chloroquine resistant *P. falciparum*. A combination with clindamycin has been suggested as an alternative treatment for mild or moderately severe infections with *Pneumocystis carinii* in acquired immune deficiency syndrome (AIDS) patients.

Preparations and dosage

Dosage: Malaria prophylaxis, see specialist guidelines.
Limited availability in the UK.

Further information

Pukrittayakamee S, Vanijanonta S, Chantra A, Clemens R, White N J 1994 Blood stage antimalarial efficacy of primaquine in *Plasmodium vivax* malaria. *Journal of Infectious Diseases* 169: 932–935

Vilde J L, Remington J S 1992 Role of clindamycin with or without another agent for treatment of pneumocystosis in patients with AIDS. *Journal of Infectious Diseases* 166: 694–695

Wernsdorfer H, Trigg P I (eds) 1987 Primaquine: pharmacokinetics, metabolism, toxicity and activity. WHO/Wiley, Chichester

World Health Organization 1990 Practical chemotherapy of malaria. Technical report series 805. WHO, Geneva

QUININE

A quinolinemethanol from the bark of the *Cinchona* tree. A laevorotatory stereo-isomer of quinidine.

Antimicrobial activity

It inhibits the erythrocytic stages of human malaria parasites at <1 mg/l, but not the liver stages. It is also active against the gametocytes of *P. vivax*, *P. ovale* and *P. malariae*, but not *P. falciparum*. The stereo-isomer, quinidine, is more active than quinine, but epiquinine (cinchonine) and epiquinidine (cinchonidine) have much lower antimalarial activities. The mechanism of action is complex: quinine intercalates into lipid bilayers with a high affinity for the erythrocyte membrane; it also prevents haemazoin pigment formation in the parasite food vacuole possibly by inhibition of haem polymerase.

Acquired resistance

Resistance in *P. falciparum* was first reported in Brazil in 1910. It is now widespread in South-East Asia where some strains are also resistant to chloroquine, sulfadoxine–pyrimethamine and mefloquine. Cross-resistance with mefloquine has been demonstrated in *P. falciparum* in Central Africa and in laboratory studies.

Pharmacokinetics

About 80–90% of an oral dose is absorbed and peak plasma levels of 5 mg/l are achieved within 1–3 h. Plasma protein binding is about 70% in healthy humans, rising to 90% in uncomplicated malaria and 92% in cerebral malaria due to

high levels of acute-phase proteins. The volume of distribution is 1.8 l/kg. The elimination half-life is 8.7 h (18.2 h in severe malaria). There is extensive hepatic metabolism to hydroxylated derivatives. Urinary clearance is <20% of total clearance.

Toxicity and side-effects

Up to 25% of patients experience cardiac dysrhythmia, hypoglycaemia cinchonism (tinnitus, vomiting, diarrhoea, headache). Severe effects, including hypotension and hypoglycaemia, are of particular importance in children, pregnant women and the severely ill. Rarely, quinine can induce haemolytic anaemia ('blackwater fever').

Clinical use

It is used for the treatment of falciparum malaria, particularly cerebral malaria, if chloroquine resistance is suspected (Ch. 62). It is often used in combination with tetracycline (or doxycycline), clindamycin or pyrimethamine–sulfadoxine. Quinine in combination with clindamycin is also used in human babesiosis.

Preparations and dosage

Dosage: Treatment of falciparum malaria – adults, oral, 600 mg of quinine salt every 8 h for 7 days; i.v., initial loading dose of 20 mg/kg quinine salt (up to a maximum of 1.4 g) infused over 4 h, then after 8–12 h a maintenance dose of 10 mg/kg (up to a maximum of 700 mg) infused over 4 h, every 8–12 h until oral therapy can be taken to complete the 7 day course. Children, oral, 10 mg/kg of quinine salt every 8 h for 7 days.

Malaria prophylaxis, see specialist guidelines.

Widely available.

Further information

Bjorkmann A, Willcox M, Marbiah N, Payne D 1991 Susceptibility of *Plasmodium falciparum* to different doses of quinine in vivo and to quinine and quinidine in vitro in relation to chloroquine in Liberia. *Bulletin of the World Health Organization* 69: 459–465

Brasseur P, Kouamouo J, Druilhe P 1991 Mefloquine-resistant malaria induced by inappropriate quinine regimens? *Journal of Infectious Diseases* 164: 625–626

Pukrittayakamee S, Supanaranond W, Looareesuwan S, Vanijanonta S, White N J 1994 Quinine in severe falciparum malaria: evidence of declining efficacy in Thailand. *Transactions of the Royal Society of Tropical Medicine and Hygiene* 88: 324–327

Watt G, Loesuttivibool L, Shanks G D et al 1992 Quinine with tetracycline for the treatment of drug-resistant *falciparum* malaria in Thailand. *American Journal of Tropical Medicine and Hygiene* 47: 108–111

Wernsdorfer W H, Payne D 1991 The dynamics of drug resistance in *Plasmodium falciparum*. *Pharmacology and Therapeutics* 50: 95–121

White N J 1992 Antimalarial pharmacokinetics and treatment regimens. *British Journal of Clinical Pharmacology* 34: 1–10

Further information

Brasseur G, Favennec L, Perrine D, Chenu J P, Brasseur P 1994 Successful treatment of *Acanthamoeba* keratitis by hexamidine. *Cornea* 5: 459-462.

Pepin J, Milord F 1994. The treatment of human African trypanosomiasis. *Advances in Parasitology* 33: 1–47

Varga J H, Wolf T C, Parmley V C, Rowsey J J 1993 Combined treatment of *Acanthamoeba* keratitis with propamidine, neomycin and polyhexamethylene biguanide. *American Journal of Ophthamology* 115: 466–470

QUINIDINE

A quinolinemethanol from the bark of the *Cinchona* tree. The dextrarotatory stereo-isomer of quinine.

It is a blood schizonticide but with higher intrinsic antimalarial activity than quinine. It is well absorbed after oral administration and reaches peak plasma levels in 1–2 h. Blood concentrations after an equivalent dose are 30% lower than those of quinine because of a greater volume of distribution. The elimination half-life is 7 h. Quinidine is more toxic than quinine, but the injectable formulation used as an antiarrhythmic drug may be used in severe drug-resistant *P. falciparum* malaria if quinine is not available.

Further information

White N J 1992 Antimalarial pharmacokinetics and treatment regimens. *British Journal of Clinical Pharmacology* 34: 1–10

Diamidines

Stilbamidine, propamidine, pentamidine and diminazene were initially developed for the treatment of African trypanosomiasis following the identification of the trypanocidal activity of structurally related biguanidines in 1937. Pentamidine has been used extensively for early stage infections with *T. b. gambiense* and was formerly given half-yearly as part of a mass prophylaxis campaign in Central Africa. Pentamidine has acquired a new lease of life because of its efficacy in the prophylaxis and treatment of *Pneum. carinii* infections. Diminazene aceturate (Berenil) is used for cattle trypanosomiasis, but is not registered for human use. Propamidine and hexamidine have been used for ocular amoebiasis caused by *Acanthamoeba* spp.; therapeutic activity is also reported for the structurally related polyhexamethylene biguanide.

PENTAMIDINE

Synthetic bis(4'-amidino-phenoxy)pentane. Available as the isethionate (2-hydroxymethane sulphonate) salt. Production of the methanesuphonate salt (Lomidine) has been discontinued.

Antimicrobial activity

It has broad antiprotozoal activity in experimental models against *P. falciparum*, *Toxoplasma gondii*, *Leishmania* spp., *Trypanosoma* spp. and *Babesia* spp. It also has activity against *Pneum. carinii*. Binding to DNA, disruption of kinetoplast DNA, inhibition of ribosomal function and of adenosyl methionine decarboxylase, with effects on polyamine levels have all been reported. Pentamidine is accumulated by active transport but is not metabolized by trypanosomes.

Acquired resistance

Relapse rates of 7–16% have been reported in the treatment of human African trypanosomiasis in West Africa. Patients usually respond to a subsequent course of treatment with melarsoprol. Arsenic-resistant *T. brucei* are cross-resistant to diamidines, but far more so to diminazene and stilbamidine than pentamidine.

Pharmacokinetics

It is given parenterally as oral absorption is poor. Plasma levels of about 0.5 mg/l are achieved 1 h after a single intramuscular dose of 4 mg/kg. About 15–20% of the dose is excreted in the urine. The estimated volume of distribution is 3 l/kg. About 70% of the dose may be bound to serum proteins. Pentamidine is rapidly and extensively metabolized by rat liver, and high concentrations are retained in renal and hepatic tissue for up to 6 months after administration. In humans distribution is mainly in the liver, kidney, adrenals and spleen, with lower accumulation in the lung. This tissue retention is the basis for the prophylactic use of pentamidine. Critically, for the treatment of African trypanosomiasis, pentamidine is unable to cross the blood–brain barrier in sufficient quantity to be trypanocidal; <1% of the plasma concentration has been measured in the CSF of sleeping-sickness patients.

Toxicology and side-effects

It has a wide range of toxic side-effects from local irritation and sterile abscess at the site of injection, transient effects (vomiting, abdominal discomfort) to systemic effects (hypotension, effects on heart, hypoglycaemia and hyperglycaemia, leukopenia, thrombocytopenia). In a study of the treatment of South American cutaneous leishmaniasis, 17% for patients prematurely terminated treatment due to toxicity and another 30% reported side-effects. The World Health Organization (WHO) recommendations for treatment of African trypanosomiasis suggest that adrenalin, glucose and calcium should also be available.

Clinical use

It is used for the treatment of early stages of human African trypanosomiasis caused by *T. b. gambiense* before CNS involvement (p. 912). It is also a second-line drug for the treatment of leishmaniasis unresponsive to pentavalent antimonials (p. 910). There is limited evidence for the use of pentamidine in the treatment of clinical babesiosis. Currently the major use of pentamidine is in the prophylaxis and therapy of *Pneum. carinii* pneumonia (p. 669).

Preparations and dosage
Propamidine isethionate

Proprietary name: Brolene.

Preparation: Ophthalmic ointment.

Widely available.

Pentamidine isethionate

Proprietary name: Pentacarinat.

Preparation: Injection.

Dosage: Visceral leishmaniasis: adults, i.m., 3–4 mg/kg once or twice weekly until the condition resolves.

Trypanosomiasis: adults, i.m., i.v., 4 mg/kg daily or on alternate days to a total of 7–10 injections.

Widely available.

Further information

Berger B J, Henry L, Hall J E, Tidwell R 1992 Problems and pitfalls in the assay of pentamidine. *Clinical Pharmacokinetics* 22: 163–168

Bronner U, Doua F, Ericsson O et al 1991 Pentamidine concentrations in plasma, whole blood and cerebrospinal fluid during treatment of *Trypanosoma gambiense* infection in Cote d'Ivoire. *Transactions of the Royal Society of Tropical Medicine and Hygiene* 85: 608–611

Bryceson A 1987 Therapy in man. In: Peters W, Killick-Kendrick R (eds) The leishmaniases. Academic Press, London, vol II, p 847–907

Donnelly H, Bernard E M, Rothkotter H, Gold J W M, Armstrong D 1988 Distribution of pentamidine in AIDS. *Journal of Infectious Diseases* 157: 985–989

Leoung G S, Feigal D W, Montgomery A B et al 1990 Aerolized pentamidine for prophylaxis against *Pneumocystis carinii* pneumonia. *New England Journal of Medicine* 323: 769–775

Pepin J, Milord F 1994 The treatment of human African trypanosomiasis. *Advances in Parasitology* 33: 1–47

Soto J, Buffet P, Grogl M, Berman J 1994 Successful treatment of Columbian cutaneous leishmaniasis with four injections of pentamidine. *American Journal of Tropical Medicine and Hygiene* 50: 107–111

Thakur C P, Kumar M, Pandey A K 1991 Comparison of regimens of treatment of antimony resistant kala azar patients: a randomized study. *American Journal of Tropical Medicine and Hygiene* 45: 435–441

Vöhringer H F, Arasteh K 1993 Pharmacokinetic optimisation in the treatment of *Pneumocystis carinii* pneumonia. *Clinical Pharmacokinetics* 24: 388–412

Biguanides

Proguanil and chloroproguanil, are antimalarial prodrugs; their active metabolites are the triazines cycloguanil and chlorcycloguanil respectively. Proguanil is used widely as a prophylactic for malaria; chlorproguanil has therapeutic activity in combination with dapsone. These drugs, along with the diaminopyrimidines (Ch. 21), are often referred to as antifols due to their mechanism of action.

PROGUANIL

An arylbiguanide.

Proguanil

Cycloguanil

Antimicrobial activity

It may have some antiplasmodial action, but most of the useful activity is attributable to its metabolite cycloguanil, which inhibits the early erythrocytic stages of all four *Plasmodium* spp. that cause human malaria and the primary hepatic stage of *P. falciparum*. In common with trimethoprim (p. 350), cycloguanil is a potent inhibitor of dihydrofolate reductase and, like pyrimethamine (p. 348), has a high affinity for the plasmodial enzyme. Proguanil appears to act synergically with atovaquone (p. 534).

Acquired resistance

Resistance of *P. falciparum* associated with alterations in dihydrofolate reductase has been reported world-wide, although infrequently despite its use since the 1940s. Resistance in *P. vivax* and *P. malariae* has been reported in South-East Asia. Cross-resistance with pyrimethamine is not absolute, since differential resistance can arise from different point mutations on the dihydrofolate reductase gene.

Pharmacokinetics

Oral bioavailability is >90%, but absorption is slow; peak plasma levels of 0.4 mg/l are reached 2–4 h after a 100 mg dose. It is 75% protein bound and is concentrated 10- to 15-fold by erythrocytes. The elimination half-life is 10 h with 60% of the dose excreted in urine. About 20% of proguanil is metabolized to dihydrotriazene derivatives, most importantly cycloguanil, by hepatic cytochrome P450 processes. Cycloguanil is detectable 2 h after administration of proguanil. High proportions of 'non-metabolizers' have been identified in Japan and Kenya, indicating another source of resistance to this drug.

Toxicity and side-effects

It is a well tolerated drug at recommended doses. Gastro-intestinal and renal effects have been reported at doses exceeding 600 mg/day.

Clinical use

It is used only as a prophylactic antimalarial, usually in combination with chloroquine (p. 903). Combination with atovaquone is under trial for the treatment of drug-resistant falciparum malaria.

> **Preparations and dosage**
> *Proprietary name:* Paludrine.
> *Preparation:* Tablets.
> For malaria prophylaxis, see specialist guidelines.
> Widely available.

Further information

Bradley D J, Warhurst D C 1995 Malaria prophylaxis: guidelines for travellers from the United Kingdom. *British Medical Journal* 341: 848–851

Helsby N A, Watkins W M, Mberu E, Ward S A 1991 Inter-individual variation in the metabolic activation of the antimalarial biguanides. *Parasitology Today* 7: 120–123

Peterson D S, Milhous W K, Wellems T E 1990 Molecular basis of differential resistance to cycloguanil and pyrimethamine in *Plasmodium falciparum* malaria. *Proceedings of the National Academy of Sciences, USA* 87: 3018–3022

Wyler D J 1993 Malaria chemoprophylaxis for the traveler. *New England Journal of Medicine* 329: 31–37

Sesquiterpene lactones

In 1979, a research group in China described the use of a sesquiterpene peroxide, artemisinin (qinghaosu), in the treatment of malaria caused by *P. falciparum and P. vivax*. This compound, derived from a plant used in traditional Chinese medicine, *Artemisia annua*, has been used extensively in East Asia for the treatment of malaria. Since the identification of antimalarial activity artemisinin and two derivatives, artesunate and artemether, which have higher intrinsic antimalarial activity and improved formulations, have replaced quinine as a treatment of falciparum malaria in China and have been used in millions of cases in South-East Asia. These drugs are not presently available outside Asia. The WHO is developing artemether, a derivative more lipophilic and potentially less toxic than artemether. The novel antimalarial structure, with its rapid activity against the erythrocytic stage, has been the stimulus for the development of semi-synthetic and synthetic trioxane and dioxane compounds containing an endoperoxide bridge and activities against *Plasmodium* spp. and *Tox. gondii.* Although the mechanism of action is not completely understood, the endoperoxide bridge is essential for the antimalarial activity of artemisinin compounds. Haem-activated artemisinin generates free radicals which oxidize lipids and damage membranes and alkylate proteins.

Artemisinin

R = CCH$_2$CH$_2$COOH: Artesunate
‖
O

R = CH$_3$ Artemether

Further information

Davidson D E 1994 Role of arteether in the treatment of malaria and plans for further development. *Transactions of the Royal Society of Tropical Medicine and Hygiene* 88 (suppl 1): 51–52

Editorial 1992 Rediscovering wormwood: qinghaosu for malaria. *Lancet* 339: 649–651

Hien T T, White N J 1993 Qinghaosu. *Lancet* 341: 603–608

Meshnick S R, Taylor T E, Kamchonwongpaisan S 1996 Artemisinin and the antimalarial endoperoxides: from herbal remedy to targeted chemotherapy. *Microbiological Reviews* 60: 301–315

White N J 1994 Artemisinin: current status. *Transactions of the Royal Society of Tropical Medicine and Hygiene* 88 (suppl 1): 3–4

ARTEMISININ

A sesquiterpene peroxide derived from *A. annua.* Chiefly used in the form of artemether, the methyl ester synthesized from dihydroartemisinin, or artesunate, the water-soluble hemisuccinate, which is suitable for intravenous use.

Antimicrobial activity

It is active against the erythrocytic stages of chloroquine-sensitive and chloroquine-resistant strains of *P. falciparum* and other malaria parasites. Two anomers of artemether are produced on synthesis, α-artemether and β-artemether, of which the latter has higher antimalarial activity. Activity against *Tox. gondii, Leishmania major* and the helminth *Schistosoma mansoni* has been demonstrated in experimental models.

Pharmacokinetics

Artemisinin and its derivatives are concentrated by erythrocytes and rapidly hydrolysed to dihydroartemisinin. It has been suggested that oral doses are hydrolysed before they enter the systemic circulation. Artemether is usually administered by the intramuscular route, although an oral formulation is also available; artesunate can also be given intravenously. Pharmacokinetic data are limited. After injection of artemether, peak plasma concentrations of 0.2 mg/l are achieved in 4–9 h, whereas the peak plasma concentration of oral artemether is reached within 2–3 h. The elimination half-life of intravenous artesunate is <30 min and that of dihydroartemisinin 45 min, but artemether appears to have a much longer half-life of 4–11 h.

Toxicity and side-effects

Few toxic effects other than drug-induced fever and a reversible decrease in reticulocyte counts have been reported. High-dose studies in animal models have suggested a toxic metabolite which causes neurotoxicity and reproducible dose-related neuropathic lesions.

Clinical use

It is presently used exclusively in malaria, including cerebral malaria. Reported cure rates in Thailand are 65–98% for artemether and 100% for 5-day courses of artesunate. Combinations with mefloquine or doxycycline have been proposed.

Further information

Brewer T G, Peggins J O, Grate S J et al 1994 Neurotoxicity in animals due to arteether and artemether. *Transactions of the Royal Society of Tropical Medicine and Hygiene* 88 (suppl 1): 33–36

Hien T T, White N J 1993 Qinghaosu. *Lancet* 341: 603–608

Looareesuwan S 1994 Overview of clinical studies on artemisinin derivatives in Thailand. *Transactions of the Royal Society of Tropical Medicine and Hygiene* 88 (suppl 1): 9–11

Taylor T, Wills B, Kazembre P et al 1993 Rapid coma resolution with artemether in Malawian children with cerebral malaria. *Lancet* 341: 661–662

White N J, Waller D, Crawley J et al 1992 Comparison of artemether and chloroquine for severe malaria in Gambian children. *Lancet* 339: 317–321

World Health Organization 1990 Practical chemotherapy of malaria. Technical report series 805. WHO, Geneva

Miscellaneous antiprotozoal agents

ATOVAQUONE

A chlorophenyl cyclohexyl hydroxynaphthoquinone.

Antimicrobial activity

It is more active than standard antimalarials in vitro against *P. falciparum* with an IC_{50} value of about 1 nM. It is also active against both tachyzoites and cysts of *Tox. gondii* in vitro and in mice. *Pneum. carinii* is sensitive in vitro at 0.1–3.0 mg/l and high doses are effective in the rat.

In *P. falciparum* the site of action is the cytochrome bc_1 complex. Inhibition of the respiratory chain results in inhibition of dihydro-orotate dehydrogenase and the disruption of pyrimidine biosynthesis; this may explain the synergy seen with proguanil. The mechanism of action against *Pneum. carinii* has not been determined.

Acquired resistance

In clinical trials of the treatment of malaria in Thailand there was a 25% relapse rate; two patients failed to respond upon retreatment with atovaquone suggesting drug-resistant parasites were present.

Pharmacokinetics

It has poor water solubility and is highly lipophilic. It is poorly absorbed from the intestine, but bioavailablility is increased 3-fold when administered with meals. In the plasma >99.9% is protein bound. Single doses of 750 mg achieved steady-state plasma levels of 27 mg/l. The plasma elimination half-life was 70 h in healthy volunteers and 55 h in patients with AIDS. Steady-state plasma concentrations are up to 50% lower in AIDS patients than asymptomatic HIV-positive cases. Atovaquone penetrates the CSF, but the concentration is less than 1% of the plasma level. Unlike some other naphthoquinones it is not metabolized by human liver microsomes.

Toxicity and side-effects

Most clinical trials have involved patients with AIDS in whom adverse effects are often difficult to detect; however, more than 20% reported fever, nausea, diarrhoea and rashes. There were limited changes in hepatocellular function.

Clinical use

It is presently used principally for the treatment of *Pneum. carinii* pneumonia in patients intolerant of co-trimoxazole (Ch. 46). In the treatment of malaria it is unsuitable when used alone, but combinations with tetracycline and proguanil appear curative; the combination with proguanil is under trial in multiresistant falciparum malaria. It has been used in cerebral toxoplasmosis in AIDS patients but further studies are necessary.

Further information

Blanchard T J, Mabey D C W, Hunte-Cooke A et al 1994 Multiresistant falciparum malaria cured using atovaquone and proguanil. *Transactions of the Royal Society of Tropical Medicine and Hygiene* 88: 693

Hudson A T 1993 Atovaquone – a novel broad-spectrum anti-infective drug. *Parasitology Today* 9: 66–68

Hudson A T, Dickins M, Ginger C D et al 1991 566C80: a potent broad spectrum anti-infective agent with activity against malaria and opportunistic infections in AIDS patients. *Drugs in Experimental and Clinical Research* 17: 427–435

Hughes W, Leoung G, Kramer F et al 1993 Comparison of atovaquone (566C80) with trimethoprim–sulphamethoxazole to treat *Pneumocystis carinii* pneumonia in patients with AIDS. *New England Journal of Medicine* 328: 1521–1527

Kovacs J and the NIAID clinical center intramural AIDS program 1992 Efficacy of atovaquone in treatment of toxoplasmosis in patients with AIDS. *Lancet* 340: 637–638

DEHYDROEMETINE

The synthetic racemic derivative of the plant alkaloid emetine.

Antimicrobial activity

Like the parent compound, emetine, it inhibits *E. histolytica* at concentrations of 1–10 mg/l in vitro, but it is more active than the parent in animal models. It also has activity against *Leishmania* spp. in experimental models. Dehydroemetine irreversibly inhibits the translocation of peptidyl-tRNA from acceptor to donor sites during protein synthesis.

Acquired resistance

Drug-resistant *E. histolytica* is rare, differences in sensitivity have been reported.

Pharmacokinetics

It is administered parenterally. No human pharmacokinetic data are available. A half-life of 2 days, compared with 5 days for emetine, has been reported. There is selective tissue binding and accumulation in the liver, lung, spleen and kidney.

Toxicity and side-effects

Dehydroemetine is considerably less toxic than emetine, possibly because it is more rapidly eliminated. Nevertheless, nausea, vomiting, diarrhoea and abdominal cramps frequently occur. Neuromuscular effects have also been reported. More serious cardiotoxic effects can lead to electrocardiogram (ECG) changes, tachycardia and a drop in blood pressure.

Clinical use

It is a second-line drug for the treatment of severe intestinal or hepatic amoebiasis, and is sometimes given before administration of iodoquinol or chloroquine.

Preparations and dosage

Preparation: Injection.

Dosage: Adults, s.c., i.m., 1–1.5 mg/kg daily for 5 days with a maximum daily dose of 90 mg.

Limited availability.

Further information

Burchard G D, Mirelman D 1988 *Entamoeba histolytica*: virulence potential and sensitivity to metronidazole and emetine of four isolates possessing nonpathogenic zymodemes. *Experimental Parasitology* 66: 231–242

Schwartz D E, Herrero J 1965 Comparative pharmacokinetic studies of dehydroemetine and emetine in guinea pigs using spectrofluorometric methods. *American Journal of Tropical Medicine and Hygiene* 14: 78–83

DILOXANIDE

Dichloro(hydroxyphenyl)methylacetamide. Available as a furoate salt, an insoluble ester.

Antimicrobial activity

It inhibits *E. histolytica* with unusually high specificity at concentrations of 0.01–0.1 mg/l.

Acquired resistance

No resistance has been reported. Patients with dysentery have lower cure rates than cyst excreters.

Pharmacokinetics

Human pharmacokinetic data are limited. Animal data show that diloxanide furoate is rapidly absorbed from the intestine. The furoate is hydrolysed in the gut leaving high intraluminal concentrations of free diloxanide. About 75% is excreted via the kidney within 48 h, mostly as a glucuronide.

Toxicity and side-effects

It is well tolerated, but flatulence is common, and nausea and vomiting may occur.

Clinical use

It is recommended for asymptomatic intestinal (luminal) amoebiasis with cure rates of up to 95% reported.

Combinations with metronidazole and tinidazole have been used for extraintestinal amoebiasis.

Further information

Di Perri G, Strosselli M, Rondanelli E G 1989 Therapy of entamoebiasis. *Journal of Chemotherapy* 1: 113–122

Dubey M P, Gupta P S, Chuttani H K 1965 Entamide fuorate in the treatment of intestinal amoebiasis. *Journal of Tropical Medicine and Hygiene* 68: 63–66

EFLORNITHINE
α-**Difluoromethylornithine, DFMO**

$$H_2N(CH_2)_3 - \overset{\displaystyle NH_2}{\underset{\displaystyle CHF_2}{C}} - COOH$$

Antimicrobial activity

Cultured trypomastigotes of *T. brucei* are relatively insensitive, but high doses are effective against bloodstream and CNS infections of *T. b. brucei* and *T. b. gambiense* in rodents, provided a strong antibody response is also present. *T. b. rhodesiense* infections do not respond. Synergy with some arsenicals has been demonstrated. It is also active against *P. falciparum* in experimental models and against *Leishmania* promastigotes and *Giardia lamblia* in culture.

It is a selective and irreversible inhibitor of ornithine decarboxylase which catalyses the conversion of ornithine to putrescine, the first step in the biosynthesis of the polyamines spermidine and spermine.

Acquired resistance

Acquired resistance in *T. b. gambiense* in West Africa has not been reported, but *T. b. rhodesiense* strains from East Africa are innately resistant.

Pharmacokinetics

Bioavailability following a single oral dose of 10 mg/kg is 55%. Peak plasma concentrations of about 7 mg/l are achieved 4 h after ingestion. In adult sleeping sickness patients receiving 200 mg/kg intravenously, the mean serum concentration was 87.5 nmol/l. The mean elimination half-life is 3.3 h with 83% renal clearance; most is eliminated unchanged. In a study in Zaire the mean serum concentration in children under 12 years old was half that of adults, probably due to more rapid renal clearance. CNS penetration is good in adults with a CSF:plasma ratio of 0.91 at the end of administration for 14 days. However, the CSF:plasma ratio in children under 12 years old was 0.58. Relapses have been recorded in patients in whom CSF levels dropped below 50 nmol/ml at the end of treatment.

Toxicity and side-effects

Osmotic diarrhoea and bone marrow suppression are common, and up to 50% of sleeping sickness patients develop leucopenia. Reversible anaemia and thrombo-cytopenia have been observed. Convulsions and seizures, different to those observed in melarsoprol-induced encephalopathy, have been reported in 4–18% of treated sleeping sickness patients but not in patients treated for *Pneum. carinii* pneumonia. This difference might be due to the CNS inflammation associated with sleeping sickness.

Clinical use

It is effective in late stage *T. b. gambiense* infections including arsenic-resistant cases. Monotherapy is not effective against East African sleeping sickness, but trials of eflornithine plus suramin are in progress for *T. b. rhodesiense* infections. It has been used speculatively for treatment of *Pneumocystis carinii* infections in AIDS patients.

Further information

Bacchi C 1993 Resistance to clinical drugs in African trypanosomes. *Parasitology Today* 9: 190–193

McCann P P, Pegg A E 1992 Ornithine decarboxylase as an enzyme target for therapy. *Pharmacology and Therapeutics* 54: 195–215

Milord F, Loko L, Ethier L, Mpia B, Pepin J 1993 Eflornithine concentrations in serum and cerebrospinal fluid in 63 patients treated for *Trypanosoma brucei gambiense* sleeping sickness. *Transactions of the Royal Society of Tropical Medicine and Hygiene* 87: 473–477

Pepin J, Milord F 1994 The treatment of human African trypanosomiasis. *Advances in Parasitology* 33: 1–47

Vohringer H F, Arasteh K 1993 Pharmacokinetic optimisation in the treatment of *Pneumocystis carinii* pneumonia. *Clinical Pharmacokinetics* 24: 388–412

HALOFANTRINE

A phenanthrene methanol.

Antimicrobial activity

It inhibits erythrocytic stages of chloroquine-sensitive and chloroquine-resistant *P. falciparum* and other *Plasmodium* spp. in vitro at concentrations in the range of 0.4–4.0 mg/l; it is more active than mefloquine. The enantiomers of halofantrine have equivalent activity in vitro. The precise mechanism of action has not been determined although it has been shown to form complexes with haemazoin (ferriprotoporphyrin IX).

Acquired resistance

Resistance in *P. falciparum* has been reported in Central and West Africa where halofantrine has been used widely. Cross-resistance with mefloquine has been reported in Thailand where halofantrine has not been used.

Pharmacokinetics

It has extremely low aqueous solubility and absorption shows both intra- and inter-subject variability. Bioavailability is increased more than 6-fold after a fatty meal. In patients with malaria bioavailability is significantly lower than in healthy individuals. Parenteral formulations are not available. Peak plasma levels are variable and occur 6 h after administration. Halofantrine is not concentrated by infected or uninfected erythrocytes unlike many other antimalarials. About 20–30% of the dose is metabolized to a desbutyl derivative. The elimination half-life of the parent drug is 1 day and that of the metabolite 3 days. Little unchanged drug is excreted in urine.

Toxicity and side-effects

Abdominal pain, diarrhoea and pruritus are the most frequent. High doses (72 mg/kg) have been reported to be cardiotoxic, inducing prolongation of the PR and QT intervals. Mefloquine increases these changes and the drugs should not be used together.

Clinical use

Halofantrine is used for the treatment of multidrug-resistant falciparum malaria (p. 899).

> **Preparations and dosage**
> *Proprietary name:* Halfan.
> *Preparation:* Tablets.
> *Dosage:* Treatment of falciparum malaria: adults, oral, 1.5 g divided into 3 doses of 500 mg given at intervals of 6 h and repeat the course after an interval of 1 week.
> Widely available.

Further information

Brasseur P, Bittsindou P, Moyou R et al 1993 Fast emergence of *Plasmodium falciparum* resistance to halofantrine. *Lancet* 341: 901–902

Karbwang J, Bangchang K N 1994 Clinical pharmacokinetics of halofantrine. *Clinical Pharmacokinetics* 27: 104–119

Nosten F, Ter Kuile F, Luxemburger C et al 1993 Cardiac effects of antimalarial treatment of halofantrine. *Lancet* 341: 1054–1056

Shanks G, Watt G, Edstein M et al 1992 Halofantrine given with food for falciparum malaria. *Transactions of the Royal Society of Tropical Medicine and Hygiene* 86: 233–234

Ter Kuile F, Golan G, Nosten F et al 1993 Halofantrine versus mefloquine in treatment of multidrug-resistant falciparum malaria. *Lancet* 341: 1044–1049

Wilson C M, Volkman S K, Thaithong S et al 1993 Amplification of *pfmdr 1* associated with mefloquine and halofantrine resistance in *Plasmodium falciparum* from Thailand. *Molecular and Biochemical Parasitology* 57: 151–160

World Health Organization 1993 Drug Alert: halofantrine. *Weekly Epidemiological Record* 68: 269–270

MEPACRINE

Quinacrine; a synthetic acridine derivative.

Antimicrobial activity

It is active against the asexual erythrocytic stage of all four *Plasmodium* spp. that infect man and the gametocytes of *P. vivax* and *P. malariae*. The enantiomers have equal antimalarial activity. It exhibits broad antiprotozoal activity in experimental models against *T. cruzi*, *Leishmania* spp., *E. histolytica*, *Trichomonas vaginalis* and *G. lamblia*. It is also active against tapeworms. The precise mechanisms of action are unclear, although there is interaction with DNA and membrane phospholipids.

Acquired resistance

The structural resemblance to chloroquine suggests the likelihood of cross-resistance with that drug, but evidence for this is equivocal.

Pharmacokinetics

Peak plasma concentrations of 50 µg/l are reached in 1 to 3 h after an oral dose of 100 mg. Protein binding is 85%. It is eliminated slowly, with a half-life of 5 days. There is extensive tissue binding and a 6-fold concentration into leukocytes from plasma. About 10% of the daily dose is excreted in the urine.

Toxicity and side-effects

It causes dizziness, headache and gastric problems. Toxic psychoses, bone marrow depression, yellow skin and exfoliative dermatitis are described. It should not be used in combination with 8-aminoquinolines.

Clinical use

It was formerly much used in the prophylaxis of malaria and in tapeworm infections, but it has been superseded by other drugs. Use is now restricted to the oral treatment of giardiasis. Intralesional injections have been tried in cutaneous leishmaniasis. Its sclerosant effect has led to its use in the form of intravaginal pellets as a non-surgical method of female sterilization.

Preparations and dosage

Preparation: Tablets.

Dosage: Adults, oral, 100 mg three times daily. A second course of treatment after 2 weeks may sometimes be required.

Limited availability.

Further information

Davidson R A 1990 Treatment of giardiasis: the North American perspective. In: Meyer E A (ed) Giardiasis. Elsevier, Amsterdam, p 325–334

Shannon J A, Earle D P, Brodie B B, Taggart J V, Berliner R W 1944 The pharmacological basis for the rational use of atabrine in the treatment of malaria. *Journal of Pharmacology and Experimental Therapeutics* 81: 307–330

World Health Organization 1990 Control of the leishmaniases. Technical report series 793. WHO, Geneva, p 53

SURAMIN

A sulphated naphthylamine.

Antimicrobial activity

It has no significant trypanocidal activity in vitro, but is effective in animals infected with *T. brucei*. Trypanosomes take up suramin bound to plasma protein by a combination of fluid phase and receptor-mediated endocytosis. Glycolytic enzymes located in the glycosomes, a unique trypanosomatid microbody, appear to be the most important target. It acts synergically with nitroimidazoles and eflornithine in the elimination of trypanosomes from CSF of infected mice.

Acquired resistance

Relapse rates of 30–50% have been reported in Kenya and Tanzania, but it has not been possible to assess whether this was due to resistance.

Pharmacokinetics

It is poorly absorbed following oral administration and causes irritation when injected by intramuscular or subcutaneous routes; it is normally administered by slow intravenous infusion. More than 99% of the dose forms highly bound complexes with plasma proteins and can be detected in blood for 3 months. After six doses of 1 g at weekly intervals, plasma levels higher than 100 mg/l were observed for several weeks with a half-life of 44–54 days. No metabolism was observed and 80% was removed by renal clearance. Tissue distribution is high to reticulo-endothelial cells, especially liver macrophages, the adrenal glands and the kidney. Due to its large molecular size and anionic charge at physiological pH it does not enter erythrocytes and it penetrates the blood–brain barrier poorly.

Toxicity and side-effects

It is a toxic drug, especially in malnourished patients. A test dose of 200 mg has been recommended. Immediate febrile reactions (nausea, vomiting, loss of consciousness) can be avoided by slow intravenous administration. Intramuscular or subcutaneous injections are painful and irritating. These reactions can be followed by fever and urticaria. Anaphylactic shock is rare (<1 in 2000 patients). Delayed reactions include renal damage, exfoliative dermatitis, anaemia, leucopenia, agranulocytosis, jaundice and diarrhoea.

Clinical use

It is effective in early stage *T. b. gambiense* and *T. b. rhodesiense* infection. It is not used in late stage disease because of the poor penetration into the CNS. It is also used in onchocerciasis.

Preparations and dosage

Proprietary name: Suramin.

Preparation: Injection.

Dosage: The dose schedule varies depending on the stage of the disease.

Availabe in South Africa.

Further information

Pepin J, Milord F 1994 The treatment of human African trypanosomiasis. *Advances in Parasitology* 33: 1–47

Voogd T E, Vansterkenburg E L M, Wilting J, Janssen L H M 1993 Recent research on the biological activity of suramin. *Pharmacological Reviews* 45: 177–203

Willson M, Callens M, Kuntz D A, Perie J, Opperdoes F 1993 Synthesis and activity of inhibitors highly specific for the glycolytic enzymes from *Trypanosoma brucei*. *Molecular and Biochemical Parasitology* 59: 210

World Health Organization 1986 The epidemiology and control of African trypanosomiasis. Technical report series 739. WHO, Geneva

Antibacterial and other antimicrobial agents used in protozoal disease

Properties of diaminopyrimidines (Ch. 21), nitroimidazoles (Ch. 30) and nitrofurans (Ch. 29) that are widely used as antiprotozoal agents are described in the appropriate chapters. Among antibiotics, tetracyclines (Ch. 35), clindamycin (Ch. 26) and certain macrolides (Ch. 27) have a place in the treatment of some protozoal diseases. The aminoglycoside, paromomycin (Ch. 13) is sometimes used in amoebiasis and is increasingly used in leishmaniasis; it is also one of the few drugs claimed to be useful in intractable cryptosporidiosis.

Antifungal polyene and azole derivatives (Ch. 36) are increasingly used in diseases caused by protozoa. Both extracellular and intracellular forms of *Leishmania* spp. and *T. cruzi* are highly sensitive to amphotericin B in vitro at concentrations below 1 mg/l. Amphotericin B lipid formulations have proved valuable in the treatment of visceral leishmaniasis, but immunocompromised patients often relapsed after initial improvement. Amphotericin B is also used for the treatment of primarily amoebic meningo-encephalitis caused by *Naegleria fowleri*.

The imidazoles, miconazole and ketoconazole (pp. 491, 490) and the triazole itraconazole (p. 489) are also active against *Leishmania* spp. and *T. cruzi* in experimental models, but results have been equivocal in clinical trials. The anthelmintic benzimidazole albendazole (p. 514) is effective in infections caused by *G. lamblia* and is also on trial for the treatment of microsporidiosis in AIDS patients.

Further information

Das S S, Simpson A J H 1993 Therapy of protozoan infections in patients with impaired immunity. *Current Opinion in Infectious Diseases* 6: 784–793

Davidson R N, Di Martino L, Gradoni L et al 1994 Liposomal amphotericin B (AmBisome) in Mediterranean visceral leishmaniasis: a multi-centre trial. *Quarterly Journal of Medicine* 87: 75–81

De Castro S L 1993 The challenge of Chagas' disease chemotherapy: an update of drugs assayed against *Trypanosoma cruzi*. *Acta Tropica* 53: 83–98

Dietrich D T, Lew E A, Kotler D P, Poles M A, Orenstein J M 1994 Treatment with albendazole for intestinal disease due to *Enterocytozoon bieneusi* in patients with AIDS. *Journal of Infectious Diseases* 169: 178–183

Dietze R, Milan E P, Berman J D, Grogl M, Falqueto A 1993 Treatment of Brazilian kala-azar with a short course of Amphocil (Amphotericin B cholesterol dispersion). *Clinical Infectious Diseases* 17: 981–986

Edlind T 1991 Protein synthesis as a target for antiprotozoal drugs. In: Coombs G, North M (eds) Biochemical protozoology. Taylor & Francis, London, p 569–586

Lossick J G, Kent H L 1991 Trichomoniasis: trends in diagnosis and management. *American Journal of Obstetrics and Gynecology* 165: 1217–1222

Mishra M, Biswan U K, Jha D N, Khan A B 1992 Amphotericin versus pentamidine in antimony-unresponsive kala-azar. *Lancet* 340: 1256–1257

Navin T R, Arana B A, Arana F E, Berman J, Chajon J F 1992 Placebo-controlled clinical trial of sodium stibogluconate (Pentostam) versus ketoconazole for treating cutaneous leishmaniasis. *Journal of Infectious Diseases* 165: 528–534

Olliaro P L, Bryceson A D M 1993 Practical progress and new drugs for changing patterns of leishmaniasis. *Parasitology Today* 9: 323–328

Reynoldson J A, Thompson R C A, Horton R J 1992 Albendazole as a future antigiardial agent. *Parasitology Today* 8: 412–414

Scott J A G, Davidson R N, Moody A H et al 1992 Aminosidine (paromomycin) in the treatment of leishmaniasis imported into the United Kingdom. *Transactions of the Royal Society of Tropical Medicine and Hygiene* 86: 617–619

Teklemarian S, Gebre Hiwot A, Frommel D, Miko T L, Ganlov G, Bryceson A 1994 Aminosidine and its combination with sodium stibogluconate in the treatment of diffuse cutaneous leishmaniasis caused by *Leishmania aethiopica*. *Transactions of the Royal Society of Tropical Medicine and Hygiene* 88: 334–339

Antiviral agents

K. G. Nicholson

Introduction

Despite the success of public health measures, including vaccination, viruses still account for considerable morbidity, mortality and economic loss. Clinical interest in the development of antivirals has until recently been weak – primarily because many viral infections are acute and self-limiting, but also because laboratory diagnosis of viral infection has been so slow that results emerge too late to influence management. Moreover, the parasitic association of viruses and the host cell led to the belief that drugs that interfere with the viral life cycle would inevitably be toxic to the host. Developments in rapid viral diagnosis, recognition of chronic hepatitis B, C and D, the emergence of acquired immune deficiency syndrome (AIDS), and an improved understanding of viral replication have altered this picture dramatically, and many new candidate antiviral agents are undergoing laboratory testing and clinical evaluation.

Antiviral agents can act potentially at a number of points in viral replication: by directly inactivating the virus prior to cell attachment and entry; blocking attachment of virus to host-cell membrane receptors and penetration; blocking viral uncoating; preventing integration of viral DNA into the host genome; blocking transcription or translation into viral messenger RNA and proteins; and interfering with glycosylation steps, viral assembly and release. Human viral pathogens fall into four groups – single and double stranded DNA and RNA, which may vary in size, polarity and in other ways. This nucleic acid is very closely integrated with host cellular components, without which the virus cannot replicate. However, viruses do have unique requirements in order to express their genome and may contain in their genome, or code for, specific enzymes that are essential for their life cycle, e.g. the reverse transcriptase of the retroviruses.

Based on these considerations, considerable effort has gone into identifying agents that specifically inhibit one or more steps in the viral life cycle and have little or no effect on the host. Generally this approach is unlikely to produce broad-spectrum agents. As might be anticipated, a great many compounds with antiviral activity have now been identified and they fall into diverse chemical groups. Currently most interest is focused on the nucleoside and nucleotide analogues that block nucleic acid metabolism. This chapter deals first with compounds licensed for clinical use (Table 40.1) and then developmental and investigational agents and those of restricted clinical application are discussed.

Of the relatively few compounds to come into clinical use, apart from two adamantanes, one phosphonate and interferon-α, all have been nucleoside analogues.

Adamantanes

The parent compound, 1-aminoadamantane hydrochloride, is a tricyclic primary amine that was discovered in the 1960s and was found to inhibit replication of strains of influenza A. Numerous derivatives have been synthesized, but none has a better profile than rimantadine.

AMANTADINE
1-Aminoadamantane hydrochloride; 1-adamantanamine hydrochloride

A symmetrical synthetic C-10 tricyclic amine with an unusual cage-like structure.

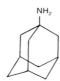

Antiviral activity

It inhibits H1N1, H2N2, H3N2 and Hsw1N1 strains of influenza type A in tissue culture at concentrations of 0.2–0.6 mg/l. It is generally accepted that both amantadine and rimantadine block the ion channel of the influenza A M2 membrane protein. This prevents acidification of the virus interior which is required for fusion of the viral envelope to the endosome leading to release of viral RNA, and thereby blocks replication.

In view of the general susceptibility of influenza type A viruses, it is reasonably anticipated that future variants, including pandemic strains, will be similarly inhibited. It has little or no activity against influenza B, and higher concentrations than can be safely achieved in man are required to inhibit rubella, parainfluenza and respiratory syncytial viruses.

Acquired resistance

Drug-resistant strains of influenza A have been recovered from man which show complete cross-resistance between amantadine and other adamantanes. Resistant strains have been recovered from nasopharyngeal specimens of approximately 30% of children, adults and the elderly in residential homes during treatment with amantadine or rimantadine. Resistant strains are transmissible, are not evidently attenuated, and are associated with mutations in amino acid positions 27, 30 and 31 in the M2 transmembrane sequence. Postexposure prophylaxis, the concomitant administration of drug to index cases and contacts, seems to favour the emergence of drug resistance. Resistance develops within several days of onset of treatment, and where treatment and prophylaxis are being undertaken concomitantly it is essential that symptomatic patients be isolated to reduce the possible transmission of resistant virus.

Pharmacokinetics

Amantadine is almost completely absorbed after oral administration, and peak plasma concentrations are seen around 4–6 h (range 2–8 h). Daily administration of 200 mg by the oral route leads within 4–7 days to steady state plasma concentrations in the range 0.4–0.9 mg/l. After oral administration respiratory secretion levels approach plasma concentrations.

It is eliminated virtually entirely by the kidney as unchanged drug with excretion of approximately 56% of a single oral dose in a subsequent 24 h urine collection.

Table 40.1 *Antiviral agents currently available for clinical use*

Agent	Uses
Adamantanes:	
Amantadine	Prophylaxis and treatment of influenza A
Rimantadine	As above
Interferon-α	Chronic hepatitis B and C infection (hairy cell and chronic myelogenous leukaemias and Kaposis' sarcoma)
Nucleosides:	
Acyclovir	Topical: ophthalmic and cutaneous HSV infection
	Oral: VZV and prophylaxis and treatment of HSV skin and mucous membrane infections
	Parenteral: severe HSV and VZV infections
Didanosine	HIV infection (second-line therapy)
Famciclovir	Treatment of shingles
Ganciclovir	Life- or sight-threatening CMV infection in the immunocompromised
Idoxuridine	Ophthalmic HSV infection
Ribavirin	Aerosol: RSV infection and influenza A and B intravenous and oral: Lassa fever and some other viral haemorrhagic fevers
Stavudine	HIV infection (second-line therapy)
Trifluridine	Ophthalmic HSV infection
Valaciclovir	Treatment of shingles
Vidarabine	Topical: ophthalmic HSV infection
	Parenteral: severe HSV and VZV infections
Zidovudine	HIV infection with a CD4 cell count of less than 500/mm³. Prevention of maternal–infant transmission
Zalcitabine	HIV infection (second-line therapy)
Phosphonates:	
Foscarnet	Life- or sight-threatening CMV infection in the immunocompromised

Altogether 90% of an oral dose is excreted in the urine with an elimination half-life of 11.8 h (range 9.7–14.5 h) in young healthy subjects with normal renal function. In elderly men (60–76 years old) the half-life is 28.9 h and in patients with renal insufficiency half-lives of 18.5 h to 33.8 days have been observed. The renal clearance is around 398 ml/min (range 112–772 ml/min), indicating active secretion as well as glomerular filtration. Less than 5% of a dose is removed during haemodialysis and average half-lives of 8.3 and 13 days have been recorded in patients on chronic haemodialysis. Extreme care must therefore be taken to ensure that the drug does not accumulate to toxic levels.

Toxicity and side-effects

It is embryotoxic and teratogenic in rats at 50 mg/kg daily, about 15 times the usual human dose. Cardiovascular maldevelopment has been observed in an infant whose mother was exposed during the first 3 months of pregnancy to 100 mg/day. Administration to women of child-bearing potential is therefore unjustified except perhaps in life-threatening influenzal pneumonia.

Minor neurological symptoms including insomnia, light-headedness, difficulty in concentration, nervousness, dizziness, and headache are reported in up to 20% of individuals receiving 200 mg. Other side-effects include anorexia, nausea, vomiting, dry mouth, constipation and urinary retention. They mostly arise during the first 3–4 days of therapy and are reversible when the drug is discontinued or the dosage is reduced. An exception to rapid onset of adverse reactions is livedo reticularis. Convulsions, hallucinations and confusion are apparently dose related, usually occurring at levels in excess of 1.5 mg/l; convulsions may occur at a lower threshold in patients with a history of epilepsy and the drug is best avoided in such patients.

Cases of deliberate overdose have occurred, and in one instance a patient who had taken an estimated 2.8 g developed an acute toxic psychosis with disorientation, visual hallucinations, aggressive behaviour, urinary retention and dilated pupils. Congestive cardiac failure and cardiac arrhythmias may also be experienced.

Amantadine may aggravate central nervous, gastrointestinal or other side-effects provoked by anticholinergic drugs or L-dopa. In one report two patients developed visual hallucinations while concurrently taking amantadine and benzhexol; these responded to a reduction of the dose of benzhexol. Observations limited to one patient indicate that either hydrochlorthiazide, triamterene or both reduce the clearance of amantadine and can produce higher plasma concentrations and toxic effects. There is no specific antidote to amantadine. Haemodialysis is not helpful because of the large volume of distribution. Physostigmine may be of value in countering amantadine-induced delirium and myoclonus.

Clinical use

It is used both in the prevention and treatment of influenza for short periods and rational use requires laboratory and epidemiological evidence of influenza A in the community. Candidates for prophylaxis include unvaccinated children and adults at high risk because of underlying disease, unvaccinated adults in essential community positions, household contacts of an index case, people unable to receive influenza vaccine because of egg sensitivity, and those living in semi-closed institutions. Indeed, a World Health Organization (WHO) Advisory Group recommends amantadine prophylaxis for elderly and high-risk people in institutional settings to augment protection afforded by vaccination. If vaccination has been overlooked, high-risk individuals can still be vaccinated after an outbreak appears locally, but the development of an immune response usually takes several weeks and this vulnerable period may be covered by chemoprophylaxis. When vaccine is unavailable, or the influenza A strain causing an epidemic differs markedly from the vaccine strain, amantadine may be given for the entire duration of the outbreak, a period of about 4–8 weeks. In view of the repeated demonstration of the efficacy of prophylactic amantadine 200 mg daily, it has been proposed that the trough amantadine plasma concentration associated with this dose in healthy adults aged 18–43 years (0.3 mg/l) should be the target trough concentration in the calculation of amantadine doses for influenza A prophylaxis in populations with different amantadine kinetics. However, there is no clear plasma concentration–effect relationship and it is suggested that protection may fail with high trough levels.

The 100 mg capsule represents too large a dose for neonates and young children. A suggested dose for children aged 1–9 years is 4–8 mg/kg body weight daily in divided doses up to a maximum of 150 mg daily. A single 100 mg capsule daily is suggested by the manufacturers for children aged 10–15 years. The drug should be used cautiously in the elderly as excretion falls with age. Concurrent cardiovascular insufficiency or confusion should also be taken into account.

Preparations and dosage

Proprietary name: Symmetrel.

Preparations: Capsules, syrup.

Dosage: Adults, oral, Influenza A treatment, 100 mg twice daily for 5–7 days. Children, 10–15 years, 100 mg/day (treatment or prophylaxis). Prophylaxis, 100 mg twice a day.

Widely available.

Further information

Aoki F Y, Stiver H G, Sitar D S, Boudreault A, Ogilvie R I 1985 Prophylactic amantadine dose and plasma concentration–effect relationships in healthy adults. *Clinical Pharmacology and Therapeutics* 37: 128–136

Horadam V W, Sharp J G, Smilack J D et al 1981 Pharmacokinetics of amantadine hydrochloride in subjects with normal and impaired renal function. *Annals of Internal Medicine* 94: 454–458

Oxford J S, Galbraith A 1980 Antiviral activity of amantadine: a review of laboratory and clinical data. *Pharmacology and Therapeutics* 11: 181–262

Soung L S, Ing T S, Daugirdas J T et al 1980 Amantadine hydrochloride pharmacokinetics in haemodialysis patients. *Annals of Internal Medicine* 93 (part 1): 46–49

RIMANTADINE
1-Methyl-1-adamantanemethylamine hydrochloride

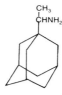

This amantadine analogue was first developed in the USA, but has been studied and used clinically in the USSR for many years. Numerous derivatives have been synthesized, but none so far with better profiles.

Antiviral activity

In ferret tracheal ciliated epithelium infected with influenza A, rimantadine is more effective than amantadine on a weight-for-weight basis. It is also more effective against experimentally induced influenza A infection in laboratory animals.

There is complete cross-resistance with amantadine.

Pharmacokinetics

Single- and multiple-dose pharmacokinetic studies in elderly patients and in young adults have shown remarkably similar results. The peak plasma concentration following 100 mg twice daily is 400–500 ng/ml and the elimination half-life is approximately 35 h. The steady-state concentration in nasal mucus develops by day 5 and the mucus concentration is approximately 1.5-fold higher than in plasma. In comparison with amantadine, the drug is found at higher concentrations in nasal mucus, in relation to plasma concentrations, than is amantadine. Despite the structural similarities between amantadine and rimantadine there are some notable differences in their pharmacokinetics and metabolism. The majority of amantadine is excreted in the urine, whereas less than 20% of rimantadine is excreted unchanged by this route. Rimantadine is metabolized by the liver, but the majority of its breakdown products are excreted in the urine. Its plasma half-life is much less affected by renal dysfunction than is that of amantadine.

Toxicity and side-effects

It is at least as effective as amantadine in the prophylaxis of influenza type A, but produces significantly fewer side-effects at equivalent doses. Indeed in one study, the central nervous system (CNS) attributable side-effects of medication were not significantly higher than placebo, but were considerably higher with amantadine. This may in part be related to differences in pharmacokinetics, since with equal doses the blood levels of amantadine are approximately twice those of rimantadine.

Clinical use

Prolonged administration is well tolerated by elderly patients in nursing homes and, on the basis of this and other information, it appears to be the drug of choice for the prophylaxis and treatment of influenza A.

Preparations and dosage

Dosage: Adults, oral, 200 mg/day in single or divided doses. Available in continental Europe and the USA.

Further information

Tominack R L, Hayden F G 1987 Rimantadine hydrochloride and amantadine hydrochloride use in influenza A virus infections. *Infectious Disease Clinics of North America* 1: 459–478

Tominack R L, Wills R J, Gustavson L E, Hayden F G 1988 Multiple dose pharmacokinetics of rimantadine in elderly adults. *Antimicrobial Agents and Chemotherapy* 32: 1813–1819

Interferons

The interferons are low-molecular-weight proteins that are produced by mammalian cells both in vitro and in vivo in response to viral infection and certain other stimuli. There are three classes of interferons: interferon-α and interferon-β, produced by lymphocytes and fibroblasts respectively, and interferon-γ, which is produced by unsensitized lymphoid cells in response to mitogens and sensitized lymphocytes when stimulated with specific antigen. Interferons are generally host-species specific and are now produced by recombinant genetic techniques.

Interferon inducers

A variety of substances has been found to excite the production or release of interferons. Some are natural macromolecules (e.g. lipopolysaccharides), others are synthetic (e.g. synthetic polynucleotides), some are microbial cells, while others are low-molecular-weight compounds (e.g. tilorone). Several such compounds have been investigated as potential antiviral agents against human immunodeficiency virus (HIV).

INTERFERON-α

Human protein, molecular weight (MW) approximately 19 kDa, produced by recombinant DNA technology in *Escherichia coli*.

Antiviral activity

It renders cells resistant to infection with a wide range of viruses and also has a number of other effects, including immunoregulatory functions, mediation of inflammation, cell multiplication inhibitory action, interaction with mixed histocompatability genes, and effects on differentiation, including the induction of the synthesis of specific proteins and enzymes. Thus it cannot be regarded as a simple antiviral, though this is probably one of its most important functions. It has no effect on extracellular virus and does not prevent virus from penetrating cells. It reversibly binds to specific cellular receptors, thereby activating cytoplasmic enzymes affecting messenger RNA translation and protein synthesis; the antiviral state takes several hours to develop but may persist for days thereafter.

Pharmacokinetics

It reaches peak plasma concentrations of 20 and 50–100 U/ml within 2–4 h of intramuscular injection of 3×10^6 and 9×10^6 U, respectively. It is cleared from the circulation with elimination half-lives of 3–8 h after intramuscular injection and 2–3 h after intravenous injection. The half-life after intranasal application is 20 min. It penetrates the cerebrospinal fluid (CSF) poorly and is not cleared by haemodialysis. Little or none is excreted in the urine, and its fate after release from the cell receptor is largely unknown.

Toxicity and side-effects

Its toxicity has become increasingly apparent with the advent of purer preparations. 'Flu'-like symptoms (fever, arthralgia, myalgia, headache, malaise, chills), which can usually be reduced or eliminated by the concurrent administration of paracetomol, and lymphocytopenia are common unwanted effects, generally arising 2–4 h after administration of several million units. Liver function test values are frequently elevated at doses above 10^7 U/day. These effects are rapidly reversible and tolerance may develop after several days. Other toxic effects include gastro-intestinal disturbances (anorexia, nausea, diarrhoea, vomiting), weight loss, local pain, severe fatigue, alopecia, paraesthesiae, confusion, dizziness, drowsiness, nervousness and bone marrow suppression. The haematological toxicity is dose dependent (threshold around 3×10^6 U/day) and readily reversible. Hypotension may develop during, or up to, 2 days after treatment, and arrhythmias and cardiac failure have been observed. Paradoxically, herpes labialis may occur. It inhibits hepatic cytochrome P_{450} systems and oxidative drug metabolism in man and may cause a modest prolongation in the half-life of drugs such as theophylline. Administration of doses greatly in excess of the recommended clinical dose to pregnant rhesus monkeys in the early to mid-trimester caused abortions. Its effect on human pregnancy is unknown and it is uncertain whether it is excreted in breast milk. Neutralizing antibodies have been reported in around a quarter of treated patients but no clinical sequelae to their presence has been documented.

Repeated application to the nasal mucosa is generally well tolerated, though at daily doses of about 10^7 U for more than 5 days some individuals develop nasal congestion, sore throat, hoarseness, nasal burning, increased nasal secretions and blood in nasal mucus, together with mucosal friability, crusts and erosions. No toxic effects have been observed from repeated topical applications to the eye or to the vagina. Intralesional administration is generally well tolerated.

Clinical use

It is available for the treatment of hairy cell leukaemia, chronic myelogenous leukaemia and Kaposi's sarcoma. It has also been found to be useful in the treatment of some patients with chronic hepatitis B and C infection. The findings of a number of studies in patients with chronic hepatitis B suggest that relatively short courses (2–6 weeks) are ineffective even at dosage levels of 100 MU/day; 3 months' treatment appears to be optimum with no further benefit from longer courses; thrice-weekly treatment is as effective as daily therapy; a dosage of 5–10 MU is optimum; heterosexuals respond better than homosexuals; orientals and those infected with HIV generally fail to respond; overall, up to 60% of patients respond to treatment. Treatment regimens are currently being evaluated in chronic hepatitis C, but preliminary studies indicate that interferon therapy for 6 months or longer may be required, and that approximately half of those who respond initially with a lowering of liver enzymes subsequently relapse.

Another area of interest has been in the prevention and treatment of respiratory viral infections. Prophylactic interferon administered as a nasal spray for 7 days as soon as family members develop symptoms of an upper respiratory tract infection, abolishes virtually all rhinovirus infections, but has little or no effect on infections caused by other respiratory viruses. Further studies are required to define the role, if any, in the prevention of respiratory viral infections in 'high-risk' groups such as those with cystic fibrosis and asthma.

Topical application, when combined with acyclovir or trifluorothymidine, accelerates healing of herpes simplex eye infections. Variable success has been obtained with intralesional interferon injections in the treatment of condyloma accuminata.

Preparations and dosage

Proprietary names: Interferon-α, Intron A, Roferon A, Wellferon, Viraferon, Interferon-γ1b, Imukin.

Preparation: Injection.

Dosage: Dose varies according to the condition being treated.

Widely available.

Further information

Alexander G J M, Brahm J, Fagan A E et al 1987 Loss of HBsAg with interferon therapy in chronic hepatitis B infection. *Lancet* ii: 66–69

Jacyna M R, Brooks M G, Lok R H T, Main J, Murray-Lyon I M, Thomas H C 1989 Randomised controlled trial of interferon alpha (lymphoblastoid interferon) in chronic non-A non-B hepatitis. *British Medical Journal* 298: 80–82

Monto A S, Albrecht J K, Schwartz S A 1988 Demonstration of dose-response relationship in seasonal prophylaxis of respiratory infections with α-2b interferon. *Antimicrobial Agents and Chemotherapy* 32: 47–50

Nucleoside analogues

Most of the compounds are purines or pyrimidines (e.g. vidarabine), are halogenated or have substituted sugars, but in acyclovir and ganciclovir, the sugar is acyclic and in ribavirin the 'nucleoside' moiety is triazole carboxamide.

Replacement of ribose or 2'-deoxyribose in nucleosides by arabinose produces compounds which inhibit viral and cellular DNA synthesis. The discovery of the naturally occurring aranucleotides, spongothymidine (Ara T) and spongouridine (Ara U) in the sponge Cryptotethya crypta *prompted the synthesis and evaluation of cytosine arabinoside (Ara C) and adenine arabinoside (Ara A) in the late 1950s and early 1960s. Ara A was later discovered to be a naturally occurring product of* Streptomyces antibioticus. *A number of aranucleosides in addition to vidarabine which is available for clinical use have been synthesized. Ara C has proven useful in the treatment of certain leukaemias and, in view of its considerable cytotoxicity, it is generally accepted that the drug does more damage to the host than to the virus. Treatment of herpetic keratitis with Ara C has been limited by unacceptable corneal toxicity.*

As with a number of other classes of antimicrobial agents, attempts have been made to improve on the properties of antiviral nucleosides by halogenation. Idoxuridine and trifluridine are currently available for topical use. Details of other halogenated nucleosides (bromovinyldeoxyuridine (BVDU) fluoroiodoaracytosine (FIAC) and fluoromethyl Arau (FMAU), which are amongst the most potent and selective of antiherpes agents) are given in the previous edition of this book.

ACYCLOVIR
Acycloguanosine; 9-(2-hydroxyethoxymethyl)guanine; ACV

A synthetic acyclic purine nucleoside analogue of the natural nucleoside 2'-deoxyguanosine.

Antiviral activity

The results of antiviral inhibitory activity vary according to the nature of the assay, the cells used, the viral strain, its multiplicity of infection and the timing of treatment in relation to infection. Herpes simplex virus (HSV) types 1 and 2, simian herpes virus B and varicella zoster viruses, which code for their own thymidine kinases, are all susceptible to concentrations readily attainable in man. The

ID_{50} for HSV types 1 and 2 is 0.1 μM, whereas that for uninfected vero cells is 300 μM. The concentration required to inhibit HSV type 1 and type 2 replication by 90 and 99% is approximately 10- and 100-fold greater than that producing 50% inhibition. The ID_{50} for varicella zoster virus (VZV) is 3 μM, while that for WI 38 cells, the line in which VZV was cultivated, is >3000 μM.

Because thymidine-kinase-negative HSV mutants and cytomegalovirus (CMV) do not code for thymidine kinase, monophosphorylation of acyclovir does not readily occur in cells infected with these viruses. Moreover, CMV DNA polymerase is not readily inhibited by acyclovir triphosphate. Although Epstein–Barr virus (EBV) may have reduced thymidine kinase activity, its DNA polymerase is susceptible to acyclovir triphosphate. Accordingly EBV shows intermediate susceptibility, whereas CMV isolates are generally resistant. Human herpes virus type 6 tends to be less susceptible than EBV. Acyclovir has little or no inhibitory activity against viruses other than those in the herpes group. Decreasing hepatitis B polymerase activity has been found in vitro in hepatoma cells exposed to increasing concentrations of acyclovir. However, two randomized trials of intravenous acyclovir have failed to show any significant effect on seroconversion, although the drug does have a transient and partial effect on hepatitis B virus (HBV) DNA polymerase activity in man.

The combination of acyclovir with interferons, ribavirin, vidarabine and trifluridine gives additive or synergistic activity against HSV, and acyclovir with interferon-α or trifluridine also gives additive or synergistic activity against VZV and CMV. Recent evidence suggests a potential benefit on survival from HIV infection of acyclovir plus zidovudine. However, this does not appear to be associated with changes in HIV p24 antigen levels or CD4 cell counts, and the role of acyclovir is unclear.

A combination of factors is responsible for the drug's high potency and low toxicity. Firstly, host-cell enzymes do not effectively phosphorylate it and phosphorylation occurs mainly in herpes-infected cells where the necessary viral enzyme is present. The resulting acyclovir monophosphate is converted by several cellular enzymes to acyclovir triphosphate, a potent and selective inhibitor of HSV DNA-polymerase and a DNA chain terminator.

Acquired resistance

HSV may become resistant by one of several different mechanisms. Mutations that involve deficient thymidine kinase production are most common; alterations in the DNA polymerase gene also result in resistance. Resistant mutants may be found in wild virus populations and mutants lacking thymidine kinase activity may be readily induced by passage of HSV in the presence of the drug. Acyclovir-resistant strains have mostly been reported in immunocompromised patients, are generally thymidine-kinase negative, and have a decrease in virulence. Resistant mutants that retain thymidine kinase activity appear to retain their virulence. Emergence of resistant HSV strains is less frequent in immunocompetent patients, occurring in about 2% of those receiving prolonged treatment.

Pharmacokinetics

Therapeutic drug levels are readily attained after both oral and intravenous administration, though only about 20% of an oral dose of 200 mg is absorbed. Oral doses of 200 mg 4-hourly give a mean peak plasma level of 2.5 μM (range 1.4–4 μM) at 1.5–1.75 h after medication; while more than 90% lower than the levels after intravenous therapy, they are still inhibitory to HSV types 1 and 2. Steady-state peak plasma concentrations after 8-hourly doses of 2.5, 5, 10 and 15 mg/kg were 30.1, 43.2, 88.9 and 91.7 μM, respectively. These levels were similar to those found after single doses, indicating that accumulation of the drug is unlikely in patients without renal dysfunction.

It is widely distributed in various tissues and body fluids. Delivery of the drug to the basal epidermis after topical administration is about 30–50% of that obtained by oral administration. Acyclovir ointment penetrates the corneal epithelium. CSF concentrations are approximately 50% of simultaneous plasma concentrations. Vesicular fluid concentrations approximate those in plasma. Its concentration in saliva is 13% of that in plasma and it is found in vaginal secretions at variable concentration. Acyclovir is actively secreted into breast milk and is found at a concentration several-fold higher than in plasma. Placental cord blood contains levels of 69–99% of maternal plasma and the drug is 3–6 times more concentrated in amniotic fluid.

The plasma half-life after intravenous administration is about 3 h and after oral administration approximately 3.3 h. Probenecid (1 g oral) increases its half-life by 18% and the plasma concentration–time curve by 40%. Mean peak plasma concentrations and the area under the curve (AUC) are significantly reduced when the drug is given with a heavy meal in comparison to a light one. It is minimally protein bound (15%) and approximately 15% of an intravenous dose is metabolized in persons with normal renal function. The only significant urinary metabolite of acyclovir is 9-carboxymethoxymethylguanine, which accounts for up to 14% of a dose in persons with normal renal function. This metabolite has virtually no activity against HSV. Less than 0.2% of the dose is recovered as the 8-hydroxylation product, 8-hydroxy-9-(2-hydroxymethoxy-methyl)guanine.

The principal route of elimination of acyclovir is in the urine and the mean percentage of a dose recovered unchanged ranges from 45% to 79%, which decreases with decreasing creatinine clearance. In patients with renal failure, mean peak plasma concentrations nearly doubled and the elimination half-life increased to 19.5 h. Dosage reductions are therefore advised for various stages of renal impairment. During haemodialysis the half-life dropped to 5.7 h and after dialysis the plasma concentration was about 60% less than the predialysis concentration. Half-lives of 12–17 h have been reported for patients undergoing continuous ambulatory peritoneal dialysis, with only 13% or less of administered drug being recovered in the 24-h dialysate. The half-life in a patient undergoing arterio-venous haemofiltration/dialysis was about 20 h.

Acyclovir does not significantly alter the pharmacokinetics of zidovudine and high doses (3200 mg/day) do not affect trough cyclosporin levels in renal transplant recipients.

Toxicity and side-effects

Few adverse reactions to topical, ocular, oral or intravenous formulations have been reported, despite extensive clinical evaluation. Allergic contact dermatitis occasionally occurs with acyclovir cream. Superficial punctate keratopathy is the most common ophthalmic adverse event, occurring in 10% of patients receiving ophthalmic ointment; stinging or burning on application occurs in 4%. Less common complications of the ophthalmic preparation include conjunctivitis, blepharitis and pain. During early trials, transient increases in blood urea and creatinine were seen in about 10% of patients given rapid bolus injections. This is analogous to the renal dysfunction seen in experimental animals with deposition of acyclovir crystals in the renal tubules: it can be largely avoided by reducing the rate of infusion, adequate hydration and dosage adjustment in renal failure. Nausea, vomiting, diarrhoea and abdominal pain occasionally occur, particularly in association with a raised creatinine concentration. Acute reversible renal failure has been reported. Reconstituted acyclovir has a pH of about 11, and severe inflammation and occasionally ulceration have been reported after extravasation of the drug at the infusion site. Encephalopathy, tremors, confusion, hallucinations, convulsions, psychiatric disorders, bone-marrow depression and abnormal liver function have occasionally arisen. Skin rashes have been reported in a few patients and resolve on discontinuation of the drug.

Acyclovir has not been shown to be embryotoxic or teratogenic to mice or rabbits, despite the presence of substantial concentrations of the drug in amniotic fluid and fetal tissue. Teratogenicity in rats has been reported. Results of mutagenicity tests in vitro and in vivo indicate that it is unlikely to pose a genetic risk to man, and the drug was not found to be carcinogenic in long-term studies in mice and rats. The Acyclovir in Pregnancy Registry has followed up 312 acyclovir-exposed pregnancies. Of these there were 24 spontaneous fetal losses, 47 induced abortions, 159 births without congenital deformity and 9 with congenital abnormalities. Among the 73 second- and third-trimester births one infant was born with a congenital abnormality. There was no consistent pattern to any of the abnormalities. Of the cases followed prospectively the congenital abnormality rate was 4.1%, which is similar to the rate of 3% in the general population of live-born infants. Until further information is available, the use of acyclovir in pregnancy is only recommended for the treatment of life-threatening maternal HSV infection.

Clinical use

It is used for topical treatment of herpes simplex keratitis and lesions of the skin and mucous membranes; oral treatment of herpes zoster and treatment and prophylaxis of herpes simplex lesions of the skin and mucous membranes; and intravenous treatment of more severe HSV infections in the immunocompromised and immunocompetent, including primary genital herpes, herpes simplex encephalitis, and neonatal herpes; the intravenous preparation is also used for prophylaxis of HSV infections in the severely immunocompromised.

Preparations and dosage

Proprietary name: Zovirax.

Preparations: Tablets, suspension, i.v. infusion, cream, ophthalmic.

Dosage: Adults, children, oral, dose varies according to the condition being treated. I.v. infusion, adults, herpes simplex or recurrent varicella-zoster, 5 mg/kg every 8 h, doubled in primary and recurrent varicella-zoster in the immunocompromised and in simplex encephalitis. Children ≤3 months, 10 mg/kg every 8 h; 3 months to 12 years, 250 mg/m^2 every 8 h; dose doubled in the immunocompromised and simplex encephalitis.

Widely available.

Further information

Alexander G J M, Fagan E A, Heagerty J E et al 1987 Controlled clinical trial of acyclovir in chronic hepatitis B infection. *Journal of Medical Virology* 21: 81–87

Dugadzig R M, Skettris I S, Belitsky P, Schlech W F, Givner M L 1991 Effect of coadministration of acyclovir and cyclosporine on kidney function and cyclosporine concentrations in renal transplant recipients. *Annals of Pharmacotherapy* 25: 316–317

Galle P R, Theilmann L 1990 Inhibition of hepatitis B virus polymerase activity by various agents. Transient expression of hepatitis B virus DNA in hepatoma cells as novel system for evaluation of antiviral drugs. *Arzneimittel-Forschung* 40: 1380–1382

Goday J, Aguirre A, Gil Ibarra N, Eizaguirre X 1991 Allergic contact dermatitis from acyclovir. *Contact Dermatitis* 24: 380–381

Grant D M 1987 Acyclovir (Zovirax) ophthalmic ointment: a review of clinical tolerance. *Current Eye Research* 6: 231–235

Haefeli W, Schoenberger R A Z, Weiss P 1993 Acyclovir-induced neurotoxicity: concentration side-effect relationship in acyclovir overdose. *American Journal of Medicine* 94: 212–215

Hernandez E, Praga M, Moreno F, Montoyo G 1991 Acute renal failure induced by oral acyclovir. *Clinical Nephrology* 36: 155–156

Jones T, Alderman C 1991 Acyclovir clearance by CAVHD. *Intensive Care Medicine* 17: 125–126

MacDiarmaid-Gordon A R, O'Connor M, Bearman M, Ackrill P 1992 Neurotoxicity associated with oral acyclovir in patients undergoing dialysis. *Nephron* 62: 280–283

O'Brien J J, Campoli-Richards D M 1989 Acyclovir: an updated review of its antiviral activity, pharmacokinetic properties and therapeutic efficacy. *Drugs* 37: 233–309

Parry G E, Dunn P, Shah V P, Pershing L P 1992 Acyclovir bioavailability in human skin. *Journal of Investigative Dermatology* 98: 856–863

Proceedings of a symposium on acyclovir 1988 *American Journal of Medicine* 85 (suppl 2A)

Stahlman R, Klug S, Lewandowski C et al 1987 Teratogenicity of acyclovir in rats. *Infection* 15: 261–262

Stein D S, Graham N M H, Park L P et al 1994 The effect of the interaction of acyclovir with zidovudine on progression to AIDS and survival. *Annals of Internal Medicine* 121: 100–108

Wagstaff A J, Faulds D, Goa K L 1994 Aciclovir: a reappraisal of its antiviral activity, pharmacokinetic properties and therapeutic efficacy. *Drugs* 47: 153–205

Wilson C G, Washington N, Hardy J G, Bond S W 1987 The influence of food on the absorption of acyclovir: a pharmacokinetic and scintigraphic assessment. *International Journal of Pharmaceutics* 38: 221–225

DIDANOSINE
2',3'-Dideoxyinosine; ddI

A synthetic purine nucleoside analogue.

Antiviral activity

The concentrations required to inhibit HIV infection in vitro vary greatly depending upon the assay, virus inoculum, laboratory performing the test, and cells used. The ID_{50} ranges from 2.5 to 10 μM (1 μM = 0.24 mg/l) in T cells, and 0.01–0.1 μM in monocyte/macrophage cell cultures. Expression of HIV p24 gag protein in H9 cells was blocked by 10 μM didanosine, but concentrations of >10 μM were required to block completely the cytopathic effects in ATH8 cells. ID_{50} values of 2.1 μM for HIV-1 and 5.6 μM for HIV-2 were obtained in a plaque reduction assay in HT4-6C cells.

Acquired resistance

The presence of clinically-significant resistance to didanosine pre- and posttherapy is under investigation. Two of 14 pretherapy isolates in one study had ID_{50} values of 30 and 50 μM. Comparison of pre- and posttherapy sensitivities of HIV-1 isolates from 14 patients on long-term didanosine revealed a decrease in sensitivity of 15-fold in one patient, 6-fold in three patients, and was not significantly different in the remainder. The mechanism for didanosine resistance involves mutations of codons 65, 74 or 184 in the gene for reverse transcriptase. However, most data indicate that the codon 74 mutation is the primary mutation responsible for didanosine resistance. Eight of 9 patients who received 11–25 months of didanosine monotherapy in studies at the US National Cancer Institute developed a mutation at position 74, implying that development of resistance is common. In a further study, 36 of 64 (56%) patients with advanced HIV, who were switched from zidovudine to didanosine, developed the didanosine resistance mutation at codon 74 by 24 weeks. The patients who developed the codon 74 mutation had a greater decline in CD4 cells after the development of the mutation and a greater serum virus burden than patients without the mutation. Resistance to zidovudine and didanosine involves mutations at different loci and zidovudine-resistant HIV-1 strains remain sensitive to didanosine.

Pharmacokinetics

Didanosine is poorly soluble at low pH. At gastric pH levels it is rapidly degraded into 2',3'-deoxyribose and the free base. It is therefore administered as a buffered chewable dispersible tablet or buffered powder for oral solution for maximal absorption. Oral bioavailability is dose dependent and was 27% when given once daily and 36% when given twice daily in phase I trials in patients with AIDS-related complex or AIDS. Oral bioavailability was 43% for doses of <5.1 mg/kg daily given in two divided doses. Didanosine is about 20–25% more bioavailable from tablet formulation compared to the solution. There are considerable inter-patient differences in bioavailability in both adults and children, which may have both toxicologic and therapeutic implications. In children the bioavailability of doses of 20–180 mg/m² ranged from 2 to 81% (mean 31%).

Mean peak serum concentrations after a 375 mg dose of the powder and two 150 mg tablets were 1.6 mg/l (range 0.4–2.9 mg/l) and 1.6 mg/l (range 0.5–2.6 mg/l), respectively. Food alters the peak plasma concentration and AUC values by approximately 50%. Studies with didanosine tablets in eight asymptomatic HIV patients revealed a mean peak plasma concentration of 2.8 mg/l (range 1.1–4.2 mg/l) in the fasting state, and 1.3 mg/l (range 0.7–2.2 mg/l) after a meal. The effect of food can be minimized if medication is given 30–60 min before or 2 h after a meal. Intravenous infusion of 0.2–6.4 mg/kg revealed a volume of distribution of 1.01 l/kg. Limited studies in man indicate that the drug penetrates the CSF with a CSF/plasma ratio of 0.21 at 1 h after a 1.5 l infusion. In children, the concentrations of didanosine in CSF ranged from 0.04 to 0.12 mg/l at 1.5–3.5 h after a single oral or intravenous dose. The CSF concentration corresponded to a mean of 46% (range 12–85%) of a simultaneous plasma sample. Passage of didanosine across the placenta has been reported.

About 50% of a dose is excreted unchanged in the urine by glomerular filtration and active tubular secretion. Studies in laboratory animals suggest that the remainder is metabolized to hypoxanthine, xanthine and uric acid. The metabolic fate of the dideoxyribose moiety is unknown.

Its serum elimination half-life ranges from 0.8 to 2.7 h in adults after oral administration. In children it is 0.5–1.0 h after an oral dose. The intracellular half-life of dideoxy-adenosine triphosphate is reported to be 8–24 h in vitro, which contrasts with 3 h or less for zidovudine and zalcitabine. Plasma clearance of didanosine is reduced in patients with impaired creatinine clearance, and such patients may be at greater risk of toxicity. Moreover, the magnesium and aluminium content of each buffered tablet (15.7 and 25.3 mEq, respectively) may present an excessive load. Didanosine is removed by haemodialysis, but the amount cleared by dialysis is low and supplemented dosing is not required. The pharmacokinetics of didanosine have not been studied in those with hepatic impairment.

Toxicity and side-effects

A major problem associated with the administration of didanosine is its toxicity. The most common dose-related toxic effects are peripheral neuropathy and pancreatitis. At 'high' doses (375 mg twice daily for patients ≥60 kg; and 250 mg twice daily for patients <60 kg), the 1-year rate of pancreatitis was 13% and at the current 'recommended' dose (250 mg buffered powder twice daily for patients ≥60 kg; 167 mg twice daily for patients <60 kg) the incidence was 7%. At doses >12.5mg/kg/day the incidence of pancreatitis was 27%. Suspension of didanosine therapy should be considered when treatment with other drugs known to cause pancreatitis is required. At 'high' and 'recommended' doses the 1-year rates of peripheral neuropathy in 609 patients was 14% and 13%, respectively. In a German study using the same 'high' dose, but lower doses of 100 and 67 mg twice daily for patients ≥60 and <60 kg, respectively, the incidence of neuropathy was 20% and 13%, respectively, at 10 months. In phase I studies of doses of >12.5 mg/kg per day, the incidence of neuropathy was 51%, and 34% had neuropathy severe enough to require dose modification. Diarrhoea is a common adverse effect. Other reported adverse effects include nausea and vomiting, rashes, diabetes mellitus, headache, leuko-penia, granulocytopenia, thrombocytopenia, anaemia, hyperuricaemia and liver function abnormalities. Co-administration of drugs that are known to cause peripheral neuropathy or pancreatitis may increase the likelihood of these adverse events. Because the plasma protein binding of didanosine is less than 5%, drug interactions involving binding-site displacement are unlikely.

No evidence of mutagenicity was observed in Ames salmonella mutagenicity assays or in *Esch. coli*. In a mammalian cell gene mutation assay didanosine was weakly positive at 2000 mg/l. Chromosome aberrations occurred in human peripheral lymphocytes at concentrations of ≥500 mg/l. No long-term carcinogenicity studies of didanosine in animals have been reported. No harmful effects on rat or rabbit fetuses have been observed at doses of up to 12 and 14 times the estimated human exposure based on plasma levels. Didanosine crosses the placenta of rats.

Clinical use

Didanosine is currently indicated for the treatment of adult patients with advanced HIV infection who have previously received prolonged therapy with zidovudine. It is also indicated for the treatment of adults and children with advanced HIV infection who are intolerant of zidovudine or who have developed clinical or immunological deterioration during zidovudine therapy. These indications are based on changes in HIV surrogate markers seen in clinical studies and by decreases in the rate of progression of HIV infection.

The AIDS Clinical Trials Group study 116B/117 showed that patients treated previously with zidovudine reached morbidity and mortality end-points less frequently if they were treated with didanosine rather than continue with zidovudine. Similar findings were also noted among patients treated for ≥6 months with zidovudine who manifested signs of progressive disease, such as new clinical syndromes or a marked decrease in CD4 counts. These observations support the common practice of using new clinical signs or a change in CD4 count as an indication for changing therapy from zidovudine to didanosine.

Alternating or simultaneous regimens of zidovudine and didanosine have been studied in the quest for treatment schedules that retard the emergence of drug-resistance. Simultaneous zidovudine with didanosine evidently provides more sustained elevation in CD4 cells than alternating therapy with both agents and provides a greater decrease in viraemia over the first 2–3 months of therapy. Emergence of didanosine-related mutations at position 74 is evidently blocked by alternating or simultaneous zidovudine and didanosine. In contrast, mutations at codon 215, which confers resistance to zidovudine, occurs in virtually all patients receiving alternating or simultaneous regimens of zidovudine or didanosine over a period of 2 years.

Preparations and dosage

Proprietary name: Videx.

Preparation: Tablets.

Dosage: Oral, adults <60 kg, 125 mg every 12 h; adults ≥60 kg, 200 mg every 12 h.

Available in the USA and the UK.

Further information

Balis F M, Pizzo P A, Butler K M et al 1992 Clinical pharmacology of 2',3'-dideoxyinosine in human immunodeficiency virus-infected children. *Journal of Infectious Diseases* 165: 99–104

Cooley T P, Kunches L M, Saunders C A et al 1990 Once daily administration of 2',3'-dideoxyinosine (ddl) in patients with the acquired immunodeficiency syndrome or AIDS-related complex: a phase I trial. *New England Journal of Medicine* 322: 1340–1345

Hartman N R, Yarchoan R, Pluda J M et al 1990 Pharmacokinetics of 2',3'-dideoxyadenosine and 2',3'-dideoxyinosine in patients with severe human immunodeficiency virus infection. *Clinical Pharmacology and Therapeutics* 47: 647–654

Jablonowski H, Arasteh K, Staszewski S et al 1995 A dose comparison study of didanosine in patients with very advanced HIV infection who are intolerant to or clinically deteriorate on zidovudine. *AIDS* 9: 463–469

Knupp C A, Shyu W C, Dolin R et al 1991 Pharmacokinetics of didanosine in patients with acquired immunodeficiency syndrome or acquired immunodeficiency syndrome-related complex. *Clinical Pharmacology and Therapeutics* 49: 523–535

Knupp C A, Milbrath R, Barbhaiya R H 1993 Effect of time of food administration on the bioavailability of didanosine from chewable tablet formulation. *Journal of Clinical Pharmacology* 33: 568–573

Kojioma E, Shirasaka T, Anderson B D et al 1995 Human immunodeficiency virus type 1 (HIV-1) viremia changes and development of drug-related mutations in patients with symptomatic HIV-1 infection receiving alternating or simultaneous zidovudine and didanosine therapy. *Journal of Infectious Diseases* 171: 1152–1158

Kozal M J, Kroodsma K, Winters M A et al 1994 Didanosine resistance in HIV-infected patients switched from zidovudine to didanosine monotherapy. *Annals of Internal Medicine* 121: 263–268

Lambert J S, Sedlin M, Reichman R C et al 1990 2',3'-Dideoxyinosine (ddl) in patients with the acquired immunodeficiency syndrome or AIDS-related complex: a phase I trial. *New England Journal of Medicine* 322: 1333–1340

McGowan J J, Tomaszewski J E, Cradock J et al 1990 Overview of the preclinical development of an antiretroviral drug, 2',3'-dideoxyinosine. *Reviews in Infectious Diseases* 12 (suppl 5): S513–S520

Pons J C, Boubon M C, Taburet A M et al 1991 Fetoplacental passage of 2',3'-dideoxyinosine [letter]. *Lancet* 337: 732

Shuy W C, Knupp C A, Pitman K A, Dunkle L, Barbhaiya R H 1991 Food-induced reduction in bioavailability of didanosine. *Clinical Pharmacology and Therapeutics* 50: 503–507

Singlas E, Taburet A M, Lebas F B et al 1992 Didanosine pharmacokinetics in patients with normal and impaired renal function: influence of hemodialysis. *Antimicrobial Agents and Chemotherapy* 36: 1519–1524

Spruance S L, Pavia A T, Peterson D et al 1994 Didanosine compared with continuation of zidovudine in HIV-infected patients with signs of clinical deterioration while receiving zidovudine. *Annals of Internal Medicine* 120: 360–368

Yarchoan R, Pluda J M, Thomas R V et al 1990 Long term toxicity/activity profile of 2',3'-dideoxyinosine in AIDS or AIDS-related complex. *Lancet* ii: 526–529

FAMCICLOVIR
9-(4-Acetoxy-3-acetoxymethylbut-1-yl)guanine, FMV

A pro-drug: the diacetyl ester of the active antiviral agent 6-deoxypenciclovir. It is a synthetic acyclic purine nucleoside analogue which, after oral administration, undergoes rapid first-pass metabolism to produce penciclovir.

Famciclovir

Penciclovir

Antiviral activity

Famciclovir is converted to penciclovir (PCV) which is active against members of the herpes virus family. Penciclovir and aciclovir have similar inhibitory activities against clinical isolates of HSV-1 and HSV-2, and VZV, but the relative activities of these compounds depends upon the cells used and the type of assay. Penciclovir has greatest activity against HSV-1 (mean $ID_{50} \approx 1.6$ μM), somewhat less activity against HSV-2 (mean $ID_{50} \approx 6.0$ μM), and less activity against VZV (mean $ID_{50} \approx 12$ μM). The ID_{50} values for acyclovir in the same cells were 0.9, 2.7 and 17 μM, respectively. CMV is relatively resistant to penciclovir and EBV has intermediate susceptibility. Penciclovir, like acyclovir, inhibits hepatitis B virus activity in vitro.

In cells infected with HSV-1, HSV-2 and VZV, PCV is monophosphorylated by virus-encoded thymidine kinase, phosphorylation proceeding more efficiently than that of acyclovir in herpes-infected cells. Cellular enzymes then phosphorylate PCV further to PCV triphosphate. Although PCV triphosphate has less affinity for viral DNA polymerases than acyclovir triphosphate, it has a much longer half-life, thereby facilitating less frequent oral dosing. PCV triphosphate is structurally similar to deoxyguanosine triphosphate (dGTP), a substrate for viral DNA polymerase. PCV-triphosphate competes with dGTP for incorporation into DNA by viral DNA polymerase, and its incorporation blocks chain extension.

Combinations of penciclovir with human interferons-α, -β and -γ, have synergistic activity against HSV-1 and HSV-2. The combination of foscarnet and penciclovir is synergistic against HSV-1 and additive against HSV-2. However, the combination of penciclovir and zidovudine at high concentrations resulted in diminished activity against HSV types 1 and 2.

Acquired resistance

Development of resistance to PCV has not yet been identified in clinical isolates. PCV is inactive against thymidine-kinase-deficient strains of herpes simplex. Occasional strains of HSV-1 and VZV that are resistant to acyclovir retain sensitivity to PCV. Foscarnet-resistant HSV isolates also appear to retain sensitivity to both PCV and acyclovir.

Pharmacokinetics

Famciclovir is readily absorbed and, following absorption, is converted rapidly by enzyme-mediated deacetylation and oxidation to the active antiviral metabolite, penciclovir, since little unchanged famciclovir is detected in plasma. Its bioavailability is 77% and peak plasma concentrations of 2.7–4.0 mg/l are found in fasting subjects after an oral dose of famciclovir of 500 mg. Penciclovir itself has a bioavailability of only 5%.

Penciclovir shows linear pharmacokinetics with respect to maximum plasma concentration and AUC. Following oral doses of famciclovir of 125, 250, 500 and 750 mg, peak plasma concentrations of penciclovir were 0.8, 1.6, 3.3 and 5.1 mg/l, respectively; the percentages recovered in the urine were 50.9, 56.5, 59.9 and 60.4%, respectively, confirming the high bioavailability. The time to peak plasma concentration, urinary recovery, renal clearance and plasma half-life are similar with increasing dose. The volume of distribution is approximately 1.5 l/kg. The pharmacokinetics in elderly subjects are similar to those seen in younger subjects, although small increases in AUC and plasma half-lives were seen, consistent with slightly decreased renal clearance. Food does not lead to any significant change in the availability or elimination of penciclovir.

Renal excretion is the major route of elimination. Following intravenous infusion, approximately 70% is excreted unchanged in the urine. Following oral administration, the major metabolite is penciclovir, which accounts for 82% of urinary drug-related material. The remainder includes metabolites of famciclovir, of which the largest is the 6-deoxy precursor of penciclovir. Renal clearance exceeds glomerular filtration, indicating renal tubular secretion. The mean plasma elimination half-life after single oral doses of famciclovir is 2.1–2.7 h.

Since famciclovir undergoes considerable presystemic metabolism, there is a potential for drug interactions between famciclovir and other drugs that are metabolized by hepatic enzymes. There is no evidence of clinically significant pharmacokinetic interactions between famciclovir and allopurinol, cimetidine, theophylline, digoxin or zidovudine.

Toxicity and side-effects

In clinical trials the incidence of adverse events after famciclovir, acyclovir and placebo were similar, the most common adverse events being headache and nausea.

Clinical use

It is currently indicated for treatment of herpes zoster infections and genital herpes.

Preparations and dosage

Proprietary name: Famvir.

Preparation: Tablets.

Dosage: Adults, oral, 250 mg three times daily for 7 days. Widely available.

Further information

Boyd M R, Bacon T H, Sutton D, Cole M 1987 Antiherpes activity of 9-(4-hydroxy-3-hydroxymethylbut-1-yl)guanine (BRL 39123) in cell culture. *Antimicrobial Agents and Chemotherapy* 31: 1238–1242

Boyd M R, Safrin S, Kern E R 1993 Penciclovir: a review of its spectrum of activity, selectivity, and cross-resistance pattern. *Antiviral Chemistry and Chemotherapy* 4 (suppl 1): 3–11

Daniels S, Schentag J J 1993 Drug interaction studies and safety of famciclovir in healthy volunteers: a review. *Antiviral Chemistry and Chemotherapy* 4 (suppl 1): 57–64

Hodge R A V 1993 Famciclovir and penciclovir. The mode of action of famciclovir including its conversion to penciclovir. *Antiviral Chemistry and Chemotherapy* 4: 67–84

Pue M A, Benet L Z 1993 Pharmacokinetics of famciclovir in man. *Antiviral Chemistry and Chemotherapy* 4 (suppl 1): 47–55

Sutton S, Taylor J, Bacon T H 1992 Activity of penciclovir in combination with azido-thymidine, ganciclovir, aciclovir, foscarnet, and human interferons against herpes simplex replication in cell culture. *Antiviral Chemistry and Chemotherapy* 3: 85–94

GANCICLOVIR

9-(1,3-Dihydroxy-2-propoxymethyl) guanine; DHPG

A synthetic 2'-deoxyguanosine nucleoside analogue.

Antiviral activity

Ganciclovir (DHPG) is phosphorylated to DHPG monophosphate by a cellular deoxyguanosine kinase more rapidly in infected cells than in uninfected cells. HSV and VZV induce their own thymidine kinase and effectively monophosphorylate DHPG. DHPG monophosphate is further metabolized to the triphosphate (active form) by cellular enzymes. The UL97 open-reading frame of CMV encodes a protein (phosphonotransferase) which is capable of regulating phosphorylation of ganciclovir and in CMV-infected cells there is approximately a 10-fold higher concentration of DHPG triphosphate than in uninfected cells. DHPG triphosphate competes with guanosine triphosphate for incorporation into viral DNA, and incorporated drug suppresses viral DNA replication.

HSV-1 and HSV-2 are inhibited by 0.2–8.0 μM (0.05–2.0 mg/l). Its activity is similar to that of acyclovir against HSV-1 in vitro, but is slightly superior against HSV-2. The ID_{50} for CMV ranges from 0.5 to 11 μM (0.125–2.75 mg/l). EBV is inhibited by 1–4 μM and VZV by 4 to 40 μM. Although it inhibits CMV replication during acute infection in a mouse model, latency is not prevented and CMV can be reactivated by immunosuppression.

Ganciclovir and foscarnet act synergistically in inhibiting cytomegalovirus. It is also synergistic in vitro in combination with several investigational compounds – HPMPA (S)-9-(3-hydroxy-2-phosphonylmethoxypropyl)-adenosine, HPMPC (S)-9-(3-hydroxy-2-phosphonylmethoxypropyl)-cytosine and 2-acetylpyridine-5-[(dimethylamino)thiocarbonyl]-thio-carbonohydrazone. It gives additive in vitro inhibitory activity in combination with an anti-CMV monoclonal antibody. Its CMV activity may be reduced in the presence of zidovudine, and the anti-HIV activity of zidovudine and didanosine also appear to be lessened by ganciclovir.

Acquired resistance

The use of prolonged repeated courses of ganciclovir leads to the selection of resistant strains. Such strains are not uncommon, being found in 8% of patients receiving ganciclovir for >3 months, and have been identified in some cases of treatment failure. Studies of laboratory-derived ganciclovir-resistant strains indicate that drug resistance can result from alterations in the phosphonotransferase encoded by the gene region UL 27, the viral DNA polymerase (gene region UL 54), or both.

Pharmacokinetics

Its pharmacokinetic behaviour after intravenous administration appears to be similar to that of acyclovir in terms of its half-life, peak serum levels and renal excretion. After an initial infusion of 5 mg/kg, the plasma half-life was 2.9 h in patients with normal renal function. The plasma level at the end of a 1 h infusion averaged 33.2 μM, and after 11 h it was 2.2 μM. After repeated 5 mg/kg doses every 8 h, the mean peak serum levels were 25 μM and mean trough levels were 3.6 μM. Thus when the drug is administered at a dose of 5 mg/kg, levels in plasma are in excess or in the same range as the CMV ID_{50}. In patients treated for 8–22 days with 1 or 2.5 mg/kg every 8 h, the mean steady-state plasma concentrations after a 1 h infusion of 1 mg/kg ranged from 7.2 μM immediately after infusion to 0.8 μM after 8 h. Corresponding values after a dose of 2.5 mg/kg were 19.6 and 3.2 μM, respectively.

Oral bioavailability ranges between 5.4 to 7.1% (mean 6%). Multiple dosing with oral ganciclovir 1000 mg three times daily resulted in peak levels of 1.13 mg/l (≈4.3 μM) and a trough of 0.52 mg/l (≈2.1 μM). These plasma concentrations are less than those found after intravenous therapy and given the breakthrough that occurs with intravenous therapy, the oral pharmacokinetic data suggest that breakthrough and development of resistance may be more common with oral administration.

There are only limited data on its distribution. The levels of the drug in CSF are estimated to be 24–67% of those in plasma. Mean intravitreal ganciclovir levels of ~4 μM were reported for samples taken a mean of 12 h after therapy with a mean dose of 6 mg/kg daily. However, no significant correlations were found by other investigators between time after the last dose and intravitreal concentration. The observed mean value in the eye is below the concentration of ganciclovir required to achieve 50% or 90% inhibition of CMV plaque formation by clinical isolates, which may explain the difficulty in controlling CMV retinitis. Using in vitro experimental methods, it has been shown that ganciclovir is concentrated at the human maternal placental surface and then crosses passively into the fetal compartment.

Approximately 80% of the drug is eliminated unchanged in the urine within 24 h. Probenicid, as well as other drugs that may inhibit renal tubular secretion or absorption, may reduce its renal clearance. In severe renal impairment, the mean plasma half-life was 28.3 h. It must therefore be given in reduced dosage in patients with impaired renal function. Plasma levels of the drug were reduced in one study by approximately 50% by haemodialysis, and in another by 90%. The half-life on dialysis is approximately 4 h, with a mean blood flow rate of 250 ml/min. Patients undergoing dialysis should be given 1.25 mg/kg daily; therapy should also be administered after dialysis.

It is only 1–2% bound to plasma proteins and drug interactions involving binding site displacement are not anticipated. No significant pharmacokinetic interaction occurs when ganciclovir and foscarnet are given as concomitant or daily alternate therapy. However, recent studies indicate a significant two-way pharmacokinetic interaction between ganciclovir and didanosine. Ganciclovir also increases the AUC for AZT.

Toxicity and side-effects

The IC_{50} for human bone marrow colony-forming cells is 39 ± 73 μM; for other cell lines it ranges from 110 to 2900 μM. Toxicity frequently limits therapy. Marrow suppression in man may develop on as little as 5 mg/kg on alternate days. In one study, neutropenia of <1000/mm³ occurred in nearly 40% of recipients and <500/mm³ in 16%; in another study, 34% of those given induction therapy of 10 mg/kg daily for 14 days, followed by 5 mg/kg daily, developed neutropenia of <500/mm³. Neutropenia is usually reversible and tends to develop during the early treatment or maintenance phase, but may occur later. Thrombocytopenia of <20 000/mm³ and <50 000/mm³ develops in about 10 and 19% of patients, respectively. Frequent monitoring of the full blood count is recommended.

Adverse effects on the CNS, including confusion, convulsions, psychosis, hallucinations, tremor, ataxia, coma, dizziness, headaches and somnolence occur in approximately 5%. Liver function abnormalities, fever and rash occur in about 2%. Intraocular injection of ganciclovir is associated with intense pain, and occasionally amaurosis lasting for 1–10 min afterwards.

Animal studies indicate that inhibition of spermatogenesis and suppression of female fertility can occur. It is also potentially embryolethal, mutagenic and teratogenic and is contraindicated during pregnancy or lactation. Ganciclovir can cause local tissue damage and should not be administered intramuscularly or subcutaneously; patients should be adequately hydrated during treatment and infusion into veins should be ensured with adequate flow allowing rapid dilution and distribution.

Synergistic marrow toxicity can be expected with concomitant use of zidovudine. Convulsions have been reported in patients taking ganciclovir and imipenem–cilastin concomitantly.

Clinical use

Due to its toxicity, it is indicated only for the treatment of life- or sight-threatening CMV infections in immuno-compromised individuals. Ganciclovir is also available for prevention of CMV disease in patients receiving immuno-suppressive therapy for organ transplantation.

Preparations and dosage

Proprietary name: Cymevene.

Preparations: Capsules, i.v. infusion.

Dosage: Adults, treatment, 5 mg/kg every 12 h for 14–21 days for prevention. Maintenance dose, i.v., 6 mg/kg daily on 5 days per week *or* 5 mg/kg every day. Oral, 1 g three times daily or 500 mg six times daily, following at least 3 weeks i.v. therapy.

Widely available.

Further information

Boulieu R, Bastien O, Bleyzac N 1993 Pharmacokinetics of ganciclovir in heart transplant patients undergoing continuous venovenous haemodialysis. *Therapeutic Drug Monitoring* 15: 105–107

Chow S, Erice A, Jordan M C et al 1995 Analysis of the UL97 phosphonotransferase coding sequence in clinical cytomegalovirus isolates and identification of mutations conferring ganciclovir resistance. *Journal of Infectious Diseases* 171: 576–583

Drew W L, Felsenstein D, Hirsch M S 1985 Sensitivity of clinical isolates of human cytomegalovirus to 9-(1,3-dihydroxy-2 propoxymethyl)guanine. *Journal of Infectious Diseases* 152: 833–834

Drew W L, Miner R C, Busch D F et al 1991 Prevalence of resistance in patients receiving ganciclovir for serious cytomegalovirus infection. *Journal of Infectious Diseases* 163: 716–719

Feng J S, Crouch J Y, Tian P Y et al 1993 Zidovudine antagonises the antiviral effects of ganciclovir against cytomegalovirus infection in cultured cells and in guinea pigs. *Antiviral Chemistry and Chemotherapy* 4: 19–25

Fletcher C, Sawchuk R, Chinnock B, De Miranda P, Balfour H H 1986 Human pharmacokinetics of the antiviral drug DHPG. *Clinical Pharmacology and Therapeutics* 40: 281–286

Henderson G I, Hu Z Q, Yang Y et al 1993 Ganciclovir transfer by human placenta and its effect on rat foetal cells. *American Journal of Science* 306: 151–156

Katzenstein D A, Crane R T, Jordan M C 1986 Successful treatment of murine cytomegalovirus disease does not prevent latent virus infection. *Journal of Laboratory and Clinical Medicine* 108: 155–160

Kupperman B D, Quiceno J I, Flores-Aguilar M et al 1993 Intravitreal ganciclovir concentration after intravenous administration in AIDS patients with cytomegalovirus retinitis. *Journal of Infectious Diseases* 168: 1506–1509

Lake K D, Fletcher C V, Love K R, Brown D C, Joyce L D, Pritzker M R 1988 Ganciclovir pharmacokinetics during renal impairment. *Antimicrobial Agents and Chemotherapy* 32: 1899–1900

Littler E, Stuart E, Chee M S 1992 Human cytomegalovirus UL97 open reading frame encodes a protein that phosphorylates the antiviral analogue ganciclovir. *Nature* 358: 160–162

Manischewitz J F, Quinnan G V, Lane H C et al 1990 Synergistic effect of ganciclovir and foscarnet on cytomegalovirus replication in vitro. *Antimicrobial Agents and Chemotherapy* 34: 373–375

Markham A, Faulds D 1994 Ganciclovir. An update of its therapeutic use in cytomegalovirus infection. *Drugs* 48: 455–484

Medina D J, Hsuing G D, Mellors J W 1992 Ganciclovir antagonises the anti-human immunodeficiency virus type 1 activity of zidovudine and didanosine in vitro. *Antimicrobial Agents and Chemotherapy* 36: 1127–1130

Nokta M, Tolpin M D, Nadler P I, Pollard R B 1994 Human monoclonal anti-cytomegalovirus (CMV) antibody (MSL 109): enhancement of an in vitro foscarnet and ganciclovir-induced inhibition of CMV replication. *Antiviral Research* 24: 17–26

Sommadasi J-P, Bevan R, Ling T et al 1988 Clinical pharmacokinetics of ganciclovir in patients with normal and impaired renal function. *Reviews in Infectious Diseases* 10: S507–S514

IDOXURIDINE
5-Iodo-2'-deoxyuridine; IDU

A synthetic halogenated pyrimidine analogue originally synthesized as an anticancer agent.

Antiviral activity

It inhibits several enzymes concerned with the biosynthesis of DNA (thymidine kinase, thymidylate kinase DNA polymerase) and competes with thymidine for incorporation into viral and cellular DNA. There is also alteration of gene expression subsequent to its incorporation into DNA.

Its activity is largely limited to DNA viruses, primarily HSV-1 and HSV-2 and VZV. HSV-1 plaque formation in BHK 21 cells is sensitive to 6.25–25 mg/l; type 2 microplaques required 62.5–125 mg/l. RNA viruses are not affected, with the exception of oncogenic RNA viruses such as Rous sarcoma virus.

Drug resistance is easily generated in vitro, and may be an obstacle to treatment. However, there is little or no cross-resistance with newer nucleoside analogues.

Pharmacokinetics

It is poorly soluble in water, and aqueous solutions are ineffective against infections other than those localized to the eye. Dimethylsulphoxide, a powerful solvent, augments cutaneous penetration of idoxuridine, but is itself teratogenic and causes ocular damage in certain animal species. In animals, therapeutic levels are achieved in the cornea within 30 min of ophthalmic application and persist for 4 h. Penetration is otherwise poor, with only the biologically inactive dehalogenated metabolite uracil entering the eye. In man, intravenously administered idoxuridine is rapidly metabolized to iodouracil and uracil and has a plasma half-life of about 30 min. It is not active orally and does not cross the blood–brain barrier.

Toxicity and side-effects

It is too toxic for systemic use and causes contact dermatitis, punctate epithelial keratopathy, follicular conjunctivitis, ptosis, stenosis and occlusion of the puncta and keratinization of the lid margins in up to 14% of those receiving ophthalmic preparations. Trials of its use in herpes simplex encephalitis have produced liver function abnormalities and serious bone marrow toxicity.

Clinical use

It was the first widely used antiviral agent after the demonstration in 1962 of its beneficial effect in herpes keratitis. It has had only limited success in the treatment of ocular herpes simplex infections and shingles. It has now largely been superseded by acyclovir.

Preparations and dosage

Proprietary names: Idoxene, Herpid, Iduridin, Virudox.
Preparations: Topical, ophthalmic.
Widely available.

Further information

Gold J A, Stewart R C, McKee J 1965 The epidemiology and chemotherapy of herpes simplex keratitis and herpes simplex skin infections. *Annals of the New York Academy of Science* 130: 209–212

Nicholson K G 1984 Respiratory infections, genital herpes and herpetic keratitis. *Lancet* ii: 617–621

Nicholson K G 1984 Antiviral therapy: varicella zoster virus infections, herpes labialis and mucocutaneous herpes, and cytomegalovirus infections. *Lancet* ii: 677–682

RIBAVIRIN
1-β-ᴅ-Ribofuranosyl-1,2,4-triazole-3-carboxamide

A synthetic nucleoside consisting of ᴅ-ribose attached to a 1,2,4-triazole carboxamide.

It differs from other analogues in that it is neither a pyrimidine nor a purine. Stereochemical studies indicate that it is a guanosine analogue. It is phosphorylated in cells and is an inhibitor of inosine monophosphate dehydrogenase which is involved in the synthesis of guanosine triphosphate. Decrease in intracellular thymidine triphosphate has also been noted.

Antiviral activity

Both in vitro and in vivo laboratory tests indicate that, of the DNA viruses, the herpes viruses are the most sensitive. Of the human RNA viruses, good activity has been noted with the Orthomyxoviridae (influenza types A and B), Paramyxoviridae (parainfluenza virus types 1, 2 and 3, mumps, measles, respiratory syncytial virus (RSV)), Arenaviridae (Lassa fever, Machupo), and Bunyaviridae (Rift Valley fever, sandfly fever, Hantaan viruses); variable or negative findings have been observed with Picornaviridae (polio, coxsackie, rhinoviruses), Reoviridae (rotaviruses) and Togaviridae (equine encephalitis viruses, Chikungunya, yellow fever viruses). RSV plaques are reduced by 85–98% by 16 mg/l.

Recent attention has focused on the ability of ribavirin to inhibit HIV, it is believed by interfering with the guanylation step required for 5'-capping of mRNA. Anti-HIV activity has been noted in primary infected human adult T lymphocytes at levels of 50–100 mg/l (205–410 μM/l); treatment studies of Lassa fever in man indicate that such levels can be tolerated for short periods. Attention has also focused on its ability to inhibit hepatitis C virus (HCV). During ribavirin therapy significant reductions have been noted in alanine transaminase levels and HCV RNA titre, although the effects have been rather transient. Recent preliminary data indicate that ribavirin and interferon-β may act synergistically in chronic HCV infection. Combination therapy with ribavirin and interferon-α has been associated with sustained reduction in alanine transaminase levels and loss of HCV RNA in 40% of patients who failed to respond to interferon previously.

The antiviral activity of ribavirin appears to be mediated by several mechanisms, including the depletion of nucleotide pools, blocking of cap formation of mRNA, and inhibition of viral RNA-dependent RNA polymerases. In most cell lines in which antiviral testing has been performed, the antiviral activity is usually distinct from the cytostatic dose, which ranges from 200 to 1000 mg/l. In contrast to other antivirals, development of ribavirin-resistant virus strains has not been demonstrated.

Pharmacokinetics

It is rapidly absorbed after oral administration with peak plasma concentrations of 4.1–8.2 μM/l within 60–90 min of a 3 mg/kg dose. Oral bioavailability after 600, 1200 and 2400 mg was 36, 52 and 46%, respectively. Mean peak ribavirin concentrations after 1 week of oral ribavirin 200, 400 and 800 mg every 8 h were 5.0, 11.1 and 20.9 μmol/l, respectively. Trough levels 9–12 h after the final dose after 2 weeks' therapy were 5.1, 13.2 and 18.4 μmol/l, respectively, indicating continued accumulation of the drug. Drug was still detectable 4 weeks after discontinuation of oral dosing. Mean peak plasma ribavirin concentrations after intravenous doses of 600, 1200 and 2400 mg were 43.6, 72.3 and 160.8 μmol/l, respectively; at 8 h the mean plasma concentrations were 2.1, 5.6 and 10.2 μmol/l. Ribavirin is not bound to plasma proteins. After intravenous administration 19.4% of the dose was eliminated during the first 24 h as compared with 7.3% after an oral dose – the difference reflecting the bioavailability.

Ribavirin is rapidly degraded by deribosylation or amide hydrolysis, and together with its metabolites is slowly eliminated by the kidney as the principal route of elimination. About 50% of the drug or its metabolites appears in the urine within 72 h: about 15% is excreted in the stools; the remainder seems to be retained in body tissues, principally in red blood cells which concentrate the drug or metabolites to a peak at 4 days, the half-life in red cells being about 40 days. The plasma half-life is about 24 h.

Aerosolized ribavirin (6 g in 300 ml distilled water) has generally been administered at a rate of 12–15 ml/h using a Collison jet nebulizer, the estimated dosage being 1.8 mg/kg per h for infants and 0.9 mg/kg per h for adults. When ribavirin was administered by small-particle aerosol for 2.5–8 h, plasma concentrations ranged from 0.44 to 8.7 μmol/l.

Toxicity and side-effects

It is generally well tolerated, though adverse reactions appear to be related to dose and duration of therapy. Minor adverse reactions include metallic taste, dry mouth sensation and increased thirst, flatulence, fatigue and CNS complaints including headache, irritability and insomnia. Daily doses of 1 g may cause unconjugated bilirubin levels to double and the reticulocyte count to increase. Haemoglobin concentrations may decrease with prolonged treatment or higher dosages; thus with doses of 3.9–12.6 g/day, a drop in haemoglobin was noted by day 7–13 of treatment, which was generally 'rapidly' reversible on withdrawal of the drug, but in some instances necessitated blood transfusion.

Aerosol administration of about 2 g in 36 or 39 h during 3 days is well tolerated, does not affect results of pulmonary function tests, and seems non-toxic. Ribavirin is both teratogenic and embryotoxic in laboratory animals, so precautions must be observed in women of child-bearing age.

Clinical use

Aerosolized ribavirin is licensed for RSV infections in infants and there is a good case for its use in those with severe RSV infections during the first few months of life, especially those with congenital heart disease or severe combined immunodeficiency disease. The vast majority of infants and children with RSV have either no lower respiratory tract disease or disease that is mild and self-limited, and does not require hospitalization. Of those with mild lower respiratory tract involvement, many will need brief hospitalization for a period shorter than that required for a full course of therapy (3–7 days). Hence the decision to treat with ribavirin aerosol should be based on the severity of the infection.

Aerosolized ribavirin accelerates the resolution of fever and illness and reduces virus shedding due to influenza infection, but the improvements are generally modest and insufficient to justify treatment in otherwise healthy subjects. It is highly effective in Lassa fever when initiated within the first 6 days of treatment and has been shown to reduce mortality from Hantaan virus, the agent responsible for the haemorrhagic fever with renal syndrome.

Preparations and dosage

Proprietary name: Virazid.

Preparation: Inhalation.

Dosage: By aerosol inhalation or nebulization (via small-particle aerosol generator) of solution containing 20 mg/ml for 12–18 h for at least 3 days and a maximum of 7 days.

Widely available.

Further information

Brillanti S, Garson J, Foli M et al 1994 A pilot study of combination therapy with ribavirin plus interferon alpha for interferon alpha resistant chronic hepatitis C. *Gastroenterology* 107: 812–817

Di Bisceglie A M, Shindo M, Fong T L et al 1992 A pilot study of ribavirin therapy for chronic hepatitis C. *Hepatology* 16: 649–654

Kakumu S, Yoshioka K, Wakita T et al 1993 A pilot study of ribavirin and interferon beta for the treatment of chronic hepatitis C. *Gastroenterology* 105: 507–512

Laskin O L, Longstreth J A, Hart C C et al 1987 Ribavirin disposition in high-risk patients for acquired immunodeficiency syndrome. *Clinical Pharmacology and Therapeutics* 41: 546–555

Nicholson K (ed) 1988 HIV and other highly pathogenic viruses. International congress and symposium series No. 145. Royal Society of Medicine, London

Patterson J L, Fernandez-Larsson R 1990 Molecular mechanisms of action of ribavirin. *Reviews of Infectious Diseases* 12: 1139–1146

Reichard O, Andersson J, Schvarz R, Welland O 1991 Ribavirin treatment for chronic hepatitis C. *Lancet* 337: 1058–1061

Roberts R B, Laskin O L, Laurence J et al 1987 Ribavirin pharmacokinetics in high-risk patients for acquired immunodeficiency syndrome. *Clinical Pharmacology and Therapeutics* 42: 365–373

Smith R A, Kirkpatrick W (eds) 1980 Ribavirin. A broad spectrum antiviral agent. Academic Press, New York

Stapleton T (ed) 1986 Studies with a broad spectrum antiviral agent. International congress and symposium series No. 108. Royal Society of Medicine, London

STAVUDINE
2',3'-Didehydro-3'-deoxythymidine; d4T

Like zidovudine, stavudine is a 2',3'-dideoxynucleotide analogue. It is a pyrimidine nucleoside in which the 3'-hydroxyl group of the sugar moiety is blocked by dehydrogenation into a double carbon–carbon bond instead of substitution by an azido group as in zidovudine.

Antiviral activity

Stavudine and zidovudine are structurally close analogues of thymidine and have similar in vitro potency against HIV replication in different cell systems. The concentrations required to inhibit HIV infection in vitro vary greatly depending upon the time between virus infection and treatment, size of virus inoculum, type of assay and cells employed. The ID_{50} in T cells (MT4, ATH8 and CEM cells), peripheral blood mononuclear cells and monocyte/macrophages are 0.002–0.92, 0.002–0.009 and 0.0132–0.112 mg/l, respectively. Like zidovudine, stavudine is activated by cellular thymidine kinase, thymidylate kinase and pyrimidine diphosphate kinase into its 5'-active triphosphate. The intracellular half-life of stavudine (and zidovudine) 5'-triphosphate derivatives is 3–4 h. Stavudine triphosphate inhibits HIV replication by two mechanisms. It inhibits HIV reverse transcriptase by competing with the natural substrate deoxythymidine triphosphate, and it inhibits viral DNA synthesis by acting as a chain terminator since it lacks the 3'-hydroxyl group necessary for chain elongation.

In vitro studies have been used to assess the activity of stavudine in combination with other antiretroviral agents. The combination of stavudine and zidovudine at a molar ratio of 20 showed an antagonistic antiviral effect; at molar ratios of 100 and 500 an additive effect was apparent. The combination of stavudine with didanosine at molar ratios of 0.05, 0.1, 0.16 and 0.5 revealed an additive effect. The competing activities of stavudine and zidovudine with thymidine kinase may explain the observed inhibition of intracellular phosphorylation of stavudine by zidovudine and hinders the potential combination of these two agents. Both drugs are minimally phosphorylated in resting or quiescent cells because of their low thymidine kinase activity. Accordingly, stavudine and zidovudine exhibit decreased anti-HIV activity in such cells.

In patients with HIV infection, stavudine transiently increases median CD4 lymphocyte counts at doses of 0.5 and 2.0 mg/kg per day. Treatment with 0.5 and 2.0 mg/kg daily for 10 weeks decreased estimated HIV concentrations by 12 and 77%, respectively, and platelet counts also improved transiently at the two dosage levels. There was little or no effect on these parameters at a dosage of 0.1 mg/kg daily.

Acquired resistance

Development of resistance has been studied using isolates obtained from 13 patients after 18–22 months of treatment. Three of 11 post-treatment isolates showed 4- to 12-fold reduction in sensitivity to stavudine, and 9- to 176-fold reduction in sensitivity to zidovudine. Three of 11 post-treatment isolates also became resistant to didanosine. A stavudine-resistant isolate from one patient was cross-resistant to both zidovudine and didanosine. Genotypic analysis of pre- and post-treatment isolates identified multiple mutations in the reverse transcriptase gene.

Pharmacokinetics

Oral bioavailability is almost complete at doses of 0.25–4 mg/kg, but may be reduced with doses exceeding 200 mg. Peak serum concentrations after oral ingestion of 0.67, 1.33, 2.62 and 4.0 mg/kg were 1.19, 1.56, 3.49 and 4.15 mg/l, respectively, and occurred ≤1 h after dosing. Ingestion with food prolongs the time to peak serum concentrations from 0.6 to 1.5 h and, although it reduces the peak concentrations by approximately half, the AUC is similar. Thus it appears that stavudine may be taken without regard to meals. Intravenous infusion of 1 mg/kg over 1 h revealed a volume of distribution of 0.53 l/kg. The volume of distribution is independent of dose and does not correlate with body weight. Limited studies in man shows that the drug penetrates the CSF. In 7 patients, CSF concentrations ranged from 0.01 to 0.12 mg/l at 2–3 h after treatment with 0.125–1 mg/kg, corresponding to 16–97% (mean 55%) of the concentration in plasma.

Stavudine is apparently excreted by renal and non-renal routes. About 40% of a dose is excreted as unchanged drug by the kidney, both by glomerular filtration and renal tubular excretion. The fate of the remaining drug is unknown, but studies in non-human primates suggest that the sugar moiety is cleaved from the base forming thymine which is degraded to β-aminoisobutyric acid. Its serum elimination half-life is about 1 h in man. The mean (± SD) terminal elimination half-life in patients with creatinine clearances of 25–50 and 9–25 ml/min was 3.5 ± 2.5 h and 4.8 ± 0.8 h, respectively. The pharmacokinetics of stavudine have not been studied in the elderly or those with hepatic insufficiency. In rats the drug crosses the placenta and is readily excreted into breast milk.

Toxicity and side-effects

Its principal toxic effect is peripheral neuropathy which is dose and duration related and generally resolves after drug discontinuation. In phase I trials, the rate of neuropathy per 100 patient-years was 21 at 0.5 mg/kg per day, 21 at 1 mg/kg per day and 66 at 2 mg/kg per day. In the phase II trial it was 6 at 0.1 mg/kg per day, 17 at 0.5 mg/kg per day and 41 at 2 mg/kg per day. There is a low frequency of neuropathy during the first 12 weeks of treatment and an abrupt increase between 12 and 24 weeks. Neuropathy resolved after discontinuation of the drug in 55% of patients and the median time to resolution was dose related: 1 week in patients given 0.1 mg/kg daily, 1.4 weeks in patients given 0.5 mg/kg daily, and 3 weeks in those given 2.0 mg/kg daily. Risk factors for the development of neuropathy include a low baseline CD4 lymphocyte count and a prior history of neuropathy. The appearance of neuropathy does not preclude further therapy at a lower dosage.

Macrocytosis of >100 μm³ was seen in 68% of patients receiving <2.0 mg/kg per day, was dose related and was not associated with anaemia. Stavudine does not appear to cause myelosuppression or impair hepatic or renal function. Aspartate aminotransferase levels may increase among patients receiving 0.5 and 2.0 mg/kg per day, but are not associated with other liver enzyme abnormalities and may not require treatment modification. Possible adverse effects include abdominal cramps, nausea and vomiting, diarrhoea, flatulence, malaise, insomnia, depression, headaches, myalgia, nervousness and rash.

No evidence of mutagenicity was observed in the Ames test or in *Esch. coli* reverse mutation and CHO/HGPRT mammalian cell gene mutation assays. Long-term carcinogenicity studies in animals have not been completed. At concentrations of 25–250 mg/l stavudine was associated with an increased frequency of chromosome aberrations in human lymphocytes. It produced positive results in the in vitro human lymphocyte clastogenesis and mouse fibroblast assays. In in vivo studies it was clastogenic in bone marrow cells following oral administration to mice at doses of 600–2000 mg/kg daily for 3 days. No evidence of teratogenicity has been observed in rats and rabbits given up to 399 and 183 times, respectively, the exposure of that at a clinical dosage of 1 mg/kg per day. In rats the concentration of drug in fetal tissue was approximately half the concentration in maternal plasma.

Clinical use

Stavudine has recently been approved by the US Food and Drugs Administration for use in adults with advanced HIV disease who are intolerant of approved therapies having proven clinical benefit, have experienced significant clinical or immunologic deterioration while receiving such therapy, or for whom such therapy is contraindicated. Approval was based on changes in HIV surrogate markers seen in clinical studies. No long-term data on clinical efficacy in terms of reduction in opportunistic infections or increased survival are currently available.

Preparations and dosage

Proprietary name: Zerit.

Preparation: Capsules.

Dosage: 40 mg orally every 12 h for persons weighing >60 kg, and 30 mg every 12 h for persons weighing <60 kg.

Further information

Dudley M N 1995 Clinical pharmacokinetics of nucleoside antiretroviral agents. *Journal of Infectious Diseases* 171 (suppl 2): S99–S112

Dudley M N, Graham K, Kaul S et al 1992 Pharmacokinetics of stavudine in patients with AIDS or AIDS-related complex. *Journal of Infectious Diseases* 166: 480–485

Murray H W, Squires K E, Weiss W et al 1995 Stavudine in patients with AIDS and AIDS-related complex: AIDS clinical trials group 089. *Journal of Infectious Diseases* 171 (suppl 2): S123–S130

Petersen E A, Ramirez-Ronda C H, Hardy W D et al 1995 Dose-related activity of stavudine in patients infected with human immunodeficiency virus. *Journal of Infectious Diseases* 171 (suppl 2): S131–S139

Skowron G 1995 Biologic effects and safety of stavudine: overview of phase I and II clinical trials. *Journal of Infectious Diseases* 171 (suppl 2): S113–S117

Zhu Z, Ho H T, Hitchcock M J M et al 1990 Cellular pharmacology of 2',3'-didehydro-2',3'-dideoxythymidine (d4T) in human peripheral blood mononuclear cells. *Biochemistry and Pharmacology* 39: R15–R19

TRIFLURIDINE
5-Trifluoromethyl-2'-deoxyuridine; trifluorothymidine; TFT

A synthetic halogenated pyrimidine nucleoside analogue, first synthesized in the early 1960s as an antitumour agent. It inhibits enzymes of the DNA pathway and is incorporated into both cellular and progeny viral DNA causing faulty transcription of late messenger RNA and the production of incompetent virion protein. It does not require a viral thymidine kinase for phosphorylation to the monophosphate derivative and it is therefore far less selective and more toxic than other analogues. It is active against HSV-1 and HSV-2, vaccinia virus, CMV and possibly adenovirus. When applied as a 1% ophthalmic solution, it rapidly gains entry into the aqueous humour of HSV-infected rabbit's eyes but is cleared within 60–90 min. It causes sister chromatid exchange – an indicator of mutagenicity – at 0.5 mg/l in human lymphocytes and fibroblasts. It is teratogenic to chick embryos when injected directly into the yolk sac and its principal adverse effects in man following systemic administration include leucopenia, anaemia, fever and hypocalcaemia. Accordingly, it is restricted to topical ophthalmic use. In man ophthalmic 1% aqueous solution produces occasional punctate lesions visible with Bengal rose; other side-effects are said to be similar to those of idoxuridine and vidarabine but to arise less frequently.

Preparations and dosage
Proprietary name: Viroptic.
Preparation: Ophthalmic drops.
Limited availability, including the UK and the USA.

Further information

Heidelberger C 1979 Trifluorothymidine. *Pharmacology and Therapeutics* 6: 427–442

VALACICLOVIR
9-(4-Acetoxy-3-acetoxymethylbut-1-yl)guanine

A pro-drug, the L-valyl ester, of acyclovir.

It is a synthetic acyclic purine (guanine) nucleoside analogue which, after oral administration, undergoes rapid first-pass intestinal and hepatic metabolism by enzymatic hydrolysis to produce acyclovir.

Antiviral activity

Its activity is that of acyclovir (p. 551).

Pharmacokinetics

It is readily absorbed and, following absorption, is converted rapidly to the active antiviral metabolite, acyclovir, since little unchanged valaciclovir is detected in plasma. The absolute bioavailability of acyclovir following 1000 mg valaciclovir (54%), is unaffected by food, and peak plasma concentrations of 22 µM are found in subjects after an oral dose of 1000 mg valaciclovir four times daily. Oral doses of valaciclovir 1000 mg four times daily give comparable systemic acyclovir exposure to that of intravenous acyclovir 5 mg/kg every 8 h.

The peak plasma concentration and AUC show a less than proportional increase with increasing dose of valaciclovir, presumably due to reduced absorption with increasing doses. The time to peak acyclovir concentration also displays dose dependency, ranging from 0.9 to 1.8 h after single oral doses of 100–1000 mg. Estimates of aciclovir half-life were approximately 2.5–3 h. Less than 1% of a dose of valaciclovir is recovered as unchanged drug in the urine. In multidose studies the amount of acyclovir recovered across dose levels ranged from about 40 to 50%. Similarly, about 7–12% of the dose was found as the acyclovir metabolite 9-[(carboxymethoxy)methyl]guanine (CMMG). Overall, acyclovir accounts for about 80–85% of total urinary recovery.

Toxicity and side-effects

In clinical trials, the most common adverse events were headache and nausea, which occurred in a similar frequency in subjects taking placebo.

Clinical use

It is indicated for treatment of herpes zoster infections.

Preparations and dosage

Proprietary name: Valtrex.

Preparation: Tablets.

Dosage: Adults, oral, 1000 mg three times daily for 7 days.

Available in the UK.

Further information

Beauchamp K M, Orr G F, de Miranda P, Burnette T, Krenitsky T A 1992 Amino acid ester prodrugs of acyclovir. *Antiviral Chemistry and Chemotherapy* 3: 157–164

Weller S, Blum M R, Doucette M et al 1993 Pharmacokinetics of the acyclovir prodrug valaciclovir after escalating single- and multiple-dose administration to normal volunteers. *Clinical Pharmacology and Therapeutics* 54: 595–605

VIDARABINE

9-β-D-Arabinofuranosyladenine; adenine arabinoside; Ara A

A purine nucleoside analogue, originally synthesized in 1960 as an anti-cancer drug.

Antiviral activity

It must be phosphorylated to active nucleotide, which acts mainly by inhibiting DNA-polymerase. It has been suggested that it also acts as a chain terminator in herpes simplex DNA synthesis but not in cellular DNA synthesis. Its antiviral spectrum includes all the herpesviruses and several poxviruses (vaccinia and myxoma). Polyoma and adenoviruses are only slightly sensitive. Amongst RNA viruses, it is active against Rous sarcoma virus, murine leukaemia virus, rabies virus and vesicular stomatitis virus. It also inhibits hepatitis B DNA polymerase.

Pharmacokinetics

It is poorly soluble in water and for systemic use is usually administered in large volumes over 24 h. The monophosphate is much more soluble and may be given intramuscularly. It is rapidly deaminated to hypoxanthine arabinoside (Ara-Hx), a compound that is more soluble than its parent but much less active. This rapid inactivation has made it difficult to study its biological and pharmacological properties. Deaminase inhibitors are known, and although they greatly increase its antiviral activity, they also increase the toxicity.

Intravenous infusion of 10–20 mg/kg over 12 h produces within a few hours mean serum concentrations of about 3.0–4.1 mg/l of vidarabine equivalents, mostly Ara-Hx, which has a plasma half-life of around 3.5 h. About 50% of a daily 12 h infusion appears in the urine as Ara-Hx within 24 h, and about 2% as unchanged drug. Renal dysfunction allows high serum concentrations of Ara-Hx to develop and neurological deterioration has been reported. It should be given at reduced dosage or avoided in such patients. Concurrent administration of interferon seems to raise the level of ara-Hx and thus increase toxicity.

Ara-Hx is widely distributed in tissues, and levels in the brain and CSF are about the same as plasma levels. When applied topically to the eye it does not penetrate; Ara-Hx can sometimes be found in the aqueous, but not at effective concentrations.

Toxicity and side-effects

Gastro-intestinal symptoms develop in roughly 20% of patients receiving 10 mg/kg i.v. per day; they usually arise several days after the start of therapy, are dose related and tend to diminish after 1–4 days despite continued treatment. Effects on the CNS such as hallucinations, tremors, ataxia, dysarthria, weakness, abnormal electroencephalograms (EEGs), myoclonus, confusion and coma develop in 2–10% of patients given 10—20 mg/kg daily, and the incidence rises when interferon is given in addition. Some of these reactions can take weeks to resolve and are occasionally fatal. Marrow toxicity may also develop. Other side-effects include modest rises in bilirubin and aspartate transaminase, rash, pruritis and thrombophlebitis and pain at the site of infusion. It causes chromosomal damage in human blood preparations, and in some species of animals it is reportedly teratogenic, carcinogenic and mutagenic. It should therefore be used with exceptional care in women of child-bearing age, and a less toxic alternative should be used whenever possible. The ophthalmic preparation may cause lacrimation, foreign-body sensation, burning, irritation, superficial punctate keratitis, pain, photophobia, punctal occlusion and sensitivity.

Clinical use

It is available as an ophthalmic ointment and is indicated for the treatment of herpes keratoconjunctivitis. Many ophthalmologists now prefer to use acyclovir. Before the introduction of acyclovir, the parenteral form was used to treat severe herpes infections and HSV and VZV infections in the immunocompromised.

Preparations and dosage

Proprietary name: Vira-A.

Preparations: Ophthalmic, i.v. infusion.

Dosage: Adults, i.v. infusion: herpes simplex,, 15 mg/kg daily for 10 days; varicella-zoster; 10 mg/kg daily for 5 days. Limited availability.

Further information

Whitley R, Alford C, Hess F, Buchanan R 1980 Vidarabine: a preliminary review of its pharmacological properties and therapeutic use. *Drugs* 20: 267–282

VIDARABINE MONOPHOSPHATE
9-β-D-Arabinofuranosyladenine monophosphate; adenine arabinoside monophosphate; Ara AMP

The potential usefulness of vidarabine is restricted by its poor solubility and rapid deamination. Since its deamination occurs at the nucleoside level, a means of overcoming this problem might be to utilize the nucleotide Ara AMP, which is the first product in the series of reactions which converts Ara A to the active triphosphate form, Ara ATP. Although Ara AMP is more soluble, its rate of take-up by cells is only 3–5% of the parent. It is evidently deaminated following initial dephosphorylation and its major advantage is thus its greater solubility. Its antiviral spectrum is evidently identical to that of vidarabine.

Further information

Weller I V D, Lok A S F, Mindel A et al 1985 Randomised controlled trial of adenine arabinoside 5'-monophosphate (ARA-AMP) in chronic hepatitis B infection. *Gut* 26: 745–751

Whitley R J, Tucker B C, Kinkel A W et al 1980 Pharmacology, tolerance, and antiviral activity of vidarabine monophosphate in humans. *Antimicrobial Agents and Chemotherapy* 18: 709–715

ZALCITABINE
2',3'-Dideoxycytidine; ddC

A synthetic analogue of the pyrimidine nucleoside 2'-deoxycytidine in which the 3'-hydroxyl group of the sugar moiety is replaced by hydrogen.

Antiviral activity

Zalcitabine inhibits HIV-1 and HIV-2, among a broad range of retroviruses, and has activity against human and duck HBV. Following cell uptake, zalcitabine is phosphorylated by cellular deoxycytidine kinase to the 5'-monophosphate. This is in turn converted into the diphosphate and then into the active triphosphate compound which inhibits HIV reverse transcriptase. Because the triphosphate lacks a 3'-hydroxyl group, no further nucleosides can be attached to the chain following the addition of dideoxycytidine triphosphate, i.e. the drug acts as a chain terminator. HIV reverse transcriptase evidently has a higher affinity for the 2',3'-dideoxynucleosides than for endogenous nucleotides as substrates.

The concentrations of zalcitabine required to inhibit HIV infection in vitro vary greatly depending upon the assay and cells used, the interval between virus infection and treatment, and the multiplicity of infection. In human T-cell lines the concentration required to block replication by 50% (ID_{50}) is generally in the range 30–500 nM (1 nM = 0.21 ng/ml); the ID_{90} is 100–1000 nM zalcitabine. Virus-induced cytopathic effects are blocked by concentrations of 30–300 nM and in assays measuring p24 antigen inhibition, the ID_{50} is 1–500 nM and the ID_{90} is 500–1000 nM. Comparative studies of anti-HIV activity of zalcitabine against HIV-1 and HIV-2 revealed no significant differences in sensitivity. Granulocyte-macrophage colony stimulating factor enhances HIV replication and reduces zalcitabine efficacy by approximately 10-fold in monocyte/macrophage cell cultures.

Acquired resistance

Emergence of HIV variants resistant to zalcitabine has been reported. The mechanism of resistance involves mutations of codons 65, 69, 74, 75, 184 and 215 in the *pol* gene encoding reverse transcriptase. Mutations at positions 74, 75 and 184 are also associated with resistance to didanosine, that at position 75 to stavudine, and those at positions 65 and 184 to lamivudine. Combination therapy with zidovudine does not appear to prevent the emergence of zidovudine-resistant strains. Combination of zidovudine and zalcitabine has additive to synergistic inhibitory activity against HIV in vitro, and viral isolates resistant to zidovudine remain susceptible to zalcitabine in vitro. Synergistic effects have been noted in vitro when zalcitabine was combined with recombinant interferon-α, soluble CD4, dextran sulphate and dipyridamole. In contrast ribavirin antagonizes the antiviral activity of zalcitabine.

Pharmacokinetics

Zalcitabine has an oral bioavailability in adults in excess of 85%, and peak plasma concentrations are found 1–2 h after oral dosing with 0.25 mg/kg. Limited studies in children using oral doses of 0.03 and 0.045 mg/kg revealed a bioavailability of 54%. Co-administration of a dose with food resulted in a 39% reduction in peak plasma concentrations, a doubling in the time taken to reach peak plasma concentration, and a 14% reduction in absorption, as reflected by the AUC. At a dose of 0.5 mg, the mean plasma concentration was 7.6 ng/ml (range 4.6–11.4 ng/ml). Intravenous infusion of 0.5 mg revealed a volume of distribution of 0.64 l/kg (range 0.59–0.69 l/kg). The mean concentration in CSF samples obtained 2–3.5 h after initiation of intravenous therapy was 20% (range 9–37%) of that in simultaneously obtained plasma.

About 75% of an intravenous dose and 62% of a single oral dose is excreted unchanged in the urine. It does not undergo significant metabolism by the liver and the primary metabolite of zalcitabine, dideoxyuridine, accounts for less than 15% of an oral dose in urine and faeces. Clearance appears to be independent of dose over the range 0.03–0.5 mg/kg. Renal clearance exceeds glomerular filtration indicating renal tubular secretion. Zalcitabine has an elimination half-life of 1–2 h in adults after oral and intravenous administration. The half-life was prolonged by up to 8.5 h in patients with impaired renal function (creatinine clearance of <55 ml/min) in comparison to patients with normal renal function. It is not known whether the drug is excreted in human breast milk or crosses the human placenta.

No significant pharmacokinetic interactions occurred when zidovudine and zalcitabine, or zalcitabine and loperamide, were co-administered to 12 HIV-positive patients. Both probenecid and cimetidine increase the AUC of zalcitabine (by 50 and 36%, respectively), whereas co-magaldrox and metaclopramide reduce the AUC by 25 and 10%, respectively.

Toxicity and side-effects

A major problem associated with the administration of zalcitabine is its toxicity. Peripheral neuropathy is twice as common in patients taking zalcitabine as in those taking didanosine, occurring at a rate of 45.1 per 100 patient-years in a cohort of 237 subjects taking 0.75 mg zalcitabine orally three times daily. Peripheral neuropathy, which is dose related, with electrophysiological studies being consistent with the presence of axonal degeneration, is sensorimotor. It may progress to severe pain requiring narcotic analgesics, may worsen for several weeks after the drug is stopped, and can be irreversible. Because of the frequency and severity of the neuropathy, concomitant use of zalcitabine with drugs that have the potential to cause neuropathy is not recommended. Because the plasma protein binding is less than 4%, drug interactions involving binding site displacement are unlikely.

Pancreatitis, which has been fatal in some cases, has been seen in approximately 1% of patients. Of 528 patients with a prior history of pancreatitis or increased serum amylase, 5.3% developed pancreatitis, and 4.4% asymptomatic elevated serum amylase. Oral ulceration has been reported at a rate of 4.7 per 100 patient-years. A dose-dependent maculopapular rash may occur within the first few weeks of therapy and is associated with mouth ulcers and, occasionally, fever. Other frequent adverse effects include anorexia, nausea, vomiting, abdominal pain, diarrhoea, malaise, headache, dizziness, myalgia and arthralgia. Cardiomyopathy, anaphylaxis, lactic acidosis and liver failure have been reported in a few cases. Laboratory tests may reveal anaemia, leukopenia, neutropenia, eosinophilia, thrombocytopenia and elevations of the transaminases and alkaline phosphatase.

No evidence of mutagenicity was observed in Ames assays using 7 different tester strains. An in vitro mammalian cell transformation assay was positive at doses of 500 mg/l. Dose-related chromosomal aberration was seen with human peripheral blood lymphocytes exposed to zalcitabine at 1.5 mg/l and higher. Oral doses of 2500 and 4500 mg/kg were clastogenic in the mouse micronucleus assay. Carcinogenicity studies in animals have not yet been reported. Zalcitabine is teratogenic in mice at plasma concentrations estimated to be 1365 and 2730 times the maximum recommended human dose (MRHD) and in rats at 2142 times the MRHD. Hydrocephalus in the F1 offspring has been related to the treatment of rats with 1071 times the MRHD. Increased embryolethality has been observed in both rats and mice given high doses.

Clinical use

Zalcitabine monotherapy is currently indicated for the management of adult patients with advanced HIV infection who are intolerant of zidovudine or who have disease progression while receiving zidovudine. These indications are based on changes in surrogate markers and by the demonstration that zalcitabine was at least as effective as didanosine in terms of time to an AIDS-defining event or death.

Preparations and dosage

Proprietary name: Hivid.

Preparation: Tablets.

Dosage: Adults, optimal dosage regimen is unknown; based on controlled trials a dose of 0.75 mg three times daily is recommended. Children, no recommendations are available.

Further information

Abrams D I, Goldman A I, Launer C et al 1994 A comparative trial of didanosine or zalcitabine after treatment with zidovudine in patients with human immunodeficiency virus infection. *New England Journal of Medicine* 330: 657–662

Baba M, Pauwels R, Balzarini J et al 1987 Ribavirin antagonises inhibitory effects of pyrimidine 2',3'-dideoxynucleosides but enhances inhibitory effects of purine 2',3'-dideoxynucleosides on replication of human immunodeficiency virus in vitro. *Antimicrobial Agents and Chemotherapy* 31: 1613–1617

Dubinski R M, Yarchoan R, Dalakas M, Broder S 1989 Reversible axonal neuropathy from the treatment of AIDS and related disorders with 2',3'-dideoxycytidine (ddC). *Muscle and Nerve* 12: 856–860

Eron J J, Johnson V A, Merrill D P, Chou T C, Hirsch M S 1992 Synergistic inhibition of replication of human immunodeficiency virus type 1, including that of a zidovudine-resistant isolate, by zidovudine and 2',3'-dideoxycytidine in vitro. *Antimicrobial Agents and Chemotherapy* 36: 1559–1562

Gustavson L E, Fukuda E K, Rubio J A, Dunton A W 1990 A pilot study of the bioavailability and pharmacokinetics of 2',3'-dideoxycytidine in patients with AIDS or AIDS-related complex. *Journal of the Acquired Immunodeficiency Syndrome* 3: 28–31

Klecker R W, Collins J M, Yarchoan R C et al 1988 Pharmacokinetics of 2',3'-dideoxycytidine in patients with AIDS and related disorders. *Journal of Clinical Pharmacology* 28: 837–842

Larder B A, Chesebro B, Richman D D 1990 Susceptibilities of zidovudine-susceptible and -resistant human immunodeficiency virus isolates to antiviral agents determined by using a quantitative plaque-reduction assay. *Antimicrobial Agents and Chemotherapy* 34: 436–441

Merigan T C, Skowron G, Bozzette S A et al 1989 Circulating p24 antigen levels and responses to dideoxycytidine in human immunodeficiency virus (HIV) infections. *Annals of Internal Medicine* 110: 189–194

Mitsuya H, Broder S 1987 Strategies for antiviral therapy in AIDS. *Nature* 325: 773–778

Pizzo P A, Butler K, Balis K et al 1990 Dideoxycytidine alone and in an alternating schedule with zidovudine in children with symptomatic human immunodeficiency virus infection. *Journal of Pediatrics* 117: 799–808

Schaumburg H H, Arezzo J, Berger A et al 1990 Dideoxycytidine (ddC) neuropathy in human immunodeficiency virus infections: a report of 52 patients [abstract]. *Neurology* 40 (suppl 1): 1133P

Shelton M J, O'Donnell A M, Morse G D 1993 Zalcitabine. *Annals of Pharmacotherapy* 27: 480–489

Whittington R, Brogden R N 1992 Zalcitabine. A review of its pharmacology and clinical potential in acquired immunodeficiency syndrome. *Drugs* 44: 656–683

Yarchoan R, Perno C F, Thomas R V et al 1988 Phase I studies of 2',3'-dideoxycytidine in severe human immunodeficiency virus infection as a single agent and alternating with zidovudine. *Lancet* i: 76–81

Yokota T, Mochzuki S, Konno K et al 1991 Inhibitory effects of selected antiviral compounds on human hepatitis B virus DNA synthesis. *Antimicrobial Agents and Chemotherapy* 35: 394–397

ZIDOVUDINE
3'-Azido-3'-deoxythymidine; azidothymidine, AZT

3'-Azido-3'-deoxythymidine, a synthetic pyrimidine (thymidine) analogue, originally developed in 1964 as a potential anticancer agent.

Antiviral activity

It is a potent inhibitor of HIV replication in vitro in a range of human T-cell lines and peripheral blood monocytes. Its activity can be measured in terms of cytopathic effects, antigen expression, reverse transcriptase activity, replication and viral particle release. The concentrations of zidovudine producing 50% inhibitory activity vary depending upon the cells and viruses used, the size of the inoculum, the timing of drug exposure and duration of the assay. There is no standardized assay and the relationship between in vitro activity and response to therapy is unclear.

The plaque-formation ID_{50} for most clinical isolates from untreated individuals ranges between 0.01 and 0.05µM (mean 0.03 µM) and the ID_{95} is generally below 1 µM. Inhibition of the multiplication of uninfected lymphocytes occurs at concentrations of >1 mM. It inhibits numerous other animal retroviruses, both in vitro and in vivo. Complete inhibition of replication of feline leukaemia virus (FeLV) was achieved at a concentration of 52.4 µM; 90% at 10.1 µM; and 50–75% at 1.1 µM. Murine Harvey sarcoma virus, SL3/3 (another murine retrovirus), avian leukosis virus, equine infectious anaemia virus, and simian lymphotrophic virus type III are also exquisitely susceptible. It is inactive against HSV-1, human CMV, adenovirus type 5, coronavirus, influenza A virus, respiratory syncytial virus, measles virus, rhinovirus 1B, bovine rota virus and yellow fever virus. It is active against EBV for which the MIC_{50} is 1–10 µM/l.

It also has potent bactericidal activity against many Enterobacteria (including strains of *Esch. coli, Salmonella typhimurium, Klebsiella pneumoniae, Shigella flexneri and Enterobacter aerogenes*) and vibrios, but no activity against *Pseudomonas aeruginosa*, Gram-positive bacteria, anaerobic bacteria, *Mycobacterium tuberculosis*, non-tuberculous mycobacteria, or most pathogenic fungi.

Additive or synergistic activity against HIV-1 has been demonstrated in vitro with recombinant interferon-α, recombinant interferon-β, acyclovir, didanosine, zalcitabine, stavudine, foscarnet, nevirapine, carbovir, catanospermine, ampligen, amphotericin B methyl ester, dextran sulphate and granulocyte–monocyte colony-stimulating factor. In contrast, ribavirin antagonizes its effect on HIV-1, the responsible mechanism appearing to be inhibition of zidovudine phosphorylation.

Zidovudine (AZT) is phosphorylated in both infected and non-infected cells to AZT monophosphate (AZTMP) by cellular thymidine kinase. This is subsequently converted by cellular thymidylate kinase into a diphosphate form and by other cellular enzymes into its active triphosphate form. The rate of phosphorylation may be low in some cells, which may account for its variable antiviral effect. Its apparent retroviral selectivity results from its action as an inhibitor of and substrate for the viral reverse transcriptase. It binds preferentially to HIV-reverse transcriptase, and its incorporation into the growing DNA strand results in chain termination. Competition by AZT-triphosphate for HIV reverse transcriptase is approximately 100-fold greater than for cellular DNA polymerase α.

Acquired resistance

Extensive data have confirmed the emergence of zidovudine-resistant isolates of HIV at all stages of HIV infection after treatment for periods of several months or longer. Resistance has been reported after therapy for only 2 months, and many patients have resistant strains at 6 months. At 12 months, resistance has been noted significantly more often in patients with 'late-stage' (89%) as compared with 'early-stage' (31%) HIV disease. Resistance is described as 'high-level' ($IC_{50} \geq 1.0$ µM) or 'moderate' ($IC_{50} > 0.2$ µM and < 1.0 µM). High level resistance is more common among those with < 50 CD4 cells/mm^3 than among those with $\geq$ 50 CD4 cells/mm^3. High level resistance predicts disease progression when other confounding variables are allowed for. High level resistance is associated with a sequential accumulation of mutations in the HIV *pol* gene which codes for reverse transcriptase. These mutations occur at amino acids 41, 67, 70, 215 and 219, and occur in step-wise fashion. The syncitium inducing viral biologic phenotype of HIV appears to be associated with a poor response to zidovudine. Zidovudine-resistant strains may occasionally revert to zidovudine-susceptible phenotype when the drug is withdrawn or changed to another agent. In such instances, sensitivity may be regained after several months. Resistance is less likely to develop when other antiretroviral agents are used, but combination therapy does not necessarily prevent the development of resistance. Resistance appears to develop more readily with zidovudine than with didanosine or zalcitabine

Pharmacokinetics

Zidovudine is well absorbed from the gut with a bioavailability of 60–70%. Bioavailability was reduced to 44% in patients with mild diarrhoea and was also reduced in patients with low CD4 cell counts. Peak plasma concentrations vary from about 1.5 to 18 µM/l in a linear fashion with single and multiple doses of 1–10 mg/kg and occur 0.5–1.5 h after administration. Peak plasma concentrations after an oral dose of 250 mg was 2.3 µmol/l. Recent studies have revealed considerable interpatient variability in AUC after a fixed oral dose with between-patient coefficients of variation of up to 50%. The AUC in a fed state is 78% of that in a fasting state and is more variable, but liquid-based 25 g protein meals do not affect overall absorption of zidovudine.

With intravenous dosing the mean terminal plasma half-life is 1.5 h. Its pharmacokinetics in pregnancy and in the intrapartum and postpartum periods were found to be similar to those in non-pregnant women in two studies, but in a third the volume of distribution and clearance were both increased. In infants ≤14 days of age, total body clearance of zidovudine is reduced and the half-life prolonged to over 3 h. In contrast the pharmacokinetic parameters in infants aged >14 days were comparable to those reported in adults. The neonates were found to have reduced formation of zidovudine glucuronide suggesting that gestational age may need to be taken into account in dosing.

Plasma protein binding is relatively low (34–38%) and so drug interactions involving binding-site displacement are not anticipated. Zidovudine is widely distributed with a mean volume of distribution of about 1.5–1.8 l/kg. It is concentrated in the semen, and levels in saliva are approximately 68% of those in plasma. CSF/plasma ratios are strongly related to the time after ingestion and range from less than 0.1 to 2.05. Levels in the CSF seem to be independent of daily dose in the range 200–1200 mg and are much less variable than those in plasma. It crosses the human placenta and is found in human amniotic fluid and neonatal blood. Intracellular phosphorylated zidovudine concentrations correlate poorly with dosage and plasma concentrations.

It is primarily eliminated by renal excretion, either as unchanged drug (10–20%) or as the inactive metabolite 5'-O-ether glucuronide (50–80%). The majority of the glucuronidation occurs in the liver by a uridine diphospho-glucuronosyltransferase, but the kidney also plays an important role. An additional metabolite of zidovudine, aminothymidine, is formed in the liver by the cytochrome P_{450} system; only a small proportion is excreted as this metabolite, but it may be responsible for some of the haematological toxicity. Since glucuronidation occurs predominantly in the liver, accumulation of zidovudine is likely to occur in patients with hepatic impairment, leading to increased risk of toxicity. Renal clearance of zidovudine greatly exceeds creatinine clearance indicating that significant tubular secretion takes place. Accumulation of zidovudine and its metabolites is likely to occur in the presence of renal impairment and increases the risk of toxicity.

Removal of zidovudine by peritoneal dialysis or haemodialysis is negligible. However, zidovudine glucuronide is cleared by about 50% by dialysis. Peak serum concentrations are elevated and the half-life prolonged when oral zidovudine is given to patients with cirrhosis. Probenecid inhibits glucuronidation and reduces tubular secretion of some drugs; it significantly reduces zidovudine clearance and the AUC can be doubled. Paracetomol is glucoronidated in the liver, but there is no evidence that it effects zidovudine pharmacokinetics. However, there is an increased risk of anaemia and neutropenia during concomitant use of zidovudine and paracetomol, but the

cause is uncertain. Naproxen, a potent inhibitor of glucuronidation, was found to have no effect on zidovudine pharmacokinetics. Acyclovir does not influence the pharmacokinetics of zidovudine, but it does have a favourable effect on survival. No pharmacokinetic interactions have been found with concomitant use of zidovudine with ganciclovir, zalcitabine, didanosine or foscarnet. Trimethoprim alone or in combination with sulphamethoxazole reduces renal clearance of zidovudine by about half, and zidovudine glucuronide by about a quarter possibly due to reduced tubular secretion. Dapsone in combination with zidovudine is associated with a greater likelihood of anaemia, neutropenia and thrombocytopenia but it is uncertain whether it has an effect on zidovudine pharmacokinetics. Clarithromycin inhibits the absorption of zidovudine resulting in lower peak levels and AUC. Rifampicin and rifabutin both appear to reduce zidovudine AUC values. Interferon-β increases the plasma half-life of zidovudine, but the preliminary data show no evidence of an interaction with interferon-α. Valproic acid which, like zidovudine, is metabolized by glucuronidation, increases the plasma AUC two-fold and increases the amount of unconjugated zidovudine two-fold.

Toxicity and side-effects

Anaemia, usually occurring after 6 weeks of therapy, neutropenia, usually occurring at any time after 4 weeks therapy, and leucopenia, usually secondary to neutropenia, are common adverse effects, particularly in patients with AIDS rather than ARC, and especially those with CD4 counts of <100/mm³. Increases in the mean corpuscular volume occur almost invariably. Neutropenia is more common in patients with pre-existing neutropenia, anaemia or low vitamin B_{12} levels, and those taking paracetomol concomitantly. Fortnightly blood tests are recommended during the first 3 months of therapy and monthly tests thereafter. Particular care should be taken in patients with pre-existing bone-marrow impairment, i.e. haemoglobin less than 9.0 g/dl or neutrophil count less than 1.0×10^9/l. Dosage adjustments are recommended for patients with haematological toxicity. Discontinuation of therapy is suggested if the haemoglobin falls below 7.5 g/dl or the neutrophil count falls to less than 0.75×10^9/l. Marrow recovery is usually observed within 2 weeks, after which time therapy at a reduced dosage may be reinstituted. After a further 2–4 weeks the dose may be gradually increased, depending upon patient tolerance, until the original dose is reached.

Frequent adverse effects include nausea, occurring in about 20–30%, vomiting, headache, rash, abdominal pain, anorexia, fever, myalgia, paraesthesia, insomnia and malaise; but, apart from nausea, myalgia and insomnia, the incidence of these effects is only slightly higher than in placebo recipients. Less commonly reported, and less clearly associated adverse effects, include nail, skin and oral mucosal pigmentation, asthenia, somnolence, diarrhoea, dizziness, paraesthesia, sweating, dyspnoea, dyspepsia, flatulence, bad taste, chest pain, loss of mental acuity, confusion, anxiety, depression, urinary frequency, generalized pain, chills, cough, urticaria, pruritis, influenza-like syndrome and liver function abnormalities.

No evidence of mutagenicity has been observed in the Ames test, but it is weakly mutagenic in the L5178Y mouse lymphoma cell assay at concentrations of >4000 mg/l, and in a cytogenetics study performed in cultured human lymphocytes, dose-related chromosomal alterations were noted at concentrations of >3 mg/l. Chromosomal damage has not been observed in rats. In laboratory rodents, the median lethal dose was greater than 750 mg/kg intravenously and greater than 3000 mg/kg orally. There was no evidence of teratogenicity in rats or rabbits given the drug during gestation.

Clinical use

Zidovudine is indicated for patients with advanced HIV disease, including those with AIDS and AIDS-related complex. It is also indicated for early symptomatic patients with CD4 counts of <500/mm³, and in asymptomatic patients with markers indicating progressive disease including CD4 counts of <200/mm³, or counts between 500 and 200/mm³ which are falling rapidly. It is indicated for HIV-infected children aged >3 months who have HIV-related symptoms or who are asymptomatic, but have markers indicating HIV-related immune suppression. Zidovudine has been shown to reduce the rate of maternal–fetal transmission and should be considered for use in HIV-positive pregnant women (over 14 weeks gestation) and their newborn infants.

Preparations and dosage

Proprietary name: Retrovir.

Preparations: Capsules, syrup, injection.

Dosage: Adults, oral: Various dosages including 500–600 mg daily in 2–5 divided doses or 1 g daily in two divided doses. Children >3 months, oral: initially 180 mg/m² every 6 h. Intravenouse infusion, adults, 2.5 mg/kg every 4 h for a maximum of 2 weeks.

The following dosage regimen has been shown to be effective in reducing maternal–fetal transmission. Pregnant women (over 14 weeks gestation): 100 mg five times daily until the beginning of labour. During labour and delivery zidovudine is administered intravenously at 2 mg/kg body weight over 1 h followed by a continuous infusion at 1 mg/kg per hour until the umbilical cord is clamped. Infants unable to receive oral dosing are given zidovudine intravenously at 1.5 mg/kg infused over 30 min every 6 h. Widely available.

Further information

Birch C, Tachedjian G, Lucas C R, Gust I 1988 In vitro effectiveness of a combination of zidovudine and ansamycin against human immunodeficiency virus. *Journal of Infectious Diseases* 158: 895

Boucher F D, Modlin J F, Weller S et al 1993 Phase I evaluation of zidovudine administered to infants exposed at birth to the human immunodeficiency virus. *Journal of Pediatrics* 122: 137–144

Burger D M, Meenhorst P L, Koks C H W, Beijnen J H 1993 Drug interactions with zidovudine. *AIDS* 7: 445–460

Chaisson R E, Allain J P, Leuther M, Volberding P A 1986 Significant changes in HIV antigen level in the serum of patients treated with azidothymidine. *New England Journal of Medicine* 315: 1610–1611

Connor E M, Sperling R S, Gelber R et al 1994 Reduction of maternal–infant transmission of human immunodeficiency virus type I with zidovudine treatment. *New England Journal of Medicine* 331: 1173–1180

Dudley M N 1995 Clinical pharmacokinetics of nucleoside antiretroviral agents. *Journal of Infectious Diseases* 171 (suppl 2): S99–S112

Elwell L P, Ferone R, Freeman G A et al 1987 Antibacterial activity and mechanism of action of 3'-azido-3'-deoxythymidine (BW A509U). *Antimicrobial Agents and Chemotherapy* 31: 274–280

Hartshorn K L, Vogt M W, Chou T C et al 1987 Synergistic inhibition of human immunodeficiency virus in vitro by azidothymidine and recombinant alpha A interferon. *Antimicrobial Agents and Chemotherapy* 31: 168–172

Jackson G G, Paul D A, Kalk L A et al 1988 Human immunodeficiency virus (HIV) antigenaemia (p24) in the acquired immunodeficiency syndrome (AIDS) and the effect of treatment with zidovudine (AZT). *Annals of Internal Medicine* 108: 175–80

Klecker R W, Collins J M, Yarchoan R et al 1987 Plasma and cerebrospinal fluid pharmacokinetics of 3'-azido-3'-deoxythymidine: a novel pyrimidine analog with potential application for the treatment of AIDS and related diseases. *Clinical Pharmacology and Therapeutics* 41: 407–412

Larder B A, Darby G, Richman D D 1989 HIV with reduced sensitivity to zidovudine (AZT) isolated during prolonged therapy. *Science* 243: 1731–1734

Lotterer B, Ruhnke M, Trautman M, Beyer R, Bauer F E 1991 Decreased and variable systemic availability of zidovudine in patients with AIDS if administered with a meal. *European Journal of Clinical Pharmacology* 40: 305–308

Macnab K A, Gill M J, Sutherland L R, De Boer Visser N, Church D 1993 Erratic zidovudine bioavailability in HIV seropositive patients. *Journal of Antimicrobial Chemotherapy* 31: 421–428

O'Sullivan M J, Boyer P J, Scott G B et al 1993 The pharmacokinetics and safety of zidovudine in the third trimester of pregnancy for women infected with the human immunodeficiency virus and their infants: phase I acquired immunodeficiency syndrome clinical trials group study (protocol 082). *American Journal of Obstetrics and Gynecology* 168: 1510–1516

Reiss P, Lange J M A, Boucher C A, Danner S A, Goudsmit J 1988 Resumption of HIV antigen production during continuous zidovudine treatment. *Lancet* i: 421

Richman D D, Fischl M A, Grieco M H et al 1987 The toxicity of azidothymidine (AZT) in the treatment of patients with AIDS and AIDS-related complex. A double-blind, placebo-controlled trial. *New England Journal of Medicine* 317: 192–197

Rolinski A, Wintergerst U, Matusschke A, Fuessl H, Goebel F O 1991 Evaluation of saliva as a specimen for monitoring zidovudine therapy in HIV-infected patients. *AIDS* 5: 885–888

Sahai J, Gallicano K, Garber G et al 1992 The effect of a protein meal on zidovudine pharmacokinetics in HIV-infected patients. *British Journal of Clinical Pharmacology* 33: 657–660

Singlas E, Pioger J C, Taburet A M, Colin J N, Fillastre J P 1989 Zidovudine disposition in patients with severe renal impairment: influence of haemodialysis. *Clinical Pharmacology and Therapeutics* 46: 190–197

Smith M S, Brian E L, Pagano J S 1987 Resumption of virus production after human immunodeficiency virus infection of T lymphocytes in the presence of azidothymidine. *Journal of Virology* 61: 3769–3773

Sommadosi J P 1993 Nucleoside analogues: similarities and differences. *Journal of Infectious Diseases* 16 (suppl 1): S7–S15

Sperling R S, Roboz J, Dische R et al 1992 Zidovudine pharmacokinetics during pregnancy. *American Journal of Perinatology* 9: 247–249

Stretcher B N, Pesce A J, Murray J A et al 1991 Concentrations of phosphorylated zidovudine (ZDV) in patients leukocytes do not correlate with ZDV dose or plasma concentrations. *Therapeutic Drug Monitoring* 13: 325–331

Taburet A M, Naveau S, Zorza G et al 1990 Pharmacokinetics of zidovudine in patients with liver cirrhosis. *Clinical Pharmacology and Therapeutics* 47: 731–739

Terasaki T, Pardridge W M 1988 Restricted transport of 3'-azido-3'-deoxythymidine and dideoxynucleosides through the blood–brain barrier. *Journal of Infectious Diseases* 158: 630–632

Vogt M W, Hartshorn K L, Furman P A et al 1987 Ribavirin antagonises the effect of azidothymidine on HIV replication. *Science* 235: 1376–1379

Watts D H, Brown Z A, Tartaglione T et al 1991 Pharmacokinetic disposition of zidovudine during pregnancy. *Journal of Infectious Disease* 163: 226–232

Phosphonic acids

This group includes the two aliphatic compounds: phosphonoformic acid and phosphonoacetic acid. Phosphonoacetate forms a six-ring chelate with metal ions and similar five-ring chelates would be expected for phosphonoformate. It is probable that this chelating activity is responsible for the effect of these agents on a wide range of polymerases and nucleases. Only phosphonoformic acid has been licensed for clinical use.

Foscarnet

Phosphonoformic acid; trisodium phosphonoformate; PFA

A synthetic non-nucleoside pyrophosphate analogue.

Antiviral activity

It inhibits the RNA polymerase of influenza A virus, the DNA polymerases of HSV-1 and HSV-2, CMV, EBV, VZV and HBV more efficiently than host-cell DNA polymerases. Foscarnet concentrations of about 6–55 μM are required to inhibit

CMV plaque formation by 50% (ID_{50}), but clinical isolates are generally 1.5–8 times less sensitive. In vitro inhibition of CMV replication is reversed by withdrawal of the drug. Most strains of HSV that are resistant to acyclovir are susceptible in vitro and in vivo to foscarnet. However, when treatment is stopped there is a high frequency of relapse. Foscarnet acts as a non-competitive inhibitor for substrates and templates of reverse transcriptases from various animal retroviruses in doses ranging from 0.7 to 100 µM. It inhibits HIV reverse transcriptase in concentrations ranging from 0.1 to 5.0 µM, but 680 µM was required to block replication of the virus in H9 cell cultures. The mean ID_{50} of foscarnet against HIV isolates in peripheral blood mononuclear cells was 29.7 µM/l (range 1–100 µM/l). In p24-antigen-positive patients, intravenous therapy resulted in a 55% mean reduction of p24 antigen concentration, although maintenance therapy saw an increase in some antigen levels to 54–77% of the baseline value. In three trials, HIV was isolated from peripheral blood mononuclear cells in 80–100% of cultures obtained before therapy, compared with 27–53% of cultures obtained at the end of therapy.

Foscarnet exerts additive or synergic activity in vitro against CMV with zidovudine and ganciclovir. Synergy or additive activity against HIV replication has been documented with interferon-α, zidovudine and dideoxythymidine.

Acquired resistance

Resistance to foscarnet has been generated in vitro, and CMV strains have occasionally been recovered from man that are resistant to both ganciclovir and foscarnet. Changes in HIV-1 reverse transcriptase that have led to resistance to foscarnet have been identified in vitro. Amino acid changes at position 89 in HIV-1 reverse transcriptase may be important in acquisition of resistance.

Pharmacokinetics

The solubility of foscarnet in water at pH 7 is only about 5% (w/w). Oral bioavailability is poor, approximately 17%. Mean peak and trough levels on day 14 of intravenous therapy with 60 mg/kg 8-hourly were 557 and 155 µM, respectively. A wide range of plasma concentrations was noted (75–500 µM/l) during 3–21 days of continuous intravenous infusion of 0.14–0.19 mg/kg per min. During continuous intravenous therapy the concentrations reached a plateau on day 3. Various investigators have noted considerable differences of steady-state plasma concentrations between individuals. The mean volume of distribution following intravenous infusion has been estimated at 0.52–0.74 l/kg. Several studies in man indicate that the drug penetrates the CSF: in one study, the mean concentration of 68.5 µmol/l was 43% of the mean plasma concentration; in another, the mean CSF concentrations 1 h after 90 mg/kg under steady-state conditions were 131 mg/l (436 µmol/l) and 308 mg/l (1023 µmol/l) in 26 patients with HIV; the penetration coefficient was 0.66 and the CSF concentrations were virustatic.

Elimination of foscarnet appears to be triphasic, with two initially short half-lives of 0.5–1.4 h and 3.3–6.8 h, followed by a long terminal phase of 88 h. About 88% of the cumulative intravenous dose is recovered unchanged in the urine within a week of stopping an infusion, indicating that the drug is not metabolized to any significant extent. Non-renal clearance accounts for about 14–18% of total clearance and is believed to relate to uptake into bone. Plasma foscarnet clearance decreases markedly with decreased renal function and the elimination half-life may be increased by up to 10-fold. However, a preliminary report indicates that 27% of a dose can be removed by conventional dialysis and 58% by high-flux dialysis.

Concomitant foscarnet and zidovudine therapy does not affect the pharmacokinetics of either drug. No significant pharmacokinetic interaction occurs when ganciclovir and foscarnet are given as concomitant or daily alternating therapy.

Toxicity and side-effects

Compared to ganciclovir, the use of foscarnet is more frequently limited by toxicity, but greater survival benefits have been noted. Renal toxicity is the most common dose-limiting adverse event. Of 188 AIDS patients treated with foscarnet, 27% developed impaired renal function and 2% developed acute renal failure. A two- to three-fold increase in serum creatinine levels occurred in 20–60% (mean 45%) patients given 130–230 mg/kg daily as a continuous intravenous infusion. Renal impairment usually develops within the first few weeks of treatment and is generally reversible within several weeks of discontinuing therapy. Foscarnet chelates metal ions, and serum electrolyte abnormalities, predominantly hypocalcaemia, hypomagnesaemia, hypokalaemia, and hypophosphataemia are common, occurring in about 30, 15, 16 and 8% of patients, respectively. Convulsions occur in about 10–15%. Other side-effects include anaemia (25–50%), penile or vulval ulceration (3–9%), nausea and vomiting (20–30%), local irritation and thrombophlebitis at the infusion site, abdominal pain and occasional pancreatitis, headache (~25%), dizziness, involuntary muscle contractions, tremor, hypoaesthesia, ataxia, neuropathy, anxiety, nervousness, depression and confusion, and skin rash. Nephrogenic diabetes insipidus has been reported. In comparative studies of foscarnet and ganciclovir, patients are more likely to discontinue foscarnet because of adverse events, than vice versa.

In view of its nephrotoxicity, coadministration of foscarnet with potentially nephrotoxic drugs (e.g. aminoglycosides, amphotericin B, pentamidine, cyclosporin) should be avoided. Foscarnet is contraindicated in pregnancy. Topical application does not result in dermal toxicity similar to that produced by phosphonacetic acid.

Clinical use

Foscarnet is currently indicated for the treatment of CMV retinitis in patients in whom ganciclovir is contraindicated, inappropriate or ineffective. It is also appropriate for other symptomatic cytomegalovirus infections in the immunocompromised. In view of results in AIDS patients which favour foscarnet, its anti-HIV activity, the toxicities of both ganciclovir and foscarnet, and the synery between the two agents, there is increasing interest in concomitant or alternating therapy with ganciclovir and foscarnet in AIDS. Foscarnet is also potentially of value in the treatment of acyclovir-resistant HSV infection.

Preparations and dosage

Proprietary name: Foscavir.

Preparation: Intravenous infusion.

Dosage: Adults, 20 mg/kg over 30 min, then 21–200 mg/kg daily, according to renal function, for 2–3 weeks.

Widely available.

Further information

Aweeka F, Gambertoglio J, Mills J, Jacobson M A 1989 Pharmacokinetics of intermittently administered intravenous foscarnet in the treatment of acquired immunodeficiency syndrome patients with serious cytomegalovirus retinitis. *Antimicrobial Agents and Chemotherapy* 33: 742–745

Aweeka F, Gambertoglio J G, van der Horst C, Raasch R, Jacobson M A 1992 Pharmacokinetics of concomitantly administered foscarnet and zidovudine in treatment of human immunodeficiency virus infection (AIDS Clinical Trials Group Program 053). *Antimicrobial Agents and Chemotherapy* 36: 1773–1778

Aweeka F, Gambertoglio J G, Kramer F et al 1995 Foscarnet and ganciclovir pharmacokinetics during concomitant or alternating maintenance therapy for AIDS-related cytomegalovirus retinitis. *Clinical Pharmacology and Therapeutics* 57: 403–412

Cox S W, Aperia K, Sandström E et al 1994 Cross-resistance between AZT, ddI, and other anti-retroviral drugs in primary isolates of HIV-1. *Antiviral Chemistry and Chemotherapy* 5: 7–12

Farthing C F, Dalgleish A G, Clark A, McClure M, Chanas A, Gazzard B G 1987 Phosphonoformate (foscarnet): a pilot study in AIDS and AIDS related complex. *AIDS* 1: 21–25

Hartshorn K L, Sandstrom E G, Neumeyer D et al 1986 Synergistic inhibition of human T-cell lymphotrophic virus type III replication in vitro by phosphonoformate and recombinant alpha-A interferon. *Antimicrobial Agents and Chemotherapy* 30: 1889–1891

Hengge U R, Brockmeyer N H, Malessa R, Ravens U, Goos M 1993 Foscarnet penetrates the blood–brain barrier: rationale for therapy of cytomegalovirus encephalitis. *Antimicrobial Agents and Chemotherapy* 37: 1010–1014

Jacobson M A, Crowe S, Levy J et al 1988 Effect of foscarnet therapy on infection with human immunodeficiency virus in patients with AIDS. *Journal of Infectious Diseases* 158: 862–865

Jacobson M A, Causey D, Polsky B et al 1993 A dose ranging study of daily maintenance intravenous foscarnet therapy for cytomegalovirus retinitis in AIDS. *Journal of Infectious Diseases* 168: 444–448

Knox K K, Drobyski W R, Carrigan W R 1991 Cytomegalovirus isolate resistant to ganciclovir and foscarnet from a marrow transplant patient [letter]. *Lancet* 337: 1292–1293

Leport C, Paget S, Pepin J M et al 1993 CMV retinitis resistant to foscarnet. A case with clinicovirologic correlation [abstract No. 175]. *Antiviral Research* 20 (suppl 1): 137

Safrin S, Crumpacker C, Chatis P et al 1991 A controlled trial comparing foscarnet with vidarabine for acyclovir-resistant mucocutaneous herpes simplex in the acquired immunodeficiency syndrome. *New England Journal of Medicine* 325: 551–555

Sjövall J, Karlsson A, Ogenstad S, Sandström E, Saarimaki M 1988 Pharmacokinetics and absorption of foscarnet after intravenous and oral administration to patients with human immunodeficiency virus. *Clinical Pharmacology and Therapeutics* 44: 65–73

Sjövall J, Bergdahl S, Movin G, Ogenstad S, Saarimati M 1989 Pharmacokinetics of foscarnet and distribution to cerebrospinal fluid after intravenous infusion in patients with human immunodeficiency virus infection. *Antimicrobial Agents and Chemotherapy* 33: 1023–1031

Song Q, Yang G, Goff S P et al 1992 Mutagenesis of the Glu-89 residue in human immunodeficiency virus type 1 (HIV-1) and HIV-2 reverse transcriptase: effects on nucleoside analogue resistance. *Journal of Virology* 66: 7568–7571

Studies of Ocular Complications of AIDS Research Group, in collaboration with the AIDS Clinical Trials Group 1995 Morbidity and toxic effects associated with ganciclovir or foscarnet therapy in a randomised cytomegalovirus retinitis trial. *Archives of Internal Medicine* 155: 65–73

Tatrowicz W A, Lurain N S, Thompson K D 1992 A ganciclovir resistant clinical isolate of human cytomegalovirus exhibiting cross-resistance to other DNA polymerase inhibitors. *Journal of Infectious Diseases* 166: 904–907

Wagstaff A J, Bryson H M 1994 Foscarnet. A reappraisal of its antiviral activity, pharmacokinetic properties and therapeutic use in immunocompromised patients with viral infections. *Drugs* 48: 199–226

Compounds in development

Large numbers of compounds have been investigated over the years for antiviral activity and potential therapeutic use. Many that showed initial promise have not progressed. Details of a number of such compounds can be found in the previous edition of this book, including: the chelating agent β-diketone; the immunomodulator, thiopentin; the interferon inducers, ampligen and pyrimidone; together with assorted other compounds including antimoniotungstate, catanospermine, certain oligopeptides and peptide T, rifabutin, some sulphated polysaccharides, suramin and the thiosemicarbizone, methisazone.

Some interest continues in CD4 analogues and in the immunomodulator immuthiol, and several new chemical entities have emerged.

CD4 ANALOGUES

Recombinant technology has been used to produce soluble CD4 analogues which like the CD4 molecule of T lymphocytes have a high affinity for the gp 120 envelope protein of HIV. Soluble CD4 neither inhibits replication nor destroys HIV, but has been shown to neutralize the infectivity of HIV in vitro, probably by acting as a competitive inhibitor. Preliminary studies in the chimpanzee have failed to show any adverse immunological effects.

Quantities of synthetic CD4 oligopeptides ranging from 200 to 10 mg/ml inhibit binding of HIV-1 in CD4 positive cell lines and block viral replication and syncitia formation. Synthetic CD4 has an antiviral effect in rhesus monkeys infected with simian immunodeficiency virus. In vitro it acts synergistically with zidovudine.

Several groups have undertaken phase I/II trials of recombinant soluble CD4. A serum half-life of approximately 45 min has been reported. Repeated daily intramuscular injections of 30 mg CD4 give steady-state serum levels of 50–300 ng/ml. Mean p24 antigen levels declined to 23% of baseline levels after 28 days' therapy. The short half-life of soluble CD4 has led to attempts to make recombinant CD4-

immunoglobulin G, which has a half-life of about 2 days after intravenous administration.

Side-effects of soluble CD4 include local irritation at injection sites and fever. Neither soluble CD4 nor CD4-immunoglobulin G have given convincing results in patients with AIDS or ARC.

Further information

Fisher R A, Bertonis J M, Meier W et al 1988 HIV infection is blocked in vitro by recombinant soluble CD4. *Nature* 331: 76–78

Hodges T L, Kahn J O, Kaplan L D et al 1991 Phase I study of recombinant CD4-immunoglobulin G therapy of patients with AIDS and AIDS-related complex. *Antimicrobial Agents and Chemotherapy* 35: 2580–2586

Hussey R E, Richardson N E, Kowalski M et al 1988 A CD4 protein selectively inhibits HIV replication and syncitium formation. *Nature* 331: 78–81

Johnson V A, Barlow M A, Chou T-C et al 1989 Synergistic inhibition of human immunodeficiency virus type 1 (HIV-1) replication in vitro by recombinant soluble CD4 and 3'-azido-3'-deoxythymidine. *Journal of Infectious Disease* 159: 837–844

Schooley R T, Merigan T C, Gaut P et al 1990 A phase I/II escalating dose trial of recombinant soluble CD4 therapy in patients with AIDS or AIDS-related complex. *Annals of Internal Medicine* 112: 247–253

IMUTHIOL
Sodium diethyldithiocarbamate; ditiocarb; DTC

A metal-chelating agent that induces T-cell differentiation and maturation. It also inhibits HIV-1 expression and reverse transcriptase activity in peripheral blood lymphocytes from patients with HIV and has antistaphylococcal and antifungal activity. It can be given orally and intravenously. A dose response study in patients with ARC or AIDS showed that doses up to 400 mg/m^2 administered once weekly were not toxic, whereas 800 mg/m^2 either once or twice a week had side-effects. A metallic taste is a common side-effect; it lasts a few hours after intravenous administration and for up to a day after oral treatment. Disulfiram effects have been noted, and chest pain, nausea, fever, dyspnoea and skin rash occur at a high-dose level of 800 mg/m^2. In preliminary trials in patients with HIV-1 in Walter–Reed stages 2–4, diminished progression rates were noted and the decline in CD4 count was reduced. However, it had no effect on the virus load of the patients. It was administered in a placebo-controlled study to 389 symptomatic HIV-infected patients, with or without zidovudine, and was associated with a reduction in new opportunistic infections over a 24-week period.

Further information

Hersch E, Brewton G, Abrams D et al 1991 Ditiocarb sodium (diethylcarbamate) therapy in patients with symptomatic HIV infection and AIDS. *Journal of the American Medical Association* 265: 1538–1544

Reisinger E C, Kern P, Ernst M et al 1990 Inhibition of HIV progression by dithiocarb. *Lancet* 335: 679–682

New chemical entities

Activity in the field of antiviral agents remains intense and many promising new compounds have been identified. Some, like cidofir and lamivudine, are nucleoside or nucleotide analogues, but most fall into a chemically diverse group of non-nucleoside reverse-transcriptase inhibitors including atevirdine; the pyrimidone derivative L697661; nevirapine; and the substituted benzodiazepine, TIBO and its derivatives. Others, like MK639 and saquinavir, are protease inhibitors.

Nucleosides and nucleotides

CIDOFIR

(S)-1-[3-Hydroxy-2-(phosphonylmethoxy)propyl]cytosine

A new class of antiviral agent containing a phosphonate group enabling it to mimic a nucleotide and bypass initial virus-dependent phosphorylation. Cellular enzymes are responsible for serial conversion to the diphosphate and triphosphate, which is the active intracellular compound. It has in vitro and in vivo activity against CMV and other herpes viruses including acyclovir-resistant herpes simplex. Oral hairy leukoplakia resolved on therapy, suggesting that it has activity against EBV.

Peak plasma concentrations were 7.7 and 23.0 mg/l at doses of 3 and 10 mg/kg respectively. The intracellular half-life of the diphosphate is 17–65 h. The volume of distribution was about 0.6 l/kg and the elimination half-life was about 3 and 4 h at doses of 3 and 10 mg/kg, respectively.

Nephrotoxicity was a dose-limiting adverse effect which was heralded by proteinuria and occurred at weekly doses of ≥3 mg/kg in 2 of 5 patients after 6 and 14 consecutive weeks of therapy. Two of 5 patients given 10 mg/kg developed nephrotoxicity after only two doses, which

manifested as a Fanconi-like syndrome with proteinuria, glucosuria, bicarbonaturia, phosphaturia, polyuria and increased creatinine. Biopsy revealed proximal tubular effects. Prehydration and extended dosing intervals seems to be nephroprotective.

A prolonged and dose-dependent anti-CMV effect was noted in HIV patients at doses ≥3 mg/kg per week given intravenously.

Further information

Lalezari J P, Drew W L, Glutzer E et al 1995 (S)-1-[3-Hydroxy-2-(phosphonylmethoxy)propyl]cytosine (Cidofir): results of a phase I/II study of a novel antiviral nucleotide analogue. *Journal of Infectious Diseases* 171: 788–796

LAMIVUDINE
2'-Deoxy-3'-thiacytidine; 3TC

The laevorotatory enantiomer of a cytosine dideoxy-nucleoside analogue.

Antiviral activity

Lamivudine has been identified as a potent inhibitor of HIV-1 and HIV-2 in vitro as well as of hepatitis B virus and duck hepatitis B virus. Its anti-HIV activity occurs through reverse transcriptase inhibition and chain termination. In established HIV infected cell lines, IC_{50} and IC_{90} values measured by various techniques have been found in the ranges 0.004–1.14 and 0.032–3.5 μM, respectively. It exhibits additive or synergic in vitro activity with zidovudine and is active against zidovudine-resistant isolates.

Acquired resistance

A mutation at codon 184 (in a highly conserved domain coding for the reverse transcriptase of HIV-1, that encodes for low level resistance to didanosine and zalcitabine) confers high level resistance to lamivudine. In vitro selection procedures have resulted in HIV-1 variants with as great as 1000-fold resistance to lamivudine after as few as 10 passages. In addition, virus isolates during the first few months of treatment showed the same amino acid change at codon 184, indicating that the mutation may occur rapidly. Lamivudine-resistant isolates retain sensitivity to zidovudine, didanosine and zalcitabine.

Pharmacokinetics

Oral bioavailability is 69–95% for doses between 0.35 and 8.0 mg/kg. Bioavailability tends to decrease with increasing dose. Ingestion of drug with food prolongs the time to peak and reduces the peak serum levels, but has no significant effect on drug absorption. Peak serum concentrations after oral ingestion of doubling doses in the range 0.25–8.0 mg/kg were 227, 1263, 1725, 2646 and 5815 ng/ml, respectively. Intravenous infusions over 1 h of doubling doses in the same range gave peak serum concentrations of 386, 1615, 3301, 5620 and 10 560 ng/ml, respectively, with a volume of distribution of 1.3 l/kg.

Its serum elimination half-life is 2.5 h. Concomitant administration of zidovudine for 3 days did not alter the pharmacokinetics of lamivudine. In patients given 8.0–20.0 mg/kg per day, the mean CSF/serum ratio 2 h after a dose was 0.06 (range 0.04–0.08). The CSF concentrations ranged from 0.41 to 1.43 μM/l (94–328 ng/l).

About 68–71% of an oral or intravenous dose is excreted unchanged in the urine. Renal clearance greatly exceeds creatinine clearance, indicating renal tubular secretion.

Toxicity and side-effects

More than 5000 patients have been treated in clinical studies. It is generally well tolerated at doses of 0.5–20.0 mg/kg daily administered in two equal doses every 12 h. Diarrhoea, headache, fatigue, nausea and abdominal pain are reported most frequently and are usually mild and transient. Neutropenia, thrombocytopenia, pancreatitis and elevations of hepatic enzymes and bilirubin occasionally develop.

Clinical use

Efficacy against HIV is currently being evaluated as monotherapy and in combination with zidovudine in controlled clinical trials. It is also being administered on an open-label programme and currently being assessed in the treatment of chronic hepatitis B infection.

Further information

Angel J B, Hussey E K, Hall S T et al 1993 Pharmacokinetics of 3TC (GR 109714X) administered with and without food to HIV-infected patients. *Drug Investigations* 6: 70–74

Boucher C A B, Cammack N, Schipper P et al 1993 High-level resistance to (–) enantiomer 2'-deoxy-3'-thiacytidine in vitro is due to one amino acid substitution in the catalytic site of human immunodeficiency virus type I reverse transcriptase. *Antimicrobial Agents and Chemotherapy* 37: 2231–2234

Gao Q, Gu Z, Parniak M A et al 1993 The same mutation that encodes low level human immunodeficiency virus type I resistance to 2',3'-dideoxyinosine and 2',3'-dideoxy-cytidine confers high-level resistance to the (–) enantiomer of 2',3'-dideoxy-3'-thiacytidine. *Antimicrobial Agents and Chemotherapy* 37: 1390–1392

Horton C, Yuen G, Mikolich D et al 1994 Pharmacokinetics of lamivudine administered alone and with zidovudine in asymptomatic patients with human immunodeficiency virus infection [abstract]. *Clinical Pharmacology and Therapeutics* 55: 198

van Leeuwen R, Katlama C, Kitchen V et al 1995 Evaluation of safety and efficacy of 3TC (Lamivudine) in patients with asymptomatic or mildly symptomatic human immuno-deficiency virus infection: a phase I/II study. *Journal of Infectious Diseases* 171: 1166–1171

van Leeuwen R, Lange J M A, Hussey E K et al 1992 The safety and pharmacokinetics of a reverse transcriptase inhibitor, 3TC, in patients with HIV infection: a phase I study. *AIDS* 6: 1471–1475

Wainberg M A, Salomon H, Gu Z et al 1995 Development of HIV-I resistance to (–)-2'-deoxy-3'-thiacytidine in patients with AIDS or advanced AIDS-related complex. *AIDS* 9: 351–357

Non-nucleoside reverse transcriptase inhibitors

ATEVIRDINE
U-87201E

A *bis*(heteroaryl)piperazine (BHAP) compound that is a non-nucleoside reverse transcriptase inhibitor of HIV-1 with an IC_{50} of about 0.1–1 μM. HIV-1 strains resistant to nevirapine or pyridinones have mutations at residue 181 and are resistant to TIBO derivatives (p. 575) and the BHAPs. In addition, passage in the presence of atevirdine and other BHAPs produces resistant strains of HIV-1 with an RT mutation at position 236.

In view of the high likelihood of acquisition of resistance to atevirdine, pilot studies were undertaken in healthy volunteers and in a group of zidovudine naive HIV-1 infected patients who received concomitant zidovudine therapy. Administration of 600 mg every 8 h yielded a trough plasma concentration at 96 h of 2.4–13 μM. Trough plasma concentrations of the *N*-dealkylated metabolite and the ratio of atevirdine to this metabolite showed considerable interpatient variation. Additional studies in healthy adult volunteers have revealed non-linear pharmacokinetics.

HIV-1 sensitivity testing showed development of resistance by HIV-1 strains from 38% of patients after 12–24 weeks of concomitant zidovudine therapy. The combined therapy was generally well tolerated, though 2 of 20 patients developed a rash, with fever and hepatitis in one.

In comparison with placebo, atevirdine decreases viral

load as assessed by fresh plasma culture at week 4, and increases CD4 cell counts above baseline at weeks 8–12. However, 7 of 30 patients receiving 600 mg every 8 h developed an adverse event necessitating discontinuation of medication; 5 developed rash; one developed acute hepatitis and renal failure at week 3.

Further information

Reichman R C, Morse G D, Demeter L M et al 1995 Phase I study of Atevirdine, a non-nucleoside reverse transcriptase inhibitor, in combination with zidovudine for human immunodeficiency virus type I infection. *Journal of Infectious Diseases* 171: 297–304

Romero D L, Busso M, Tan C-K et al 1991 Non-nucleoside reverse transcriptase inhibitors that potently and specifically block human immunodeficiency virus type I replication. *Proceedings of the National Academy of Sciences of the USA* 88: 8806–8810

NEVIRAPINE

11-Cyclopropyl-5,11-dihydro-4-methyl-6*H*-dipyrido-[3,2-b:2',3'-e] [1,4]diazepin-6-one; BI-RG 587

A non-nucleoside reverse transcriptase inhibitor of HIV. It is a dipyridodiazepinone that inhibits HIV reverse transcriptase by binding to tyrosines at amino acid residues 181 and 188, which are located near the catalytic site. It has an in vitro IC_{50} for HIV of 0.04 µmol/l and is toxic to cells at 321 µM/l. Passage in the presence of the drug in vitro rapidly led to the selection of virus that was 400-fold less susceptible. Nevirapine is synergic with zidovudine and is active against zidovudine-resistant HIV. It is inactive against HIV strains resistant to TIBO (p. 575) suggesting that its mechanism of action is similar.

Phase I single-dose pharmacokinetic studies revealed that doses as low as 12.5 mg achieved plasma concentrations in excess of the IC_{50} for HIV isolates. It is readily absorbed with a mean peak plasma concentration after the first dose of 12.8 µM occurring at 4 h. Steady-state peak and trough concentrations were 27.1 and 15.8 µM, respectively.

Macular rash is a common adverse reaction, which is accompanied by fever and myalgia in some patients. Headache, nausea and vomiting and liver enzyme abnormalities are also common.

In clinical trials using 12.5, 50 and 200 mg, decline in p24 antigen levels were observed for periods of 1–2 weeks when nevirapine-resistant strains emerged with mutations at residue 181 of the RT gene. A further study using 400 mg/day revealed a rapid reduction in HIV p24 antigen and RNA concentrations in all patients, but nevirapine-resistant HIV strains were recovered from all patients by week 12. It

evidently selects for resistant virus much more rapidly than current nucleoside analogues, and a single mutation selects for high-level resistance. Combination therapy with zidovudine failed to prevent the development of resistance. The plasma levels achieved exceeded the IC_{50} levels of resistant virus and large phase III trials are underway.

Further information

Cheeseman S H, Hattox S E, McLaughlin M M et al 1993 Pharmacokinetics of nevirapine: initial single rising dose study in humans. *Antimicrobial Agents and Chemotherapy* 37: 178–182

Havlir D, Cheeseman S H, McLaughlin M et al 1995 High-dose nevirapine: safety, pharmacokinetics, and antiviral effect in patients with human immunodeficiency virus infection. *Journal of Infectious Diseases* 171: 537–545

Merluzzi V J, Hargrave K D, Labadia M et al 1990 Inhibition of HIV-1 replication by a non-nucleoside reverse transcriptase inhibitor. *Science* 250: 1411–1413

Richman D D, Havlir D, Corbeil J et al 1994 Nevirapine resistance mutations of human immunodeficiency virus type I selected during therapy. *Journal of Virology* 68: 1660–1666

PYRIDONE

L 697 661; [3-([(4,7-dichloro-1,3-benzoxazol-9-yl)methyl]amino)-5-ethyl-6-methylpyridin-2-(1*H*)-one]

A pyridone derivative, one of a structurally diverse group of non-nucleoside reverse transcriptase inhibitors. Foscarnet displaces L697 639 – a related compound – from reverse transcriptase. The IC_{50} of L 697 661 for HIV-1 in cell culture was 0.012–0.2 µM/l depending on the virus and cell system used. Zidovudine-resistant virus is sensitive to L 697 661, and zidovudine and L 697 661 display synergic activity in cell culture. Patients receiving monotherapy with L 697 661 harbour virus strains with significantly reduced susceptibility (2- to >30-fold) within 6 weeks of beginning treatment. The resistance is mediated in vitro and in vivo by amino acid substitutions at RT residue 103 or 181. The latter substitution alone is associated with a greater than 100-fold loss in sensitivity.

A peak plasma concentration of 2.56 µmol/l was observed after 200 mg orally. At doses of 100 or 200 mg every 8 h the drug was well tolerated.

Monotherapy exerts a transient effect on CD4 cell counts and p24 antigen levels, the loss of effect correlating temporally with selection of resistant virus variants. Monotherapy has been compared with zidovudine monotherapy and with combination therapy in zidovudine-naive patients with CD4 cell counts of 200–500/mm³. Cohorts from each group were evaluated for the development of resistance. By week 7 all patients in the L 697 661 monotherapy group had developed resistance. Resistance was delayed in the group receiving combination therapy, but had developed in all patients by weeks 16–32. The study was of insufficient statistical power to identify any meaningful differences between groups with respect to CD4 cell counts, p24 antigen, neopterin or β_2-microglobulin levels. However, the decrease in CD4 cell counts in the L 697 661 monotherapy group provides evidence of a lack of sustained activity of monotherapy alone.

Further information

Goldman M E, Nunberg J H, O'Brien J A et al 1991 Pyridinone derivatives: specific human immunodeficiency virus type I reverse transcriptase inhibitors with antiviral activity. *Proceedings of the National Academy of Sciences of the USA* 88: 6863–6867

Nurnberg J H, Schleif W A, Boots E J et al 1992 Viral resistance to human immunodeficiency virus type I specific pyridinone reverse transcriptase inhibitors. *Journal of Virology* 65: 4887–4892

Saag M S, Emini E A, Laskin O L et al 1993 A short-term clinical evaluation of L-697 661, a non-nucleoside inhibitor of HIV-I reverse transcriptase. *New England Journal of Medicine* 329: 1065–1072

Sardana V V, Emini E A, Gotlib L et al 1992 Functional analysis of HIV-I reverse transcriptase amino acids involved in resistance to multiple non-nucleotide inhibitors. *Journal of Biological Chemistry* 267: 17526–17530

Stuszewski S, Massari F E, Kober R et al 1995 Combination therapy with zidovudine prevents selection of human immunodeficiency virus type I variants expressing high-level resistance to L-697 661, a non-nucleoside reverse transcriptase inhibitor. *Journal of Infectious Diseases* 171: 1159–1165

TIBO AND TIBO DERIVATIVES
Tetrahydroimadazo-(4,5,1-*jk*)-(1,4)-benzodiazepin-2-(*I,H*)-one; R-14458

TIBO compounds are non-competitive inhibitors of HIV-1 reverse transcriptase. The ID_{50} of TIBO derivative R-829123 is 1.5 nmol/l to 0.65 µM/l, depending upon the virus and system used. Oral bioavailability of R-829123 is low, but inhibitory plasma concentrations are achieved. A phase I study of intravenous medication has been performed in patients with AIDS. There was a transient decrease in p24

antigen, but there was no clear antiviral effect and antiviral resistance developed rapidly. The drug was well tolerated.

Further information

Pauwels R, Andries K, Desmyter J et al 1990 Potent and selective inhibition of HIV-I replication in vitro by a novel series of TIBO derivatives. *Nature* 343: 470–474

Protease inhibitors

The HIV protease enzyme is a *pol* gene product which mediates the processing of viral precursor polyproteins and is essential for the production of infectious virus. Accordingly, it is a primary target in the treatment of HIV infection. Potent inhibitors have been developed and their interactions with the viral protease have been studied by X-ray crystallography. A few compounds have reached clinical trials.

MK 639
L 735 524; *N*-[2(*R*)-hydroxy-1(*S*)-indanyl]-5-[2(*S*)-(1,1-dimethylethylaminocarbonyl)-4[(pyridin-3-yl)methyl]piperazin-1-yl]-4(*S*)-hydroxy-2(*R*)-phenylmethylpentanamide

A potent and selective inhibitor of the HIV-1 protease with an IC_{95} concentration of about 50 nM in vitro. It is also effective against viruses resistant to various reverse transcriptase inhibitors. Phenotypic resistance in strains from treated patients correlated with substitutions of valine at position 82, but mutations at this point alone were insufficient for resistance and required interactions with other amino acid substitutions. These observations indicate the common nature of the protease inhibitors' target and suggest that combination with multiple protease inhibitors may still yield resistant virus.

Pharmacokinetic studies have been undertaken and the metabolites in urine have been described. The major metabolic pathways have been identified as: glucuronidation at the pyridine nitrogen to yield a quaternized ammonium conjugate; pyridine-*N*-oxidation; *para*-hydroxylation of the phenyl methyl group; 3'-hydroxylation of the indan; and *N*-depyridomethylation. Urinary excretion of the drug and its metabolites represent a minor pathway of elimination, but in urine the parent compound seems to be the major component.

Preliminary studies in man suggest that it has an acceptable safety profile and an antiviral effect associated with an increase in the number of CD4 cells. However, many treated patients yield resistant viral variants containing multiple amino acid substitutions. These variants expressed striking cross-resistance to five other structurally diverse protease inhibitors tested.

Further information

Balani S K, Arison B H, Mathai L et al 1995 Metabolites of L-735 524, a potent HIV-1 protease inhibitor, in human urine. *Drug Metabolism and Disposition* 23: 266–270

Condra J H, Schlief W A, Blahy O M et al 1995 In vivo emergence of HIV-1 variants resistant to multiple protease inhibitors. *Nature* 374: 569–671

Vacca J P, Dorsey W A, Schlief R B et al 1994 L 735 524, an orally bioavailable HIV-1 protease inhibitor. *Proceedings of the National Academy of Sciences of the USA* 91: 4096–4100

SAQUINAVIR
Ro 31-8959

A transition stage analogue of an HIV proteinase cleavage site developed through computer-led rational design based on the three-dimensional structure of HIV proteinase. It inhibits the proteinases of both HIV-1 and HIV-2 in vitro, acting by inhibiting proteolysis of the Gag and Gag-pol proteins and leading to the formation of non-infectious particles. The IC_{50} and IC_{90} are 2.2 and 16.1 nmol/l, respectively, and antiviral activity occurs at 1000-fold lower concentrations than those causing cytotoxicity or inhibiting human aspartyl proteinases. Clinical isolates, including zidovudine-resistant HIV, are almost as sensitive as laboratory strains. Promising results were obtained in infected cell cultures. After several months of treatment the cultures remained free from infection, suggesting that the drug blocked the production of infectious virus, and the infected cells died.

Resistance to saquinavir has been generated in laboratory strains of HIV by repeated passage in the presence of the drug. Several point mutations have been associated with resistance. Resistant isolates, with a 10-fold loss in sensitivity, were recovered from all four patients after approximately 50 weeks of therapy with 600 mg three times daily.

A 600 mg dose of saquinavir resulted in mean peak plasma concentrations several fold higher than the IC_{90} for laboratory strains. A phase I study of oral saquinavir revealed an oral bioavailability of only 4%. The half-life was 12 h.

Dose-ranging studies showed that saquinavir monotherapy, and combination with zidovudine, were well tolerated. Treatment was associated with increases in CD4 counts and inhibition of HIV, which was greatest in combination with zidovudine.

Further information

Craig J C, Duncan I B, Hockley D et al 1991 Antiviral properties of Ro-31-8959, an inhibitor of human immunodeficiency virus (HIV) proteinase. *Antiviral Research* 16: 295–305

Vella S 1994 Update on a proteinase inhibitor. *AIDS* 8 (suppl 3): S25–S29

Treatment

Septicaemia

J. Cohen

Introduction

Experienced clinicians agree that septic shock is a diagnosis easily made at the bedside. Agreement on how to define the condition has been more difficult.

It is not the purpose of this chapter to describe in detail the clinical or pathological features of sepsis. In summary, it is a multisystem disease occurring in the context of severe infection, and characterized by microvascular insufficiency often leading to multiple organ failure. This syndrome has in the past been called 'septicaemia', but this is an imprecise term which should no longer be used. What to use as an alternative has been the subject of considerable controversy. The following terms occur frequently in the literature (formal definitions are given in Box 41.1):

Bacteraemia. *This is an unambiguous term which has no pathophysiological or clinical connotations, and should be reserved to denote the presence of bacteria in the bloodstream.*

Systemic inflammatory response syndrome (SIRS) and multiorgan dysfunction syndrome (MODS). *The inflammatory response is remarkably similar, irrespective of the nature of the injury. Patients with severe burns or acute pancreatitis can appear very similar to a 'septic' patient (i.e. one who is ill secondary to infection). SIRS and MODS were conceived as a way of recognizing that the pathological processes may be the same in all these cases.*

Sepsis. *The inflammatory response to infection. This has been further modified by referring to the sepsis syndrome (sepsis with evidence of altered organ perfusion) or severe sepsis (sepsis associated with organ dysfunction, hypoperfusion abnormality or hypotension). Septic shock is a subset of severe sepsis and is associated with a worse prognosis. The critical difference between SIRS and sepsis is the requirement for evidence of infection.*

Box 41.1 *Diagnostic criteria for conditions associated with bacteraemia and sepsis*

Bacteraemia
The presence of viable bacteria in the bloodstream

Systemic inflammatory response syndrome (SIRS)
Two or more of the following criteria:
- Temperature >38°C or <36°C
- Heart rate >90 beats/min
- Respiratory rate >20 breaths/min or P_aCO_2 < 32 mmHg
- White blood cell count >12 × 10⁹/l or <4 × 10⁹/l

Multiple organ dysfunction syndrome (MODS)
Presence of altered organ function in an acutely ill patient such that homeostasis cannot be maintained without intervention

Sepsis
Two or more of the following criteria occurring as a result of infection:
- Temperature >38°C or <36°C
- Heart rate >90 beats/min
- Respiratory rate >20 breaths/min or P_aCO_2 < 32 mmHg
- White blood cell count >12 × 10⁹/l or <4 × 10⁹/l

Severe sepsis
Sepsis associated with organ dysfunction, defined as follows:
- *Cardiovascular*: BP ≤ 90 mmHg, or a fall in systolic BP > 40 mmHg for >1 h in the presence of adequate filling pressures, or the patient is unresponsive to at least 500 ml saline infused over 1 h
- *Respiratory*: P_aO_2 ≤ 70 mmHg (room air). If the primary diagnosis is pneumonia, special considerations apply
- *Renal*: urine output ≤0.5 ml/kg per hour for at least 1 h
- *Central nervous system*: significant alteration in mental status (a decrease of at least 2 points on the Glasgow Coma Score)

Septic shock
Sepsis associated with hypotension despite adequate fluid resuscitation, and perfusion abnormalities which may include, but are not limited to, lactic acidosis, oliguria, or an acute alteration in mental status

Adapted from Hebert et al (1993) and Bone et al (1992).

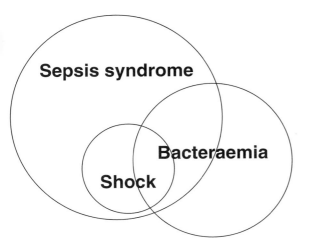

Fig. 41.1 A diagram illustrating the overlapping relationships between bacteraemia, sepsis and septic shock.

Table 41.1 Representative distribution of microbial causes of bacteraemia. (Adapted from Bamberger & Gurley (1994), Ispahani et al (1987) and Forgacs et al (1986).)

	%
Gram-positive bacteria	
Staph. aureus	20
Str. pneumoniae	10
Ent. faecalis	10
Staph. epidermidis	5
Total	45
Gram-negative bacteria	
Esch. coli	20
K. aerogenes	10
Proteus spp.	10
Ps. aeruginosa	7
Other	5
Total	52
Other	
Yeasts, anaerobes, etc.	3
Total	100

This confusing nomenclature has arisen because sepsis is not a single disease but a syndrome which can result from diverse causes, and with a spectrum of severity which ranges from fever associated with transitory hypotension through to profound shock and high mortality. Furthermore, the same clinical picture is seen in some non-infective conditions. Identifying subgroups and giving them labels is worthwhile only if by doing so one can design better treatment or predict outcome more accurately. In fact, there is a good correlation between sepsis, the number of organ failures and outcome. Further studies will be necessary to determine if treatment too should be modified on the basis of these criteria.

At present, the most useful terms are bacteraemia, the sepsis syndrome and septic shock, and these will be used in the remainder of this chapter. It is helpful to remember that these terms are not synonyms, but represent partially overlapping subgroups (Fig. 41.1).

Epidemiology

BACTERAEMIA

Clinically significant bacteraemia occurs with a frequency of about 5–10 per 1000 hospital admissions, a figure that has been rising slowly during the last 10 years largely due to an increasing number of nosocomial infections. Table 41.1 shows the typical distribution of microbial causes of bacteraemia. Several interesting points emerge: first, Gram-positive organisms are almost as common as Gram-negative

bacteria and, indeed, in many more recent series there is a clear trend towards a preponderance of Gram-positive bacteraemia. For instance, sequential studies in one institution over the 10-year period 1979–1989 showed a fall in the proportion of Gram-negative bacteraemias from 49.2 to 43.1%, while Gram-positive infections rose from 49.6 to 53.7% (Geerdes et al 1992). This change probably partly reflects the earlier use of prophylactic (or 'pre-emptive') antibiotics when serious Gram-negative infection is suspected. As a result, bacteraemia is less common. Equally important has been the rise in the number of cases of bacteraemia caused by coagulase-negative staphylococci, a direct consequence of the increased use of indwelling vascular lines. Infections caused by these organisms can be difficult to assess; there is no doubt that they can be pathogens and that they cause fever and systemic symptoms, especially in immunocompromised patients (see below), but in my experience they rarely cause *shock*. Yet precisely because coagulase negative bacteraemia occurs in patients who have multiple instrumentation (and hence are often in a high-risk category for developing the sepsis syndrome) it is difficult to dismiss them as contaminants. This can be a considerable problem in the clinical-trial setting; one recent report concluded that coagulase-negative staphylococci were the single commonest microbial cause of the sepsis syndrome (Kieft et al 1993), a finding which is probably misleading.

Another emerging epidemiological trend has been the resurgence of severe infections caused by *Streptococcus pyogenes*. During the 1980s a number of reports appeared of septic shock developing in previously healthy individuals, often associated with necrotizing fasciitis. The isolates of *Str. pyogenes* were usually of the M1 type and produced the exotoxin SPEA (streptococcal pyrogenic exotoxin A) (Stevens 1992). The condition was in many ways similar to the staphylococcal toxic shock syndrome, and it has been called the 'toxic strep syndrome'. These infections are still uncommon, but quite why they should be increasing in frequency is unknown.

A second point which is less easy to appreciate in Table 41.1 is the variation in epidemiology between populations. For instance, studies of bacteraemia in intensive care unit patients reveal a rather higher incidence of *Pseudomonas* infections and of candidaemia than in the general hospital population (Forgacs et al 1986). On the other hand, in neutropenic patients the excess of infections caused by *Escherichia coli, Pseudomonas aeruginosa* and other Gram-negative bacteria that was the pattern 15 years ago has been replaced by coagulase negative staphylococci, and interestingly, viridans streptococci (Ch. 43).

SITES OF INFECTION

Typically, fewer than one-third of all patients with the sepsis syndrome will be bacteraemic; in the remainder, a microbial aetiology will be inferred on the basis of cultures from a specific organ or site (e.g. lower respiratory tract), or cultures will be negative or non-contributory. Hence a knowledge of the microbiology of the underlying primary sites of infection can be invaluable in guiding empirical therapy. Table 41.2 lists the typical distribution of primary sites of infection in patients with the sepsis syndrome. It is apparent that the lower respiratory tract is frequently identified as the underlying source, although it must be admitted that the basis upon which such judgements are made are rather vague. A full discussion of the microbiological criteria for identifying the site of infection in septic patients is beyond the scope of this chapter (see for instance Lynn & Cohen (1995a)). From the practical point of view, the isolation of a microorganism (even a potential pathogen)

from a non-sterile site in a patient with sepsis syndrome does not necessarily implicate that organism as the cause of the patient's illness.

SEPSIS, SHOCK AND MORTALITY

The incidence of shock depends on which population is examined and which definition is used. For instance, in one UK study, 20% of patients with 'true' bacteraemia developed shock, and in this group the mortality was about 50% (Ispahani et al 1987). In contrast, if one starts with a population defined clinically as having the sepsis syndrome, only about 45% will be bacteraemic, but 30% overall will be shocked on admission and a further 24% of patients will develop shock (Bone et al 1987). In this study, the mortality in patients who did not develop shock was 13%, but it rose to over 40% in those who developed shock during admission. Bacteraemia is a risk factor for developing shock: 47% of bacteraemic patients developed shock compared to 30% of non-bacteraemic patients.

The relationships between SIRS, sepsis, shock and death is well illustrated by a recent prospective study of nearly 4000 patients admitted to intensive care units in the USA (Rangel-Frausto et al 1995). The incidence density of SIRS on surgical intensive care units was 857 episodes per 1000 patient-days, and the mortality of these patients was just 7%, emphasizing that SIRS is a very sensitive definition. However, in the small proportion (4%) who developed septic shock, mortality was 46% (Table 41.3).

The simplest way to appreciate the overall mortality associated with bacteraemia and sepsis is to examine the placebo mortality rates in the several large clinical trials carried out during the last 3 years (see below). These studies have all used a rather similar definition of the sepsis syndrome as the entry criterion for the trial, and in most of them the mortality in the placebo arm of the trial has been 35–45%. Several estimates suggest that in the USA alone there are 100 000–300 000 cases of the sepsis syndrome

Table 41.2 *Representative data showing distribution of the primary site of infection in patients with the sepsis syndrome (Adapted from Knaus et al (1993) and Kieft et al (1993).)*

Site of origin of sepsis syndrome	%
Lower respiratory tract	50
Gastro-intestinal tract	15
Surgical wound/skin	10
Urinary tract	8
Intravenous line	8
Miscellaneous	5
Unknown site of origin	4

Table 41.3 *The natural history of the systemic inflammatory response syndrome (SIRS) (Adapted from Rangel-Frausto et al (1995).)*

	Complications of SIRS (%)		
	Sepsis	Severe sepsis	Shock
Progression from SIRS to	26	18	4
Incidence of bacteraemia	17	25	69
Mortality	16	20	46

annually, which therefore represents perhaps 50 000–100 000 deaths. It is these figures which have provided the impetus to trying to develop new approaches to treatment based on a better understanding of the basic pathophysiology of the disease.

Pathophysiology

MICROBIOLOGICAL FACTORS

In order to cause an infection a microorganism must first come into contact with a susceptible host, attach to the surface (often by a specialized and specific mechanism), penetrate the outer host defences and evade the immune response. All these processes are, strictly speaking, micro-biological factors which contribute to the pathogenesis of septic shock, but a detailed discussion of the cellular and molecular mechanisms involved is beyond the remit of this chapter. However, certain factors are very specifically associated with the development of shock; the best example is endotoxin (lipopolysaccharide (LPS)).

Endotoxin

LPS is situated in the outer part of the cell wall of Gram-negative bacteria (Fig. 41.2). The outer (O) side-chain consists of a series of oligosaccharides which confer serotypic specificity on a particular strain, and thus demonstrate considerable variability. In contrast, the core oligosaccharides which are situated internal to the O side-chain show a much more limited range of structure. Bound to the inner surface of the core is a lipid molecule, lipid A. The structure of lipid A is highly conserved amongst Gram-negative bacteria; furthermore, studies with synthetic lipid A have confirmed that it is responsible for almost all the toxicity of LPS. Knowing this, it is not difficult to understand why septic shock caused by *Escherichia coli* bacteraemia, for example, is clinically indistinguishable from that caused by *Klebsiella* spp.

The evidence that LPS is responsible for many of the features of septic shock is persuasive, and has been reviewed in detail by Morrison et al (1994). LPS which has been prepared from Gram-negative bacteria, and even synthetic lipid A can reproduce many of the clinical and pathological signs associated with sepsis. Minor chemical modification of lipid A in specific areas of the molecule will abrogate the toxicity. Substances which can bind and neutralize LPS (for instance the antibiotic polymyxin B or the neutrophil granule protein called bactericidal/permeability increasing protein (BPI)) are very effective, both in vitro and in vivo, at preventing the effects of LPS. Finally, bacteria naturally shed LPS during growth and division, and in some specific cases (e.g. meningococcal bacteraemia), there is a direct quantitative relationship between plasma levels of LPS on admission and the clinical outcome. Although endotoxaemia is associated with more severe manifestations of shock, 'endotoxaemia' and 'bacter-aemia' are not synonymous. In a study of 100 patients with shock, endotoxaemia was detected in 43 patients and bacteraemia in 37 (Danner et al 1991). Of these 37 patients, the 23 who had endotoxaemia had a mortality of 39%, compared to 7% in the 14 non-endotoxaemic group.

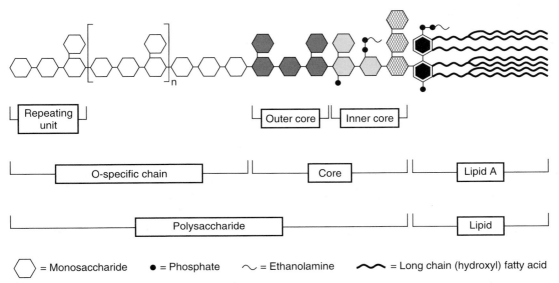

Fig. 41.2 *A schematic diagram of the biochemical structure of endotoxin.*

One subject of considerable controversy is the extent to which antibiotic-induced endotoxin release might represent a clinically significant risk. There is no doubt that, in vitro, certain classes of antibiotics (particularly those which have a rapid bactericidal effect) cause LPS release in parallel with bacterial cell death. What is not known is whether this means that such antibiotics should be avoided in clinical practice because of the risk that the initial contact between the antibiotic and a large population of organisms might cause a sudden release of LPS and clinical deterioration, comparable with the Jarisch–Herxheimer reaction seen with the penicillin treatment of syphilis. At present, there are no convincing clinical data which suggest that, for most common Gram-negative infections, the issue of possible LPS release should influence antibiotic choice. Nevertheless, this is an area of great interest and trials addressing this question are likely to begin soon.

The mechanism by which LPS binds to or interacts with host cell surfaces has always been something of an enigma. Recently it has been learnt that rather than binding directly via an 'LPS receptor', LPS binds to a naturally occurring acute-phase serum protein called lipopolysaccharide-binding protein (LBP). The LPS–LBP complex then serves as the ligand for a cell surface receptor called CD14 (Ziegler-Heitbrock & Ulevitch 1993). Binding of LPS–LBP to CD14 on the surface of macrophages activates the cell and signal transduction leads to the elaboration of cytokines and other mediators.

Products of Gram-positive bacteria

The cell wall of Gram-positive bacteria lacks endotoxin, but there are a number of other structural components which might be implicated in pathogenesis. Principal amongst these is lipoteichoic acid, which is certainly able to initiate some of the mediator cascades associated with sepsis (see below).

Of more importance are the extracellular toxins produced in large number by many of the Gram-positive bacteria associated with shock. Several of these are well characterized – they include the staphylococcal toxic shock toxin (TSST-1) and the pyrogenic exotoxins produced by *Str. pyogenes* (Bohach et al 1990). Although these toxins can be identified by their effects on cell cultures in vitro, it is only recently that there has been some understanding of the mechanisms of pathogenicity in vivo. Many of these exotoxins have the ability to act as superantigens, and it has been suggested that this underlies their association with shock (Kotb 1992, Johnson et al 1992, Schlievert 1993, Sissons 1993). Unlike conventional peptide antigens (which interact in a very specific way with the major histocompatibility complex (MHC) class II on antigen presenting cells and the T-cell receptor), superantigens can bind rather promiscuously to so-called Vβ domains on the outside of the

peptide binding groove of the T-cell receptor. This binding results in activation of the T-cell and, so it is argued, massive stimulation of T-cell cytokines and hence shock. The best clinical example of this is the proposed role of streptococcal pyrogenic exotoxin A in the 'toxic strep syndrome'.

HOST FACTORS

Mediators

Endotoxin and other bacterial components induce a broad array of mediators from macrophages and other cells, particularly endothelial cells. Numerous humoral mediators have been identified, and it is likely many more will be found (Box 41.2). Although it is convenient to discuss them in turn, in reality they act through a complex network of synergistic and antagonistic interactions (Fig. 41.3).

Complement. The anaphylatoxins C3a and C5a are produced following activation of the alternative pathway of complement by LPS or some Gram-positive bacterial cell wall components, or by activation of the classical pathway, typically by immune complexes. Complement components induce vasodilatation and increased vascular permeability, aggregation of platelets, and aggregation and activation of neutrophils, all processes which have been implicated in the pathogenesis of the adult respiratory distress syndrome (ARDS). The subsequent release of arachidonic acid derivatives, cytotoxic products of molecular oxygen and lysosomal enzymes exert additional local vasoactive effects on the microvasculature and cause endothelial cell cytotoxicity resulting in capillary leakage. Complement activation has been associated with a fatal outcome in both Gram-positive and Gram-negative shock (McPhaden & Whaley 1985).

Coagulation factors. Coagulopathy is a well-recognized feature of the sepsis syndrome (Colman 1989, Bone 1992a). Factor XII (Hageman factor) has long been known to play a central role in the pathogenesis of septic shock. It is activated equally effectively by peptidoglycan residues and

Box 41.2

Mediators of sepsis

- Complement
- Vasoactive mediators
- Arachidonic acid derivatives
- Kinins
- Platelet activating factor (PAF)
- Histamine
- Endothelins
- Endorphins
- Coagulation factors
- Reactive oxygen species
- Cytokines

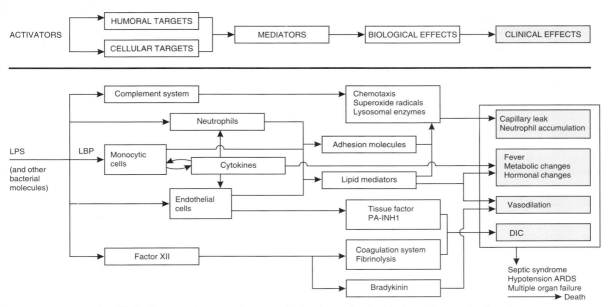

Fig. 41.3 *Diagram illustrating the network of pathways involved in the pathogenesis of sepsis.*

teichoic acid from the cell wall of Gram-positive bacteria, as well as by LPS. Through activation of factor XI, Hageman factor triggers the production of tissue factor both by the intrinsic coagulation pathway and by endothelial cells and macrophages; in turn, tissue factor activates the extrinsic coagulation pathway. Uncontrolled stimulation of these pathways leads to the so-called 'disseminated intravascular coagulopathy' which occurs to varying degrees in many septic patients. Moreover, activation of the contact system by LPS-activated factor XII results in the conversion of prekallikrein to kallikrein. This in turn cleaves high-molecular-weight kininogen to release bradykinin, a potent hypotensive agent.

Platelet activating factor (PAF). This is a potent phospholipid that leads to autocatalytic amplification of cytokine release. Although first identified because of its effects on platelets, it is now clear that it can be produced by a wide variety of cell types in response to injury, and that it has marked inflammatory effects (Bone 1992b). Elevated levels of PAF have been found in animal models of LPS-induced lung injury and shock, and experimental inhibitors of PAF are protective in these models.

Cytokines. The physiological role of cytokines is to act as a means of communication within the immune system. They form a complex network of regulatory pathways, and there is considerable structural and functional redundancy within the system. Not surprisingly, cytokines play a key role in natural host defence mechanisms against infection, particularly with intracellular organisms such as *Listeria* and *Leishmania* spp. But there are good data suggesting

that uncontrolled production of cytokines leads to many of the pathological features seen in sepsis.

The evidence implicating cytokines in sepsis can be summarized as follows:

● LPS and other microbial products are potent inducers of cytokines in vitro
● Injection of LPS in human volunteers elicits a cytokine response which is coincident with the physiological changes that occur
● In some conditions, levels of cytokines on admission to hospital correlate with the severity of the disease, and with outcome
● Anticytokine antibodies can protect experimental animals from LPS- or bacterial-induced death.

It is helpful to think of LPS-induced cytokines falling into two groups. The pro-inflammatory cytokines (often called T_H1 cytokines because they are associated with a particular phenotype of mouse T helper lymphocytes) include tumour necrosis factor (TNF), interleukin-1 (IL-1), IL-6, IL-8, and interferon-γ. In contrast, T_H2 cytokines such as IL-4, IL-10 and transforming growth factor β (TGF-β) are regulatory proteins which act to counterbalance the inflammatory effects of the T_H1 group. It is important to emphasize that LPS will induce both groups, and it is only when the natural balance between them is sufficiently disturbed that the damaging inflammatory effects occur.

Cytokines act by binding to specific cellular receptors. Many of these receptors have been identified and they share some common features. For instance, many are transmembrane proteins and under physiological conditions the extracellular part of the molecule can be shed into the circulation. These 'soluble receptors' appear to act as a means of modulating the responses to the cytokine: TNF bound to soluble TNF-receptor, for instance, can no longer activate cells. Cytokine receptors are also of interest as potential therapeutic targets in sepsis (see below).

A detailed discussion of the functions of different cytokines is beyond the scope of this chapter (for reviews see Rees (1991), Dinarello & Wolff (1993) and Molloy et al (1993)). It will be apparent from Figure 41.3 that they occupy a pivotal role, interacting with many of the effector pathways which lead to tissue injury and organ damage in sepsis. Of particular importance, pro-inflammatory cytokines have a powerful effect in activating neutrophils and mediating the process by which neutrophil–endothelial interactions lead to inflammation.

Neutrophils and the endothelium

Neutrophils play a key role in the pathogenesis of septic shock. Once activated by LPS and/or cytokines, they damage tissues by releasing toxic oxygen metabolites and lysosomal enzymes or may aggregate and cause microemboli. Before neutrophils migrate into tissues their progress within the blood vessels must be slowed, and they must be induced to adhere to the vascular endothelium. This complex process depends on the expression of a series of adhesion molecules which first tether the neutrophil lightly to the endothelium, then cause it to roll along the surface until it is firmly bound and can begin to traverse the barrier (Cohen 1994). The expression of these adhesion molecules is upregulated by cytokines, and blocking of the adhesion process by monoclonal antibodies reduces neutrophil-mediated inflammation.

The role of the endothelium itself in sepsis has only very recently been appreciated. Not only is it a target for injury, but it can respond to LPS by producing in turn a range of mediator and effector molecules. One example is PAF, discussed above. An effector which has received much attention is nitric oxide.

Nitric oxide was first recognized as endothelium-derived relaxing factor (EDRF), an extremely potent vasodilator. Nitric oxide-induced vasodilatation is unresponsive to pressor agents, a situation reminiscent of the 'vasoplegia' seen in the profoundly shocked patient. Furthermore, LPS and cytokines can induce nitric oxide formation in vitro, and in some animal models TNF-induced hypotension can be attenuated by inhibitors of nitric oxide synthase (NOS), the enzyme which converts L-arginine to nitric oxide. It is now known that there are three different NOSs: two of which are constitutively expressed, endothelial NOS and neuronal NOS; and an inducible enzyme (iNOS), which is found in many cell types. It has been proposed that, whereas continuous background production of endothelial nitric oxide is necessary to maintain vascular patency, inappropriate activity of iNOS (induced by LPS or other bacterial products) leads to profound vasodilatation and shock. Therapeutic manipulation of this pathway is the subject of much current work (see below).

Treatment

GRAM-POSITIVE BACTERIA

Streptococcus pyogenes

β-Haemolytic streptococci remain predictably susceptible to penicillin, and the treatment of choice is still benzylpenicillin 1.2 g, 4–6 hourly, by intravenous injection for 10–14 days. Despite this, epidemiological studies reveal that streptococcal bacteraemia has a high case mortality, and this is in part due to the rapidity with which this infection progresses from what may appear a relatively trivial cellulitis caused by a superficial abrasion, to a fulminating shock-like syndrome. Shock as a complication has been recognized for many years; it was sometimes called 'septic scarlet fever' and this continues to be reported (Shaunak et al 1988); there is some evidence that the incidence of these complications is rising (Hoge et al 1993). Recently, however, the similarities between streptococcal sepsis and the staphylococcal toxic shock syndrome (see below) have led to the introduction of the rather inelegant term 'streptococcal toxic shock like syndrome' (The Working Group on Severe Streptococcal Infections 1993). These patients need intensive supportive care and may benefit from adjunctive therapies which are currently under investigation (see below). Another manifestation of severe streptococcal sepsis is necrotizing fasciitis (Chelsom et al 1994). As in other causes of extensive toxin-mediated soft tissue damage, early and extensive surgical debridement is an essential part of the management. The very large numbers of organisms present in the tissues in these cases led some to speculate that penicillin might be relatively ineffective – the so-called 'Eagle effect'. In an animal model, clindamycin, a protein synthesis inhibitor, was more effective than penicillin (Stevens et al 1988), and this has led to the recommendation to treat severe streptococcal sepsis with both penicillin and clindamycin.

Viridans streptococci

In neutropenic patients, viridans streptococci can gain entry to the bloodstream from the mucosa damaged by cytotoxic chemotherapy. It has emerged that in some patients, infection (particularly when caused by *Streptococcus mitis*) can lead to fulminating shock and ARDS (Watanakunakorn & Pautelakis 1993, Bochud et al 1994). These strains are susceptible to penicillin, but antimicrobial therapy alone is often inadequate. The pathogenesis of this syndrome remains unknown. The treatment of bacterial endocarditis caused by viridans streptococci is described elsewhere (Ch. 49).

Group B streptococci (*Streptococcus agalactiae*)

Group B streptococcal bacteraemia is of most importance in infancy (Ch. 49), but lately it has been appreciated that it may cause serious infection in adults, particularly the elderly or debilitated (Farley et al 1993). Interestingly, group B streptococci appear not to cause a shock syndrome. Although penicillin-susceptible, the minimum inhibitory concentration (MIC) of group B strains is 5–10 times higher than those of group A, and these infections are best treated by high-dose penicillin (6 g/day in divided doses) or a combination of penicillin and an aminoglycoside. Like other streptococci, group B strains are resistant to amino-glycosides given alone. Vancomycin or teicoplanin are suitable alternatives in patients intolerant of penicillin.

Streptococcus pneumoniae

Somewhat surprisingly, a study of bacteraemia conducted between 1975 and 1980 found that *Str. pneumoniae* was the third most commonly reported isolate; only *Esch. coli* and *Staphylococcus aureus* were more common (Young 1982). Approximately 20% of cases of pneumococcal pneumonias are complicated by bacteraemia, and this is the commonest cause of pneumococcal bacteraemia in adults. Generally there is an underlying condition such as alcoholism, chronic chest disease, HIV infection or cirrhosis (Gransden et al 1985). In contrast, most children with pneumococcal bacteraemia seem to be healthy before the infection and do not have pneumonia (Gruer et al 1984). The overall case mortality in these populations is 15–30%, and is higher in elderly patients with co-morbidities. In addition, there is a specific association between severe pneumococcal sepsis and patients with no spleen, or with functional hyposplenia. In these patients, pneumococcal infection presents as a fulminating shock syndrome and the case mortality is 50% or more. Most isolates of *Str. pneumoniae* remain very sensitive to penicillin and can be treated with benzylpeni-cillin 1.2–2.4 g/day. However, in some areas penicillin resistance has emerged to a degree which means that presumptive treatment (e.g. in splenectomised patients) must now be broadened; a suitable regimen is a combination of vancomycin and cefotaxime. If the isolate is fully sensitive then treatment can be modified accordingly (Jacobs 1992).

Enterococci

Enterococci cause 5–10% of nosocomial bacteraemias. The commonest portals of entry are the urinary tract, the abdominal and pelvic cavities, wounds (such as decubitus ulcers) and the biliary tree. At least a third of enterococcal bacteraemias are polymicrobial; less than 5% of cases are associated with endocarditis (Ch. 49). Enterococcal bacteraemia is associated with significant mortality, but it is not clear how much of this is attributable to the fact that many such infections occur in patients with serious underlying diseases; shock is not a feature of enterococcal bacteraemia. The rising incidence of enterococcal infections seems in the main to reflect nosocomial acquisition, and is closely correlated with prior use of antibiotics (especially cephalosporins). Antimicrobial resistance in enterococci represents one of the most difficult emerging problems of the last 10 years.

Enterococci exhibit intrinsic resistance to β-lactams and trimethoprim–sulphamethoxazole, as well as low-level aminoglycoside resistance. For *Enterococcus faecalis* the typical MIC_{90} values to penicillin and ampicillin are 4 and 1 mg/l, respectively; for *Enterococcus faecium* the figures are 64 and 32 mg/l. Cephalosporins have no role in the treatment of these infections. More disturbingly, enterococci have acquired resistance to a wide range of antimicrobial agents from several different classes. Many isolates have developed high-level resistance to both β-lactams and aminoglycosides, and resistance to fluoroquinolones, macro-lides and rifampicin is widespread. For many years, vancomycin was the 'reserve agent' used to treat serious infections caused by these multiresistant strains, but during the last 5 years vancomycin resistance has emerged, both in Europe and in the USA. Infections caused by these strains can be virtually untreatable. (For a fuller discussion of the mechanisms of resistance in enterococci see Ch. 3.)

The standard treatment for patient with enterococcal endocarditis is a combination of a cell-wall active agent (penicillin or ampicillin) with an aminoglycoside (usually streptomycin or gentamicin) (Ch. 49). Whether combination treatment is appropriate in the absence of endocarditis is less clear. For uncomplicated infections (e.g. of the urinary tract) ampicillin can be used alone, but for bacteraemia the evidence is conflicting. Gullberg et al (1989) described 75 episodes of enterococcal bacteraemia; only 5 had endocar-ditis. Thirty-eight patients were treated with two antibiotics (usually ampicillin and gentamicin), and 90% responded. Eighteen patients received treatment with one antibiotic; 89% responded. Perhaps most surprisingly, 19 patients received no treatment at all, and only four died (in two cases of other causes before the blood culture results were reported). In the other cases the isolates were either thought to be contaminants, or were overlooked; the patients survived without complications. However, in contrast to this paper, Hoge et al (1991) concluded that treatment of enterococcal bacteraemia did improve the outcome. They retrospectively reviewed 81 episodes, and found 41 which met a strict case definition. Among this group with clinically significant infection, antibiotic therapy directed against enterococci was associated with a statistically significant reduction in the in-hospital mortality. My personal practice is to use ampicillin and gentamicin for all serious enterococcal infections. Vancomycin will substitute for ampicillin if necessary.

Treatment of serious infections due to vancomycin-resistant enterococci is extremely difficult. Careful and detailed susceptibility testing of the isolate is mandatory. Preliminary clinical experience with quinupristin/dalfopristin has been encouraging (Lynn et al 1994), but much more work is necessary.

Staphylococcus aureus

In a study of 400 episodes, Gransden et al (1984) reported that *Staph. aureus* accounted for 17.5% of all cases of bacteraemia over a 14-year period. The mortality was 24%, and in most cases the source of the infection was readily discerned, most often being an indwelling vascular catheter site. However, the picture painted by this report is in some senses misleading: bacteraemic *Staph. aureus* can cause a spectrum of illness from a relatively benign condition requiring short-course treatment to fulminating staphylococcal endocarditis needing emergency surgery. This wide spectrum has caused controversy about the correct management.

Only about 10% of episodes of staphylococcal bacteraemia are associated with endocarditis (Mylotte et al 1987), and not all cases of bacteraemia have to be treated as though endocarditis was present. That said, there are two important caveats: firstly, endocarditis must always be considered, and if necessary reconsidered, since it is potentially life-threatening and may need urgent surgical intervention. (The detailed management of staphylococcal endocarditis is discussed in Ch. 49.) Secondly, *Staph. aureus* bacteraemia always requires treatment. This statement may seem unnecessary, but the regular experience of patients who have had little or no treatment in the belief that the condition was benign, only to later develop serious metastatic complications, leaves me in no doubt that this point requires emphasis.

A multivariate analysis of patients with staphylococcal bacteraemia identified four parameters which significantly predicted endocarditis: (a) absence of a primary site of infection, (b) community acquired infection, (c) metastatic complications and (d) valvular vegetations seen on echocardiography (Bayer et al 1987). Of these, the lack of an identifiable focus is probably the most helpful feature. Patients at low risk of endocarditis can probably be given a shorter period of treatment (Sheagren 1984). This is usually taken to mean 2 weeks of parenteral therapy, and in my opinion this should not be reduced further.

Few strains of *Staph. aureus* are now sensitive to benzylpenicillin. For uncomplicated staphylococcal bacteraemia the drug of first choice is flucloxacillin (nafcillin in the USA) at a dose of not less than 2 g every 6 h. Vancomycin is a suitable alternative for the penicillin-allergic patient. The controversy surrounding the possible benefit of using combination therapy is discussed in full in the section on endocarditis; however, it should be noted that, despite the common practice of using two drugs, there are no data demonstrating a superior outcome with this policy.

Staphylococcal toxic shock syndrome is caused by strains which produce the exotoxin TSST-1 (see above). The antimicrobial therapy is no different from that of other serious staphylococcal infections. Supportive care follows the same lines as for Gram-negative septic shock (see below).

Coagulase-negative staphylococci

These organisms are now the leading cause of hospital-acquired bacteraemia. Once thought to be 'contaminants', it is now apparent that they are genuine pathogens and cause significant morbidity, although in my experience they rarely cause shock. The one exception to this is the neutropenic patient, in whom coagulase-negative staphylococci are the single most common blood culture isolate and in whom more severe illness, and even death, may occur.

Most blood culture isolates of coagulase-negative staphylococci are methicillin resistant, and the majority are also resistant to many other antibiotics, including erythromycin, clindamycin, tetracycline and chloramphenicol. However, there are individual differences and, particularly in difficult cases, the susceptibility pattern should be investigated in detail. In most instances the antibiotic of choice is vancomycin, although some strains of *Staphylococcus haemolyticus* are vancomycin resistant. Teicoplanin is an alternative to vancomycin, but these antibiotics are not absolutely interchangeable and specific sensitivity results should be obtained. It has become common practice to use rifampicin in combination with a glycopeptide to treat serious infections, particularly endocarditis. Although supported by anecdotal data and personal experience, there are no good trials which confirm that adding rifampicin is beneficial.

In the general hospital population most infections are associated with indwelling devices or catheters, and these can be some of the most indolent and difficult infections to treat (Lowy & Hammer 1983). A recurring dilemma is the need to remove the offending device in order to cure the infection. Advice differs widely; surprisingly, there are no good prospective trials which directly compare the two strategies. There is no doubt that in 'uncomplicated' bacteraemias related to infection of indwelling vascular catheters (even permanent catheters of the Hickman type), antibacterial therapy alone is sometimes sufficient, and there is often no need to remove the catheter if it is still needed (Raad & Bodey 1992). Equally clearly, however, infections of deep-seated devices such as prosthetic joints or heart valves are rarely cured by antibiotics alone.

GRAM-NEGATIVE BACTERIA

Enterobacteria and *Pseudomonas aeruginosa*

Aerobic Gram-negative bacilli are the most common cause of hospital bacteraemia, typically accounting for about 40% of positive blood cultures. The contribution of different species to this total varies with the type of hospital, notably in the proportion caused by *Ps. aeruginosa*, which is more common in hospitals with oncology and burns units.

Antibiotic choice can be difficult for a number of reasons. The organisms concerned vary widely in their antibiotic susceptibility, and indeed the patterns can change with time. Furthermore, it is rarely possible to accurately predict the results of the blood culture; indeed, sepsis caused by Gram-negative bacteria cannot reliably be distinguished from that caused by Gram-positive organisms. Finally, a significant number of bacteraemic episodes are polymicrobial. These issues are discussed in more detail below in considering the empirical choice of antibiotics for sepsis. Here we will consider the treatment of bacteriologically confirmed infections.

The landmark studies by McCabe & Jackson, and later by Kreger et al showed clearly that the use of appropriate antibiotic therapy (defined as at least one antibiotic active in vitro against the causative strain) significantly improved the outcome of patients with Gram-negative bacillary bacteraemia (reviewed in Calandra & Cornetta 1991). Later studies also pointed out the importance of using an adequate dose, a particular problem with aminoglycosides which have often been underdosed for fear of causing toxicity. More recently, the enormous choice of effective and safe antibiotics with a broad spectrum of activity against most of the common causes of Gram-negative bacteraemia has meant that the principal issue in choosing an antibiotic is the susceptibility pattern of the local strains. Clinicians need to be familiar with the data for their own region (ideally their own hospital) as the basis of guiding therapy. Indeed, so effective are the new β-lactams, such as the extended-spectrum cephalosporins and monobactams, and the quinolones, that it would be impossible to mount a trial of 'uncomplicated' bacteraemia and expect to find a significant difference in outcome or toxicity. In contrast, such trials are done in patients with impaired immunity, particularly in neutropenic patients, and some important differences have emerged (Ch. 43).

The main debate in this field over the last 10–15 years has concerned the need for combination therapy in treating Gram-negative bacteraemia. It needs to be emphasized that most of the debate (and virtually all of the data) have focused on neutropenic patients. Here I will try and restrict the discussion to the non-neutropenic patient.

The case for using combination therapy rests on three planks. (a) Two (or more) drugs will provide a broader spectrum, and hence it is less likely that the initial therapy will 'miss' the causative strain; this applies to empirical therapy when the causative organism is still unknown (see below). (b) Two drugs will provide synergy against the causative strain, and synergy in vitro can be correlated with improved survival of the patient. (c) By analogy with antituberculous chemotherapy, the use of two drugs will lessen the risk of developing resistance. Let us examine the validity of these latter two arguments.

Studies conducted in neutropenic patients 15–20 years ago with combinations such as carbenicillin and gentamicin showed that the outcome was better if one could demonstrate synergy in vitro against the infecting strain, although this was only present in about 50% of cases. In fact, synergy was the in vitro correlate of enhanced bactericidal activity, and the clinical association was that survival was improved in patients in whom bactericidal activity in the serum against the specific strain was greater than 1 in 16 (Sculier & Klastersky 1984). With the advent of newer antibiotics the bactericidal activity achieved in the serum with these single agents proved to be equal or greater than that obtained in the past with the combination of antibiotics. Thus the rationale for using 'synergistic' combinations is now weaker. Only one recent paper has attempted to address this issue in non-neutropenic patients. Korvick et al (1992) carried out a prospective study of 230 patients with Klebsiella bacteraemia: half received a β-lactam plus an aminoglycoside, and the other half monotherapy with a cephalosporin. Overall, the 14-day mortality did not differ between the two groups, but in a subgroup who had hypotension early in their course the mortality was 24% in the combination group compared to 50% in the monotherapy group.

The second argument, that two agents will lessen the chance of the emergence of resistance, was investigated in a recent study by Siebert et al (1993). They evaluated 76 patients with Gram-negative bacteraemia who had received a single antibiotic (usually a cephalosporin) and had survived at least 48 h. Resistance during treatment developed in just one case, an isolate of *Ps. aeruginosa* which was probably being treated inappropriately.

In general then, in patients with uncomplicated Gram-negative bacteraemia in which the organism and its susceptibility pattern is known, there is scant evidence that two antibiotics are better than one. Infections caused by *Ps. aeruginosa* require special comment. Because of the higher case mortality, and perhaps also because these infections more frequently occur in patients with compromised host defences, it has become common practice to treat with a combination of a suitable penicillin and an aminoglycoside at maximum doses. It must be acknowledged that there is a body of literature based on both in vitro data (Chandrasekar et al 1987) and clinical trials (Verhagen et al 1986) which argues that this is unnecessary but, despite this, combination therapy is still probably the standard of care for these infections.

The treatment of typhoid fever is discussed on page 711.

Bacteraemia caused by other Gram-negative bacteria

Campylobacter. Campylobacter most often cause an enteritis, but in a proportion of cases (reportedly less than 10%, although this is probably an underestimate) there is an accompanying bacteraemia. Sometimes this is transient and clinically silent; such patients resolve spontaneously without treatment. More sustained infections require antibiotics. Infections due to *Campylobacter jejuni* are treated with erythromycin; ciprofloxacin is an alternative, but some strains are resistant. There are no good data on treating serious bacteraemic infections, but on the basis of susceptibility testing it has been suggested that gentamicin, imipenem or cefotaxime would be appropriate. More recently it has become apparent that immunocompromised patients can develop severe bacteraemic infections with other species of campylobacter, including *C. fetus*, *C. upsaliensis* and *C. hyointestinalis*. Experience is still very limited, but a combination of ampicillin and gentamicin is recommended.

Brucellosis. This is discussed in Chapter 61.

Meliodosis. This is a systemic infection caused by *Pseudomonas pseudomallei*. It is endemic in Thailand and South-East Asia where it is one of the commonest causes of community acquired bacteraemia, but occasional cases have been reported from parts of Africa, Central America and Europe. The commonest clinical manifestation is pneumonia, but an acute septicaemic form of the disease is well described; it presents as septic shock and, if untreated, has a mortality of 90%. Although co-trimoxazole is active against some strains there is now widespread resistance in Thailand, and the treatment of choice is now ceftazidime 120 mg/kg daily for 2 weeks followed by not less than 2 months of oral treatment with ampicillin clavulanate.

Capnocytophaga canimorsus. This is the name now given to an organism previously referred to as DF-2, and associated with dog bites. In immunosuppressed individuals, especially those who are asplenic or receiving corticosteroids, it can cause a fulminating shock-like illness associated with disseminated intravascular coagulation. Since isolation and characterization of the organism will usually be delayed, treatment must start immediately on clinical suspicion. The treatment of choice is benzylpenicillin given intravenously in high dose. The organism is sensitive in vitro to van-comycin, which is an alternative in the truly penicillin-allergic patient.

ANAEROBIC INFECTIONS

Bacteroides fragilis is the commonest anaerobic isolate from blood cultures, perhaps because it is one of the least fastidious and easily grown. Patients with *Bacteroides* sepsis are often seriously ill with underlying bowel or pelvic disease or intra-abdominal abscesses. For this reason it is unusual to have 'pure' anaerobic sepsis; infections are usually polymicrobial and may include enteric Gram-negative bacilli and enterococci. Even if *B. fragilis* alone is isolated it is wise to assume that there are other more fastidious species present. Surgical drainage of collections is at least as important a part of the management as is antibiotic therapy.

The drug used most widely for the treatment of anaerobic infections is metronidazole; until relatively recently this was not approved in the USA, and for this reason clindamycin was often used as an alternative. Direct comparisons between the two drugs are relatively rare, but since metronidazole causes less serious side-effects is usually preferred. The one exception is in anaerobic pleuro-pulmonary infection, where clindamycin seems to be superior (Perlino 1981) (Ch. 48).

Several other antimicrobial agents have useful antianaerobic activity; these include benzylpenicillin (which is active against many anaerobic organisms with the notable exception of *B. fragilis*), ampicillin–clavulanate, piperacillin, cefoxitin and imipenem.

Because of the polymicrobial nature of many of these infections it is uncommon (and probably unwise) to use a narrow-spectrum antianaerobic agent alone. Combinations such as a β-lactam agent plus gentamicin plus metronidazole, or clindamycin plus gentamicin provide safe cover. In complicated postoperative infections in which anaerobic sepsis is a concern, imipenem is a useful drug; ampicillin–clavulanate is a good alternative if enterococci are likely to be present.

Sepsis and septic shock

Early recognition is essential if the high mortality of septic shock is to be avoided. Identifying patients and starting treatment before they have become profoundly hypotensive and have evidence of multiple organ failure offers the best chance of preventing death. The management of septic patients can be arbitrarily divided into three components: (a) supportive care, aimed at optimizing oxygenation of the tissues; (b) treatment aimed at the infection (which will include antimicrobial therapy as well as appropriate surgical drainage); and (c) so-called adjunctive therapy, which is concerned with modulating the host response. A detailed discussion of fluid and oxygen management is beyond the scope of this chapter; I will confine myself to aspects of the antimicrobial treatment, and briefly discuss the current status of adjunctive agents for sepsis and septic shock.

EMPIRICAL ANTIBIOTIC THERAPY

The high mortality and rapid progression of septic shock mandates the use of antibiotics before the results of blood cultures are available. However, empirical therapy need not mean 'blind' therapy, as it is sometimes called. While it is very rarely possible to be so certain about the microbiological diagnosis that narrow-spectrum agents can be used, it is equally wrong to have a 'standard' regimen which is used for all septic patients, irrespective of the clinical setting. The following points are helpful in assessing a patient and choosing a regimen:

- The history and clinical setting: Is this a postoperative infection and, if so, was it a thoracic, intra-abdominal or pelvic procedure? Was the bowel breached? Is there a history of trauma? Are there clues from the history as to the likely focus of the infection?
- Is this a community acquired or hospital acquired infection? Is there a recent history of foreign travel?
- What is the underlying disease? Is there renal impairment? Is the patient on dialysis, or neutropenic?
- What is the recent microbiological and antibiotic history? Although one cannot rely on a recent isolate as being causative in the current episode of sepsis, it is certainly important to know if, for example, the patient is colonized with *Pseudomonas*. Equally, it is important to be aware if the patient has been receiving antibiotics for some time, in part because one must presume that whatever is causing the current infection is resistant to those

drugs, but also because this raises the spectre of fungal infection.

This basic information can be assembled quickly, and an appropriate regimen chosen; cultures should be obtained and treatment started. Sometimes urgent laboratory investigations will be helpful: the value of a blood film or a rapid Gram stain of skin lesions cannot be underestimated, but therapy should not be delayed while these are done. Occasionally, the clinical picture is so unambiguous that the treatment is obvious, as in the patient with meningococcal shock for instance. The neutropenic patient with fever is a special case, and haematology units will have a standard regimen used for instituting treatment (Ch. 43). In most patients, however, the clinician will need to consider all the information available and then choose the most suitable combination of agents.

Table 41.4 illustrates one approach to this process. Clearly the table only points out the principles of antibiotic choice; in each case there are many alternatives, depending in part on the factors noted above. In the penicillin-allergic patient, for instance, vancomycin will often be a satisfactory substitute, and ampicillin clavulanate is a useful alternative to imipenem. If a *Pseudomonas* infection is suspected then it will be important to include a drug with appropriate activity, usually ceftazidime or ciprofloxacin, with or without the addition of an aminoglycoside. Thus the reader will readily appreciate how difficult – and indeed inappropriate – it is to generalize in suggesting a regimen for the empirical therapy of sepsis. Finally, it is important to emphasise that the recommendations in Table 41.4 are designed for patients with sepsis or shock originating from the site indicated, *not* necessarily for infections localized to that site. For instance, a serious community acquired chest infection would normally be treated with amoxycillin and erythromycin; it is only when the patient has signs of systemic sepsis that some modification might be required (e.g. to treat a possible staphylococcal pneumonia).

The drugs chosen should be prescribed at the maximum dosage and are usually administered parenterally for 2

Table 41.4   *The principles of antibiotic choice for patients with sepsis and shock*

Presumed site of infection	Initial treatment	
	Community acquired	Hospital acquired
Urinary tract	Cephalosporin or ciprofloxacin	
Biliary tract	Ampicillin + gentamicin	Piperacillin + gentamicin
Respiratory tract	Flucloxacillin + gentamicin	Cephalosporin + gentamicin
Skin and soft tissue	Penicillin + flucloxacillin	Flucloxacillin + gentamicin
Lower gut or pelvis	Piperacillin + gentamicin + metronidazole *or* clindamycin + gentamicin *or* imipenem ± gentamicin	

weeks, but this statement too is a generalization which bears closer scrutiny. Recommendations for the optimum duration of treatment for bacteraemia are largely based on precedent and clinical experience rather than comparative data. Two weeks is a typical time, but there is little doubt that in some cases it can be safely shortened. Unfortunately, there is no easy formula for identifying patients for whom, say, 7 days' treatment would suffice, and inadequate treatment can lead to relapse. However, one recent approach has been to suggest that patients who respond promptly to 1 week of intravenous therapy can safely be converted to oral therapy (usually with the same drug) for a further 1–2 weeks, and this has much to commend it.

Another controversial issue is that of the wisdom of modifying the antibiotic therapy as soon as the susceptibility of the causative organism is known. Here again some judgement is required: if blood cultures reveal a *Staph. aureus* or pneumococcus, for instance, then it is clearly possible to use a rather specific regimen. On the other hand, consider a patient who has been on an intensive care unit for 2 weeks following major bowel surgery, who has received many antibiotics during that time, and who has become septic after returning from a second operative procedure. Let us suppose that the patient was treated empirically with ceftazidime, gentamicin and metronidazole and responded very rapidly to that treatment, but 24 h later the laboratory reports *Esch. coli* sensitive to cefuroxime in the blood cultures. It would be possible to change to cefuroxime alone, but this would be unwise because in such a complex situation one can never be certain that other organisms were not involved, and because in such an ill patient one may not get a 'second chance'. Ultimately it is the patient's response which is the best guide.

ADJUNCTIVE TREATMENT

The high mortality of septic shock and the unravelling of much of the pathophysiology of the disease has prompted an intense effort to try and identify alternative therapeutic targets. This has spawned a huge literature and scores of different agents have been investigated, some of which have reached clinical trial. Thus far, however, none of these treatments have regulatory approval so here I will briefly review the different strategies and concentrate on those which look most likely to reach clinical practice soon. A detailed review of all adjunctive therapies has recently been published (Lynn & Cohen 1995b) which contains the primary references to all the data discussed below.

Strategies aimed at microbial products

The most obvious candidate is endotoxin, since this is the component of Gram-negative bacteria which initiates the process of shock, and because it is common to all Gram-negative bacteria. By immunizing animals with cell-wall deficient mutants of Gram-negative bacteria, investigators produced antibodies which reacted with the core glycolipid of endotoxin (see above), and at least in some animal models these antibodies were protective. This work led to the development of monoclonal antibodies to endotoxin and to two drugs in particular, Centoxin and E5, despite the fact that there was much debate as to how these particular antibodies worked and whether the protective effect was reproducible. Following the first phase III trial of Centoxin (which demonstrated a survival benefit in the subset of patients with Gram-negative bacteraemia and shock) many questions were asked about the trial methodology and the statistical analysis, and when eventually a second trial was done the beneficial effects could not be confirmed and the drug was withdrawn. The position with E5 is a little more complicated since the three phase III trials have all been a little different in design and in each case an apparent benefit identified in subsets of the population were not subsequently confirmed. E5 remains in clinical development.

Meanwhile, an alternative approach to neutralizing endotoxin has been based on a molecule called bactericidal/permeability increasing factor (BPI), a natural product of human neutrophils which has the extraordinary ability both to bind and neutralize endotoxin and also to kill Gram-negative bacteria. Clinical trials with recombinant BPI are just beginning.

Strategies aimed at mediators

Experimental data indicated that the pro-inflammatory cytokines, and in particular IL-1 and TNF, were very attractive potential targets. In the case of IL-1, it emerged that there was a natural inhibitor called IL-1 receptor antagonist (IL-1ra) which competed for receptor occupancy but when bound did not cause signal transduction. A phase III trial of IL-1ra suggested that it conferred a survival advantage on a subgroup of the more seriously ill patients, but this was a retrospective analysis which was not confirmed following a second trial. The approach to TNF was a little different, and the first strategy was to use a neutralizing monoclonal antibody. Two phase III trials suggested that once again, it was the more ill patients who benefited in terms of shock reversal; a third trial is in progress to determine if this effect can be confirmed. Another way of neutralising TNF is to take advantage of the soluble (extracellular) fragments of the natural TNF receptors. There are two such receptors, called p55 and p75 based on their size. Their extracellular components are very similar, and in vitro both bind TNF very well. Shedding of the extracellular part of the receptor seems to be part of normal physiological control mechanisms for TNF, and by cloning these parts and then joining them to the Fc piece of immunoglobulin G (IgG) it was possible to make a soluble TNF receptor–IgG:Fc (sTNFR:Fc) complex which could be injected and would bind and neutralize TNF. However, when a clinical trial was done with a p75 sTNFR:Fc the mortality was higher in the treated group than in the placebo group. The reason for this is still not clear; one possible explanation is that the drug was too effective, and that neutralizing all the TNF is harmful. The episode is a good example of the possible hazards of manipulating the highly complex network of mediators, the primary purpose of which is, of course, to integrate the immune response, not least in response to infection.

Among many other mediators that have been examined, most clinical experience has been gained with drugs that inhibit PAF (see above). Once again the experimental data were encouraging, and the first phase III trial showed benefit to the subset of patients with Gram-negative sepsis. However, this was not confirmed in a follow-up study, and further trials are in progress.

Limiting tissue injury

This is the most 'distal' part of the pathway, and again there are concerns that modifying neutrophil responses or the expression of adhesion molecules, for instance, could be a two-edged sword, since these are important components of host defences. The recognition that excess production of nitric oxide may be the major cause of the hypotension of sepsis has led to attempts to inhibit selectively the enzyme responsible, inducible nitric oxide synthase (iNOS), with drugs such as N^G-monomethyl-L-arginine. The difficulty is that too complete a shutdown of nitric oxide production might lead to complications such as vascular collapse (because nitric oxide is responsible for the background vasodilatation which maintains vascular patency), or secondary infections (because it is an important effector of microbial killing in macrophages). Clinical trials with these drugs are just beginning.

References

Bamberger D M, Gurley M B 1994 Microbial etiology and clinical characteristics of distributive shock. *Clinical Infectious Diseases* 18: 726–730

Bayer A S, Lam K, Ginzton L, Norman D C, Chiu C, Ward J I 1987 *Staphylococcus aureus* bacteremia. Clinical, serologic, and echocardiographic findings in patients with and without endocarditis. *Archives of Internal Medicine* 147: 457–462

Bochud P, Eggiman P, Calandra T, van Melle G, Saghafi L, Francioli P 1994 Bacteremia due to viridans streptococcus in neutropenic patients with cancer: clinical spectrum and risk factors. *Clinical Infectious Diseases* 18: 25–31

Bohach G A, Fast D J, Nelson R D, Schlievert P M 1990 Staphylococcal and streptococcal pyrogenic toxins involved in toxic shock syndrome and related illnesses. *CRC Critical Reviews in Microbiology* 17: 251–272

Bone R C 1992a Modulators of coagulation. A critical appraisal of their role in sepsis. *Archives of Internal Medicine* 152: 1381–1389

Bone R C 1992b Phospholipids and their inhibitors: a critical evaluation of their role in the treatment of sepsis. *Critical Care Medicine* 20: 884–890

Bone R C, Fisher J C J, Clemmer T P, Slotman G J, Metz C A, Balk R A 1987 A controlled clinical trial of high-dose methyl-prednisolone in the treatment of severe sepsis and septic shock. *New England Journal of Medicine* 317: 653–658

Bone R C, Balk R A, Cerra F B et al 1992 Definitions for sepsis and organ failure and guidelines for the use of innovative therapies in sepsis. The ACCP/SCCM Consensus Conference Committee. American College of Chest Physicians/Society of Critical Care Medicine. *Chest* 101: 1644–1655

Calandra T, Cometta A 1991 Antibiotic therapy for Gram-negative bacteremia. *Infectious Diseases Clinics of North America* 5: 817–834

Chandrasekar P H, Crane L R, Bailey E J 1987 Comparison of the activity of antibiotic combinations in vitro with clinical outcome and resistance emergence in serious infection by *Pseudomonas aeruginosa* in non-neutropenic patients. *Journal of Antimicrobial Chemotherapy* 19: 321–329

Chelsom J, Halstensen A, Haga T, Høiby E A 1994 Necrotising fasciitis due to group A streptococci in western Norway: incidence and clinical features. *Lancet* 344: 1111–1115

Cohen M S 1994 Molecular events in the activation of human neutrophils for microbial killing. *Clinical Infectious Diseases* 18 (suppl 2): S170–S179

Colman R W 1989 The role of plasma proteases in septic shock. *New England Journal of Medicine* 320: 1207–1209

Danner R L, Elin R J, Hosseini J M, Wesley R A, Reilly J M, Parrillo J E 1991 Endotoxemia in human septic shock. *Chest* 99: 169–175

Dinarello C A, Wolff S M 1993 The role of interleukin-1 in disease. *New England Journal of Medicine* 328: 106–113

Farley M M, Harvey R C, Stull T et al 1993 A population-based assessment of invasive disease due to group B streptococcus in nonpregnant adults. *New England Journal of Medicine* 328: 1807–1811

Forgacs I C, Eykyn S J, Bradley R D 1986 Serious infection in the intensive therapy unit: a 15 year study of bacteraemia. *Quarterly Journal of Medicine* 60: 773–779

Geerdes H F, Ziegler D, Lode H et al 1992 Septicemia in 980 patients at a university hospital in Berlin: prospective studies during 4 selected years between 1979 and 1989. *Clinical Infectious Diseases* 15: 991–1002

Gransden W R, Eykyn S J, Philips I 1984 *Staphylococcus aureus* bacteraemia: 400 episodes in St Thomas's Hospital. *British Medical Journal* 288: 300–303

Gransden W R, Eykyn S J, Philips I 1985 Pneumococcal bacteraemia: 325 episodes diagnosed at St Thomas's hospital. *British Medical Journal* 290: 505–508

Gruer L D, McKendrick M W, Geddes A M 1984 Pneumococcal bacteraemia – a continuing challenge. *Quarterly Journal of Medicine New Series* 53: 259–270

Gullberg R M, Homann S R, Phair J P 1989 Enterococcal bacteremia: analysis of 75 episodes. *Reviews of Infectious Diseases* 11: 74–85

Hebert P C, Drummond A J, Singer J, Bernard G R, Russell J A 1993 A simple multiple system organ failure scoring system predicts mortality of patients who have sepsis syndrome. *Chest* 104: 230–235

Hoge C W, Adams J, Buchanan B, Sears S D 1991 Enterococcal bacteremia: to treat or not to treat, a reappraisal. *Reviews of Infectious Diseases* 13: 600–605

Hoge C W, Schwartz B, Talkington D F, Breiman R F, MacNeill E M, Englender S J 1993 The changing epidemiology of invasive group A streptococcal infections and the emergence of streptococcal toxic shock-like syndrome. A retrospective population-based study. *Journal of American Medicine Association* 269: 384–389

Ispahani P, Pearson N J, Greenwood D 1987 An analysis of community and hospital-acquired bacteraemia in a large teaching hospital in the United Kingdom. *Quarterly Journal of Medicine* 63: 427–440

Jacobs M R 1992 Treatment and diagnosis of infections caused by drug-resistant *Streptococcus pneumoniae*. *Clinical Infectious Diseases* 15: 119–127

Johnson H M, Russell J K, Pontzer C H 1992 Superantigens in human disease. *Scientific American* April: 42–73

Kieft H, Hoepelman A I, Zhou W, Rozenberg-Arska M, Struyvenberg A, Verhoef J 1993 The sepsis syndrome in a Dutch university hospital. Clinical observations. *Archives of Internal Medicine* 153: 2241–2247

Knaus W A, Harrell F E, Fisher J C J et al 1993 The clinical evaluation of new drugs for sepsis. A prospective study design based on survival analysis. *Journal of the American Medicine Association* 270: 1233–1241

Korvick J A, Bryan C S, Farber B et al 1992 Prospective observational study of Klebsiella bacteremia in 230 patients:

outcome for antibiotic combinations versus monotherapy. *Antimicrobial Agents and Chemotherapy* 36: 2639–2644

Kotb M 1992 Role of superantigens in the pathogenesis of infectious diseases and their sequelae. *Current Opinion in Infectious Diseases* 5: 364–374

Lowy F D, Hammer S M 1983 *Staphylococcus epidermidis* infections. *Annals of Internal Medicine* 99: 834–839

Lynn W A, Cohen J 1995a Microbiological requirements for studies of sepsis. In: Sibbald W J, Vincent J (eds) Clinical trials for the treatment of sepsis. Update in emergency medicine and intensive care 19. Springer, Berlin, p 71–85

Lynn W A, Cohen J 1995b Adjunctive therapy for septic shock: a review of experimental approaches. *Clinical Infectious Diseases* 20: 143–158

Lynn W A, Clutterbuck E, Want S et al 1994 Treatment of CAPD-peritonitis due to glycopeptide-resistant *Enterococcus faecium* with quinupristin/dalfopristin. *Lancet* 344: 1025–1026

McPhaden A R, Whaley K 1985 The complement system in sepsis and trauma. *British Medical Bulletin* 41: 281–286

Molloy R G, Mannick J A, Rodrick M L 1993 Cytokines, sepsis and immunomodulation. *British Journal of Surgery* 80: 289–297

Morrison D C, Danner R L, Dinarello C A et al 1994 Bacterial endotoxins and pathogenesis of Gram-negative infections: current status and future direction. *Journal of Endotoxin Research* 1: 71–83

Mylotte J M, McDermott C, Spooner J A 1987 Prospective study of 114 consecutive episodes of *Staphylococcus aureus* bacteremia. *Reviews of Infectious Diseases* 9: 891–907

Perlino C A 1981 Metronidazole vs clindamycin treatment of anaerobic pulmonary infection. Failure of metronidazole therapy. *Archives of Internal Medicine* 141: 1424–1427

Raad I I, Bodey G P 1992 Infectious complications of indwelling vascular catheters. *Clinical Infectious Diseases* 15: 197–210

Rangel-Frausto M, Pittet D, Costigan M, Hwang T, Davis C S, Wenzel R P 1995 The natural history of the systemic inflammatory response syndrome (SIRS). A prospective study. *Journal of American Medicine Association* 273: 117–123

Rees R C 1991 Cytokines: their role in regulating immunity and the response to infection. *Reviews in Medical Microbiology* 3: 9–14

Schlievert P M 1993 Role of superantigens in human disease. *Journal of Infectious Diseases* 167: 997–1002

Sculier J P, Klastersky J 1984 Significance of serum bactericidal activity in Gram-negative bacillary bacteremia in patients with and without granulocytopenia. *American Journal of Medicine* 76: 429–435

Shaunak S, Wendon J, Monteil M, Gordon A M 1988 Septic scarlet fever due to *Streptococcus pyogenes* cellulitis. *Quarterly Journal of Medicine* 69: 921–925

Sheagren J N 1984 *Staphylococcus aureus*. The persistent pathogen [second of two parts]. *New England Journal of Medicine* 310: 1437–1442

Siebert J D, Thompson Jr J B, Tan J S, Gerson L W 1993 Emergence of antimicrobial resistance in Gram-negative bacilli causing bacteremia during therapy. *American Journal of Clinical Pathology* 100: 47–51

Sissons J G 1993 Superantigens and infectious disease. *Lancet* 341: 1627–1629

Stevens D L 1992 Invasive group A streptococcus infections. *Clinical Infectious Diseases* 14: 2–13

Stevens D L, Gibbons A E, Bergstrom R, Winn V 1988 The Eagle effect revisited: efficacy of clindamycin, erythromycin, and penicillin in the treatment of streptococcal myositis. *Journal of Infectious Diseases* 158: 23–28

The Working Group on Severe Streptococcal Infections 1993 Defining the group A streptococcal toxic shock syndrome. Rationale and consensus definition. *Journal of the American Medicine Association* 269: 390–391

Verhagen C, de Pauw B E, Donnelly J P, Williams K J, de Witte T, Janssen J T 1986 Ceftazidime alone for treating *Pseudomonas aeruginosa* septicaemia in neutropenic patients. *Journal of Antimicrobial Chemotherapy* 13: 125–131

Watanakunakorn C, Pantelakis J 1993 Alpha-hemolytic streptococcal bacteremia: a review of 203 episodes during 1980–1991. *Scandinavian Journal of Infectious Diseases* 25: 403–408

Young S E 1982 Bacteraemia 1975–1980: a survey of cases reported to the PHLS Communicable Diseases Surveillance Centre. *Journal of Infection* 5: 19–26

Ziegler-Heitbrock H W, Ulevitch R J 1993 CD14: cell surface receptor and differentiation marker. *Immunology Today* 14: 121–125

Abdominal and other surgical infections

E. W. Taylor

Introduction

Surgical wound infection remains a common postoperative complication and much work has been done to define the optimum prophylactic antibiotic regimen which will reduce the incidence of infection. Other infective complications such as intra-abdominal abscess, pneumonia, urinary tract infections and septicaemia may lead to the death of the patient, and it has been estimated that over half of the patients who die in surgical intensive care units die of infective complications.

Many patients present to surgeons with community acquired infection or the infective complications of naturally occurring pathology such as appendicitis, diverticulitis or cholecystitis. It is important to segregate these from subsequent, hospital acquired infection when auditing the incidence of postoperative infections. Audit of surgical wound infection has been proposed as a hospital quality-assurance indicator, but this remains problematic, especially as there is no universally acceptable definition. Some have relied upon culture of the infecting organism, but this presupposes that a suitable specimen for culture is always sent, that laboratory facilities are available to confirm the infection, and that the isolation of an organism equates to clinical infection. This is clearly not so and others feel that the diagnosis should be made on clinical grounds alone in most circumstances (Peel & Taylor 1991).

The duration of surveillance is also important. The increasing trend towards early discharge from hospital means that the signs and symptoms of an infection may only develop after the patient has left hospital.

Law et al (1990) found a clean wound infection rate of 1.3% in hospital, but an additional 4% of patients developed infection after leaving hospital. With prosthetic implants infections may not present for up to 1 year after operation and the classical signs of infection may never be apparent.

In addition many patients have other diseases or are taking drugs which represent risk factors for infection. Any audit of postoperative infection must take these risk factors into account.

Whilst wound infection may be a primary event, the discharge of pus from the wound may be secondary to some other underlying complication. Thus a haematoma, seroma, collection of bile or gastro-intestinal content, urine or cerebrospinal fluid (CSF) beneath the wound may discharge through the wound, and from this bacteria will be isolated. However these 'wound infections' represent an infection secondary to the underlying complication rather than a primary wound infection.

FACTORS DETERMINING THE INCIDENCE OF POSTOPERATIVE INFECTION

The risk of infection after an operation is a balance between the bacterial contamination of the operating field, the extent to which tissue damage occurs or foreign bodies are implanted at the time of the operation, and the ability of the patient's body to resist these threats.

Bacterial contamination

Bacteria contaminating the wound or deep tissues of the body at operation may be either exogenous or endogenous in origin. Exogenous contamination may be airborne or by transfer from the surgical team at operation. Many of the rituals and practices within the operating theatre have evolved as surgeons have attempted to prevent exogenous contamination. This preventative approach perhaps reached its peak with the development of the laminar air-flow systems with high efficiency particle air (HEPA) bacterial filters, total body exhaust systems and no-touch technique favoured in some orthopaedic units where ultra-clean, prosthetic implant surgery is performed. However, there is little scientific evidence to show that the use of caps, masks, gloves or overshoes alters the infection rate after most non-implant operations. There is little doubt that most post-operative infections are caused by organisms endogenous to the patient.

Man is host to 10^{14} bacteria of some 500 different species and, whenever one of the spaces or tracts in the body normally colonized by bacteria is opened, some contamination of the tissues is inevitable. These include the sinuses and antra of the skull, the gastro-intestinal tract, the upper trachea and pharynx, the genito-urinary tracts and the biliary tract. Although generally considered exogenous, bacteria carried in from the skin to contaminate the tissues are derived from the patient's normal flora, and therefore cannot truly be considered exogenous.

The type of organism contaminating the wound also influences the incidence of infection. Some are more pathogenic and virulent than others. Endogenous bacteria rarely proliferate in normal tissue (Polk & Miles 1973) but grow readily in the presence of damaged tissue or foreign bodies. In addition, bacteria may act synergistically to create abscesses; the presence of both aerobic and anaerobic bacteria promote abscess formation, whereas each alone cause little morbidity (Onderdonk et al 1976).

The wound

The proliferation of endogenous bacteria is dependent upon a degree of tissue damage, which will vary greatly from wound to wound, operation to operation and perhaps more importantly, from surgeon to surgeon. The importance of delicate handling of the tissues and competent surgical technique cannot be overemphasized. A wound containing a seroma or haematoma provides an ideal culture medium for bacterial growth as does tissue traumatized by overtight sutures, for example.

Many operations use prosthetic, non-absorbable materials which radically reduce the number of organisms necessary to create infection (Elek & Conen 1957). Suction or open drains inserted into the wound or into body cavities to drain fluids probably increase the risk of infection, both by providing a portal of entry for bacteria and by acting as foreign bodies (Simchen et al 1990).

Host resistance

The ability of the patient to resist the bacterial contamination that occurs at operation is the other major determinant of postoperative infection. Some of the many factors which influence host resistance are shown in Box 42.1. The role of blood transfusion in reducing immunocompetence has recently been documented; it has long been known that blood transfusion reduces rejection after renal transplantation and

Box 42.1 *Factors reducing host resistance*

- Extremes of age
- Obesity
- Malnutrition
- Cirrhosis
- Uraemia
- Diabetes mellitus
- Malignancy
- Burns
- Splenectomy
- Corticosteroids
- Cytotoxic drugs
- AIDS
- Acute infections
- Foreign bodies
- Blood transfusion

there is evidence that transfusion increases the risk of recurrent tumour after cancer operations (Burrows & Tartter 1982, George & Marello 1987, McClinton et al 1990). The influence on postoperative infection, however, was first highlighted by Tartter (1988, 1989), while Jensen et al (1990) reported 28% incidence of infection after colorectal surgery if the patient received a perioperative blood transfusion compared with 2% if no blood was transfused. This effect occurred when whole blood was transfused but not with red cell concentrates. Braga et al (1992) found transfusion of more than 1000 ml of blood to be an independent risk factor for infection in 285 patients undergoing operations for gastro-intestinal cancer.

Incidence of infection

The classification of operations into clean, clean-contaminated, contaminated and dirty has become internationally accepted and the audit by Cruse and Foord documents the influence this has on infection (Table 42.1) (Cruse 1992). However, this classification only takes into account the presumed bacterial contamination and the distinction between clean-contaminated and contaminated can become arbitrary and subjective. Haley et al (1985) assessed a large number of risk factors in 59 352 patients and compared the results with the standard classification. They found only

Table 42.1 *Influence of bacterial contamination on postoperative infection (Cruse 1992)*

Category	No. of patients	Patients infected	
		No.	%
Clean	73 589	1002	1.4
Clean-contaminated	14 018	879	6.3
Contaminated	9 085	1211	13.3
Dirty	3 038	1310	39.9
Total	100 000	4412	4.4

four significant risk factors: operations lasting more than 2 h, abdominal operations, operations classified as contaminated or dirty, and patients who had three or more recorded concomitant diagnoses. There was better correlation between the incidence of infection and the number of patient risk factors than with the standard classification of bacteriological contamination. Culver et al (1991), in a further assessment of risk factors in 84 961 patients, showed that the duration of operation at which risk increased was dependent on the type of surgery performed, and showed that it was possible to replace concomitant diagnoses with the American Society of Anesthesiology's grading of fitness for operation. This analysis of risk in such large cohorts of patients suggests that some assessment of patient risk factors should be introduced into all future trials or audits of postoperative infection.

COST OF INFECTION

Postoperative infection has a financial cost, both to the health service and to the patient in addition to the cost in terms of morbidity and mortality. Patients experience discomfort and inconvenience at the time of surgery, undergo repeated visits to hospital, and not infrequently require additional surgery. In 1986, it was reported in the UK Parliament that infection resulted in an average of 4 days' extra stay in hospital (Hansard 1986). This is an underestimate. Bremmelgaard et al (1989) reported the average postoperative stay to be 20.5 days longer in infected patients, while patients undergoing colorectal surgery who developed an infection were in hospital an average of 11 more days (Taylor et al 1994). In the UK, where the cost of a bed-day in the NHS (1995) is approximately £150, the incidence of postoperative infection assumed to be approximately 5% and the increased hospital stay is realistically estimated to be 7–8 days, then the cost to the health service approaches £200 million per annum. This excludes the additional nursing, dressings and possibly antibiotics after discharge.

ANTIBIOTIC PROPHYLAXIS

The role of antibiotic prophylaxis is to reduce the incidence of postoperative infection when bacterial contamination of the tissues at operation is inevitable or occurs unexpectedly. It has generally been considered that the role of prophylaxis is to prevent the occurrence of wound infection, yet other forms of operation-related infection, particularly intra-abdominal abscess, may also be reduced. The evidence that antibiotics reduce the incidence of respiratory and urinary tract infections is not so impressive.

Prophylaxis must be distinguished from therapy. Patients presenting with an infective problem for which an urgent operation is performed require antibiotic therapy to treat the established infection. Antibiotics may reduce the incidence of wound infection, but this is a secondary benefit. The type of antibiotic, the regimen and route of administration should all be chosen to treat the original infection and should be considered therapeutic, not prophylactic.

Selection of antibiotic

The prophylactic antibiotic should be active against those organisms most likely to contaminate the wound. As stated, whilst *Staphylococcus aureus* and other skin organisms represent the main contaminating organism from the environment, it is usually the organisms colonizing the body tract or opened cavity which cause postoperative infection, and it is these organisms that determine the antibiotic regimen.

The choice of antibiotic regimen will depend upon the site of operation and the likely bacterial contaminants (Table 42.2). Some suggest that the prophylactic regimen should differ from antibiotics used for a subsequent postoperative infection (Stuckey & Gross 1990). Thus in the USA cephalothin and cefoxitin are widely used for prophylaxis, retaining cefotaxime, ceftazidine, piperacillin and the carbapenems for therapy. This is based on the assumption that subsequent infections are likely to be caused by organisms resistant to the antibiotic used for prophylaxis. However, there is little evidence to support this view, which would be more credible if prolonged prophylactic courses of antibiotics were adopted, thus selecting out resistant strains; changes in susceptibility patterns of subsequent postoperative infections have not been documented where single-dose prophylaxis is used.

The cost of the antibiotic is important, but must be seen in the context of cost versus benefit. If a cheaper antibiotic is less effective, the cost of the consequent infections may far outweigh the cost of a more expensive but more effective agent. Lazorthes et al (1982) randomized 162 patients undergoing groin-hernia repair to receive a single dose of cefamandole and 162 patients to receive placebo. No patient receiving the antibiotic (which cost approximately US $500) developed infection, whereas 7 of the placebo patients developed wound infections for which the treatment cost was approximately US $5000. However, if 3–5 days' 'prophylaxis' had been given instead of single dose this cost–benefit would have been lost.

The other major factor in the choice of the prophylactic antibiotic regimen is safety. Penicillin sensitivity and its cross-sensitivity with the cephalosporins, aminoglycoside renal and ototoxicity, and the development of pseudomembranous colitis with the third-generation cephalosporins are examples. Once again, the incidence of these complications is minimal with the use of single-dose prophylaxis.

Table 42.2   *Antibiotic prophylaxis*

Type of operation	Principal pathogens	Antibiotic recommended	Dose*
Clean operations			
Cardiac	Staph. aureus	Cefuroxime	1.5 g i.v. (±750 mg at 8 and 16 h)
Neurosurgery	Staph. epidermidis	Co-amoxiclav	1 g i.v. (±1 g at 8 and 16 h)
Implant	GNAB if operation below	Vancomycin if MRSA	500 mg i.v. infusion over 60 min
(? Other clean	waist	suspected	(±6 hourly)
operations	Streptococci		
	MRSA		
Clean contaminated operations			
Head and neck	Streptococci	Cefuroxime	1.5 g i.v. (±750 mg at 8 and 16 h)
(if sinus, nasal, oral	Staphylococci	Co-amoxiclav	1 g i.v. (±1 g at 8 and 16 h)
or pharyngeal mucosa	Oral anaerobes		
breached)			
Thoracic			
Bronchial	Streptococci	Cefuroxime	1.5 g i.v. (±750 mg at 8 and 16 h)
	Staphylococci		
Oesophageal	Staphylococci	Cefuroxime	1.5 g i.v. (±750 mg at 8 and 16 h)
	GNAB	Ciprofloxacin	200 mg i.v. (±100 mg at 8 and 16 h)
	Oral anaerobes	Co-amoxiclav	1 g i.v. (±1 g at 8 and 16 h)
		Piperacillin	2 g i.v. (±2 g at 8 and 16 h)
Upper gastro-intestinal			
Gastric	Gram +ve cocci	Cefuroxime	1.5 g i.v. (±750 mg at 8 and 16 h)
	GNAB	Co-amoxiclav	1 g i.v. (±1 g at 8 and 16 h)
		Ciprofloxacin	200 mg i.v. (+100 mg at 8 and 16 h)
Biliary	GNAB	Piperacillin	2 g i.v. (±2 g at 8 and 16 h)
Laparotomy/cholecystomy	Enterococci		
ERCP			
Urology			
TURP	GNAB	Cefuroxime	1.5 g i.v. (±750 mg at 8 and 16 h)
	Enterococci	Co-amoxiclav	1 g i.v. (±1 g at 8 and 16 h)
		Piperacillin	2 g i.v. (±2 g at 8 and 16 h)
		Ciprofloxacin	200 mg i.v. (±100 mg at 8 and 16 h)
Clean contaminated operations			
Obstetrics and gynaecology	GNAB	Cefuroxime	1.5 g i.v. (±750 mg at 8 and 16 h)
Hysterectomy	β-Haemolytic streptococci	Cefotaxime	2 g i.v. (±1 g at 8 and 16 h)
	Bacteroides spp.	Piperacillin	2 g i.v. (±2 g at 8 and 16 h)
Caesarean section	Enterococci	Co-amoxiclav	1 g i.v. (±1 g at 8 and 16 h)
	Staphylococci		
	? *Chlamydia* spp.		
Amputation	*Clostridia* spp.	Benzyl penicillin	600 mg i.v. (±600 mg 6-hourly for 5 days)
Contaminated operations			
Colorectal	GNAB	Cefotaxime	2 g i.v. (±2 g at 8 and 16 h)
Elective	*Bacteroides* spp.	Piperacillin	2 g i.v. (±2 g at 8 and 16 h)
Emergency	Other anaerobes	Co-amoxiclav	1 g i.v. (±1 g at 8 and 16 h)
	? Enterococci	Gentamicin +	80 mg for an adult patient
		metronidazole	500 mg i.v. or 1 g
Intestinal obstruction			
Trauma (within 4 h)			

ERCP, endoscopic retrograde cholangiopancreatogram; GNAB, Gram-negative aerobic bacteria; MRSA, methicillin-resistant *Staph. aureus*; TURP, trans-urethral prostatectomy.
* The evidence would suggest that single-dose prophylaxis is adequate. However, many surgeons continue to administer 24 h antibiotic prophylaxis and this is shown in brackets.

Time of administration

The antibiotic should be administered so that there is a high circulating blood level at the time of the operation. In practice this means the antibiotic should be given either intramuscularly with any premedication 1 h before surgery, or intravenously on induction of anaesthesia. Should contamination occur unexpectedly during the course of the operation, additional appropriate antibiotic(s) should be administered immediately. The importance of timing of administration of prophylaxis on the incidence of infection has been demonstrated by Classen et al (1992). Where the antibiotic was administered more than 2 h preoperatively (3.8% infection) or more than 3 h postoperatively (3.3% infection), the infection rates were significantly higher than when the antibiotic was given perioperatively (0.4% infection).

Duration of prophylaxis

The duration of antibiotic prophylaxis has proved controversial. Increasing evidence suggests that single-dose prophylaxis is adequate for all operations, except where there is blood loss in excess of 2 l for an adult patient, or the operation lasts for more than 2 h. Rowe-Jones et al (1990) randomized 943 patients to receive cefotaxime 1 g i.v. with metronidazole 0.5 g i.v. on induction of anaesthesia, or cefuroxime 1.5 g i.v. with metronidazole 0.5 g i.v. preoperatively followed by two further doses at 8 and 16 h postoperatively. The mortality was 5.5 and 6.6%, respectively, and the incidence of wound infection was 7.1 and 7.3%. Strachan et al (1977) showed no difference between one dose and 5 days' prophylaxis in biliary-tract surgery, Turano et al (1992) no difference between one and three doses of cefotaxime in 273 patients having abdominal, gynaecological and urological operations, Bates et al (1992) no difference between one and three doses of co-amoxiclav in patients undergoing at-risk abdominal surgery, and Jensen et al (1990) no difference between one and three doses in colorectal surgery. A number of other studies have confirmed that a single dose is as effective as multidose prophylaxis, even in implant surgery (Di Piro et al 1986, Scher et al 1986, Periti et al 1989, University of Melbourne Colorectal Group 1989).

The effect of the duration of operation on the incidence of infection has been investigated extensively by Culver et al (1991) and varies from operation to operation, but a time longer than 2 h is a good general indicator. This is governed by the half-life of many antibiotics or, where there is extensive blood loss, by falling drug concentrations. Even in the severely immunocompromised there is no evidence that more prolonged antibiotic prophylaxis is of benefit (Moesgaard & Lukkegaard-Neilsen 1989). Prolonged prophylaxis is one of the major areas of antibiotic misuse and contributes to

the development of drug resistance. Strict adherence to well-constructed antibiotic policies is important for its control.

Route of administration

Antibiotics for prophylaxis are usually administered intravenously and occasionally intramuscularly, but have also been given subcutaneously in the area of the incision (Dixon et al 1984, Taylor et al 1985). This route certainly provides a high level of the antibiotic in the region of the wound, but there is little evidence that this is more effective than giving the antibiotic parenterally. It has also been suggested that a suitable antibiotic can be given orally (McAardle et al 1991) for some operations. This may well be less expensive than parenteral antibiotic prophylaxis, but presumes that the antibiotic is given on time, a compliant patient, satisfactory absorption of the drug and that the operating list runs to time.

Which patients should receive antibiotic prophylaxis?

It has been traditional teaching that patients should receive antibiotic prophylaxis only when a bacterially colonized tract or cavity will be involved in the surgical activities. In addition, those patients undergoing prosthetic implant procedures or neurosurgical operations often receive antibiotic prophylaxis since, although the incidence of infection is low, any resulting infection can be quite catastrophic. However, this teaching has been challenged by Platt et al (1990) who assessed cefonicid against placebo in patients undergoing non-implant breast surgery and groin hernia repairs in a large multicentre study. Although the incidence of postoperative infection was low (4.5% versus 8.1%) the outcome favoured the group receiving the antibiotic; the study was sufficiently large (1218 patients) to render the difference in the incidence of infection statistically significant ($p < 0.01$). Should these findings be confirmed, these results could lead to major changes in clinical practice.

Selective decontamination of the digestive tract

Selective decontamination of the digestive tract (SDD) was developed in an attempt to reduce the incidence of morbidity and mortality resulting from nosocomial infection by Gram-negative aerobic bacilli (GNAB) in patients treated in intensive care units. The intention was to remove the GNAB and yeasts from the oropharynx and upper and lower gastro-intestinal tract using non-absorbable antibiotics, thus reducing the colonization and infection of the lungs and other tissues by these organisms. The topic is discussed in more detail in Chapter 44. Whilst the incidence of nosocomial pneumonia has been shown to be reduced by this regimen, a reduction in overall mortality has not been satisfactorily demonstrated (Ramsay 1992, SDD Trialists Collaborative Group 1993). The difficulty would appear to be related to the time it takes to eradicate the GNAB from the gastro-intestinal tract. In these very sick patients this can take 5–10 days, by which time these organisms have already caused the infections from which the patients die. Nevertheless, SDD has been advocated for use prophylactically (Donnelly 1993) with some persuasive literature, although failure to demonstrate clear evidence for a reduction in mortality has been the cause of much controversy.

Most organisms causing postoperative wound and other nosocomial infections arise from the gastro-intestinal tract. Certainly the organisms responsible for the development of septicaemia, multiple organ failure and overwhelming sepsis would appear to derive from the colon, which has been described as the 'motor' of multiple organ failure (Carrico et al 1986). The colonic flora contains both aerobic and anaerobic organisms which act synergistically to produce postoperative intra-abdominal infection. Eradication of the anaerobic bacteria from the colon would probably not be possible in view of the large numbers involved, and is not desirable because of the influence these organisms have on colonization resistance (Tetteroo et al 1994). However, the smaller number of GNAB in the colon can be eradicated, or greatly suppressed, by standard SDD therapy or by the 4-fluoroquinolone antibiotics (Maschmeyer et al 1988), and thus cannot cause infection either by direct contamination of the tissues, by synergy with anaerobic organisms or by bacterial translocation. This approach has been favourably assessed in oesophageal surgery (Tetteroo et al 1990), liver transplantation (Weisner 1990, Bion et al 1994), small-bowel transplantation (Beath et al 1994) and, more recently, in colorectal surgery (Taylor et al 1994) (p. 603).

ANTIBIOTIC THERAPY

Many emergency surgical procedures are undertaken in patients who present with primary infective pathology. In some situations surgical treatment of this infection is all that is required and, particularly in patients with superficial or deep abscesses, drainage of the abscess alone without antibiotic therapy may suffice. Antibiotics may be required when there is contamination of peritoneal or pleural cavities, cellulitis, lymphangitis or septicaemia. In these situations an empirical 'best guess' antibiotic regimen is necessary (Evans et al 1994), and can be modified subsequently in the light of laboratory information.

As with antibiotic prophylaxis, there is increasing evidence that short-course, high-dose therapy is at least as effective as the prolonged 7–14 day therapy previously administered. This is particularly so where the focus of infection has been dealt with surgically; as in patients with appendicitis, perforated colon, or penetrating or blunt abdominal trauma in whom the lesion has been removed. In the case of abdominal trauma 12–24 h therapy is adequate; Oreskovich et al (1982) compared 12 h with 5 day antibiotic therapy with penicillin G and doxycycline in 81 evaluable patients, and found no difference in the average number of days with fever, the need for additional antibiotics or infective complications. Fabian et al (1993) also compared 1-day with 5-day therapy in a randomized study of 285 patients who had sustained abdominal trauma. The colon had been injured in 15% of patients. There was no difference in the mortality (3% in each group) or in the incidence of abdominal infections (8% and 10%). Where the infective pathology cannot or has not been surgically eliminated, such as in patients with cholangitis or diverticulitis, longer courses of therapy may be necessary.

HEAD AND NECK SURGERY

Operations which breach the mucosa of the mouth or pharynx or which enter the antra or paranasal sinuses expose the tissues to the normal flora of these spaces. The commonest pathogens are streptococci, staphylococci, GNAB and anaerobic bacteria. Head and neck operations have been classified according to the risk of postoperative wound infection as in Box 42.2. GNAB have been reported in 29–82% of infected wounds (Swift et al 1984) and probably contaminate the tissues via the nasogastric tube. Because of the wide range of infecting organisms, many different antibiotic prophylactic regimens have been adopted. A second-generation cephalosporin with metronidazole or co-amoxiclav would seem a reasonable option. Clearly, antibiotic prophylaxis would be indicated for clean-contaminated and contaminated operations, and antibiotic therapy may be necessary following the drainage of a neck abscess.

Box 42.2 *Classification of head and neck operations (Swift 1992)*

Clean
Radical neck dissection
Parotidectomy
Submandibular gland excision
Thyroidectomy
Excision of uninfected branchial cyst

Clean-contaminated
Laryngeal fissure
Excision laryngocoele

Contaminated
Total laryngectomy
Laryngo-pharyngectomy
Glossectomy
Hemi-mandibulectomy

Dirty
Drainage of neck abscess

Head and neck infections

The neck structures are surrounded by fascial layers between which lie a number of potential spaces which, if infected, may result in potentially serious or fatal complications such as airway obstruction from soft tissue swelling, mediastinitis, septicaemia, carotid artery haemorrhage, jugular vein thrombosis, meningitis or even cavernous sinus thrombosis. Acute bacterial parotitis is uncommon, but may occur in the elderly or with dehydration. *Staph. aureus* is the most common pathogen, but many organisms have been isolated and either flucloxacillin, cefuroxime or co-amoxiclav would be an appropriate choice of drug.

Peritonsillar abscess or quinsy may form between the tonsil or capsule and the superior constrictor muscle of the pharynx. Again, a mixed bacterial flora is usual, which includes anaerobes; incision and drainage is often required, although high-dose penicillin G, clindamycin or co-amoxiclav may be effective in reducing the risk of spread to fascial planes. Adequate drainage with appropriate antibiotic therapy has also reduced the need for subsequent tonsillectomy.

A parapharyngeal abscess may follow dental infection, tonsillitis or a quinsy, and should be drained via a collar incision at the level of the hyoid bone and treated with an antibiotic regimen similar to one used to manage peritonsillar abscess.

Ludwig's angina is a severe, acute cellulitis of the sublingual space and floor of the mouth and is frequently caused by poor dental hygiene. While the mortality has fallen from 50% to 10% since the advent of antibiotic therapy, the condition remains serious and life-threatening (Fritsch & Klein 1992). Frequently there is little or no pus, but when organisms have been cultured these are streptococci, staphylococci or anaerobic organisms. The flora is frequently mixed and antibiotic therapy is essential. A parenteral broad-spectrum agent such as cefotaxime and metronidazole or clindamycin and gentamicin would be appropriate choices.

CARDIOTHORACIC SURGERY

The oesophagus is normally colonized by organisms from the oropharynx and the upper respiratory tract. Many oesophageal operations are combined with gastric surgery; these and oesophageal strictures may lead to overgrowth of both aerobic and anaerobic organisms with Enterobacteriaceae, enterococci and streptococci (Findlay 1982). Single-dose prophylaxis with cefuroxime, cefotaxime or piperacillin, possibly with the addition of metronidazole for malignant problems, or alternatively co-amoxiclav is recommended.

The lower respiratory tract is normally sterile. However, pulmonary pathology for which surgery is performed may well change this situation and antibiotic prophylaxis is standard in most thoracic units. The common infecting organisms are streptococci, staphylococci, GNAB and oral anaerobes. This is true also of empyema and lung abscesses (Bartlett et al 1974). The same antibiotics as for oesophageal surgery are recommended; single dose for prophylaxis, but prolonged therapy for up to 6–8 weeks may be necessary in the treatment of lung abscess (Ch. 48).

Cardiac surgery

Before the advent of antibiotics, infective endocarditis (Ch. 49) had a mortality of 100%. This has been reduced to 30% by the introduction of antimicrobial agents and improved surgical techniques. The common organisms responsible are usually *Staph. aureus*, streptococci and coagulase-negative staphylococci, and occasionally yeasts. Surgery on the infected valve should always be covered by appropriate antimicrobial therapy (Ch. 49) and efforts made to eliminate any predisposing forms of infection such as dental disease.

Surgical technique is paramount in preventing early postoperative infection of prosthetic valves, although it is recognized that intravascular lines, pacing wires and urinary catheters provide other portals of infection. *Staph. aureus*, coagulase-negative staphylococci, streptococci and occasionally GNAB predominate (Ch. 49). Late infection of prosthetic valves may follow subsequent bacteraemia, particularly from dental procedures. The role of prophylactic regimens are discussed in Chapter 49.

Sternotomy wound infections and mediastinitis

Minor wound infections may occur in up to 16% of patients following sternotomy (Wilson et al 1988) and deep infections in 0.5–4.5% of patients (Bor et al 1983). The latter can produce mediastinitis, osteomyelitis, pericarditis, septicaemia, disruption of coronary artery grafts, wound dehiscence, infection of prosthetic valves and possibly death. *Staph. aureus* is frequently isolated but coagulase-negative staphylococci can be an important pathogen in the sternotomy site which may contain bone debris, haematomata, bone wax and suture wires.

Superficial infections should be drained and treated with an antistaphylococcal agent such as flucloxacillin until microbiological information is available. Deeper infections may require aggressive surgical debridement and high-dose, long-term antibiotic therapy based on the bacterial cultures from the deep tissues and local sensitivity patterns.

Mediastinitis may complicate cardiac surgery, oesophageal surgery, penetrating trauma and spontaneous or instrumental perforation. The surgical management depends upon the underlying cause and may involve thoracotomy with drainage of the mediastinum. The insertion of drains and irrigation with povidone iodine is favoured by some (Angelini et al 1990), but not others (Ko et al 1992). Whatever surgical management is instituted the use of broad-spectrum antibiotic therapy covering both aerobic and anaerobic organisms (e.g. cefotaxime and metronidazole, imipenem or co-amoxiclav) is mandatory.

Infections associated with cardiac pacemakers

Approximately a quarter of a million cardiac pacemakers are implanted each year. Infection may occur in the pocket created to hold the pacemaker, the subcutaneous electrodes, or in the tissues surrounding the leads. As might be expected the incidence of infection is higher for temporary external pacemakers (1–5%), than for permanent pacemakers (1%) (Sugarman & Young 1989). *Staph. aureus* and *Staph. epidermidis* are the predominant pathogens. *Staph. aureus* is more common within 2 weeks of operation, whereas *Staph. epidermidis* (coagulase-negative staphylococci) is more commonly associated with late infection (Lewis et al 1985). Fungal infections are rare and usually fatal (Wilson et al 1993).

Pacemaker pocket abscess causes swelling, erythema and discharge of pus or extrusion of the prosthesis. Bacteria, usually *Staph. aureus*, can be isolated from the blood in some patients. Mural endocarditis may ensue. Management generally requires removal of both pacemaker and leads (Lewis et al 1985). Thirty-two of 75 patients with infected pacemakers were treated conservatively with antibiotics, debridement and irrigation or aspiration of infected sites. All but one patient failed such therapy and required pacemaker removal. In the remaining 43 patients the infected pacemaker was treated primarily by removal, with successful resolution of the infection in all cases. Removal of the pacemaker is not a minor surgical procedure and may necessitate open heart surgery with cardiopulmonary bypass or inflow occlusion (Frame et al 1993).

Whilst prophylactic antibiotics are widely used when implanting a pacemaker, evidence for the efficacy is difficult to obtain. The infection rate is low (around 1%) and statistically valid trials are therefore virtually impossible to undertake. Bluhm et al (1986) compared flucloxacillin with placebo in a prospective double-blind trial of 106 patients and found no infection in either group with a follow-up of up to 35 months. Similarly, Ramsdale et al (1984) found no difference between patients who did and who did not receive antibiotic prophylaxis. However, like other implant procedures, although the incidence of infection is low the complications when they do occur can be life-threatening. Therefore it would seem wise to continue the normal practice to administer single-dose prophylaxis. Flucoxacillin or co-amoxiclav are suitable agents.

VASCULAR SURGERY

Arterial disease is on the increase. Consequently, the repertoire of vascular surgical procedures and range of materials from which the implanted grafts are made has increased. Graft infections are a major problem with considerable cost implications (Sugarman & Young 1989). Grafts to or below the groin are most vulnerable, particularly when there is distal tissue necrosis or infection.

Graft infection can be difficult to diagnose and culture of perigraft fluid is often unrewarding. The role of coagulase-negative staphylococci and other organisms when present within a biofilm bound to the prosthesis are often protected from antibiotic inactivation. Culture of these organisms may only be successful after graft removal and ultrasonication, which releases the organism.

The serious consequences of graft infection have quite reasonably led to almost universal prescribing of perioperative antibiotic prophylaxis. Those active against both *Staph. aureus* and *Staph. epidermidis* and, if the operation extends to or below the groin, against the Enterobacteriaceae, are recommended. There is little evidence to indicate that more than single-dose prophylaxis is necessary (Strachan 1992).

ABDOMINAL OPERATIONS

Prophylaxis

Although surgery for benign peptic ulceration has become uncommon, that for gastric malignancy continues unabated. In normal health the stomach is essentially sterile because of the high acid secretion. However, with gastric carcinoma and situations where the acidity is neutralized bacterial overgrowth readily occurs. The stomach becomes colonized with the Enterobacteriaceae and oral bacteria so that perioperative broad-spectrum antibiotic prophylaxis, with a second- or third-generation cephalosporin, ureidopenicillin or co-amoxiclav is indicated. This is also true for small bowel surgery. Anaerobic organisms may also be found in all these sites, especially the distal small bowel, and so metronidazole is usually added to regimens that lack anaerobic activity.

Splenectomy

The problems of overwhelming postsplenectomy sepsis (OPSI) are well recognized and are described in Chapter 11. In addition to the long term risk of infection there is increasing evidence that splenectomy increases the risk of immediate postoperative infection and, in 1982, Standage & Goss reported an incidence of 29% morbidity, mostly infective and 9.4% mortality in a series of 277 patients who underwent splenectomy. The majority of the deaths were from infective complications. Operative mortality occurred in 15% of patients after incidental splenectomy, which was markedly higher than the incidence after splenectomy for other pathologies. The fact that it is common surgical practice to place a drain in the splenic bed at operation may have increased the incidence of infection (Rao 1988). Despite the findings of Standage & Goss the incidence of infective complications would appear to be higher in those patients undergoing splenectomy for malignant disease than when splenectomy was performed for trauma.

Biliary tract operations

Bacterial colonization of the bile occurs with increasing age, acute cholecystitis, gallstones and strictures of the common bile duct, be they benign or malignant. The Enterobacteriaceae and faecal streptococci predominate; anaerobes are uncommon. Endoscopic retrograde choledochopancreatography (ERCP) is commonly performed in situations in which the bile may be colonized, and antibiotic prophylaxis is indicated to prevent septicaemia occurring during the injection of contrast media. Occasionally, pseudomonas septicaemia has been recorded from organisms contaminating the bridge of the endoscope.

Patients with colonized bile are at a higher risk of postoperative infection and have been recommended to receive prophylactic antibiotics. This hypothesis was tested in 644 patients who received preoperative prophylaxis with sulbactam–ampicillin. The bile was found to be colonized in 121 (19% of patients) and the incidence of infection in this group was 22% compared with 2% in patients with sterile bile ($p < 0.001$). However, more than half of the patients who had colonized bile (65 of 121) had no high-risk factor (Wells et al 1989). For this reason, it is recommended that single-dose antibiotic prophylaxis be given to all patients undergoing open cholecystectomy, which is the standard practice in most surgical units (Cahill & Payne 1988).

The advent of laparoscopic surgery has led to a reappraisal of the need for prophylaxis. In large series of laparoscopic cholecystectomies, the incidence of infection is exceptionally low (0.5%), and is mainly infection of the umbilical port hole, through which the gallbladder is removed (Southern Surgeons Club 1991, Peters et al 1991, Litwin et al 1992). The reason for this difference in the incidence of infection is not clear. There is considerable evidence that postoperative infection after open cholecystectomy is caused by organisms which colonize the bile (Edwards et al 1990), and it could be anticipated that bile contamination would be at least as high during a laparoscopic operation. However, the degree of wound tissue damage is different. Because of the low incidence of infective complications the role of antibiotic prophylaxis for laparoscopic cholecystectomy remains uncertain. Until studies clearly show that prophylaxis is not indicated, single-dose

prophylaxis is recommended for elective cholecystectomy, however this is performed.

Appendicectomy

Appendicectomy remains a commonly performed abdominal operation either electively, for acute appendicitis, 'en passant' to another intra-abdominal procedure, or at an interval event after the resolution of an appendix abscess. When performed for acute appendicitis the appendix ranges from normal to perforated with the release of faecoliths into the peritoneal cavity. Histological examination of the removed appendix often shows that surgical assessment of the state of the appendix at operation is unreliable – an apparently normal appendix may have mucosal appendicitis, an inflamed appendix may be histologically perforated and an apparently purulent, perforated appendix may not in fact show transmural perforation or infarction.

Infection is more common in patients with perforated or gangrenous appendices, and antibiotic therapy rather than prophylaxis is indicated. Pieper et al (1982), in a retrospective series of more than 1000 appendicectomies, showed an overall incidence of infective complications of 11.5%. This ranged from 5% in patients with a normal appendix to 33.6% for those with a perforated appendix. Some have contended that wound infection should be uncommon in low risk patients such as children and those from whom a normal appendix is removed (Kizilcan et al 1992). Krukowski et al (1988), in a meta-analysis of antibiotic prophylaxis studies in appendicectomy, showed a 10.4% incidence of infection in low-risk and 34.9% infection in high-risk patients in the control (no antibiotic) groups. Thus current opinion favours the use of antimicrobial prophylaxis in all operations for acute appendicitis.

Anaerobic organisms, particularly *Bacteroides* spp., are common in wound infections after appendicectomy and this has led to the widespread use of metronidazole in Europe and similar antianaerobic agents in North America. However, the results with metronidazole are not always favourable. Bates et al (1992) reported 15.7% infection in low-risk and 31.8% infection in high-risk patients with rectal metronidazole and Krukowski's meta-analysis shows an incidence of 7.4% infection in low-risk and 31.9% in high risk patients when metronidazole alone is used, either intravenously or rectally. Many studies were subsequently performed to assess metronidazole in combination with another antibiotic active against the aerobic flora. This same meta-analysis suggests that an infection rate of 3.8% in low-risk and 15% in high-risk patients is then achieved. Wilson et al (1987) assessed the value of a single perioperative dose of cefotetan 2 g to a 5-day regimen of metronidazole per rectum. Fourteen (9.5%) of 148 patients receiving the metronidazole alone developed postoperative infection, whereas 3 (2.1%) of 141 patients who received the cefotetan did so ($p < 0.05$). The second- and third-generation cephalosporins as well as the cephamycin antibiotics have become popular prophylaxis for appendicectomy, and again Krukowski's meta-analysis has shown an infection of 2.9% in low-risk and 21.2% in high-risk patients when these agents are used.

Many studies do not separate high- and low-risk patients: al-Dhohayan et al (1993) have shown co-amoxiclav to be at least as effective as metronidazole and gentamicin; Salam et al (1994) have shown piperacillin to be as effective as cefoxitin; Pokorny et al (1991) found ticarcillin–clavulanate (Timentin) to be as effective as triple therapy with ampicillin, gentamicin and clindamycin, while Uhari et al (1992) showed that imipenem–cilastatin was as effective as tobramycin and metronidazole for appendicitis in children.

Coldham et al (1993) have suggested that single-dose prophylaxis is appropriate and cost-effective for appendicectomy, and many surgeons would be happy to consider this for low-risk patients. The duration of therapy required for high-risk patients with perforated or gangrenous appendicitis remains to be determined. Provided the infected focus has been adequately extirpated, with or without peritoneal toilet, it is likely that 24 or 48 h therapy will be as effective, although 5 days' treatment is usually administered.

It remains to be seen what effect minimally invasive techniques for appendicitis will have on postoperative infection (Wilson 1995). If infection rates are significantly lowered, as has become apparent following laparoscopic cholecystectomy, then current practice may need to be reassessed. However, it should be remembered that appendicectomy is normally performed for an acute, infective episode, whereas cholecystectomy is performed in an elective, non-infected situation.

Colorectal surgery

The colon, particularly the descending colon and rectum contain the largest number of bacteria and surgery to these sites is associated with the highest incidence of postoperative infection and associated mortality. With good surgical technique the contamination of the tissues during colorectal resection should be no greater than when operating on other areas of the gastro-intestinal tract, although synergistic interaction of aerobes and anaerobes increases the risk of infection.

Bowel preparation

Most surgeons would accept that preoperative bowel preparation is a sensible if not essential part of the preparation of a patient for elective colorectal surgery. This view has been challenged (Irving & Scrimgeour 1987, Santos et al 1994) since there is little evidence to support the concept that adequate bowel preparation reduces the

bacterial contamination of the tissues at the time of operation. Indeed, some forms of bowel preparation, such as the osmotic cathartic mannitol 10%, have been shown to increase the viable bacterial count of the residual flora in the mucus of the colon (Keighley et al 1981). Nevertheless, it remains normal practice in many countries to attempt to remove the bulk of faecal material from the colon preoperatively. The use of oral antibiotics has become an important part of this preparation in the USA (see below). When operating on the obstructed colon the faecal contents can be evacuated by irrigation, on the operating table, using a Foley catheter via the appendix stump and disposable anaesthetic trunking inserted into the cut distal end of the colon, to lead the irrigation fluid away from the operative field.

Oral antibiotics

Attempts have been made to reduce the perioperative bacterial contamination that occurs when the colon is transected by reducing the bacterial load in the gut using antibiotics preoperatively. The Nichols–Condon regimen of antibiotic prophylaxis favoured in the USA is neomycin 1 g and erythromycin base 1 g given at 13.00, 14.00 and 23.00 h on the day prior to operation (Nichols et al 1972). Erythromycin base is used because, like neomycin, it is poorly absorbed. However, this route of antibiotic administration has not found favour in Europe (Keighley et al 1979, Weaver et al 1986) and, in practice, most colorectal surgeons in the USA and some in Europe combine preoperative oral administration with perioperative parenteral prophylaxis (Solla & Rothenberger 1990).

Selective decontamination to remove or suppress the GNAB in the colon preoperatively has been advocated on the basis that such contamination that did occur would be with the anaerobes only, thus preventing the synergistic interaction necessary for postoperative wound and intra-abdominal infections. Oral ciprofloxacin has been shown to remove selectively GNAB from the gastro-intestinal tract within 24 h using a cathartic agent in addition to the quinolone (Taylor et al 1990). In a subsequent large multi-centre study to investigate the efficacy of this form of bowel preparation after elective colorectal surgery, the incidence of wound infection was 11% in the antibiotic group and 23% in the controls ($p = 0.007$). All patients received the same parenteral antibiotic; piperacillin 4 g i.v. on induction of anaesthesia. When all operation-related infections were taken into account, the group receiving oral ciprofloxacin had a 14.5% incidence of infection compared with 33% in the group that did not ($p = 0.0002$) (Taylor et al 1994).

Despite this evidence that a form of selective decontamination of the colon may be of benefit preoperatively, other attempts to assess this form of antibiotic use have yielded mixed results. Lazorthes et al (1982), in a small study of 90 patients undergoing elective colorectal operations, gave 30 patients kanamycin and metronidazole orally, a further 30 patients the same drugs parenterally on induction of anaesthesia and a further group of 30 patients the same drugs preoperatively by mouth as well as parenterally at operation. Despite the small numbers, the difference in the incidence of infection in each of the groups (30%, 23%, 3.3%) was statistically significant ($p < 0.01$). However, Lau et al (1988), in a study of 194 patients undergoing elective colorectal surgery for carcinoma, randomized patients to receive oral neomycin and erythromycin base, systemic metronidazole and gentamicin or a combination of both regimens. Postoperative septic complications occurred in 27.4%, 11.9% and 12.3%, respectively. They concluded that systemic was preferable to oral prophylaxis, but that a combination of both added no special benefit. Stellato et al (1990), in a similar study, randomized 146 evaluable patients to receive oral neomycin and erythromycin, parenteral cefoxitin or a combination of both. The incidence of infective complications was 11.4%, 11.7% and 7.8%. These differences were not statistically significant and they concluded that no advantage was gained by combining oral and parenteral antibiotic prophylaxis. Playforth et al (1988) reported wound infection rates of 27.6% in patients who received no oral antibiotic and 13.9% in the group that did ($p = 0.04$). They concluded that it was important in colorectal operations to ensure not only adequate tissue levels of parenteral antimicrobials but also to reduce the risk of endogenous bacterial infection by partial decontamination of the bowel.

Whilst it is not normal practice in Europe, it is likely that a combination of preoperative oral and perioperative parenteral antibiotic prophylaxis is likely to reduce the incidence of infection to its lowest level in this form of surgery.

Parenteral antibiotics

The work of Willis and others in the 1970s established the importance of activity against the anaerobes, particularly *Bacteroides* spp., of the antibiotic regimen used for prophylaxis in appendicectomy and colorectal surgery (Willis et al 1976, 1977). Although a number of drugs such as clindamycin, cefoxitin and tinidazole have activity against the anaerobes, metronidazole has been the mainstay of both therapy and prophylaxis in this area. Metronidazole can be given intravenously, orally or rectally, and all routes have been shown to be effective. Parenteral metronidazole is by far the most expensive formulation.

However, it is not only the anaerobes which cause infection after appendicectomy or colorectal surgery, and hence it is common practice to add an agent active against the aerobic flora of the gastro-intestinal tract. More recently, it has become apparent that this cover should include both Gram-positive and Gram-negative organisms. The incidence of staphylococcal infection should not be underestimated. In a study of infection after elective colorectal operations in which patients received either piperacillin or gentamicin and metronidazole, Walker et al (1988) found 25% of the wound infections to be staphylococcal. Similarly, Morris et al (1990) found a high incidence of Gram-positive organisms in particular *Staph. aureus*, in infections after patients had received aztreonam with metronidazole. They concluded that the antibacterial combination chosen for prophylaxis in elective colorectal surgery must include adequate cover against Gram-positive organisms.

The literature is replete with clinical trials of the efficacy of various antibiotics for prophylaxis in elective colorectal surgery. Most studies have shown no or little difference between the agents used. Although it is no longer ethical to conduct placebo-controlled studies in colorectal surgery, it is of considerable interest to note the wide variation in the infection rates from different centres. They vary from approximately 5% infection in Scandinavia, where the use of doxycycline is popular (Bergman & Solhaug 1987), to 26% in the UK (Karran et al 1993). Such differences cannot reflect the influence of the antibiotic chosen alone. There are many factors which determine the incidence of infection, of which the preoperative condition of the patient as well as the surgical expertise and degree of tissue damage is paramount.

As emphasized previously, there is no evidence that multiple-dose prophylaxis confers any benefit over a single-dose regimen. Broad-spectrum activity against both anaerobes and aerobes, both Gram positive and Gram negative, is essential. Traditionally, a combination of gentamicin and metronidazole, with or without the addition of ampicillin to improve the activity against *Enterococcus faecalis*, has been considered to be the 'gold standard'. However, the possible toxic effect of gentamicin has encouraged the use of alternative regimens such as a second- or third-generation cephalosporin or a ureido-penicillin plus metronidazole. Co-amoxiclav or imipenem are also used, without the addition of metronidazole.

PERITONITIS

Peritonitis is a generalized or localized inflammation of the peritoneum leading to formation of a serous exudate which rapidly becomes infected and purulent. Non-bacterial causes of peritonitis, usually chemical peritonitis, may be caused by the leakage of sterile gastric juices, bile, urine or pancreatic fluid into the peritoneal cavity. Meconium peritonitis may occur after intrauterine perforation of the gastro-intestinal tract, while granulomatous peritonitis may result from sarcoidosis or tuberculosis. Occasionally, drugs, such as isoniazid, practolol and intraperitoneal cytolytics for malignant disease, may cause acute or chronic peritonitis. Starch peritonitis from talc on surgical gloves is a historical cause.

Primary peritonitis

Primary or spontaneous bacterial peritonitis (SBP) is unusual. It may occur in children who have undergone splenectomy or with the nephrotic syndrome, but is more commonly seen in adult patients with cirrhosis and ascites. In this latter group the prevalence has been estimated as 8–27% with a resultant mortality of 48–57%.

The route by which bacteria gain access to the peritoneal cavity is not clear. Bacteria could gain access to the ascitic fluid by translocation from the colon, although bacteraemia occurring in the presence of abnormal host resistance, intrahepatic shunting and impaired opsonic activity of ascitic fluid is probably more likely. Bacteraemia is, in itself, more likely to occur in these patients because of compromized neutrophil and reticulo-endothelial function in cirrhotic patients. The usual pathogens are *Escherichia coli*, streptococci, and *Klebsiella pneumoniae*. A single organism is usually cultured. In one-third of patients no organism is isolated (culture-negative neutrocytic ascites). Peritonitis is diagnosed by the presence of an ascitic fluid neutrophil count greater than $0.5 \times 10^9/l$, negative ascitic fluid culture, no other cause of intra-abdominal infection, no prior antibiotic treatment within 30 days and no alternative explanation for the elevated white cell count.

Antibiotic therapy should be guided by laboratory data. Because anaerobic organisms are unusual, cefotaxime, piperacillin or co-amoxiclav continued for 10–14 days are usually adequate.

SBP recurrence is common, and has a high mortality. Prophylactic measures include reduction of ascitic fluid by diuretic therapy as well as more specific management of any precipitating disease. Some have recommended prolonged use of antibiotics such as ciprofloxacin, which selectively removes the GNAB from the gastro-intestinal tract, although long-term morbidity or the frequency of hospitalization is unaltered (Bhuva et al 1994).

Secondary peritonitis

There are many causes of bacterial peritonitis, ranging from initially sterile collections of gastric fluid or bile, which subsequently become infected, to perforation of colonic diverticulae or carcinoma, leading to faecal peritonitis. The more distal the lesion is in the gastro-intestinal tract the heavier the bacterial load. Wherever the lesion, the Enterobacteriaceae, acting either alone or in synergy with anaerobic bacteria, predominate. The role of enterococci and *Pseudomonas aeruginosa* as primary pathogens remains controversial. The former is frequently isolated from intra-abdominal infection but rarely as a single isolate, and pseudomonal infections are more common in repeat laparotomies than as a primary pathogen. Peritonitis following blunt or penetrating abdominal trauma may introduce exogenous infection, although the organisms from the injured viscus are most likely to be the pathogens.

The management of bacterial peritonitis involves adequate preoperative resuscitation, laparotomy with repair or resection of the damaged viscera with or without faecal diversion, and appropriate antibiotic therapy such as cefotaxime and metronidazole or clindamycin and gentamicin. Since many of these patients will be seriously ill, the points discussed in Chapter 41 should also be considered. Saline or antibiotic peritoneal lavage is thought to have some merit, but the use of intraperitoneal drains should be minimized.

The antibiotic regimen should include activity against both aerobic and anaerobic organisms. In most situations 5 days' high-dose therapy is sufficient. In future, other forms of supportive therapy, such as monoclonal antibodies against endotoxin, TNF and interleukin receptors, may prove helpful, but at present they are unproven.

Peritoneal lavage

The use of antibiotic solutions to lavage the infected peritoneal cavity has had some advocates who have used parenteral tetracycline together with a tetracycline solution (1 mg/ml saline) with impressive results (Stewart 1978, Krukowski et al 1986). However, the meticulous technical protocol used by these workers cannot be ignored, and whether the excellent results can be attributed to tetracycline lavage or to their expertise has been questioned (Sauven et al 1986). Anxieties that the lavage will spread bacterial contamination to the remaining 'uncontaminated' peritoneal cavity, or that intra-abdominal adhesions may result seem unfounded. The lavage certainly removes debris from the peritoneal cavity which would otherwise function as a foreign body. Silverman et al (1986) reported infection in 25 (34%) of 74 patients who had saline lavage compared with 15 (18%) of 85 patients whose peritoneal cavity was lavaged with tetracycline solution ($p < 0.05$), which counters the argument, suggesting that it is not purely the mechanical debridement which is of benefit.

Pancreatitis

Pancreatitis remains a common cause of acute peritonitis. The diagnosis is usually straightforward and, with appropriate resuscitation and analgesia, most patients recover. However, 5–10% die from the initial attack, and infection leading to septicaemia and multiple organ failure is one of the more common causes. Acute pancreatitis causes necrosis of the peripancreatic parenchyma, while inflammation of the pancreas may lead to duct necrosis. There is considerable oedema of the retroperitoneal and adjacent tissues (the retroperitoneal 'burn'), including the stomach, colon and upper small bowel.

Why and by what route the necrotic pancreas becomes infected is not clear. Pancreatitis frequently occurs in the presence of gallstones and here the bile is frequently colonized. It is most probable that passage of bacteria from the bowel lumen or from the bile into the pancreatic duct is the route of infection, although bacterial translocation through the colonic wall into the lymphatics and retroperitoneal inflammatory oedema is also possible. The value of antibiotics used from the onset of the attack remains debatable. Many trials report too few patients and use possibly inappropriate antibiotics such as ampicillin or cephalothin. The incidence of infection has certainly not been altered by these antibiotics (Finch et al 1976, Stone & Fabian 1980); perhaps broader spectrum antibiotics may have resulted in a different outcome. In a recent study in which 74 patients with necrotizing pancreatitis were randomized to imipenem–cilastatin 0.5 g i.v. for 2 weeks or no antibiotic, there was a significant benefit in favour of the antibiotic group (12.2% v 30.3% sepsis, p < 0.01) (Pederzoli et al 1993). A similarly beneficial result has been reported by Widdison et al (1994) using cefotaxime in an experimental study of infected pancreatitis in cats.

The diagnosis of infection in acute pancreatitis can be very difficult. The onset of sepsis and multiple organ failure may occur despite the fact that no organism can be isolated from the necrotic pancreatic tissue. A sudden deterioration in a patient's condition may be associated with infection and ultrasound or computed-tomography guided fine-needle aspiration of the peripancreatic tissues may define whether the collection is infected or not. However, when deterioration occurs debridement and drainage of the pancreatic tissues may be indicated, whether or not the tissues are infected. Antibiotics are usually administered.

Abdominal trauma

Approximately 50% of deaths after major injuries occur within a few minutes of the accident and are caused by brain stem, spinal cord, cardiac or major blood vessel injury. Other patients die within 2 h of respiratory failure or haemorrhage into body cavities or brain tissue, but approximately 20% of deaths after major injury occur over the next 20 weeks and some 80% die of organ failure and infection. This infection may not be caused by the trauma but may be associated with endotracheal intubation, blood transfusion, catheterization, intensive care unit management, or nasogastric suction, all of which increase the risk of infection following trauma (Oller 1990). The risk of infection after abdominal trauma depends on the mechanism of injury, and the organs involved. The interval between

injury and treatment is an important factor as is the occurrence of hypovolaemic shock, particularly when associated with vascular injury.

Weigelt et al (1987) in a review of 949 patients showed a higher incidence of infection after shotgun injuries (20–25%) than after gunshot wounds (3.6–16%) or stab injuries (4–4.7%). Similarly, Dellenger et al (1984) showed that 42 (30%) of 140 patients sustaining gunshot wounds developed infection compared with 31 (16%) of 190 patients who sustained stab wounds. The incidence of infection was higher when the colon was injured (35%) than when there was no colonic injury (18%).

Weigelt et al (1987) also showed that the incidence of infection increased when four or more intra-abdominal organs were injured. In a review of injuries after vascular trauma Wilson et al (1989) correlated the incidence of intra-abdominal infection with the blood pressure on admission to the accident and emergency department. Where the blood pressure was initially unrecordable, 40% of those surviving developed intra-abdominal infection; the incidence of intra-abdominal infection was 25% when the blood pressure was below 70 mmHg, 23% where the blood pressure was 70–90 mmHg and 11% where the blood pressure was in excess of 90 mmHg. It was initially postulated that bacterial translocation occurred more commonly in patients with hypovolaemic shock. Bacterial translocation does occur after traumatic injury but may be independent of haemorrhagic shock and its clinical significance remains in some doubt (Brathwaite et al 1993).

As might be expected, infection is more common after colonic injury. In a multicentre review of 54 361 patients, 2739 (5%) required laparotomy and the colon was injured in 195 (11%) of these patients (Ross et al 1992). This was the organ most commonly injured, with small bowel injury occurring in 4%, liver injury in 3% and splenic injury in 3%. The factor most closely associated with the development of infection after trauma is peritoneal contamination by intestinal contents. In addition, the presence of a stoma is a significant risk factor and this has led to a re-evaluation of primary repair of the colon following such injuries. In the civilian context, the majority of colon injuries can be managed by repair or resection with primary anastomosis. Ivatury et al (1993), in a multiple regression analysis of risk factors in 252 patients sustaining penetrating injuries of the colon, found the abdominal trauma index and the presence of a colostomy as the significant independent risk factors associated with the occurrence of intra-abdominal abscess. Demetriades et al (1992) studied prospectively 100 patients with bullet injuries of the colon. Seventy-six per cent had primary repair of the colon, with 11.8% developing abdominal sepsis. This compared with 29.2% sepsis in the remaining 24 patients. In a review of 137 patients with intraperitoneal colonic injury, George et al (1988) reported an 18% complication rate in the 88 patients managed by primary closure and 42% in the 37 patients managed by end colostomy or ileostomy.

Nutrition is as important in the traumatized patient as in other patients requiring major surgery, particularly when the integrity of the gastro-intestinal tract has been disturbed. Much has been written about the role played by individual elements of the diet, which is beyond the scope of this chapter. Nevertheless, there is increasing evidence to suggest that enteral is preferable to parenteral nutrition, and may reduce the incidence of postoperative septic complications. Kudsk et al (1994) studied protein levels in 68 severely injured patients with abdominal trauma indexes of 15 or more, randomized to enteral or parenteral feeding. They concluded that patients fed enterally showed lower levels of acute phase proteins, primarily caused by septic complications after severe trauma, and higher levels of constitutive proteins. Moore et al (1992) conducted a meta-analysis of trials to compare enteral with parenteral feeding postoperatively and assess the incidence of septic complications; 118 patients receiving enteral and 112 patients receiving parenteral nutrition were evaluable. There were significantly ($p = 0.01$) fewer enteral patients (18%) with septic complications than those receiving parenteral nutrition (35%).

Clearly these patients require parenteral antibiotic therapy and it might be thought that SDD (Ch. 44) might be of value in this situation. However, in 72 patients who had sustained multiple trauma with chest injuries requiring intermittent positive pressure ventilation, and who had a mean injury severity score of 29.5, Hammond et al (1994) reported no difference in the number of patients infected (11 receiving SDD vs 11 receiving placebo), the number of infections (17 vs 16) or deaths (5 vs 3). The duration of stay both in the intensive care unit and in the hospital were also similar.

Infection following abdominal trauma which involves the gastro-intestinal tract is caused by both aerobic and anaerobic bacterial flora. Brook (1988) has shown that infection is biphasic with the Enterobacteriaceae as the major pathogens in the peritonitis stage and anaerobes, particularly *Bacteroides fragilis* in the later abscess stage. For this reason, the antibiotic(s) must be active against both aerobic and anaerobic organisms.

The pharmacokinetics of antibiotics in trauma patients may be important. Reed et al (1992) have shown a significant expansion in the apparent volume of distribution for amikacin, which correlated with fluid resuscitation. They previously noted failure to achieve adequate levels using standard regimens (Ericsson et al 1989) and believed this was due to apparent underdosing. In their original study they found no difference between 72 and 24 h treatment with amikacin and clindamycin in 150 abdominal trauma patients requiring laparotomy (19% vs 21%). Their data suggested that higher doses of the antibiotic were more effective than longer courses in reducing infection in these patients.

There is increasing evidence that short-course, high-dose therapy is indicated in these patients, provided there has been adequate surgical elimination of the source of infection. Oreskovich et al (1982) showed no difference between 24 and 5 days' antibiotic administration in patients with penetrating abdominal trauma nor did Fabian et al (1992) when they compared 24 h with 5 days in 500 traumatized patients. Nichols et al (1993) has suggested that patients can be stratified into those requiring short-term therapy and those who may benefit from longer term therapy, although he showed no difference between short-term therapy of 2 days and a similar group of 145 historical control subjects who received 5 days of antibiotic therapy. The Surgical Infection Society of North America has recently published guidelines on the treatment of intra-abdominal infection. They recommend that prolonged antibiotic therapy is not required in patients sustaining traumatic enteric perforations if they are operated on within 12 h of injury (Bohnen et al 1992).

LIVER ABSCESS

Liver abscess is uncommon in the West and tends to be diagnosed in the more elderly population (Branum et al 1990). However, it can occur in any age group and may be difficult to diagnose. Two types of abscess are well recognized – pyogenic and amoebic; both need to be differentiated from other cystic conditions in the liver.

Pyogenic abscess

Pyogenic abscess used to more commonly follow portal pyaemia associated with acute appendicitis. However, with the widespread use of antibiotics in managing appendicitis, pyogenic abscess is now more common in the elderly where malignancy, biliary sepsis and diverticulitis disease are more common. A pyogenic abscess may be single or multiple, and is most often found in the right lobe of the liver. Patients with compromised host defences are more susceptible. For example, unusual pathogens such as *Mycobacterium avium/intracellulare* in patients with acquired immune deficiency syndrome (AIDS) (Cappell 1991) and *Yersinia enterocolitica* associated with cirrhosis, diabetes mellitus, alcoholism or malnutrition have been reported (Elliott & Partridge 1991). In over half of patients no cause is found.

The organism responsible for pyogenic abscess often reflects the aetiology. Abscesses are usually polybacterial. Anaerobes are particularly important (Brook & Fraizer 1993). *Streptococcus milleri* is a microaerophilic commensal of the gastro-intestinal tract and has recently emerged as an important cause of hepatic abscesses (Allison et al 1984, Molina et al 1991). *Klebsiella* and *Esch. coli* and occasionally *Proteus vulgaris* and *Pseudomonas* spp. are commonly responsible.

The diagnosis can be difficult. The classic features of abdominal pain, pyrexia, anorexia, malaise and weight loss are less common, particularly in older persons. A high white cell count and raised erythrocyte sedimentation rate are common. The chest X-ray may show a sympathetic pleural effusion or an air/fluid level within the liver; the latter carries a worse prognosis (Chou et al 1995). Ultrasound scans or a computerized tomography (CT) scan are usually diagnostic. A CT scan with enhancement can detect an abscess of 1 cm diameter (Halvorsen et al 1984).

Treatment of pyogenic liver abscess relies upon adequate drainage and appropriate antibiotic therapy (Krige 1995). Drainage may be either open or percutaneous needle aspiration. The insertion of a catheter under ultrasonic or CT guidance is now widely practised (Hashimoto et al 1995). Although antibiotics have been instilled via the needle or irrigated via the catheter this is not usually required. Where radiographic expertise is lacking, or when needle aspiration or catheter drainage fails, open transperitoneal drainage should be performed (Chou et al 1994). This is more likely in multiloculated or multiple abscesses. Moore et al (1994) have suggested that left lobe abscesses in children are best treated by elective early open surgical drainage.

Antibiotic therapy is essential and, until culture and sensitivity results are available, broad-spectrum therapy active against aerobes and anaerobes should be given. A combination of penicillin, gentamicin and metronidazole is appropriate, while vancomycin can be of use in the penicillin allergic patient. Therapy should be guided by response and repeat ultrasound examination. Short-course therapy of 10–14 days may suffice for those abscesses drained adequately, while up to 4 weeks or more may be necessary for less rapidly responding infections. *Streptococcus milleri* infections are resistant to metronidazole, and penicillin is the drug of choice. Cefotaxime is a better choice than gentamicin in the elderly with reduced renal function.

References

al-Dhohayan A, Alsebayl M, Shibl A, Al Eshalwy S, Kattan K, Al Saleh M 1993 Comparative study of augmentin versus metronidazole/gentamicin in the prevention of infections after appendicectomy. *European Surgical Research* 25: 60–64

Allison H F, Immelman E J, Forder A A 1984 Pyogenic liver abscess caused by *Streptococcus milleri*. *South African Medical Journal* 65: 432–425

Angelini G D, Lamarra M, Azzu A A, Bryan A J 1990 Wound infection following early repeat sternotomy for postoperative bleeding. An experience utilizing intraoperative irrigation with povidone iodine. *Journal of Cardiovascular Surgery Torino* 31: 793–795

Bartlett J G, Gorbach S L, Thadepalli H, Finegold S M 1974 Bacteriology of empyema. *Lancet* i: 338–340

Bates T, Roberts J V, Smith K, German K A 1992 A randomized trial of one versus three doses of augmentin as wound prophylaxis in at-risk abdominal surgery. *Postgraduate Medical Journal* 68: 811–816

Beath S V, Kelly D A, Booth I W, Freeman J, Buckels J A C, Mayer A D 1994 Post-operative care of children undergoing small bowel and liver transplantation. *British Journal of Intensive Care* 4: 302–308

Bergman L, Solhaug J H 1987 Single dose chemoprophylaxis in elective colorectal surgery: comparison between doxycycline plus metronidazole and doxycycline. *Annals of Surgery* 205: 77–81

Bhuva M, Ganger D, Jensen D 1994 Spontaneous bacterial peritonitis: an update on evaluation management and prevention. *American Journal of Medicine* 97: 169–175

Bion J F, Badger I, Crosby H A et al 1994 Selective decontamination of the digestive tract reduces Gram-negative pulmonary colonization but not systemic endotoxemia in patients undergoing elective liver transplantation. *Critical Care Medicine* 22: 40–49

Bluhm G, Nordlander R, Ransjo U 1986 Antibiotic prophylaxis in pacemaker surgery: a prospective double blind trial with systemic administration of antibiotic versus placebo at implantation of cardiac pacemakers. *Pacing and Clinical Electrophysiology* 9: 720–726

Bohnen J M, Solomkin J S, Dellinger E P, Bjornson H S, Page C P 1992 Guidelines for clinical care: antiinfective agents for intra-abdominal infection: a Surgical Infection Society policy statement. *Archives of Surgery* 127: 83–89

Bor D H, Rose R M, Modlin J F, Weintraub R, Friedland G H 1983 Mediastinitis after cardiovascular surgery. *Reviews of Infectious Diseases* 5: 885–897

Braga M, Vignali A, Radaelli G, Gianotti L, Di Carlo V 1992 Association between perioperative blood transfusion and postoperative infection in patients having elective operations for gastrointestinal cancer. *European Journal of Surgery* 158: 531–536

Branum G D, Tyson G S, Branum M A, Meyers W C 1990 Hepatic abscess. Changes in etiology, diagnosis and management. *Annals of Surgery* 212: 655–662

Brathwaite C E M, Ross S E, Nagele R, Mure A J, O'Malley K F, Garcia-Perez F A 1993 Bacterial translocation occurs in humans after traumatic injury: evidence using immuno-fluorescence. *Journal of Trauma* 34: 586–590

Bremmelgaard A, Raahave D, Beier-Holgersen R, Pedersen J V, Andersen S, Sorensen A I 1989 Computer aided surveillance of surgical infections and identification of risk factors. *Journal of Hospital Infection* 13: 1–18

Brook I 1988 Management of infection following intra-abdominal trauma. *Annals of Emergency Medicine* 17(6): 626–632

Brook I, Fraizer E H 1993 Role of anaerobic bacteria and liver abscesses in children. *Paediatric Infectious Disease Journal* 12: 743–747

Burrows L, Tartter P 1982 Effect of blood transfusion on colonic malignancy rates. *Lancet* ii: 662

Cahill C J, Payne J A 1988 Current practice in biliary surgery. *British Journal of Surgery* 75: 1169–1172

Cappell M S 1991 Hepatobiliary manifestations of the acquired immune deficiency syndrome. *American Journal of Gastro-enterology* 86: 1–15

Carrico C J, Meakins J L, Marshall J C, Fry D, Maier R V 1986 Multiple-organ-failure syndrome. *Archives of Surgery* 121: 196–208

Chappuis C W, Frey D J, Dietzen C D, Panetta T P, Buechter K J, Cohn I 1991 Management of penetrating colon injuries. A prospective randomized trial. *Annals of Surgery* 213: 492–497

Chou F F, Sheen-Chen S M, Chen Y S, Chen M C, Chen F C, Tai D I 1994 Prognostic factors for pyogenic abscess of the liver. *Journal of the American College of Surgeons* 179: 727–732

Chou F F, Sheen-Chen S M, Chen Y S, Lee T Y 1995 The comparison of clinical course and results of treatment between gas-forming and non gas-forming pyogenic liver abscess. *Archives of Surgery* 130: 401–405

Classen D C, Evans R S, Pestotnik S L, Horn S D, Menlove R L, Burke J P 1992 The timing of prophylactic administration of antibiotics and the risk of surgical wound infection. *New England Journal of Medicine* 326: 281–286

Coldham G J, Mickleson J C, Ali P G 1993 Antibiotic protocol for appendicectomy – costs and benefits of single dose therapy. *New Zealand Medical Journal* 106: 13–14

Cruse P J E 1992 Classification of operations and audit of infection. In: Taylor E W (ed) Infection in surgical practice. Oxford University Press, Oxford

Culver D H, Horan T C, Gaines R P et al 1991 Surgical wound infection rates by wound class, operative proce-dure, and patient risk index. National Nosocomial Infections Surveillance System. *American Journal of Medicine* 91 (suppl 3B): 152S–157S

Dellinger E P, Oreskovich M R, Wertz M J, Hamasaki V, Lennard E S 1984 Risk of infection following laparotomy for penetrating abdominal injury. *Archives of Surgery* 119: 20–27

Demetriades D, Charalambides D, Pantanowitz D 1992 Gunshot wounds of the colon: role of primary repair. *Annals of the Royal College of Surgeons* 74: 381–384

Di Piro J T, Chung R P F, Bowden T A, Mannsburger J A 1986 Single dose antibiotic prophylaxis of surgical wound infec-tions. *American Journal of Surgery* 152: 552–559

Dixon J M, Armstrong C P, Duffy S W, Chetty U, Davies G C 1984 A randomized prospective trial comparing the value of intravenous and preincisional cefamandole in reducing postoperative sepsis after operations upon the gastro-intestinal tract. *Surgery, Gynecology and Obstetrics* 158: 303–307

Donnelly J P 1993 Selective decontamination of the digestive tract and its role in antimicrobial prophylaxis. *Journal of Antimicrobial Chemotherapy* 31: 813–829

Edwards G F S, Lindsay G, Taylor E W, West of Scotland Surgical Infection Study Group 1990 Bacteriological assessment of ampicillin with sulbactam as antibiotic pro-phylaxis in patients undergoing biliary tract operations. *Journal of Hospital Infection* 16: 249–255

Elek S D, Conen P E 1957 The virulence of *Staphylococcus pyogenes* for man. A study of the problems of wound infection. *British Journal of Experimental Pathology* 38: 573–586

Elliott T B, Partridge B W 1991 Multiple hepatic abscesses due to *Yersinia enterocolitica*. *Australian and New Zealand Journal of Surgery* 61: 708–710

Ericsson C D, Fischer R P, Rowlands B J, Hunt C, Miller-Crotchett P, Reed L 1989 Prophylactic antibiotics in trauma: the hazards of underdosing. *Journal of Trauma* 29: 1356–1361

Evans R S, Classen D C, Pestotnik S L, Lundsgaarde H P, Burke J P 1994 Improving empiric antibiotic selection using computer decision support. *Archives of Internal Medicine* 154: 878–884

Fabian T C, Croce M A, Payne E W, Minard G, Pritchard F E, Kudsk K A 1992 Duration of antibiotic therapy for penetrating abdominal trauma: a prospective trial. *Surgery* 112: 788–794

Fabian T C 1993 Prevention of infections following penetrating abdominal trauma. *American Journal of Surgery* 165 (suppl 2A): 14S–19S

Finch W T, Sawyers J L, Schenker S 1976 A prospective study to determine the efficacy of antibiotics in acute pancreatitis. *Annals of Surgery* 183: 667–670

Findlay I G, Wright P A, Menzies T, McCardle C S 1982 Microbial flora in carcinoma of oesophagous. *Thorax* 37: 181–184

Frame R, Brodman R F, Furman S, Andrews C A, Gross J N 1993 Surgical removal of infected transvenous pacemaker leads. *Pacing and Clinical Electrophysiology* 16: 2343–2348

Fritsch D E, Klein D G 1992 Ludwig's angina. *Heart and Lung* 21: 39–46

George C D, Marello P J 1987 Immunological effect of blood transfusion upon renal transplantation tumour operation and bacterial infections. *American Journal of Surgery* 152: 329–337

George S M, Fabian T C, Mangiante E C 1988 Colon trauma: further support for primary repair. *American Journal of Surgery* 156: 16–20

Haley R W, Culver D H, Morgan W M et al 1985 Identifying patients at risk of surgical wound infection. A simple multivariate index of patient susceptibility and wound contamination. *American Journal of Epidemiology* 121: 206–215

Halvorsen R A, Korookin M, Foster W L, Silverman P M, Thomson W M 1984 The variable CT appearance of hepatic abscesses. *American Journal of Roentgenology* 142: 941–946

Hammond J M J, Potgieter P D, Saunders G L 1994 Selective decontamination of the digestive tract in multiple trauma patients – Is there a role? Results of a prospective, double-blind, randomized trial. *Critical Care Medicine* 22: 33–39

Hansard 1986 Written answers 2 July, column 573

Hashimoto L, Hermann R, Grundfest-Broniatowski S 1995 Pyogenic hepatic abscess; results of current management. *American Surgeon* 61: 407–411

Irving A D, Scrimgeour D 1987 Mechanical bowel preparation for colonic resection and anastomosis. *British Journal of Surgery* 74: 580–581

Ivatury R R, Gaudino J, Nallathambi M N, Simon R J, Kazigo Z J, Stahl W M 1993 Definitive treatment of colon injuries: a prospective study. *American Journal of Surgery* 59: 43–49

Jensen L S, Andersen A, Fristrup S C, Holme J B, Hvid H M, Kraglund K 1990 Comparison of one dose versus three doses of prophylactic antibiotics and the influence of blood transfusion on infectious complications after acute and elective colorectal surgery. *British Journal of Surgery* 77: 513–518

Karran S J, Sutton G, Gartell P, Karran S E, Thinnes D, Blenkensopp J 1993 Imipenem prophylaxis in elective colorectal surgery. *British Journal of Surgery* 80: 1196–1198

Keighley M R B, Arabi Y, Alexander-Williams J, Youngs D, Burden D W 1979 Comparison between systemic and oral antimicrobial prophylaxis in colorectal surgery. *Lancet* 28: 894–897

Keighley M R B, Taylor E W, Hares M M et al 1981 Influence of oral manitol bowel preparation on colonic microflora and the risk of explosion during endoscopic diathermy. *British Journal of Surgery* 68: 554–556

Kizilcan F, Tanyel F C, Buyukpamukcu N, Hicsonmez A 1992 The necessity of prophylactic antibiotics in uncomplicated appendicitis during childhood. *Journal of Pediatric Surgery* 27: 586–588

Ko W, Lazenby W D, Zelano J A, Isom O W, Krieger K H 1992 The effects of shaving methods and intraoperative irrigation on suppurative mediastinitis after bypass operations. *Annals of Thoracic Surgery* 53: 301–305

Krige J E J 1995 The changing pattern of pyogenic liver sepsis. *Current Opinion in Surgical Infections* 3: 25–32

Krukowski J H, Koruth N M, Matheson N A 1986 Antibiotic lavage in emergency surgery for peritoneal sepsis. *Journal of the Royal College of Surgeons, Edinburgh* 31: 1–6

Krukowski J H, Irwin S T, Denholm S, Matheson N A 1988 Preventing wound infection after appendicectomy: a review. *British Journal of Surgery* 75: 1023–1033

Kudsk K A, Croce M A, Fabian T C et al 1992 Enteral versus parenteral feeding. Effects on septic morbidity after blunt and penetrating abdominal trauma. *Annals of Surgery* 215: 503–511

Kudsk K A, Minard G, Wojtysiak S L, Croce M A, Fabian T C, Brown R O 1994 Visceral protein response to enteral versus parenteral nutrition and sepsis in patients with trauma. *Surgery* 116: 516–523

Lau W Y, Chu K W, Poon G P, Ho K K 1988 Prophylactic antibiotics in elective colorectal surgery. *British Journal of Surgery* 75: 782–785

Law D J W, Mishriki S F, Jeffrey P J 1990 The importance of surveillance after discharge from hospital in the diagnosis of post-operative wound infection. *Annals of the Royal College of Surgeons, England* 72: 207–209

Lazorthes F, Legrand G, Monrozies X et al 1982 Comparison between oral and systemic antibiotics and their combined use for the prevention of complications in colorectal surgery. *Diseases of the Colon and Rectum* 25: 309–311

Lewis A B, Hayes D L, Holmes D R, Vlietstra R E, Pluth J R, Osborne M J 1985 Update on infections involving permanent pacemakers. Characterisation and management. *Journal of Thoracic and Cardiovascular Surgery* 89: 758–763

Litwin D E, Girotti M J, Poulin E C, Mamazza J, Negy A G 1992 Laparoscopic cholecystectomy: trans Canada experience with 2201 cases. *Canadian Journal of Surgery* 35: 291–296

Maschmeyer G, Haralambie E, Gaus W et al 1988 Ciprofloxicin and norfloxicin for selective decontamination in patients with severe granulocytopenia. *Infection* 16: 98–104

McArdle C S, Morran C G, Pettit L, Gemmell C G, Sleigh J D, Tillotson G S 1991 The value of oral antibiotic prophylaxis in biliary tract surgery. *Journal of Hospital Infection* 19 (suppl C): 59–64

McClinton S, Moffat L E, Scott S, Urbaniak S J, Kerridge D F 1990 Blood transfusion and survival following surgery for prostatic carcinoma. *British Journal of Surgery* 77: 140–142

Moesgaard F, Lukkegaard-Neilsen M 1989 Pre-operative cell mediated immunity and duration of antibiotic prophylaxis in relation to post-operative infective complications. A controlled trial in biliary gastroduodenal and colorectal surgery. *Acta Chirurgia Scandinavica* 155: 281–286

Molina J M, Leport C, Bure A, Wolff M, Michon C, Vilde J L 1991 Clinical and bacterial features of infections caused by *Streptococcus milleri*. *Scandinavian Journal of Infectious Diseases* 23: 659–666

Moore F A, Moore E E, Jones T N, McCroskey B L, Peterson V M 1989 TEN versus TPN following major abdominal trauma – reduced septic morbidity. *Journal of Trauma* 29: 916–922

Moore F A, Feliciano D V, Andrassy R J 1992 Early enteral feeding, compared with parenteral, reduces postoperative septic complications. The results of a meta-analysis. *Annals of Surgery* 216: 172–183

Moore S W, Millar A J, Cywes S 1994 Conservative initial treatment for liver abscesses in children. *British Journal of Surgery* 81: 872–874

Morris D L, Rodgers-Wilson S, Payne J et al 1990 A comparison of aztreonam/metronidazole and cefotaxime/metronidazole in elective colorectal surgery: antimicrobial prophylaxis must include Gram-positive cover. *Journal of Antimicrobial Chemotherapy* 95: 273–278

Nichols R L, Condon R E, Gorbach S L, Nyhus L M 1972 Efficacy of preoperative antimicrobial preparation of the bowel. *Annals of Surgery* 176: 227–232

Nichols R L, Smith J W, Robertson G D et al 1993 Prospective alterations in therapy for penetrating abdominal trauma. *Archives of Surgery* 128: 55–64

Oller D W 1990 Infection in victims of trauma. *Problems in Critical Care* 4: 3–20

Onderdonk A B, Bartlett J G, Louie T, Sullivan-Seigler N, Gorbach S L 1976 Microbial synergy in experimental intra-abdominal abscess. *Infection and Immunology* 13: 22–26

Oreskovich M R, Dellinger E P, Lennard E S, Wertz M, Carrico C J, Minshew B H 1982 Duration of preventive antibiotic administration for penetrating abdominal trauma. *Archives of Surgery* 117: 200–205

Pederzoli P, Bassi C, Vesentini S, Campedelli A 1993 A randomized multi-centre clinical trial of antibiotic prophylaxis of septic complications in acute necrotising pancreatitis with imipenem. *Surgery, Gynecology and Obstetrics* 176: 480–483

Peel A L G, Taylor E W 1991 Proposed definitions for the audit of post operative infection: a discussion paper. *Annals of the Royal College of Surgeons, England* 73: 385–388

Periti P, Mazzei T, Tonelli F 1989 Single dose cefotetan versus multi dose cefoxitin antimicrobial prophylaxis in colorectal surgery. *Diseases of the Colon and Rectum* 32: 121–127

Peters J H, Gibbons G D, Innes J T et al 1991 Complications of laparoscopic cholecystectomy. *Surgery* 110: 769–777

Pieper R, Kazer L, Nasman P 1982 Acute appendicitis. *Acta Chirurgia Scandinavica* 148: 51–62

Platt R, Zaleznik D F, Hopkins C C et al 1990 Perioperative antibiotic prophylaxis for hernia and breast surgery. *New England Journal of Medicine* 322: 153–160

Playforth M J, Smith G M R, Evans M, Pollock A V 1988 Antimicrobial bowel preparation – oral, parenteral or both? *Diseases of the Colon and Rectum* 31: 90–93

Pokorny W J, Kaplan S L, Mason E O 1991 A preliminary report of ticarcillin and clavulanate versus triple antibiotic therapy in children with ruptured appendicitis. *Surgery, Gynecology and Obstetrics* 172 (suppl): 54–56

Polk H C, Miles A A 1973 The decisive period in the primary infections of muscle by *Escherichia coli*. *British Journal of Experimental Pathology* 54: 99–101

Ramsay G 1992 The role of selective decontamination of the digestive tract. In: Taylor E W (ed) Infection in surgical practice, Oxford University Press, Oxford

Ramsdale D R, Charles R G, Roland D B, Singh S S, Gautam P C, Faragher E B 1984 Antibiotic prophylaxis for pacemaker implantation: a prospective randomized trial. *Pacing and Clinical Electrophysiology* 7: 844–849

Rao G N 1988 Predictive factors in local sepsis after splenectomy for trauma in adults. *Journal of the Royal College of Surgeons Edinburgh* 33: 68–70

Reed R L, Ericsson C D, Wu A, Miller-Crotchett P, Fischer R P 1992 The pharmacokinetics of prophylactic antibiotics in trauma. *Journal of Trauma* 32: 21–27

Ross S E, Cobean R A, Hoyt D B et al 1992 Blunt colonic injury – a multi-centre review. *Journal of Trauma* 33: 379–384

Rowe-Jones D C, Peel A L G, Shaw J F L, Teasdale C, Cole D S 1990 Single dose cefotaxime plus metronidazole versus three doses cefuroxime plus metronidazole as prophylaxis against wound infection in colorectal surgery: a multicentre prospective randomized study. *British Medical Journal* 300: 18–22

Salam I M, Abu Galala K H, El Ashaal Y I, Chandran V P, Asham N N, Sim A J 1994 A randomized prospective study of cefoxitin versus pipericillin in appendicectomy. *Journal of Hospital Infection* 26: 133–136

Santos J C M, Batista J, Sirimarco M T, Guimaraes A S, Levy C E 1994 Prospective randomized trial of mechanical bowel preparation in patients undergoing elective colorectal surgery. *British Journal of Surgery* 81: 1673–1676

Sauven P, Playforth M J, Smith G M, Evans M, Pollock A V 1986 Single dose antibiotic prophylaxis of abdominal surgical wound infection; a trial of pre-operative latamoxef against per-operative tetracycline lavage. *Journal of the Royal Society of Medicine* 79: 137–141

Schein M, Assalia A, Bachus H 1994 Minimal antibiotic therapy after emergency abdominal surgery: a prospective study. *British Journal of Surgery* 81: 989–991

Scher K S, Wroczynski A F, Jones C W 1986 Duration of antibiotic prophylaxis. An experimental study. *American Journal of Surgery* 151: 209–212

Selective Decontamination of the Digestive Tract Trialists' Collaborative Group 1993 Meta-analysis of randomised controlled trials of selective decontamination of the digestive tract. *British Medical Journal* 307: 525–532

Silverman S H, Ambrose N S, Youngs D J, Sheperd A F, Roberts A P, Keighley M R 1986 The effect of peritoneal lavage with tetracycline solution on postoperative infection. A prospective, randomized, clinical trial. *Diseases of the Colon and Rectum* 29: 165–169

Simchen E, Rozin R, Wax Y 1990 The Israeli study of surgical infection of drains and the risk of wound infection in operations for hernia. *Surgery, Gynecology and Obstetrics* 170: 331–337

Solla J A, Rothenberger D A 1990 Pre-operative bowel preparation. Survey colon and rectal surgeons. *Diseases of the Colon and Rectum* 33: 154–159

Southern Surgeons Club 1991 A prospect of analysis of 1518 laparoscopic cholecystectomies. *New England Journal of Medicine* 324: 1073–1078

Standage B A, Goss J C 1982 Outcome and sepsis after splenectomy in adults. *American Journal of Surgery* 143: 545–548

Stellato T A, Danzigger L H, Gordon N et al 1990 Antibiotics in elective colon surgery. A randomized trial of oral and oral/systemic antibiotics for prophylaxis. *American Surgeon* 56: 251–254

Stewart D J 1978 Antibiotic lavage in the prevention of intraperitoneal sepsis. *Annals of the Royal College of Surgeons, England* 60: 240–243

Stone H M, Fabian T C 1980 Peritoneal analysis in the treatment of acute alcoholic pancreatitis. *Surgery, Gynecology and Obstetrics* 150: 878–882

Strachan C J L 1992 Infection in vascular surgery. In: Taylor E W (ed) Infection in surgical practice. Oxford University Press, Oxford

Strachan C J L, Black J, Powers S J A et al 1977 Prophylactic use of cephazolin against wound sepsis after cholecystectomy. *British Medical Journal* i: 1254–1256

Stuckey J, Gross R J 1990 Infectious disease. In: Kammerer W S, Gross R J (eds) Medical consultation. Williams & Wilkins, Baltimore

Sugarman B, Young E J 1989 Infections associated with prosthetic devices: magnitude of the problem. *Infectious Diseases Clinics of North America* 3: 187–198

Swift A C 1992 Infection in ENT surgery. In: Taylor E W (ed) Infection in surgical practice. Oxford University Press, Oxford

Swift A C, Bartzokas C A, Corkill J E 1984 The gastro-oral pathway of intestinal bacteria after head and neck cancer surgery. *Clinical Otolaryngology* 1: 263–269

Tarrter P I 1988 Blood transfusion and infectious complications following colorectal cancer surgery. *British Journal of Surgery* 75: 789–792

Tarrter P I 1989 Blood transfusion and postoperative infection. *Transfusion* 29: 456–459

Taylor E W, Lindsay G, West of Scotland Surgical Infection Study Group 1994 Selective decontamination of the colon before elective colorectal operations. *World Journal of Surgery* 18: 926–931

Taylor E W, Lindsay G, Helyar A G 1990 Pre-operative selective decontamination of the colon by ciprofloxicin and mechanical catharsis in patients undergoing elective colorectal operations. *Surgical Research Communications* 7: 351–355

Taylor T V, Dawson D L, De Silva M, Shaw S J, Durrans D, Makin D 1985 Preoperative intraincisional cefamandole reduces wound infection and postoperative inpatient stay in upper abdominal surgery. *Annals of the Royal College of Surgeons, England* 67: 235–237

Tetteroo G W M, Wagenvoort J H T, Castelein A, Tilanus H W, Ince C, Bruining H A 1990 Selective decontamination to reduce Gram-negative colonization and infections after oesophageal resection. *Lancet* 335: 704–707

Tetteroo G W M, Wagenvoort J H T, Bruining H A 1994 Bacteriology of selective decontamination: efficacy and rebound colonization. *Journal of Antimicrobial Chemotherapy* 34: 139–148

Turano A 1992 Multicentre Study Group. New clinical data on the prophylaxis of infections in abdominal, gynecologic and urologic surgery. *American Journal of Surgery* (suppl 4a): 16S–20S

Uhari M, Seppanen J, Heikkinen E 1996 Imipenem–cilastatin versus tobramycin and metronidazole for appendicitis related infections. *Paediatric Infectious Diseases Journal* 11: 445–450

University of Melbourne Colorectal Group 1989 A comparison of single dose systemic timentin with mezlocillin for prophylaxis of wound infection in colorectal surgery. *Diseases of the Colon and Rectum* 32: 940–943

Walker A J, Taylor E W, Lindsay G, Dewar E P 1988 A multicentre study to compare piperacillin with a combination of netilmycin and metronidazole in prophylaxis in elective colorectal surgery undertaken in district general hospitals. *Journal of Hospital Infection* 11: 340–348

Weaver M, Burdon D W, Youngs D J, Keighley M R B 1986 Oral neomycin and erythromycin compared with single dose systemic metronidazole and ceftriaxone prophylaxis in elective colorectal surgery. *American Journal of Surgery* 151: 437–442

Weigelt J L, Haley R W, Seibert B 1987 Factors which influence the risk of wound infection in trauma patients. *Trauma* 27: 774–781

Weisner R H 1990 The incidence of Gram-negative bacterial and fungal infections in liver transplant patients treated with selective decontamination. *Infection* 18 (suppl 1): 19–21

Wells G R, Taylor E W, Lindsay G, Morton L, West of Scotland Surgical Infection Study Group 1989 The relationship between bile colonization, high risk factors and postoperative sepsis in patients undergoing biliary tract operations while receiving a prophylactic antibiotic. *British Journal of Surgery* 76: 374–377

Widdison A L, Karanjia N D, Reber H A 1994 Antimicrobial treatment of pancreatic infection in cats. *British Journal of Surgery* 81: 886–889

Willis A T, Ferguson I R, Jones P H et al 1976 Metronidazole in prevention and treatment of bacteroides infections after appendicectomy. *British Medical Journal* 1: 318–321

Willis A T, Ferguson I R, Jones P H et al 1977 Metronidazole in prevention and treatment of bacteroides infections in elective colonic surgery. *British Medical Journal* 1: 607–610

Wilson A P, Gruneberg T N, Treasure T, Sturridge M F 1988 *Staphylococcus epidermidis* as a cause of postoperative wound infection after cardiac surgery: An assessment of pathogenicity and a wound scoring method. *British Journal of Surgery* 75: 168–170

Wilson R F, Wiencek R G, Balog M 1989 Predicting and preventing infection after abdominal vascular injuries. *Trauma* 29: 1371–1375

Wilson A P R 1995 Antibiotic prophylaxis and infection control measures in minimally invasive surgery. *Journal of Antimicrobial Chemotherapy* 36: 1–5

Wilson H A, Downes T R, Julian J S, White W L, Haponik E F 1993 *Candida* endocarditis. A treatable form of pacemaker infection. *Chest* 103: 283–284

Wilson R G, Taylor E W, Lindsay G et al 1987 A comparative study of cefotetan and metronidazole against metronidazole alone to prevent infection after appendectomy. *Surgery, Gynecology and Obstetrics* 164: 447–451

Working Party of the British Society for Antimicrobial Chemotherapy 1985 Antibiotic treatment of streptococcal and staphylococcal endocarditis. *Lancet* ii: 815–817

43

Infections associated with neutropenia and transplants

C. C. Kibbler

Introduction

Neutropenic patients and those undergoing transplantation are among the most profoundly immunosuppressed encountered in clinical practice. Whilst many pathogens are common to both these groups of patients, their propensity to cause infection and the incidence, severity, mortality and treatment vary considerably. None of these patients suffers from a single specific immunological deficit, there being a subtle blend of physical and immunological defects which evolve with time. Hence judgements about therapy need to be based upon knowledge of the balance of these defects and the timing of the infection.

The past three decades have seen large numbers of clinical trials of antimicrobial therapy or prophylaxis performed in neutropenic patients. On the other hand, there have been few prospective, randomized studies of antimicrobial agents in organ-transplant recipients and most published work has reported experiences from single centres in series of patients. This may reflect a difference in emphasis and priority given to infections by those managing these patients, as well as a real qualitative and quantitative difference in infections between the two groups. For all of these reasons and because neutropenic and transplant patients are managed by different clinicians this chapter will consider the two groups separately.

Infections in neutropenic patients

There is an inverse relationship between the numbers of circulating neutrophils and the risk of infection (Bodey et al 1966). This effect becomes apparent when the absolute neutrophil count is less than $1.0 \times 10^9/l$. The risk increases considerably as the count falls below $0.5 \times 10^9/l$ and all patients with a count of less than $0.1 \times 10^9/l$ for more than 3 weeks have been found to develop an infective episode (Bodey et al 1966).

CAUSES OF NEUTROPENIA

Most neutropenic patients have a low neutrophil count as a consequence of chemotherapy for leukaemia. A proportion of leukaemic patients will present with neutropenia before chemotherapy. It should also be appreciated that the neutrophils of leukaemic patients, particularly those with acute myeloid leukaemia, often have impaired microbicidal activity (Cline 1973a, b).

Patients undergoing chemotherapy for lymphoma or for solid tumours may also suffer a reduction in circulating neutrophils, but this is rarely less than $0.1 \times 10^9/l$ and is often not below $0.5 \times 10^9/l$. Further, the duration of neutropenia is often less than 7 days. The degree and duration of neutropenia differ. Among those with aplastic anaemia or bone marrow transplant (BMT) recipients who fail to engraft, neutropenia is often profound and prolonged.

Patients undergoing bone marrow transplantation behave essentially like neutropenic patients during their early post-transplant phase, but remain immunosuppressed for up to 2 years, even without complications such as graft-versus-host disease.

Other causes of neutropenia are shown in Box 43.1.

FACTORS PREDISPOSING TO INFECTION

The pathogenesis of infection is multifactorial and is often the consequence of a breach in the skin or oral mucosa plus the defects in cellular or humoral immunity.

Box 43.1 *Non-malignant causes of neutropenia*

Congenital
- Cyclical neutropenia
- Chronic benign neutropenia
- Severe congenital neutropenia

Acquired
- Drug-induced
  - Cytotoxic chemotherapy (the commonest cause of neutropenia)
  - Antimicrobial associated:
    chloramphenicol
    β-lactams
    sulphonamides
    trimethoprim
    nitrofurantoin
    flucytosine
  - Other drugs (e.g. phenothiazines, tolbutamide)
- Alcohol
- Megaloblastic anaemia
- Auto-immune neutropenia

Certain defects appear to predispose to specific infections (Table 43.1). Lymphopenia, as a consequence of lymphoid malignancy or treatment, is associated with reactivation of intracellular organisms such as mycobacteria, the herpes viruses, *Toxoplasma gondii* and *Pneumocystis carinii*. Patients with chronic lymphoid malignancies and those receiving immunosuppressive chemotherapy, such as BMT recipients, have impaired antibody production which

Table 43.1 *Factors predisposing to infection in the neutropenic patient*

Immune defect/risk factor	Example of opportunistic organisms
Neutropenia	*Streptococcus oralis* *Pseudomonas aeruginosa* *Candida* spp. *Aspergillus* spp.
Lymphoid cell defect	*Mycobacterium* spp. *Toxoplasma gondii* Herpes viruses *Pneumocystis carinii*
Humoral	*Streptococcus pneumoniae*
Mucosal barrier (e.g. HSV/ chemotherapy-induced mucositis)	*Streptococcus oralis* Enterobacteriaceae Fungi
Vascular access	Coagulase-negative staphylococci Fungi
Foreign travel/ethnic origin	*Mycobacterium* spp. *Strongyloides stercoralis*
Anatomical defect/reservoir (e.g. chronic sinusitis)	*Pseudomonas* spp.
Splenectomy	*Streptococcus pneumoniae*

HSV, herpes simplex virus.

predisposes to infection with encapsulated organisms such as *Streptococcus pneumoniae*. The use of indwelling central venous catheters and mucosal damage caused by chemotherapy and herpes simplex virus (HSV) infection (Hann et al 1983) allows penetration by commensal flora. In recent years changes in cytotoxic chemotherapy have rendered the oropharynx a major portal of entry for α-haemolytic streptococci. Likewise, splenectomy undertaken as treatment or for diagnosis renders the patient susceptible to infection with encapsulated organisms such as *Str. pneumoniae*. Others have pre-existing sites of chronic infection such as middle ear disease or bronchiectasis, which may act as reservoirs of infection with organisms such as *Pseudomonas aeruginosa*. Ethnic origin and foreign travel may increase exposure to infections such as tuberculosis, malaria or strongyloidiasis.

CAUSATIVE ORGANISMS

Approximately 30% of febrile episodes in neutropenic patients can be confirmed microbiologically, and of these most are due to bacteraemia. Over the past two decades, infections with Gram-positive bacteria, especially the coagulase-negative staphylococci and α-haemolytic streptococci, have increased in frequency. In the EORTC participatory centres the incidence of bacteraemia due to Gram-positive organisms have increased from 29% in the first trial (The EORTC International Antimicrobial Therapy Project Group 1978) to 69% in the seventh (The International Antimicrobial Therapy Project Cooperative Group of the EORTC 1993). This increase correlates to some extent with the escalating use of central venous catheters, the development of alternative high-dose chemotherapy with attendant mucositis, and better prevention of Gram-negative infections.

Gram-negative bacteria continue to cause the most serious episodes of sepsis. Infections caused by the Enterobacteriaceae and *Ps. aeruginosa* carry a mortality of 40–60% (Schimpff et al 1974, Bodey et al 1985). Oropharyngeal candidosis is extremely common, while invasive candidosis and aspergillosis accounts for 20–30% of fatal infections when treating acute leukaemia (DeGregorio et al 1982, Bodey et al 1992). Other important infective agents are listed in Box 43.2.

CHEMOPROPHYLAXIS

Much emphasis should be placed on the prevention of infections, particularly those carrying a high mortality such as Gram-negative bacteraemia or invasive aspergillosis. Strategies for preventing acquisition of organisms, such as the use of filtered room air, appear important in some

Box 43.2 *Important infectious agents in neutropenic patients*

Bacteria
Staphylococci
Streptococci
Enterobacteriaceae
Pseudomonads
Mycobacterium spp.
Legionella spp.
Clostridium septicum
Clostridium difficile
Stomatococci

Fungi
Candida spp.
Aspergillus spp.
Zygomycetes
Cryptococcus neoformans
Trichosporon beigelii
Pneumocystis carinii

Viruses
Herpes simplex virus
Varicella zoster virus
Cytomegalovirus
Epstein–Barr virus
Hepatitis A, B, C viruses
Parvovirus
Adenovirus
Polyomavirus
Measles virus

Protozoa/parasites
Toxoplasma gondii
Strongyloides stercoralis

profoundly neutropenic patients at risk from aspergillosis, but detailed discussion is not possible here.

In the 1970s, various trials examined the efficacy of non-absorbable antibiotics. Unfortunately, there was considerable variation in the stringency of patient decontamination, the duration of neutropenia, the nature of the anticancer chemotherapy regimens used and the use of liquid versus capsule or tablet formulations of antibiotics among the studies. However, several controlled trials of oral non-absorbable antibiotics only showed a benefit when they were combined with a protective environment (Jameson et al 1971, Levine et al 1973, Yates & Holland 1973, Schimpff et al 1975, Dietrich et al 1977, Storring et al 1977, Rodriguez et al 1978, Buckner et al 1978, Bodey 1979).

Co-trimoxazole was first used in patients with acute leukaemia to prevent *Pneumocystis carinii* pneumonitis, but it also reduced the incidence of bacterial infection (Hughes et al 1973). Further studies have shown variable results, although greatest benefit has been shown in patients with prolonged neutropenia, among whom a consistent reduction in Gram-negative bacterial infections has been found (Gurwith et al 1979, Dekker et al 1981, Wade et al 1981, EORTC 1984). However, the incidence of side-effects

(including bone marrow suppression) and the selection of multiresistant organisms has caused some concern.

Oral ciprofloxacin, ofloxacin and norfloxacin have been compared in a number of studies with placebo, co-trimoxazole and non-absorbable antibiotics. In the majority of these the 4-quinolone treated patients had significantly fewer Gram-negative bacterial infections, a delayed onset of fever and a reduction in the number of days of fever. Ciprofloxacin (500 mg twice-daily) and norfloxacin (400 mg twice-daily) have been compared in a multicentre randomized trial in 801 patients with haematological malignancy or BMT (GIMENA Infection Program 1991). Ciprofloxacin significantly reduced the number of febrile episodes, microbiologically documented infections (17% vs 24%) and neutropenic episodes requiring empirical antibacterial therapy. A more recent study (Donnelly et al 1992) comparing ciprofloxacin (500 mg twice-daily) with co-trimoxazole (960 mg three times daily) plus colistin (200 mg four times daily) demonstrated statistical superiority for the latter regimen in terms of fewer infective complications (31% vs 18%), febrile days (5.9 vs 8.2), infectious episodes (0.9 vs 1.2) and a greater delay in the onset of fever (19 vs 14 days). However, in the co-trimoxazole/colistin group, bacteraemias due to resistant Gram-negative organisms occurred whereas there was none in the ciprofloxacin-treated patient group.

On balance, the benefits in using the 4-quinolones (particularly ciprofloxacin or ofloxacin) and, to a lesser extent, co-trimoxazole in higher dose in combination with colistin outweigh the disadvantages. Certainly during the 8 years that ciprofloxacin has been in use on our haematology unit, serious pseudomonal sepsis has been almost exclusively confined to those, such as paediatric patients, who have not received it.

The issue of antifungal prophylaxis is more controversial. Early attempts to eradicate or suppress fungi in the gut and oropharynx by means of the oral polyenes met with variable success. Nystatin, in doses up to 12×10^6 units/day had little effect on the incidence of invasive candidosis in neutropenic patients (DeGregorio et al 1982), whereas amphotericin B, as suspension, tablets or lozenges, was superior to placebo in preventing the disease (Odds 1988).

While most invasive fungal infections gain entry via the gut (Odds 1988), non-absorbable antifungal agents do not protect against fungal infections at other sites, namely the skin, intravenous catheter sites and the respiratory tract. The oral, systemically active azoles have the potential to control colonization as well as preventing dissemination.

Ketoconazole, in daily doses of 200–600 mg, reduces yeast carriage and the incidence of both local and systemic candidosis versus placebo or non-absorbable agents (Odds 1988). However, absorption is impaired in neutropenic patients, particularly in BMT recipients (Hann et al 1982) and breakthrough infections have occurred (Hansen et al

1987). There is also the problem of elevated cyclosporin A levels as a result of activity on hepatic P450 enzymes (p. 626) (Hawkins & Armstrong 1984).

Fluconazole, in daily doses of 50–400 mg reduces colonization and mucosal thrush as well as reducing the number of disseminated yeast infections (Brammer 1990, Wingard et al 1991, Goodman et al 1992). Unfortunately, its use in some centres has been associated with an increase in colonization and infection with *Candida krusei* which is intrinsically resistant to fluconazole (Wingard et al 1991). Fluconazole is also inactive against the important invasive moulds which affect this population, especially *Aspergillus* species and the Zygomycetes. In contrast, itraconazole has activity against the moulds, particularly *Aspergillus* species (Ch. 60).

Amphotericin B administered as a nasal spray has produced conflicting results in preventing invasive aspergillosis (Meunier 1987, Jorgensen et al 1989) although when aerosolized it has had greater success (Conneally et al 1990, Myers et al 1992).

Prophylaxis against *Pneum. carinii* infection has proved remarkably effective in those undergoing treatment for acute lymphoblastic leukaemia (Hughes et al 1973) and for the first 6 months post-BMT. Co-trimoxazole three times weekly is preferred, although nebulized pentamidine is often used in adults during bone marrow engraftment to avoid the myelosuppressive effects of co-trimoxazole.

Most virus infections in the neutropenic patient are due to reactivation of the human herpes viruses. Acyclovir, 200 mg 8-hourly to 800 mg 12-hourly, is effective as prophylaxis against herpes simplex virus (HSV) infection in HSV seropositive patients with leukaemia undergoing chemotherapy, or in BMT recipients (Zaia 1990, Wade 1993).

Chemoprophylaxis against cytomegalovirus (CMV) infection has only been investigated in detail in BMT recipients, although disease also occurs in patients with acute leukaemia receiving chemotherapy. High-dose acyclovir has been shown to be partially effective in preventing CMV infection and disease post-BMT. A recent multi-centre randomized trial compared 500 mg/m^2 intravenously 8-hourly for 1 month followed by 800 mg 6-hourly by mouth for 6 months, with 200 or 400 mg 6-hourly orally for 1 month followed by placebo (Prentice et al 1994). There was a reduced incidence of CMV infection and increased survival by day 210 post-BMT, although the rates of CMV pneumonia were similar in the two groups.

The use of ganciclovir as prophylaxis against CMV infection has shown some benefit in reducing the incidence of CMV disease but with no effect on survival during the first 4 months post-BMT (Goodrich et al 1993, Winston et al 1993). When used as pre-emptive therapy following detection of CMV infection, improved survival at 100 and 180 days post-transplant has been demonstrated (Goodrich et al 1991). The difference in these two approaches may be due to the myelosuppressive effects of ganciclovir causing a higher number of deaths from non-viral infections when used as prophylaxis, as well as failure to prevent CMV pneumonia. It would seem more appropriate to use ganciclovir as

Table 43.2 *Current antimicrobial prophylactic regimens*

Prophylaxis	Agent	Dosage	Duration
Antibacterial	Ciprofloxacin	500 mg 12-hourly	During period of neutropenia
Antifungal	Fluconazole	100 mg once daily	During period of neutropenia 6 months post-BMT
	Amphotericin B suspension	500 mg 6-hourly	During period of neutropenia 6 months post-BMT
Anti-*Pneum. carinii*	Co-trimoxazole	960 mg 12-hourly 3 times/week	1 week pre- and 6 months post-BMT Throughout treatment in ALL
	(Nebulized pentamidine in adults)	(150 mg fortnightly)	During period of neutropenia
Antituberculous*	Isoniazid	5 mg/kg daily	During period of neutropenia 6 months post-BMT
Herpes simplex virus†	Acyclovir	400–800 mg 4–5 times/day	During period of neutropenia
Cytomegalovirus‡	Seronegative blood products		
	Acyclovir	High dose	Not yet established
	Ganciclovir		Not yet established

* At-risk patients only.
† Seropositive patients only.
‡ BMT patients only.

pre-emptive therapy, particularly now that tests for antigenaemia and the CMV polymerase chain reaction (PCR) allow even earlier detection of infection (Einsele et al 1991, Boeckh et al 1992, Kidd et al 1993). A summary of prophylactic regimens is shown in Table 43.2.

EMPIRICAL THERAPY

It is now accepted that empirical antibiotic therapy should be given as soon as a neutropenic patient becomes febrile, because to await microbiological diagnosis is associated with a high mortality, particularly in patients with Gram-negative bacteraemia. The regimen should be active against the common organisms likely to result in overwhelming sepsis or death, and be influenced by local antibiotic sensitivity patterns, the incidence of particular infections, the specific needs of the patient and the prophylactic regimen used. Traditionally the significant organisms have been the Enterobacteriaceae and *Ps. aeruginosa* which carry a mortality of 40–60% (Schimpff et al 1974, Bodey et al 1985). Earlier regimens included an aminoglycoside in combination with a β-lactam antibiotic in an attempt to achieve broad-spectrum and synergic activity against organisms such as *Ps. aeruginosa*. However, the potential renal, auditory and vestibular toxicity associated with prolonged and repeated courses of aminoglycosides has resulted in many studies of non-aminoglycoside containing regimens. These have consisted of combinations of two β-lactam agents (the 'double β-lactam combination') or a

single broad-spectrum agent such as ceftazidime, cefoperazone, cefpirome, a quinolone or a carbapenem ('monotherapy'). The advantages and disadvantages of these different regimens are shown in Table 43.3.

The first studies of double β-lactam therapy gave results inferior to aminoglycoside containing regimens (Bodey et al 1977, EORTC 1978, Gurwith et al 1978). Subsequently, studies using ceftazidime, latamoxef and cefoperazone in combination with a ureidopenicillin were performed (Winston et al 1984, Winston et al 1988, Kibbler et al 1989a). These all concluded that such combinations were of equal efficacy and less nephrotoxic than aminoglycoside containing regimens. However, it was unclear whether they were any better than β-lactam monotherapy. There have been many randomized controlled trials of ceftazidime monotherapy which have shown no difference in efficacy from aminoglycoside containing regimens. A recent meta-analysis of carefully selected studies has shown that combination therapy is not significantly different from ceftazidime alone, even in patients who were bacteraemic (Sanders et al 1991). In addition, this analysis has shown no apparent benefit for adding an aminoglycoside empirically.

Besides ceftazidime monotherapy, a number of other regimens have been studied (Box 43.3). Of these, the most frequently studied monotherapy regimen has been with imipenem which has been compared with several regimens including cefoperazone plus piperacillin, ceftazidime alone, ceftazidime plus vancomycin or amikacin, and gentamicin plus cefuroxime or cephalothin (Winston et al 1988, Liang

Table 43.3 *Options for initial empirical therapy*

Regimen	Advantages	Disadvantages
Aminoglycoside + betalactam	Broad spectrum Proven efficacy Synergy vs Gram-negative bacteria and streptococci	Poor activity vs coagulase-negative staphylococci Nephro- and oto-toxic Serum assays required
Double β-lactam therapy	Broad spectrum Avoids aminoglycoside toxicity No monitoring required	No more effective than single-agent therapy Possible prolongation of neutropenia Electrolyte imbalance Possible antagonism
Monotherapy	Broad spectrum Avoids aminoglycoside toxicity Avoids antagonism No monitoring required Cheaper	Lack of synergy (? less effective vs *Ps. aeruginosa*) Less active vs Gram-positive bacteria (with ceftazidime) Risk of resistance Potential CNS toxicity (with imipenem)
Single agent + glycopeptide	Broad spectrum including coagulase-negative staphylococci and α-haemolytic streptococci No monitoring required (with teicoplanin)	Expensive Unnecessary in some units Nephro- and oto-toxicity (with vancomycin) Monitoring required (with vancomycin) Risk of glycopeptide resistance

Box 43.3 *Representative antibiotic regimens that have been evaluated for empirical therapy in febrile neutropenic patients (after Bodey 1986)*

Penicillin and aminoglycoside combinations
Carbenicillin and gentamicin/amikacin/sissomicin
Ticarcillin and gentamicin/tobramycin/amikacin/netilmicin
Mezlocillin and tobramycin
Piperacillin and gentamicin/amikacin
Azlocillin and amikacin
Piperacillin/tazobactam and amikacin

Cephalosporin and aminoglycoside combinations
Cephalothin and gentamicin
Latamoxef and gentamicin/amikacin
Cefotaxime and amikacin
Ceftazidime and tobramycin/amikacin
Cefoperazone and amikacin
Ceftriaxone and amikacin

Double β-lactam combinations
Carbenicillin and cephalothin
Carbenicillin and cephamandole
Ceftazidime and flucloxacillin
Ticarcillin and latamoxef
Piperacillin and latamoxef
Ceftazidime and azlocillin
Ceftazidime and piperacillin

Triple agent combinations
Carbenicillin, cephalothin and gentamicin
Carbenicillin, cefazolin and amikacin
Cefotaxime, piperacillin and netilmicin

Monotherapy regimens
Latamoxef
Ceftazidime
Cefoperazone
Imipenem
Meropenem
Ciprofloxacin

Other agents and drugs under investigation
Vancomycin
Teicoplanin
Cotrimoxazole
Aztreonam
Ticarcillin/clavulanate
Cefpirome

et al 1990, Riikonen 1991, Cornelissen et al 1992, Rolston et al 1992). Outcome has been at least as good as with ceftazidime monotherapy, double β-lactam regimens and aminoglycoside plus β-lactam combinations, although some failures, of Gram-positive infections, have occurred. There have also been reports that *Stenotrophomonas (Xanthomonas) maltophilia* is selected out by imipenem to which it is intrinsically resistant (Kerr et al 1990). In addition, there have been concerns over central nervous system (CNS) toxicity with high-dose imipenem (Winston et al 1988) or ciprofloxacin prophylaxis (McWhinney et al 1991).

One advantage of imipenem is its activity against the α-haemolytic streptococci (McWhinney et al 1993a), allowing it to be used alone without the need for early glycopeptide therapy. This is shared by meropenem, another newly introduced carbapenem recently evaluated by the EORTC, which appears to lack CNS toxicity (Cometta et al 1995). The current excess of Gram-positive infections indicates that empirical therapy should contain a broad-spectrum anti-Gram-positive agent. Glycopeptides have been widely promoted, but clinical trials have provided conflicting evidence as to whether and when to add such an agent.

In centres where there are significant numbers of Gram-positive infections, initial vancomycin or teicoplanin has increased response rates and reduced morbidity (Karp et al 1991, Chow et al 1993), although no study has shown a reduction in mortality. In addition, vancomycin is associated with increased toxicity (Ramphal et al 1992, Chow et al 1993). However, with a lower incidence of Gram-positive infection the use of initial vancomycin is not significantly beneficial and can be reserved for documented infections (Pizzo et al 1991, Ramphal et al 1992).

The increasing isolation of vancomycin resistant enterococci is giving cause for concern in many centres (Shlaes et al 1993, Handwerger et al 1993) and has prompted the Centers for Disease Control (CDC) to issue guidelines on the use of vancomycin which specifically exclude its use as empirical therapy in the neutropenic patient (Centers for Disease Control and Prevention 1994). This seems prudent and is endorsed.

The duration of treatment has never been stringently examined. Since the first EORTC trial the evidence has suggested that prolonged treatment is associated with more superinfections, often fungal, but without an improved outcome. Whilst the consensus is now against continuing treatment until the patient is no longer neutropenic, the minimum duration has not been defined. There appears little difference between response rates and relapse rates in trials requiring 10 days' therapy for microbiologically documented infections (Kibbler et al 1989a) and others requiring a minimum of 7 days. Current EORTC trials are conducted on the basis of discontinuing antibiotics after 7 days minimum treatment and four consecutive afebrile days.

MANAGEMENT OF THE PATIENT WITH PERSISTENT PYREXIA

Before quinolones were used as prophylaxis approximately 20–30% of febrile patients who remained persistently neutropenic failed to respond to apparently appropriate antibiotic therapy. Some remain febrile until recovery of their neutrophil counts irrespective of the antimicrobial therapy administered. Many patients with persistent fever will have an occult fungal infection. The likelihood of fungal infection increases with the number of preceding febrile episodes; in one study 44% of patients suffering their fourth bout of fever had a fungal infection as the cause (Barnes & Rogers 1988). In view of the difficulties in diagnosis the use of empirical antifungal therapy has been advocated and shown to be effective. The largest study examined the effect of amphotericin B (0.6 mg/kg daily) in patients remaining febrile 4 days after empirical therapy (Anonymous 1989). Whilst more responded in the amphotericin B treated group, the effect was only significant in patients not given antifungal prophylaxis (78% vs 45%; p = 0.04).

A most difficult therapeutic challenge is the patient who continues to deteriorate during the first 48 h of empirical therapy. It is important that there be no gaps in the spectrum of the selected regimen. Deterioration may be due to Gram-negative organisms or Gram-positive organisms such as α-haemolytic streptococci which may cause similar features of sepsis syndrome (including ARDS) and septic shock or enterococci. Gram-negative activity (including antipseudomonal activity) is essential. Consequently, the addition of an aminoglycoside to initial β-lactam monotherapy is recommended and a glycopeptide should also be considered. The above approach is summarized in Figure 43.1.

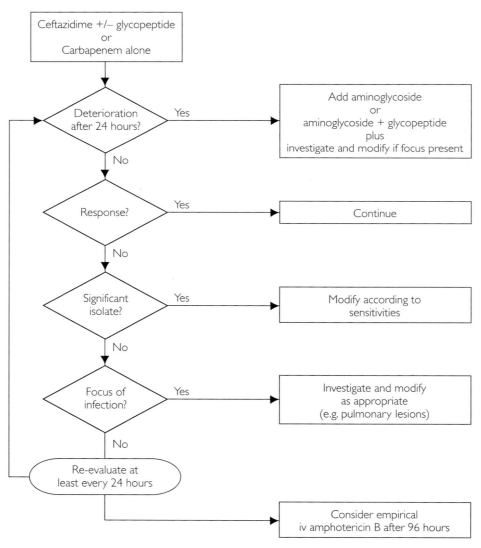

Fig. 43.1 *An algorithm for the initial management of febrile neutropenic patients receiving quinolone prophylaxis.*

ASPECTS OF THERAPY FOR SPECIFIC ORGANISMS AND INFECTIONS

Catheter-associated infections

The majority of neutropenic patients undergoing treatment have an indwelling central line and these commonly become infected. The predominant pathogens are coagulase-negative staphylococci, followed by *Staphylococcus aureus* (Winston et al 1983). Others include *Candida* spp., coryneforms, *Acinetobacter, Stenotrophomonas* and *Pseudomonas* spp. (Bodey 1986). Ideally, infected catheters should be removed, but coagulase-negative staphylococcal infections may be effectively suppressed or eliminated with antibiotics administered via the catheter, until neutropenia has resolved (Pizzo et al 1981). A high percentage of coagulase-negative staphylococci isolated on haematology units are resistant to methicillin and other β-lactams and hence a glycopeptide (most frequently vancomycin) is recommended, with the chance of success being more than 50%. Similar response rates can be obtained with coryneform infections but those due to *Candida* spp., Enterobacteriaceae, *Staph. aureus* and *Ps. aeruginosa* require removal of the catheter, and appropriate antimicrobial therapy.

Pulmonary infections of unknown cause

Pulmonary infiltrates occurring in a febrile neutropenic patient are common and have a number of causes, especially in the BMT recipient. Causes include non-infective conditions such as pulmonary oedema, alveolar haemorrhage and the idiopathic pneumonitis syndrome. Focal lesions are more indicative of fungal infection, and computed tomography (CT) or magnetic resonance imaging (MRI) scanning may reveal characteristic features of these. However, in most cases treatment has to be given empirically.

Initial therapy should certainly include agents effective against common respiratory pathogens such as *Str. pneumoniae* and *Haemophilus influenzae* as well as Gram-negative organisms including *Ps. aeruginosa* and hence a carbapenem or ceftazidime, with or without an aminoglycoside, is recommended.

Atypical pneumonias are extremely uncommon in this population and, unless there are particular clinical or epidemiological reasons to suggest Legionnaires' disease, erythromycin can be omitted from the initial therapy. Mycobacterial infections may occasionally complicate haemotological malignancies. Patients with lymphoid malignancy and BMT recipients who have not been receiving co-trimoxazole prophylaxis are at risk of *Pneum. carinii* pneumonitis and empirical high-dose co-trimoxazole therapy (120 mg/kg daily in divided doses) is warranted in such patients. BMT recipients are particularly at risk of CMV pneumonitis post-transplant. However, the latter two infections usually present a month or so post-transplant when the patient is no longer neutropenic, so that the timing of the presentation should be taken into account when decisions are being made regarding empirical therapy. The treatment of CMV pneumonitis is with ganciclovir (5 mg/kg i.v. twice daily) plus i.v. immunoglobulin 200–400 mg/kg on alternate days for 14–21 days (Emanuel et al 1988, Reed et al 1988, Ljungman et al 1992). Despite this, mortality from this infection is still in excess of 50% in BMT patients. Further, the myelosuppressive effect of ganciclovir can present a particular problem in these patients.

Invasive aspergillosis

Intravenous amphotericin B (1.0–1.5 mg/kg daily) has long been the treatment of choice for invasive aspergillosis. The mortality is high (60–70%) in neutropenic patients despite the use of this agent, and successful outcome is dependent upon early treatment (Aisner et al 1977) and, to a considerable extent, on bone marrow recovery (Fisher et al 1981).

Itraconazole has been used with success in this population (Denning et al 1989) and the drug is being increasingly used for completion therapy, once a patient has responded to intravenous amphotericin B. Lipid preparations of amphotericin B have given good results (Mills et al 1994), although none of these agents has been compared with conventional amphotericin B in treating aspergillosis. The therapy of fungal infection is considered in detail in Chapter 60.

The development of mycotic lung sequestra (which have been mistakenly termed mycetomas) requires additional therapy. These lesions appear once the bone marrow is regenerating. Patients are at risk of life-threatening haemoptysis (Kibbler et al 1988). In addition, patients who require further chemotherapy or bone marrow transplantation are at considerable risk of relapse of the original infection. For both these problems we now recommend to proceed rapidly to resection unless this is absolutely contraindicated (McWhinney et al 1993a). Regrettably, this strategy appears of less benefit to BMT recipients.

ADDITIONAL THERAPIES

Growth factors

In recent years, haematopoietic growth factors have been extensively used to treat neutropenic patients. Studies have consistently shown that granulocyte colony stimulating factor (G-CSF) reduces the duration of neutropenia. However, the reduction in infectious complications has been modest and most trials have been unable to demonstrate a reduction in infectious morbidity and mortality (Demetri & Antman 1992, Glaspy & Golde 1992, Pettengell et al 1992). This is probably because the major effect of G-CSF is to accelerate the recovery of neutrophils, whereas the critical lag period of profound neutropenia is not affected (Singer 1992).

Growth factors are likely to prove more beneficial in priming peripheral blood stem cells prior to harvesting and reinfusion into neutropenic hosts. Another area where growth factors with macrophage stimulating activity (granulocyte–macrophage colony stimulating factor and macrophage colony stimulating factor) are showing promise is in the treatment of invasive fungal infections in these patients (Bodey et al 1993).

Granulocyte transfusions

Transfusions of circulating white cells have been used to augment antimicrobial therapy in neutropenic patients with unresponsive infection. However, their use has now largely been abandoned, although benefit had been demonstrated in children in whom it is possible to achieve significant increases in neutrophil counts. Renewed interest is now being shown in this modality coupled with improved methods of harvesting and increased yield following the use of growth factors.

Immunoglobulin therapy

Passive immunotherapy has been used both for prevention of infection and for treatment. However, it has been proven to have a significant benefit in a few conditions only. The addition of intravenous immunoglobulin to ganciclovir improves survival in CMV pneumonitis.

Routine prophylactic use of intravenous immunoglobulin in leukaemia therapy does not reduce viral infections, although an immunoglobulin M (IgM) enriched preparation (Pentaglobin) has reduced endotoxin-related infections and prevented infectious deaths in BMT recipients (Poynton et al 1992). Post-exposure immunoglobulin is indicated for the prevention of hepatitis A, measles and varicella-zoster infection (with hyperimmune immunoglobulin).

Infections in transplant recipients

IMMUNOSUPPRESSIVE THERAPY

Developments in surgery and better control of rejection and infective complications has transformed organ transplantation over the past three decades. In 1993, the 1-year graft survival for single-lung allografts in the USA was 52% (with 54% patient survival) and 90% (with 97% patient survival) for living related renal allografts (UNOS 1993). The results are similar for Europe. The key change in immunosuppressive regimens has been the introduction of cyclosporin and the reduction in corticosteroids which this has allowed.

Most transplant units use a triple regimen of azathioprine, cyclosporin A and prednisone (Table 43.4). Azathioprine is a purine analogue which inhibits both B- and T-cell proliferation. As a consequence both cell-mediated immunity (CMI) and humoral immunity is inhibited – the primary response being inhibited more than the secondary response. The drug may take weeks or months to exert its full effect. Cyclosporin arrests the lymphocyte cell cycle in the resting phase, having most effect on CD4 positive T cells and a minimal effect on B cells. This results in effective suppression of CMI, little effect on humoral immunity and no effect on phagocytosis. The inflammatory response is preserved.

Corticosteroids in high dose have a very broad immunosuppressive action. There is a marked but transient lymphocytopenia and monocytopenia which is maximal at 4–6 h after administration, with a return to normal peripheral counts after 24 h. This effect is greatest on circulating T cells and appears to be the result of redistribution of lymphocytes to the extravascular pool, particularly to the bone marrow. In addition, there is a reduction in antigen-stimulated proliferation and a blunting of the primary antibody response. Corticosteroids also inhibit

Table 43.4 *Transplant immunosuppression regimens*

Regimen	Dose
Background immunosuppression	
Cyclosporin	≤6 mg/kg per day (may be higher initially)
Azathioprine	≤3 mg/kg per day
Prednisone	≤200 mg per day initially (reducing to <40 mg/day)
Treatment of acute rejection	
Methyl prednisolone	1 g/day for up to 72 h
Further antirejection therapy	
Antilymphocyte globulin	
Antithymocyte globulin	
OKT3 panlymphocyte monoclonal antibody	

neutrophil chemotaxis and monocyte phagocytosis, dramatically reducing inflammatory responses at high dosage and disguising the presence of infection.

The aim of these regimens is to achieve a balance between graft rejection and risk of infection. Episodes of subsequent acute rejection require considerable immunosuppression and are accompanied by an increased risk of opportunistic infections. Rejection episodes are usually treated with high-dose methylprednisolone or various antibody preparations such as polyclonal antithymocyte globulin (ATG), antilymphocyte globulin (ALG) or the pan-T-cell monoclonal antibody OKT3. It should be remembered that patients requiring a second or third graft are usually even more immunosuppressed.

Tacrolimus (FK506), has been recently licensed and substituted for cyclosporin for certain indications; several studies have demonstrated fewer infective complications (Torre-Cisneros et al 1991, Sakr et al 1992, Kusne et al 1992, European FK506 Multicentre Liver Study Group 1994), which may be a consequence of the need for less antirejection therapy. A number of investigational agents under development may permit more targeted therapy with a further reduction in infective complications.

The immunosuppressive therapy for bone marrow transplantation is somewhat different and consists of two components: the 'conditioning' regimen and the anti-graft-versus-host regimen. Most conditioning regimens contain high-dose cyclophosphamide together with either total body irradiation or another agent such as busulphan. Post-transplant regimens may include corticosteroids, methotrexate or cyclosporin A for the first 100 days. T-cell depletion may obviate the need for such regimens. As a consequence, the BMT recipient has an initial phase of neutropenia, lasting approximately 3 weeks, followed by a period of gradually resolving, but relatively profound, lymphocyte-mediated immune deficiency. Immune reconstitution may take up to 2 years to recover.

TIME COURSE OF INFECTION POST-TRANSPLANT

There is a sequential pattern to the infectious complications following any transplantation procedure. Knowledge of this is helpful in guiding duration of prophylaxis and establishing a diagnosis through appropriate investigations and in administering treatment when infection is suspected.

In the first month post-transplant, infections are largely those associated with the transplant surgical procedure. Some infections are transmitted with the allograft or are present in the recipient prior to transplantation. Between 1 and 6 months post-transplantation the most important infections are caused by the herpes group viruses (especially CMV), *Listeria monocytogenes, Pneum. carinii* and other

fungi. Subsequent infections are usually the result of community acquired organisms. A few patients will have chronic viral infections affecting the graft, while others who have been intensively immunosuppressed remain at risk of opportunistic infections.

CAUSATIVE ORGANISMS

Bacterial infections

Bacterial infections occur in 50–70% of transplantation procedures (Eickhoff et al 1972, Montgomery et al 1973, Kirby et al 1987, Kusne et al 1988, Colonna et al 1988, Paya et al 1989, George et al 1991), and in some series patients have suffered at least one bacterial infection in the post-transplant period (George et al 1991). The common infections are: intra-abdominal abscess, cholangitis, bacteraemia, wound infection, lower respiratory tract infection and urinary tract infection, with intra-abdominal infection responsible for approximately 30% in liver transplantation (Kusne et al 1988, Colonna et al 1988, Paya et al 1989, George et al 1991). The overall mortality is less than 5%, but varies according to site and organ transplanted (Colonna et al 1988, Paya et al, 1989, George et al 1991).

Representative organisms isolated from infected patients in the postoperative period are shown in Box 43.4. Bacteria isolated from the graft perfusion fluid differ in their propensity to cause post-transplantation infection. Positive cultures have been found in up to 40% of cases in renal transplantation, but most of these have been due to Gram-positive skin bacteria and do not seem to have serious consequences (McCoy et al 1975, Majeski et al 1982, Nelson et al 1984). However, the isolation of the Enterobacteriaceae and *Ps. aeruginosa* correlate with vascular infection and postoperative sepsis (Fernando et al 1976, Weber et al 1979, Nelson et al 1984) and warrant systemic antibiotic therapy following transplantation.

Box 43.4 *Organisms causing post-transplant infections*

Gram-positive bacteria	**Fungi**
Coagulase-negative staphylococci	*Candida* spp.
Staphylococcus aureus	*Aspergillus* spp.
Enterococci	*Pneumocystis carinii*
Streptococci	*Cryptococcus neoformans*
Listeria monocytogenes	
Nocardia spp.	**Viruses**
	HSV
Gram-negative bacteria	CMV
Enterobacteriaceae	HBV
Pseudomonas spp.	HCV
Stenotrophomonas maltophilia	Varicella-zoster virus
Legionella spp.	Polyoma viruses
Anaerobic bacteria	**Others**
Bacteroides spp.	*Mycobacterium* spp.
Clostridium spp.	*Toxoplasma gondii*

Infections due to *Nocardia* spp. are important late complications following transplantation, usually occurring after the first month and which correlate with the degree of immunosuppression. Outbreaks in renal transplant units have been described (Leaker et al 1989).

Fungal infections

As with most immunocompromised patients colonization with yeasts is common, although the incidence varies according to the number and frequency of sites sampled and the use of antifungal prophylaxis. Infection rates vary with the type of transplant, being least for renal transplant recipients (approximately 5%) and most for liver transplant recipients (>20%) (Paya 1993). The majority of infections are severe, although those associated with renal transplantation are often due to catheter-related sepsis or mucosal infection. The majority of infections are caused by *Candida* spp. (approximately 80%) with *Aspergillus* spp. accounting for the majority of remainder (Wajszczuk et al 1985, Paya 1993). *Pneum. carinii* pneumonitis occurs in about 10% of liver, kidney and heart transplant recipients, and in more than 80% of heart–lung and lung transplant recipients not receiving prophylaxis (Gryzan et al 1988). It is closely linked with CMV disease.

Although occurring very infrequently, disseminated aspergillosis is the most common cause of focal brain infection in solid organ transplant patients ((Martinez & Ahdab-Barmada 1993, Singh et al 1994b) and *Cryptococcus neoformans* is the most frequent cause of meningitis.

Severe fungal infections carry a high mortality. Candidal infections are associated with death in more than 50% and invasive aspergillosis is almost universally fatal in this group (Paya 1993).

The majority of fungal infections occur in the first 2 months post-transplant (Paya 1993), although *Pneum. carinii* infection tends to be delayed and cryptococcosis may well affect patients in the late transplant period. The management of these infections is discussed further in Chapter 60.

Viral infections

CMV is the major virus causing morbidity and mortality in these patients and is responsible for the greatest number of all types of infection. The incidence varies from 45% (Umana et al 1992) to 100% (Mollison 1993), reflecting the incidence of seropositivity amongst the recipient population and the numbers of seropositive to seronegative transplantations. Overall, 25–30% of those infected develop disease (Umana et al 1992, Mollison et al 1993, Mustafa 1994), although of those at highest risk (seropositive to seronegative transplants) 50–60% will develop clinical disease (Rubin 1994). About 3% of those affected will develop CMV pneumonitis (Mustafa 1994).

Post-transplant hepatitis occurs in more than 10% of solid organ transplant recipients overall. The most common cause is hepatitis C virus (HCV). In liver transplant patients the majority of these infections occur as a result of reinfection in patients who have been transplanted for HCV related cirrhosis. PCR techniques have shown that virtually all infected patients suffer reinfection post-transplant. Before universal screening of blood donors and awareness of donor status, primary HCV infections occurred in more than 35% (Wright et al 1992); the incidence is now much lower. In one study, 95% of those with pretransplant infection developed post-transplant hepatitis and the majority were found to be due to HCV.

Reinfection with hepatitis B virus (HBV) following liver transplantation is almost inevitable unless long-term immunoprophylaxis is used. The highest recurrence is seen in those who are HBV-DNA positive pretransplant (Samuel et al 1993).

Epstein–Barr virus reactivation post-transplant is probably underdiagnosed. The most important complication of this is post-transplant lymphoproliferative disorder (PTLD). The overall incidence of this condition is approximately 1% (Rostaing et al 1993). In a large series of various solid organ graft recipients, viraemia was found in 3.9%, and 75% of those with primary viraemia developed PTLD compared with 11% of secondary viraemia cases (Rostaing et al 1993).

Before the advent of acyclovir, HSV infections (almost exclusively the consequence of reactivation) were responsible for clinical disease in approximately 50% of seropositive patients (Rubin 1994). HSV infections are now much less clinically significant than other herpes group infections.

Infections due to other organisms

The incidence of toxoplasmosis varies according to the type of transplant (most common in heart transplant recipients), the seroprevalence of the infection (20% in the UK, higher in other countries such as France) and the serological status of donor and recipient, where the highest rate and most severe infections occur when transplanting a seropositive donor to a seronegative recipient.

The overall incidence of mycobacterial infection in the transplant population is 1%, more than 50-fold greater than the incidence in the general population (Rubin 1994).

CHEMOPROPHYLAXIS

Most prophylactic regimens used in transplant patients are based on the risk of infection and likely organisms. Regimens shown to be effective in the neutropenic patient or in surgical prophylaxis have been adopted, yet few have been subject to randomized comparative trials. A short course of prophylactic antibiotics is probably appropriate to prevent wound infection.

Several studies have demonstrated the benefit of long-term prophylaxis for urinary tract infections (UTIs) in renal transplant recipients. Both co-trimoxazole (960 mg nightly) and ciprofloxacin have been effective, although co-trimoxazole has the additional benefit of preventing *Pneum. carinii* infection (Tolkoff-Rubin et al 1982, Fox et al 1990).

The issue of mycobacterial prophylaxis remains controversial and policies vary internationally. There is a significant risk of isoniazid hepatic toxicity and so this drug should be used selectively. Patients in whom such treatment is justified are those of Asian or other high-risk ethnic origin, those with a past history of tuberculosis and those with chest X-ray changes suggesting past infection. In the USA the tuberculin skin test is often used as a determinant for prophylaxis.

The high risk of fungal infection in liver transplant recipients has led to the administration of antifungal agents in the post-transplant period. Non-absorbable agents such as amphotericin B or nystatin, sometimes in combination with oral antibiotics such as gentamicin and polymyxin B, are widely used (Ch. 60). Recently, a working party has recommended the use of fluconazole as prophylaxis in liver transplantation, unless there is a high institutional incidence of invasive aspergillosis, when itraconazole is recommended (Working Party of the British Society for Antimicrobial Chemotherapy 1993).

Several randomized comparative studies have demonstrated the superior efficacy of early (first 14 days or until discharge) post-transplant ganciclovir, with (Kakazato et al 1993) or without (Martin 1993) gammaglobulin in preventing CMV symptomatic infection in the liver transplant setting, when compared with various doses of acyclovir. Symptomatic infection was reduced to 5–9%. Acyclovir in high dose appears to be effective in comparison with no antiviral prophylaxis (Mollison et al 1993). Pre-emptive prophylaxis has recently been studied in transplant patients. This targets patients at highest risk of disease and limits duration of drug administration, reducing toxicity and cost. Hence kidney–pancreas transplant patients receiving OKT3 pan-T-cell monoclonal antibody therapy and CMV-shedding liver transplant recipients have both been shown to benefit from pre-emptive prophylaxis with ganciclovir (Hopt et al 1994, Singh et al 1994a).

TREATMENT

Whilst transplant recipients are severely immunocompromised, they do not have the same paucity of signs as neutropenic patients in the face of serious sepsis, and, indeed, in the immediate postoperative period behave more like patients with surgical sepsis. Consequently, the concept of early empirical therapy in response to fever has not been applied to these patients.

All attempts should be made to identify a focus of sepsis or the non-infective cause for fever in a transplant patient. Antimicrobial therapy may reasonably be withheld if the patient is otherwise well and there is no identifiable infective cause, but this should be kept under review. If empirical treatment is deemed necessary the choice of antimicrobials should be governed by the timing of the infection (and hence the likely organisms), the type of transplant and the site of sepsis, as discussed previously.

ASPECTS OF THERAPY FOR SPECIFIC INFECTIONS

Pulmonary infections of unknown cause

Patients presenting with pulmonary infiltrates and fever 1 month or more post-transplant are most likely to have CMV or *Pneum. carinii* infection (unless they are receiving co-trimoxazole prophylaxis). These should be managed as in the bone marrow transplant patient (see above).

Post-transplant lymphoproliferative disorder

The incidence of PTLD is 1–2% in renal transplant recipients (Cockfield et al 1993, Strauss et al 1993), and is related to the degree of immunosuppression (it is seen particularly in patients receiving OKT3) and is more likely in primary EBV infection. At present, the mainstay of therapy is the reduction of immunosuppression together with intravenous acyclovir (10 mg/kg 8-hourly). However, many patients will require local resection or radiotherapy of affected tissue and/or antilymphoma chemotherapy. There are continuing developments in this field, including the possibility of immunotherapy by means of donor leucocyte infusions (Papadopoulos 1994).

DRUG INTERACTIONS DURING TREATMENT OF INFECTION

Cyclosporin interacts with a large number of antimicrobial agents (Table 43.5). Levels of the drug may be altered by the induction or inhibition of the hepatic cytochrome P450 enzyme system and it is essential that cyclosporin levels are measured to prevent cyclosporin toxicity, as well as to avoid inadequate or excessive immunosuppression, with the consequences of either rejection or infection. Rifampicin is a potent inducer of the P450 enzyme system and causes increased metabolism of cyclosporin. Erythromycin, some of the newer macrolides, and the azole antifungal agents, particularly ketoconazole (and itraconazole and fluconazole

Table 43.5 *Potential drug interactions during management of infections in organ transplant recipients*

Antimicrobial agent	Immunosuppressive agent	Effect
Aminoglycosides	Cyclosporin	Exacerbation of nephrotoxicity
Amphotericin B	Cyclosporin	Exacerbation of nephrotoxicity
Co-trimoxazole	Cyclosporin	Possible exacerbation of nephrotoxicity
Co-trimoxazole (i.v.)	Cyclosporin	Reduced levels of cyclosporin
Doxycycline	Cyclosporin	Increased cyclosporin levels
Erythromycin	Cyclosporin	Increased cyclosporin levels
Fluconazole	Cyclosporin	Increased cyclosporin levels
Ganciclovir	Azathioprine	Possible exacerbation of myelosuppression
Itraconazole	Cyclosporin	Increased cyclosporin levels
Ketoconazole	Cyclosporin	Increased cyclosporin levels
Pentamidine (i.v.)	Cyclosporin	Possible exacerbation of nephrotoxicity
Rifampicin	Cyclosporin	Reduced levels of cyclosporin
	Prednisone	Reduced levels of prednisone
Sulphonamides	Azathioprine	Possible exacerbation of myelosuppression
Trimethoprim	Azathioprine	Possible exacerbation of myelosuppression
Vancomycin	Cyclosporin	Exacerbation of nephrotoxicity

at high doses), competitively inhibit this pathway, thus increasing levels of cyclosporin. The levels of corticosteroids may be reduced by rifampicin and so doses should be increased during treatment of tuberculosis in the transplant patient.

Renal function is often impaired in the transplantation setting and there may be a complex interaction between cyclosporin (itself potentially nephrotoxic, particularly during initial therapy) and nephrotoxic antimicrobial agents such as the aminoglycosides, high-dose co-trimoxazole, vancomycin and amphotericin B. Therapeutic drug monitoring is mandatory (with the exception of amphotericin B) to prevent additional toxicity. Alternative agents should be chosen whenever possible.

Conclusion

In managing infective complications in the neutropenic and organ transplant patient the emphasis should always be placed on prevention. Despite the advent of antimicrobials with good activity against the infecting agents, the mortality from many of these infections remains high. It is also clear that, once established, various cytokine pathways and immunopathological mechanisms are activated so that much more than an antimicrobial agent is required to control the infection and restore the host's equilibrium.

References

Aisner J, Schimpff S C, Wiernik P H 1977 Treatment of invasive aspergillosis: relationship of early diagnosis and treatment to response. *Annals of Internal Medicine* 86: 539 –543

Anonymous 1989 Empiric antifungal therapy in febrile granulocytopenic patients. EORTC International Antimicrobial Therapy Cooperative Group. *American Journal of Medicine* 86: 668–672

Barnes R A, Rogers T R 1988 Response rates to a staged antibiotic regimen in febrile neutropenic patients. *Journal of Antimicrobial Chemotherapy* 22: 759–763

Bodey G P 1979 Treatment of acute leukemia in protected environment units. *Cancer* 44: 431–436

Bodey G P 1986 Infection in cancer patients. A continuing association. *American Journal of Medicine* 81 (suppl 1A): 11–26

Bodey G P, Buckley M, Sathe Y S, Freireich E J 1966 Quantitative relationships between circulating leucocytes and infection in patients with acute leukaemia. *Annals of Internal Medicine* 64 (2): 328–340

Bodey G P, Buckley Valdivieso M, Feld R, Rodriguez V, McCredie K 1977 Carbenicillin plus cephalothin or cefazolin as therapy for infections in neutropenic patients. *American Journal of Medical Sciences* 273: 309–318

Bodey G P, Jadeja J, Elting L 1985 Pseudomonas bacteremia. Retrospective analysis of 410 episodes. *Archives of Internal Medicine* 145: 1621–1629

Bodey G P, Bueltmann B, Duguid W et al 1992 Fungal infections in cancer patients – an international autopsy survey. *European Journal of Clinical Microbiology* 11: 99–109

Bodey G P, Anaissie E, Gutterman J, Vadhan-Raj S 1993 Role of granulocyte-macrophage colony-stimulating factor as adjuvant therapy for fungal infection in patients with cancer. *Clinical Infectious Diseases* 17: 705–707

Boeckh M, Bowden R A, Goodrich J M et al 1992 Cytomegalovirus antigen detection in peripheral blood leukocytes after allogeneic marrow transplantation. Blood 80: 1358–1364

Brammer K W 1990 Management of fungal infection in neutropenic patients with fluconazole. Haematologie und Bluttransfusion 33: 546–550

Buckner C D, Clift R A, Sanders J E et al 1978 Protective environment for marrow transplant recipients. Annals of Internal Medicine 89: 893–901

Calandra T, Zinner S H, Viscoli C et al 1993 Efficacy and toxicity of single daily doses of amikacin and ceftriaxone versus multiple daily doses of amikacin and ceftazidime for infection in patients with cancer and granulocytopenia. Annals of Internal Medicine 119: 584–593

Castaldo P, Stratta R J, Wood R P et al 1991a Fungal infections in liver allograft recipients. Transplantation Proceedings 23: 1967

Castaldo P, Stratta R J, Wood R P et al 1991b Clinical spectrum of fungal infections after orthotopic liver transplantation. Archives of Surgery 126: 149–156

Centers of Disease Control and Prevention 1994 Preventing the spread of vancomycin resistance: report from the hospital infection control practices advisory committee. Federal Register 59: 25 757

Chow A W, Jewesson P J, Kureishi A, Phillips G L 1993 Teicoplanin versus vancomycin in the empirical treatment of febrile neutropenic patients. European Journal of Haematology 51: 18–24

Cline M J 1973a A new white cell test which measures individual phagocyte function in a mixed leukocyte population. I. A neutrophil defect in acute myelocytic leukemia. Journal of Laboratory and Clinical Medicine 81: 311–316

Cline M J 1973b Defective mononuclear phagocytic function in patients with myelomonocytic leukemia and in some patients with lymphomas. Journal of Clinical Investigation 52: 2815–2190

Cockfield S M, Preiksatis J K, Jewell L D, Parfrey N A 1993 Post-transplant lymphoproliferative disorder in renal allograft recipients. Transplantation 56: 88–96

Colonna J O, Winston D J, Brill J E et al 1988 Infectious complications in liver transplantation. Archives of Surgery 123: 360–364

Cometta A, Zinner S, De Bock R et al 1995 Piperacillin–tazobactam plus amikacin as empiric therapy for fever in granulocytopenic patients with cancer. Antimicrobial Agents and Chemotherapy 39: 445–452

Cometta A, Calandra T, Gaya H et al 1996 Monotherapy with meropenem versus combination therapy with ceftazidime plus amikacin as empiric therapy for fever in granulo-cytopenic patients with cancer. Antimicrobial Agents and Chemotherapy 40: 1108–1115

Conneally E, Cafferkey M T, Daly P A et al 1990 Nebulized amphotericin B as prophylaxis against invasive aspergillosis in granulocytopenic patients. Bone Marrow Transplantation 5: 403–406

Cornelissen J J, De Graeff A, Verdonck L F et al 1992 Imipenem versus gentamicin combined with either cefur-oxime or cephalothin as initial therapy for febrile neutropenic patients. Antimicrobial Agents and Chemotherapy 36: 801–807

DeGregorio M W, Lee W M F, Linker C A et al 1982 Fungal infections in patients with acute leukemia. American Journal of Medicine 73: 543–548

Dekker A W, Rozenberg-Arska M, Sixma J J et al 1981 Prevention of infection by trimethoprim-sulfamethoxazole plus amphotericin B in patients with acute nonlymphocytic leukemia. Annals of Internal Medicine 95: 555–559

De Pauw B E, Deresinski S C, Feld R et al 1994 Ceftazidime compared with piperacillin and tobramycin for the empiric treatment of fever in neutropenic patients with cancer – a multicenter randomized trial. Annals of Internal Medicine 120: 834–844

Demetri G D, Antman K H S 1992 Granulocyte–macrophage colony-stimulating factor (GMCSF): preclinical and clinical investigations. Seminars in Oncology 19: 362–385

Denning D W, Tucker R M, Hanson L H, Stevens D A 1989 Treatment of invasive aspergillosis with itraconazole. American Journal of Medicine 86: 791–800

Dietrich M, Gaus W, Vossen J et al 1977 Protective isolation and antimicrobial decontamination in patients with high susceptibility to infection. A prospective co-operative study of gnotobiotic care in acute leukemia patients. I. Clinical results. Infection 5: 107–114

Donnelly J P, Maschmeyer G, Daenen S 1992 Selective oral antimicrobial prophylaxis for the prevention of infection in acute leukaemia – ciprofloxacin versus co-trimoxazole plus colistin. European Journal of Cancer 28A: 873–878

Eickhoff T C, Olin D B, Anderson R J et al 1972 Current problems and approaches to diagnosis of infection in renal transplant recipients. Transplantation Proceedings 4: 693–697

Einsele H, Steidle M, Vallbracht A et al 1991 Early occurrence of human cytomegalovirus infection after bone marrow transplantation as demonstrated by polymerase chain reaction technique. Blood 77: 1104–1110

Emanuel D, Cunningham I, Jules-Elysee K et al 1988 Cytomegalovirus pneumonia after bone marrow trans-plantation successfully treated with the combination of ganciclovir and high-dose intravenous immune globulin. Annals of Internal Medicine 109: 777–782

EORTC International Antimicrobial Therapy Project Group 1984 Trimethoprim–sulfamethoxazole in the prevention of infection in neutropenic patients. *Journal of Infectious Diseases* 150: 372–379

EORTC International Antimicrobial Therapy Group 1987 Ceftazidime combined with a short or long course of amikacin for empirical therapy of Gram-negative bacteraemia in cancer patients with granulocytopenia. *New England Journal of Medicine* 317: 1692–1628

European FK506 Multicentre Liver Study Group 1994 Randomised trial comparing tacrolimus (FK506) and cyclosporin in prevention of liver allograft rejection. *Lancet* 344: 423–428

Fernando O N, Higgins A F, Moorhead J F 1976 Secondary haemorrhage after renal transplantation. *Lancet* ii: 368

Fisher B D, Armstrong D, Yu B, Gold J W 1981 Invasive aspergillosis: progress in early diagnosis and treatment. *American Journal of Medicine* 71: 571–577

Fox B C, Sollinger H W, Belzer F O et al 1990 A prospective, randomized, double-blind study of trimethoprim–sulfamethoxazole for prophylaxis of infections in renal transplantation: clinical efficacy, absorption of trimethoprim–sulfamethoxazole, effects on the microflora, and the cost benefit of prophylaxis. *American Journal of Medicine* 89: 255

George D L, Arnow P M, Fox A S et al 1991 Bacterial infection as a complication of liver transplantation: epidemiology and risk factors. *Reviews of Infectious Diseases* 13: 387–396

GIMENA Infection Program 1991 Prevention of bacterial infection in neutropenic patients with hematologic malignancies. A randomized multicenter trial comparing norfloxacin with ciprofloxacin. *Annals of Internal Medicine* 115: 7–12

Glaspy J A, Golde D W 1992 Granulocyte colony-stimulating factor (GCSF): preclinical and clinical investigations. *Seminars in Oncology* 19: 386–394

Goodman J L, Winston D J, Greenfield R A et al 1992 A controlled trial of fluconazole to prevent fungal infections in patients undergoing bone marrow transplantation. *New England Journal of Medicine* 326: 845–851

Goodrich J M, Mori M, Gleaves C A et al 1991 Prevention of cytomegalovirus disease after allogeneic marrow transplantation by early treatment with ganciclovir. *New England Journal of Medicine* 325: 1601–1607

Goodrich J M, Bowden R A, Fisher L et al 1993 Ganciclovir prophylaxis to prevent cytomegalovirus disease after allogeneic marrow transplant. *Annals of Internal Medicine* 118: 173–178

Gryzan S, Paradis I L, Zaavi A et al 1988 Unexpectedly high incidence of *Pneumocystis carinii* infection after lung-heart transplantation: implications for lung defense and allograft survival. *American Reviews of Respiratory Diseases* 137: 1268–1274

Gurwith M, Brunton J L, Lank B et al 1978 Granulocytopenia in hospitalised patients. II. A prospective comparison of two antibiotic regimens in the empiric therapy of febrile patients. *American Journal of Medicine* 64: 127–132

Gurwith M J, Brunton J L, Lank B L et al 1979 A prospective controlled investigation of prophylactic trimethoprim-sulfamethoxazole in hospitalized granulocytopenic patients. *American Journal of Medicine* 66: 248–256

Handwerger S, Rancher B, Alterac D et al 1993 Outbreak due to *Enterococcus faecium* highly resistant to vancomycin, penicillin, and gentamicin. *Clinical Infectious Diseases* 16: 750–755

Hann I M, Corringham R, Keaney M et al 1982 Ketoconazole versus nystatin plus amphotericin B for fungal prophylaxis in severely immunocompromised patients. *Lancet* i: 826–829

Hann I, Prentice H G, Blacklock H A et al 1983 Acyclovir prophylaxis against herpes virus infections in severely immunocompromised patients: randomised double blind trial. *British Medical Journal* 287: 384–388

Hansen R M, Reinerio N, Sohnle P G et al 1987 Ketoconazole in the prevention of candidiasis in patients with cancer. A prospective, randomized, controlled, double-blind study. *Archives of Internal Medicine* 147: 710–712

Hawkins C, Armstrong D 1984 Fungal infections in the immunocompromised host. *Clinics in Haematology* 13 (3): 599–630

Hopt U T, Pfeffer F, Schareck W, Busing M, Ming C 1994 Ganciclovir for prophylaxis of CMV disease after pancreas/kidney transplantation. *Transplantation Proceedings* 26: 434–435

Hughes W T, Price R A, Kim H K et al 1973 *Pneumocystis carinii* pneumonia in children with malignancies. *Journal of Pediatrics* 82: 404–415

Jameson B, Gamble D R, Lynch J, Kay H E M 1971 Five-year analysis of protective isolation. *Lancet* i: 1034–1040

Jorgensen C J, Dreyfus F, Vaixeler J et al 1989 Failure of amphotericin B spray to prevent aspergillosis in granulocytopenic patients. *Nouvelle Revue Francaise d'Hematologie* 31: 327–328

Kakazato P Z, Burns W, Moore P, Garcia-Kennedy R, Cox K, Esquivel C 1993 Viral prophylaxis in hepatic transplantation: preliminary report of a randomized trial of acyclovir and ganciclovir. *Transplantation Proceedings* 25: 1935–1937

Karp J E, Merz W G, Dick J D, Saral R 1991 Strategies to prevent or control infections after bone marrow transplants. *Bone Marrow Transplantation* 8: 1–6

Kerr K G, Hawkey P M, Child J A, Norfolk D R, Anderson A W 1990 *Pseudomonas maltophilia* infections in neutropenic patients and the use of imipenem. *Postgraduate Medical Journal* 66: 1090

Kibbler C C, Milkins S R, Bhamra A et al 1988 Apparent pulmonary mycetoma following invasive aspergillosis in neutropenic patients. *Thorax* 43: 108–112

Kibbler C C, Prentice H G, Sage R J et al 1989a A comparison of double beta-lactam combinations with netilmicin/ureidopenicillin regimens in the empirical therapy of febrile neutropenic patients. *Journal of Antimicrobial Chemotherapy* 23: 759–771

Kibbler C C, Prentice H G, Sage R J et al 1989b Do double beta-lactam combinations prolong neutropenia in patients undergoing chemotherapy or bone marrow transplantation for haematological disease? *Antimicrobial Agents and Chemotherapy* 33 (4): 503–507

Kidd M, Fox J C, Pillay D et al 1993 Provision of prognostic information in immunocompromised patients by routine application of the polymerase chain reaction for cytomegalovirus. *Transplantation* 56: 867–871

Kirby R M, McMaster P, Clements D et al 1987 Orthotopic liver transplantation: postoperative complications and their management. *British Journal of Surgery* 74: 3–11

Klastersky J, Glauser M P, Schimpff S C, Gaya H 1986 Antimicrobial Therapy Project Group for Research on Treatment of Cancer. Prospective randomised comparison of three antibiotic regimens for empirical therapy of suspected bacteremic infection in febrile granulocytopenic patients. *Antimicrobial Agents and Chemotherapy* 29: 263–270

Kusne S, Dummer J S, Singh N et al 1988 Infections after liver transplantation. An analysis of 101 consecutive cases. *Medicine Baltimore* 67: 132–143

Kusne S, Fung J, Alessiani M et al 1992 Infections during a randomized trial comparing cyclosporine to FK506 immunosuppression in liver transplantation. *Transplantation Proceedings* 24: 429–430

Leaker B, Hellyar A, Neild G H et al 1989 Nocardia infection in a renal transplant unit. *Transplantation Proceedings* 21: 2103–2104

Levine A S, Siegal S E, Schreiber A D et al 1973 Protected environments and prophylactic antibiotics. A prospective controlled study of their utility in the therapy of acute leukemia. *New England Journal of Medicine* 288: 477–483

Liang R, Yung R, Chiu E et al 1990 Ceftazidime versus imipenem–cilastatin as initial monotherapy for febrile neutropenic patients. *Antimicrobial Agents and Chemotherapy* 34: 1336–1341

Ljungman P, Engelhard D, Link H et al 1992 Treatment of interstitial pneumonitis due to cytomegalovirus with ganciclovir and intravenous immune globulin: experience of European Bone Marrow Transplant Group. *Clinical Infectious Diseases* 14 (4): 831–835

Majeski J A, Alexander J W, First M R et al 1982 Transplantation of microbially contaminated cadaver kidneys. *Archives of Surgery* 117: 221–224

Martin M 1993 Antiviral prophylaxis for CMV infection in liver transplantation. *Transplantation Proceedings* 25 (suppl 4): 10–14

Martinez A J, Ahdab-Barmada M 1993 The neuropathology of liver transplantation: comparison of main complications in children and adults. *Modern Pathology* 6: 25–32

McCoy G C, Loening S, Braun W E et al 1975 The fate of cadaver renal allografts contaminated before transplantation. *Transplantation* 20: 467–472

McWhinney P H M, Kibbler C C, Prentice H G et al 1991 A prospective trial of imipenem versus ceftazidime/vancomycin as empirical therapy for fever in neutropenic patients. 17th International Congress of Chemotherapy, Berlin, abstract 1276

McWhinney P H, Patel S, Whiley R A et al 1993a Activities of potential therapeutic and prophylactic antibiotics against blood culture isolates of viridans group streptococci from neutropenic patients receiving ciprofloxacin. *Antimicrobial Agents and Chemotherapy* 37: 2493–2495

McWhinney P H, Kibbler C C, Hamon M D et al 1993b Progress in the diagnosis and management of aspergillosis in bone marrow transplantation: 13 years' experience. *Clinical Infectious Diseases* 17: 397–404

Meunier F 1987 Prevention of mycoses in immunocompromised patients. *Reviews in Infectious Diseases* 9: 408–416

Mills W, Chopra R, Linch D C, Goldstone A H 1994 Liposomal amphotericin B in the treatment of fungal infections in neutropenic patients: a single-centre experience of 133 episodes in 116 patients. *British Journal of Haematology* 86: 754–760

Mollison L C, Richards M J, Johnson P D et al 1993 High dose oral acyclovir reduces the incidence of cytomegalovirus infection in liver transplant recipients. *Journal of Infectious Diseases* 168: 721–724

Montgomery J R, Barrett F F, Williams T W Jr 1973 Infectious complications in cardiac transplant patients. *Transplantation Proceedings* 5: 1239–1243

Mustafa M M 1994 Cytomegalovirus infection and disease in the immunocompromised host. *Pediatric Infectious Diseases* 13: 249–259

Myers S E, Devine S M, Topper R L et al 1992 A pilot study of prophylactic aerosolized amphotericin B in patients at risk for prolonged neutropenia. *Leukemia and Lymphoma* 8: 229–233

Nelson P W, Delmonico F L, Tolkoff-Rubin N E et al 1984 Unsuspected donor *Pseudomonas* infection causing arterial disruption after renal transplantation. *Transplantation* 37: 313–314

Odds F C 1988 *Candida* and candidosis, 2nd edn. Baillière Tindall, London

Papadopoulos E B, Ladanyi M, Emanuel D et al 1994 Infusions of donor leukocytes to treat Epstein–Barr virus-associated lymphoproliferative disorders after allogeneic bone marrow transplantation. *New England Journal of Medicine* 330: 1185–1191

Paya C V 1993 Fungal infections in solid-organ transplantation. *Clinical Infectious Diseases* 16: 677–688

Paya C V, Hermans P E, Washington J A et al 1989 Incidence, distribution and outcome of episodes of infection in 100 orthotopic liver transplantations. *Mayo Clinic Proceedings* 64: 555–564

Pettengell R, Gurney H, Radford J A et al 1992 Granulocyte colony-stimulating factor to prevent dose-limited neutropenia in non-Hodgkin's lymphoma: a randomized controlled trial. *Blood* 80: 1430–1436

Pizzo P A, Commers J, Cotton D et al 1984 Approaching the controversies in the antibacterial management of cancer patients. *American Journal of Medicine* 76: 436–449

Pizzo P A, Hathorn J W, Hiemenz J et al 1986 A randomised trial comparing ceftazidime alone with combination antibiotic therapy in cancer patients with fever and neutropenia. *New England Journal of Medicine* 315: 552–558

Pizzo P A, Rubin M, Freifeld A, Walsh T J 1991 The child with cancer and infection. I. Empiric therapy for fever and neutropenia, and preventive strategies. *Journal of Pediatrics* 119: 679–694

Poynton C H, Jackson S K, Fegan C, Barnes R A, Whittaker J A 1992 Use of IgM enriched immunoglobulin (Pentaglobin) in bone marrow transplantation. *Bone Marrow Transplant* 9: 451–457

Prentice H G, Gluckman E, Powles R L et al 1994 Impact of long-term acyclovir on cytomegalovirus infection and survival after allogeneic bone marrow transplantation. European Acyclovir for CMV Prophylaxis Study Group. *Lancet* 343: 749–753

Ramphal R, Bolger M, Oblon D J et al 1992 Vancomycin is not an essential component of the initial empiric treatment regimen for febrile neutropenic patients receiving ceftazidime: a prospective randomized study. *Antimicrobial Agents and Chemotherapy* 36: 1062–1067

Reed E C, Bowden R A, Dandliker P S, Lilleby K E, Meyers J D 1988 Treatment of cytomegalovirus pneumonia with ganciclovir and intravenous cytomegalovirus immunoglobulin in patients with bone marrow transplants. *Annals of Internal Medicine* 109: 783–788

Riikonen P 1991 Imipenem compared with ceftazidime plus vancomycin as initial therapy for fever in neutropenic

children with cancer. *Pediatric Infectious Disease Journal* 10: 918–923

Rodriguez V, Bodey G P, Freireich E J et al 1978 Randomized trial of protected environment prophylactic antibiotics in 145 adults with acute leukemia. *Medicine* 57: 253–266

Rolston K V I, Berkey P, Bodey G P et al 1992 A comparison of imipenem ceftazimide with or without amikacin as empiric therapy in febrile neutropenic patients. *Archives of Internal Medicine* 152: 283–291

Rostaing L, Icart J, Durand D et al 1993 Clinical outcome of Epstein–Barr viraemia in transplant patients. *Transplant Proceedings* 25: 2286–2287

Rubin R H 1994 Infection in the organ transplant recipient. In: Rubin R H, Young L S (eds) Clinical approach to infection in the compromised host, 3rd edn. Plenum, New York, p 629–705

Sakr M, Hassanein T, Gaveler J et al 1992 Cytomegalovirus infection of the upper gastrointestinal tract following liver transplantation: incidence, location and severity in cyclosporin and FK506 treated patients. *Transplantation* 53: 786–791

Samuel D, Muller R, Alexander G 1993 Liver transplantation in European patients with the hepatitis B surface antigen. *New England Journal of Medicine* 329: 1842–1847

Sanders J W, Powe N R, Moore R D 1991 Ceftazidime monotherapy for empiric treatment of febrile neutropenic patients: a meta-analysis. *Journal of Infectious Diseases* 164: 907–916

Schimpff S C, Greene W H, Young V W, Wiernik P H 1974 Significance of *Pseudomonas aeruginosa* in the patient with leukemia or lymphoma. *Journal of Infectious Diseases* 130: S24–S31

Schimpff S C, Greene W H, Young V W et al 1975 Infection prevention in acute nonlymphocytic leukemia. Laminar air flow room reverse isolation with oral nonabsorbable antibiotic prophylaxis. *Annals of Internal Medicine* 82: 351–358

Schroter G P J, Hoelscher M, Putnam C W, Porter K A, Starzl T E 1977 Fungus infections after liver transplantation. *Annals of Surgery* 186: 115–122

Shenep J L, Hughes W T, Roberson P K et al 1988 Vancomycin, ticarcillin, and amikacin compared with ticarcillin–clavulanate and amikacin in the empirical treatment of febrile, neutropenic children with cancer. *New England Journal of Medicine* 319: 1053–1058

Shlaes D M, Binczewski B, Rice L B 1993 Emerging antibiotic resistance and the immunocompromised host. *Clinical Infectious Diseases* 17 (suppl 2): 5527–5536

Singer J W 1992 Role of colony-stimulating factors in bone marrow transplantation. *Seminars in Oncology* 19: 27–31

Singh N, Yu V L, Mieles L et al 1994a High-dose acyclovir compared with short-course preemptive ganciclovir therapy to prevent cytomegalovirus disease in liver transplant recipients: a randomized trial. *Annals of Internal Medicine* 120: 375–381

Singh N, Yu V L, Gayowski T 1994b Central nervous system lesions in adult liver transplant recipients – clinical review with implications for management. *Medicine* 73: 110

UNOS 1993 Statistics from United Network for Organ Sharing

Storring R A, Jameson B, McElwain T J, Wiltshire E 1977 Oral nonabsorbed antibiotics prevent infection in acute non-lymphoblastic leukaemia. *Lancet* ii: 837–840

Strauss S E, Cohen J I, Tosato G et al 1993 Epstein–Barr virus infection: biology, pathogenesis, and management. *Annals of Internal Medicine* 118: 45–58

The EORTC International Antimicrobial Therapy Project Group 1978 Three antibiotic regimens in the treatment of infection in febrile granulocytopenic patients with cancer. *Journal of Infectious Diseases* 137: 14–29

The International Antimicrobial Therapy Project Cooperative Group of the European Organization for Research and Treatment of Cancer 1993 Efficacy and toxicity of single daily doses of amikacin and ceftriaxone versus multiple daily doses of amikacin and ceftazidime for infection in patients with cancer and granulocytopenia. *Annals of Internal Medicine* 119: 584–593

Tolkoff-Rubin N E, Cosimi A B, Russell P S et al 1982 A controlled study of trimethoprim–sulfamethoxazole prophylaxis of urinary tract infections in renal transplant recipients. *Reviews of Infectious Diseases* 4: 614–618

Torre-Cisneros J, Manez R, Kusne S, Alessiani M, Martin M, Starzl T E 1991 The spectrum of aspergillosis in liver transplant patients: comparison of FK506 and cyclosporin immunosuppression. *Transplantation Proceedings* 23: 3040–3041

Umana J P, Mutimer D J, Shaw J C et al 1992 Cytomegalovirus surveillance following liver transplantation: does it allow presymptomatic diagnosis of CMV disease? *Transplantation Proceedings* 24: 2643

Viviani M A, Tortorano A M, Malaspina C et al 1992 Surveillance and treatment of liver transplant recipients for candidiasis and aspergillosis. *European Journal of Epidemiology* 8: 433–436

Wade J C 1993 Management of infection in patients with

acute leukemia. *Hematology/Oncology Clinics of North America* 7: 293–315

Wade J C, Schimpff S C, Hargadon M T et al 1981 A comparison of trimethoprim–sulfamethoxazole plus nystatin with gentamicin plus nystatin in the prevention of infections in acute leukemia. *New England Journal of Medicine* 304: 1057–1062

Wajszczuk C P, Dummer J S, Ho M et al 1985 Fungal infections in liver transplant recipients. *Transplantation* 40: 347–353

Weber T R, Freier D T, Turcotte J F 1979 Transplantation of infected kidneys. *Transplantation* 27: 63–65

Wingard J R, Merz W G, Rinaldi M G et al 1991 Increase in *Candida krusei* infection among patients with bone marrow transplantation and neutropenia treated prophylactically with fluconazole. *New England Journal of Medicine* 325: 1274–1277

Winston D J, Dudnick D V, Chapin M et al 1983 Coagulase-negative staphylococcal bacteremia in patients receiving immunosuppressive therapy. *Archives of Internal Medicine* 143: 32–36

Winston D J, Barnes R C, Ho W G et al 1984 Moxalactam plus piperacillin versus moxalactam plus amikacin in febrile granulocytopenic patients. *American Journal of Medicine* 77: 442–450

Winston D J, Ho W G, Bruckner D A, Gale R P, Champlin R E 1988 Controlled trials of double beta-lactam therapy with cefoperazone plus piperacillin in febrile granulocytopenic patients. *American Journal of Medicine* 85 (suppl 1A): 21–30

Winston D J, Ho W G, Bartoni et al 1993 Ganciclovir prophylaxis of cytomegalovirus infection and disease in allogeneic bone marrow transplant recipients. Results of a placebo-controlled, double-blind trial. *Annals of Internal Medicine* 118: 179–184

Working Party of the British Society for Antimicrobial Chemotherapy 1993 Chemoprophylaxis for candidosis and aspergillosis in neutropenia and transplantation: a review and recommendation. *Journal of Antimicrobial Chemotherapy* 32: 5–21

Wright T L, Donegan E, Hsu H H et al 1992 Recurrent and acquired hepatitis C viral infection in liver transplant recipients. *Gastroenterology* 103: 317–322

Yates J W, Holland J F 1973 A controlled study of isolation and endogenous microbial suppression in acute myelocytic leukemia patients. *Cancer* 32: 1490–1498

Zaia J A 1990 Viral infections associated with bone marrow transplantation. *Hematology/Oncology Clinics of North America* 4: 603–623

Infections in intensive care patients

M. G. Thomas

Introduction

Infection is a common reason for admission to an intensive care unit (ICU) and a common complication of stay in an ICU. A recent study of 10 038 patients in 1417 ICUs in 17 European countries found that 44.8% of ICU patients had one or more infections (Vincent et al 1995). Another study found an infection rate of 23.5% in the 5189 patients admitted to a medical/surgical ICU of a Massachusetts hospital during a 3-year period from 1981 to 1983 (Brown et al 1985).

The presence of infection in patients in ICU is an important risk factor for increased mortality and morbidity. A recent prospective study (Chandrasekar et al 1986) found a 10–20 times increased risk of death in ICU patients with infection. Infection on admission to the ICU and nosocomial intra-abdominal infection have been shown to be independently predictive of fatality, after allowing for other variables such as acute physiology (APACHE) score or the use of steroids or chemotherapy (Craven et al 1988).

Approximately half the infections present in ICU patients are acquired before admission to the ICU, and usually before admission to hospital (Brown et al 1985, Vincent et al 1995). Community acquired infection is common in paediatric and adult medical and surgical ICUs but infrequent in neonatal and cardiac surgical ICUs (Brown et al 1985). The nature of community acquired infections is influenced by the population which the hospital serves. For example, the presence in the community of large numbers of immigrants from developing countries, injecting drug users, or human immunodeficiency virus (HIV) infected persons will increase the incidence of malaria, endovascular infection and acquired immune deficiency syndrome (AIDS) in the patients admitted to the ICU.

Approximately half the infections present in ICU patients are acquired following admission to the ICU. Nosocomial infection rates are particularly high in surgical ICUs, but are also high in medical and combined medical/surgical ICUs (Table 44.1). The most important sites of nosocomial infection in ICU patients are the respiratory tract, the urinary tract and surgical wounds (Table 44.2). The

Table 44.1 *Nosocomial infection rates* in ICUs*

	Study				
	Vincent et al (1995)	Brown et al (1985)	Chandrasekar et al (1986)	Donowitz et al (1982)	Craven et al (1988)
Total No. of infections	2485	1840	66	440	678
Type of ICU (%)					
Medical/surgical	20.6	11.2	–	18	–
Medical	–	–	14	–	35
Surgical	–	–	35	–	62
Coronary	–	1.8	–	–	–
Paediatric	–	6.2	–	–	–
Cardiothoracic surgery	–	0.8	–	–	–
Burns	–	–	30	–	–

* Total number of infections/100 admissions.

Table 44.2 Site of nosocomial infection in ICUs*

	Study			
	Vincent et al (1995)	Brown et al (1985)	Donowitz et al (1982)	Craven et al (1988)
Total No. of infections	2485	1840	440	490
Site of infection (%)				
Respiratory tract	65	36	25	23
Genito-urinary tract	18	26	25	35
Wound	7	4	8	18
Intra-abdominal	5	10	–	3
Bacteraemia	12	3	29	17
Skin	5	5	–	–
Central nervous system	–	5	–	2
Other	10	12	13	–

* Infection at each site as a proportion of total infection rate.

Table 44.3 Organisms isolated from nosocomial infections in ICUs

	Study			
	Vincent et al (1995)	Brown et al (1985)	Donowitz et al (1982)	Craven et al (1988)
Total No. of isolates		1826	120	656
Organisms (%)				
Staph. aureus	30	9	14	8
Staph. epidermidis	19	–	14	–
Enterococci	12	6	6	5
Esch. coli		13	6	13
Klebsiella/ Enterobacter/ Serratia spp.	} 34	} 14	22	24
Pseudomonas	29	9	11	13
Candida	17	9	6	7
Other	–	28	22	30
No isolate	–	12	–	2

spectrum of organisms responsible for infections acquired in the ICU differs from that causing community acquired infections. Thus Haemophilus influenzae *is the major cause of community acquired infection in patients admitted to a paediatric ICU (Brown et al 1985), and* Neisseria meningitidis *and* Streptococcus pneumoniae *are important causes of community acquired infection in adults (Khoo et al 1992). These organisms are unusual causes of ICU acquired infection.* Escherichia coli, Klebsiella *spp.,* Enterobacter *spp.,* Serratia *spp.,* Pseudomonas aeruginosa *and* Staphylococcus aureus *are responsible for almost half of all nosocomial ICU infections (Table 44.3).*

Pneumonia

Pneumonia (Ch. 48) is a common reason for admission to the ICU and the most common nosocomial infection in patients in the ICU. Both community acquired and nosocomial pneumonia have a high mortality in ICU patients, and management of these conditions is complicated by difficulties with diagnosis and antimicrobial treatment. Many ICUs have attempted to improve the outcome for their patients by using prophylactic regimens which attempt to reduce the incidence of pneumonia (see below). Differences in pathogenesis, and microbial aetiology are responsible for the different treatments recommended for community acquired and nosocomial pneumonia.

COMMUNITY ACQUIRED PNEUMONIA

Str. pneumoniae, Staph. aureus, H. influenzae, Legionella pneumophila and *Mycoplasma pneumoniae* are the most commonly identified bacterial causes of community acquired pneumonia in patients admitted to the ICU (Table 44.4). Influenza viruses and cytomegalovirus have been found to be important causes of pneumonia in some studies (Ortqvist et al 1985, Marrie et al 1989, British Thoracic Society 1992). It seems likely that *Str. pneumoniae* is the aetiological agent for many patients in whom no microbial cause can be proven (Marrie et al 1989, Fang et al 1990, Potgieter & Hammond 1992). Aerobic Gram-negative bacilli, particularly *Ps. aeruginosa* and *Klebsiella pneumoniae*, are uncommon causes of community acquired pneumonia in patients admitted to the ICU, but are associated with a mortality of 50–75% (British Thoracic Society 1986, Torres et al 1991, Potgieter & Hammond 1992), in contrast to an overall mortality of 20–50% (Ortqvist et al 1985, Torres et al 1991, British Thoracic Society 1992, Potgieter & Hammond 1992).

Unfortunately, the clinical presentation is usually an unreliable guide to the aetiology of community acquired pneumonia (Torres et al 1991, Potgieter & Hammond 1992, American Thoracic Society 1992), and thus initial treatment will often need to cover the most common pathogens. Occasionally the clinical features on admission may provide useful clues to the aetiology. For example, a history of chronic respiratory disease, alcoholism, immunosuppression or bronchiectasis should alert the doctor to the possibility that the pneumonia is due to an aerobic Gram-negative bacillus (Fang et al 1990, Torres et al 1991, British Thoracic Society 1992, American Thoracic Society 1993). Other clues to a specific diagnosis include the presence of an epidemic due to mycoplasma or influenza. During an influenza epidemic secondary infection with *Staph. aureus* should be suspected. The admission radiographic findings in patients hospitalized with pneumonia usually do not allow a reliable discrimination between the various possible aetiologies (Macfarlane et al 1984). However, an infiltrate which spreads within the same lobe, to other lobes of the same lung, or to the opposite lung is found more frequently in follow-up radiographs from patients with pneumonia due to *Legionella pneumophila* or bacteraemic *Str. pneumoniae* than with pneumonia due to non-bacteraemic *Str. pneumoniae* or *Mycoplasma pneumoniae* (Macfarlane et al 1984).

Sputum Gram stain suggests the aetiology in approximately 10% of patients (British Thoracic Society 1992), while sputum culture and blood culture are diagnostic in 12–44% (Ortqvist et al 1985, British Thoracic Society 1992) and 10–35% (Ortqvist et al 1985, British Thoracic Society 1992, Potgieter & Hammond 1992), respectively. Sorenson et al (1989) have suggested that fibre-optic bronchoscopy with protected brush sampling from the areas of radiological abnormality can increase the chances of obtaining a microbiologic diagnosis. However, this technique provided a positive culture result in only 50% of patients in whom it was performed, and the overall mortality in this small series (36 patients) was 22%, which is comparable to that in other similar studies. Other studies which have used invasive methods (e.g. bronchoscopy with protected brush sampling or broncho-alveolar lavage or percutaneous lung aspiration with ultrathin needles) have not demonstrated an improvement in outcome as a result of these investigations (Torres et al 1991, Potgieter & Hammond 1992). The use of bronchoscopy with broncho-alveolar lavage should at present be reserved for selected patients (e.g. those in whom infection with *Mycobacterium tuberculosis*, *Pneumocystis carinii* or cytomegalovirus is thought likely).

Because infection with *L. pneumophila* and *M. pneumoniae* are common causes of community acquired infection in the ICU, treatment with erythromycin is widely considered an essential component of the initial antimicrobial regimen (British Thoracic Society and Public Health Laboratory Service 1986, Fang et al 1990, Torres et al 1991, British Thoracic Society 1992, American Thoracic Society 1993). Since erythromycin has limited in vitro activity against *H. influenzae* and lacks activity against Gram-negative bacilli and many strains of *Staph. aureus*, treatment with this agent

Table 44.4 *Aetiology of community acquired pneumonia in ICU patients*

	Study				
	BTS (1992)	Ortqvist et al (1985)	Marrie et al (1989)	Torres et al (1991)	Potgieter & Hammond (1992)
Total No. of patients	60	53	133	92	95
Organism (%)					
Str. pneumoniae	18	28	13	15	33
Staph. aureus	5	2	9	0	8
H. influenzae	12	0	6	0	13
L. pneumophila	12	0	2	14	5
M pneumoniae	7	6	3	7	1
Viruses	12	11	17	0	1
'Aspiration'	0	0	17	0	0
Other	0	6	3	16	22
Unknown	42	47	26	48	25

should be combined with a second- or third-generation cephalosporin or β-lactam–β-lactamase inhibitor combination (such as amoxycillin–clavulanic acid). A regimen of erythromycin 1 g 6-hourly plus cefuroxime 0.75–1.5 g 8-hourly is appropriate treatment for most patients with community acquired pneumonia admitted to the ICU, but should be modified in a minority of patients. Patients whose initial sputum (or tracheal aspirate) Gram stain suggests infection due to aerobic Gram-negative bacilli should be treated with erythromycin plus ceftriaxone (or ceftazidime) plus gentamicin. If high-level penicillin resistance is common in community isolates of *Str. pneumoniae* then vancomycin should be added to the usual regimen (Friedland & McCracken 1994). Finally, in patients with suspected or proven anaerobic infection clindamycin or metronidazole should be added to the usual regimen (Gudiol et al 1990).

NOSOCOMIAL PNEUMONIA

Nosocomial pneumonia is the most common ICU acquired infection (Brown et al 1985, Vincent et al 1995). In patients ventilated for more than 48 h the incidence of pneumonia is approximately 20% with an associated mortality of 40–60% (Craven et al 1986, Rello et al 1991). Despite the high incidence of nosocomial pneumonia and its high mortality it remains a diagnostic and therapeutic dilemma. Pneumonia can be diagnosed with certainty in a minority of patients in whom it is suspected, the pathogen(s) responsible for pneumonia are often uncertain, and the outcome is poor despite aggressive antibiotic treatment (Seidenfeld et al 1986). It seems likely that nosocomial pneumonia in ICU patients is frequently a marker of terminal illness rather than an independently important cause of death (Bryan & Reynolds 1984a, Craven et al 1986).

Aspiration of oropharyngeal secretions is considered the usual route of acquiring lung infection. Impaired consciousness, the presence of endotracheal and nasogastric tubes, and tracheostomies all increase the risk of aspiration and the incidence of pneumonia. The organisms aspirated into the lungs reflect those present in the oropharynx and stomach. Following admission to the ICU the oropharynx and stomach become increasingly colonized with aerobic Gram-negative bacilli. Thus aspiration of oropharyngeal secretions at the onset of the illness or injury which leads to ICU admission will result in pneumonia due to a different spectrum of organisms from aspiration, occurring a week or more after admission to the ICU. Langer et al (1989) have drawn attention to the high incidence of pneumonia in the first week after admission to the ICU and have demonstrated that Gram-negative organisms are progressively more common causes of nosocomial pneumonia with increased duration of ICU stay.

Diagnosis

Diagnosis of pneumonia in ICU patients, particularly those who are being ventilated, is extremely difficult. While fever, leucocytosis, purulent sputum, radiological evidence of new pulmonary infiltrates and the presence of pathogenic bacteria in the tracheobronchial secretions are all strongly suggestive of pneumonia, these clinical features may all be present in its absence. Postmortem studies of patients dying with acute respiratory distress syndrome show high false-positive and false-negative rates for the clinical diagnosis of pneumonia (Andrews et al 1981, Bell et al 1983). Because the organisms responsible for causing nosocomial pneumonia in ICU patients are commonly derived from those colonizing the oropharynx, the use of sputum or tracheal aspirates to identify the causative organism(s) is hampered by the problem of distinguishing between contaminants and true pathogens. A variety of techniques, including transtracheal aspiration, transthoracic aspiration and bronchoscopy with sampling by broncho-alveolar lavage or protected specimen brush, have been evaluated, but none has gained widespread acceptance (Cook et al 1994).

Gram-negative enteric bacilli, *Staph. aureus*, *Str. pneumoniae* and *H. influenzae* are the pathogens most commonly responsible for nosocomial pneumonia. In one study of 168 patients with bacteraemic nosocomial pneumonia the organisms isolated from blood cultures were members of the Klebsiella–Enterobacter–Serratia family (26%), *Ps. aeruginosa* (13%), *Esch. coli* (8%), other aerobic Gram-negative organisms (8%), *Staph. aureus* (23%), *Str. pneumoniae* (11%) and other Gram-positive organisms (10%) (Bryan & Reynolds 1984a). Polymicrobial bacteraemia, most commonly with *Staph. aureus*, *K. pneumoniae* or *Ps. aeruginosa*, occurred in 10% of episodes.

Treatment

Treatment of nosocomial pneumonia should be with an agent or combination of agents that covers this spectrum of pathogens. Occasionally, the prior consistent isolation of a pathogen from surveillance cultures of the patient's sputum may assist with selection of an antibiotic regimen. Similarly, the knowledge that *H. influenzae* and *Staph. aureus* are much more likely to cause pneumonia in a patient who has not recently received antibiotic therapy and that *Ps. aeruginosa* is a particularly common cause in patients who have received prior antibiotic therapy (Rello et al 1993) can assist with antibiotic selection. Finally, the occurrence of endemic or epidemic transmission of a nosocomial pathogen within the ICU may need to be considered.

The combination of an aminoglycoside plus a third-generation cephalosporin or a broad-spectrum penicillin have been the regimens most commonly recommended for initial treatment of nosocomial pneumonia in the ICU (Scheld & Mandell 1991, La Force 1992). These regimens have been selected on the basis of having adequate activity against the usual spectrum of pathogens, plus optimal activity against *Ps. aeruginosa* because of the especially high mortality associated with pneumonia due to this organism. The poor penetration of aminoglycosides into pulmonary secretions is a significant problem in the treatment of severe nosocomial pneumonia. This is illustrated by the finding that the outcome in patients with Gram-negative pneumonia treated with gentamicin or tobramycin is significantly improved if the initial maximal peak serum concentrations are greater than 7 mg/l (Moore et al 1984). The increasing use of once-daily dosing with aminoglycosides, which usually produces peak gentamicin concentrations of 10–20 mg/l, should enhance the efficacy of these drugs in the treatment of pneumonia. Another method of attempting to achieve adequate local concentrations of aminoglycoside has been to supplement parenteral therapy with aminoglycoside therapy delivered directly into the endotracheal tube. However, in one randomized double-blind study the administration of 40 mg tobramycin every 8 h via the endotracheal tube did not improve the clinical outcome in patients with Gram-negative pneumonia, all of whom were treated systemically with either cefazolin or piperacillin (Brown et al 1990).

Concern about the nephrotoxicity and ototoxicity associated with aminoglycoside therapy has led to the use of regimens in which aztreonam is substituted for the aminoglycoside. Aztreonam lacks activity against Gram-positive organisms and generally should be used in combination with another agent with Gram-positive activity such as clindamycin, vancomycin or cloxacillin. Rodriguez & Ramirez-Ronda (1985) found clindamycin plus aztreonam (2 g 8-hourly) to be as efficacious as clindamycin plus tobramycin (80 mg 8-hourly) in the treatment of lower respiratory tract infections caused by aerobic Gram-negative bacilli. Another trial comparing aztreonam (1–2 g every 8–12 h) with tobramycin in the treatment of nosocomial pneumonia in ICU patients, most of whom were treated with additional antibiotics, found a better clinical and micro-biological outcome in the aztreonam-treated group (Schentag et al 1985).

Ceftazidime, imipenem–cilastatin, ciprofloxacin and a number of other agents have been evaluated as monotherapy for nosocomial pneumonia. Ceftazidime monotherapy (2 g 8-hourly) was comparable to tobramycin plus cefazolin (Mandell et al 1987) and tobramycin plus ticarcillin (Cone et al 1985) in two small studies of hospitalized patients with pneumonia. Ceftazidime (2 g 12-hourly) and imipenem (500 mg 6-hourly) had similar efficacy in a large study of nosocomial pneumonia (Norrby et al 1993). Imipenem–cilastatin monotherapy (1.5–3.0 g/day) resulted in a clinical cure in 26/29 patients with nosocomial pneumonia (Salata et al 1985). Ticarcillin plus clavulanic acid given in a dose of 3–5 g ticarcillin plus 200 mg clavulanic acid 8-hourly, was associated with a clinical cure rate of 96% in patients

with nosocomial bronchopulmonary infections in ICUs (Schwigon et al 1986). Ciprofloxacin 200 mg 12-hourly i.v. (Peloquin et al 1989) and pefloxacin 800–1200 mg/day (Martin et al 1988) have been used as monotherapy for nosocomial pneumonia in ventilated patients. However, the clinical failure rate was 26% with pefloxacin and 47% with ciprofloxacin. None of the monotherapy regimens evaluated was adequate treatment for pneumonia due to *Pseudomonas* spp. Persistent infection during treatment, development of resistance to the agent used, and clinical failure of monotherapy, occasionally with an improved response when a second agent was added to the regimen, were common problems with pseudomonas pneumonia with all the monotherapy regimens. While the overall outcome of monotherapy is similar to that of combination therapy (La Force 1989), pneumonia known or suspected to be caused by *Ps. aeruginosa* (or by *Enterobacter* or *Serratia* spp.) should be treated with a combination regimen.

The initial treatment of the patient in ICU with a nosocomial pneumonia should usually be with a broad-spectrum cephalosporin (e.g. cefuroxime) or penicillin (e.g. amoxycillin–clavulanate) plus an aminoglycoside. In patients in whom infection with pseudomonas is more likely (e.g. those who have had a prolonged ICU stay plus prior antibiotic therapy) a β-lactam with activity against pseudo-monas (e.g. ceftazidime) should be used. Erythromycin should be added to the regimen in hospitals experiencing epidemic or endemic infection with legionella. Treatment may be modified on the basis of the microbiology results, for example to include flucloxacillin or vancomycin in the regimen if staphylococcal infection is demonstrated. Treatment should be continued for 2–3 weeks depending on clinical response.

Selective decontamination of the digestive tract

The use of selective decontamination of the digestive tract (SDD) to reduce the incidence of infection in multiple trauma patients was first reported by Stoutenbeek et al (1984). The regimen used for SDD is commonly a mixture of polymyxin, tobramycin (or gentamicin) and amphotericin B. This mixture is applied as a paste to the oral mucosa, and a liquid suspension is swallowed or administered via a nasogastric tube four times daily. The regimen is intended to eliminate fungi and aerobic Gram-negative bacteria from the gastro-intestinal tract but to have little effect on the predominant anaerobic flora and thus maintain 'colonization resistance' due to their continued growth. The purpose of SDD is to reduce the rate of pneumonia and other serious infections caused by pathogenic organisms originating from the gastro-intestinal tract. In a subsequent modification of SDD the topical oral and enteric regimen used throughout the ICU stay has been supplemented by the addition of a systemic broad-spectrum antibiotic (usually cefotaxime) for the first 4 days of the ICU stay. This selective parenteral and enteral anti-sepsis regimen (SPEAR) is intended to improve upon the efficacy of SDD by treating occult or incubating infections present at admission to ICU. Even when regimens have included an initial period of systemic antimicrobial therapy the acronym SDD is most frequently used to describe this form of chemoprophylaxis.

Colonization of the oropharynx, stomach and rectum is dramatically affected by SDD regimens. Aerobic Gram-negative bacilli are eliminated from the oropharynx and stomach within 3–4 days of starting SDD. In contrast, they continue to be isolated from these sites in approximately 20–50% of control patients not given SDD. The proportion of patients with aerobic Gram-negative bacilli present in rectal swabs also declines from approximately 60–90% to 10–20% over a period of 10–14 days (Ledingham et al 1988, Hammond et al 1992, Hamer & Barza 1993).

The reduction in colonization of the upper gastro-intestinal tract by aerobic Gram-negative bacilli is associated in most studies with a marked reduction in the incidence of nosocomial infection, especially pneumonia. Thus two recent meta-analyses of controlled trials of SDD (Vandenbroucke-Grauls & Vandenbroucke 1991, Selective Decontamination of the Digestive Tract Trialists Collaborative Group 1993) have demonstrated a 64–80% reduction in the incidence of respiratory tract infections. The beneficial effect of SDD appears to be largely due to the topical antimicrobial therapy as trials which included a systemic agent showed similar efficacy to those which used only the topical regimen. This conclusion is supported by the finding that systemic prophylaxis with penicillin or cefoxitin given for the first 24 h of ICU admission does not significantly affect the incidence of early onset pneumonia (Mandelli et al 1989).

Despite reducing the incidence of respiratory tract infections, SDD regimens have minimal effect on overall mortality. The odds ratio for risk of death in all patients treated with SDD was 0.90 (95% confidence interval (CI) 0.79–1.04) in one meta-analysis (Selective Decontamination of the Digestive Tract Trialists Collaborative Group 1993) and 0.70 (95% CI 0.45–1.09) in the other (Vandenbroucke-Grauls & Vandenbroucke 1991). Subgroup analysis in the former trial demonstrated a small but statistically significant benefit in overall mortality for those patients treated with SDD plus systemic antimicrobial therapy (odds ratio 0.80; 95% CI 0.67–0.97). As mortality rates in control patients were approximately 30%, a 20% reduction in the risk of death in the patients given SDD means that approximately 17 patients would need to be treated to prevent one death. The discrepancy between the highly significant effect on the

incidence of respiratory tract infection and the lack of a significant effect on mortality is not unexpected. A number of studies have failed to demonstrate an independent association between nosocomial pneumonia and mortality in ICU patients (Craven et al 1986, Leu et al 1989, Rello et al 1991). While pneumonia is a common terminal event in severely ill patients, these studies suggest that such patients frequently die with pneumonia rather than because of the pneumonia. In this context it is not surprising that prevention of pneumonia fails to reduce mortality.

The adverse effects of SDD regimens include the significantly increased expenditure on antibiotics (Gastinne et al 1992, Hammond et al 1992) and the potential for increased antibiotic resistance in the endemic bacterial flora of the ICU due to the selective pressure exerted by the SDD regimen (Webb 1992). At present SDD should be regarded as a prophylactic regimen which requires further study to determine whether it is cost-effective in selected subgroups (e.g. trauma and burn patients). While some ICUs will continue to use SDD, concern about the contribution it is likely to make to increasing antimicrobial resistance will remain an important argument against its use (European Society of Intensive Care Medicine 1992).

While the role of SDD in the prevention of nosocomial pneumonia and other infections in ICU patients remains open to question, other approaches to the prevention of nosocomial pneumonia deserve equal or greater attention. A recent meta-analysis (Tryba 1991) has reviewed several trials which compared the incidence of pneumonia in ICU patients treated with either sucralfate, or H_2 antagonists, or antacids as prophylaxis against stress-induced gastric ulceration. Prophylaxis with sucralfate was associated with a significantly lower rate of pneumonia than prophylaxis either with H_2 antagonists (odds ratio 0.50; 95% CI 0.32–0.78), or with antacids (odds ratio 0.40; 95% CI 0.24–0.69). Short-term mortality from all causes was less in the sucralfate treated patients than in the patients treated with H_2 antagonists or antacids. The contributions made by a variety of infection control practices, including cleaning and sterilization of equipment, performance of surveillance cultures and change of ventilator circuits, to the prevention of nosocomial pneumonia have been well reviewed by Tablan et al (1994), and a recent study by Valles et al (1995) has demonstrated that continuous aspiration of subglottic secretions can reduce the incidence of ventilator-associated pneumonia by 50%.

Urinary tract infection

Infection of the urinary tract is an uncommon reason for admission to ICU but a very common complication of care in an ICU. In two large studies, urinary tract infection was the second most common nosocomial infection in ICU patients (Brown et al 1985, Vincent et al 1995). In these studies urinary tract infection occurred in 6–18% of ICU patients. In the majority of ICU patients urinary tract infection is a relatively insignificant complication of urinary catheterization which resolves on removal of the catheter. In a minority it is the cause of systemic illness and in a few it may contribute to mortality. Antimicrobial treatment is not indicated in the majority of patients and should be reserved for those patients who have evidence of systemic sepsis.

Urinary tract infection in ICU patients almost always follows insertion of a urinary catheter or some other instrumentation of the urinary tract. Colonization of the urethral meatus frequently precedes urinary tract infection (Garibaldi et al 1980, Daifuku & Stamm 1984), and contamination of the urethral meatus with organisms transmitted between patients on the hands of nursing and medical staff appears to play a significant role in the pathogenesis of both epidemic and endemic nosocomial urinary tract infections (Schaberg et al 1976, 1980). After migrating in the peri-urethral mucous sheath surrounding the urinary catheter the bacteria reach the bladder and multiply rapidly, usually reaching bacterial counts of >10^5 cfu/ml within 1 day of the onset of infection (Stark & Maki 1984).

The incidence of urinary tract infection following insertion of a urinary catheter is approximately 5% per day of catheterization with a cumulative incidence of about 50% after catheterization for 10 or more days (Garibaldi et al 1974). Krieger et al (1983a) found 33 episodes of bacteraemia in 1233 patients with nosocomial urinary tract infections to give a rate of bacteraemia secondary to nosocomial urinary tract infection of 2.7%. Bryan & Reynolds (1984b) detected bacteraemia in 3.9% of patients with nosocomial urinary tract infection and found a 31% overall mortality rate in patients with nosocomial bacteraemic urinary tract infection. However, the mortality rate attributed directly to the urinary tract infection was 13% and most deaths occurred in patients with rapidly fatal or ultimately fatal underlying diseases. Platt et al (1982) found that nosocomial urinary tract infection was associated with a three times greater risk of death in catheterized patients and that reduction of the incidence of infection is associated with reduction in mortality (Platt et al 1983). Nosocomial urinary tract infection may also be the source for infection at other sites, including the respiratory tract and surgical wounds (Bryan & Reynolds 1984b, Krieger et al 1983b). Preventive measures have been outlined by Garibaldi (1993) and Stamm (1992).

The diagnosis of urinary tract infection commonly depends on the detection of >10^5 cfu/ml urine. While some investigators have used >10^2 or 10^3 cfu/ml as criteria for infection it appears that in catheterized patients low-level bacteriuria almost always progresses rapidly to concen-

Table 44.5 *Aetiology of nosocomial urinary tract infections in ICU patients*

	Study	
	Craven et al (1988)	Norrby et al (1993)
Total No. of isolates	217	57
Organism (%)		
Esch. coli	19	37
Klebsiella, Enterobacter, Serratia spp.	31	21
Ps. aeruginosa	12	14
Ent. faecalis	5	0
Staph. aureus	1	0
Staphylococcus spp.	–	7
C. albicans	15	–
Other	16	21

trations >10^5 cfu/ml unless the patient is being treated with an antibacterial to which the pathogen is susceptible (Stark & Maki 1984). The organisms responsible for nosocomial urinary tract infection in ICU patients are shown in Table 44.5. In many patients the pathogen will have been identified in a urine specimen collected before the onset of sepsis. In others sepsis may occur simultaneously with or shortly after the onset of bacteriuria and initial therapy will therefore be empirical.

A variety of different antimicrobials have been evaluated in the treatment of hospitalized patients with serious urinary tract infection. The most important requirement of a regimen is adequate activity against aerobic Gram-negative bacilli, including pseudomonas. Gentamicin, or another aminoglycoside, has long been considered the standard parenteral treatment for pyelonephritis (Platt 1983), but concerns about nephrotoxicity and ototoxicity have prompted the assessment of other agents.

Aztreonam, ceftazidime, imipenem, ciprofloxacin and a host of other agents have demonstrated generally similar efficacy to the aminoglycosides (Sattler et al 1984, Fang et al 1991, Cox 1993). The selection of initial empiric therapy is influenced more by the relative costs of these agents than by any differences in clinical efficacy. Once the urinary pathogen has been identified treatment can often be modified to use a cheaper narrow-spectrum agent. Treatment for 7–10 days is usually adequate. The management of urinary tract infection is discussed in Chapter 56.

Intravascular catheter-associated infections

Infections of intravascular cannulae are an important and

underdiagnosed cause of morbidity and mortality in ICU patients. These infections may range in severity from asymptomatic colonization of the cannula hub or skin insertion site to suppurative thrombophlebitis. Bacteraemia is a common complication of severe catheter-associated infection, and in ICU patients is associated with a significantly increased mortality (Smith et al 1991). The incidence of intravascular catheter-associated sepsis is particularly affected by the spectrum and density of bacterial colonization of the skin at the insertion site, the duration of catheterization and the type of catheter used. Maki (1992) has recently estimated the rates of primary bacteraemia to be approximately 0.2% for peripheral intravenous cannulae, 1% for arterial catheters used for haemodynamic monitoring and 3–5% for short-term non-cuffed central venous catheters. Infection rates in patients with burns are commonly much higher (Pruitt et al 1980). The organisms most commonly responsible for catheter-associated sepsis in ICU patients are *Staph. aureus* (30%), *Staphylococcus epidermidis* (30%), Gram-negative bacilli (30%), *Enterococcus faecalis* (5%) and *Candida albicans* (5%) (Collignon et al 1988, Richet et al 1990, Pittet et al 1994).

Catheter-associated infection should be suspected in all febrile patients who lack an identified source of sepsis. Infection of central venous catheters is not usually associated with any signs of sepsis at the insertion site. In contrast, insertion-site inflammation may be a useful sign of infection associated with peripheral venous and arterial catheters. However, the majority of patients with insertion-site inflammation do not have significant infection and sepsis may occur in the absence of local inflammation. In one study of 130 arterial catheters bacteraemia occurred in 3/14 patients with inflammation at the site of catheter insertion and 2/116 patients without local inflammation (Band & Maki 1979).

The management of catheter-associated infection is discussed in detail in Chapter 45.

The optimal duration of treatment for intravascular catheter-associated sepsis is uncertain. Jernigan & Farr (1993) reviewed 11 studies of short-course therapy of catheter-related *Staph. aureus* bacteraemia and concluded that treatment should be for more than 2 weeks. However, it seems likely that judicious adjustment of treatment duration on the basis of the severity of the catheter-associated infection, the infecting organism and the initial response to treatment will usually ensure a good outcome. Thus patients who have clinical evidence of suppurative thrombophlebitis or perivascular abscess, or infection which fails to respond clinically within a few days of catheter removal and antibiotic treatment, should receive treatment for at least 2 weeks. In these patients adjunctive treatment with heparin, surgical removal of the infected vein, or drainage of a perivascular abscess may be necessary for cure (Verghese et al 1985). In patients with less severe infection who

become afebrile within a few days of starting treatment a total duration of 10–14 days is very likely to be adequate. All patients with intravascular catheter-associated sepsis, especially those with infection due to *Staph. aureus*, should be carefully evaluated for the development of distant foci of infection (e.g. endocarditis, epidural abscess, septic arthritis). While these complications most commonly occur during the first 14 days after onset of the catheter-associated infection (Arnow et al 1993) they may present as late as 2 months after the completion of antibiotic treatment (Jernigan & Farr 1993).

Intra-abdominal infection

Intra-abdominal infection (Ch. 42) is a common important cause of sepsis in the ICU. In a study conducted by Brown et al (1985) intra-abdominal infection was the third most common infection and comprised 14% of all infections in a combined medical–surgical ICU. The mortality of patients with severe generalized peritonitis or abdominal abscess(es), the most common intra-abdominal infections in the ICU, is 30–60% (Bohnen et al 1983, 1988). Intra-abdominal infections associated with an especially high mortality include spontaneous bacterial peritonitis (Mbopi Keou et al 1992), generalized peritonitis not originating from appendicitis or a perforated duodenal ulcer (Bohnen et al 1983), postoperative peritonitis (Bohnen et al 1983) and infected pancreatic necrosis (Schein 1992). The presence of multiorgan dysfunction, as measured by APACHE II or other similar scoring systems, also is an important determinant of outcome. The mortality in patients with intra-abdominal sepsis and an APACHE II score of <10, 10–20, and >20 was <10%, 10–50% and 50–90%, respectively, in two large prospective trials (Bohnen et al 1988, Solomkin et al 1990).

The organisms responsible for intra-abdominal sepsis are dependent on the source of infection. Spontaneous bacterial peritonitis is usually a monomicrobial infection. *Esch. coli*, *K. pneumoniae* and Gram-positive cocci are the usual pathogens. Anaerobes are rarely present (Mbopi Keou et al 1992). Peritonitis secondary to contamination by intestinal contents usually results in a polymicrobial mixed aerobic and anaerobic infection with *Bacteroides fragilis* and *Esch. coli* the most commonly isolated species (Gorbach 1993). Tertiary peritonitis, which occurs in severely ill patients following prior laparotomy, and which is not usually associated with peritoneal contamination by intestinal contents, is often monomicrobial and commonly due to *Staph. epidermidis*, *Enterococcus* spp., *Enterobacter* spp., *Pseudomonas* spp. and *C. albicans* (McClean et al 1994).

Runyon et al (1991) treated spontaneous bacterial peritonitis with cefotaxime 2 g 8-hourly for 5 days, with no deaths due to infection and a 93% microbiologic cure rate. As spontaneous bacterial peritonitis is usually due to community acquired infection with relatively sensitive organisms it seems likely that very similar results could be achieved with cefuroxime 0.75 g 8-hourly. A ureidopenicillin or co-amoxyclav would also be appropriate forms of treatment.

Peritonitis following contamination of the peritoneal cavity should be treated with a regimen active against enteric Gram-negative bacilli and anaerobes. Regimens which combine an aminoglycoside (e.g. gentamicin or tobramycin) with an anti-anaerobic agent (e.g. metronidazole or clindamycin) have been widely used for intra-abdominal sepsis. However, concerns about the toxicity, efficacy and inconvenience of aminoglycoside therapy have stimulated the investigation of alternative regimens. Aztreonam plus clindamycin was found to have similar efficacy to tobramycin (or gentamicin) plus clindamycin in five recent clinical trials reviewed by Di Piro & Fortson (1993). Monotherapy with imipenem, piperacillin plus tazobactam, cefotetan or cefoxitin is as effective as combination treatment with aminoglycoside plus an anti-anaerobic drug (Ho & Barza 1987, Solomkin et al 1990, Eklund et al 1993) and is associated with significantly less nephrotoxicity. These data have led Gorbach (1993) to suggest that aminoglycoside-containing regimens should not be used routinely for the initial treatment of uncomplicated intra-abdominal infection. Enterococci are frequently present in polymicrobial intra-abdominal infections but are uncommonly found alone. Treatment with an agent active against enterococci (e.g. amoxycillin) is rarely required (Nichols & Muzik 1992, Gorbach 1993). Monotherapy with cefoxitin, combination therapy with cefuroxime plus metronidazole, or gentamicin plus metronidazole (or clindamycin) are cheap, widely used alternatives for treatment of intra-abdominal infection. New, more expensive alternatives such as imipenem, or piperacillin plus tazobactam should be reserved for patients with complicated infections. Patients with generalized peritonitis or localized abdominal abscess should ordinarily be treated for 5–7 days (Bohnen et al 1992). Antimicrobial therapy, other than brief perioperative prophylaxis, is not necessary either in patients with peritoneal contamination without infection (e.g. gastroduodenal ulcer perforation operated on within 24 h of onset) or in patients in whom a localized infectious process is treated by excision (e.g. acute suppurative appendicitis, simple acute cholecystitis and ischaemic bowel without perforation).

Tertiary peritonitis and infected pancreatic necrosis should initially be treated with amoxycillin, gentamicin and metronidazole, but treatment should be modified when appropriate microbiology results are available. When infection is due to *Candida* spp. other antimicrobial agents should be discontinued and foreign bodies removed if possible and treatment with amphotericin B given for at least 4 weeks (British Society for Antimicrobial Chemotherapy Working Party 1994).

Sinusitis

Sinusitis (Ch. 47), particularly affecting the maxillary sinuses, is a common occult cause of fever in ICU patients. Two large prospective studies found microbiologically proven sinusitis in 18% (Holzapfel et al 1993) and 30% (Rouby et al 1994) of ICU patients. Complications of sinusitis include bronchopneumonia, septicaemia and subdural empyema.

Sinusitis should be suspected in all febrile mechanically ventilated patients, but especially in those patients who have endotracheal and gastric tubes inserted through the nares (Holzapfel et al 1993, Rouby et al 1994). Purulent rhinorrhoea and middle ear effusion(s) (detected by pneumatic otoscopy) are useful clinical associations with sinusitis (Borman et al 1992). Partial or complete opacification of the sinuses has been demonstrated in 30–60% of patients admitted to an ICU for at least 7 days (Holzapfel et al 1993, Rouby et al 1994). However, in approximately half of these patients the maxillary sinus fluid does not grow significant numbers ($>10^3$ cfu/ml) of organisms. The demonstration of fluid in the sinuses (by computerized tomography (CT) X-ray or ultrasound) should not therefore be regarded as proof of the presence of purulent sinusitis. In those patients who do have purulent sinusitis the infection is commonly polymicrobial with Gram-negative bacilli present in most patients. *Candida* and anaerobes are occasional causes of sinusitis.

The initial treatment of sinusitis should include removal of any nasal tubes and treatment with a broad-spectrum antibiotic such as cefoxitin. In patients with persistent fever, radiological evidence of significant sinus opacification and no other focus of infection, the affected sinuses should be surgically drained and lavaged and treatment modified on the basis of culture results.

Infections due to multiresistant bacteria

Colonization and infection with bacteria resistant to commonly used antibiotics is a rapidly evolving problem in ICU patients. Recent reports have described resistance to gentamicin in 40% of isolates of *Ps. aeruginosa* from ICUs in Germany (Shah et al 1991), resistance to cefotaxime, ceftriaxone and aztreonam in 20–30% of isolates of *K. pneumoniae* from ICUs in France (Sirot et al 1992) and resistance to vancomycin in 14% of enterococcal isolates from ICUs in the USA (Centers for Disease Control 1993). Potential adverse consequences of colonization or infection with multiresistant strains include failure of antimicrobial therapy, increased expense of antimicrobial therapy, spread of infection to other patients, and transfer of resistance to other bacterial species. Epidemics of multiresistant bacteria in ICU patients are often followed by spread to patients in other parts of the hospital and then the community. The ICU commonly is both a source and a reservoir of multiresistant bacteria. When formulating policies for antibiotic use in the ICU doctors should be influenced by the distant effects of their antibiotic choices and avoid unnecessary prescription of those agents most likely to facilitate the selection of multiresistant strains (Ch. 2).

Colonization and infection with multiresistant bacteria may result from acquisition of endemic or epidemic strains following admission to the ICU. However, selection of resistant strains from the patient's endogenous flora appears to be the usual source (Weinstein 1991). A variety of factors including greater severity of the underlying illness, prolonged stay in the ICU, the use of invasive devices, and the prolonged use of broad-spectrum antimicrobial therapy increase the rate of infection with these organisms (Pittet et al 1992). Resistance of a bacterial isolate to commonly tested antibiotics (e.g. methicillin resistance in *Staph. aureus*, vancomycin resistance in enterococci, aminoglycoside and third-generation cephalosporin resistance in Gram-negative bacilli) frequently serves as a marker of an epidemic of nosocomial infection which might otherwise remain unsuspected. Such epidemics are of importance in themselves, but should also be regarded as the visible tip of an iceberg of undetected nosocomially transmitted infection.

Pseudomonas, *Klebsiella*, *Enterobacter*, *Serratia* and *Acinetobacter* spp., methicillin-resistant *Staph. aureus* and enterococci are the most commonly reported causes of epidemics of nosocomial bacteraemia in ICU patients (Pittet 1993). Such epidemics usually last less than 3 months, affect an average of 10 patients per outbreak, commonly arise from contaminated medical equipment, and often depend on transmission of infection by the hands of ICU staff. Similar factors no doubt contribute to the much larger problem of endemic nosocomial infection, but are less easily identified because the organisms responsible often lack unusual antibiotic resistance patterns.

METHICILLIN-RESISTANT *STAPH. AUREUS*

Methicillin-resistant *Staph. aureus* (MRSA) is a common cause of epidemics of infection in ICUs. Burns, surgical wounds, prolonged ICU stay, and prolonged courses of multiple antibiotics all increase the risk of MRSA infection. While persistent colonization of hospital staff has been suspected as the source of infection in some MRSA

outbreaks, this is not found in the majority of outbreaks. However, transient contamination of the hands is common in those staff directly involved in the care of patients with MRSA infection, and is presumed to be the most common mode of transmission of infection between patients (Thompson et al 1982). Control and, not infrequently, termination of epidemics of MRSA can be achieved by surveillance of patients for MRSA colonization or infection, strict isolation of colonized or infected patients, consistent use of handwashing between patients and appropriate treatment to minimize colonization or eradicate infection in affected patients and staff.

MRSA colonization may be reduced or eliminated by stopping antibiotic treatment of other conditions whenever possible, effective treatment of underlying skin disorders, application of mupirocin ointment of colonized sites, and washing with an antiseptic (Duckworth 1990). Infection with MRSA is treated with intravenous vancomycin, or oral clindamycin or fusidic acid supplemented by oral rifampicin.

RESISTANT ENTEROCOCCI

Enterococci (especially *Ent. faecalis* and *Enterococcus faecium*) resistant to gentamicin, ampicillin or vancomycin have recently emerged as an important cause of nosocomial infection in ICUs (Frieden et al 1993, Handwerger et al 1993). Prolonged ICU stay, persistent intra-abdominal infections, and prolonged broad-spectrum antimicrobial therapy with agents inactive against enterococci are common features in patients with enterococcal infection. Faeces and urine of colonized patients are the usual sources of infection, and transmission on the hands of hospital staff is presumed to be the major route of cross-infection. The urinary tract, bloodstream and surgical wounds are the most common sites of infection; enterococcal pneumonia is rare (Schaberg et al 1991, Frieden et al 1993).

Bacteraemia due to enterococci highly resistant to gentamicin (minimum inhibitory concentration (MIC) >1000 mg/l), but susceptible to ampicillin or vancomycin, may be successfully treated with amoxycillin (or ampicillin) or vancomycin monotherapy (Watanakunakorn & Patel 1993, Graninger & Ragette 1992). This is in contrast to enterococcal endocarditis which requires combination treatment with amoxycillin or vancomycin plus an aminoglycoside for cure. Optimal treatment of infection with enterococci resistant to ampicillin, vancomycin and aminoglycosides is at present unclear. Animal models suggest that ampicillin–sulbactam or teicoplanin may be useful (Eliopoulos et al 1992).

The rapid emergence of multiresistant enterococci, the difficulties posed by treatment of these infections, and the spectre of transfer of resistance to *Staph. aureus* are important reasons to limit the use of vancomycin as much as possible. Vancomycin should not ordinarily be used for perioperative prophylaxis, initial treatment of antibiotic-associated colitis, initial empirical treatment of febrile neutropenic patients, selective decontamination of the digestive tract, or eradication of MRSA colonization. Guidelines for the prevention and control of nosocomial transmission of vancomycin resistant enterococci have been published recently (Hospital Infection Control Practices Advisory Committee 1995).

K. PNEUMONIAE

Since their first appearance in 1983, *K. pneumoniae* resistant to broad-spectrum cephalosporins and aminoglycosides have caused epidemics of infection in ICUs worldwide (Philippon et al 1989). Resistance is due to readily transmissible plasmids which encode for extended spectrum β-lactamases and for aminoglycoside and quinolone resistance. The β-lactamases are susceptible to inhibitors such as clavulanic acid and sulbactam which may assist with identification of these strains in the laboratory (Sirot et al 1992). Outbreaks of infection may involve multiple strains of *K. pneumoniae* and may spread to involve other bacteria such as *Esch. coli, Citrobacter freundii, Serratia marcescens* and *Enterobacter aerogenes* (Sirot et al 1988).

Infection with multiresistant *K. pneumoniae* usually involves the urinary tract, the respiratory tract or wounds (Brun-Buisson et al 1987). Enteric colonization and transmission on the hands of hospital staff appear to contribute to epidemic spread. Treatment with cefotaxime or related cephalosporins may be effective against urinary tract infections due to multiresistant *K. pneumoniae*, but these agents will not be adequate for the treatment of major infections at other sites (Brun-Buisson et al 1987). Imipenem, cephamycins such as cefoxitin, and piperacillin plus tazobactam or ticarcillin plus clavulanate, are active against most broad-spectrum β-lactamase-producing *K. pneumoniae*. Despite resistance to many other aminoglycosides, sensitivity to gentamicin is often retained.

Another important source of infection due to multiresistant Gram-negative bacilli is the selection of organisms with chromosomally encoded class I β-lactamase production. *Pseudomonas, Enterobacter, Citrobacter* and *Serratia* spp. are the organisms which most frequently produce class I β-lactamase. Induction of enzyme production or selection of stably derepressed mutant cells which constitutively manufacture class I β-lactamase at a high level, may lead to development of resistance to β-lactams during treatment (Livermore 1991, Snydman 1991). Enzyme production is strongly induced when organisms are exposed to first-generation cephalosporins, cefoxitin or imipenem, but is only weakly induced by exposure to second- and third-generation cephalosporins, ureidopenicillins and monobactams. Induced

enzyme production ceases promptly when treatment with the inducing antibiotic is stopped. Selection of stably derepressed mutants constitutively producing large amounts of β-lactamase occurs when inducible strains (especially *Ps. aeruginosa* and *Enterobacter cloacae*) are exposed to broad-spectrum cephalosporins, ureidopenicillins or monobactams. Resistance persists even when treatment with the antibiotic responsible for selecting the mutant strain is stopped. Development of resistance during treatment occurs in approximately 10–20% of patients (Snydman 1991, Shah et al 1991), and spread within the ICU may result in multi-resistance in 30% of ICU isolates of *E. cloacae* (Livermore 1991).

Imipenem, despite being a strong inducer of class I β-lactamase, is not susceptible to the enzyme's action. Alternative regimens include imipenem monotherapy or combination therapy with imipenem plus an aminoglycoside or fluoroquinolone selected on the basis of careful susceptibility testing (Meyer et al 1993). Patients treated with a broad-spectrum cephalosporin, ureidopenicillin or monobactam for an infection due to an initially sensitive strain should be carefully observed for the emergence of resistant mutants during treatment.

MULTIRESISTANT *ACINETOBACTER CALCOACETICUS*

Multiresistant *A. calcoaceticus* is an occasional cause of epidemics of infection in ICU patients. Epidemic strains are resistant to many broad-spectrum cephalosporins, and have variable susceptibility to aminoglycosides. Colonization and infection of the respiratory tract in artificially ventilated patients is a common feature of epidemics. Improvements in the methods used to sterilize ventilator equipment has led to termination of epidemics (Hartstein et al 1988). In most patients *A. calcoaceticus* merely colonizes the respiratory tract; however, it may be responsible for pneumonia and other serious infections. Imipenem alone, or in combination with an aminoglycoside, is often appropriate treatment.

A frequent theme for many epidemics caused by multiresistant bacteria has been the widespread use of antibiotics in response to increased resistance in other commonly isolated bacterial species. For example, vancomycin resistance in enterococci has emerged following increased use of vancomycin to treat suspected or proven MRSA (and methicillin-resistant *Staph. epidermidis* (MRSE)) infections. Similarly, epidemics of infection due to multiresistant *K. pneumonia* and *A. calcoaceticus* have followed increased use of third-generation cephalosporins and imipenem (Meyer et al 1993). Thus the increased use of potent antibiotics with ever broader spectra of activity acts as a stimulus to the evolution of new epidemics of ever more resistant pathogens. The effect is to mortgage the future of antibiotic treatment to pay for our present practices. While there is no one solution to this problem which can be applied to all ICUs, the use of prescribing guidelines which encourage the use of older narrow-spectrum antibiotics and limit the use of new broad-spectrum antibiotic agents should prolong the life-expectancy of these new drugs, delay the emergence of resistant strains and set a better example for prescribing patterns in the rest of the hospital (Neu 1993). (Ch. 12).

References

American Thoracic Society 1993 Guidelines for the initial management of adults with community-acquired pneumonia: diagnosis, assessment of severity, and initial antimicrobial therapy. *American Review of Respiratory Disease* 148: 1418–1426

Andrews C P, Coalson J J, Smith J D, Johanson W G 1981 Diagnosis of nosocomial bacterial pneumonia in acute, diffuse lung injury. *Chest* 80: 254–258

Arnow P M, Quimosing E M, Beach M 1993 Consequences of intravascular catheter sepsis. *Clinical Infectious Diseases* 16: 778–784

Band J D, Maki D G 1979 Infections caused by arterial catheters used for hemodynamic monitoring. *American Journal of Medicine* 67: 735–741

Bell R C, Coalson J J, Smith J D, Johanson W G 1983 Multiple organ system failure and infection in adult respiratory distress syndrome. *Annals of Internal Medicine* 99: 293–298

Bohnen J, Boulanger M, Meakins J L, McLean A P H 1983 Prognosis in generalized peritonitis. Relation to cause and risk factors. *Archives of Surgery* 118: 285–290

Bohnen J M A, Mustard R A, Oxholm S E, Schouten B D 1988 APACHE II score and abdominal sepsis. A prospective study. *Archives of Surgery* 123: 225–229

Bohnen J M A, Solomkin J S, Dellinger E P, Bjornson H S, Page C P 1992 Guidelines for clinical care: anti-infective agents for intra-abdominal infection. *Archives of Surgery* 127: 83–89

Borman K R, Brown P M, Mezera K K, Jhaveri H 1992 Occult fever in surgical intensive care unit patients is seldom caused by sinusitis. *American Journal of Surgery* 164: 412–416

British Society for Antimicrobial Chemotherapy Working Party 1994 Management of deep *Candida* infection in surgical and intensive care unit patients. *Intensive Care Medicine* 20: 522–528

British Thoracic Society and the Public Health Laboratory Service 1987 Community-acquired pneumonia in adults in British hospitals in 1982–1983: a survey of aetiology, mortality, prognostic factors and outcome. *Quarterly Journal of Medicine* NS62: 195–220

British Thoracic Society Research Committee and the Public Health Laboratory Service 1992 The aetiology, management and outcome of severe community-acquired pneumonia on the intensive care unit. *Respiratory Medicine* 86: 7–13

Brown R B, Hosmer D, Chen H C et al 1985 A comparison of infections in different ICUs within the same hospital. *Critical Care Medicine* 13: 472–476

Brown R B, Kruse J A, Counts G W et al 1990 Double-blind study of endotracheal tobramycin in the treatment of Gram-negative bacterial pneumonia. *Antimicrobial Agents and Chemotherapy* 34: 269–272

Brun-Buisson C, Legrand P, Philippon A, Montravers F, Ansquer M, Duval J 1987 Transferable enzymatic resistance to third-generation cephalosporins during nosocomial outbreak of multi-resistant *Klebsiella pneumoniae*. *Lancet* ii: 302–306

Bryan C S, Reynolds K L 1984a Bacteremic nosocomial pneumonia. Analysis of 172 episodes from a single metropolitan area. *American Review of Respiratory Disease* 129: 668–671

Bryan C S, Reynolds K L 1984b Hospital-acquired bacteremic urinary tract infection: epidemiology and outcome. *Journal of Urology* 132: 494–498

Centers for Disease Control 1993 Nosocomial enterococci resistant to vancomycin – United States, 1989–1993. *Morbidity and Mortality Weekly Report* 42: 597–599

Chandrasekar P H, Kruse J A, Mathews M F 1986 Nosocomial infection among patients in different types of intensive care units at a city hospital. *Critical Care Medicine* 14: 508–510

Collignon P, Soni N, Pearson I, Sorrell T, Woods P 1988 Sepsis associated with central vein catheters in critically ill patients. *Intensive Care Medicine* 14: 227–231

Cone L A, Woodard D R, Stoltzman D S, Byrd R G 1985 Ceftazidime versus tobramycin–ticarcillin in the treatment of pneumonia and bacteremia. *Antimicrobial Agents and Chemotherapy* 28: 33–36

Cook D J, Brun-Buisson C, Guyatt G H, Sibbald W J 1994 Evaluation of new diagnostic technologies: bronchoalveolar lavage and the diagnosis of ventilator associated pneumonia. *Critical Care Medicine* 22: 1314–1322

Cox C E 1993 Comparison of intravenous fleroxacin with ceftazidime for treatment of complicated urinary tract infections. *American Journal of Medicine* 94 (suppl 3A): 118S–125S

Craven D E, Kunches L M, Kilinsky V, Lichtenberg D A, Make B J, McCabe W R 1986 Risk factors for pneumonia and fatality in patients receiving continuous mechanical ventilation. *American Review of Respiratory Disease* 133: 792–796

Craven D E, Kunches L M, Lichtenberg D A et al 1988 Nosocomial infection and fatality in medical and surgical intensive care unit patients. *Archives of Internal Medicine* 148: 1161–1168

Daifuku R, Stamm W E 1984 Association of rectal and urethral colonization with urinary tract infection in patients with indwelling catheters. *Journal of the American Medical Association* 252: 2028–2030

DiPiro J T, Fortson N S 1993 Combination antibiotic therapy in the management of intra-abdominal infection. *American Journal of Surgery* 165 (suppl 2A): 82S–88S

Donowitz L G, Wenzel R P, Hoyt J W 1982 High risk of hospital-acquired infection in the ICU patient. *Critical Care Medicine* 10: 355–357

Duckworth G 1990 Revised guidelines for the control of epidemic methicillin-resistant *Staphylococcus aureus. Journal of Hospital Infection* 16: 351–377

Eklund A-E, Nord C E, Swedish Study Group 1993 A randomized multicenter trial of piperacillin/tazobactam versus imipenem/cilastatin in the treatment of severe intra-abdominal infections. *Journal of Antimicrobial Chemotherapy* 31 (suppl A): 79–85

Eliopoulos G M, Thauvin-Eliopoulos C, Moellering R C 1992 Contribution of animal models in the search for effective therapy for endocarditis due to enterococci with high-level resistance to gentamicin. *Clinical Infectious Diseases* 15: 58–62

European Society of Intensive Care Medicine 1992 Selective decontamination of the digestive tract in intensive care patients. *Infection Control and Hospital Epidemiology* 13: 609–611

Fang G-D, Fine M, Orloff J et al 1990 New and emerging etiologies for community-acquired pneumonia with implications for therapy. *Medicine* 69: 307–316

Fang G, Brennen C, Wagener M et al 1991 Use of ciprofloxacin versus use of aminoglycosides for therapy of complicated urinary tract infection: prospective, randomized clinical and pharmacokinetic study. *Antimicrobial Agents and Chemotherapy* 35: 1849–1855

Frieden T R, Munsiff S S, Low D E et al 1993 Emergence of vancomycin-resistant enterococci in New York City. *Lancet* 342: 76–79

Friedland I R, McCracken G H 1994 Management of infections caused by antibiotic-resistant *Streptococcus pneumoniae. New England Journal of Medicine* 331: 377–382

Garibaldi R A 1993 Hospital-acquired urinary tract infections. In: Wenzel R P (ed) Prevention and control of nosocomial infections, 2nd edn. Williams & Wilkins, Baltimore, p 600–613

Garibaldi R A, Burke J P, Dickman M L, Smith C B 1974 Factors predisposing to bacteriuria during indwelling urethral catheterization. *New England Journal of Medicine* 291: 215–219

Garibaldi R A, Burke J P, Britt M R, Miller M A, Smith C B 1980 Meatal colonization and catheter-associated bacteriuria. *New England Journal of Medicine* 303: 316–318

Gastinne H, Wolff M, Delatour F, Faurisson F, Chevret S 1992 A controlled trial in intensive care units of selective decontamination of the digestive tract with nonabsorbable antibiotics. *New England Journal of Medicine* 326: 594–599

Gorbach S L 1993 Treatment of intra-abdominal infections. *Journal of Antimicrobial Chemotherapy* 31 (suppl A): 67–78

Graninger W, Ragette R 1992 Nosocomial bacteraemia due to *Enterococcus faecalis* without endocarditis. *Clinical Infectious Diseases* 15: 49–57

Gudiol F, Manresa F, Pallares R et al 1990 Clindamycin vs penicillin for anaerobic lung infections. *Archives of Internal Medicine* 150: 2525–2529

Hamer D H, Barza M 1993 Prevention of hospital-acquired pneumonia in critically ill patients. *Antimicrobial Agents and Chemotherapy* 37: 931–938

Hammond J M J, Potgieter P D, Saunders G L, Forder A A 1992 Double-blind study of selective decontamination of the digestive tract in intensive care. *Lancet* 340: 5–9

Handwerger S, Raucher B, Altarac D et al 1993 Nosocomial outbreak due to *Enterococcus faecium* highly resistant to vancomycin, penicillin, and gentamicin. *Clinical Infectious Diseases* 16: 750–755

Hartstein A I, Rashad A L, Liebler J M et al 1988 Multiple intensive care unit outbreak of *Acinetobacter calcoaceticus* subspecies *anitratus* respiratory infection and colonization associated with contaminated, reusable ventilator circuits and resuscitation bags. *American Journal of Medicine* 85: 624–631

Ho J L, Barza M 1987 Role of aminoglycoside antibiotics in the treatment of intra-abdominal infection. *Antimicrobial Agents and Chemotherapy* 31: 485–491

Holzapfel L, Chevret S, Madinier G et al 1993 Influence of long-term oro- or nasotracheal intubation on nosocomial maxillary sinusitis and pneumonia: results of a prospective, randomized, clinical trial. *Critical Care Medicine* 21: 1132–1138

Hospital Infection Control Practices Advisory Committee 1995 Recommendations for preventing the spread of vancomycin resistance. *Infection Control and Hospital Epidemiology* 16: 105–113

Jernigan J A, Farr B M 1993 Short-course therapy of catheter-related *Staphylococcus aureus* bacteremia: a meta-analysis. *Annals of Internal Medicine* 119: 304–311

Khoo S H, Creagh-Barry P, Wilkins E G L, Pasvol G 1992 Fulminant community acquired infections admitted to an intensive care unit. *Quarterly Journal of Medicine* NS83: 381–388

Krieger J N, Kaiser D L, Wenzel R P 1983a Urinary tract etiology of bloodstream infections in hospitalized patients. *Journal of Infectious Diseases* 148: 57–62

Krieger J N, Kaiser D L, Wenzel R P 1983b Nosocomial urinary tract infections cause wound infections post-operatively in surgical patients. *Surgery, Gynaecology and Obstetrics* 156: 313–318

La Force F M 1989 Systemic antimicrobial therapy of noso-comial pneumonia: monotherapy versus combination therapy. *European Journal of Clinical Microbiology and Infectious Diseases* 8: 61–68

La Force F M 1992 Lower respiratory tract infections. In: Bennett J V, Brachman P S (eds) Hospital infections, 3rd edn. Little, Brown and Co., Boston, p 611–639

Langer M, Mosconi P, Cigada M, Mandelli M, Intensive Care Unit Group of Infection Control 1989 Long term respira-tory support and risk of pneumonia in critically ill patients. *American Review of Respiratory Disease* 140: 302–305

Ledingham I M, Alcock S R, Eastaway A T, McDonald J C, McKay I C, Ramsay G 1988 Triple regimen of selective decontamination of the digestive tract, systemic cefotaxime, and microbiological surveillance for prevention of acquired infection in intensive care. *Lancet* i: 785–790

Leu H-S, Kaiser D L, Mori M, Woolson R F, Wenzel R P 1989 Hospital-acquired pneumonia: attributable mortality and morbidity. *American Journal of Epidemiology* 129: 1258–1267

Livermore D M 1991 Mechanisms of resistance to β-lactam antibiotics. *Scandinavian Journal of Infectious Diseases* (suppl 78): 7–16

Macfarlane J T, Miller A C, Roderick Smith W H, Morris A H, Rose D H 1984 Comparative radiographic features of community acquired legionnaires disease, pneumococcal pneumonia, mycoplasma pneumonia, and psittacosis. *Thorax* 39: 28–33

McClean K L, Sheehan G J, Harding G K M 1994 Intra-abdominal infection: a review. *Clinical Infectious Diseases* 19: 100–116

Maki D G 1992 Infections due to infusion therapy. In: Bennett J V, Brachman P S (eds) Hospital infections, 3rd edn. Little, Brown and Co., Boston, p 849–898

Mandell L A, Nicolle L E, Ronald A R et al 1987 A prospective randomized trial of ceftazidime versus cefazolin/tobramycin in the treatment of hospitalized patients with pneumonia. *Journal of Antimicrobial Chemotherapy* 20: 95–107

Mandelli M, Mosconi P, Langer M, Cigada M, Intensive Care Unit Group of Infection Control 1989 Prevention of pneumonia in an intensive care unit: a randomized multicenter clinical trial. *Critical Care Medicine* 17: 501–505

Marrie T J, Durant H, Yates L 1989 Community-acquired pneumonia requiring hospitalization: 5-year prospective study. *Reviews of Infectious Diseases* 11: 586–599

Martin C, Gouin F, Fourrier F, Junginger W, Prieur B L 1988 Pefloxacin in the treatment of nosocomial lower respiratory tract infections in intensive care patients. *Journal of Antimicrobial Chemotherapy* 21: 795–799

Mbopi Keou F-X, Bloch F, Buu Hoi A et al 1992 Spontaneous peritonitis in cirrhotic hospital in-patients: retrospective analysis of 101 cases. *Quarterly Journal of Medicine* NS 83: 401–407

Meyer K S, Urban C, Eagan J A, Berger B J, Rahal J J 1993 Nosocomial outbreak of *Klebsiella* infection resistant to late-generation cephalosporins. *Annals of Internal Medicine* 119: 353–358

Moore R D, Smith C R, Lietman P S 1984 Association of aminoglycoside plasma levels with therapeutic outcome in Gram-negative pneumonia. *American Journal of Medicine* 77: 657–662

Neu H C 1993 Antimicrobial agents: role in the prevention and control of nosocomial infections. In: Wenzel R P (ed) Prevention and control of nosocomial infections, 2nd edn. Williams & Wilkins, Baltimore, p 406–419

Nichols R L, Muzik A C 1992 Enterococcal infections in surgical patients: the mystery continues. *Clinical Infectious Diseases* 15: 72–76

Norrby S R, Finch R G, Glauser M, European Study Group 1993 Monotherapy in serious hospital-acquired infections: a clinical trial of ceftazidime versus imipenem/cilastatin. *Journal of Antimicrobial Chemotherapy* 31: 927–937

Ortqvist A, Sterner G, Nilsson J A 1985 Severe community-acquired pneumonia: factors influencing need of intensive care treatment and prognosis. *Scandinavian Journal of Infectious Diseases* 17: 377–386

Peloquin C A, Cumbo T J, Nix D E, Sands M F, Schentag J J 1989 Evaluation of intravenous ciprofloxacin in patients with nosocomial lower respiratory tract infections. *Archives of Internal Medicine* 149: 2269–2273

Philippon A, Labia R, Jacoby G 1989 Extended-spectrum β-lactamases. *Antimicrobial Agents and Chemotherapy* 33: 1131–1136

Pittet D 1993 Nosocomial bloodstream infections. In: Wenzel R P (ed) Prevention and control of nosocomial infections, 2nd edn. Williams & Wilkins, Baltimore, p 512–555

Pittet D, Herwaldt L A, Massanari R M 1992 The intensive care unit. In: Bennett J V, Brachman P S (eds) Hospital infections, 3rd edn. Little, Brown and Co., Boston, p 405–439

Pittet D, Tarara D, Wenzel R P 1994 Nosocomial bloodstream infection in critically ill patients. Journal of the American Medical Association 271: 1598–1601

Platt R 1983 Diagnosis and empiric therapy of urinary tract infection in the seriously ill patient. Reviews of Infectious Diseases 5 (suppl 1): S65–S73

Platt R, Polk B F, Murdock B, Rosner B 1982 Mortality associated with nosocomial urinary-tract infection. New England Journal of Medicine 307: 637–642

Platt R, Polk B F, Murdock B, Rosner B 1983 Reduction of mortality associated with nosocomial urinary tract infection. Lancet i: 893–897

Potgieter P D, Hammond J M J 1992 Etiology and diagnosis of pneumonia requiring ICU admission. Chest 101: 199–203

Pruitt B A, McManus W F, Kim S H, Treat R C 1980 Diagnosis and treatment of cannula-related intravenous sepsis in burn patients. Annals of Surgery 191: 546–554

Rello J, Quintana E, Ausina V et al 1991 Incidence, etiology and outcome of nosocomial pneumonia in mechanically ventilated patients. Chest 100: 439–444

Rello J, Ausina V, Ricart M, Castella J, Prats G 1993 Impact of previous antimicrobial therapy on the etiology and outcome of ventilator-associated pneumonia. Chest 104: 1230–1235

Richet H, Hubert B, Nitemberg G et al 1990 Prospective multicenter study of vascular-catheter-related complications and risk factors for positive central-catheter cultures in intensive care unit patients. Journal of Clinical Microbiology 28: 2520–2525

Rodriguez J R, Ramirez-Ronda C H 1985 Efficacy and safety of aztreonam versus tobramycin for aerobic Gram-negative bacilli lower respiratory tract infections. American Journal of Medicine 78 (suppl 2A): 42–43

Rouby J-J, Laurent P, Gosnach M et al 1994 Risk factors and clinical relevance of nosocomial maxillary sinusitis in the critically ill. American Journal of Respiratory and Critical Care Medicine 150: 776–783

Runyon B A, McHutchison J G, Antillon M R, Akriviadis E A, Montano A A 1991 Short-course versus long-course antibiotic treatment of spontaneous bacterial peritonitis. Gastroenterology 100: 1737–1742

Salata R A, Gebhart R L, Palmer D L et al 1985 Pneumonia treated with imipenem/cilastatin. American Journal of Medicine 78 (suppl 6A): 104–109

Sattler F R, Moyer J E, Schramm M, Lombard J S, Appelbaum P C 1984 Aztreonam compared with gentamicin for treatment of serious urinary tract infections. Lancet i: 1315–1318

Schaberg D R, Weinstein R A, Stamm W E 1976 Epidemics of nosocomial urinary tract infection caused by multiply resistant Gram-negative bacilli: epidemiology and control. Journal of Infectious Diseases 133: 363–366

Schaberg D R, Haley R W, Highsmith A K, Anderson R L, McGowan J E 1980 Nosocomial bacteriuria: a prospective study of case clustering and antimicrobial resistance. Annals of Internal Medicine 93: 420–424

Schaberg D R, Culver D H, Gaynes R P 1991 Major trends in the microbial etiology of nosocomial infection. American Journal of Medicine 91 (suppl 3B): 72S–75S

Schein M 1992 Management of severe intra-abdominal infection. Surgery Annual 24: 47–68

Scheld W M, Mandell G L 1991 Nosocomial pneumonia: pathogenesis and recent advances in diagnosis and therapy. Reviews of Infectious Diseases 13 (suppl 9): S743–S751

Schentag J J, Vari A J, Winslade N E et al 1985 Treatment with aztreonam or tobramycin in critical care patients with nosocomial Gram-negative pneumonia. American Journal of Medicine 78 (suppl 2A): 34–41

Schwigon C D, Hulla F W, Schulze B, Maslak A 1986 Timentin in the treatment of nosocomial bronchopulmonary infections in intensive care units. Journal of Antimicrobial Chemotherapy 17 (suppl C): 115–122

Seidenfeld J J, Pohl D F, Bell R C, Harris G D, Johanson W G 1986 Incidence, site, and outcome of infections in patients with the adult respiratory distress syndrome. American Review of Respiratory Disease 134: 12–16

Selective Decontamination of the Digestive Tract Trialists Collaborative Group 1993 Meta-analysis of randomised controlled trials of selective decontamination of the digestive tract. British Medical Journal 307: 525–532

Shah P M, Asanger R, Kahan F M 1991 Incidence of multi-resistance in Gram-negative aerobes from intensive care units of 10 German hospitals. Scandinavian Journal of Infectious Diseases (suppl 78): 22–34

Sirot D L, Goldstein F W, Soussy C J et al 1992 Resistance to cefotaxime and seven other β-lactams in members of the family Enterobacteriaceae: a 3-year survey in France. Antimicrobial Agents and Chemotherapy 36: 1677–1681

Sirot J, Chanal C, Petit A, Sirot D, Labia R, Gerbaud G 1988 *Klebsiella pneumoniae* and other enterobacteriaceae producing novel plasmid-mediated β-lactamases markedly active against third-generation cephalosporins: epidemiologic studies. *Reviews of Infectious Disease* 10: 850–859

Smith R L, Meixler S M, Simberkoff M S 1991 Excess mortality critically ill patients with nosocomial bloodstream infections. *Chest* 100: 164–167

Snydman D R 1991 Clinical implications of multi-drug resistance in the intensive care unit. *Scandinavian Journal of Infectious Diseases* (suppl 78): 54–63

Solomkin J S, Dellinger E P, Christou N V, Busuttil R W 1990 Results of a multicenter trial comparing imipenem/cilastatin to tobramycin/clindamycin for intra-abdominal infections. *Annals of Surgery* 212: 581–591

Sovenson J, Forsberg P, Hakanson E et al 1989 A new diagnostic approach to the patient with severe pneumonia. *Scandinavian Journal of Infectious Diseases* 21: 33–41

Stamm W E 1992 Nosocomial urinary tract infections. In: Bennett J V, Brachman P S (eds) Hospital infections, 3rd edn. Little, Brown and Co., Boston, p 597–610

Stark R P, Maki D G 1984 Bacteriuria in the catheterized patient. What quantitative level of bacteriuria is relevant? *New England Journal of Medicine* 311: 560–564

Stoutenbeek C P, van Saene H K F, Miranda D R, Zandstra D F 1984 The effect of selective decontamination of the digestive tract on colonisation and infection rate in multiple trauma patients. *Intensive Care Medicine* 10: 185–192

Tablan O C, Anderson L J, Arden N H et al 1994 Guideline for prevention of nosocomial pneumonia. *American Journal of Infection Control* 22: 247–292

Thompson R L, Cabezudo I, Wenzel R P 1982 Epidemiology of nosocomial infections caused by methicillin-resistant *Staphylococcus aureus*. *Annals of Internal Medicine* 97: 309–317

Torres A, Serra-Batlles J, Ferrer A et al 1991 Severe community-acquired pneumonia. *American Review of Respiratory Disease* 144: 312–318

Tryba M 1991 Sucralfate versus antacids or H_2 antagonists for stress ulcer prophylaxis: a meta-analysis on efficacy and pneumonia rate. *Critical Care Medicine* 19: 942–949

Valles J, Artigas A, Rello J et al 1995 Continuous aspiration of subglottic secretions in preventing ventilator-associated pneumonia. *Annals of Internal Medicine* 122: 179–186

Vandenbroucke-Grauls C M J E, Vandenbroucke J P 1991 Effect of selective decontamination of the digestive tract on respiratory tract infections and mortality in the intensive care unit. *Lancet* 338: 859–862

Verghese A, Widrich W C, Arbeit R D 1985 Central venous septic thrombophlebitis – the role of medical therapy. *Medicine* 64: 394–400

Vincent J-L, Bihari D J, Suter P M et al 1995 The prevalence of nosocomial infection in intensive care units in Europe – the results of the EPIC study. *Journal of the American Medical Association* 274: 639–644

Watanakunakorn C, Patel R 1993 Comparison of patients with enterococcal bacteremia due to strains with and without high-level resistance to gentamicin. *Clinical Infectious Diseases* 17: 74–78

Webb C H 1992 Antibiotic resistance associated with selective decontamination of the digestive tract. *Journal of Hospital Infection* 22: 1–5

Weinstein R A 1991 Epidemiology and control of nosocomial infections in adult intensive care units. *American Journal of Medicine* 91 (suppl 3B): 179S–184S

Infections associated with implanted devices

R. Bayston

Introduction

Since the introduction of hydrocephalus shunts and total hip replacements in the 1950s and 1960s, the number of implantable devices in use has increased enormously. They can be considered to fall into three categories: short-term, such as peripheral venous access cannulae; medium-term, such as central venous access devices; and long-term, such as total joint replacements, hydrocephalus shunts and prosthetic heart valves.

Implants are constructed from biocompatible materials, and these must also satisfy the mechanical requirements for use. Large joint replacements are made of steel, titanium, high-density polyethylene, or a combination of these, and may or may not utilize acrylic bone cement to enhance load-bearing capacity. Cardiac pacemaker leads and their generator packs are not biocompatible and are therefore encapsulated in silicone elastomer. Most other long- and medium-term implants are constructed from silicone elastomer, while other polymers including polyurethane are often used for those implanted for relatively short periods. Despite the fact that these materials are biocompatible, they are not bioinert. They are extremely rapidly coated with proteins and glycoproteins which include albumin, immuno-globulins, fibrin and fibrinogen, fibronectin, collagen and laminin. With regard to infective complications it is to this 'conditioning film' rather than to the biomaterial surface that infecting organisms attach. The organisms most commonly involved in implant-related infections are Staphylococcus aureus, coagulase-negative staphylococci (CoNS), coryneforms, streptococci, and Acinetobacter and Candida spp. Almost all organisms capable of causing implant-related infection are able to establish themselves as a biofilm. This consists of a matrix of microbial cells, their exopolymers, and host-derived material firmly anchored via the conditioning film to the biomaterial surface. The biofilm mode of microbial existence has important clinical implications. The organisms are surviving under conditions of nutrient and oxygen depletion. This leads to extremely low cell turnover rates and expression of phenotypes which are not only optimal for survival under such adverse conditions but which cause many antimicrobials to be ineffective (Brown et al 1990). The minimum inhibitory concentration (MIC) for an antimicrobial against an organism in the biofilm mode is usually at least three orders of magnitude higher than for the same organism grown under conventional laboratory conditions (Evans & Holmes 1987). This makes the eradication of implant-related infection so difficult, and often leads to eventual surgical removal of the implant.

Amongst the organisms causing implant-related infections, most attention has been paid to the biofilms of Staphylococcus epidermidis, which produces an exopolysaccharide (slime). To date, laboratory detection of slime has not been useful in determining clinical management or outcome of therapy (West et al 1986, Kotilainen 1990). Other organisms such as coryneforms and acinetobacter also produce an exopolysaccharide (Peters et al 1981, Bayston et al 1994).

Arteriovenous fistulae for haemodialysis

Haemodialysis for the management of end-stage renal disease requires reliable access to the vascular system. Modern fistulae, which anastomose the radial artery and cephalic vein, employ either bovine heterografts or grafts of expanded PTFE (Teflon, Gore Tex) or polyester (Dacron). These have a lower rate of associated thrombosis and infection than earlier materials, although the latter is still a considerable problem.

Organisms may be introduced at operation to create the fistula, and haematogenous infection may occur from a distant site, but the major risk is from repeated use. The organism causing most infections is *Staph. aureus*, which is often derived from the patient's own skin and mucous membranes (Cheesbrough et al 1986). *Pseudomonas aeruginosa* is also frequently responsible. While local signs and abscess formation are common in such infections, these are absent in about a third of cases. Bacteraemia is common and endocarditis is a risk (Cross & Steigbigel 1978).

The superior biocompatibility and functional properties of Dacron or expanded Teflon are outweighed by their propensity to act as a matrix for biofilm-associated infections. Not surprisingly, therefore, management of such an infection usually involves graft removal as well as administration of antimicrobials. The agents of choice for staphylococcal infection are the glycopeptides; in the case of vancomycin therapeutic drug monitoring is essential and dosage is 1 g i.v. at approximately weekly intervals depending on plasma levels. Aminoglycosides for *Ps. aeruginosa* and other Gram-negative bacilli must be similarly monitored. Ceftazidime is also useful for *Ps. aeruginosa* infections.

The use of 'high-flux' haemodialysis using polysulphone membranes leads to special problems of dosage for both glycopeptides and aminoglycosides. Up to 50% of the antimicrobial is removed during the procedure, and it is common practice to administer a 'top-up' dose after completion of dialysis. However, there is considerable redistribution of antimicrobial, which rapidly restores the 'lost' plasma concentration (Hastelson et al 1987, Pollard et al 1994) so that no postdialysis dose is required. However, in the case of ceftazidime, where the half-life of the drug has been shown to decrease by 90% in patients on haemodialysis, a further 1 g dose at the end of the dialysis session is recommended (Nikolaidis & Tourkantonis 1985, van Dalen et al 1986). For patients on low-flux haemodialysis, the dose and frequency of ceftazidime should be determined in conjunction with serum creatinine/creatinine clearance determinations, but the maintenance dose is usually 0.5 g i.v. every 48 h.

In patients known to be at risk from infective endocarditis, prolonged treatment may be necessary and if required, a new graft can be inserted before the end of the course of antimicrobials if the local infection has been eradicated.

Prophylaxis at the time of insertion of the graft should be aimed at the staphylococci and Gram-negative bacilli including *Ps. aeruginosa*, and ceftazidime 1 g i.v. and vancomycin 1 g i.v. should be given.

Vascular grafts

Two types of graft are in use for the replacement of a vascular segment. These include a homograft of vascular tissue taken from elsewhere in the body or, more commonly, a prosthetic graft manufactured from Dacron or Teflon (Gore Tex) fabric. Early experimental studies showed that, when infection occurs, homografts may rapidly disrupt leading to life-threatening blood loss, whereas prosthetic grafts usually retain their integrity although infection often persists. Only prosthetic grafts will be considered here.

Infection may be acquired haematogenously or more usually at the time of insertion. The causative organisms vary depending on the site of the graft. In most sites, *Staph. aureus* predominates, closely followed by CoNS (Bandyk 1992). However, in abdominal vascular grafts *Escherichia coli* predominates, and polymicrobial infections can occur. Most late infections are due to CoNS, and there is increasing evidence that most of these are introduced at implantation (Bandyk et al 1984). The incidence of graft infection also varies with site, the highest incidence being found in those in the groin. Reported incidences vary between 1% and 5% (O'Brien & Collin 1992).

Treatment

The seriousness of vascular graft infection cannot be overemphasized. The graft must be removed but the distal vascular supply must be maintained through a temporary extracorporeal bypass. The mortality rate and morbidity, including limb loss, are high. Simultaneous graft replacement can only be considered if there is no frank infection external to the graft.

Treatment

Initial treatment is directed against staphylococci. Vancomycin is the drug of choice. Teicoplanin is easier to administer, but occasional resistant strains of CoNS are seen. In the case of abdominal grafts or whenever *Esch. coli* infection is suspected, gentamicin or a cephalosporin (cefuroxime or cefotaxime) must be added. If graft erosion or an enteral fistula is suspected, metronidazole should also be given. Opinion varies as to the duration of therapy after successful regrafting of infected cases, but at least 6 weeks is recommended. When glycopeptides are used, renal function and plasma drug levels should be carefully monitored.

Prophylaxis

Antimicrobial prophylaxis, directed at staphylococci and aerobic Gram-negative bacilli, should be used in all vascular graft procedures. In a double-blind study, Worning et al (1986) compared methicillin plus netilmicin with a placebo, giving the first dose at induction and the second and third doses at 8 and 16 h. However, they considered the results disappointing. Hasselgren et al (1984) thought that this could have been due to the administration of only one dose to some patients. It is essential that the prophylactic antimicrobials are given intraoperatively as well as preoperatively, in view of the long duration of operation and inevitable blood loss, in order to maintain blood and tissue levels. Vancomycin and either cefuroxime or cefotaxime should be used.

Vascular access catheters

Access to the peripheral vascular system is useful for short-term administration of drugs, fluids and blood products and for the longer term administration of, for instance, parenteral nutrition fluids or cytotoxic drugs requiring central access.

PERIPHERAL CANNULATION

The annual number of patients receiving peripheral cannulation in USA has been estimated as approximately 25 million, with an infection rate of about 4% (Maki et al 1988). An estimate of the number of peripheral cannulae used in British hospitals can be made from a multicentre European study (Nyström et al 1983), in which 15 British hospitals took part. Of the 3865 surgical patients enrolled, 1543 (40%) had a peripheral intravenous catheter inserted. The incidence of bacteraemia is very low, though local infection and thrombophlebitis is more common (Tully et al 1981, Hoffmann et al 1988, Maki & Ringer 1991). Some reports suggest that the use of steel rather than plastic or Teflon needles leads to fewer infections (Maki et al 1973, Tully et al 1981), but when they are inserted under controlled conditions by trained personnel there appears to be no significant difference (Williams et al 1982), especially with the newer catheter materials (Maki & Ringer 1991). However, after 48 h the risk of infection and bacteraemia increases with all types of cannulae (Maki et al 1973). If a cut-down is required the incidence of infection rises considerably.

There is no indication for the use of antimicrobial prophylaxis in peripheral cannulation. Almost all local infections and most bacteraemias resolve with cannula removal alone, though in practice a short course (24–48 h) of an antimicrobial such as flucloxacillin or oxacillin or, for resistant strains, vancomycin should be prescribed. If pyrexia does not settle, or if there is abscess formation, a full course of treatment should be given.

CENTRAL VASCULAR CANNULATION

The catheters in common use for central vascular access are arterial lines for monitoring haemodynamic perfor-

mance, and the Hickman and Broviac for administration of drugs or parenteral nutrition fluids. Each of the latter has a subcutaneous Dacron cuff to anchor it in place, and is tunnelled surgically from its cutaneous exit site to the venous entry site, its tip usually lying in the superior vena cava or right atrium. The cuffed catheters are made from silicone elastomer. A conditioning film forms on the outer surface and for a few millimetres inside the distal tip, and it is not unusual to find a thrombus adherent to the outer surface of the intravascular or intracardiac portion. Usually no such film forms on the inner surface. As intended, fibroblasts infiltrate the Dacron cuff and serve to anchor it, though if infection occurs early this process may fail.

Swan–Ganz catheters for haemodynamic monitoring have been shown to have a relatively low risk of infection as they are usually not left in place for more than 4 days (Mermel & Maki 1994), but centrally placed venous catheters often remain in place for weeks or months and have a higher infection rate than peripheral cannulae. In the multicentre study by Nyström et al (1983), the incidence of central venous catheter-related bacteraemia was 5.9%. Where double- or, particularly, triple-lumen catheters are used, the infection rate can be as high as 32% (Weightman et al 1988). However, the risk of catheter-related bacteraemia in single-lumen catheters has been found in a prospective study to be 0.8% (Pittet et al 1991). The risk of bacteraemia from an exit site infection can be eliminated by the use of a Portacath or Mediport, which have an injection port placed subcutaneously. Drugs and fluids are administered by percutaneous injection into the port. However, luminal infections of these devices by staphylococci and other organisms are not uncommon, and abscess formation around the injection port due to *Staph. aureus* is a well-recognized problem.

While some infections may be introduced at the time of placement of the catheter, most occur later due either to contamination of the lumen by organisms gaining access when the line is disconnected to change bags or when injections are made, or from extension of exit site and track infections. The commonest infecting organisms are staphylococci, with CoNS predominating. Other organisms include coryneforms and enterococci. Cytotoxic infusions used have antimicrobial activity, and most parenteral nutrition fluids are inhospitable to bacteria, having a high osmolality and low pH (Crocker et al 1984). An exception are lipid emulsions such as Intralipid, which are associated with infection by lipophilic yeasts. Coryneforms and particularly *Corynebacterium jeikeium* are an important cause of bacteraemia complicating central venous catheters. Not only are these organisms multiresistant to antimicrobials, but they also produce an extracellular slime similar to that produced by CoNS (Bayston et al 1994). Therapeutically they pose identical problems to those of CoNS with regard to difficulty of eradication. Other important causes of central catheter-related sepsis, particularly those receiving total parenteral nutrition (TPN), are pseudomonads (Ps. *aeruginosa* and *Burkholderia* (*Pseudomonas) cepacia*) and *Candida* spp. While all such organisms may be present on the skin of a seriously ill patient exposed to broad-spectrum antimicrobials, *B. cepacia* has been particularly associated with contaminated infusion fluids.

Treatment of established central-catheter-related infection is controversial, some recommending catheter removal and some discouraging it. The majority of luminal CoNS infections can be eradicated with antibiotics, though Raad et al (1992) found a 20% relapse rate. In a retrospective study of *Staph. aureus* central catheter infections, a significant risk of secondary complications emerged even when the catheters were removed as part of the management (Raad & Sabbagh 1992). Among the risks are endocarditis and disseminated sepsis (Verghese et al 1985, Terpenning et al 1988).

The difficulties associated with removal and replacement of a cuffed catheter are such that attempts at salvage are usually made unless there is persistent track infection or a known risk of endocarditis. This latter risk is real, as illustrated by Fang et al (1993) who found that, of 18 patients having prosthetic heart valves inserted and who developed hospital-acquired staphylococcal endocarditis, a third could be directly attributed to central venous catheter infection.

Initial empirical treatment should consist of a glycopeptide and a third-generation cephalosporin such as ceftazidime or a quinolone. The regimen should then be modified when culture results become available. If *Candida* is isolated amphotericin B or fluconazole should be used. Vancomycin is the drug of choice for staphylococcal, enterococcal or coryneform infections. However, strains of enterococci showing resistance to both vancomycin and teicoplanin are increasing, and pose a serious therapeutic problem. Teicoplanin-resistant staphylococci are uncommon, but include *Staphylococcus haemolyticus* and a few strains of *Staph. epidermidis* (Vedel et al 1990, Tripodi et al 1994). A randomized prospective comparison of vancomycin and teicoplanin for the treatment of Hickman catheter infections, all caused by staphylococci, enterococci or coryneforms, showed no significant difference between the two drugs in terms of efficacy (Smith et al 1989). Interestingly, no catheters in this study had to be removed. There were more adverse effects in the vancomycin group (25%) than the teicoplanin group (8%), though these could be minimized with slower infusions. *Ps. aeruginosa* infections should be treated with either gentamicin or ceftazidime, either alone or in combination, according to severity. *B. cepacia* and other pseudomonads which are resistant to aminoglycosides are usually susceptible to ceftazidime. While the majority of *Ps. aeruginosa* are susceptible to ciprofloxacin in vitro, this cannot always be relied upon when treating serious infections. Regimens for other aerobic Gram-negative bacilli should be based on susceptibility test results, though the empirical combination of vancomycin or teicoplanin with ceftazidime will cover most isolates. *Candida* infections can be treated with a combination of amphotericin B and 5-fluorocytosine or fluconazole alone (Ch. 60). In the case of pseudomonads and *Candida* spp., catheter removal is recommended whenever possible in view of the grave risks of metastatic infection, including endocarditis.

The prophylactic administration of antimicrobials to cover the insertion of central venous catheters has not been shown to be useful. Indeed, those most at risk from procedure-related infection, that is those already having been in hospital for prolonged periods or those requiring a cut-down, are almost always already receiving antimicrobials.

In an attempt to prevent exit-site infection in peripheral catheters, topical polymyxin, neomycin and bacitracin ointment has been used with marginal benefit but an increase in candida infection (Maki & Band 1981). Mupirocin ointment has been used to prevent exit site infection in central venous catheters, and a significant reduction in staphylococcal infection was seen without any selection of candida (Hill et al 1990). However, mupirocin is selective for coryneforms (Bayston & Higgins 1986) and might therefore lead to an increase in *Coryn. jeikeium* infections. There are also increasing reports of mupirocin resistance in *Staph. aureus* (Baird & Cola 1987, Gilbart et al 1993). There is general agreement that among the measures to prevent catheter infection one of the most important is strict adherence to aseptic technique during insertion and use.

Continuous ambulatory peritoneal dialysis

Continuous ambulatory peritoneal dialysis (CAPD) has proved a successful treatment for end-stage renal disease. The disadvantages of haemodialysis are overcome and dialysis continues while the patient leads a fairly normal life. Dialysis fluid is introduced through an indwelling catheter into the peritoneal cavity and after either a 6-h or overnight dwell time the fluid is drained into the same bag. Patients are trained to change their bags using rigorous aseptic technique.

The Tenckhoff catheter is in almost universal use. This is tunnelled through the abdominal wall to separate the cutaneous exit site from the site of entry into the peritoneal cavity. The catheter has either one or two Dacron cuffs, one of which is sited in the subcutaneous tunnel and the other at the site of entry into the peritoneal cavity.

Two types of infective complication are seen: the exit site

may become infected, with erythema, purulent exudate and local pain and this may affect the whole track; or the lumen of the catheter may become colonized, with the introduction of bacteria into the peritoneal cavity giving rise to acute peritonitis. Both exit-site/track infection and peritonitis may occur together, and one may lead to the other. The presence of an exit-site infection has been shown to be a significant risk factor for the development of peritonitis (Churchill et al 1989). Causative organisms are usually those of the patient's own flora (Horsman et al 1986, Lye et al 1994), though Hanslik et al (1994) found no relationship between nasal colonization with *Staph. aureus* and exit-site infection. Peritonitis is often a consequence of a break in aseptic technique during bag change. The incidence of peritonitis varies between units and within units. Patients with a low risk due to good compliance and other factors might experience one episode every one to 2 years, though 'high-risk' patients can remain free of peritonitis for less than a few weeks at a time (Bailie et al 1993). Exit-site infections are more common, while track infections may be present without external signs. True exit-site and track infections are difficult to eradicate and often lead to catheter removal.

The most common cause of peritonitis is *Staph. epidermidis* (40–60%) with *Staph. aureus* and Gram-negative bacilli accounting for approximately 7–12% each. Occasional infections are due to coryneforms or fungi, mixed infections suggesting intestinal perforation.

Antimicrobial prophylaxis is not recommended at catheter insertion or on a continuous basis during dialysis (Eremin & Marshall 1969, Vas et al 1981, Vas 1994). Even though procedures such as colonoscopy are occasionally associated with cases of CAPD peritonitis (Holley et al 1987), the risk is very small and there is probably no indication for prophylaxis. Improvements in techniques and catheter design have been studied in an attempt to reduce the incidence of peritonitis, with variable results. Tofte-Jensen et al (1994) assessed a system in which fresh bags were used and iodine was used as a 'clamp' at exchange. While the fresh-bag technique produced a fall in numbers of cases of peritonitis, the 'iodine clamp' had no effect. Other similar alterations in device design have been investigated. Maiorca et al (1983) carried out a randomized controlled trial to compare a conventional set with a design incorporating a Y-connector which was filled with sodium hypochlorite during the dwell time. The incidence of peritonitis was reduced to one-third of that in those using the conventional design, confirming earlier non-randomized studies. However, accidental introduction of the hypochlorite intraperitoneally, causing severe pain, occurred in some patients. Churchill et al (1989) confirmed the reduction in peritonitis in a multi-centre randomized trial. However, the incidence of exit-site infections was not affected, and accidental aspiration of hypochlorite occurred in 25% of patients. Balteau et al (1991) investigated a Y-connector system without disinfectant

which used a fresh bag for the dialysate, but required only one connection. In their hands, the incidence of peritonitis was reduced.

Treatment

The management of peritonitis, exit-site or track infection, and those cases where both are present differs. In addition, there is little international agreement on the most appropriate regimens. For the treatment of peritonitis the reader is referred to the guidelines of the British Society for Antimicrobial Chemotherapy (Bint et al 1987) and the updated guidelines of the international Ad Hoc Advisory Committee on Peritonitis Management (Keane et al 1993). These state that there is no advantage in giving antimicrobials by both parenteral and intraperitoneal routes, and that the latter is preferred and the intraperitoneal route is more convenient, allowing outpatient treatment. However, the frequency of doses varies considerably, from one dose in each exchange to one dose weekly. A variety of antimicrobials have been used, and so long as their antimicrobial spectra are appropriate they appear to be equally successful. In view of the likely causative organisms, activity against Gram-positive and Gram-negative organisms, including *Ps. aeruginosa*, is initially required. Vancomycin is preferred for Gram-positive bacteria, and has been used successfully as initial treatment with ceftazidime (Gray et al 1985) or an aminoglycoside for Gram-negative bacteria. Once culture results become known, one or other of the drugs should be discontinued (Box 45.1). It should be remembered that the majority of *Staph. epidermidis* are now methicillin resistant, and also insusceptible to cephalosporins. One report suggests that cephalosporins are inactivated by peritoneal dialysate (Appleby & John 1982), and β-lactamases of tissue origin are known, though this does not appear to be of clinical significance. The combination of vancomycin plus an aminoglycoside has the advantage that, in the event of an enterococcus being isolated, it can be continued, whereas the combination of vancomycin plus ceftazidime would be less likely to be successful. Occasional enterococci will be resistant to vancomycin and teicoplanin can be substituted, but some strains are resistant to both glycopeptides. Lynn et al (1994) successfully treated three cases of CAPD-related peritonitis caused by multi-resistant *Enterococcus faecium* with quinupristin/dalfopristin, a pristinamycin derivative. Only one patient required catheter removal. This drug, which belongs to the streptogramins, is as yet unlicensed. Most teicoplanin-resistant staphylococci are *Staph. haemolyticus*, but resistant strains of *Staph. epidermidis* have also been reported (Grant et al 1986). For candida peritonitis, a combination of flucytosine and fluconazole is recommended (Keane et al 1993) as this is less toxic than amphotericin B and has comparable success rates (Millikin et al 1991).

Box 45.1   *Treatment schema for CAPD peritonitis (modified from Keane et al (1993) and Vas (1994)), based on a 2-l exchange and a 6-h dwell time*

Initial treatment

Vancomycin 2 g i.p. (body weight >40 kg)
1 g i.p. (body weight ≤40 kg)

+

Ceftazidime 500 mg/l
or
Gentamicin 1.7 mg/kg i.p.

Then:

Culture negative
Continue vancomycin 1–2 g i.p.
1 dose weekly for 2 weeks
Stop ceftazidime/gentamicin

Culture: Gram-positive cocci (except Staph. aureus)
Continue vancomycin 1–2 g i.p.
1 dose weekly for 2 weeks
Stop ceftazidime/gentamicin

Culture: Staph. aureus
Continue vancomycin 1–2 g i.p.
1 dose weekly for 2 weeks
Stop ceftazidime/gentamicin
Add rifampicin 300 mg p.o. twice daily

Culture: Gram-negative bacilli
Continue ceftazidime 125 mg/l each exchange
or:
Gentamicin 8 mg/l each exchange
or:
20 mg/l one exchange per day
Stop vancomycin

For treatment of exit-site infections where erythema alone is present, topical application of mupirocin or another antiseptic is recommended (Keane et al 1993). However, external signs of infection are often accompanied by more extensive, though sometimes occult, infection around the catheter, and the risk of progressive track infection and peritonitis are such that topical treatment alone should not always be relied upon. The spectrum of bacteria causing exit-site infections is a little different from that of peritonitis; *Staph. aureus* and Gram-negative bacilli outnumber *Staph. epidermidis*. With this in mind, and depending on susceptibility test results, a cephalosporin such as cefuroxime may be used. If *Staph. aureus* alone is present, oral flucloxacillin (250 mg four times daily) or equivalent should be used. A 2-week course is recommended.

The two main reasons for removal of the Tenckhoff catheter are persistent exit-site or track infection and relapsing peritonitis. However, in the presence of either type of infection due to *Ps. aeruginosa* or *candida*, early removal of the catheter is usually justified (Vas 1983). Relapsing peritonitis due to *Staph. epidermidis* is often associated with biofilm formation in the catheter lumen, and though intraperitoneal vancomycin will often clear the infection, failures occur even if oral rifampicin is added. This is also true of difficult *Staph. aureus* exit-site infections where a combination of cefuroxime or flucloxacillin with rifampicin, continued for 4–6 weeks, has been recommended (Keane et al 1993). If this fails, catheter removal may be necessary. Some have advocated the immediate replacement of a new catheter at the same operation, with antimicrobial cover and the use of a new tunnel site (Paterson et al 1986). This has to be carried out with great care to be successful, but has major advantages by avoiding interruption of dialysis and further surgery to insert a replacement catheter once the infection has cleared. Cancarini et al (1994) found the method successful except in the case of refractory peritonitis due to *Ps. aeruginosa* and *Mycobacterium*, *Enterococcus* and *Acinetobacter* spp.

When *Staph. aureus* peritonitis relapses in the absence of an overt exit-site or track infection, covert infection at these sites should be considered. The use of intraperitoneal antimicrobials will often eradicate catheter-lumen colonization and peritonitis, but plasma and tissue concentrations are probably insufficient to clear the organisms from the track or, particularly, the Dacron cuffs. In such cases, oral flucloxacillin (250 mg four times daily) with or without rifampicin (300 mg twice daily) should be considered, and continued for 4–6 weeks.

Central nervous system implants

Devices implanted into the central nervous system include hydrocephalus shunts, external ventricular drains, ventricular access reservoirs, pressure monitors and pumps for long-term delivery of intraspinal chemotherapy. Most are constructed from silicone elastomer, some having metal or thermoplastic components in addition. Shunts are used to provide long-term control of cerebrospinal fluid (CSF) pressure in hydrocephalus, which is caused by failure of the intracranial absorption pathways due to trauma, previous sepsis, congenital anomaly or tumour. They are totally implanted, and intended to remain in place permanently. External ventricular drains provide short-term CSF pressure relief in cases of temporary increase such as in subarachnoid haemorrhage, or as part of the management of a shunt infection. They resemble shunts except that only the intracranial portion is internal, and the fluid drains into a sterile bag. Pressure transducers ('bolts') are implanted to enable intracranial pressure to be monitored continuously for a few hours to a few days. They are inserted through a burr hole, the internal portion remaining extradural.

Intraspinal drug delivery devices such as those for central control of spasticity consist of a catheter implanted in the lumbar theca, and connected to a battery-driven pump and rechargeable reservoir.

HYDROCEPHALUS SHUNT INFECTIONS

The placement of a CSF shunt is among the commonest neurosurgical procedures performed. There are two main routes of drainage for CSF shunts: either from the cerebral ventricle to the right atrium (ventriculoatrial (VA)) or, more usually, from the cerebral ventricle to the peritoneal cavity (ventriculoperitoneal (VP)). In addition, some drain from the spinal theca to the peritoneal cavity (lumboperitoneal (LP)) and a few drain into the pleural space (ventriculopleural (VPl)).

Soon after the introduction of CSF shunting for hydrocephalus, infective syndromes were reported (Anderson 1959, Carrington 1959). These were in VA shunts and the symptoms were of bacteraemia and sometimes meningitis. In long-standing cases, immune-complex glomerulonephritis is recognized (Black et al 1965, Stauffer 1970, Bayston & Swinden 1979). However, there has been a gradual adoption of the VP route, and this now constitutes the majority. Here the infection usually does not present as a bacteraemia but as an obstruction of the distal catheter resulting in reappearance of signs of raised intracranial pressure. There may also be abdominal pain and fever. Later, erythema may appear over the catheter track on the trunk. LP shunt infections also present similarly, while VPl infections may give rise to chest pain and respiratory distress. There is no significant difference in infection rate between VA and VP shunts, a survey of the literature showing that the ranges are 3%–23% and 6%–22%, respectively (Bayston 1989).

The most common causative organisms are the CoNS, though *Staph. aureus* and coryneforms together account for about 10%, Gram-negative bacilli and candida being less frequent. Most CSF-shunt infections result from organisms introduced during implantation, and though most VP, VPl and LP infections become apparent within weeks or months of surgery, some VA infections appear years later (Schimke et al 1961, Shurtleff et al 1971, Bayston & Swinden 1979). A separate less common group, representing true late infections, are usually due to a different spectrum of organisms and may arise from the alimentary or respiratory tracts or erosion of the skin over the shunt (Shapiro et al 1988).

Treatment

The three most common organisms involved in shunt infection, CoNS, *Staph. aureus* and coryneforms, are all capable of growing as biofilms inside the shunt tubing. Even in those shunt infections where meningoventriculitis is present, the inflammatory response is not usually marked, and is unlikely to have a significant effect on the biofilm organisms. Most parenterally administered antimicrobials fail to reach the CSF in therapeutic concentrations in the absence of a vigorous inflammatory response, and the exopolymers in the biofilm might also further impair their activity against the bacterial cells. It is not surprising, therefore, that attempts to treat shunt infections in the same way as other, extracranial, staphylococcal infections are likely to fail. Early experience (Callaghan et al 1961) has shown that, even when methicillin is administered by both intravenous and intraventricular routes for over 50 days, the infection relapses and the shunt must be removed to eradicate the infection. This experience has been repeatedly confirmed with a variety of antimicrobials given by various routes, and without shunt removal the results have been disappointing. James et al (1980) compared antibiotics (intravenous and intraventricular) and shunt removal with antibiotics alone and showed that all those with shunt removal were cured while only a third of those who retained their shunts recovered (two deaths occurred in this group).

As most shunt infections are due to Gram-positive cocci, and in view of the high likelihood of resistance to β-lactam antimicrobials among CoNS, vancomycin has been considered. Intravenous vancomycin has not proved successful for pharmacological reasons, although Visconti & Peters (1979) gave the drug intraventricularly in two cases with success which has been confirmed by others (Young et al 1981). A subsequent trial of intraventricular vancomycin and shunt removal showed impressive success rates, with no relapses and shortened duration of therapy and hospital stay (Bayston et al 1987). In this trial either flucloxacillin or rifampicin was given parenterally in addition. Others have confirmed the benefit of adding rifampicin (Archer et al 1978, Ring et al 1979, Gombert et al 1981). It is therefore recommended that treatment for shunt infections caused by Gram-positive cocci is shunt removal, external drainage, intraventricular vancomycin and oral or intravenous rifampicin, 15 mg/kg daily in 2–3 doses for children and 300 mg twice daily for adults (Bayston et al 1995). The vancomycin should be given in a daily dose of 20 mg, decreasing this to 10 mg only if the ventricular volume is known to be small. In infants with very small ventricular volumes, the dose may be decreased to 5 mg. Assessment of ventricular volumes should be carried out radiologically, but is somewhat arbitrary. The drug is safe when administered in this way and there has been no evidence of local or systemic toxicity, though it must be pointed out that this use of the drug remains unlicensed. Clinical and microbiological response is usually evident within 3–4 days, and reshunting can usually be carried out after 7–10 days, with the last dose of vancomycin being given perioperatively. Rifampicin should also be stopped at this time since the use of rifampicin alone leads to rapid development of resistance and must be avoided (Mandell & Moorman 1980).

The shunt should also be removed in the case of infection with Gram-negative bacilli, and ceftazidime 1 g 8-hourly (100 mg/kg daily in three doses for children) or gentamicin 60–80 mg 8-hourly (2 mg/kg 8-hourly for children) be given intravenously for 14 days, subject to susceptibility tests. CSF white cell count and culture should be carried out periodically during therapy to ensure that there is a satisfactory response.

Candida shunt infections also require shunt removal, with the administration of amphotericin B and flucytosine, though success has been reported with intravenous fluconazole 6 mg/kg daily for 13 days in a premature neonate (Cruciani et al 1992). Should community-acquired bacterial meningitis occur in a shunted patient, the temptation to remove the shunt should be resisted. Meningococci, pneumococci and haemophili do not appear to be capable of colonizing the shunt and therefore do not interfere with treatment, which should proceed as for non-shunted patients (Rennels & Wald 1980, Leggiadro et al 1984, Stern et al 1988, O'Keefe & Bayston 1991). Indeed, the presence of a shunt appears to be associated with a milder illness and more rapid recovery, possibly due to regulation of intracranial pressure (Shurtleff et al 1971).

Notwithstanding the poor results widely experienced with attempts to treat shunt infections due to Gram-positive cocci without shunt removal, there is some hope that a regimen might be developed by which some functioning shunts can be saved. Brown & Jones (1995) have pointed to the effectiveness of the regimen of intraventricular vancomycin and oral rifampicin with shunt retention, and have successfully treated 15 patients with CoNS infections, but not *Staph. aureus* infections. Further experience is awaited with interest.

Prophylaxis

Published studies of antimicrobial prophylaxis in shunt surgery have almost always been flawed in some way. Most do not distinguish true shunt infection from the far less common external infections which are, in reality, wound infections complicated by the presence of biomaterial. In the latter, it may be safe to assume that conventional antimicrobial prophylaxis (intravenous administration of a suitable agent at induction of anaesthesia) will be of benefit. The majority of external shunt infections are due to *Staph. aureus*, and in most cases antistaphylococcal cover alone with flucloxacillin or equivalent will be adequate. A few are caused by Gram-negative bacilli, and if additional cover is felt desirable cephradine or cefuroxime should suffice.

True shunt infection, which primarily involves the shunt lumen, is not amenable to such a regimen. Firstly, the most common causative organisms, CoNS, are often resistant to

flucloxacillin and, therefore, to cephalosporins; and, secondly, therapeutic antibacterial concentrations of most parenterally administered antimicrobials, including cephalosporins, are not achievable in the CSF in the absence of inflamed meninges. Many neurosurgeons nevertheless use some form of antimicrobial prophylaxis for shunting procedures, but there is considerable doubt as to its effectiveness. Thirdly, published studies of prophylaxis are all either uncontrolled, retrospective, sequential, or too small to allow valid analysis (Brown et al 1994). Currently there is no evidence to support the view that antimicrobial prophylaxis for shunt surgery, even using intraventricular vancomycin (Bayston et al 1990), has any beneficial effect, and it therefore cannot be recommended.

EXTERNAL VENTRICULAR DRAINAGE

When external drainage devices are used to control CSF pressure during treatment of a shunt infection, they must be carefully managed to avoid secondary infection. If it occurs this is often due to Gram-negative bacilli. Antimicrobials will already be in use to treat the shunt infection, and prophylaxis is therefore inappropriate. When external drainage is used to manage non-infective intracranial conditions such as subarachnoid haemorrhage, ascending infection is still a risk and staphylococci predominate. Again, prophylaxis is inappropriate and will merely encourage a resistant flora. When secondary infection occurs, the external drain should be replaced and appropriate antimicrobials administered according to the results of susceptibility tests. Care should be taken to ensure that the diagnosis of secondary intracranial infection is correct, and that the organisms isolated are not merely colonizing the distal portions of the tubing.

OMMAYA RESERVOIRS

These and similar reservoirs have a variety of applications, ranging from the intraventricular administration of antimicrobials for CSF-shunt infection or for fungal meningitis, to cytotoxic therapy for intracranial lymphoma or leukaemic meningitis. Injections are given percutaneously into the reservoir. Organisms which cause reservoir infection are usually introduced in this way, and are mainly *Staph. epidermidis*, *Staph. aureus* and coryneforms. The infection rate is estimated to be about 10–15%. In a series of 15 patients reported by Chamberlain and Dirr (1993) there were two reservoir infections, with some patients receiving over 400 injections into the reservoir for chemotherapy for acquired immune deficiency syndrome (AIDS) related lymphoma, emphasizing the potential for introducing infection into these devices.

Treatment

In many cases, removal of the reservoir and intraventricular administration of vancomycin using a freshly placed device will suffice to eradicate the infection, though some have successfully used the same reservoir for treatment (Hirsch et al 1991). In some cases the infection is refractory to intravenous antimicrobials even when the device is removed (Lishner et al 1991), and the use of intraventricular vancomycin offers the best chance of success.

Prophylaxis

Antimicrobial prophylaxis is unlikely to be helpful and is not recommended.

PUMPS FOR INTRASPINAL THERAPY FOR SPASTICITY

Intraspinal administration of drugs for intractable pain and the treatment of spasticity has been made more controllable by the use of programmable implantable pumps. The pump reservoir is refilled percutaneously every few weeks, with a slight but obvious risk of infection. Infection of the tissue pocket in which the pump and its reservoir are located sometimes occurs, and is usually due to *Staph. aureus.* Internal microbial colonization of the pump reservoir has occurred leading to meningitis and this is usually due to CoNS. If treated early, pocket infections can be eradicated using systemic flucloxacillin, but in the case of reservoir infections this is ineffective. Introduction of vancomycin into the reservoir has led to eradication in some cases, though in others the device has had to be removed. Published information is limited. In one report of meningitis (Bennett et al 1994), the reservoir became colonized with *Staph. epidermidis* soon after insertion despite prophylactic intravenous ceftazidime and vancomycin. After unsuccessful attempts to treat the infection with oral and intravenous antibiotics, vancomycin 50 mg/ml was introduced into the reservoir and the pump programmed to deliver 5 mg/day intrathecally. The patient became apyrexial after 2 days; vancomycin was administered for a total of 30 days at a reduced daily dose of 2.5 mg. CSF vancomycin concentrations reached 54 mg/l without toxicity. The infection was eradicated without pump removal. The authors considered, in retrospect, that a much shorter course would have been successful.

Peritoneovenous shunts for ascites

Shunts such as the LeVeen or the Denver, which resemble CSF shunts, are commonly used to treat ascites complicating cirrhosis or malignancy by draining the ascitic fluid from the peritoneal cavity to the venous system. The route taken by the catheter is from the peritoneal cavity via a subcutaneous track to the internal jugular vein and thence to the right atrium. However, their use remains controversial (Schumaker et al 1994) due to the high rate of complications, notably obstruction, and infection caused by staphylococci or Gram-negative bacilli, which presents as peritonitis or septicaemia or both.

Treatment

The little published experience indicates clearly the need for removal of an infected shunt and the administration of intravenous antimicrobials determined by the causative bacteria and their antimicrobial susceptibilities. In view of the likely intraperitoneal and intravascular suppuration, a course of 3–4 weeks is recommended.

Prophylaxis

Because of the seriousness and frequency of infection, prophylaxis would appear to be warranted. A variety of antimicrobials have been given at shunt insertion. Smajda & Franco (1985) gave oral oxacillin for 10 days postoperatively to 54 patients, but infections still occurred. Four of these appeared soon after operation and were due to *Staph. aureus.* A further eleven appeared later and were due to *Staph. aureus, Esch. coli, Klebsiella* and *Enterococcus* spp. Meakins et al (1989) found that a two-dose regimen controlled early but not late infections. Oral ofloxacin or intravenous cefotetan were used by Hillaire et al (1993) in a series of 56 patients, eight of whom nevertheless developed peritonitis postoperatively. Though there is little evidence to support the effectiveness of prophylaxis, cefuroxime is recommended for prevention of early infections, but prophylaxis is probably impractical for late infections.

Recent developments in prevention

In the case of many implantable devices, systemic antimicrobial prophylaxis is of little or no benefit, and this has led to alternative approaches. Buchholz & Engelbrecht (1970) used antibiotic-loaded bone cement to reduce the incidence of infection in total hip replacement. Controversy continued regarding the release of antimicrobials from the cement, and the case was addressed by Bayston & Milner (1982) who showed that different antimicrobials were released at different rates from different brands of cement, and that the physicochemical properties of the drugs were important determinants.

Attempts have also been made to develop infection-resistant vascular grafts by coating the grafts with antibiotic-loaded collagen (Moore et al 1981). Greco et al (1982) bonded benzalkonium chloride and oxacillin to a PTFE graft. These studies both showed encouraging results in animal infection models. Kamal et al (1991) have carried out a clinical trial of cationic-detergent-coated vascular access catheters with bonded cefazolin and showed a reduction in luminal colonization but no effect on exit site infection at 1 week. Silver impregnation, either alone or with an antimicrobial, has shown a significant reduction in exit-site-associated central venous catheter infections with a silver-impregnated cuff (Maki et al 1988), while in dogs vascular grafts coated with silver and norfloxacin have been shown to be protective (Modak et al 1987). A number of other experimental approaches are in hand which will hopefully be successful in contributing to the control of infection in implanted medical devices (Bayston & Milner 1981, Bayston et al 1989, Costerton et al 1994, Bayston 1995).

References

Anderson F M 1959 Ventriculo-auriculostomy in the treatment of hydrocephalus. *Journal of Neurosurgery* 16: 551–557

Appleby D H, John J F 1982 Effect of peritoneal dialysis solution on the antimicrobial activity of cephalosporins. *Nephron* 30: 341–344

Archer G L, Tenebaum M J, Haywood H B 1978 Rifampicin therapy of *Staphylococcus epidermidis*. *Journal of the American Medical Association* 240: 751–753

Bailie G R, Rasmussen R, Eisele G, Luscombe D K 1993 Peritonitis rates in CAPD patients using the UVXD and O-set systems. *Renal Failure* 15: 225–230

Baird D, Cola J 1987 Mupirocin resistance in *Staphylococcus aureus*. *Lancet* ii: 387–388

Balteau P R, Peluso F P, Coles G A et al 1991 Design and testing of the Baxter Integrated Disconnect Systems (IDS). *Peritoneal Dialysis International* 11: 131–136

Bandyk D F 1992 Diagnosis and treatment of biomaterial-associated vascular infections. *Infectious Diseases Clinics of North America* 6: 719–729

Bandyk D F, Berni G A, Thiele B L, Towne J B 1984 Aorto-femoral graft infection due to *Staphylococcus epidermidis*. *Archives of Surgery* 119: 102–108

Bayston R 1989 Hydrocephalus shunt infections. Chapman & Hall, London

Bayston R 1995 Protection of CSF shunts against infection by impregnation with antimicrobial agents. Further in-vitro studies. Abstracts of 39th Annual Scientific Meeting of the Society for Research into Hydrocephalus and Spina Bifida, Bristol

Bayston R, Higgins J 1986 Biochemical and cultural characteristics of 'JK' coryneforms. *Journal of Clinical Pathology* 39: 654–660

Bayston R, Milner R D G 1981 Antimicrobial activity of silicone rubber used in hydrocephalus shunts, after impregnation with antimicrobial substances. *Journal of Clinical Pathology* 34: 1057–1062

Bayston R, Milner R D G 1982 The sustained release of antimicrobial drugs from bone cement. *Journal of Bone and Joint Surgery* 64B: 460–464

Bayston R, Swinden J 1979 The aetiology and prevention of shunt nephritis. *Zeitschrift für Kinderchirurgie* 28 (4): 377–384

Bayston R, Hart C A, Barnicoat M 1987 Intraventricular vancomycin in the treatment of ventriculitis associated with cerebrospinal fluid shunting and drainage. *Journal of Neurology, Neurosurgery and Psychiatry* 50: 1419–1423

Bayston R, Grove N, Siegel J, Lawellin D, Barsham S 1989 Prevention of hydrocephalus shunt catheter colonisation in vitro by impregnation with antimicrobials. *Journal of Neurology, Neurosurgery and Psychiatry* 52: 605–609

Bayston R, Bannister C M, Boston V et al 1990 A prospective randomised controlled trial of antimicrobial prophylaxis in hydrocephalus shunt surgery. *Zeitschrift für Kinderchirurgie* 45 (suppl 1): 5–7

Bayston R, Compton C, Richards K 1994 Production of extracellular slime by coryneforms colonising hydrocephalus shunts. *Journal of Clinical Microbiology* 32: 1705–1709

Bayston R, De Louvois J, Brown E M, Hedges A J, Johnston R A, Lees P 1995 Treatment of infections associated with shunting for hydrocephalus: Working Party on the Use of Antibiotics in Neurosurgery of the British Society for Antimicrobial Chemotherapy. *British Journal of Hospital Medicine* 53: 368–373

Bennett M I, Tai Y M, Symonds J M 1994 Staphylococcal meningitis following Synchromed pump implant: a case report. *Pain* 56: 243–244

Bint A J, Finch R G, Gokal R, Goldsmith H J, Junor B, Oliver D 1987 Diagnosis and management of peritonitis in continuous ambulatory peritoneal dialysis. Report of a working party of the British Society for Antimicrobial Chemotherapy. *Lancet* i: 845–848

Black J A, Challacombe D N, Ockenden B G 1965 Nephrotic syndrome associated with bacteraemia after shunt operations for hydrocephalus. *Lancet* ii: 921–924

Brown E M, Jones E M 1995 Non-surgical management of CSF shunt infections. Abstracts of 39th Annual Scientific Meeting of the Society for Research into Hydrocephalus and Spina Bifida, Bristol, UK

Brown E M, De Louvois J, Bayston R, Hedges A J, Johnston R A, Lees P 1994 Antimicrobial prophylaxis in neurosurgery and after head injury: British Society for Antimicrobial Chemotherapy Working Party Report on Use of Antibiotics in Neurosurgery. *Lancet* 344: 1547–1551

Brown M R W, Collier P J, Gilbert P 1990 Influence of growth rate on susceptibility to antimicrobial agents: modification of cell envelope and batch and continuous culture studies. *Antimicrobial Agents and Chemotherapy* 34: 1623–1628

Buchholz H W, Engelbrecht H 1970 Über die depotwirkung einiger Antibiotica bei Vermischung mit dem Kunstharz Palacos. *Chirurgie* 41: 511–515

Callaghan R P, Cohen S J, Stewart G T 1961 Septicaemia due to colonisation of Spitz–Holter valves by *Staphylococcus.* *British Medical Journal* 1: 860–863

Cancarini G C, Manili L, Brunori G et al 1994 Simultaneous catheter replacement–removal during infectious complications in peritoneal dialysis. *Advances in Peritoneal Dialysis* 10: 210–213

Carrington K W 1959 Ventriculovenous shunting using the Holter valve as a treatment of hydrocephalus. *Journal of the Michigan Medical Society* 58: 373–376

Chamberlain M C, Dirr L 1993 Involved-field radiotherapy and intra-Ommaya methotrexate/cytarabine in patients with AIDS-related lymphomatous meningitis. *Journal of Clinical Oncology* 11: 1978–1984

Cheesbrough J S, Finch R G, Burden R P 1986 A prospective study of the mechanisms of infection associated with haemodialysis catheters. *Journal of Infectious Diseases* 154: 579–589

Churchill D N, Taylor D W, Vas S I et al 1989 Peritonitis in continuous ambulatory peritoneal dialysis: a multicenter randomised clinical trial comparing the Y-Connector Disinfectant System to standard systems. *Peritoneal Dialysis International* 9: 159–163

Costerton J W, Ellis B, Lam K, Johnson F, Khoury A 1994 Mechanism of electrical enhancement of efficacy of antibiotics in killing biofilm bacteria. *Antimicrobial Agents and Chemotherapy* 38: 2803–2809

Crocker K S, Noga R, Filibeck D J, Krey S H, Markovic M, Steffee W P 1984 Microbial growth comparisons of five commercial parenteral lipid emulsions. *Journal of Parenteral and Enteral Nutrition* 8: 391–395

Cross A S, Steigbigel R T 1978 Infective endocarditis and access site infections in patients on hemodialysis. *Medicine (Baltimore)* 55: 453–466

Cruciani M, Di Perri G, Molesini M, Vento S, Concia E, Bassetti D 1992 Use of fluconazole in the treatment of *Candida albicans* hydrocephalus shunt infection. *European Journal of Microbiology and Infectious Diseases* 11: 957

Eremin J, Marshall J C 1969 The place of prophylactic antibiotics in peritoneal dialysis. *Australian Annals of Medicine* 18: 264–265

Evans R C, Holmes C J 1987 Effect of vancomycin hydrochloride on *Staphylococcus epidermidis* biofilm associated with silicone elastomer. *Antimicrobial Agents and Chemotherapy* 31: 889–894

Fang G, Keys T F, Gentry L O et al 1993 Prosthetic valve endocarditis resulting from nosocomial bacteremia. A prospective multicenter study. *Annals of Internal Medicine* 119: 560–567

Gilbart J, Perry C R, Slocombe B 1993 High level mupirocin resistance in *Staphylococcus aureus*: evidence for two distinct isoleucyl-tRNA synthetases. *Antimicrobial Agents and Chemotherapy* 37: 32–38

Gombert M E, Landesman S H, Corrado M L, Stein S C, Melvin E T, Cummings M 1981 Vancomycin and rifampicin therapy for *Staphylococcus epidermidis* associated with CSF shunts. *Journal of Neurosurgery* 55: 633–636

Grant A C, Lacey R W, Brownjohn A M, Turney J H 1986 Teicoplanin-resistant coagulase-negative staphylococcus. *Lancet* ii: 1166–1167

Gray H H, Goulding S, Eykyn S J 1985 Intraperitoneal vancomycin and ceftazidime in the treatment of CAPD peritonitis. *Clinical Nephrology* 23: 81–84

Greco R S, Harvey R A, Smilow P C, Tesoriero J V 1982 Prevention of vascular prosthetic infection by a benzalkonium–oxacillin bonded polytetrafluoroethylene graft. *Surgery, Gynecology and Obstetrics* 155: 28–32

Hanslik T M, Newman L N, Tessman M J, Morrisey A, Friedlander M A 1994 Lack of correlation between nasal cultures positive for *Staphylococcus aureus* and the development of Staph. aureus exit site infections: results unaffected by routine mupirocin treatment of nasal Staph. aureus carriage. *Advances in Peritoneal Dialysis* 10: 158–162

Hasselgren P, Ivarsson L, Risberg B, Seeman T 1984 Effects of prophylactic antibiotics in vascular surgery. A prospective randomised double blind study. *Annals of Surgery* 200: 86–92

Hastelson C E, Berkseth R O, Mann H J, Matzke G R 1987 Aminoglycoside redistribution phenomenon after haemodialysis: netilmicin and tobramycin. *International Journal of Clinical Pharmacology, Therapeutics and Toxicology* 25: 50–55

Hill R L R, Fisher A P, Ware R J, Wilson S, Casewell M W 1990 Mupirocin for the reduction of colonisation of internal jugular cannulae – a randomised controlled trial. *Journal of Hospital Infection* 15: 311–321

Hillaire S, Labianca M, Borgonovo G, Smajda C, Grange D, Franco D 1993 Peritoneovenous shunting of intractable ascites in patients with cirrhosis: improving results and predictive factors of failure. *Surgery* 113: 373–379

Hirsch B E, Amodio M, Einzig A L, Halevy R, Soeiro R 1991 Instillation of vancomycin into a cerebrospinal fluid reservoir to clear infection: pharmacokinetic considerations. *Journal of Infectious Diseases* 163: 197–200

Hoffmann K K, Western S A, Kaiser D L, Wenzel R P, Groschel D H 1988 Bacterial colonization and phlebitis – associated risk with transparent polyurethane film for peripheral intravenous site dressings. *American Journal of Infection Control* 16: 101–106

Holley J, Seibert D, Moss A 1987 Peritonitis following colonoscopy and polypectomy: a need for prophylaxis? *Peritoneal Dialysis Bulletin* 7: 105–106

Horsman G B, MacMillan L, Amatnieks Y, Rifkin O, Vas S 1986 Plasmid profile and slime analysis of coagulase-negative staphylococci from CAPD patients with peritonitis. *Peritoneal Dialysis Bulletin* 6: 195–198

James H E, Walsh J W, Wilson H D, Connor J D, Bean J R, Tibbs P A 1980 Prospective randomised study of therapy in cerebrospinal fluid shunt infection. *Neurosurgery* 7: 459–463

Kamal G D, Pfaller M A, Rempe L E, Jebson P J R 1991 Reduced intravascular catheter infection by antibiotic bonding. *Journal of the American Medical Association* 265: 2364–2368

Keane W F, Everett E D, Golper T A et al 1993 Peritoneal dialysis-related peritonitis treatment recommendations – 1993 update. *Peritoneal Dialysis International* 13: 14–28

Kotilainen P 1990 Association of coagulase-negative staphylococcal slime production and adherence with the development and outcome of adult septicemias. *Journal of Clinical Microbiology* 28: 2779–2785

Leggiadro R J, Atluru V L, Katz S P 1984 Meningococcal meningitis associated with cerebrospinal fluid shunts. *Pediatric Infectious Diseases* 3: 489–490

Lishner M, Scheinbaum R, Messner H A 1991 Intrathecal vancomycin in the treatment of Ommaya reservoir infection by *Staphylococcus epidermidis*. *Scandinavian Journal of Infectious Diseases* 23: 101–104

Lye W C, Leong S O, van der Straaten J, Lee E J C 1994 *Staphylococcus aureus* CAPD-related infections are associated with nasal carriage. *Advances in Peritoneal Dialysis* 10: 163–165

Lynn W A, Clutterbuck E, Want S et al 1994 Treatment of CAPD peritonitis due to glycopeptide-resistant *Enterococcus faecium* with quinopristin/dalfopristin. *Lancet* 344: 1025–1026

Maiorca R, Cantaluppi A, Cancarini G et al 1983 Prospective controlled trial of a Y-connector and disinfectant to prevent peritonitis in continuous ambulatory peritoneal dialysis. *Lancet* ii: 642–644

Maki D G, Band J D 1981 A comparative study of polyantibiotic and iodophor ointments in prevention of catheter related infection. *American Journal of Medicine* 70: 739–744

Maki D G, Ringer M 1991 Risk factors for infusion-related phlebitis with small peripheral venous catheters. A randomized controlled trial. *Annals of Internal Medicine* 114: 845–854

Maki D G, Goldman D A, Rhame F S 1973 Infection control in intravenous therapy. *Annals of Internal Medicine* 79: 867–887

Maki D G, Cobb L, Garman J K, Shapiro J M, Ringer M, Helgerson R B 1988 An attachable silver-impregnated cuff for prevention of infection with central venous catheters: a prospective randomised multicentre trial. *American Journal of Medicine* 85: 307–314

Mandell G L, Moorman D R 1980 Treatment of experimental staphylococcal infections: effect of rifampicin alone and in combination on development of rifampicin resistance. *Antimicrobial Agents and Chemotherapy* 17: 658–662

Meakins J L, Hillaire S, Vons C, Smajda C, Franco D 1989 Perioperative antibiotics (2 doses) control early but not late infectious complications of peritoneo-venous shunts. *Surgical Research Communications* 5: 55–58

Mermel L A, Maki D G 1994 Infectious complications of Swan–Gantz pulmonary artery catheters. Pathogenesis, epidemiology, prevention and management. *American Journal of Respiratory and Critical Care Management* 149: 1020–1036

Millikin S P, Matzke G R, Keane W F 1991 Antimicrobial treatment of peritonitis associated with continuous ambulatory peritoneal dialysis. *Peritoneal Dialysis International* 11: 252–260

Modak S M, Sampath L, Fox C L, Benvenisty A, Nowygrod R, Reemstmau K 1987 A new method for the direct incorporation of antibiotic in prosthetic vascular grafts. *Surgery, Gynecology and Obstetrics* 164: 143–147

Moore W S, Chvapil M, Seiffert G, Keown K 1981 Development of an infection-resistant vascular prosthesis. *Archives of Surgery* 116: 1403–1407

Nikolaidis P, Tourkantonis A 1985 Effect of hemodialysis on ceftazidime pharmacokinetics. *Clinical Nephrology* 24: 142–146

Nyström B, Olesen-Larsen S, Dankert J et al 1983 Bacteraemia in surgical patients with intravenous devices: a European multicentre incidence study. *Journal of Hospital Infection* 4: 338–349

O'Brien T, Collin J 1992 Prosthetic vascular graft infection. *British Journal of Surgery* 79: 1262–1267

O'Keeffe P T, Bayston R 1991 Pneumococcal meningitis in a child with a ventriculo-peritoneal shunt. *Journal of Infection* 22: 77–79

Paterson A D, Bishop M C, Morgan A G, Burden R P 1986 Removal and replacement of Tenckhoff catheter at a single operation: treatment of resistant peritonitis in continuous ambulatory peritoneal dialysis. *Lancet* 2: 1245–1247

Peters G, Locci R, Pulverer G 1981 Microbial colonisation of prosthetic devices. II. Scanning electron microscopy of naturally infected intravenous catheters. *Zentralblatt für Bakteriologie, Mikrobiologie und Hygiene I Abteilung Orig B* 173: 293–299

Pittet D, Chouard C, Rae AC, Auckenthaler R 1991 Clinical diagnosis of central venous catheter line infections: a difficult job. [Abstract]. *Interscience Conference on Antimicrobial Agents and Chemotherapy (ICAAC)* 31: 174

Pollard T A, Lampasona V, Akkerman S et al 1994 Vancomycin redistribution: dosing recommendations following high-flux hemodialysis. *Kidney International* 45: 232–237

Raad I, Sabbagh M F 1992 Optimal duration of therapy for catheter-related *Staphylococcus aureus* bacteremia: a study of 55 cases and review. *Clinical Infectious Diseases* 14: 75–82

Raad I, Davis S, Khan J, Tarrand L, Elting L, Bodey G P 1992 Impact of central venous catheter removal on the recurrence of catheter-related coagulase-negative staphylococcal bacteremia. *Infection Control and Hospital Epidemiology* 13: 215–221

Rennels M B, Wald E R 1980 Treatment of *Haemophilus influenzae* type b meningitis in children with cerebrospinal fluid shunts. *Journal of Pediatrics* 97: 424–426

Ring J C, Cates K L, Belani K K, Gaston T L, Sveum R J, Marker S C 1979 Rifampicin for CSF shunt infections caused by coagulase-negative staphylococci. *Journal of Pediatrics* 95: 317–319

Schimke R T, Black P H, Mark V H, Schwartz M N 1961 Indolent *Staphylococcus albus* or *aureus* bacteraemia after ventriculo-atriostomy. *New England Journal of Medicine* 264: 264–270

Schumaker D L, Saclarides T J, Storen E D 1994 Peritoneovenous shunts for palliation of the patient with malignant ascites. *Annals of Surgical Oncology* 1: 378–381

Shapiro S, Boaz J, Kleiman M, Kalsbeck J, Mealey J 1988 Origin of organisms infecting ventricular shunts. Neurosurgery 22: 868–872

Shurtleff D B, Foltz E L, Christie D 1971 Ventriculo-auriculostomy-associated infection: a 12-year study. *Journal of Neurosurgery* 35: 686–694

Smajda C, Franco D 1985 The LeVeen shunt in the elective treatment of intractable ascites in cirrhosis. A prospective study on 140 patients. *Annals of Surgery* 210: 488–493

Smith S R, Cheesbrough J, Spearing R, Davies J M 1989 Randomised prospective study comparing vancomycin with teicoplanin in the treatment of infections associated with Hickman catheters. *Antimicrobial Agents and Chemotherapy* 33: 1193–1197

Stauffer U G 1970 Shunt nephritis: diffuse glomerulonephritis complicating ventriculoatrial shunts. *Developmental Medicine and Child Neurology* (suppl 22): 161–164

Stern S, Bayston R, Hayward R J 1988 Haemophilus influenzae meningitis in the presence of cerebrospinal fluid shunts. *Child's Nervous System* 4: 164–165

Terpenning M A, Buggy B P, Kauffman C A 1988 Hospital-acquired infective endocarditis. *Archives of Internal Medicine* 148: 1601–1603

Tripodi M-F, Attanasio V, Adinolfi L E et al 1994 Prevalence of antibiotic resistance among clinical isolates of methicillin-resistant staphylococci. *European Journal of Clinical Microbiology and Infectious Diseases* 13: 148–152

Tofte-Jensen P, Nielsen PK, Llem S, Hemmingsen C 1994 Peritonitis incidence on a disconnect CAPD system with or without the use of iodine clamp shields. *Advances in Peritoneal Dialysis* 10: 150–153

Tully J L, Friedland G H, Baldini L M, Goldmann D A 1981 Complications of intravenous therapy with steel needles and Teflon catheters. A comparative study. *American Journal of Medicine* 70: 702–706

van Dalen R, Vree T B, Baars A M, Termond E 1986 Dosage adjustment for ceftazidime in patients with impaired renal function. *European Journal of Clinical Pharmacology* 30: 597–605

Vas S I 1983 Microbiological aspects of chronic ambulatory peritoneal dialysis. *Kidney International* 23: 83–92

Vas S I 1994 Infections associated with the peritoneum and hemodialysis. In: Bisno A, Waldvogel F A (eds) Infections associated with indwelling medical devices, 2nd edn. ASM Press, Washington, DC, p 309–346

Vas S I, Low D E, Oreopoulos D G 1981 Antibiotic prophylaxis in CAPD patients. In: Atkins R C, Thompson N M, Farrell P C (eds) Peritoneal dialysis. Churchill Livingstone, Edinburgh, p 320–326

Vedel G, Leruez M, Lemann F, Hraoui E, Ratovohery D 1990 Prevalence of *Staphylococcus aureus* and coagulase-negative staphylococci with decreased sensitivity to glycopeptides as assessed by determination of MICs. *European Journal of Clinical Microbiology and Infectious Diseases* 9: 820–822

Verghese A, Widrich W C, Arbeit R D 1985 Central venous septic thrombophlebitis – the role of medical therapy. *Medicine* 64: 394–400

Visconti E B, Peters G 1979 Vancomycin treatment of cerebrospinal fluid shunt infections. Report of two cases. *Journal of Neurosurgery* 51: 245–246

Weightman N C, Simpson E M, Speller D C, Mott M G, Oakhill A 1988 Bacteraemia related to indwelling central venous catheters: prevention, diagnosis and treatment.

European Journal of Clinical Microbiology and Infectious Diseases 7: 125–129

West T E, Walsh J J, Krol C P, Amsterdam D 1986 Staphylococcal peritonitis in patients on continuous ambulatory peritoneal dialysis. *Journal of Clinical Microbiology* 23: 809–812

Williams D N, Gibson J, Vos J, Kind A C 1982 Infusion thrombophlebitis and infiltration associated with intravenous cannulae: a controlled study comparing three different cannula types. *National Intravenous Therapy Association* 5: 379–382

Worning I M, Frimodt-Møller N, Ostri P, Nilsson T, Højholdt K, Frimodt-Møller C 1986 Antibiotic prophylaxis in vascular reconstructive surgery: a double-blind placebo-controlled study. *Journal of Antimicrobial Chemotherapy* 17: 105–113

Young E J, Ratner R E, Clarridge J E 1981 Staphylococcal ventriculitis treated with vancomycin. *Southern Medical Journal* 74: 1014–1015

46

HIV and AIDS

T. Peto

Introduction

The acquired immunodeficiency syndrome (AIDS) was first described in New York and California in 1981. By 1983, the aetiological agent was identified as a retrovirus which has since been named as human immunodeficiency virus (HIV). Two strains, HIV-1 and HIV-2, have since been isolated: HIV-1 is the predominant strain world-wide, while HIV-2 is largely found in West Africa. The virus invades cells which express the CD4+ antigens: these comprise CD4+ lymphocytes, some macrophages and neuroglial cells. The pathophysiology of AIDS can be elegantly explained by the properties of the HIV virus. After the initial infection, some patients have a seroconversion syndrome consisting of fever, lymphadenopathy and rash, possibly associated with neurological symptoms. This usually resolves after about 3 weeks. Thereafter there is a long asymptomatic phase of the infection. Patients remain well but examination of the blood shows a slow deterioration of their circulating CD4 cells. As the disease progresses and the CD4 count falls, the patient becomes more susceptible to infections. The most common infections and tumours and their relationship to CD4 counts are shown in Box 46.1. Apart from intercurrent infections, patients with progressive disease can develop the symptoms of 'ARC' (AIDS-related complex), which commonly consist of fevers, sweats, malaise, weight loss and unexplained diarrhoea. These symptoms are often accompanied by oral candida. With late advanced HIV disease, patients develop extreme weight loss and malaise. They may also develop HIV-associated neurological complications such as dementia or spinal cord dysfunction.

GENERAL APPROACH TO THE TREATMENT OF HIV PATIENTS

A large part of the challenge of the treatment of HIV infection

lies away from the technical problems in using antiviral therapy or treating the medical complications of infection.

Box 46.1 *Staging of HIV disease: relationship to complications and CD4 count*

Seroconversion syndrome

Asymptomatic infection (CD4 count >500/µl)

Late asymptomatic disease (CD4 count 200–500/µl)
- Increased susceptibility to:
  - tuberculosis
  - pneumococcal infection
  - salmonellosis
  - shingles
  - antibiotic induced oral candidiasis
- Skin rashes
- Thrombocytopaenia
- Early Kaposi's sarcoma (originally considered an AIDS-defining diagnosis)

AIDS-related complex (CD4 count 100–300/µl)
- Recurrent oropharyngeal
- Unexplained fevers, diarrhoea and weight loss
- Oral hairy leukoplakia
- Multidermatomal shingles
- Recurrent salmonellosis

AIDS-defining illness (CD4 count <200/µl)
- *Pneumocystis carinii* pneumonia
- Toxoplasmosis
- Cryptococcal meningitis or other disseminated fungaemias
- Persistent diarrhoea caused by cryptosporidium or isospora
- Oesophageal candidiasis
- Mucocutaneous herpes simplex
- Progressive multifocal leukoencephalopathy
- Primary CNS lymphoma

Advanced AIDS (CD4 count <50 µl)
- Severe weight loss (HIV wasting syndrome)
- Cytomegalovirus retinitis
- Disseminated *Mycobacterium avium* complex
- Recurrent pneumocystosis in spite of chemoprophylaxis
- Visceral Kaposi's sarcoma
- HIV dementia or spinal cord myelopathy

Patients need to be allowed to come to terms with the diagnosis, to decide how and when to inform sexual partners at risk from infection and family and friends. The slow progress of the disease, even after an episode of an AIDS-defining illness, means that patients need to be supported for many years. This chapter describes the current methods of modifying the progress of the disease with antiviral chemotherapy, the treatment of specific opportunistic infections and their prevention by chemoprophylaxis. Although the treatment and prevention of specific opportunistic infection is very effective, the reader should realize that current specific anti-HIV antiviral drugs have only a limited impact on the overall progression of the disease, and therefore their use should only be considered to be relatively indicated. Some patients may choose to avoid the nuisance and potential toxicity of current anti-HIV drugs, while others prefer the hope that these drugs bring with them.

Apart from the direct effect of the virus, the gradual increase in immunosuppression leads the patient increasingly vulnerable to opportunistic infections and secondary tumours. These complications of HIV infection therefore need to be treated on their merits.

ANTIVIRAL THERAPY AS PROPHYLAXIS AGAINST HIV INFECTION

The use of antiviral therapy after accidental parenteral exposure of HIV-infected blood is controversial. There is no good evidence that postexposure zidovudine alters the chances of seroconversion, although a recent case-control suggests it does have some protective effect (*Mortality & Morbidity Weekly Report* 1995). Anecdotal case reports describe HIV seroconversion after needlestick injuries in spite of prompt postexposure treatment with zidovudine. The increase in the prevalence of resistance to a number of different drugs makes the use of postexposure prophylaxis even less attractive. There is insufficient data on the use of other agents alone or in combination to provide any clear guidance (Tokars et al 1993). It is reasonable, therefore, not to offer routine treatment after accidental exposure. However, because zidovudine is relatively non-toxic in healthy people, the use of postexposure zidovudine (250 mg twice daily for 4 weeks) may be used on an individual basis.

In contrast to accidental exposure to HIV, zidovudine can reduce the chance of materno-fetal transmission (Connor et al 1994). In a randomized controlled study of over 300 pregnant women with no prior experience of anti-HIV treatment, zidovudine given for 6 weeks before delivery, intravenously during delivery with caesarean section and 6 weeks postnatally showed that the zidovudine-treated group had only 13 HIV-infected infants compared to 40 in the untreated control group. Studies are now being planned to determine whether a simpler schedule would be as

effective. It is still unclear whether the rate of materno-fetal transmission is affected by the mode of delivery and trials comparing caesarian section with vaginal delivery are being conducted.

SEROCONVERSION SYNDROME

About one-half of patients accurately infected with HIV report an infectious mononucleosis-like syndrome. The illness lasts about 3 weeks and is usually self-limiting. Patients should be treated conservatively as there is no evidence, as yet, to demonstrate that specific anti-HIV treatment affects the long-term natural history of the disease. In some cases, acute seroconversion can be associated with neurological symptoms, which anecdotal reports suggest can be treated symptomatically with high dose zidovudine (1500 mg/day). On rare occasions, patients become transiently and profoundly immunodeficient, resulting in secondary infections with opportunistic infections that require treatment on their merits. However, once patients recover, all treatment can be stopped.

Clinical treatment of established HIV infection

The optimum use of the present anti-HIV antiviral drugs is unclear and there is a wide range of clinical practice reflecting these uncertainties. Fashions in treatment are likely to change over the next few years as new drugs and combinations are advocated and then tested in clinical trials. Treatment decisions, at present, focus on the issues of when to start treatment, what initial regimen should be given, and when treatment should be changed. Finally, as the disease progresses in spite of antiviral therapy, the possibility of reducing the toxicity of treatment by stopping antiviral treatment should be considered.

ANTIVIRAL TREATMENT

A number of different nucleoside analogues have been tested in clinical trials and a number have been licensed for use. There is much controversy as to how the clinical efficacy of these drugs should be assessed. Clearly, the randomized clinical trials using mortality as an end-point provide the 'gold-standard' for assessing new regimens. Unfortunately, such studies often need to include large numbers of patients or need to continue for many years before reliable results are obtained. In order to obtain quicker answers, many trials use early clinical evidence of disease progression or simply measure peripheral CD4+ lymphocytes as an index of HIV disease progression. Recently, advances in the quantitative measurements of circulating viraemia have allowed changes in viral load to be used as a measure of antiviral activity. Although these new assays for drug activity are superficially attractive and may well be a valid measure of biological activity, they should not be used as a reliable index of therapeutic efficacy. Furthermore, recent advances in the detection of viral resistance patterns in viral strains isolated have allowed the possibility that drug treatments can be changed in response to changes in viral resistance. The few large-scale mortality studies so far completed have shown that a simple interpretation of changes in lymphocyte counts, viral load or viral resistance, or short-term changes in the rate of disease progression, do not extrapolate to changes in overall survival. Therefore, there is little reliable data on the role of anti-HIV drugs in the treatment of HIV disease.

Zidovudine

Zidovudine (AZT; 3'-azido-3'-deoxythymidine) was first reported in 1985 to be active in vitro against HIV. Intracellularly, the drug is phosphorylated to form the triphosphate which is the active metabolite. It inhibits the reverse transcriptase of HIV. Within 6 months it was first administered in man, and by 1986 the results of the first placebo-controlled clinical trial were reported (Fischl et al 1987). Zidovudine was given to patients with symptomatic HIV disease (AIDS related complex (ARC) or AIDS) for 4 months. Zidovudine reduced the mortality and the progression of HIV disease: out of 146 patients in each group only 1 died in the treatment group compared to 19 in the placebo group. Zidovudine has also been shown in a number of other studies to slow the progression of HIV disease over 12 months. The effect of zidovudine in asymptomatic HIV-infected patients (with CD4 counts $< 500/\mu l$) was compared to placebo (Volberding et al 1990). After about 12 months' treatment, zidovudine slowed the rate of progression to symptomatic disease (ARC or AIDS) compared to placebo. In addition, anecdotal reports and small studies suggest that zidovudine, in the short term, can increase the patient's weight and their feeling of well-being. Zidovudine is also reported to reverse HIV-associated thrombocytopenia, neurological complications of HIV infection and HIV-related dementia (Gray et al 1994).

Unfortunately, the effect of the drug appears to be limited. Observational studies have shown that, in spite of zidovudine, the mortality of patients with AIDS is still very high. The Anglo-French study, 'Concorde' compared the effects of a policy of 'immediate zidovudine', where asymptomatic patients were given zidovudine immediately after randomization, with 'deferred zidovudine', where patients were given placebo and only given zidovudine when they showed signs of clinical progression (Concorde 1994). In

the deferred arm, of those who took zidovudine, about 80% did so either when they developed ARC or AIDS or when their CD4 counts dropped below $250/\mu l$. Patients were followed for up to 4 years. Apart from a small difference in the rate of progression to ARC in the first year of treatment, there was no difference during the 4 years of the trial between the groups in terms of rates of progression to ARC, to AIDS or to death. Patients in the Concorde trial and in other small long-term trials are being followed to determine whether there are any small differences in overall survival in the longer term.

In conclusion, although zidovudine provides some clinical benefit over about a year, the sustained use of zidovudine as monotherapy does not seem to provide any greater benefit. It is likely that the failure of long-term zidovudine is due to the development of drug resistance. HIV strains isolated from patients taking zidovudine for more than 6 months develop reverse transcriptase mutations conferring zidovudine resistance (Erice & Balfour 1994). These strains are transmissible with increasing reports of zidovudine resistant strains being isolated from individuals who have never taken zidovudine (Erice et al 1993).

Zidovudine has important side-effects, but fortunately nearly all of them are reversible. Nausea, myalgia, insomnia and headaches are common reversible reasons for zidovudine intolerance. Anecdotal reports suggest that nausea can be reduced by initiating zidovudine therapy at low doses and increasing the dose gradually over 1–2 weeks. Haematological changes are the most common laboratory abnormalities. After only a few weeks a macrocytosis usually develops but is harmless. The most important adverse event is anaemia which develops in about a third of patients with AIDS. The anaemia is dose dependent and reversible if the drug is stopped. Smaller numbers of patients develop serious neutropenia, which again is reversible and dose dependent. The incidence of side-effects increases with disease progression. The Concorde study showed that fewer than 5% stopped zidovudine because of haematological toxicity, compared to 0.2% of controls. The incidence of life-threatening or irreversible adverse events is very small and not easily attributable to zidovudine. Patients started on zidovudine should have routine full blood counts measured monthly for the first 6 months of treatment.

The optimum dose of zidovudine is still controversial. The early studies used high dosage regimens (250 mg 4-hourly) which were based on a theoretical extrapolation from the blood levels of zidovudine. No attempt was made to consider the intracellular pharmacokinetics of the drug. Because of the toxicity of this dosage and the difficulties of patients following a 4-hourly regimen, later studies compared the efficacy of lower drug doses. Randomized studies, with short-term clinical outcomes suggest that there is a U-shaped dose–response curve with 500–600 mg/day being superior to 1200 or 1500 mg/day (Fischl et al 1990). However, the pharmacological basis for this relationship remains unclear. Subsequent studies using CD4 responses as a basis for comparing different dosing schedules has shown that giving zidovudine 8-hourly or even 12-hourly is reasonable. In view of the limited effect of zidovudine on overall survival it might seem prudent to give a lower dose of zidovudine (e.g. 200 mg three times daily or 250 mg twice daily) to most patients in order to avoid dose-dependent toxicity. Higher doses (1500 mg/day) are often preferred for the treatment of HIV encephalopathy or myelopathy (Portegies et al 1993).

Didanosine

Dideoxyinosine (ddI) is subject to acid-mediated hydrolysis and must therefore be administered with a buffer in the form of a sachet or chewable tablet. Because of the long intracellular half-life of the active metabolite (ddI triphosphate), the drug does not need to be given more frequently than twice daily. Didanosine decreases viral antigenaemia and increases circulating CD4 counts (Drusano et al 1992). However, the clinical significance of these changes is unclear. Unfortunately no large-scale placebo-controlled trials of monotherapy have yet been completed, although the drug has been widely used in patients who are intolerant to zidovudine. The MRC/ANRS European–Australian 'Alpha trial' of didanosine in 1700 symptomatic patients intolerant of zidovudine compared the effect of high-dose (750 mg twice daily) with low-dose (200 mg twice daily) didanosine (Alpha International Co-ordinating Committee, 1996). Although the trial was very powerful, there was no difference between the two doses in the rate of development of AIDS, HIV encephalopathy or mortality. In spite of the lack of clinical effect (two-thirds of patients died), high-dose didanosine increased CD4 counts relative to the low dose. Smaller trials have compared the clinical effect of didanosine with zidovudine (Kahn et al 1992, Dolin et al 1995). In subgroups of patients, particularly those who have taken zidovudine for some time, it appears that didanosine is superior to zidovudine. However, the relevance of zidovudine resistance in explaining the differential effect is unclear. As with zidovudine, patients on didanosine monotherapy develop viral strains which are drug resistant. More information from clinical trials is required to determine the role of didanosine monotherapy in treatment.

In contrast to efficacy, the toxicity of didanosine is well characterized. Pancreatitis is the most important adverse event. It is dose dependent: about 1% of patients on 750 mg twice daily suffer fatal pancreatitis, while pancreatitis is much less frequent at lower doses. In order to detect pancreatitis early, it is prudent to monitor serum amylase regularly. However, it is unclear how effective monitoring is in avoiding attacks of severe pancreatitis. Diarrhoea is the most common cause of patient intolerance to didanosine, but fortunately reverses on stopping treatment. The rate of peripheral neuropathy may have been overestimated in early studies and with careful clinical monitoring can be usually avoided.

Zalcitabine

Dideoxycytidine (ddC) is well absorbed. As with zidovudine and didanosine it decreases circulating viral antigen and increases CD4 counts. Its main dose-limiting toxicity is peripheral neuropathy. If the drug is not stopped promptly, the neuropathy may not be reversible and may even worsen before it declines. There have been no placebo-controlled studies of zalcitabine; comparisons of zalcitabine monotherapy with zidovudine, in zidovudine-experienced patients and with didanosine in zidovudine-intolerant patients, have not shown any great difference in clinical outcome (Fischl et al 1993, Abrams et al 1994). It is likely that its main hope for use is in combination with other nucleoside analogues.

Stavudine

Stavudine (4TC), a fourth nucleoside analogue, has been licensed in the USA. It has been assessed on the basis of its effect on CD4 counts and viral load (Murray et al 1995). Preliminary results of a clinical trial of patients with prolonged zidovudine therapy compared continuing zidovudine with switching to stavudine suggests that patients who switched had fewer episodes of clinical progression to AIDS. The main toxicity reported was peripheral neuropathy, which occurred in about 8% of patients treated with stavudine.

Combination therapy

The development of drug resistance together with the clinical failure of monotherapy has prompted great interest in combination treatments in the hope that they will prevent the development of resistance. Recently a number of clinical trials comparing zidovudine monotherapy with zidovudine + zalcitabine and zidovudine + didanosine in several thousand patients have been completed (Delta Co-ordinating Committee 1996, and the US trials ACTG 175 and the CPCRA trials). Patients were either asymptomatic with circulating CD4 counts below 350/μl or had symptomatic disease or AIDS with a CD4 count above 50/μl. The Delta trial has shown a 38% reduction in mortality over 2–3 years with combination treatment in patients who had not taken antiretroviral drugs previously. Similar reductions were seen in the progression to AIDS or new AIDS defining events. Combination treatment was equally effective in patients at all stages of disease progression tested. Overall there was some suggestion that the didanosine/zidovudine combination was superior to the zidovudine/zalcitabine combination. It appears that these combinations are less effective in patients who have previously taken AZT for several months.

The toxicity of these combinations were low. There was no evidence of enhancement of toxicity by combining the drugs.

Experimental drugs

Although experimental drugs are screened for their effect on circulating viral load, on circulating CD4 counts and on the development of viral resistance, the clinical relevance of these changes remains unclear. The results of longer term trials measuring clinical end-points are needed before the place of these new drugs can be determined.

Lamivudine (3TC) ((–)2'-deoxy-3'-thiacytidine) is another nucleoside analogue. It appears to be relatively non-toxic and its use in combination with zidovudine has led to an apparently larger increase in CD4 counts than with zidovudine therapy alone (Eron et al 1995). Non-nucleoside reverse transcriptase inhibitors (e.g. nevaripine and loviride (2-acetyl-4-methylphenyl)amino-2,6-dichlorobenzeneacetamide)) are also being tested in clinical trials.

Protease inhibitors, a different class of antiviral therapy, offer an exciting new hope. Small-scale trials suggest that they are intrinsically more active than the reverse transcriptase inhibitors, causing very large rises in circulating CD4 counts and profound falls in viral load (Danner et al 1995). Unfortunately, these changes appear to be only transient because of the rapid development of viral resistance. The development of combination therapies, which include protease inhibitors, is therefore awaited with great interest. Recently, three protease inhibitors, saquinavir, ritonavir and indinavir have been licensed.

There have been some trials which suggest that acyclovir may be effective in reducing the rate of progression of HIV disease. The interpretation of these trials remains controversial, mainly because the trials were only designed to reduce the impact of disease from herpes viruses and not to demonstrate a direct effect on HIV disease. It is therefore highly possible that these results are not repeatable.

The efficacy of other classes of drugs, such as CD4 receptor blocking agents, immunomodulators and immunostimulating agents, have so far proved disappointing.

When to start treatment

There is much controversy about the optimum time for starting treatment. It is unclear whether progressive HIV disease is associated with irreversible damage to the immune system or whether the immunodepression is potentially reversible with really effective treatment. The results of the Concorde trial clearly show that early treatment with zidovudine monotherapy provides no additional benefit to deferring treatment until patients develop symptomatic disease (Concorde 1994). The relevance of the Concorde result to the optimum timing of the initiation of combination treatment is unclear.

Advocates for early treatment argue that the best hope for asymptomatic patients may be for them to gamble that new treatments, as yet untested, will become available as salvage treatment before their disease progresses on existing therapy. Patients adopting such a policy may be disadvantaged in that they may suffer unnecessary toxicity or they may develop resistant viral strains to drugs which would otherwise be more effective as part of newer and better combination treatments.

Which treatment?

Until recently, zidovudine was the only drug shown to prolong life in HIV disease and zidovudine monotherapy was therefore the mainstay of anti-HIV treatment. Recent reports that combination treatment of zidovudine with didanosine or zalcitabine show improved survival is likely to change clinical practice radically. A reasonable policy is to start patients with a combination of zidovudine (250 mg twice daily) and didanosine (200 mg three times daily) and to switch from didanosine to zalcitabine (75 mg three times daily) if they are intolerant to didanosine. The role of nucleoside analogues in the initiation of treatment must await the results of clinical trials. The best method for treating patients who are zidovudine intolerant or whose HIV disease is clearly progressing in spite of treatment is unclear. Some enthusiastic clinicians will switch to stavudine and/or lamivudine, while others may wish to wait for further evidence that the efficacy of treatment justifies the drug toxicity. Indeed, on present evidence it is still possible that the best policy is to discontinue all anti-HIV therapy after failure of the initial drug combination. There is urgent need to study these questions with further randomized controlled trials.

The use of other drugs (as yet unlicensed) or drug combinations should await the result of controlled clinical trials. The use of unproven treatment simply for the sake of 'doing something' should be avoided if possible.

In the future, as virological monitoring of the infection becomes better established, it may be possible to individualize antiviral treatment to the patient's own changes in viral load and to their own resistance patterns.

Treatment of opportunistic infections

Apart from the use of specific anti-HIV therapy, the main aim of treatment is the treatment of its complications – namely, the opportunistic infections and tumours (Gallant et al 1994). Most of the infections are due to reactivation of latent organisms in the host or, in some cases, to

Table 46.1 *Treatment of HIV-associated infections*

Infection	First-line treatment/maintenance
Viral	
Herpes simplex	Acyclovir
Varicella-zoster	Acyclovir
CMV	Ganciclovir
EBV	No treatment
Progressive multifocal leukoencephalopathy	No treatment
Fungal	
Pneumocystis carinii	Co-trimoxazole
Candida spp.	Fluconazole
Histoplasmosis	Amphotericin B/itraconazole
Coccidioidomycosis	Amphotericin B/fluconazole
Penicillium marneffei	Fluconazole
Protozoa	
Toxoplasmosis	Pyrimethamine/sulfadiazine
Cryptosporidium	No treatment
Isospora belli	Co-trimoxazole
Microsporidium	No proven treatment
Leishmania	Stibogluconate
Mycobacterium avium/Mycobacterium intracellulare complex	Rifabutin/ethambutol/clarithromycin

environmental organisms to which the patient is exposed. In general, the treatment (see Table 46.1) of these infections suppresses rather than eradicates the organisms, so relapse is common when treatment is stopped. The side-effects and interactions between many of the drugs used complicate the long-term treatment that is needed.

VIRAL INFECTIONS

Herpes simplex and varicella zoster virus

Severe mucocutaneous and systemic infections with herpes simplex virus are best treated with acyclovir (200 mg five times daily for 5–7 days). Prophylaxis with acyclovir (200–400 mg three times daily) is used after severe infection and in patients with chronic HIV infection and increasing severity and frequency of recurrences. These recurrences can be a prelude to the chronic persistent mucocutaneous ulceration which may require long-term treatment with 'prophylactic' doses of acyclovir. It is in this setting that acyclovir resistance can develop.

Varicella-zoster virus infections are usually treated for about 5–7 days with oral acyclovir (800 mg five times daily) or, alternatively, the newer better-absorbed agents (valacyclovir or famciclovir) can be used. In severe cases, intravenous acyclovir (100 mg/kg three times daily) may be required. Treatment should be continued beyond 1 week if fresh lesions develop after the initial treatment has finished.

Acyclovir-resistant herpes simplex and varicella-zoster viral infections are emerging as clinically important

problems. Both resistant infections have been successfully treated with foscarnet. Topical trifluorothymidine is also effective in resistant herpes infection.

Cytomegalovirus

Reactivation of cytomegalovirus (CMV) infection tends to occur when CD4 cell counts are persistently below 50/μl. Ganciclovir (an acyclic analogue of deoxyguanosine) and foscarnet (phosphonoformate, a pyrophosphate analogue which inhibits polymerase enzymes) are both used for the treatment of CMV retinopathy and gastro-intestinal disease. Both drugs arrest progression of retinitis in most patients but maintenance treatment is required to delay the time to further relapse. The role of treatment in gastro-intestinal disease is less clear, although trials have shown that anti-CMV treatment have shown a reduction in symptomatic dysphagia, abdominal pain, and diarrhoea in patients with biopsy-proven CMV disease. However, a slow response is common. The role of CMV treatment in pulmonary and central nervous system (CNS) disease without evidence of retinal or gastro-intestinal infection is unclear.

Patients presenting with visual symptoms with typical signs of CMV infection on fundoscopy should be immediately treated with intravenous ganciclovir (5 mg/kg 12-hourly) or foscarnet (60 mg/kg every 8 h) for 14–21 days, depending on the response to treatment. Lesions will recur if there is no further treatment, so many clinicians favour the routine use of maintenance treatment with ganciclovir (5 mg/kg daily for 5 days per week) or foscarnet (90–120 mg/kg daily). Insertion of a permanent indwelling central venous line can allow patients to treat themselves at home. Ganciclovir is usually recommended for first-line treatment because of its better toxicity profile, ease of administration and greater experience. However, although a single study comparing ganciclovir with foscarnet for initial treatment and long-term maintenance in CMV retinitis found no difference between the drugs in their ability to prevent progression of disease, there was an apparent and unexpected survival advantage in those patients treated with foscarnet (Murray et al 1995). The reasons for this are unclear, and the findings need repeating before it should influence clinical practice. Ganciclovir is active against herpes simplex virus so patients with frequently recurring herpes simplex infections do not require concurrent acyclovir treatment. Recently, oral ganciclovir has been used for maintenance therapy, in spite of its relatively poor bioavailability. This route should only be considered when long-term intravenous therapy is not practical.

The major side-effect of ganciclovir treatment is neutropenia, which precludes the concomitant administration of zidovudine in the treatment period, but a small proportion of patients will tolerate low doses during maintenance treatment. Granulocyte colony stimulating factor (GCSF) can be used to counteract the severe neutropenia associated with ganciclovir induction therapy. Intravitreal ganciclovir 200 µg twice weekly for 3 weeks followed by 200 µg weekly has also been used, but there may be an increased risk of retinal detachment and this localized delivery of the drug would not be expected to have activity against CMV infection elsewhere, including disease in the other eye. Foscarnet is not as well tolerated as ganciclovir and it produces reversible renal failure and electrolyte disturbances if not given with vigorous saline hydration before drug infusion. Careful and frequent monitoring is required, which complicates outpatient management. Other side-effects include penile ulceration.

In spite of vigorous treatment, CMV disease can still progress, presumably due to the development of viral resistance. Severe visual disability, however, is uncommon as most patients die of their HIV disease before they become blind.

Epstein–Barr virus

Epstein–Barr virus (EBV) rarely causes overt disease in HIV patients. However, it is implicated in the causation of oral hairy leukoplakia and some lymphomas, particularly those derived from B cells. As yet there is no indication to attempt to EBV infections directly. The treatment of lymphomas is disappointing. Conventional chemotherapy is sometimes useful, especially in patients with less advanced HIV disease.

Kaposi sarcoma virus

Recent evidence suggests that Kaposi's sarcoma is caused by an EBV-like herpes virus. At present the virus has not been fully isolated or cultured in vitro, and therefore the susceptibility of the virus to existing antiviral drugs is unknown. It is therefore unclear whether effective antiviral agents will be clinically superior to the present policy of treating Kaposi's sarcoma with radiotherapy and chemotherapy.

BACTERIAL INFECTIONS

Pneumonia

Bacterial pneumonia is more frequent in HIV-positive persons than in seronegative controls. The risk is highest amongst those with CD4 lymphocyte counts below 200 per cubic millimetre and also among those who are injecting drug users (Hirschtick et al 1995). Infections are frequently caused by encapsulated organisms such as *Str. pneumoniae* and *Haem. influenzae*. Bacteraemic infection is also more common. Other pathogens that have been encountered include *Staphylococcus aureus* and *Klebsiella pneumoniae*. This stresses the importance of prompt investigation to establish the microbial nature of the infection whilst also excluding other infections common to this population, in particular *Pneumocystis carinii* and *Mycobacterium tuberculosis*. The latter may occur early or later in the course of HIV infection; atypical presentations are more likely with advanced disease (see Ch. 59).

The management of pneumonia in this population follows the same principles as in the non-HIV population. Prevention should also be considered. Pneumococcal and *H. influenzae* vaccine is used in many centres in the hope of reducing the risks of infection. However, the immunogenicity of these vaccines is often impaired in the HIV infected and in turn their protective efficacy. However, if administered early in the course of HIV infection more favourable response can be anticipated.

Mycobacterium avium/Mycobacterium intracellulare complex (MAC)

Patients with disseminated *Mycobacterium avium/Mycobacterium intracellulare* (MAC) infection (Benson & Ellner 1993) commonly present with unexplained fever sometimes accompanied by gastro-intestinal symptoms or weight loss. Diagnosis is often made empirically by exclusion of other causes, particularly lymphoma, of fever in patients with low (<100/µl) CD4 cells. Evidence of colonization with MAC is commonly found by stool culture, but definitive evidence of systemic infection depends on isolation of MAC from blood cultures or tissue biopsy. Symptoms are often relieved with specific treatment. Most isolates of MAC are resistant to the first- and second-line antituberculous drugs. If single-drug therapy is used resistance occurs quickly. In a placebo-controlled study clarithromycin had clear activity alone in vivo but resistance occurred within weeks. Various combinations of drugs have been shown to decrease mycobacteraemia and improve symptoms in uncontrolled studies but the infection is not eliminated. There is little evidence that the treatment of MAC significantly prolongs survival in AIDS. Four, three and even two drug regimens are being assessed in clinical trials. Effective drugs include clarithromycin (1 g twice daily) ciprofloxacin (500–750 mg twice daily), rifamycin derivatives (rifampicin (10 mg/kg daily, maximum dose 600 mg/day) or rifabutin (450–600 mg/day), and ethambutol (15 mg/kg to a maximum 1 μg/day). Other drugs which are used include clofazimine (100–200 mg/day) and amikacin (7.5–15 mg/kg daily) which has to be given intravenously. Treatment is usually continued for life. Another macrolide azithromycin, a quinolone (sparfloxacin) and liposomal amikacin are also being assessed.

It is our practice to start empirical treatment in patients with proven MAC septicaemia or in patients with low CD4 counts with unexplained persistent fever. Initial treatment is with a triple combination of rifabutin, clarithromycin and ethambutol for several weeks. Regimens are changed if there is drug toxicity or if there is clear evidence of treatment failure. Intravenous amikacin, in combination with other drugs, is usually reserved for resistant symptomatic disease which is proved to be due to MAC. Although relapse is common if treatment is discontinued, remissions from symptomatic disease, rather than from bacteriological disease, can be prolonged. In some cases of resistant fever, in late HIV disease, symptomatic relief can best be achieved with the use of corticosteroids.

Rifabutin has been shown to be effective in the primary prophylaxis of MAC. A randomized placebo-controlled study of rifabutin 300 mg/day in over 500 patients with AIDS and CD4 cell counts < 200/μl has shown that there is a significantly longer time to the development of mycobacteraemia and possibly a longer period free of symptoms, but no survival advantage has yet been demonstrated (Nightingale et al 1993). The role of primary MAC prophylaxis in the management of HIV patients remains controversial.

FUNGAL DISEASES

Pneumocystis carinii pneumonia

Pneumocystis carinii pneumonia (PCP) usually presents with breathlessness and fever associated with cough in patients who are taking routine anti-PCP chemoprophylaxis. The onset is often insidious, so patients who have not been forewarned of the symptoms can often present late in the course of the disease severely hypoxic. The incidence of PCP as a first 'AIDS-defining illness' is much reduced by chemoprophylaxis, although the disease can break through standard prophylaxis in advanced HIV disease.

Treatment. The standard treatment for acute PCP infection is high dose co-trimoxazole (trimethoprim 15 mg/kg daily and sulphamethoxazole 75 mg/kg daily) divided into 3 or 4 doses/day for 3 weeks (Klein et al 1992). Although the intravenous route is preferred for severely ill patients, the drug is absorbed and the drug can be given orally if there is no gastro-intestinal disturbance. Patients should improve within 4–8 days, although they can first deteriorate over the first few days. Adjuvant therapy with corticosteroids (e.g. intravenous hydrocortisone or prednisolone 60 mg/day reducing over 7 days) has been shown to reduce the need for ventilation in patients with severe hypoxia ($Po_2 < 70$ mmHg) (Consensus Report 1990). Mortality in patients who require mechanical ventilation within 48 h of presentation is about 50%, whereas only about 5% of patients survive mechanical ventilation if intubated after 5 days of adequate therapy. Steroids should be used in patients with severe disease who require supplementary oxygen. After recovery, patients should be continued on maintenance therapy (secondary prophylaxis) with low-dose co-trimoxazole.

The standard treatment is often complicated by drug intolerance. Co-trimoxazole commonly causes nausea and vomiting which can be reduced by lowering the dose. About a third of patients develop a skin rash after about 7 days of therapy. The incidence of life-threatening Stevens–Johnson syndrome appears to be rare in patients with AIDS. Other common side-effects include neutropenia which is partly a dose dependent phenomenon. Although desensitization to co-trimoxazole has been advocated, it is usually more convenient to change to second-line agents. Intravenous pentamidine (16 mg/kg daily) or clindamycin plus primaquine are both satisfactory while trimethoprim–dapsone or atovaquone should be reserved for mild to moderate disease.

The role of salvage treatment for *Pneumocystis carinii* infection is unclear. There is little evidence that failure of therapy is due to resistance of the organism to the antibiotic; it is more likely that the failure is due to the development of acute respiratory distress syndrome. The use of trimetrexate as salvage treatment is therefore controversial.

Prophylaxis. There are good trials comparing the efficacy of different regimens for both secondary and primary prophylaxis. One double-strength co-trimoxazole daily (trimethoprim 160 mg plus sulphamethoxazole 800 mg) appears to be superior to aerosolized pentamidine (Hardy et al 1992). Other studies have shown that dapsone (50 mg/day) plus pyrimethamine (50 mg weekly) is equivalent to pentamidine (Girard et al 1993). Another study has shown dapsone 100 mg/day to be equivalent to co-trimoxazole but superior to aerosolized pentamidine (Bozzette et al 1995).

The main problem with prophylaxis is drug hypersensitivity. In about two-thirds of cases, dapsone is not tolerated in patients with hypersensitivity to sulphamethoxazole. Aerosolized pentamidine (300 mg monthly) is well tolerated. Nebulizers are available (e.g. Respigard II) which deliver varying amounts of drug with different particle sizes, so comparison between trials is difficult. The major adverse effect is bronchial irritation leading to cough and wheeze. This can be prevented by keeping particle size small and by using bronchodilators beforehand. Upper lobe recurrences, extrapulmonary *Pneumocystis carinii* infections and spontaneous pneumothorax have all been reported in patients receiving inhaled nebulized pentamidine. Alternative methods of prophylaxis include monthly intravenous pentamidine, which has been associated with hypotension and occasionally the development of hypoglycaemia.

Cryptococci

Cryptococcal meningitis can be treated with either fluconazole (400 mg/day) or amphotericin B (0.7–1.0 mg/day). Treatment needs to be continued for about 4–8 weeks. A large comparative study has shown that the overall mortality was similar in both treatment groups (Saag et al 1992). However, there were more early deaths in the fluconazole group, and amphotericin B sterilized the cerebrospinal fluid more rapidly. Fluconazole was better tolerated. There was a 20% mortality and the factors predictive of death were an abnormal mental state, a cryptococcal antigen titre above 1024 and a white cell count below $0.02 \times 10^9/l$ in the cerebrospinal fluid. For patients with severe disease, amphotericin B is probably the drug of choice, while in less severe disease fluconazole is probably more convenient. It is likely that itraconazole is as effective as fluconazole, but it has not been as widely studied. With a 20% mortality irrespective of what treatment is used, it is clear that improvements in therapy are required. The potential benefits of adding in flucytosine is unclear.

Maintenance treatment is required after initial treatment: about 50% relapse without treatment, possibly because cryptococci lie dormant in the prostate. Fluconazole (200 mg/day) was more effective than amphotericin B (1 mg/kg weekly) in a large randomized study. The comparative efficacy of higher doses of amphotericin B maintenance therapy is unknown. Liposomal preparations of amphotericin B are being assessed, as are higher doses of fluconazole, and combinations of antifungal drugs.

Candida infections

Candida spp. infection is a common and troublesome problem in HIV-infected patients. It often presents as oropharyngeal candidosis following antibiotic treatment or spontaneously causing recurrent problems. In women, vaginal candidosis is common. As the HIV disease progresses, the candida can spread to cause invasive disease and, in particular, oesophageal candidiasis which presents with dysphagia and retrosternal pain.

Oral candidosis is often asymptomatic and does not require treatment. Although treatment of symptomatic oral candidosis is possible with topical therapy (nystatin or amphotericin B), systemic use of imidazoles (ketoconazole, fluconazole or itraconazole) is more satisfactory. In patients with severe oropharyngeal candidosis or oesophageal candidosis, a systemic imidazole is preferred. There is more controversy as to whether treatment should be prolonged after the initial control of symptoms in an attempt to reduce the incidence of relapses. Longer term treatment has the advantage of reducing morbidity from early relapse, and for which the imidazoles are relatively free of side-effects. The disadvantage of prolonged treatment is the expense and the fear that it will promote the development of drug resistance.

With prolonged infection there is an increasing incidence of resistant infection. There is a slowing of the speed of clinical response to imidazoles and a need to increase the dose. Eventually complete resistance occurs. Sometimes patients will respond to adopting alternative imidazole drugs. However, eventually, resistance to imidazoles is so severe that intravenous amphotericin B is required. The role of flucytosine in resistant candidosis is unclear.

Histoplasmosis

In patients living in the southern states of the USA, the Caribbean and Latin America, histoplasmosis is a common complication of HIV. Patients present with non-specific systemic symptoms, commonly with mucocutaneous ulcers or papular lesions. Diagnosis is best made by microscopy and culture of bone marrow, biopsy specimens and blood cultures. Severe illness should be initially treated with amphotericin B. Milder disease can be treated with oral itraconazole (300 mg twice daily for 3 days followed by 200 mg/day). Long-term maintenance therapy with itraconazole (200 mg/day) is required to prevent relapse.

Penicillium marneffei

This is a common pathogen in HIV patients who have lived in South-East Asia. Patients present with systemic disease and skin nodules. Diagnosis can be made by microscopy and culture of biopsies taken from skin lesions or bone marrow. The fungus is very sensitive to fluconazole, but long-term maintenance therapy is required.

PROTOZOAL INFECTIONS

Toxoplasmosis

Toxoplasmosis commonly presents with a headache or focal neurological signs. Its prevalence is dependent on the geographical distribution of toxoplasmosis in the community. For instance it is more common in France than in the UK. Computed tomographic brain scans commonly show signs of ring-enhancing lesions, although magnetic resonance imaging is more sensitive. In some cases the scans remain negative for some weeks after presentation. The main differential diagnosis is CNS lymphoma and formal confirmation of toxoplasmosis requires a brain biopsy. In practice, brain biopsies are rarely performed. Most clinicians start empirical treatment for toxoplasmosis and rely on a therapeutic response to confirm the diagnosis. The condition responds well if treatment is started early, and a combination of sulphadiazine 4–6 g/day and pyrimethamine 50–100 mg/day (both by mouth in divided doses) for 3–6 weeks, together with folinic acid 15 mg/day, is the treatment of choice. Side-effects may prevent continued use of sulphadiazine in about a third of patients.

Clindamycin 600–1200 mg four times daily with pyrimethamine has been shown in controlled studies to be an effective alternative. Atovaquone 750 mg four times daily and the new macrolides clarithromycin 2 g/day and azithromycin, both given with pyrimethamine 75 mg/day, have also been used in small uncontrolled studies.

Corticosteroids are sometimes used in addition to first-line treatment to reduce symptomatic cerebral oedema, but their use has not been validated in controlled trials. One disadvantage of the adjunctive use of corticosteroids is that it interferes with the diagnostic value of a therapeutic trial which would otherwise distinguish cerebral toxoplasmosis from a lymphoma.

Relapse of cerebral toxoplasmosis is common after treatment is stopped, and maintenance treatment should continue indefinitely. The most appropriate regimen for maintenance treatment or secondary prophylaxis has not been determined, but treatment doses of either sulphadiazine and pyrimethamine or clindamycin and pyrimethamine are usually halved.

Primary prophylaxis of toxoplasmosis is often achieved as part of routine PCP prophylaxis. Controlled trials comparing prophylaxis with co-trimoxazole, dapsone plus pyrimethamine and nebulized pentamidine for *Pneum. carinii* pneumonia show that both co-trimoxazole and dapsone prevent toxoplasmosis compared with pentamidine. Pyrimethamine monotherapy appears to be ineffective.

Cryptosporidiosis

Cryptosporidiosis usually presents with diarrhoea, although occasionally it can cause an ascending cholangitis. Diagnosis is made by direct microscopy of the stool or of endoscopic samples. Symptoms and excretion of cysts may be intermittent. There is still no known effective therapy for cryptosporidiosis in spite of testing a large number of anti-infective agents. Critical review has failed to support

evidence that spiramycin is effective. Responses have been described after treatment with a variety of agents including γ-hyperimmune bovine colostrum, paromomycin and azithromycin. The interpretation of open studies is difficult, as symptoms can resolve spontaneously. Symptomatic treatment with codeine phosphate, loperamide and other drugs together with fluid, electrolyte and nutritional support may be the only effective measures. Empirical treatment with possibly active agents is reasonable in severe intractable cases.

Other gastro-intestinal protozoa

Gastro-intestinal symptoms can occasionally be caused by *Giardia lamblia* and, more rarely, by *Isospora belli* or microsporidia. Giardiasis can be treated conventionally with metronidazole, while isospora is sensitive to trimethoprim–sulphamethoxazole (trimethoprim 160 mg; sulphamethoxazole 800 mg 6-hourly for 7–10 days). Chronic suppressive therapy is often required. Microsporidia is more difficult to treat; anecdotal reports suggest symptomatic improvement with albendazole (400 mg twice daily) or metronidazole 500 mg three times daily).

Leishmaniasis

This is a common infection in HIV infected patients who have lived in endemic parts of the Mediterranean area, North Africa and the Middle East. Patients present with fever and systemic symptoms. The diagnosis is usually made by examination of the bone marrow. Treatment is with intravenous pentostam. Recent evidence suggests that liposomal amphotericin B is very effective against visceral leishmaniasis in immunocompetent patients; there is no evidence of improved efficacy of liposomal amphotericin B in HIV-infected patients.

PROPHYLAXIS IN HIV DISEASE

Although it is often stated that it is better to prevent rather than treat symptoms, the evidence that primary prophylaxis against opportunistic infection prolongs life is lacking. However, it is reasonable to assume that prevention of PCP might reduce the incidence of life-threatening pneumonia. The alternative strategy of advising patients to present early with respiratory symptoms has not been formally tested. Nevertheless, there is ample evidence that the use of prophylactic antibiotics is successful in preventing various infections. The aim of reducing morbidity, and therefore increasing the quality of life, has thus become a main aim of HIV care (Kaplan & Holmes 1995).

Prophylaxis should therefore be aimed at preventing the most common life-threatening infections. These vary according to the patient's environment. In northern Europe and North America, the most common infections include PCP and toxoplasmosis. The use of systemic anti-PCP drugs which are also effective against toxoplasmosis (e.g. co-trimoxazole) is therefore very attractive. Prophylaxis should start when the CD4 count falls below 200/µl.

The routine use of systemic azole anti-fungals is not recommended for prevention of cryptococcal meningitis because of the possible development of resistance of *Candida* spp. to these drugs. However, it is noteworthy that patients taking intermittent systemic azole drugs for candidosis seem to present with less cryptococcal disease. The prevention and treatment of tuberculosis should follow the experience in HIV-negative patients. There is no evidence that primary prophylaxis is indicated against tuberculosis in patients at high risk of tuberculosis.

The role of primary prophylaxis against atypical mycobacterial infections with rifabutin or cytomegalovirus disease with oral ganciclovir is still unclear. Although there is some evidence that primary prophylaxis against these infections may delay the onset of early disease, there is no evidence that this delay will translate into effective prevention of severe disease. Indeed it is possible that the extensive use of these drugs for prophylaxis will induce the development of resistance which will make treatment of overt disease more difficult.

The efficacy of other methods of prophylaxis, although attractive, have not been proven. For example, the use of vaccination against pneumococcal disease awaits the results of controlled trials. Some authorities recommend that patients should avoid drinking water fresh from the tap in order to avoid infection with cryptosporidium.

References

Abrams D, Goldman A, Launer C et al 1994 A comparative trial of didanosine or zalcitabine after treatment with zidovudine in patients with human immunodeficiency virus infection. *New England Journal of Medicine* 330: 657–662

Alpha International Co-ordinating Committee 1996 The alpha trial: European/Australian randomized double-blind trial of two doses of didanosine in zidovudine-intolerant patients with symptomatic HIV disease. *AIDS* 10: 867–880

Benson C A, Ellner J J 1993 *Mycobacterium avium* complex infection and AIDS: advances in theory and practice. *Clinical Infectious Diseases* 17: 7–20

Bozzette S A, Finkelstein D M, Spector S A et al 1995 A randomized trial of three antipneumocystis agents in patients with advanced human immunodeficiency virus infection. NIAID AIDS Clinical Trials Group. *New England Journal of Medicine* 332: 693–699

Concorde 1994 Concorde: MRC/ANRS randomised double-blind controlled trial of immediate and deferred zidovudine in symptom-free HIV infection. Concorde Coordinating Committee. *Lancet* 343: 871–881

Connor E, Sperling R, Gelbe R R et al 1994 Reduction of maternal-infant transmission of human immunodeficiency virus type I with zidovudine treatment. *New England Journal of Medicine* 331: 1173–1180

Consensus Report 1990 Consensus statement on the use of corticosteroids as adjunctive therapy for pneumocystis pneumonia in the acquired immunodeficiency syndrome. *New England Journal of Medicine* 323: 1500–1504

Danner S, Carr A, Leonard J et al 1995 A short-term study of the safety, pharmacokinetics, and efficacy of ritonavir, an inhibitor of HIV-1 protease. *New England Journal of Medicine* 333: 1528–1533

Delta Co-ordinating Committee 1996 Delta: a randomized double-blind controlled trial comparing combinations of zidovudine plus didanosine or zalcitabine with zidovudine alone in individuals with HIV infection. *Lancet* (in press)

Dolin R, Amato D A, Fischl M A et al 1995 Zidovudine compared with didanosine in patients with advanced HIV type I infection and little or no previous experience with zidovudine. AIDS Clinical Trials Group. *Archives of Internal Medicine* 155: 961–974

Drusano G, Yuen G, Lambert J 1992 Relationship between dideoxyinosine exposure, CD4 counts and p24 antigen levels in human immunodeficiency infection. *Annals of Internal Medicine* 116: 562–566

Erice A, Balfour H 1994 Resistance of human immunodeficiency virus type I to antiretroviral agents: a review. *Clinical Infectious Diseases* 18: 149–156

Erice A, Mayers D L, Strike D G 1993 Primary infection with zidovudine resistant HIV-type I. *New England Journal of Medicine* 328: 110–115

Eron J, Benoit S, Jemsek J et al 1995 Treatment with lamivudine, zidovudine, or both in HIV-positive patients with 200 to 500 CD4+ cells per cubic millimeter. *New England Journal of Medicine* 333: 1662–1669

Fischl M A, Richman D D, Grieco M H et al 1987 The efficacy of azidothymidine (AZT) in the treatment of patients with AIDS and AIDS-related complex. A double-blind, placebo-controlled trial. *New England Journal of Medicine* 317: 185–191

Fischl M A, Parker C B, Pettinelli C et al 1990 A randomized controlled trial of a reduced daily dose of zidovudine in patients with the acquired immunodeficiency syndrome. The AIDS Clinical Trials Group. *New England Journal of Medicine* 323: 1009–1014

Fischl M A, Olson R M, Follansbee S E et al 1993 Zalcitabine compared with zidovudine in patients with advanced HIV-1 infection who received previous zidovudine therapy. *Annals of Internal Medicine* 118: 762–769

Gallant J E, Moore R D, Chaisson R E 1994 Prophylaxis for opportunistic infections in patients with HIV infection. *Annals of Internal Medicine* 120: 932–944

Girard P, Landman R, Gaudebout C et al 1993 Dapsone–pyrimethamine compared with aerosolized pentamidine as primary prophylaxis against *Pneumocystis carinii* pneumonia and toxoplasmosis in HIV infection. *New England Journal of Medicine* 328: 1514–1520

Gray F, Belec L, Keohane C et al 1994 Zidovudine therapy and HIV encephalitis: a 10-year neuropathological survey. *AIDS* 8: 489–493

Hardy W D, Feinberg J, Finkelstein D M et al 1992 A controlled trial of trimethoprim–sulfamethoxazole or aerosolized pentamidine for secondary prophylaxis of *Pneumocystis carinii* pneumonia in patients with the acquired immunodeficiency syndrome. *New England Journal of Medicine* 327: 1842–1848

Hirschtick R E, Glassroth J, Jordan M C et al 1995 Bacterial pneumonia in persons infected with the human immunodeficiency virus. *New England Journal of Medicine* 333: 845–851

Kahn J O, Lagakos S W, Richman D D et al 1992 A controlled trial comparing continued zidovudine with didanosine in human immunodeficiency virus infection. The NIAID AIDS Clinical Trials Group. *New England Journal of Medicine* 327: 581–587

Kaplan J H M, Holmes K 1995 Prevention of opportunistic infections in persons infected with human immuno-deficiency virus. *Clinical Infectious Diseases* 21: S1–S140

Klein N, Duncanson F, Lenox T et al 1992 Trimethoprim–sulphamethoxazole versus pentamidine for *Pneumocystis*

carinii pneumonia in AIDS patients: results of a large prospective randomized treatment trial. *AIDS* 6: 301–305

Mortality & Morbidity Weekly Report 1995 Case-control study of HIV seroconversion in health-care workers after percutaneous exposure to HIV-infected blood. France, United Kingdom and United States, Jan 1998 – August 1994 Mortality & Morbidity Weekly Report 44. 22nd December (No 50)

Murray H W, Squires K E, Weiss W et al 1995 Stavudine in patients with AIDS and AIDS-related complex: AIDS clinical trials group 089. *Journal of Infectious Diseases* 171: S123–S130

Nightingale S, Cameron D, Gordin F et al 1993 Two controlled trials of rifabutin prophylaxis against *Mycobacterium avium* complex infection in AIDS. *New England Journal of Medicine* 329: 828–833

Portegies P, Enting R, Gans J et al 1993 Presentation and course of AIDS dementia complex: 10 years of follow up in Amsterdam, The Netherlands. *AIDS* 7: 669–675

Saag M D, Powderly W G, Cloud G A et al 1992 Comparison of amphotericin B with fluconazole in the treatment of acute AIDS-associated cryptococcal meningitis. *New England Journal of Medicine* 326: 83–89

Tokars J I, Marcus R, Culver D H et al 1993 Surveillance of HIV infection and zidovudine use among health care workers after occupational exposure to HIV-infected blood. The CDC Cooperative Needlestick Surveillance Group. *Annals of Internal Medicine* 118: 913–919

Volberding P A, Lagakos S W, Koch M A et al 1990 Zidovudine in asymptomatic human immunodeficiency virus infection. A controlled trial in persons with fewer than 500 CD4-positive cells per cubic millimeter. The AIDS Clinical Trials Group of the National Institute of Allergy and Infectious Disease. *New England Journal of Medicine* 322: 941–949

Infections of the upper respiratory tract

R. G. Finch

Introduction

The vulnerability of the upper respiratory tract to infection needs no emphasis. Despite a complex array of defence mechanisms, which include particle filtration, humidification, mucous entrapment, ciliary clearance augmented by a rich supply of lymphoid tissue and local antibody production, it is subject to repeated attacks by a plethora of viruses and bacteria and, to a lesser extent, yeasts. Factors such as age, transmissibility, crowding, immunological naievity and immunosuppression, and in the case of the middle ear and paranasal sinuses, anatomical features and a permanently damaged mucosae, contribute to this state of affairs.

The importance of upper respiratory tract infections as a cause of morbidity, working days lost, school absenteeism, but rarely mortality, is reflected in the enormous annual tonnage of antibiotics used to treat these infections, much of it inappropriate. For, while there are agents to control bacterial and fungal infections of the upper respiratory tract, the majority of infections are viral and largely unamenable to therapeutic intervention.

Apart from their local effects, infections of the upper respiratory tract may predispose to lower respiratory tract disease. It is well known that viral respiratory infections are among the triggers for an acute asthmatic attack in the predisposed. More important is the association of an infective exacerbation of chronic bronchitis or bronchiectasis in those with chronic lung disease. In those with severe chronic obstructive pulmonary disease, cor pulmonale may result. Thus the burden of upper respiratory tract infection is responsible for much morbidity and, in turn, requires selective and judicious antibiotic usage.

With a few exceptions, clinical assessment of respiratory infection does not provide a firm aetiological diagnosis, and laboratory investigations, even when available, often fail to

establish the causal organism. For this reason, infections of the respiratory tract are categorized mainly according to their epidemiology and anatomical site, apart from some clearly recognized disease syndromes.

The common cold

Most colds are of viral origin (predominantly rhinoviruses and adenoviruses) and, although some effective specific methods of preventing and treating them are beginning to emerge and are discussed later, no specific treatment is available for most of these common illnesses. Antibiotics have no role in the treatment of uncomplicated colds. The presumed, but seldom established, role of secondary bacterial infection prompted the unacceptable widespread use of antibacterial chemotherapy in these conditions.

Antibiotics are especially widely used in respiratory infections in children who receive, on average, one course of antibiotics a year in the first 6 years of life. This reflects the difficulties in establishing a clinical and microbiological diagnosis of many upper respiratory tract infections in childhood, and the recognition that coryzal symptoms may precede a number of more serious bacterial infections. The general tendency for these infections to recover rapidly without specific treatment emphasizes the importance of a restrictive antibiotic policy, but much parenteral pressure and a natural fear of bacterial complications tend to lead to non-selective prescribing. The use of antibiotics for new episodes of respiratory illness varies greatly between practitioners. Attempts to define the role of antibiotics in respiratory infections of childhood include a study by Taylor et al (1977) who, comparing amoxycillin, co-trimoxazole and placebo in 197 children with presumed viral respiratory infections, concluded that the benefits of antimicrobial treatment were marginal, and that routine prescription for this type of illness was not indicated. The common belief that prescribing antibiotics saves the general practitioner from extra work has been disproved by Howie & Hutchison (1978). Furthermore, there is world-wide concern over the rapid increase in drug resistance in the community as well as in hospitals. Thus a more rational and restrictive approach to antibiotic prescribing is recommended, especially for respiratory infections which are the predominant reason for antibiotic prescribing. This policy applies to normal individuals. It is recognized that those with chronic illness of the respiratory tract, and especially those with chronic bronchitis are more at risk of secondary bacterial complications (p. 690).

SPECIFIC TREATMENT FOR COLDS

Several trials have shown that interferon, given intranasally for 4–5 days, has a protective effect against rhinovirus colds (Scott et al 1982, Hayden & Gwaltney 1983). These prophylactic effects have been achieved both by partially purified leucocyte interferon (IFN-γ), interferon purified by monoclonal antibody, and by recombinant-DNA-produced interferon. The subjects showed no protection against respiratory infections caused by other cold viruses (influenza, parainfluenza or coronaviruses) or *Mycoplasma pneumoniae*; nor did interferon affect the course of rhinovirus colds once symptoms had developed. Intranasal administration for a few days was harmless, but attempts at longer term prophylaxis for 2 weeks often led to local symptoms of nasal irritation, including crusting and blood-stained mucus discharge.

Another approach that has shown some benefit has been to treat family contacts prophylactically (Hayden et al 1985, Douglas et al 1986). However, at present more widespread use of interferon in relation to the common cold is unlikely. The logistics and cost of treatment would be prohibitive for a largely self-limiting condition.

Synthetic antivirals have also been used in volunteer studies of the common cold. Enviroxime, given either by mouth or intranasally, reduced symptoms but had no effect on virus shedding or antibody response. Other compounds, including dichloroflavan and an antiviral chalcone which acts as a pro-drug, have also been tried, but with disappointing results (Philpotts & Tyrrell 1985, Scott 1986, Sperber & Hayden 1988) (Ch. 40).

Acute sore throat

Most acute sore throats are caused by virus infections, but an important group is caused by *Streptococcus pyogenes* (group A β-haemolytic streptococci), which accounts for a quarter to one-third of acute sore throats seen in many studies in general practice. In some countries diphtheria remains important and has re-emerged in the former USSR as a result of failures in immunization policy. *Arcanobacterium* (*Corynebacterium*) *haemolyticum* is an established cause of acute sore throat and scarlatiniform rash in children and young adults (Editorial 1987). Other less common bacterial causes include *Neisseria gonorrhoeae*, *Neisseria meningitidis*, *Yersinia enterocolitica* and *Mycoplasma pneumoniae*. The role of groups C and G streptococci remains unclear, although they can be isolated from symptomatic patients. Vincent's angina is found especially, but not exclusively, in association with gingival sepsis. Clinical signs are often unreliable as a guide to aetiology. Haemolytic streptococci are more likely to be found in association with high fever, follicular tonsillitis, tender anterior cervical glands and neutrophilia in the peripheral blood, but may be grown profusely from patients with mild sore throat or, indeed, from symptomless carriers. Conversely, bad sore throat, even with pharyngeal exudate, may be viral in origin when it is caused by Epstein–Barr virus, herpes simplex virus and, occasionally, enteroviruses or adenoviruses. For these reasons antibiotic treatment of acute sore throat is most satisfactory if based on examination of a throat swab. The use of suitable transport medium and simple rapid diagnostic tests makes this practicable in the hospital, but still presents problems in community practice in many countries.

The conventional treatment for streptococcal sore throat is penicillin. This can be given orally as phenoxymethyl penicillin 250 mg four times daily. Because of erratic taking of medicine more satisfactory results may be achieved by initiating treatment with one injection of procaine penicillin or fortified procaine penicillin (containing 300 mg of procaine penicillin and 60 mg benzylpenicillin per unit volume), continuing treatment thereafter with phenoxymethyl penicillin by mouth. In order to ensure eradication of streptococci in a high proportion of patients, it is necessary to continue penicillin for 10 days (Peter 1992). This is uncommonly achieved in practice, since patients feel well again in a few days and do not complete the course.

For many years it has been held that, despite early evidence to the contrary, treatment makes little or no difference to the rate at which symptoms subside and that the aim of therapy is to eradicate β-haemolytic streptococci from the pharynx. Recent trials have shown that antibiotic therapy does have a role in alleviating the illness of streptococcal pharyngitis, while it is known that treatment within 1 week of the onset of symptoms will prevent the now rare complication of acute rheumatic fever. Krober et al (1985) showed significant differences in resolution of fever and other markers of clinical activity between patients given penicillin and those given placebo. In a larger trial involving 260 children, Randolph et al (1985) showed that significantly fewer children given phenoxymethyl penicillin or cephadroxil showed persistence of fever or a number of local signs at 18–24 h after treatment was started than those given placebo. The trial patients were initially selected for a high probability of streptococcal infection and, indeed, 75% of them had positive throat cultures for this organism. No doubt a less highly selected group of patients with acute pharyngitis would show less benefit from antistreptococcal therapy and, even for patients with positive cultures for *Str. pyogenes*, the earlier view that penicillin had little effect on clinical course has been supported by the trial of Middleton et al (1988) which showed a modest beneficial effect on sore throat but none on fever, malaise or the abnormal signs in the throat. The necessity for 10 days therapy has been confirmed in more recent studies comparing 5 and 10 days penicillin therapy.

Alternative drugs for streptococcal sore throat include a number of oral cephalosporins such as cefaclor and cephalexin, erythromycin and other macrolides, more notably azithromycin and clarithromycin. Penicillin allergy, real or supposed, is the most common reason for alternative treatment. Of growing interest is the repeated observation in clinical trials that various oral cephalosporins appear to offer superior bacteriological efficacy to penicillin in the treatment of streptococcal pharyngitis. However, whether this is truly the situation or a reflection of the power of individual studies has been thoroughly reviewed in a meta-analysis of the many studies (Pichichero & Margolis 1991). The overall cure rate for the penicillins was 89% compared with 95% for the cephalosporins. There was no significant difference with regard to adverse events. At present, penicillin remains the most cost-effective agent for the management of the vast majority of streptococcal sore throats (Pichichero 1992).

The possibility that treatment failure with penicillin may sometimes be caused by the presence of β-lactamase-producing bacteria in the pharynx has attracted attention. Brook (1984) reviews the evidence that β-lactamase-resistant aerobic and anaerobic flora frequently emerge during penicillin treatment and may spread to household contacts. In a trial involving 45 patients of whom 93% had β-lactamase-producing organisms in the pharynx before treatment, penicillin eradicated *Str. pyogenes* in only 2 of 15, erythromycin was successful in 6 of 15 and clindamycin in 14 of 15.

For those working in circumstances that do not allow bacteriological examination in cases of sore throat, it is useful to have a policy for the use of penicillin which includes most patients likely to have streptococcal infection, but avoids its widespread use in predominantly viral syndromes. In these circumstances penicillin can be given on the following indications:

- Scarlet fever. Its exact aetiology is implicit in the diagnosis, so that pencillin is indicated.
- Follicular tonsillitis with fever and tender anterior cervical glands
- Bacterial complications of acute pharyngitis such as peritonsillar abscess (quinsy), otitis media, sinusitis, mastoiditis and suppurative cervical lymphadenitis.
- Acute sore throat in a family or community in which there is known to be a high prevalence of streptococcal infection.

STREPTOCOCCAL CARRIAGE

Although an uncommon requirement in most developed countries, the prevention of streptococcal throat infections in patients subject to rheumatic fever is best achieved with penicillin. The most successful method is a monthly injection of benzathine penicillin. Two disadvantages of this method are the need for repeated injections, albeit infrequently, and the likelihood that any allergic reactions will be of long duration. In many countries the most widely used method is oral phenoxymethylpenicillin 250 mg twice daily, but benzathine penicillin every 3 or 4 weeks may be preferable where streptococcal infection is prevalent.

Diphtheria

Antibiotics are an essential part of treatment but do not obviate the need for antitoxin. *Corynebacterium diphtheriae* is moderately susceptible to penicillin, and is also susceptible to ampicillin, erythromycin and clindamycin. Erythromycin remains the most widely used for treatment and apart from a few strains of the *mitis* biotype is still highly active (Wilson 1995). A variety of regimens are effective in the treatment of carriers including benzathine penicillin by intramuscular injection, erythromycin or clindamycin by mouth for 7 days. Some carriers will later relapse and cultures should be repeated 2 or 3 weeks after treatment. In managing outbreaks it is essential to confirm successful eradication of the pathogen.

Acute epiglottitis

This rapidly progressive and life-threatening illness is encountered mainly in children, but has also been increasingly recognized in adults. It is caused by infection with *Haemophilus influenzae* type b which may often be cultured from the blood as well as from the local lesion. The favourable impact of conjugate vaccines on *H. influenzae* meningitis is also fortunately reducing the incidence of acute epiglottitis in childhood. Treatment is as much concerned with maintaining the airway as with control of the infection. Chloramphenicol and ampicillin have both been used, and the relative rarity of the condition does not allow an objective judgement to be made between them, but the advance in ampicillin-resistance among strains of *H. influenzae* (Ch. 3) now bars the use of ampicillin or analogous drugs. Although resistance to chloramphenicol is less widespread, its well recognized association with marrow aplasia has led to a decline in its use. A cephalosporin such as cefotaxime is now widely preferred on account of β-lactamase stability, high potency and excellent safety record.

The differential diagnosis of acute croup includes not only laryngotracheobronchitis (largely viral (RSV, parainfluenza) but also, occasionally, bacterial (*M. pneumoniae*)), acute epiglottitis, diphtheria and many non-infectious conditions, but also another bacterial disease known as pseudo-membranous croup, in effect a severe bacterial tracheitis (Donnelly et al 1990). *Staphylococcus aureus* is most commonly involved, although sometimes in association with other organisms (Henry et al 1983), and treatment should include a β-lactamase-resistant penicillin.

achieved, perhaps because the low P_{O_2} and high P_{CO_2} tension of purulent sinus secretions can increase bacterial resistance to some antimicrobial agents. Treatment of severe acute sinusitis is probably best achieved by initial parenteral administration of penicillin or ampicillin followed by oral amoxycillin. An assessment of treatment options is provided by Gwaltney et al (1992). Erythromycin is a satisfactory alternative achieving inhibitory concentrations in the sinus fluid for pneumococci and *Str. pyogenes* but of marginal efficacy, as in the middle ear for *H. influenzae*. One of the newer macrolides such as azithromycin may have advantages (Felstead et al 1991). Co-trimoxazole or an oral cephalosporin such as cefaclor are commonly used alternatives. For example, Wald et al (1984) found cefaclor and amoxycillin to be equally effective in the treatment of acute maxillary sinusitis in childhood.

Acute sinusitis occurring in patients admitted to intensive care units is now increasingly recognized. This is predisposed to by impaired sinus drainage, nasogastric intubation, repeated aspiration used in airways toilet, but especially nasotracheal intubation (Kulber et al 1991). Its importance lies in its predisposing to lower respiratory tract infection, and in particular pneumonia which may have serious consequences in patients in the intensive care unit (Ch. 44).

Acute sinusitis

Most episodes of acute sinusitis complicate viral upper respiratory tract infections. *H. influenzae* are the most common isolates in acute sinusitis, but detailed studies have shown a greater variety of potential pathogens. A thorough quantitative study made at the University of Virginia of 65 needle punctures in 81 adults with acute infections of the antrum by Hamory et al (1979) showed *H. influenzae* and *Streptococcus pneumoniae* as the most common isolates, with occasional high counts of staphylococci. *Moraxella catarrhalis*, α-haemolytic streptococci, anaerobes and viruses. Ampicillin, amoxycillin and co-trimoxazole were all effective in treatment. The incidence of β-lactamase-producing isolates of *M. catarrhalis* is high and that for *H. influenzae* increasing. Agents such as amoxycillin/clavulanate and clarithromycin may therefore be considered. Anaerobic isolates are common in chronic sinus infections; heavy pure cultures of anaerobes were found in 23 or 83 specimens removed aseptically at operation (Frederick & Braude 1974). As with otitis media, results of treatment have generally correlated well with antibiotic concentrations in the sinus secretion; but even with high concentrations, as judged by conventionally determined minimum inhibitory concentrations (MICs), eradication of bacteria is not easily

Acute otitis media

The aetiology of acute otitis media can be reliably established only by myringotomy or tympanocentesis, but these procedures are rarely performed outside Scandinavia and parts of the USA, and indeed are not indicated in the great majority of patients with tympanocentesis as entry criteria and provide the only available evidence on the current causes of otitis. The predominant organisms are *Str. pneumoniae* and *H. influenzae*; the latter was formerly thought to affect mainly children less than 5 years old, but it is now known that it can cause otitis at all ages. *M. catarrhalis* has been isolated in pure culture in a small but significant proportion of exudates. *Str. pyogenes*, formerly important, is now rarely found, and *Staph. aureus*, enterobacteria and *Pseudomonas* spp. are usually associated with contamination by organisms in the external meatus. Milder forms of otitis media often resolve without chemotherapy. Much depends on the diagnostic criteria. Some authors have questioned the need for antibiotic treatment as a general policy in otitis. Van Buchen et al (1981) studied 239 infections in 171 children. All were given analgesics and decongestants. Four groups were given either no additional treatment, amoxycillin alone, amoxycillin with myringotomy or myringotomy without amoxycillin. No difference was found between any of the groups in rate of resolution of pain, temperature, ear discharge, otoscopic appearance or rate of recurrence. They suggest that initial treatment should be symptomatic only and other measures reserved for those with persistent symptoms. In a later study, van Buchen et al (1985) showed that more than 90% of 4860 children diagnosed as having otitis media recovered uneventfully with symptomatic treatment. A severe course, defined as persistent illness, high temperature and/or severe pain after 3 or 4 days were experienced by only 126 (2.7%), 30 of these with *Str. pyogenes* infection. In the same study, a trial of 100 severe cases showed that amoxycillin alone or with myringotomy was superior to myringotomy alone. Considering that the question of myringotomy was still unsettled, Engelhard et al (1989) conducted a trial in 105 infants in which the recovery rate in those treated with antibiotic, with or without myringotomy was 60%, compared with 23% in those receiving myringotomy with placebo. Completeness of recovery at follow-up was judged by otoscopic findings.

Browning et al (1983) found no benefit from antibiotics in adults with active chronic otitis, although patients with polyps or cholesteatomas were excluded.

Most recently attention has focused on the pharmaco-economic aspects of the management of acute otitis media. However, the wide variation in disease severity, approaches to clinical management and choice and duration of antibiotic therapy do not lend themselves to simple conclusions (Sagraves & Maish 1994).

Most practitioners and paediatricians are generally unwilling to forego antibiotics for otitis media, but many make distinctions based on physical signs. For example, antibiotic treatment of acute otitis with bulging drum would still be almost universally practised, whereas many doctors would not treat patients with minor signs of inflammation of the tympanic membrane.

As to antibiotic choice, amoxycillin is preferred (Klein 1994). It is active against all the relevant organisms, but its value has diminished with the spread of ampicillin resistance in *H. influenzae* (Michaels 1981). *M. catarrhalis* is a less common cause of acute otitis media, yet the majority of strains are β-lactamase producers. Amoxycillin shows excellent penetration into the middle-ear fluid (Krause et al 1982). The traditional 7–10 day course of treatment is probably too long. Chaput de Saintonge et al (1982) showed equal results in 84 patients given 3- or 10-day courses, with five primary treatment failures in the 3-day treatment group and three failures in the 10-day group. A randomized trial (Bain et al 1985) between 7-day and 2-day amoxycillin treatment showed no difference in any criterion of resolution or in unwanted effects between the two groups. Alternative drugs have been extensively tested. The published experience has been comprehensively reviewed by Bluestone & Klein 1987.

Co-trimoxazole has been widely used and shown to be about as effective as ampicillin/amoxycillin, and erythromycin has also been used, especially where there is suspicion of penicillin allergy. Of the cephalosporins, cefaclor has attracted particular interest because of its good activity in vitro against *H. influenzae*. A dose of 40 mg/kg day is evidently as effective given in a twice-daily regimen as three times daily. Comparisons between cefaclor and amoxycillin have often shown similar benefit, although in one trial (John & Valle-Jones 1983) cefaclor-treated patients showed a significantly more rapid rate of improvement. One comparison of cefaclor with co-trimoxazole (Feldman et al 1982), without bacteriological confirmation showed equal efficacy between the two drugs, but a large study which included an initial tympanocentesis repeated at 3–6 days in patients whose initial cultures were positive, showed cefaclor less effective than co-trimoxazole in eradicating *H. influenzae* and perhaps also in eradicating *Str. pneumoniae* (Marchant et al 1984). No difference in symptom score, recurrence or rates of persistent effusion were found. Negative cultures of middle-ear fluid were achieved at 3–6 days in 10 of 18 patients on cefaclor and 13 of 14 on co-trimoxazole whose initial cultures grew *H. influenzae*. The corresponding results for pneumococcal otitis were 16 of 20 on cefaclor and 19 of 19 on co-trimoxazole. All the patients with *M. catarrhalis* became negative on either regimen. Another trial including tympanocentesis showed five failures in 60 patients given cefaclor, while there were no failures in patients receiving amoxycillin/clavulanic acid (co-amoxiclav) (Odio et al 1985).

A number of oral cephalosporins, other than cefaclor, are also licensed for acute otitis media. These include cefpodoxime proxetil, loracarbef, cefuroxime axetil and cefixime, although the latter's marginal activity against penicillin-sensitive pneumococci suggests this is not an ideal choice. They provide an alternative choice when other agents are contraindicated.

Among the newer macrolides, both clarithromycin and azithromycin have proved effective in comparison with amoxycillin, co-amoxiclav, and each other (Price 1994).

We conclude that ampicillin (or amoxycillin or pivampicillin) remains the agent of first choice for acute otitis media. Erythromycin and co-trimoxazole provide valid alternatives for the penicillin-allergic patient, while amoxycillin–clavulanate (co-amoxiclav) would be of particular value if β-lactamase-producing strains of *H. influenzae* or *M. catarrhalis* are prevalent (Odio et al 1985, Engelhard et al 1989). Antibiotic treatment is unnecessary in many mild cases. Recurrent acute otitis media in childhood presents a difficult problem. Adenoidectomy is often the treatment of choice, but in some children recurrent attacks justify a trial of long-term antibiotic prophylaxis, usually with ampicillin or amoxycillin. Limited trial evidence supports this concept (Bonati et al 1992). For example,

Maynard et al (1972) showed a reduction in attacks of otitis media in 47% (67% in good compliers) in Eskimo children with a high incidence of otitis by the use of ampicillin in a dose of 125 or 250 mg/day.

References

Bain J, Murphy E, Ross F 1985 Acute otitis media: clinical course among children who received a short course of high dose antibiotic. *British Medical Journal* 291: 1243–1246.

Bernstein D I, Reuman P D, Sherwood J R, Young E C, Schiff G M 1988 Ribavirin small particle aerosol treatment of influenza B virus infection. *Antimicrobial Agents and Chemotherapy* 32: 761–764

Bluestone C D, Klein J O (eds) 1987 Otitis media in infants and children. W B Saunders, Philadelphia

Bonati M, Marchetti F, Pistotti V et al 1992 Meta-analysis of antimicrobial prophylaxis for recurrent otitis media. *Clinical Trials and Meta-analysis* 28: 39–50

Breese Hall C, McBridge J T, Gale C L, Hildreth S W, Schnnabel K C 1985 Ribavirin treatment of respiratory syncytial virus infection in infants with underlying cardiopulmonary disease. *Journal of the American Medical Association* 254: 3047–3051

Brook I 1984 The role of beta-lactamase producing bacteria in the persistence of streptococcal tonsillar infection. *Review of Infectious Diseases* 6: 601–607

Browning G G, Picozzi G L, Calder I T, Sweeney G 1983 Controlled trial of medical treatment of active chronic otitis media. *British Medical Journal* 287: 1024

Chaput de Saintonge D M, Levine D F, Temple Savage I et al 1982 Trial of 3 day and 10 day courses of amoxycillin in otitis media. *British Medical Journal* 284: 1078–1081

Conrad D A, Christenson J C, Waner J L, Marks M I 1987 Aerolised ribavirin treatment of RSV infection in infants hospitalised during an epidemic. *The Pediatric Infectious Diseases Journal* 6: 152–158

Donnelly B W, McMillan J A, Weiner L B 1990 Bacterial tracheitis: report of eight new cases and review. *Reviews in Infectious Diseases* 12: 729–735

Douglas R M, Moore B W, Miles H B et al 1986 Prophylactic efficacy of intranasal alpha$_2$-interferon against rhinovirus infections in the family setting. *New England Journal of Medicine* 314: 65–70

Editorial 1986 Ribavirin and respiratory syncytial virus. *Lancet* i: 362–363

Editorial 1987 Bacterial pharyngitis. *Lancet* i: 1241–1242

Engelhard D, Cohen D, Strauss N, Sacks T G, Jorcak-Sarni L, Shapiro M 1989 Randomised study of myringotomy, amoxycillin/clavulanate or both for acute otitis media in infants. *Lancet* ii: 141–143

Feldman W, Richardson H, Rennie B, Dawson P 1982 A trial comparing cefaclor with co-trimoxazole in the treatment of acute otitis media. *Archives of Diseases of Childhood* 57: 594–596

Felstead S, Daniel R, European Azithromycin Study Group 1991 Short-course treatment of sinusitis and other upper respiratory tract infections with azithromycin: a comparison with erythromycin and amoxycillin. *Journal of Int Med Research* 19: 363–372

Fernandez H, Banks G, Smith R 1986 Ribavirin: a clinical overview. *European Journal of Epidemiology* 2: 1–14

Frederick J, Braude A I 1974 Anaerobic infection of the para-nasal sinuses. *New England Journal of Medicine* 290: 135–137

Gwaltney J M Jr, Scheld W M, Sande M A et al 1992 The microbial etiology and antimicrobial therapy of adults with acute community-acquired sinusitis: a fifteen-year experience at the University of Virginia and review of other selected studies. *Journal of Allergy and Clinical Immunology* 90: 457–462

Hamory B H, Sande M A, Sydnor A, Seale D L, Gwaltney J M 1979 Etiology and antimicrobial therapy of acute maxillary sinusitis. *Journal of Infectious Diseases* 139: 197–202

Hayden F G, Gwaltney J M Jr 1983 Intranasal interferon for prevention of rhinovirus infection and illness. *Journal of Infectious Diseases* 148: 543

Hayden F G, Gwaltney J M Jr, Johnson M E 1985 Prophylactic efficacy and tolerance of low-dose intranasal interferon-alpha$_2$ in natural respiratory viral infections. *Antiviral Research* 5: 11–15

Henry R L, Mellis C M, Benjamin B 1983 Pseudomembranous croup. *Archives of Diseases of Childhood* 58: 180–183

Howie J G R, Hutchison K R 1978 Antibiotics and respiratory illness in general practice: prescribing policy and work load. *British Medical Journal* 2: 1342

John W B, Valle-Jones J C 1983 Treatment of otitis media in children: a comparison between cefaclor and amoxycillin. *Practitioner* 227: 1805–1809

Klein J O 1994 Otitis media. *Clinical Infectious Diseases* 19: 823–833

Krause P J, Owens M J, Nightingale C H, Klimek J J, Lehmann W B, Quintiliani R 1982 Penetration of amoxyl, cefaclor, erythromycin–sulfasoxazole and trimethoprim–sulpha-methoxazole into the middle ear fluid of patients with otitis media. *Journal of Infectious Diseases* 145: 815–821

Krober M S, Bass J W, Michels G N 1985 Streptococcal pharyngitis. Placebo-controlled double-blind evaluation of clinical response to penicillin therapy. *Journal of the American Medical Association* 253: 1271–1274

Kulber D A, Santora T A, Shabot M M, Hiatt J R 1991 Early diagnosis and treatment of sinusitis in the critically ill trauma patient. *American Surgeon* 57: 775–779

Marchant C D, Shurin P A, Turcyzk V A et al 1984 A randomised control trial of cefaclor compared with trimethoprim–sulfamethoxazole for treatment of acute otitis media. *Journal of Pediatrics* 105: 633–638

Maynard J E, Fleshman J K, Tschopp C F 1972 Otitis media in Alaskan Eskimo children: prospective evaluation of chemoprophylaxis. *Journal of the American Medical Association* 219: 597–599

Michaels R H 1981 Ampicillin-resistant *H. influenzae* and otitis media. *American Journal of Diseases of Childhood* 135: 403–405

Middleton D B, D'Amico F, Merenstein J H 1988 Standardized symptomatic treatment versus penicillin as initial therapy for streptococcal pharyngitis. *Journal of Pediatrics* 113: 1089–1094

Odio C M, Kinsmierz H, Shelton S, Nelson J D 1985 Comparative treatment trial of augmentin versus cefaclor for acute otitis media with effusion. *Pediatrics* 75: 819–826

Peter G 1992 Streptococcal pharyngitis: current therapy and criteria for evaluation of new agents. *Clinical Infectious Diseases* 14 (suppl): S218–S223, S231–S232

Philpotts R J, Tyrrell D A J 1985 Rhinovirus colds. *British Medical Journal* 41: 386–390

Pichichero M E, Margolis P A 1991 A comparison of cephalosporins and penicillin in the treatment of group A beta-hemolytic streptococcal pharyngitis: meta-analysis supporting the concept of microbial copathogenicity. *Pediatric Infectious Diseases Journal* 10: 275–281

Pichichero M E 1993 Cephalosporins are superior to penicillin for the treatment of streptococcal tonsillopharyngitis: is the difference worth it? *Pediatric Infections Diseases Journal* 12: 268–274

Price E 1994 Azithromycin in the treatment of upper respiratory tract infections. *Reviews of Contemporary Pharmacotherapy* 5: 341–349

Randolph M F, Gerber M A, De Meo K K, Wright L 1985 Effect of antibiotic therapy on the clinical course of streptococcal pharyngitis. *Journal of Pediatrics* 106: 870–875

Rodriguez W J, Kim H W, Brandt C D et al 1987 Aerosolized ribavirin in the treatment of patients with respiratory syncytial virus disease. *Pediatric Infectious Diseases Journal* 6: 159–163

Sagraves R, Maish W 1994 Therapy of acute otitis media. Clinical and economic aspects. *Pharmacoeconomics* 6: 202–214

Scott G 1986 Interfering with the real cold. *British Medical Journal* 292: 1413–1414

Scott G M, Phillpotts R J, Wallace J et al 1982 Purified interferon as protection against rhinovirus infections. *British Medical Journal* 284: 1822–1825

Smith D W, Frankel L R, Mathers L H, Tang A T S, Ariagno R L, Prober C G 1991 A controlled trial of aerosolized ribavirin in infants receiving mechanical ventilation for severe respiratory virus infection. *New England Journal of Medicine* 325: 24–29

Sperber S, Hayden F G 1988 Chemotherapy of rhinovirus colds [mini review]. *Antimicrobial Agents and Chemotherapy* 32: 409–419

Taylor B, Abbott G D, Kerr M McK, Ferguson D M 1977 Amoxicillin and co-trimoxazole in presumed viral respiratory infections of childhood; placebo-controlled trial. *British Medical Journal* 2: 552–554

Van Buchen F, Birk J H M, Van't Hof M A 1981 Therapy of acute otitis media; myringotomy, antibiotics or neither? *Lancet* ii: 883–887

Van Buchen F L, Peeters M F, Van't Hof M A 1985 Acute otitis media; a new treatment strategy. *British Medical Journal* 290: 1033–1037

Wald E R, Reilly J S, Casselbrant M et al 1984 Treatment of acute maxillary sinusitis in childhood: a comparative study of amoxycillin and cefaclor. *Journal of Pediatrics* 104: 297–302

Wilson A P R 1995 Treatment of infection caused by toxigenic and non-toxigenic strains of *Corynebacterium diphtheriae*. *Journal of Antimicrobial Chemotherapy* 35: 717–720

Infections of the lower respiratory tract

H. P. Lambert

Introduction

Lower respiratory infections are a dominant cause of morbidity and mortality from infective causes throughout the world. In developing countries these infections exceed even diarrhoeal disease as a cause of death in infancy, and in wealthier countries too respiratory infection takes precedence as a cause of death at the extremes of age. The spread of the relevant pathogen by the airborne route makes control especially difficult, a problem bought into sharp relief by the increasing importance of nosocomial respiratory infections, for example, following colonization of the respiratory tract by environmental organisms in an intensive care unit or the spread of respiratory syncytial virus in children's wards.

At the other end of the clinical spectrum, respiratory infections, largely of viral origin, are a dominant cause of absence from work and from school through sickness.

With a few exceptions, clinical assessment of respiratory infection does not provide a firm aetiological diagnosis, and laboratory investigations, even when available, often fail to establish the causal organism. For this reason, infections of the respiratory tract are categorized mainly according to their epidemiology and anatomical site.

Pneumonia

The antibiotic management of pneumonia presents special difficulties arising from the wide variety of possible causal organisms and the problems of establishing an early diagnosis. The combination of clinical and radiographic evidence may provide a characteristic diagnostic picture; for example, a florid illness, lobar distribution and neutro-

philia favour a pneumococcal cause. But viruses, *Mycoplasma pneumoniae* and other organisms may also cause severe illness and lobar consolidation, while the features of bacterial pneumonia are often modified by previous antibiotic treatment. Early laboratory investigation may give fruitful information. The utility of sputum examination is much disputed, but some value can be derived from a carefully taken purulent specimen, notably a high positive predictive value for pneumococcal disease when a dominance of lanceolate diplococci is seen in the Gram-stained preparation. In addition, direct staining methods are valuable in the diagnosis of infection by mycobacteria, *Pneumocystis carinii*, legionellosis and some fungi. Antigen-detection methods, especially latex agglutination, can be used on sputum, blood and urine. Reagents are readily available for a number of organisms, particularly a multivalent serum for the detection of most pneumococcal serotypes. Blood as well as sputum should be cultured, since an appreciable number of patients with pneumococcal pneumonia have positive blood cultures. Molecular methods are available for a number of pathogens, but at present have their main value in epidemiological investigations rather than in clinical diagnosis. More invasive methods of diagnosis using material obtained at bronchoscopy (aspirates, brushing and transbronchial biopsy), lung puncture and transtracheal aspiration are used to a very variable extent in different centres. They can provide direct information about the flora of the lower respiratory tract, but these invasive tests should only be used in centres with continued experience of them. It is often impossible to achieve a confident causal diagnosis in pneumonia soon after the patient has presented for medical attention, and this leads to the need for empirical treatment while further evidence is being acquired. It is therefore necessary to have a clear idea of which organisms are common and which, although uncommon or rare, present enough danger to be considered in the initial treatment regimen. This is best done by considering the patient's age, previous state of health, the setting in which the pneumonia occurs, and any current epidemiological information.

The other principal factor in deciding empirical initial treatment policy is the assessment of severity. Prognostic factors in pneumonia have been more clearly defined in recent years; those of particular note include age >60 years, underlying disease, respiratory rate >60/min, diastolic blood pressure <60 mmHg, and serum urea >7 mmol/l.

Thus, pneumonia can best be classified, for the purpose of establishing rational antibiotic policies, into: community-acquired pneumonia of previously healthy children and adults; pneumonia in vulnerable, hospital-based and immunosuppressed patients; and pneumonia in infants. Other lower respiratory infections needing special consideration are aspiration pneumonia and lung abscess, exacerbation of chronic obstructive airways disease, bronchiectasis and cystic fibrosis.

COMMUNITY-ACQUIRED PNEUMONIA

Aetiology and epidemiology

The predominant bacterial pathogen is still *Streptococcus pneumoniae*, although its relative importance varies greatly in different reports. Until the 1960s, the pneumococcus was identified in perhaps 80% of community acquired pneumonias. Since then wide variations have been reported (0–76%), but the persistent high mortality in patients with pneumococcal pneumonia needing admission to hospital (20–30%) makes it necessary to take into account in any initial regimen. A wide-ranging study of community-acquired pneumonia (BTS 1987) examined a large number of clinical and investigative measurements in 453 adults admitted to 25 British hospitals, and established an aetiological diagnosis in 67%; *Str. pneumoniae* 34%, *M. pneumoniae* 18% and influenza A 7% were the most common. All three patients with influenza A and *Staphylococcus aureus* died, but no patient with pneumococcal, mycoplasma or staphylococcal pneumonia died who had received an appropriate antibiotic before admission. A similar proportion of pneumococcal infections (36%) was found in one of a series of studies from Nottingham (Woodhead et al 1987a), in which *Haemophilus influenzae* and influenza virus were also important. In contrast with a previous study from the same centre, Legionnaire's disease was rare, as was *M. pneumoniae*.

Other than *Str. pneumoniae*, the most commonly identified pathogen in community-acquired pneumonia is *M. pneumoniae*. The importance of *Legionella* species in community-acquired pneumonia varies greatly from place to place (0.5–15%). Other organisms are quite rare; in particular, *Staph. aureus*, except during influenza epidemics.

This relationship was confirmed in a study of 61 cases of community-acquired staphylococcal pneumonia, which also confirmed the serious nature of this infection, since 18 patients (30%) died (Woodhead et al 1987b).

Klebsiella pneumoniae is rare in the UK and in many other countries, but more common in North America, and has strong associations with alcoholism, diabetes and chronic lung disease. It is sometimes encountered, as is *Staph. aureus*, in pneumonia affecting elderly patients in nursing homes. Eighteen patients with klebsiella pneumonia seen in an intensive care unit (ICU) in Cape Town all needed ventilation (Hammond et al 1990).

One area of uncertainty is whether there are important differences in aetiology between severe pneumonia and the more common run of community-acquired lower respiratory infections. Of the pathogens identified in 60 patients with severe pneumonia in British ICUs, *Str. pneumoniae*, *Legionella pneumophila*, *H. influenzae* and *Staph. aureus* accounted for 86%, and enterobacteria were thought to be causal in only one patient (BTS 1992). At the other end of the spectrum of severity, a study of lower respiratory infections in one general practice in Nottingham found much the same variety of pathogens as those found in pneumonia (MacFarlane et al 1993). Entry criteria included productive cough and prescription of an antibiotic, so viral infections may have been underrepresented in this series.

The atypical pneumonias include, as well as *M. pneumoniae*, those caused by *Coxiella burnetii* (Q fever), *Chlamydia psittaci*, infant pneumonia caused by *Chlamydia trachomatis*, and those caused by another species, *C. pneumoniae* (strain TWAR), now established as a cause of bronchitis and pneumonia including substantial outbreaks of community-acquired pneumonia in Scandinavia. The organism is distinct in its DNA profile from *C. trachomatis* and *C. psittaci*. It is associated with bronchitis and pneumonia with varying frequency in many communities; although the majority of infections are asymptomatic or cause only minor respiratory illness, bronchitis may last for many weeks (Grayston 1992). Like *M. pneumoniae*, *C. pneumoniae* has been associated with erythema nodosum and with myocarditis, and its possible link with coronary artery disease is a topic of much interest (Cook & Honeybourne 1994).

The relative importance of different causes of pneumonia will obviously vary in different communities, so, as always, it is important to take a geographical history. For example, the recognition that pneumonia may form part of the more severe forms of scrub typhus (Editorial 1988a) would have to be taken into account in relevant areas, as would possible contact with plague (*Yersinia pestis*) or melioidosis (*Burkholderia (Pseudomonas) pseudomallei*).

Another example is the recognition, in the south-western USA, of the hantavirus pulmonary syndrome, a serious illness associated with rodent contact. There is severe

Box 48.1   *Causes of community-acquired pneumonia**

Bacteria	**Viruses**
Streptococcus pneumoniae	Influenza
Mycoplasma pneumoniae	RSV†
Haemophilus influenzae	Parainfluenza†
Moraxella catarrhalis	Measles
Staphylococcus aureus	Adenovirus
Legionella pneumophila	Hantavirus
Klebsiella pneumoniae	
Bordetella pertussis	**Fungi**
Mixed anaerobes and aerobes	*Pneumocystis carinii* (HIV)
(abscess and aspiration)	Other
Coxiella burnetii	
Chlamydia pneumoniae	
Chlamydia psittaci	
Chlamydia trachomatis‡	
Bacillus anthracis	
Yersinia pestis	

* Note that pulmonary tuberculosis sometimes presents as an acute pneumonia, and that a history of factors leading to aspiration is often missed.
  As always, a travel history should be obtained; for example, such possibilities as rickettsial pneumonia, histoplasmosis or parasitic lung infection may have to be entertained.
† Mainly in infants and children.
‡ Mainly in infants.

hypoxia with rapid progression to respiratory failure, in addition to renal failure and haematological changes which include a characteristic appearence of the peripheral blood film, with large immunoblastic lymphocytes (Levy & Simpson 1994).

Causes of community-acquired pneumonia are listed in Box 48.1.

Choice of therapy

Several dilemmas are evident in choosing initial treatment for community-acquired pneumonia. The choice of penicillin, ampicillin or amoxycillin, usually appropriate for *Str. pneumoniae,* is inappropriate for two of the important agents, legionella and *M. pneumoniae*. Where legionella is not found, it can be held that because the influence of appropriate antibiotics such as the tetracyclines or erythromycin on *M. pneumoniae* infections is marginal and that these infections are rarely life-threatening, rapid control of pneumococcal pneumonia takes precedence over other considerations. Where, however, *Legionella* has to be considered, and when *M. pneumoniae* is highly prevalent, erythromycin or another macrolide such as clarithromycin provides an attractive alternative with suitable levels of activity against all three agents. Disadvantages of erythromycin are problems with nausea and vomiting in some patients, variable absorption of some of the oral preparations (p. 383) and problems of thrombophlebitis, and rarely ototoxicity, with the intravenous preparation.

Ampicillin and amoxycillin are also appropriate for β-lactamase-negative strains of *H. influenzae*, but where resistant strains are prevalent co-amoxiclav will be used more widely. Erythromycin is also active in vitro against this organism, although concentrations achieved in blood and sputum may be inadequate to eradicate *H. influenzae*.

A double-blind trial in 91 patients with community acquired pneumonia (MacFarlane et al 1983) compared erythromycin with ampicillin/amoxycillin. In each case, 48 h of intravenous treatment was followed by oral therapy for 7 days. These patient groups formed part of the series already quoted in which *Str. pneumoniae* was the dominant pathogen. Similar progress was achieved in both groups, but unwanted effects were more common in patients treated with erythromycin. The nine patients with *Legionella* pneumonia and the eight with 'atypical' pneumonia did as well on either regimen, but it is notable that both patients with *Legionella* infection who had an uncomplicated recovery on the ampicillin/amoxycillin treatment had infection by *Legionella micdadei*, which is susceptible to ampicillin in vitro. Many of the newer cephalosporins are active against the common causes of pneumonia and have been found effective in open studies. Their role is more appropriately considered in the discussion of hospital-acquired pneumonia. A comparison of erythromycin and clarithromycin in community-acquired pneumonia showed little difference in efficacy, but a higher incidence of adverse events in the erythromycin group (Anderson et al 1991). Patients admitted to hospital are usually given parenteral treatment, but Chan et al (1995) found intravenous followed by oral co-amoxiclav, and cefotaxime followed by cefuroxime axetil equally effective in a randomized trial of 541 patients with community-acquired lower respiratory infection admitted to hospital; immunocompromise and critical illness requiring intensive care were excluded. Little microbiological information was available, and patients with and without radiological abnormalities were included. The patients treated by oral administration throughout tended to show better progress at the time of discharge and less requirement for extended treatment and there were significant savings in cost and labour.

On the borderland between community-acquired pneumonia and hospital-acquired pneumonia are the increasing number of patients with serious chronic diseases such as diabetes, hepatic cirrhosis or with long-term immunosuppression such as transplant recipients. Although developing pneumonia in the community, they must be considered at risk from the same variety of organisms as the hospital patient; as must elderly patients in nursing homes. Another special group is constituted by human immunodeficiency virus (HIV) positive patients who may first present with pneumonia caused by *Pneumocystis carinii* and in whom pneumococcal infection is more common than in the general population (Ch. 46).

Initial therapy

A general policy for the initial treatment of community-acquired pneumonia pending the acquisition of further microbiological information must obviously depend to some extent on local knowledge of prevailing pathogens, and on local antibiotic policy. In the UK, however, it is reasonable to conclude that, for patients who are not seriously ill, amoxycillin (or an equivalent drug, ampicillin or pivampicillin) or erythromycin can be chosen. For the more seriously ill patient, and especially for patients with chronic chest disease, the possibility of infection with ampicillin-resistant *H. influenzae* or *M. catarrhalis*, or other less common organisms, should be catered for, and the choice then lies mainly between a cephalosporin such as cefuroxime, or co-amoxiclav. Erythromycin should be used in addition to either of these choices if Legionnaires' disease is a possibility, and flucloxacillin if staphylococcal infection is probable. These possibilities are especially relevant if the patient is so ill as to be admitted to an ICU. The treatment of pneumonia in these units is further considered in Chapter 44. Ciprofloxacin may also be considered, but should not be used as sole agent if *Str. pneumoniae* infection is in question, although other more recently developed fluoroquinolones such as sparfloxacin may prove suitable for this purpose. Carbon (1993), reviewing the role of these agents in respiratory infections, considers that they may be considered, in combination with a β-lactam agent, for severe community-acquired pneumonia. If, either initially or at a later stage, a specific pathogen is diagnosed, treatment can be modified accordingly. Community-acquired pneumonia is usefully reviewed by Hosker at al (1994) and guidelines have been published by several national bodies, including the American Thoracic Society (Niederman et al 1993) and the British Thoracic Society (1993). Some suggestions for this initial, empirical phase of management are summarized in Box 48.2. It is of interest that both US and Canadian recommendations favour a macrolide or a tetracycline rather than a penicillin for the less severe grades of community-acquired pneumonia. Any recommended schemes must, of course, be frequently reviewed in the light of changing susceptibility patterns.

HOSPITAL-ACQUIRED PNEUMONIA

The formidable dangers of admission to hospital have been fully documented in recent years. Among them is the risk of hospital-acquired respiratory infection, third in frequency after urinary tract and skin infections, but first as the cause of death from hospital-acquired infection. The increasing importance of Gram-negative aerobic bacteria as a cause of hospital pneumonia has been fully documented and may well be related to the use of broad-spectrum antibiotics and to the greater use of assisted ventilation. Many outbreaks associated with nebulizers were reported until suitable methods were developed to prevent infection from this source. Hospital outbreaks of Legionnaires' disease have also attracted much public attention. A wide range of organisms can cause hospital pneumonia and they are listed in Box 48.3.

A still wider spectrum of possible causal agents has to be considered in more severe immunosuppression associated with neutropenia and depression of cell-mediated immunity including acquired immune deficiency syndrome (AIDS). The causes and treatment of pneumonia in these patients are discussed fully in Chapters 43 and 46.

The standard methods are used in establishing the aetiology of hospital-acquired pneumonia, relying mainly on

---

Box 48.2 *Options for initial empirical antibiotic therapy in community-acquired pneumonia*

Patient not seriously ill, <65 years old, no other risk factors*
Low risk of pneumococci with penicillin resistance
- Benzylpenicillin
- Ampicillin
- Erythromycin
- Cephalosporin (e.g. cefuroxime, cefotaxime)
- Co-amoxiclav
- Co-trimoxazole

Substantial risk of penicillin-resistant pneumococci
- High-dose amoxicillin
- Cephalosporin
- Erythromycin (penicillin allergy)

Patient seriously ill, and/or risk factors present*

- Erythromycin + cephalosporin (e.g. cefotaxime)
- Erythromycin + ampicillin + flucloxacillin
- Erythromycin + co-amoxiclav

NB: Many names of antibiotics are given as representatives of groups. Which of the group is chosen will depend on local policies.
* Risk factors include increased age, chronic respiratory disease and other chronic conditions such as diabetes, heart failure, and chronic liver or kidney disease.

Box 48.3 *Causes of hospital-acquired pneumonia*

Bacteria
Enterobacteriaceae
  (e.g. *Esch. coli, K. pneumoniae*)
Pseudomonas aeruginosa
Staphylococcus aureus
Streptococcus pneumoniae
Haemophilus influenzae
Legionella pneumophila
Moxarella catarrhalis
Polymicrobial, anaerobes

Viruses
Respiratory syncytial virus
Influenza virus

the immediate Gram stain and culture of freshly taken sputum, and on blood culture, and occasionally on more invasive methods. Diagnostic difficulties are compounded by the frequency in the respiratory tract of hospital-acquired antibiotic-resistant organisms, especially enterobacteria and pseudomonas. Indeed, colonization by these organisms in ICUs is widespread and precedes, but does not always proceed to, clinically significant infection. Treatment of hospital-acquired pneumonia must often begin, and often continue, without evidence of specific aetiology. The antibiotic regimen chosen must therefore take account especially of the Gram-negative pathogens listed in Box 48.3 and also of any local epidemiological information about pathogens prevalent in the particular unit.

Several empirical therapies have been employed in the initial treatment of hospital-acquired pneumonia, depending on local prevalence of pathogens and on local antibiotic policies. Most frequently, combination therapy with a cephalosporin or a broad-spectrum penicillin together with an aminoglycoside has been used, modified by local epidemiological or clinical information. The most important of these are the inclusion of an agent with antipseudomonal activity, such as ceftazidime, if *Pseudomonas aeruginosa* is suspected, erythromycin or clarithromycin if legionellosis is prevalent, and flucloxacillin or vancomycin if staphylococcal infection is likely.

Concern about aminoglycoside toxicity, although partly mitigated by the trend towards once-daily dosage, has led to a number of studies of single-agent treatment, with a cephalosporin such as ceftazidime, imipenem–cilastatin, or ticarcillin–clavulanate. Another combination, seldom used but worth consideration if aspiration is suspected, is that of clindamycin with an aminoglycoside. The role of quinolones is not fully defined, and resistance to ciprofloxacin is already a substantial problem, especially among strains of *Staph. aureus* and *Ps. aeruginosa*. Carbon (1993) does not favour their use, even in combination, for nosocomial pneumonia, but against this must be set the very substantial study of Fink et al (1994). Ciprofloxacin and imipenem, both in high dosage, were compared in a multicentre study in hospital patients with severe pneumonia caused by identifiable pathogens. Ciprofloxacin performed as well as imipenem, achieving somewhat higher rates of clinical response and bacteriological clearance. Adverse events included fits in 6 of 200 patients given imipenem, compared with 1 of 202 in the ciprofloxacin group. The big difference in aetiology in hospital-acquired pneumonia compared with community-acquired pneumonia (78% of the illnesses were nosocomial) is well revealed in this study, with *Ps. aeruginosa, H. influenzae, K. pneumoniae* and *Escherichia coli* being the most common isolates. Pseudomonas infections were associated with a poor response to treatment and frequent development of bacteriological resistance.

Clearly, the regimen chosen for hospital pneumonia must

be carefully chosen in the light of local factors and, as with any other severe infection, modified if evidence of specific aetiology is forthcoming. Nosocomial pneumonia is an important topic, in view of its great importance as a cause of morbidity and mortality in ICUs, and measures aimed at its prevention, together with further discussion of its epidemiology and management, are described in Chapter 44.

TREATMENT OF PNEUMONIA OF KNOWN CAUSE (Table 48.1)

Streptococcus pneumoniae

A penicillin remains the drug of choice except where penicillin resistance in *Str. pneumoniae* has become a problem. The dose of penicillin has been clarified in several studies. It is customary to give intravenous or intramuscular injections initially followed by oral treatment after a day or two if the patient's condition permits. The high doses of intravenously administered benzylpenicillin commonly used have been shown as no more effective than procaine penicillin in a moderate dose (300 mg 12-hourly). If benzylpenicillin is chosen, a dose of 1.2 g 6-hourly can be used. Similarly, amoxycillin or ampicillin have been satisfactorily used either intravenously or orally (amoxycillin 500 mg three times daily, ampicillin 500 mg four times daily) to treat patients with pneumonia who were not seriously ill. Penicillin treatment for pneumococcal pneumonia is now threatened by the emergence of resistant pneumococci. Some strains are relatively insensitive strains, with minimum inhibitory concentrations (MICs) in the range 0.1–1 mg/l, and chest infection caused by these may still be controlled by adequate penicillin dosage. More threatening are the strains of greater resistance (>1 mg/l) to penicillin, resistant also to other antibiotics including cephalothin and chloramphenicol, and which have now become widespread (Feldman et al 1985, Pallares et al 1987, Friedland 1995). At present, it appears that pneumonia caused by relatively insensitive strains can be treated by penicillin; for the highly resistant strains a cephalosporin such as cefotaxime or vancomycin should be used, pending detailed susceptibility tests. Careful surveillance for pneumococcal drug resistance is now necessary, especially as cross-resistance between penicillin and cephalosporins is now emerging.

Tetracycline is no longer suitable as a universal treatment for all pneumonias, since strains of pneumococci resistant to this drug as well as to erythromycin and to lincomycin have emerged. Resistance to co-trimoxazole has also been reported. The most suitable alternative drug for patients allergic to penicillin is erythromycin or another macrolide, but other possibilities include clindamycin, a tetracycline and, if the evidence of penicillin allergy is dubious, a suitable cephalosporin.

Table 48.1 *Treatment of pneumonia of known cause*

Pathogen	First choice*	Second choice*
Str. pneumoniae	Penicillin	Erythromycin or other macrolide
Highly penicillin resistant	Cefotaxime	Vancomycin
M. pneumoniae	Erythromycin	Tetracycline
Staph. aureus	Flucloxacillin (? + fusidate or rifampicin)	Susceptibility tests
H. influenzae Ampicillin resistant	Ampicillin Co-amoxiclav	Co-trimoxazole Cefotaxime
L. pneumophila	Erythromycin	Erythromycin + rifampicin Doxycycline + ciprofloxacin
K. pneumoniae	Cefotaxime	Susceptibility tests
Ps. aeruginosa	Antipseudomonal β-lactam + aminoglycoside	Susceptibility tests
Aspiration pneumonia	Clindamycin	Penicillin + metronidazole
Q fever	Tetracycline	
Psittacosis	Tetracycline	
C. pneumoniae	Erythromycin	Tetracycline

* Specific compounds are named as representative of their groups.
A different compound of the group may be chosen, depending on local policies.

Mycoplasma pneumoniae

A common cause of 'atypical' pneumonia, this organism falls under particular suspicion when associated with similar cases within a family or institution. The definitive diagnosis rests on serological tests, since few laboratories undertake culture of the organism. Appropriate antibiotic treatment shortens the illness and the duration of radiological abnormality. Several tetracyclines and macrolides show benefit compared with controls receiving penicillin or no antimicrobial drug. When the initial evidence leaves doubt between the pneumococcus and *M. pneumoniae*, erythromycin is suitable for both conditions except in the unlikely event of an erythromycin-resistant pneumococcus.

Haemophilus influenzae

The role of *H. influenzae* in bronchitis has been studied extensively (p. 690), but its importance as a cause of pneumonia has proved more difficult to evaluate, although it is evident that both capsulate and non-capsulate strains of *H. influenzae* can cause pneumonia. Capsulated strains are more likely to be associated with bacteraemic infant pneumonia, and non-capsulated strains with adult pneumonia. Wallace et al (1978), describing 41 adult patients with *H. influenzae* pneumonia, found that bacteraemia was nearly always associated with capsulate strains,

but capsulate and non-capsulate strains were found in pneumonia without bacteraemia. Ampicillin was formerly the drug of choice, but with increasing prevalence of ampicillin resistance, an extended-spectrum cephalosporin such as cefotaxime or co-amoxiclav is now the drug of first choice. Other treatment choices as resistance becomes more common include the newer macrolides, such as clarithromycin and some of the quinolones, such as ciprofloxacin (Powell 1991). Co-amoxiclav is generally as effective orally as parenterally (Chan et al 1995).

Legionella pneumophila

These organisms are susceptible to a large number of antimicrobial agents, but in vitro results relate poorly to efficacy in patients. Retrospective surveys of antibiotic use in outbreaks of Legionnaires' disease establish erythromycin as the agent of choice, although occasional patients apparently respond to other agents, including high-dose ampicillin, and tetracycline. Penicillin, cephalosporins and aminoglycosides are ineffective.

Custom, based on case response studies but without well established clinical trial, tends to favour large doses of erythromycin (up to 4 g/day) and the use of the intravenous route for more seriously ill patients. Some patients with Legionnaires' disease have a prolonged illness, or relapse after treatment is discontinued, and for these reasons treatment is continued for 3 weeks (Finegold 1988). Clarithromycin, either parenterally when available, or orally in a dose of 500 mg 12-hourly, may replace erythromycin where its expense is not a factor. For patients with *Legionella* infection of mild or moderate severity who are unable to take erythromycin, a tetracycline is probably the appropriate second choice. For the seriously ill patient rifampicin is used together with erythromycin; it is very active in vitro and has a good effect in experimental models. An alternative for seriously ill patients is a combination of doxycycline and ciprofloxacin, with the advantage of avoiding a drug interaction in immunosuppressed patients receiving cyclosporin (Roig et al 1993). Favourable reports have appeared suggesting a beneficial effect of imipenem. Experimental models have provided potentially valuable data on the chemotherapy of Legionnaires' disease. Edelstein et al (1984), for example, used intratracheal instillation of *L. pneumophila* in guinea-pigs, producing histological and clinical findings very similar to those found in fatal human disease. Erythromycin, rifampicin, co-trimoxazole and doxycycline all gave significant reductions in mortality, and combinations of rifampicin with erythromycin or with doxycycline produced a much more effective killing of *Legionella* than did erythromycin or doxycycline alone. Cefoxitin and gentamicin, effective in vitro, were ineffective in this model, although good concentrations in serum and lung tissue were achieved. Erythromycin and rifampicin are also effective in inhibiting multiplication of *Legionella* within human monocytes (Horwitz & Silverstein 1983). These experimental findings give general support to the foregoing recommendations for treatment. *Legionella* infections must be considered as important causes of pneumonia in the immunocompromised as well as in the normal host.

Q fever and psittacosis

These are both treated by tetracyclines. A dose of 2 g/day of tetracycline or 200 mg/day of doxycycline is continued for 14–21 days (Raoult & Marrie 1995). It is unknown whether a longer period of treatment might prevent or lessen the chance of chronic infection. The treatment of Q fever endocarditis is described in Chapter 61.

Chlamydia pneumoniae

Erythromycin or a tetracycline are given for 10–14 days (Grayston 1992), but may be replaced by the newer macrolides, clarithromycin or azithromycin. Several of the fluoroquinolones are also active against the organism (Cook & Honeybourne 1994), but clinical data is as yet limited.

Staphylococcus aureus

As already mentioned, staphylococcal pneumonia carries a serious prognosis, the mortality in two series being 30% (Woodhead et al 1987b) and 84% (Watanakunahorn 1987). A large proportion of patients with staphylococcal pneumonia have serious associated diseases or are elderly, and even appropriate and early treatment may fail. Staphylococcal pneumonia may complicate influenza and is then particularly lethal. Treatment is on the same lines as for staphylococcal septicaemia (p. 586). The principal agent is a suitable β-lactamase-resistant penicillin, in the UK usually flucloxacillin, while for the increasing number of resistant isolates vancomycin is the agent of first choice. The penicillin is often combined with rifampicin or with fusidic acid.

Hantavirus pneumonia

The main requirement in this multisystem disorder is urgent treatment in an experienced ICU. Since intravenous ribavirin has been shown effective in haemorrhagic fever with renal syndrome, administration of this antiviral drug is justifiable.

PNEUMONIA IN INFANCY

Good evidence of aetiology in infant pneumonia is rarely achieved other than in studies which include invasive diagnostic methods such as lung puncture (Shann et al 1984). Even with extensive investigation a causal diagnosis is made in only about 50% of patients (Editorial 1988b). A number of studies have, however, made evident a notable difference between infant pneumonia in well-nourished populations and those in developing countries with much poverty, poor hygiene and malnutrition. In relatively wealthy communities most pneumonias are viral in origin, but a bacterial cause is commonly assumed to avoid the risk of leaving untreated a life-threatening bacterial pneumonia. Whether antibiotic treatment has a role in most infant pneumonias in wealthy communities is uncertain. Friis et al (1984) found no significant benefit from ampicillin (for infants <2 year olds) or penicillin (for older children) in a trial of 136 children with pneumonia or bronchiolitis, although a number of children in the non-antibiotic group were subsequently given antibiotics and two developed purulent otitis media. About half the children showed evidence of viral infection, mostly with respiratory syncytial virus (RSV). These findings stand in sharp contrast to many studies in developing countries, which have been extensively reviewed by Shann (1986). Studies including lung aspiration involving a total of more than 1000 children showed a bacterial pathogen in 62%. In addition to the dominant pathogens, *Str. pneumoniae* and *H. influenzae*, other pathogens found in infant pneumonia in the developing world include *Staph. aureus*, *Pneum. carinii*, *C. trachomatis*, *M. pneumoniae* and cytomegalovirus. In series which included them, virological investigations were positive in 23% of 1200 children. It seems, therefore, that the large differences between the impact of infant pneumonia between wealthy and developing countries may lie not in any substantial differences in the nature and frequency of viral respiratory infection but rather in the frequency of bacterial pneumonia, either primary or supervening on an initial viral infection. This concept is supported by studies from the Gambia (Forgie et al 1991); a detailed analysis of a group of lower respiratory infections confirmed the dominance of *Str. pneumoniae* and *H. influenzae* as bacterial pathogens, but found evidence of RSV infection in one-third of the children, and evidence of combined bacterial and viral infection in 15% of the infants.

We suggest that in many parts of the world ampicillin or one of its congeners, or co-trimoxazole, are suitable in the initial empirical treatment of infant pneumonia. In areas where pneumococcal resistance to penicillin, or ampicillin resistance in *H. influenzae*, are present, a cephalosporin such as cefotaxime should be chosen. As in adult pneumonia, treatment should be changed appropriately if evidence of a particular aetiology is forthcoming.

Whether antibiotics, so often given in childhood upper respiratory infections, have any influence on the likelihood of subsequent lower respiratory tract infection, is an important question, since this alleged effect is a common reason given to justify their very extensive use. Gadomski (1993) has conducted a meta-analysis of trials from both developed and developing countries and, while acknowledging a number of limitations of trial design, concludes that antibiotics neither shorten the course of upper respiratory infection nor prevent the development of pneumonia.

MANAGEMENT OF CHILDHOOD PNEUMONIA IN DEVELOPING COUNTRIES

A policy for life-threatening infant pneumonia in developing countries with small health budgets is a matter of great concern. Even when diagnostic facilities are available, the causal diagnosis of pneumonia is notoriously unsatisfactory, especially in childhood, but most life-threatening respiratory infections occur in areas where there are no diagnostic facilities and where health care is available, if at all, only through primary care workers with limited training. Much attention has therefore been paid by the World Health Organization to the development and validation of simple criteria, such as respiratory rate and chest indrawing, which would help field workers to distinguish between the general run of self-limiting upper respiratory infections and the more dangerous infections of the lower tract. Analysis of these results is beyond the scope of the present discussion, but

the reader is referred to an excellent review of this topic by Simoes (1994).

At present the mainstay of treatment is often intramuscular chloramphenicol, penicillin or ampicillin for the more seriously ill patients, and oral agents, usually ampicillin or co-trimoxazole, for the less seriously ill. Campbell et al (1988) showed that in Gambian children oral co-trimoxazole was as good as, and much cheaper than, a single injection of fortified procaine penicillin followed by 5 days of oral ampicillin. On the community scale, a number of studies have been made of case management of pneumonia by health workers employing simple algorithms to aid their assessment of severity. A meta-analysis of six published trials done in various places in the Indian subcontinent and in Tanzania (with an additional review of three other studies) (Sazawal & Black 1992) suggested that these intervention trials achieved approximately a 20% reduction in infant mortality and a 25% reduction in mortality in children <5 years old. The agents used in the different trials were oral co-trimoxazole, ampicillin or penicillin. Further studies are needed to find out if the dominant role of *Str. pneumoniae* and *H. influenzae*, found in several areas, is indeed general or whether other pathogens are important enough in some parts of the world to be taken account of in treatment policies. Another increasing problem is that of antibiotic resistance, especially in pneumococci. In a group of Pakistani children with bacteraemic pneumococcal pneumonia, 9% of the blood isolates were penicillin resistant, 39% were chloramphenicol resistant, and 62% showed varying levels of resistance to co-trimoxazole. (Mastro et al 1991). The problem of pneumococcal resistance to penicillin is now widespread (Chs 15, 53). For example, of 341 isolates in one US paediatric centre, 37 were relatively resistant and 6 fully resistant (Tan et al 1993).

Pertussis

Bordetella pertussis is susceptible to many antibiotics in vitro, including ampicillin, erythromycin, tetracycline and co-trimoxazole, but none is very effective in treatment. Erythromycin greatly diminishes nasopharyngeal carriage and has a marginally beneficial effect on the course of the illness. It should be used in infants and other vulnerable subjects, and in severe pertussis. Given to contacts, erythromycin is sometimes successful in controlling outbreaks in closed communities. (Bass 1985, Steketee et al 1988).

ASPIRATION PNEUMONIA AND LUNG ABSCESS

Aspiration from the upper airway is a common event, in fact much more frequent than is indicated by gross clinical evidence. It is especially associated with impaired consciousness, with infection in the mouth or pharynx, and with impairment of the swallowing mechanism of any origin. It is therefore a common factor in pulmonary infection in ICUs (Ch. 44). Anaerobes are of dominant importance in lung abscess and aspiration pneumonia. Other important organisms in these conditions, as in suppurative pneumonia generally and in empyema, are aerobic Gram-negative species. When aspiration occurs in a patient in hospital, pathogens such as those described in the preceding section on hospital-acquired pneumonia, are often found. The infections are often polymicrobial, either with a purely anaerobic or a mixed aerobic and anaerobic flora.

Lung abscess is much less common than simple aspiration pneumonia. It may develop as a complication of aspiration, or in relation to bronchial carcinoma, or sometimes as a manifestation of pyaemia; in the latter form, abscesses are usually multiple.

Lung abscesses were for many years treated mainly by long courses of penicillin in high doses, with generally good results. The basis for this treatment was validated by modern bacteriological findings, since most of the causal organisms are susceptible to penicillin. The most common isolates are peptostreptococci, the *B. melaninogenicus* group, and *Fusobacterium nucleatum*. Although *Bacteroides fragilis*, which is penicillin resistant, is found in about 15% of specimens, patients with this organism among their isolates also evidently respond to penicillin. The other main contender is clindamycin, which is also active against most of the relevant isolates. The efficacy of metronidazole, so evident in many important anaerobic infections, is less certain in lung abscess, several authors reporting poor results with this drug (Perlino 1981).

The choice is between penicillin and clindamycin (Bartlett & Gorbach 1983). Some workers have found them equally effective, but in an important randomized study of 39 patients with community-acquired putrid lung abscess, clindamycin proved superior to penicillin in a number of respects (Levison et al 1983). No failures of treatment were seen in 19 patients given clindamycin (600 mg 8-hourly i.v., followed by 300 mg 6-hourly orally), whereas several failures of penicillin treatment were encountered, despite administration in high dosage. The average duration of fever was 7.7 days following the start of penicillin, and 4.4 days after starting clindamycin while, of the patients available for follow-up, all 13 of those treated with clindamycin, but only 8 of the 15 treated with penicillin, were cured.

The relatively poor results with penicillin may be related to the increase of penicillin-resistant isolates, including *Bacteroides* spp. other than *B. fragilis*, than was formerly found. There are many anecdotal reports of success with clindamycin after failure with penicillin, and we too have observed this sequence as well as success with clindamycin after failure with metronidazole.

We conclude that clindamycin is the treatment of first choice for lung abscess. For the less seriously ill patient in a hospital in which antibiotic-associated colitis causes concern, high-dose penicillin together with metronidazole is still a valid alternative. If penicillin or clindamycin is used in a patient who has developed lung abscess in hospital, an additional agent, preferably a cephalosporin such as cefotaxime, should be given, since aerobic Gram-negative species may in these circumstances form an important component of the abscess flora.

In contrast to the polymicrobial and often anaerobic flora associated with the sequelae of aspiration, primary lung abscess in children is often caused by *Staph. aureus*. Surgery is sometimes necessary, but most patients respond to a β-lactamase-resistant penicillin. Clindamycin is a useful alternative in the presence of allergy or poor response to penicillin. Although the chest radiograph may remain abnormal for a long time, long-term sequelae are rare.

The treatment of choice for the main varieties of pneumonia is outlined in Table 48.1.

Bronchitis

ACUTE BRONCHITIS

In a previously normal subject, acute bronchitis is most commonly viral in origin, although the assumption of secondary bacterial infection is often made if the sputum becomes purulent. There is a dearth of adequate trials, but two of them may be especially noted. The randomized controlled trial by Stott & West (1976) of 212 adults with cough and purulent sputum but without chronic chest disease or abnormal chest signs on clinical examination revealed no difference in recovery rates between those given doxycycline or a placebo, except that, oddly enough, runny nose was less persistent and subsequent upper respiratory infections less common in the group receiving the antibiotic. The identical rate of improvement in sputum purulence is notable, since this feature is commonly used as a positive indication for the prescription of an antibiotic. The most recent study (Verheij et al 1994) found clinically relevant benefit in patients aged >55 years who have frequent cough and also feel ill. A review of published work including seven randomized studies (Gonzales & Sande 1995) shows 'no major clinical role for antibiotics in uncomplicated acute bronchitis', and concludes that education of doctors and patients is needed to reduce antibiotic use for this condition. One problem about a general caveat of this nature is that, although chronic pulmonary disease is relatively easy to exclude, other conditions which should act as exclusions from a diagnosis of simple acute bronchitis, such as atypical pneumonia, or infection of the nasal sinuses, are more difficult to make. For example, infection by *M. pneumoniae*, which causes bronchitis more commonly than pneumonia, shows some benefit from antibiotics. We conclude that antibiotics are seldom indicated in acute bronchitis, but should be used in the elderly and more seriously ill. Suitable choices, depending on available epidemiological and other information, are amoxycillin, a macrolide such as erythromycin, co-amoxiclav or a cephalosporin such as cefuroxime.

CHRONIC BRONCHITIS

The role of antimicrobial drugs in chronic bronchitis has been particularly difficult to assess, since the disease varies so greatly in its rate of progress, and especially in its propensity to acute exacerbations. *H. influenzae* and the pneumococcus are the most common bacterial isolates from sputum; staphylococci may be found and *Klebsiella* and *Pseudomonas* spp. and other Gram-negative species may become predominant after antibiotic treatment.

Moraxella (*Branhamella*) *catarrhalis* infections affect mainly patients with existing chronic respiratory illness, and are also found in immunosuppressed subjects. Although many infections are community acquired, nosocomial infection is also not infrequently seen. β-Lactamase production is common. In one extensive study (Slevin et al 1984), 38 of 99 isolates produced β-lactamase. Strains are generally susceptible to tetracycline, erythromycin, co-trimoxazole, cefotaxime and the fluoroquinolones, but resistance to trimethoprim and the dubious value of sulphonamides in chronic bronchial infection make the role of co-trimoxazole uncertain (McLeod et al 1986). The frequency of β-lactamase production by *Mor. catarrhalis* has led to the use of amoxycillin–clavulanic acid (co-amoxiclav) with apparently favourable results. Ofloxacin may be a useful alternative since, of the fluoroquinolones, it does not show an interaction with theophylline. An excellent review of this organism is given by McGowan (1987).

Antibacterial drugs have been given in chronic bronchitis with three main objects: the treatment of exacerbations when they occur; long-term prophylaxis aimed at preventing exacerbations; and suppressive treatment in advanced cases with constantly purulent sputum. The benefits attained with long-term treatment have been explored in a large number of trials, the results of which were reviewed in previous editions of this book. In most studies some reduction in time off work was achieved, usually by a diminution of the duration rather than the number of exacerbations, but several long-term studies showed little or no change in the rate at which respiratory function deteriorated. A few trials gave convincing evidence to support the common view that

long-term treatment was beneficial in the small proportion of patients with chronic bronchitis who suffer frequent acute exacerbations during the winter. Treatment throughout the winter is now prescribed for few patients, but the early treatment of acute exacerbation is widely practised. In many trials, the recorded differences between treatment groups have been slight, and the choice between them will depend on the patient's previous treatment, his experience of unwanted effects of the different drugs and, occasionally, on the results of laboratory tests.

There are several possible reasons for the relatively poor results of antibiotic treatment in bronchitis exacerbations. Many exacerbations are provoked by viral infections, such as rhinoviruses and RSV, and significant bacterial superinfection is not an inevitable consequence. In others, whatever the initiating event, later outcome may be related more to airflow obstruction and other mechanical factors than to infection, and non-infective triggers such as allergy or atmospheric pollution may provoke exacerbations. In some studies no significant difference between bacterial isolation rates taken routinely or during exacerbations has been found. Possibly some of the confusion surrounding the results of antibiotic trials in bronchitis has resulted from pooling of groups of patients in very different stages of the natural history of the condition. Several trials have revealed no difference in outcome between placebo and treatment groups, whereas the extensive trials by Pines et al (1972) in a group of patients with severe chronic purulent chest disease showed clearly that antibiotic treatment was superior to a non-antibiotic regimen. The relationship of response to severity of attack emerged also in the large trial of Anthonisen et al (1987), involving 362 episodes in 173 patients over a period of $3\frac{1}{2}$ years, since failure rates in the most severe group were 54% with placebo and 34% with antibiotic, whereas there was no difference in the least severe category. Amoxycillin, co-trimoxazole and doxycycline were used according to the physician's choice.

Because the less severe episodes are managed at home, treatment choice lies between orally administered agents, of which a tetracycline, ampicillin or a similar agent, and co-trimoxazole have been most commonly used. Many comparative trials have been published, showing little to choose between these drugs in terms of efficacy. A large study by the British Thoracic Association (Mackay 1980) in 199 patients defined dose ranges for ampicillin and amoxycillin. Each drug was given orally in a dose of either 250 or 500 mg three times daily; they were equally effective at both dose ranges and no advantage was gained with the higher dose of either drug.

Erythromycin appears about as effective as ampicillin or amoxycillin, in spite of its relatively low activity against *H. influenzae*. The newer macrolides, carrying a lesser risk of adverse effects, are now used more frequently, and several trials have found clarithromycin to be as effective as ampicillin in exacerbations of bronchitis (Bachand 1991, Aldous 1991).

Tetracyclines still play a large role in the treatment of exacerbations of bronchitis, and their use over 30 years has been reviewed by Pines (1982). Because of its ease of administration, doxycycline is now often chosen. Cephalosporins have also been used. Cefaclor and cefixime are of some interest as orally administered agents with good activity against *H. influenzae*, but the latter has only marginal activity against *Str. pneumoniae*. Ciprofloxacin has also been used in successful trials, but the poor activity of presently available fluoroquinolones against Gram-positive cocci makes them a poor choice if the illness proves to be the onset of dangerous pneumococcal disease (Korner et al 1994).

Antibiotics should certainly be given in exacerbations of chronic obstructive airways disease. The choice will be partly determined by local knowledge; suitable for oral treatment are ampicillin or amoxycillin (if resistance rates are low), co-amoxiclav, doxycycline or a cephalosporin such as cefaclor. Parenteral treatment is necessary in severe exacerbations requiring treatment in hospital and in advanced cases. The most suitable agents for most situations are a cephalosporin such as cefotaxime or cefuroxime, or co-amoxiclav. If Legionnaire's disease is suspected, a macrolide should be added, as indicated in pneumonia. Chloramphenicol is also of established value in severe purulent chest infections and may be used where drug expenditure is limited. The factors which influence treatment of pneumonia in patients with chronic bronchitis are the same as in severe exacerbations, and are not greatly influenced by whether or not the patient has areas of pulmonary consolidation, when the illness is classified as a pneumonia.

BRONCHIECTASIS

H. influenzae is the most common pathogen and blind treatment is directed towards this organism. Cole et al (1983) have shown that high-dose amoxycillin, 3 g twice daily for a week, reduced sputum volume and could improve lung function, but they did not compare this treatment with conventional doses of amoxycillin. A double-blind placebo-controlled study in 38 patients with bronchiectasis showed significant improvement from long-term (32 weeks) treatment with amoxycillin 3 g/day (Currie et al 1990). As with other respiratory infections, increasing frequency of drug resistance leads to a trend towards the use of co-amoxiclav or a cephalosporin. Many patients have a mixed flora, including Gram-negative aerobes and anaerobes. A most important aspect of treatment in bronchiectasis from any cause is postural drainage – no chemotherapy can substitute for this.

Cystic fibrosis

Patients with cystic fibrosis present a particular and growing problem. They are peculiarly susceptible to respiratory infections which lead to bronchiectasis, fibrosis, airflow obstruction and progressive loss of lung function. In the younger patient, the first pathogen to be isolated from sputum or throat swab is usually *Staph. aureus*, which may be cleared by courses of flucloxacillin or erythromycin, with sodium fusidate or a cephalosporin in reserve. Clindamycin is another valuable agent, and is usually well tolerated in children. The former practice of long-term prophylaxis with flucloxacillin or cloxacillin until adolescence has been abandoned in favour of intermittent courses of antibiotics such as 14-day courses of sodium fusidate with floxacillin if *Staph. aureus* is the dominant isolate. *H. influenzae* is another common pathogen responding to several antibiotics, with cephalosporins, co-amoxiclav and the newer macrolides of special importance, and the role of ampicillin and its congeners lessening because of a high prevalence of resistance in most places.

Eventually most cystic fibrosis patients become colonized by *Ps. aeruginosa*. Once present, this organism is not eradicated for more than a few days or weeks by any form of chemotherapy, although there is some evidence that antipseudomonal aerosol treatment as soon as the organism is first isolated may delay chronic colonization (Valerius et al 1991). Treatment is based on deterioration in clinical parameters rather than on the presence or absence of the organism in sputum, although susceptibilities of the dominant strain are a guide to the selection of antibiotic. Parenteral chemotherapy with an aminoglycoside plus an antipseudomonal penicillin has been widely used. McLaughlin et al (1983) obtained similar results from three regimens, ticarcillin–tobramycin, azlocillin–tobramycin and azlocillin–placebo, with a trend to a higher incidence of drug-resistant strains in the azlocillin-only group. An alternative to combinations such as these is monotherapy with ceftazidime. Although the clinical benefits of ciprofloxacin, an orally administered drug, have proved substantial (Hodson et al 1987), so too have the problems of emerging resistance of the resident *Ps. aeruginosa* to this compound. In patients requiring frequent hospital admission, the long-term use of gentamicin and carbenicillin by aerosol has been shown to improve lung function, without either eliminating pseudomonas or inducing drug resistance (Hodson et al 1981). An important placebo-controlled trial of aerosolized tobramycin (Ramsey et al 1993), in which patients received the active agent or placebo during 28-day periods, showed clear diminution of the intensity of pseudomonas colonization during the periods of tobramycin, with no toxicity and no difference between the groups in the emergence of resistant strains. Such treatment is expensive and time-consuming and is only at present recommended in those whose condition deteriorates progressively. Antibiotic treatment of cystic fibrosis is reviewed by Michel (1988) and by Hodson & Warner (1992).

In recent years, infection by other organisms has become a problem, especially by *Burkholderia (Pseudomonas) cepacia*, often acquired in the hospital environment. Although resistant to most antibiotics in vitro, infection may apparently respond to the regimens discussed.

Although the role of antibiotics given by aerosol inhalation has recently been tested mainly in cystic fibrosis, this method of treatment can occasionally be of value in other situations, for example in some patients in ICUs who are seriously ill with pseudomonas chest infections, since adequate concentrations of aminoglycoside antibiotics can be achieved without the danger of producing high plasma concentrations.

Influenza

Treatment

Two drugs, amantadine and rimantadine, have been extensively studied as prophylactic and therapeutic agents in influenza. The former is licensed in the UK and both are available in the USA. They share great advantages in their satisfactory activity after oral administration and in their generally low toxicity, but also the disadvantage that their activity is confined to influenza A virus strains. Both reduce the duration of fever by about half and also reduce malaise, while direct evidence of their antiviral activity is shown by a significant reduction of viral shedding. A comparative trial of the two agents (Dolin et al 1982) showed a similar degree of reduction of influenza-like illness and of laboratory evidence of infection by both agents. However, in this and other studies, rimantadine was superior from the point of view of unwanted effects, which required 22% of the amantadine group to withdraw from the trial, compared with 10% of the rimantadine group and 11% of the placebo group.

The effect of these agents has been demonstrated as additional to the benefits of vaccination. Other objective evidence of benefit from these drugs included reduction of virus shedding, and an accelerated improvement in the abnormalities of peripheral airways function during the course of influenza. Amantadine is used in therapy in dose of 200 mg/day, reduced to 100 mg/day in patients over 65 years of age.

Resistant strains can be isolated within a few days of treatment by either agent, and are capable of spreading to contacts. A multicentre trial showed rimantidine to be ineffective in the prophylaxis of influenza if the index case

had been treated with the drug (Hayden et al 1989). Other methods of treatment have also been used with some success. Both amantadine and rimantadine have been given by aerosol administration. In addition, the broad-spectrum antiviral compound tribavirin (ribavirin), of unacceptable toxicity when given orally, has been used by the aerosol route in both influenza A and B infection.

Prophylaxis

Studies of amantadine in therapy were preceded by extensive investigations of its possible role in prophylaxis during outbreaks of influenza A infection. These clearly showed a diminished incidence of influenza illness and virological evidence of infection in patients receiving the drug, suggesting its possible value during the period of an influenza A epidemic. Its lack of effect on influenza B infection is a clear disadvantage, especially in closed institutions such as boarding schools in which amantadine prophylaxis has its greatest potential role. Several authors have commented on the apparently paradoxical situation that drugs of proven value both in prevention and treatment of an important respiratory infection, and of acceptably low toxicity, are in fact little used for these purposes. Perhaps the capricious nature of influenza outbreaks, and the large number of other infections giving rise to similar syndromes, is responsible for this state of affairs.

Current recommendations in the UK (Wiselka 1994) suggest the use of amantadine for prophylaxis during an influenza outbreak

- In high-risk subjects, if unvaccinated, for 2 weeks following their vaccination
- For the whole epidemic period in high-risk patients in whom vaccination is contraindicated or likely to be ineffective
- For unvaccinated health-care workers and key staff
- For residents and staff of residential homes irrespective of their vaccination status.

Dose in prophylaxis should be 100 mg/day because of the increased risk of adverse effects in these mainly elderly patients. Guidelines such as these tend to be forgotten, no doubt because of the erratic nature of influenza outbreaks, but the serious impact of influenza on vulnerable populations indicates their importance at times of high influenza prevalence.

Respiratory syncytial virus infections

RSV is an important cause of lower respiratory tract illness in infancy and childhood, in both temperate and tropical climates, producing a variety of syndromes, of which acute bronchiolitis is the most characteristic. The virus is a common cause of hospital-acquired infection in children's wards, an aspect of its epidemiology of great importance, since the mortality from these infections in immuno-compromised children and those with heart and lung disease is very much greater than in previously normal patients. In normal adults RSV is less important, chiefly causing upper tract syndromes, but the virus is a common cause of exacerbations of bronchitis, and outbreaks with high case-fatality rates have been recorded in nursing homes for elderly patients (Editorial 1986).

The activity of tribavirin (ribavirin), a broad-spectrum antiviral agent also used in the treatment of Lassa fever, has been extensively studied in RSV infection. To avoid systemic toxicity the drug has mainly been administered by aerosol, involving very long periods of treatment each day for several days. Double-blind trials showed substantial benefit in reduced cough, general well-being and arterial oxygen saturation. Benefit was found in trials involving previously normal children and also in those with bronchopulmonary dysplasia and congenital heart disease, the latter groups showing particularly notable improvement in the first day of treatment.

The results of a substantial number of trials can be illustrated, for example, by that of Rodriguez et al (1987), in which infants with RSV infection treated with aerosolized tribavirin showed significant improvements in clinical score, physical signs and oxygen saturation compared with the placebo controls. Shedding of RSV was also significantly reduced in the treated group. The expense and complexity of this treatment has tended to confine its use to infants at special risk. Breese-Hall et al (1985), in a comparative placebo-controlled trial in children with bronchopulmonary dysplasia and congenital heart disease, showed significant benefit from treatment without adverse effects; resistance to tribavirin was not demonstrated in virus isolates collected after the treatment period. Conrad et al (1987) compared 33 infants with predisposing conditions or who were severely ill with RSV infections with 97 untreated patients seen during the same epidemic. The most notable clinical improvement was seen between the first and second days of treatment. Tribavirin by the aerosol route has also been shown to be beneficial in parainfluenza virus infections, and to a lesser extent in influenza A and B, but a negative result in a double-blind trial in influenza B has also been reported by Bernstein et al (1988). The drug can be delivered by face mask or into an oxygen hood or oxygen tent. It can also be given with assisted ventilation, but filters must be replaced regularly since there is a danger that the drug may precipitate in the equipment and impede safe ventilation (Smith et al 1991).

Despite a number of trials giving favourable results, the cost and difficulty of this form of treatment have led to continued uncertainty about valid indications. We agree with the conclusions of a recent review (Rakshi & Couriel 1994) that it would be reasonable to confine its use to 'patients with proved RSV infection and cystic fibrosis, severe immunodeficiency, congenital heart disease and pulmonary hypertension, and in infants with bronchopulmonary dysplasia and pre-existing oxygen dependence'. Indications in the USA are set rather more broadly, including infants less than 6 weeks old and all those receiving mechanical ventilation (American Academy of Pediatrics 1993), but there is a growing tendency to a more restrictive use of this agent.

An additional problem with the use of tribavirin inhalation therapy is the bronchospasm and eye irritation it sometimes causes in health care workers. Englund et al (1994) found a possible solution in a trial which showed that three 2-h periods of therapy in every 24 h were as effective as the usual 18-h period.

Other aspects of treatment

The question of antibacterial drugs is often contentious. Secondary bacterial infection was noted in only 13 of 565 hospital patients with RSV infection (Breese-Hall et al 1988) and antibacterial drugs are recommended only in those patients with atypical features suggesting this possibility. Neither corticosteroids nor bronchodilators are of value in acute bronchiolitis. Warm and humidified oxygen is often essential to relieve hypoxia, and some patients require artificial ventilation.

Prevention of RSV infection

Nosocomial infection with RSV is a serious problem in paediatric units. The extent of the risk and the possibilities for prevention obviously relate to the physical facilities, staffing levels and training and other factors which vary from place to place. Despite these variables, a number of studies leave no doubt that hospital staff play an important part in causing cross-infection, especially by way of hand contamination. Cross-infection rates can be 15–30%, and many of these infections have severe or even lethal consequences for the vulnerable patient (Editorial 1992). A careful study from Scotland (Madge et al 1992) recorded a cross-infection rate of 26% when no special precautions were taken. This was significantly reduced (to 9.5%) by cohort nursing combined with wearing of gowns and gloves for all contacts; neither measure alone was effective, but many units rely only on isolation of suspected or known RSV-infected patients, and hand washing.

High-titre anti-RSV immunoglobulin gas been used successfully for prophylaxis in infants and children at high risk, but is not generally available (Groothius et al 1993). This type of prophylaxis may become more accessible with the development of RSV-specific monoclonal antibodies.

References

Aldous P M 1991 A comparison of clarithromycin with ampicillin in the treatment of out-patients with acute bacterial exacerbations of chronic bronchitis. *Journal of Antimicrobial Chemotherapy* 27 (suppl A): 101–108

American Academy of Pediatrics, Committee on Infectious Diseases 1993 Use of ribavirin in the treatment of respiratory syncytial virus infection. *Pediatrics* 92: 501–505

Anderson G, Esmonde T S, Coles S, Macklin J, Carnegie C 1991 A comparative safety and efficacy study of clarithromycin and erythromycin stearate in community-acquired pneumonia. *Journal of Antimicrobial Chemotherapy* 27 (suppl A): 117–124

Anthonisen N R, Manfreda J, Warren C P W et al 1987 Antibiotic therapy in exacerbations of chronic obstructive pulmonary disease. *Annals of Internal Medicine* 106: 196–204

Bachand R T 1991 Comparative study of clarithromycin and ampicillin in the treatment of patients with acute bacterial exacerbations of chronic bronchitis. *Journal of Antimicrobial Chemotherapy* 27 (suppl A): 91–100

Bartlett J G, Gorbach S L 1983 Penicillin or clindamycin for primary lung abscess. *Annals of Internal Medicine* 98: 546–548

Bass J W 1985 Pertussis: current status of prevention and treatment. *Pediatric Infectious Diseases Journal* 4: 615–619

Bernstein J G, Reuman P D, Sherwood J R, Young E C, Schiff G M 1988 Ribavirin small particle aerosol treatment of influenza B virus infection. *Antimicrobial Agents and Chemotherapy* 32: 761–764

Breese-Hall C, McBridge J T, Gale C L, Hildreth S W, Schnabel K C 1985 Ribavirin treatment of respiratory syncytial viral infection in infants with underlying cardiopulmonary disease. *Journal of the American Medical Association* 254: 3047–3051

Breese-Hall C B, Powell K R, Schnabel K C, Gala C L, Pincus P H 1988 Risk of secondary bacterial infection in infants hospitalised with respiratory syncytial virus infection. *Journal of Pediatrics* 113: 266–271

British Thoracic Society 1993 Guidelines for the management of community-acquired pneumonia in adults admitted to hospital. *British Journal of Hospital Medicine* 49: 346–350

British Thoracic Society and Public Health Laborarory Service 1987 Community-acquired pneumonia in adults in British hospitals in 1982–1983: a survey of aetiology, mortality, prognostic factors and outcome. *Quarterly Journal of Medicine NS* 62: 195–220

British Thoracic Society and Public Health Laboratory Service 1992 The aetiology, management and outcome of severe community-acquired pneumonia on the intensive therapy unit. *Respiratory Medicine* 86: 7–13

Campbell H, Byass P, Forgie I M et al 1988 Trial of co-trimoxazole versus procaine penicillin with ampicillin in treatment of community-acquired pneumonia in young Gambian children. *Lancet* ii: 1182–1184

Carbon C 1993 Quinolones in the treatment of lower respiratory infections in adult patients. *Drugs* 45 (suppl 3): 91–97

Chan R, Hemeryck L, O'Regan M, Clancy L, Feely J 1995 Oral versus intravenous antibiotics for community acquired lower respiratory tract infections in a general hospital: randomised controlled trial. *British Medical Journal* 310: 1360–1362

Cole P, Roberts D E, Davies S F, Knight R K 1983 A simple oral antimicrobial regimen effective in severe chronic bronchial suppuration associated with culturable *H. influenzae*. *Journal of Antimicrobial Chemotherapy* 11: 109–113

Conrad D A, Christenson J C, Waner J L, Marks M L 1987 Aerolised ribavirin treatment of RSV infection in infants hospitalised during an epidemic. *The Pediatric Infectious Diseases Journal* 6: 152–158

Cook P J, Honeybourne D 1994 Review. *Chlamydia pneumoniae*. *Journal of Antimicrobial Chemotherapy* 34: 859–873

Currie D C, Garbett N D, Chan K L et al 1990 Double-blind randomized study of prolonged higher dose oral amoxycillin in purulent bronchiectasis. *Quarterly Journal of Medicine NS* 76: 799–816

Dolin R, Reichman R C, Madore H P et al 1982 A controlled trial of amantadine and rimantadine in the prophylaxis of influenza A infection. *New England Journal of Medicine* 307: 580–584

Edelstein P H, Calarco K, Yasui V K 1984 Antimicrobial therapy of experimentally induced Legionnaire's disease in guinea-pigs. *American Review of Respiratory Diseases* 130: 849–856

Editorial 1986 Ribavirin and respiratory syncytial virus. *Lancet* i: 362–363

Editorial 1988a Scrub typhus pneumonia. *Lancet* ii: 1062–1063

Editorial 1988b Pneumonia in childhood. *Lancet* i: 741–743

Editorial 1992 Nosocomial infection with respiratory syncytial virus. *Lancet* 340: 1071–1072

Englund J A, Piedra P A, Ahu Y, Gilbert P E, Hiatt P 1994 High-dose short duration ribavirin aerosol therapy compared with standard ribavirin therapy in children with suspected respiratory syncytial virus infection. *Journal of Pediatrics* 125: 635–641

Feldman C, Kallenhach J M, Miller S D, Thorburn J R, Koornhof H J 1985 Community-acquired pneumonia due to penicillin-resistant pneumococci. *New England Journal of Medicine* 313: 615–617

Finegold S M 1988 Legionnaire's disease – still with us [Editorial]. *New England Journal of Medicine* 318: 571–573

Fink M P, Snydman D R, Niederman M S et al 1994 Treatment of severe pneumonia in hospitalized patients: results of a multi-center, randomized, double-blind trial comparing intravenous ciprofloxacin with imipenem-cilastatin. *Antimicrobial Agents and Chemotherapy* 38: 547–557

Forgie I M, O'Neill K P, Lloyd-Evans N et al 1991 Etiology of acute lower respiratory tract infections in Gambian children. I. Acute lower respiratory tract infections in infants presenting at the hospital. *Pediatric Infectious Diseases Journal* 10: 33–41

Forgie I M, O'Neill K P, Lloyd-Evans N et al 1991 Etiology of acute lower respiratory tract infections in Gambian children. II. Acute lower respiratory infection in children aged one to nine years presenting at the hospital. *Pediatric Infectious Diseases Journal* 10: 42–47

Friedland I R 1995 Treatment of pneumococcal infection in the era of increasing penicillin resistance. *Current Opinion in Infectious Diseases* 8: 213–217

Friis B, Andersen P, Brenoe E et al 1984 Antibiotic treatment of pneumonia and bronchitis, a prospective randomised trial. *Archives of Diseases in Childhood* 59: 1038–1045

Gadomski A M 1993 Potential interventions for preventing pneumonia among young children: lack of effect of antibiotic treatment for lower respiratory infections. *The Pediatric Infectious Diseases Journal* 12: 115–120

Gonzales R, Sande M 1995 What will it take to stop physicians from prescribing antibiotics in acute bronchitis? *Lancet* 345: 665–666

Grayston J T 1992 Infections caused by *Chlamydia pneumoniae* strain TWAR. *Clinical Infectious Diseases* 15: 757–761

Groothuis J R, Simoes E A F, Levin M J et al 1993 Prophylactic administration of respiratory virus immunoglobulin to high risk infants and young children. *New England Journal of Medicine* 329: 1524–1530

Hammond J M J, Potgieter P D, Linton D M, Forder A A 1990 Intensive care management of community-acquired klebsiella pneumonia. *Respiratory Medicine* 84: 11–16

Hayden F G, Belshe R B, Clover R D, Hay A J, Oakes M G 1989 Emergence and apparent transmission of rimantidine-resistant influenza A virus in families. *New England Journal of Medicine* 321: 1696–1702

Hodson M E, Warner J O 1992 Respiratory problems and their treatment (in cystic fibrosis). *British Medical Bulletin* 48: 931–948

Hodson M E, Penketh A R L, Batten J C 1981 Aerosol carbenicillin and gentamicin treatment of *Ps. aeruginosa* infections in patients with cystic fibrosis. *Lancet* ii: 1137–1139

Hodson M E, Roberts C M, Butland R J A, Smith M J, Batten J C 1987 Oral ciprofloxacin compared with conventional intravenous treatment for *Pseudomonas aeruginosa* infection in adults with cystic fibrosis. *Lancet* i: 235–237

Horwitz M A, Silverstein S C 1983 Intracellular multiplication of legionnaire's disease bacteria (*L. pneumophilia*) in human monocytes is reversibly inhibited by erythromycin and rifampicin. *Journal of Clinical Investigation* 71: 15–26

Hosker H S R, Jones G M, Hawkey P 1994 Management of community-acquired lower respiratory tract infection. *British Medical Journal* 308: 701–705

Korner R J, Reeves D S, MacGowan A P 1994 Dangers of oral fluoroquinolone treatment in community acquired upper respiratory tract infections. *British Medical Journal* 308: 191–192

Levison M E, Mangura C T, Lorder B et al 1983 Clindamycin compared with penicillin for the treatment of anaerobic lung abscess. *Annals of Internal Medicine* 98: 466–471

Levy H, Simpson S Q 1994 Hantavirus pulmonary syndrome. *American Journal of Critical Care* 149: 1710–1713

MacFarlane J T, Finch R G, Ward M J, Rose D H 1983 Erythromycin compared with a combination of ampicillin and amoxycillin as initial treatment for adults with pneumonia including Legionnaire's disease. *Journal of Infection* 7: 111–117

MacFarlane J T, Colville, Guion A, MacFarlane R M, Rose D H 1993 Prospective study of aetiology and outcome of adult lower respiratory infections in the community. *Lancet* 341: 511–514

McGowan J E 1987 Respiratory tract infections due to *Branhamella catarrhalis* and *Neisseria* species. In: Remington J S, Swartz M N (eds) Current clinical topics in infectious diseases. McGraw-Hill, New York, ch 8, p 181–203

Mackay A D 1980 Amoxycillin versus ampicillin in treatment of exacerbations of chronic bronchitis. *British Journal of Diseases of the Chest* 74: 379–384

McLaughlin F J, Matthews W J, Strider D J et al 1983 Clinical and bacteriological response to three antibiotic regimens for acute exacerbations of cystic fibrosis: ticarcillin–tobramycin, azlocillin–tobramycin and azlocillin–placebo. *Journal of Infectious Diseases* 147: 559–567

McLeod D T, Ahmad F, Capewell S, Croghan M J, Calder M A, Seaton A 1986 Increase in bronchopulmonary infection due to *Branhamelia catarrhalis*. *British Medical Journal* 292: 1103–1105

Madge P, Paton J Y, McColl J H, Mackie P L K 1992 Prospective controlled study of four infection-control procedures to prevent nosocomial infection with respiratory syncytial virus. *Lancet* 340: 1079–1083

Mastro T D, Ghafoor A, Khalid Nomani N et al 1991 Antimicrobial resistance of pneumococci in children with acute lower respiratory tract infection in Pakistan. *Lancet* 337: 156–159

Michel B C 1988 Antibacterial therapy in cystic fibrosis – a review of the literature, published between 1980 and February 1987. *Chest* 94 (suppl): S129–S140

Niederman M S, Bass J B, Campbell G D et al 1993 Guidelines for the initial management of adults with community-acquired pneumonia: diagnosis, assessment of severity and initial antimicrobial therapy. *American Review of Respiratory Diseases* 148: 1418–1421

Pallares R, Gudiol F, Linares J et al 1987 Risk factors and response to antibiotic therapy in adults with bacteremic pneumonia caused by penicillin-resistant pneumococci. *New England Journal of Medicine* 317: 18–22

Perlino C A 1981 Metronidazole vs. clindamycin treatment of anaerobic pulmonary infection. Failure of metronidazole therapy. *Archives of Internal Medicine* 141: 1424–1427

Pines A 1982 The tetracyclines in purulent exacerbations of chronic bronchitis. *Journal of Antimicrobial Chemotherapy* 9: 337–351

Pines A, Raafat H, Greenfield J S B, Linsell W 1972 Antibiotic regimens in moderately ill patients with purulent exacerbation of chronic bronchitis. *British Journal of Diseases of the Chest* 66: 107–115

Powell M 1991 Chemotherapy for infections caused by *Haemophilus influenzae*: current problems and future prospects. *Journal of Antimicrobial Chemotherapy* 27: 3–7

Rakshi K, Courciel J M 1994 Management of acute bronchiolitis. *Archives of Diseases of Childhood* 71: 463–469

Ramsey B W, Doekin H L, Eisenberg J D 1993 Efficacy of aerosolized tobramycin in patients with cystic fibrosis. *New England Journal of Medicine* 328: 1740–1746

Raoult D, Marrie T 1995 Q fever. *Clinical Infectious Diseases* 20: 489–495

Rodriguez W J, Kim H W, Brandt C D et al 1987 Aerosolized ribavirin in the treatment of patients with respiratory syncytial virus disease. *The Pediatric Infectious Diseases Journal* 6: 159–163

Roig J, Carreres A, Domingo C 1993 Treatment of Legionnaires disease: current recommendations. *Drugs* 46: 63–79

Sazawal S, Black R E 1992 Meta-analysis of intervention trials on case management of pneumonia in community settings. *Lancet* 340: 528–533

Shann F 1986 Etiology of severe pneumonia in children in developing countries. *Pediatric Infectious Diseases* 5: 247–252

Shann F, Gratten M, Germer S, Linneman V, Hazlett D, Payne R 1984 Aetiology of pneumonia in children in Goroka Hospital, Papua New Guinea. *Lancet* ii: 537–540

Simoes E A F 1994 Recognizing and diagnosing pneumonia in developing countries. *Current Opinion in Infectious Diseases* 7: 358–363

Slevin N J, Aitken J, Thornley P E 1984 Clinical and microbiological features of *Branhamella catarrhalis* bronchopulmonary infections. *Lancet* i: 782–783

Smith D W, Frankel L R, Mathers L H, Tang A T S, Ariagno R L, Prober C G 1991 A controlled trial of aerosolized ribavirin in infants receiving mechanical ventilation for severe respiratory syncytial virus infection. *New England Journal of Medicine* 325: 24–29

Steketee R W, Wassilack S L F, Adkins W N et al 1988 Evidence for a high attack rate and efficacy of erythromycin prophylaxis in a pertussis outbreak in a facility for the developmentally disabled. *Journal of Infectious Diseases* 157: 434–440

Stott N C H, West R R 1976 Randomised controlled trial of antibiotics in patients with cough and purulent sputum. *British Medical Journal* 2: 556–559

Tan T Q, Mason E O, Kaplan S L 1993 Penicillin-resistant systemic pneumococcal infection in children; a retrospective case-control study. *Pediatrics* 92: 761–767

Valerius N H, Koch C, Hoiby N 1991 Prevention of chronic *Ps. aeruginosa* colonisation in cystic fibrosis by early treatment. *Lancet* 338: 725–726

Verheij T J M, Hermans J, Mulder J D 1994 Effects of doxycycline in patients with acute cough and purulent sputum: a double blind placebo controlled trial. *British Journal of General Practice* 44: 400–404

Wallace R J, Mucher D M, Martin R R 1978 *Hemophillus influenzae* pneumonia in adults. *American Journal of Medicine* 64: 87–93

Watanakunahorn C 1987 Bacteremic *Staphylococcus aureus* pneumonia. *Scandinavian Journal of Infectious Diseases* 19: 623–627

Wiselka M 1994 Influenza: diagnosis, management and prophylaxis. *British Medical Journal* 308: 1341–1345

Woodhead M A, MacFarlane J T, McCracken J S, Rose D H, Finch R G 1987a Prospective study of the aetiology and outcome of pneumonia in the community. *Lancet* i: 671–674

Woodhead M A, Radvan J, MacFarlane J T 1987b Adult community-acquired staphylococcal pneumonia in the antibiotic era; a review of 61 cases. *Quarterly Journal of Medicine* NS 64: 783–790

Endocarditis

D. T. Durack

Introduction

The diagnosis 'infective endocarditis' (IE) refers to microbial infection of the heart valves or endocardium. This is not a single disease, but a diverse group of diseases. Many species of microorganism can infect the interior of the heart; the primary lesions can occur in a variety of locations; the pathology is variable; and the time course of the illness can range from chronic to fulminant (Box 49.1). These features can occur in many combinations. Therefore, there can be no single or simple regimen for treatment of IE. Treatment should be chosen from the long list of possible regimens after careful assessment of all available information on each individual case.

PRINCIPLES OF TREATMENT

For optimal treatment of this serious disease, certain requirements should be met. These include: accurate diagnosis of IE; assessment of the patient's cardiac status, and any complications of IE; correct choice between empirical and specific treatment; identification of the aetiological organism; reliable antibiotic susceptibility information; total eradication of the aetiological organisms; correct timing of surgical intervention, when indicated; adequate follow-up after treatment; and consideration of prophylaxis against future episodes.

Accurate diagnosis of IE

Because IE is not one but many different diseases, it is not surprising that its clinical manifestations can be numerous and confusing. The differential diagnosis is wide, and confirmation of a presumptive diagnosis of IE can be difficult. One diagnostic approach requires either surgical or autopsy proof before the diagnosis of 'definite IE' can be accepted. However, a recent revision of the diagnostic criteria for IE allows accurate diagnosis of 'definite IE' based on clinical criteria, without requiring surgery or autopsy. Alternative diagnoses such as bacteraemia without IE and other infective and non-infective conditions should be carefully considered and excluded before a secure diagnosis of IE is made.

Box 49.1   *Infective endocarditis and endarteritis: a variety of diseases*

Location	Organisms	Pathology	Progression
Native heart valve	Bacteria	Vegetations – valvular	Acute
Prosthetic heart valve	Rickettsiae	Vegetations – other sites	Subacute
Endocardium or endothelium	Chlamydiae	Perforation of valve	Chronic
Intracardiac devices (e.g. catheters, pacemakers, patches, implants)	Fungi, yeasts	Abscess	
	Fungi, moulds	Pseudoaneurysm	
Ventricular assist devices		Mycotic aneurysm	
Intravascular grafts and devices		Infected thrombus	

Accurate assessment of cardiac status and complications

Many patients with IE have new intracardiac pathology due to IE itself as well as pre-existing heart disease. There may be systemic complications such as arterial emboli, infarcts, haemorrhages, abscesses or mycotic aneurysms. To guide optimal management, all such lesions should be identified and assessed by means of appropriate tests including echo-cardiography, cardiac catheterization, and imaging by X-ray, computerized tomography or magnetic resonance imaging.

Correct choice between empirical and specific treatment

Early in the course of illness, IE may be suspected or considered, but a definitive diagnosis cannot be made at that time. Under these circumstances, the question arises of whether to give empirical therapy immediately, or to wait for blood cultures and other test results. This can best be decided by determining whether the illness is due to acute or subacute endocarditis.

Identification of the aetiological organism

Because the natural history, treatment and prognosis is highly dependent upon the infecting organism, proper speciation is desirable. For example, group D streptococcal endocarditis could be caused by either *Streptococcus bovis* or by *Enterococcus faecalis,* but the treatment and prognosis for each are quite different.

Reliable antibiotic susceptibility information

Because many different species and strains of micro-organisms can cause IE, many different patterns of antibiotic susceptibility will be found. Previously stable sensitivity patterns may change due to the spread of antibiotic resistance among species of bacteria. Dependable information on susceptibility must be available to choose the best treatment.

Total eradication of the aetiological organisms

In most bacterial and fungal infections, cure can be achieved by antibiotic treatment without necessarily killing all the aetiological organisms. Inhibition of growth or reduction in the number of organisms in infected tissues is often sufficient, because host defenses can eradicate the few remaining pathogens. This is the reason why bacteriostatic antimicrobials are often highly effective in treatment of infections, e.g. tetracyclines in some forms of pneumonia. In IE, however, host defences are partially or completely excluded from the vegetations, so that a total bactericidal effect is needed to prevent relapse.

Microbiological cure refers to the eradication of all the aetiological organisms, which is necessary but not always sufficient for *clinical cure.* For example, patients with IE may die of stroke or heart failure, or suffer other serious complications, despite being microbiologically 'cured'.

Correct timing of surgical intervention, when indicated

Surgery is indicated in up to one-third of cases of IE to achieve the best possible outcome. Selection of cases for surgery, and choice of the optimal time to intervene, are critically important aspects of management. This is a complex subject, the details of which are outside the scope of this chapter.

Adequate follow-up after treatment

Relapse after correct treatment of IE is uncommon. The actual frequency of relapse varies according to the infecting organism and associated cardiac lesions. Less than 2% of patients relapse after treatment of native valve IE due to penicillin-sensitive streptococci. This rate is less than the rate of reinfection; in other words, recurrent IE after treatment usually is more likely to be due to reinfection than to relapse. Higher rates of relapse (5–15%) follow treatment of staphylococcal, Gram-negative and prosthetic valve IE, especially if a valve-ring abscess has developed. In all cases, proper follow-up is needed to identify possible relapses. In the asymptomatic patient whose blood count, C-reactive protein (CRP) and erythrocyte sedimentation rate (ESR) are normal or returning toward normal after treatment, follow-up blood cultures are unnecessary. However, the possibility of relapse should be kept in mind; any indication (especially recurrent fever) that cure has not been achieved should lead to immediate re-evaluation, including follow-up blood cultures.

Consideration of prophylaxis against future episodes

After microbiological cure of an episode of IE, the patient is in double jeopardy for another episode. The original predisposition remains, and the cured IE itself is an additional risk factor for IE. Therefore, prophylaxis is indicated for selected future medical and dental procedures which might cause bacteraemia and possibly IE. Most important of these is dental extraction, but other medical procedures such as urinary tract instrumentation also constitute relative indications for administration of prophylactic antibiotics.

LABORATORY SUPPORT FOR TREATMENT OF ENDOCARDITIS

Information from the diagnostic microbiology laboratory is

essential for optimal management of IE because the choice of treatment depends primarily upon the identity and antibiotic sensitivities of the infecting organism. For each case, tests should be chosen which give the necessary information in a cost-effective manner.

Identification

The causative organism should be correctly characterized. The minimum information required is the type of bacteria and the relevant antibiotic sensitivity. Subacute IE caused by a fully penicillin-sensitive streptococcus could usually be cured without any further information. However, such a minimalist approach would yield little understanding of pathogenesis or portal of entry for the organism. To illustrate, a patient with IE due to a penicillin-sensitive streptococcus could be infected by either a viridans group organism originating from the mouth, or a strain of *Str. bovis* originating from the bowel. The implications are quite different: one case needs dental attention, the other investigation for a possible colonic tumour. Therefore, proper speciation of the aetiological organism is generally advisable. In special situations, further characterization by means of molecular typing may be useful. These techniques offer a reliable way to distinguish between epidemic strains, and between relapse and reinfection in patients with recurrent IE caused by similar organisms; biochemical profiles and antibiograms are no longer considered specific enough to establish that two isolates are the same.

Antimicrobial susceptibility tests

Accurate determination of susceptibility to relevant antimicrobials is needed to choose the best therapeutic regimens for IE. Currently, this has become even more critical because of increasing resistance among many of the enterococcal and staphylococcal species which commonly cause endocarditis.

Standard methods such as manual disk diffusion tests or automated systems using liquid media are acceptable for most organisms that cause IE. Measurement of both minimum inhibitory concentration (MIC) and minimum bactericidal concentration (MBC) for organisms causing IE has been recommended in the past. This arose from the well-documented observation that bactericidal antibiotics were more likely to cure IE than are bacteriostatic agents. However, convincing evidence has now accumulated showing that IE due to 'tolerant' organisms (which are inhibited but not killed by normally bactericidal antibiotics) usually can be cured effectively by these same antibiotics. This observation indicates that measurement of MBC does not provide essential information, so it is no longer routinely recommended.

In addition to antibiotic sensitivities, other relevant tests include detection or measurement of methicillin resistance among *Staphylococcus aureus* and *Staphylococcus epidermidis*, low- and high-level aminoglycoside resistance among enterococci, vancomycin resistance among enterococci, penicillinase production and serum antibiotic concentrations. Penicillinase production by enterococci can be missed by standard sensitivity assays because results are inoculum dependent; the nitrocefin assay should be used.

Measurement of serum antibiotic concentrations at appropriate intervals is needed for most patients receiving aminoglycosides or vancomycin, whether or not they have endocarditis. However, these tests are often ordered far more often than is necessary, thus wasting resources. Patients with normal renal function who are receiving once-daily doses of aminoglycosides at standard dosage (see Table 49.3) are unlikely to develop toxicity unless the duration of treatment is unusually long. Except in patients of advanced age, or with other special factors which might raise the likelihood of aminoglycoside toxicity, measuring serum creatinine two or three times weekly and aminoglycoside trough concentrations once or twice weekly is generally safe and economical.

To monitor the activity of antimicrobials during treatment, serum inhibitory and bactericidal titres (SIT and SBT) may be determined. This entails measuring the dilution of serum obtained from a patient receiving antimicrobial treatment which will inhibit (SIT) and kill (SBT) the patient's own aetiological organism. This test was popular, even routine, for monitoring of treatment of IE in the past. However, these tests are difficult to standardize, difficult to interpret, and neither necessary nor helpful in most cases of IE. If an unusual or unproven regimen is chosen, especially if treatment seems to be failing, it may occasionally be informative to measure SIT and SBT. If so, the test would be best performed by a specialized reference or research laboratory.

Treatment

Principles

The standard approach for treatment of IE is to administer one or more antimicrobials which meet two simple criteria: they can fully inhibit growth of the aetiological organism, and they have a history of proven effectiveness in treatment of IE due to the same or similar species. It is not always possible to meet these criteria. In the early stages of management of acute IE, it is usually necessary to choose empirical treatment before susceptibility results are available. This can be done by determining the most likely organisms on the basis of clinical evidence, then choosing antimicrobials which have a track record of efficacy against them. After initial tests have been completed, they may reveal that the organism is not fully susceptible to any of the standard antimicrobials. This is especially likely to occur in the case of enterococci. Finally, the aetiological organism may cause IE so rarely the there is little or no published experience available to guide treatment.

In general, the treatment regimen chosen for common bacterial pathogens should include a cell-wall active agent, i.e. a β-lactam or a glycopeptide, either alone or in combination. Because most recommended regimens recommended for treatment of IE utilize full dosages for several weeks, drug toxicity is common. Side-effects should be anticipated, and minimized by appropriate monitoring of kidney function and serum concentrations of drugs with timely dose adjustments as needed. IE is less common in children than in adults, but poses similar therapeutic problems. After suitable antimicrobials have been chosen, the doses employed for infants and small children must be carefully modified for paediatric use. Continuous intravenous infusion of antibiotics can be substituted for divided intravenous doses in any of the regimens recommended below. Antimicrobial efficacy is probably similar for both methods, but continuous infusion by means of a pump may be more convenient, especially if the patient receives part of the course of treatment as an outpatient.

EMPIRICAL THERAPY FOR IE

When a patient presents with symptoms and signs compatible with the diagnosis of IE, appropriate diagnostic tests including blood cultures and echocardiography must be ordered; then a decision must be made as to whether immediate empiric antibiotic therapy should be given before the diagnosis is confirmed. This decision depends mainly upon whether the patient has an acute or subacute endocarditis syndrome. Acute endocarditis is a rapidly progressive

disease caused by primary pathogens such as *Staph. aureus* or *Streptococcus pneumoniae*. These organisms can destroy cardiac valves rapidly; the associated septicaemia can cause severe symptoms; and they may give rise to 'metastatic' foci of infection by seeding tissues elsewhere in the body. Therefore, suspected acute endocarditis should be treated with antibiotics promptly, before the organism can be identified. Such cases should be treated as if they had staphylococcal infection, because this is one of the most likely causes of acute IE.

Subacute IE is usually caused by organisms of low virulence such as the viridans streptococci, and is more slowly progressive. This does not necessarily imply that the symptoms will be mild; a stroke or other serious complication can occur at any time. Subacute infection has usually been present for at least several weeks before the diagnosis is suspected, and antibiotics cannot immediately reverse the risk of progressive valvular damage or emboli; this takes 1–2 weeks. Therefore, in most subacute cases antibiotic therapy may be withheld for 1–2 days, awaiting the initial results of blood cultures and other diagnostic tests, and detailed interpretation of echocardiographs. This approach is advisable because, if antibiotics are given too early, the opportunity to recover the pathogen from further blood cultures may be lost. After 1–2 days initial blood culture results will often be available to confirm the diagnosis and to guide optimal choice of therapy. If after 36–48 h blood cultures remain negative but the diagnosis of subacute IE still seems likely, antibiotic treatment should not be further delayed; one additional set of blood cultures should be taken and empirical therapy begun. The antibiotic regimen should cover most species of streptococci, which are the organisms most likely to cause subacute endocarditis. The recommended regimens for empirical therapy are listed in Table 49.1.

Table 49.1 *Empirical regimens for treatment of IE when the pathogen is unknown (Durack 1990, Wilson et al 1995)*

Indication	Drug/dose	Route	Frequency	Duration	Notes
Acute endocarditis syndrome First-line regimen	Flucloxacillin or nafcillin 2 g + gentamicin 1 mg/kg + vancomycin 15 mg/kg not to exceed 2 g/day	i.v. i.v. i.v.	Every 4 h Every 8 h Every 12 h	Until pathogen is identified, or 4 weeks, whichever is longer	Serum concentrations of gentamicin and vancomycin should be monitored, and doses adjusted accordingly
Alternative regimen	Ceftazidime 2.0 g + gentamicin 1 mg/kg + vancomycin 15 mg/kg not to exceed 2 g/day	i.v. i.v. i.v.	Every 8 h Every 8 h Every 12 h	Until pathogen is identified, or 4 weeks, whichever is longer	For patients allergic to penicillins but not cephalosporin. Serum concentrations of gentamicin and vancomycin should be monitored, and doses adjusted accordingly

Table 49.1 Cont'd

Indication	Drug/dose	Route	Frequency	Duration	Notes
Subacute endocarditis syndrome First-line regimen	Ampicillin 2.0 g + gentamicin 1.5 mg/kg	i.v. i.v.	Every 4 h Every 12 h	Until pathogen is identified, or 4 weeks, whichever is longer	Serum concentrations of gentamicin should be monitored, and doses adjusted accordingly
Alternative regimen	Vancomycin 15 mg/kg not to exceed 2 g/day + gentamicin 1.5 mg/kg	i.v. i.v.	Every 12 h Every 12 h	Until pathogen is identified, or 4 weeks, whichever is longer	For patients allergic to penicillin. Serum concentrations of vancomycin and gentamicin should be monitored, and doses adjusted accordingly

STREPTOCOCCAL ENDOCARDITIS

Streptococci are the commonest cause of IE. Many different species fall under this classification, with a variety of antibiotic sensitivity patterns (Table 49.2).

Penicillin-sensitive streptococci

Most non-enterococcal streptococci are still fully penicillin sensitive, defined by an MIC for penicillin of ≤0.1 mg/l. This includes the common non-enterococcal group D species, *Str. bovis*. Several reliable regimens are available for treatment of uncomplicated IE caused by the sensitive streptococci (Table 49.4). The microbiological cure rate achieved by all these regimens against these organisms is approximately 98%, a rate so high that clinical trials have been unable to demonstrate significant differences between these regimens. The choice of regimen should be made on grounds of convenience and cost, for each case. Intravenous once-daily ceftriaxone for 4 weeks has the advantage of allowing many patients without complications or other contraindications to be discharged from hospital on outpatient parenteral therapy well before the end of treatment. If patients are properly selected, outpatient therapy is safe, popular with patients and economical.

A minority of streptococci are partially resistant to

Table 49.2 Summary of treatment options for various species and strains of streptococci that may cause IE

Group or genus	Selected species	Sensitivity	Main options for treatment
Viridans streptococci	*Str. sanguis* *Str. mutans* *Str. mitior* *Str. oralis*	Majority fully sensitive to penicillin; some intermediate; a few resistant	1. Penicillin or cephalosporin alone 2. Penicillin or cephalosporin + aminoglycoside 3. Vancomycin
Nutritionally variant strains of viridans streptococci	*Str. adjacens*	More likely to be tolerant or partially resistant to penicillin	β-Lactam + aminoglycoside
Group D Enterococci	*Ent. faecalis* *Ent. faecium* *Ent. durans* *Ent. gallinarum* *Ent. casseliflavus*	Usually resistant to penicillin; high and increasing rate of resistance to aminoglycosides and vancomycin	1. Penicillin + aminoglycoside 2. Vancomycin 3. Vancomycin + aminoglycoside
Non-enterococci	*Str. bovis* *Str. equinus*	Fully sensitive to penicillin	As for viridans group
Group B streptococci	*Str. agalactiae*	Fully sensitive to penicillin	
Group A, C, G streptococci	*Str. pyogenes*	Fully sensitive to penicillin	
Pneumococci	*Str. pneumoniae*	Majority fully sensitive to penicillin; some intermediate, a few resistant	

Table 49.3 *Recommended regimens for treatment of streptococcal (non-enterococcal) IE*

Indication	Drug/dose	Route	Frequency	Duration (weeks)	Notes
Penicillin-sensitive strains First-line regimens	Penicillin 2–4 million units (1.5–3.0 g)	i.v.	Every 6 h	4	Suitable for most patients who are not hypersensitive to penicillin
	Ceftriaxone 1–2 g	i.v. or i.m.	Once daily	4	Suitable for most patients; convenient for outpatient therapy
	Penicillin 3–4 million units (2–4 g) +	i.v.	Every 4 h	2	For patients <60 years old with no major complications
	gentamicin 3 mg/kg	i.v. or i.m.	Once daily	2	
	Ceftriaxone 1–2 g +	i.v. or i.m.	Once daily	2	For patients <60 years old with no major complications
	gentamicin 3 mg/kg	i.v. or i.m.	Once daily	2	
Alternative regimens	Ceftriaxone 2 g *followed by*	i.v. or i.m.	Once daily	2	Economical regimen; convenient for outpatient therapy
	amoxicillin 1 g	Orally	4 times daily	2	
	Vancomycin 15 mg/kg, not to exceed total dose of 2 g/day	i.v.	q. 12 h	4	For patients who cannot tolerate any β-lactam antibiotics
Partially resistant strains (MIC 0.1–1.0 mg/l) First-line regimen	Penicillin 3–4 million units (2–3 g) +	i.v.	Every 4 h	4	
	gentamicin 1 mg/kg	i.v. or i.m.	Every 8 h	4	
Alternate regimen	Vancomycin 15 mg/kg not to exceed total dose of 4 g/day +	i.v.	q. 12 h	4	For patients hypersensitive to penicillin; needs careful monitoring of serum creatinine and antibiotic concentrations to manage toxicity
	gentamicin 1 mg/kg	i.v. or i.m.	Every 8 h	4	

Table 49.4 *Regimens for IE due to enterococci and penicillin-resistant streptococci (MIC ≥1 mg/l), including prosthetic valve endocarditis caused by these species (Durade 1990, Wilson et al 1995)*

Indication	Drug/dose	Route	Frequency	Duration (weeks)	Notes
First-line regimen	Penicillin 4 million units (2–3 g) *or* ampicillin 2 g + gentamicin 1 mg/kg	i.v.	Every 4 h	4–6	For strains that do not have high-level resistance to gentamicin
Alternative regimen	Vancomycin 15 mg/kg not to exceed 2 g/day total dose +	i.v.	Every 12 h	4–6	For highly penicillin-resistant strains; monitoring for toxicity essential
	gentamicin 1 mg/kg	i.v.	Every 8 h	4–6	

penicillin, with MICs varying between 0.1 and 1.0 mg/l. IE due to these strains should be treated with a regimen which includes an aminoglycoside to ensure high cure rates (Table 49.3). Alternatively, vancomycin alone could be used (Table 49.3). Penicillin-resistant strains with MIC of more than 1.0 mg/l should be treated like enterococci (Table 49.4).

Enterococci

These important species (Table 49.2) cause 5–10% of cases of IE. Because enterococci show high rates of both intrinsic and acquired resistance to antibiotics, some cases of enterococcal IE are very difficult to treat. This problem has

Table 49.5 *Potential drugs for treatment of IE caused by highly resistant or multiresistant enterococci. In each case, the choice will be affected by the sensitivity pattern of the individual strain isolated (M. E. Levison, personal communication)*

Resistance profile	Potential therapeutic options
High-level gentamicin resistance, MIC >500 mg/l	Cell wall active drug plus streptomycin
High-level streptomycin resistance, MIC >2000 mg/l	Cell wall active agent plus gentamicin
High-level resistance to both gentamicin and streptomycin	Cell wall active drug for 12 weeks or more, plus surgery as indicated
β-Lactamase-producing organism with high-level aminoglycoside resistance	Ampicillin/sulbactam, imipenem or glycopeptide
High-level penicillin resistance, MIC >64 mg/l	Glycopeptide plus aminoglycoside
Vancomycin A resistance, penicillin sensitive	β-Lactam plus aminoglycoside
Vancomycin A resistance, high-level penicillin resistance	Fluoroquinolone, doxycycline, teichoplanin, novobiocin, pristinamycins (two or more, according to sensitivity test results)
Vancomycin B resistance, penicillin sensitive	β-Lactam or teichoplanin plus aminoglycoside
Vancomycin B resistance, high-level penicillin resistance	Teichoplanin plus aminoglycoside

recently worsened because of the appearance of strains which are vancomycin resistant (mostly *Enterococcus faecium*) or β-lactamase producing (mostly *Ent. faecalis*).

Each isolate should be tested for antibiotic sensitivity to guide choice of treatment. Standard strains of *Ent. faecalis* are killed synergistically be penicillin plus an aminoglycoside, even if standard tests show that they are partially resistant to both drugs. The combination has long been proven effective for treatment of enterococcal IE, and therefore is recommended as the first-line regimen (Tables 49.4 and 49.5). However, synergistic killing is unlikely if the strain has one or more of the following properties: high-level resistance to gentamicin and/or streptomycin (MIC >500 mg/l or >2000 mg/l, respectively), high-level intrinsic resistance to penicillin (MIC ≥64 mg/l), or β-lactamase production (MIC ≥64 mg/l). For these strains, a regimen including vancomycin (Tables 49.4 and 49.5) should be used, unless the strain is resistant to it. Unfortunately, multiple-drug resistance is common among enterococci. For example, vancomycin-resistant strains frequently have high-level intrinsic resistance to penicillins.

Because published experience with treatment of IE caused by the most resistant strains of enterococci is limited, validated treatment regimens are not available. Some potentially useful alternative antimicrobials are listed in Table 49.5. For strains resistant to both vancomycin and aminoglycosides but partially sensitive to ampicillin, treatment can be attempted with an extended course of high-dose ampicillin alone: 16–20 g/day i.v. for 12 weeks or more. For vancomycin-resistant strains which also produce penicillinase, treatment can be attempted using a combination of ampicillin plus a β-lactamase inhibitor such as sulbactam or clavulanic acid. Other antibiotics may be chosen on the basis of sensitivity testing. Potentially active

drugs include fluoroquinolones, doxycycline, teicoplanin, novobiocin and pristinamycin derivatives (Synercid). When non-standard regimens are used to treat these resistant strains treatment should be prolonged (8–12 weeks or more, if toxicity allows) and valve replacement surgery should be considered early to improve the chance of microbiological cure.

STAPHYLOCOCCI

Staphylococci are the second most common group of bacteria causing IE, after the streptococci. They cause a variety of IE syndromes, the two most important being acute IE due to *Staph. aureus* and prosthetic valve infection by *Staph. epidermidis*. The outcome of staphylococcal IE is generally less favourable than for streptococcal infections, and surgical intervention for complications, especially abscesses, is more likely to be needed. Because most strains are penicillin resistant due to β-lactamase production, the first-line treatment is a penicillinase-resistant β-lactam agent (Table 49.6). Patients who are hypersensitive to β-lactam drugs should be treated with vancomycin. Methicillin-resistant strains of *Staph. aureus* (MRSA) and *Staph. epidermidis* (MRSE) have become common (15–40% of isolates); these also require treatment with vancomycin. Because there are few satisfactory alternatives, the possibility that vancomycin resistance will emerge among staphylococci in the near future poses a serious threat to the effective treatment of IE.

Prosthetic valve infection with *Staph. epidermidis* is difficult to cure. Therefore, treatment with two or three antibiotics for at least 6 weeks is usually recommended, with surgical intervention as needed. Recommended

Table 49.6 *Regimens for treatment of IE caused by staphylococci, on native or prosthetic valves (Durack et al 1994, Wilson et al 1995)*

Indication	Drug/dose	Route	Frequency (weeks)	Duration	Notes
Staph. aureus Methicillin sensitive	Flucloxacillin or nafcillin 2 g	i.v.	Every 4 h	4–6	Neutropenia may occur. Gentamicin 3 mg/kg daily may be added for the first 3 days to achieve rapid killing by synergy, but is not of proven value
Methicillin resistant	Vancomycin 15 mg/kg not to exceed 2 g/day	i.v.	Every 12 h	4–6	
Staph. epidermidis	Vancomycin 15 mg/kg not to exceed 2 g/day +	i.v.	Every 12 h	4–6	
	gentamicin 1.5 mg/kg +	i.v.	Every 12 h	4–6	
	rifampicin 300 mg	i.v.	Twice daily	4–6	

regimens for the treatment of staphylococcal IE are listed in Table 49.6.

FASTIDIOUS GRAM-NEGATIVE (HACEK) ORGANISMS

The acronym HACEK derives from the initials of the following species: *Haemophilus* spp., *Actinobacillus actinomycetem-comitans*, *Cardiobacterium hominis*, *Eikenella* spp. and *Kingella kingae*. These are small Gram-negative bacilli which cause 3–5% of cases of IE. They usually cause subacute infection, sometimes with larger than usual vegetations; they are often nutritionally fastidious and slow-growing in blood culture. They are usually sensitive to ampicillin and cephalosporins. Ceftriaxone 2 g i.v. or i.m. plus gentamicin 3 mg/kg i.v. or i.m., both given once daily, is a convenient first-line regimen which can be completed as outpatient therapy in selected patients. Microbiological cure is usually achieved in 3–4 weeks and the overall prognosis is fairly good, although not as favourable as for subacute endo-carditis due to penicillin-sensitive streptococci.

GRAM-NEGATIVE BACILLI

Although the aerobic Gram-negative bacilli are common human pathogens which often cause bacteraemias, they seldom cause endocarditis. For example, IE caused by *Escherichia coli* or *Klebsiella* spp. is rare, even when bacteraemia occurs in a patient with pre-existing valvular disease. The most important genus is *Pseudomonas*, which occasionally causes IE in drug addicts or in patients with prosthetic valves. IE caused by *Brucella* species is important in some geographic regions, especially Spain and other countries bordering the Mediterranean.

Gram-negative bacilli tend to cause acute endocarditis, which is more difficult to cure and carries high morbidity and mortality. Treatment for each case should be chosen on the basis of antibiotic sensitivity testing of the aetiological organism. The preferred regimens combine a β-lactam antibiotic with an aminoglycoside, to be given parenterally for 6 weeks. Toxicity or drug hypersensitivity may occur during this long period of treatment, requiring either dose adjustment or change to another regimen. The rate of relapse after treatment is notably higher than for antibiotic-sensitive Gram-positive bacteria.

ENDOCARDITIS DUE TO UNUSUAL PATHOGENS

The list of organisms known to cause IE is long, but the majority are uncommon or rare. Strict anaerobes only rarely infect the heart, causing less than 1% of cases of IE. *Coxiella burnetii* causes a subacute systemic infection which may involve native or prosthetic heart valves. Microbiological cure is difficult to achieve with antimicrobials alone, so relapse is common. The highest chance of cure requires valve replacement as well as prolonged treatment with a tetracycline, for 6 months or more. If surgery cannot be done, treatment for at least 1 year is recommended; some experts suggest continuing suppressive therapy for life in these cases. *Chlamydia* spp. can cause IE, but are even more rare than *Coxiella* spp. infections. Several cases of IE caused by *Bartonella* spp. have recently been reported in patients with AIDS. The optimal treatment for this rare disease is not yet known; parenteral erythromycin for 4–6 weeks may be effective. Polymicrobial infections have been reported occasionally in drug addicts, but even in these patients cause less than 1% of cases.

FUNGAL ENDOCARDITIS

The most common form of fungal endocarditis is caused by yeasts, usually *Candida* spp. Most at risk are parenteral drug addicts, hospitalized patients, especially neonates and those on prolonged parenteral nutrition and patients with prosthetic valves. Blood cultures are less likely to be positive than in untreated bacterial endocarditis; repeated sampling will increase the chance of isolating yeasts. The best chance of cure requires valve replacement plus antifungal therapy. The disease is too rare to allow formal comparison of regimens such as amphotericin B versus imidazoles, and the optimal duration of therapy is unknown. A few cases have been cured with antifungal therapy alone when surgery could not be performed. In this situation, an imidazole such as fluconazole should be administered for 6–24 months, and possibly even longer. If the yeast is resistant to imidazoles, amphotericin B can be given until toxicity prevents its continuation. The prognosis for IE due to yeasts is worse than for bacterial endocarditis, but much better than for IE due to moulds. Either native or prosthetic valves may become infected with a mould. The most common pathogen is an *Aspergillus* species, but many other moulds have been reported as rare causes of IE. This distinct form of fungal IE is characterized by a high rate of negative blood cultures, and very poor prognosis. Surgery is the mainstay of treatment, but amphotericin B or another antifungal drug should be given according to the sensitivity of the aetiological species. Valve replacement should be performed whenever feasible, because cure without surgery is rare.

PREVENTION OF INFECTIVE ENDOCARDITIS

Although IE is an uncommon disease, prevention is desirable because of its high morbidity and significant mortality. Most

Box 49.2 *Estimates of risk for infective endocarditis related to pre-existing cardiac disorders (Durack 1995, 1997)*

Relatively high risk	**Intermediate risk**	**Low or negligible risk**
Prosthetic heart valves	Mitral valve prolapse with regurgitation	Mitral valve prolapse without regurgitation
Previous infective endocarditis	Pure mitral stenosis	Trivial valvular regurgitation by
Cyanotic congenital heart disease	Tricuspid valve disease	echocardiography without structural abnormality
Patent ductus arteriosus	Pulmonary stenosis	Isolated atrial septal defect
Aortic regurgitation*	Asymmetric septal hypertrophy	Arteriosclerotic plaques
Aortic stenosis*	Bicuspid aortic valve or calcific aortic sclerosis	Coronary artery disease
Mitral regurgitation	with minimal haemodynamic abnormality	Cardiac pacemaker
Mitral stenosis and regurgitation	Degenerative valvular disease in elderly patients	
Ventricular septal defect		
Coarctation of the aorta		
	Surgically repaired intracardiac lesions with	Surgically repaired intracardiac lesions, with
Surgically repaired intracardiac lesions with	minimal or no haemodynamic abnormality, less	minimal or no haemodynamic abnormality, more
residual haemodynamic abnormality	than 6 months after operation	than 6 months after operation

* Includes tricuspid, bicuspid and unicuspid valves.

Box 49.3 *Recommendations for use of prophylaxis for endocarditis with various procedures which may cause bacteraemia (Dajani et al 1990, Durack 1990, 1995)*

Prophylaxis recommended	**Prophylaxis not recommended**
Dental extractions, and intra-oral procedures that cause bleeding, including professional cleaning and scaling	Minor dental procedures not likely to cause bleeding, such as adjustment of orthodontic appliances, simple fillings above the gum line, root canal
Tonsillectomy, adenoidectomy and other operations that involve upper respiratory mucosa	Injection of intraoral local anaesthetic
Sclerotherapy for oesophageal varices and oesophageal dilatation	Shedding of primary teeth
Cystoscopy, urethral dilatation	Tympanostomy tube insertion
Urethral catheterization if urinary infection present	Endotracheal tube insertion
Urinary tract surgery, including prostatic surgery	Bronchoscopy with flexible bronchoscope, with or without biopsy
Incision and drainage of infected tissue	Cardiac catheterization
Vaginal delivery complicated by infection	Gastro-intestinal endoscopy with or without biopsy
Vaginal hysterectomy	Caesarian section and hysterectomy
	In the absence of infection: urethral catheterization, dilatation and curettage, uncomplicated vaginal delivery, therapeutic abortion, insertion or removal of intra-uterine device, sterilization procedures, laparoscopy

cases cannot be prevented, because the time of onset and the portal of entry for causative organisms cannot be precisely predicted. However, up to 5–7% of cases could be due to bacteria introduced during dental, surgical and diagnostic procedures. Tooth extraction appears to present a significant risk for viridans streptococcal IE in patients with predisposing cardiac conditions. For this reason, antibiotics are recommended before such procedures in an attempt to prevent some cases of IE.

Antibiotics can prevent experimental endocarditis in rabbits and rats, but have not been proven effective in humans. Therefore, this remains an empiric practice, which may have been overused in the past. Unnecessary use of antibiotics could promote emergence of resistant bacteria. Prophylaxis for IE is probably not cost-effective as a general strategy, but it may be worthwhile in selected situations.

The recommended approach is to give antibiotic to selected patients with higher risk cardiac conditions such as prosthetic valves or previous endocarditis (Box 49.2) before higher risk procedures such as tooth extraction or urinary tract surgery (Box 49.3). Prophylaxis should be considered optional for intermediate risk and unnecessary for low-risk situations.

Each patient should be given clear instruction on the procedure for notifying health-care providers of his or her condition and for obtaining antibiotic premedication. Preferably this information should be communicated in writing, in the form of a letter or printed wallet card kept by the patient. The regimen should be chosen according to standard recommendations such as those provided by the British Society for Antimicrobial Chemotherapy and the American Heart Association (Table 49.7).

Table 49.7 *Current recommendations for prophylaxis of endocarditis**

Indication	Regimen
Standard regimen	
For dental procedures; oral or upper respiratory tract surgery; minor GI or GU tract procedures	Amoxycillin 3.0 g orally 1 h before, then 1.5 g 6 h later
Special regimens	
Oral regimen for penicillin-allergic patients (oral and respiratory tract only)	Clindamycin 600 mg orally 1 h before, then 300 mg 6 h later
Parenteral regimen for high-risk patients; also for GI or GU tract procedures	Ampicillin 2 g i.v. or i.m. plus gentamicin 1.5 mg/kg i.v. or i.m. 0.5 h before
Parenteral regimen for penicillin-allergic patients	Vancomycin 1 g i.v. slowly over 1 h, starting 1 h before; add gentamicin 1.5 mg/kg i.m. or i.v. if GI or GU tract involved
Cardiac surgery including implantation of prosthetic valves	Cefazolin 2 g i.v. at induction of anaesthesia, repeated 8 and 16 h later *or* Vancomycin 1 g i.v. slowly over 1 h starting at induction, then 1 g i.v. 12 h later

GI, gastro-intestinal; GU, genito-urinary.
* Note that occasional prevention failures may occur with any regimen. These are recommendations only; clinical judgment as to safety and cost–benefit of prophylaxis should guide the decision in individual cases. One or two additional doses may be given if the period of risk for bacteraemia is prolonged. Gentamicin, 1.5 mg/kg i.v., may be given with each dose to increase activity against Gram-negative bacteria. Adapted from Dajani et al (1990), Durack (1990, 1995) and Working Party of the British Society of Antimicrobial Chemotherapy (1996).

References

Dajani A S, Bisno A L, Chung K J et al 1990 Prevention of bacterial endocarditis. Recommendations by the American Heart Association. *Journal of the American Medical Association* 264: 2919–2922

Durack D T 1997 Infective and noninfective endocarditis. In: Schlant R C (ed) The heart, 9th edn. McGraw Hill, New York, ch 82

Durack D T 1995 Prevention of infective endocarditis. *New England Journal of Medicine* 332: 38–44

Durack D T, Lukes A S, Bright D K, Duke Endocarditis Service

1994 New criteria for diagnosis of infective endocarditis: utilization of specific echocardiographic findings. *American Journal of Medicine* 96: 200–209

Wilson W R, Karchmer A W, Dajani A S et al 1995 Antibiotic treatment of adults with infective endocarditis due to viridans streptococci, enterococci, other streptococci, staphylococci, and HACEK microorganisms. *Journal of the American Medical Association* in press

Working Party of the British Society of Antimicrobial Chemotherapy 1996 Antibiotic treatment of streptococcal and staphylococcal endocarditis. *Lancet* in press

Further reading

Fowler V G, Durack D T 1994 Infective endocarditis. *Current Opinion in Cardiology* 9: 389–400

Francioli P, Etienne J, Hoigne R, Thys J P, Gerber A 1992 Treatment of streptococcal endocarditis with a single daily dose of ceftriaxone sodium for 4 weeks: efficacy and outpatient treatment feasibility. *Journal of the American Medical Association* 267: 264–267

Stamboulian D et al 1991 *Reviews of Infectious Diseases* 13 (suppl 2): S160

Infections of the gastro-intestinal tract

P. Kelly and M. J. G. Farthing

Introduction

Intestinal infections usually present with diarrhoea, sometimes accompanied by abdominal cramps, fever and vomiting. Persistent infections may be associated with anorexia and weight loss. It is rarely possible to attribute a particular illness to a specific enteropathogen on the basis of signs and symptoms, but in any given geographical area and patient population it will be possible to establish which infections are prevalent, together with their likely antibiotic sensitivities. These patterns of illness may change rapidly with the progress of epidemics, particularly in developing countries. The treatment of gastro-intestinal infections is often empirical, and thus the principles of management rely on the identification of the common clinical syndromes, namely: acute watery diarrhoea, dysentery, persistent diarrhoea with or without malabsorption, and the enteric fever pattern of illness. Travellers' diarrhoea is now a well-defined clinical infective diarrhoea syndrome in which antimicrobial chemotherapy is sometimes recommended for treatment and prevention.

Approaches to management of gastro-intestinal infections

ACUTE WATERY DIARRHOEA

Self-limiting, acute watery diarrhoea is the most common type of infective diarrhoeal illness. The range of organisms responsible for acute watery diarrhoea is shown in Box 50.1. The development of oral rehydration therapy (ORT) has revolutionized the treatment of acute infective diar-

Box 50.1 *Microbial enteropathogens responsible for acute watery diarrhoea*

Bacteria
Enterotoxigenic *Escherichia coli*
Salmonella enteritidis
Shigella spp. (early phase of infection)
Vibrio cholerae
Vibrio parahaemolyticus

Viruses
Rotavirus
Enteric adenovirus (types 40 and 41)
Norwalk and related viruses

Protozoa
Cryptosporidium parvum
Giardia lamblia

rhoea, and may well represent one of the greatest therapeutic advances of the century (Farthing 1994a) given that diarrhoea ranks third in world causes of morbidity and mortality (World Bank 1993).

It is usually unnecessary to make a specific microbiological diagnosis in acute diarrhoea as ORT is frequently all that is required for management. In children, the morbidity and mortality from acute diarrhoeal disease results largely from the ensuing dehydration and acidosis. Thus, at the onset of diarrhoea it is wise to begin treatment to prevent dehydration. This can now be achieved simply by administering an oral glucose–electrolyte solution which promotes absorption of water and sodium despite a secretory state in the proximal small intestine as occurs in cholera or infection with enterotoxigenic *Escherichia coli* or when there is mucosal damage as a result of rotavirus infection. The solution recommended by the World Health Organization (WHO) is now widely available throughout the world and has saved millions of lives during the past 10 years. This solution, however, is not widely used in Europe and North America because of the high sodium concentration (90 mmol/l) and the fear of hypernatraemia. In industrialized countries, lower sodium concentrations (50–60 mmol/l) are usually used. The efficacy of simple glucose–electrolyte ORS has been improved by replacing glucose with complex carbohydrate substrates such as rice powder or other cereals. These preparations reduce stool volume and the duration of diarrhoea compared to glucose–electrolyte ORS, and probably work better because of their low osmolality. Recent work suggests that it may be possible to improve the efficacy of simple glucose–electrolyte ORS by reducing the concentration of some of the constituents, notably glucose and sodium and thereby reducing osmolality (International Study Group 1995).

Antimicrobial chemotherapy is not routinely required for acute watery diarrhoea with the exception of cholera (see below). However, the severity and duration of acute watery diarrhoea in travellers often due to enterotoxigenic *Esch. coli*, can be reduced by administration of short courses of broad-spectrum antibiotics such as doxycycline, co-trimoxazole and the 4-fluoroquinolones.

Some cases of acute watery diarrhoea, particularly food-borne, are caused by preformed toxins, which may cause disease without infection by the bacterium. Such toxins are produced by *Staphylococcus aureus, Bacillus cereus* and *Clostridium perfringens*.

DYSENTERY (DIARRHOEA WITH BLOOD)

Dysentery is a clinical syndrome of bloody diarrhoea, often associated with abdominal cramps and fever. It is due to inflammation often with ulceration of the colonic mucosa following infection with an invasive enteropathogen such as *Shigella* spp., *Entamoeba histolytica* or entero-invasive *Esch. coli* (Box 50.2). As with acute watery diarrhoea, ORT

Box 50.2 *Enteropathogens causing bloody diarrhoea*

Bacteria
Shigella spp.
Salmonella spp.
Enteroinvasive *Escherichia coli* (EIEC)
Enterohaemorrhagic *Escherichia coli* (EHEC)
Campylobacter jejuni
Yersinia enterocolitica
Mycobacterium tuberculosis

Protozoa
Entamoeba histolytica
Balantidium coli
Cytomegalovirus (immunocompromised)

Helminths
Schistosoma spp.
Trichuris trichiura

is frequently important in management, especially in children, although fluid and electrolyte losses are usually less than in watery diarrhoea. The use of antibiotics reduces duration and severity of illness (Mahoney et al 1993), and in many instances has a major impact on mortality. Antibiotics are mandatory for dysenteric shigellosis and amoebiasis, and are probably useful in dysentery due to other organisms such as enterohaemorrhagic *Esch. coli*, *Salmonella* spp. and possibly *Campylobacter jejuni*.

PERSISTENT DIARRHOEA AND MALABSORPTION SYNDROMES

Infections such as Whipple's disease, intestinal tuberculosis, giardiasis and many infections in the undernourished or immunocompromised host may become chronic and lead to profound weight loss (Box 50.3). In such cases the diarrhoea is often intermittent and variable, even from day to day. It is important to identify the infecting organism to guide treatment, although this may be difficult. In certain situations such as human immune deficiency virus (HIV) infection or acquired immune deficiency syndrome (AIDS), it may be prudent to treat on an empirical basis, taking into account local patterns of infection in relevant patients. Where undernutrition has predisposed to infection or followed from it, nutritional support may be required. Specific malabsorption syndromes such as lactase deficiency may complicate intestinal infection. Treatment is by withdrawal of the malabsorbed nutrient from the diet with a view to attempted reintroduction after a period of months has elapsed.

Box 50.3 *Causes of persistent diarrhoea*

Protozoa
Giardiasis
Amoebiasis
Cryptosporidiosis
Microsporidiosis
Isosporiasis
Balantidium coli
Cyclospora cayatenensis

Bacteria
Salmonella spp. infection*
Campylobacter spp. infection*
Intestinal tuberculosis/*Mycobacterium avium* complex
Trophyrema whippelii (Whipple's bacillus)

Helminths
Strongyloides
Colonic schistosomiasis

Miscellaneous
Inflammatory bowel disease
Tropical sprue
Postinfectious irritable bowel

*Mostly acute illness, but may be prolonged.

ENTERIC FEVER

Typhoid, or enteric fever, is primarily a systemic bacter-aemic infection with a gastro-intestinal portal of entry, and with important intestinal complications. Infection is classically with *Salmonella typhi* and *paratyphi*, but enteric-fever-like illnesses may also occur with other penetrating organisms such as *C. jejuni* and *Yersinia enterocolitica*. Treatment requires systemic antibiotics after culture of the organism from blood or bone marrow and confirmation of antibiotic sensitivity.

TRAVELLERS' DIARRHOEA

Travellers' diarrhoea is now recognized to be an infectious disease caused by a variety of enteropathogens. Diarrhoea in travellers to the tropics from industrial countries is usually due to enterotoxigenic *Esch. coli* (ETEC); other bacterial, viral and protozoal causes are shown in Table 50.1. A variety of broad-spectrum antibiotics given for 3–5 days have been shown to reduce the severity and duration of travellers' diarrhoea. Recently, treatment with single-dose (500 mg) ciprofloxacin has also been shown to be effective in reducing the duration and severity of the illness (Salam et al 1994). Further studies will be needed to establish whether ultra-short courses of antibiotics lead to the

development of resistance. The issue of whether to recommend antibiotic prophylaxis for travellers is controversial, but any recommendations should take into account the fact that most diarrhoeal illness in travellers is self-limiting and the adverse effects of prophylaxis will often outweigh its potential benefit. This topic has recently been reviewed in detail (Farthing et al 1994b).

ANTIDIARRHOEAL DRUGS AND INFECTIVE DIARRHOEA

Four drugs are widely used for the treatment of infective diarrhoea: codeine phosphate, loperamide, diphenoxylate and kaolin–morphine mixtures. None of these agents is recommended for infants and young children with acute diarrhoea because of concerns about respiratory depression and of precipitating paralytic ileus. Over-the-counter formulations of three of these agents are available for use by travellers, but their value is questionable. In acute diarrhoea of moderate severity, they may cause abdominal bloating which can be as unpleasant as diarrhoea. These agents are useful for unavoidable journeys by rail, air, etc., while afflicted. Loperamide and codeine are undoubtedly useful in chronic diarrhoea, particularly in HIV-related diarrhoea, when correction of the fundamental derangement or infection is often impossible. A recent study from

Table 50.1 *Prevalence of microbial enteropathogens in travellers' diarrhoea*

Enteropathogen	Reported isolation rate (%)	Estimated prevalence (%)
Bacteria		
ETEC	20–75	40*
Salmonella spp.	0–16	3
Shigella spp.	0–30	8
Campylobacter jejuni	1–11	5*
Aeromonas and *Plesimonas* spp.	1–57	5
Vibrio parahaemolyticus	1–16	1*
EIEC	5–7	2
Protozoa		
Giardia lamblia	0–9	2
Entamoeba histolytica	0–9	<1
Cryptosporidium parvum	1–10	1†
Microsporidia, Cyclospora	?	?
Helminths		<1
Viruses		
Rotavirus	0–36	10
Norwalk virus family		
Multiple pathogens	9–22	20
No pathogen isolated	15–55	20

EIEC, entero-invasive *Escherichia coli*; ETEC, enterotoxigenic *Escherichia coli*.
* Seasonal variation.
† Marked regional variation.

Indonesia showed that in bacillary dysentery in adults loperamide shortened the duration of symptoms when used in conjunction with ciprofloxacin, compared to ciprofloxacin alone (Murphy et al 1993). However, clinicians have for many years been concerned by the observation that dysentery in experimental animals is worsened by the administration of opiates and in patients, excretion of dysenteric enteropathogens may be prolonged and the risk of colonic dilatation increased.

Bacterial gastro-intestinal infections

CHOLERA

Cholera is a life-threatening high volume, watery diarrhoea due to the action of cholera toxin, a secretory enterotoxin liberated by *Vibrio cholerae* strains O1 or O139. The keystone of therapy is fluid replacement, either intravenously or with ORT. Antibiotics are useful in reducing the duration of the disease and in reducing the infectivity of the diarrhoeal faeces. Fluid replacement may involve extremely large volumes, up to 40 l in some cases. Intravenous replacement is necessary in shocked patients, and replacement fluid should consist of: 150 mmol/l sodium chloride with 20–30 mmol/l potassium and adequate bicarbonate. Fluid should be given to restore blood pressure, urine output, skin turgor and mental function, and then followed by sufficient maintenance fluid to replace continuing fluid losses.

As soon as practicable, treatment with an antibiotic should begin, since the fluid requirements are substantially lessened if an appropriate antibiotic is also given. Standard treatment is with tetracycline 250 mg four times daily for 3–5 days. Antibiotic prophylaxis has also been shown to diminish the attack rate in contacts of the disease. As in treatment, a tetracycline has usually been employed, but resistance has emerged as a major problem. Tetracycline resistance increased from 15% to 95% of isolates between two epidemics in Zambia in less than a year (N. Luo, unpublished observations). Antibiotic treatment during an epidemic will always require monitoring of *V. cholerae* isolates for patterns of resistance, and antibiotic choices may need to be revised. *V. cholerae* is usually also sensitive to doxycycline, ampicillin, chloramphenicol, trimethoprim–sulphamethoxazole, furazolidone, and the fluoroquinolones. In the epidemic in Peru, ciprofloxacin in a dose of 250 mg/day for 3 days proved as effective as tetracycline in treatment (Gotuzzo et al 1995). A single dose of 250 mg did not prevent transmission in household contacts, but had a marginal effect on severity in contacts who were already infected (Echeverria et al 1995).

INFECTION WITH *SALMONELLA TYPHI*

Chloramphenicol is the most widely used treatment for *Salm. typhi* infection and remains the standard with which other agents must be compared. The usual dose is 2 g/day in four divided doses, given orally, or intravenously if the patient is seriously ill. Defervescence takes 3–5 days in most cases, but may take as long as 12 days. Treatment should be continued for 14 days. Parenterally administered chloramphenicol, whether given by the intravenous or intramuscular route, is not fully utilized and treatment should be given orally as soon as is practicable. Blood cultures remained positive in 60% of patients after the third day despite adequate doses in one study from Bangladesh (Islam et al 1993). In vitro resistance to chloramphenicol does not necessarily mean that treatment will fail: a study from India found that 3 of 15 patients with chloramphenicol-resistant typhoid were still cured by chloramphenicol (Chakravorty et al 1993).

Alternatives to chloramphenicol include amoxycillin (1 g four times daily for 2 weeks) and co-trimoxazole (960 mg twice daily for 2 weeks). Pillay et al (1975) found amoxycillin to have similar efficacy to chloramphenicol, but defervescence was more rapid with amoxycillin. Butler et al (1982) found co-trimoxazole to be as effective as chloramphenicol, but with more rapid blood culture clearance. Co-trimoxazole is associated with adverse effects in 10–15% of patients. Trimethoprim alone has also been used, but is probably less effective. In a retrospective review, chloramphenicol, amoxycillin and co-trimoxazole were found to be of equal efficacy (Fallon et al 1988). However, resistance has become widespread; resistance to all three drugs was found in 44% of cases in Qatar (Uwaydah et al 1992) and in 83% of cases in Calcutta (Arora et al 1992).

Recently, attention has focused on treatment with third-generation cephalosporins and the fluoroquinolones. Several cephalosporins, including cefotaxime, cefoperazone, ceftriaxone and cefixime, have been shown to be effective. Randomized comparisons of ceftriaxone against chloramphenicol show ceftriaxone 4 g i.v. once daily for 3 days to be as good (Lasserre et al 1991), ceftriaxone 4 g i.m. daily for 5 days to be superior (Girgis et al 1990), and 4 g i.v. daily for 5 days to be slightly less effective (Islam et al 1993). An open study of cefixime (20 mg/kg orally daily for 12 days) in children showed 100% cure rate in the short term, with only 2 out of 50 patients relapsing over 8 weeks (Girgis et al 1993). In this study, 88% of patients had multiply resistant isolates. A randomized trial of ciprofloxacin (500 mg twice daily orally for 7 days) against ceftriaxone (3 g parenterally daily for 7 days) in adults showed 27% failure in the ceftriaxone group, but none in the ciprofloxacin group. Ciprofloxacin can be given in a dose of 500 mg twice daily for 7 days orally (Uwaydah et al 1992, Mathai et al 1993). Another fluoroquinolone, fleroxacin, has been shown to be superior to chloramphenicol (Arnold et al 1993).

Children present a special problem in multiresistant typhoid, as fluoroquinolones have caused articular damage in growing animals, and are relatively contraindicated. Review revealed 36 cases of reversible arthralgia in 1113 children with cystic fibrosis treated with ciprofloxacin, but there was no evidence of cartilage damage, and generally the drug was effective and non-toxic (Kubin 1993). Ceftriaxone has been found to be effective (Navqi et al 1992), but treatment failures do occur. Dutta et al (1993) obtained cure in 17 of 18 children with ciprofloxacin, and found no evidence of toxicity during a 3 month follow-up period. The same authors also found furazolidone to be at least as good as chloramphenicol (Dutta et al 1993), but this was not a study of multiply-resistant isolates. Aztreonam (150 mg/kg daily i.v. for 15 days) was found to be as effective as chloramphenicol (Tanaka-Kido et al 1990).

In summary, chloramphenicol remains an agent of first choice in typhoid where the organism is susceptible, especially in developing countries with limited health budgets. Fluoroquinolones and cephalosporins are, however, now frequently indicated because of problems of drug resistance. Anxiety about the use of ciprofloxacin in children has been much allayed by increased experience.

Steroid therapy is indicated in severe typhoid with shock. Hoffman et al (1984) showed a reduction in mortality with high dose (11 mg/kg over 48 h) dexamethasone (2/20 deaths with dexamethasone compared to 10/18 with placebo).

Lower doses did not have significant benefit in a study from Papua New Guinea (Rogerson et al 1991). Cerebellar dysfunction in three patients following typhoid was reported to resolve after a dexamethasone and antibiotic combination (Girgis et al 1993).

Chronic carriage of *Salm. typhi* in the biliary tract can be eradicated with ciprofloxacin 750 mg twice daily for 28 days (Ferrecio et al 1988) or norfloxacin (Gotuzzo et al 1988). Amoxycillin is probably less effective, and co-trimoxazole less still.

SHIGELLOSIS

Infection with *Shigella* spp. may cause acute self-limiting watery diarrhoea or dysentery. It is only in the case of dysentery that antibiotic therapy is warranted (see above). Four species are pathogenic for humans: *S. dysenteriae* (cause of the most severe dysentery), *S. flexneri*, *S. boydii* and *S. sonnei*.

The rapid rise of antibiotic resistance in *Shigella* spp. is due to their potential for acquiring plasmid-borne resistance genes, which can be transferred from other species such as *Esch. coli* (Bratoeva et al 1994). This makes it imperative to follow the changes in antibiotic resistance during an epidemic, or over time in endemic areas. Problems with antibiotic resistance are such that few isolates are still sensitive to ampicillin or co-trimoxazole, and in some areas these agents are now totally ineffective, both in developing countries and in the industrial world. Recently reported rates of resistance vary (Table 50.2), but in some geographic locations it is difficult to choose an inexpensive drug.

Table 50.2 *Resistance of* Shigella *isolates to commonly used antibiotics in several studies conducted from 1985 onwards*

Country	n	Resistance*(%)				Reference
		AMP	CTX	TET	NLX	
Bangladesh	520	51	48		58	Bennish et al (1992a)
Canada	598	>90	38	>90		Harnett (1992)
Chile (children)	94	42	45	8		Boehme et al (1992)
Djibouti	140	42	52	97	0	Cavallo et al (1993)
Germany	255		66	54		Aleksic et al (1993)
Kenya (AIDS)	41	54	95	100	2	Kruse et al (1992)
Netherlands		53	25			Voogd et al (1992)
Nigeria	108	100		100		Eko et al (1991)
Saudi Arabia (UN military forces)	113	21	85	68		Hyams et al (1991)
Saudi Arabia	234	54	72	77		Kagalwalla et al (1992)
Zambia	91	100	98	100	0	N. Luo (pers. comm.)

* AMP, ampicillin; CTX, co-trimoxazole; TET, tetracycline; NLX, nalidixic acid.

Experience with fluoroquinolones and third-generation cephalosporins is growing, but already there is evidence that resistance to ciprofloxacin, pefloxacin and enoxacin may become a problem (Thirunarayanan et al 1993). Bhattacharya et al (1992) reported a randomized trial of norfloxacin against nalidixic acid. No difference was observed, despite 14% in vitro resistance to nalidixic acid. A trial of single- or dual-dose ciprofloxacin in *Shigella* dysentery showed that a single dose of 1 g ciprofloxacin was an effective cure unless the infecting organism was *S. dysenteriae* type 1, in which case the failure rate was 10%. These patients require 5 days of treatment with 500 mg ciprofloxacin twice daily, and this regimen had no failures (Bennish et al 1992b). Bennish et al (1990) also reported a randomized trial of ciprofloxacin (500 mg twice daily for 5 days) against ampicillin (500 mg four times daily for 5 days) in adult men with dysentery in Bangladesh. They found complete resolution or improvement in 95% of the ciprofloxacin-treated group, and 62% of the ampicillin group. However, analysis of the ampicillin group showed favourable responses in 23 of 26 patients with ampicillin-sensitive isolates, and in 15 of 35 patients with ampicillin-resistant isolates. Although ciprofloxacin is clearly superior, ampicillin resistance does not preclude a response.

Concern about fluoroquinolone safety in children has prompted interest in cephalosporins. In an Israeli study in an area of high (82%) resistance to co-trimoxazole, cefixime (8 mg/kg daily) was surprisingly not superior to co-trimoxazole. Another Israeli study found ceftriaxone for 2 days to be as effective as a 5-day course (Eidlitz-Marcus et al 1993). A trial from Guatemala of ceftibuten against co-trimoxazole in children with dysentery due to Shigella or to enteroinvasive *Esch. coli* (EIEC) found ceftibuten to be equally efficacious unless resistance to co-trimoxazole was present, in which patients the cephalosporin was superior (Prado et al 1992).

The choice of antibiotic to be used for bacillary dysentery will depend on local sensitivities of isolates of *Shigella* and, if possible, EIEC.

NON-TYPHOID SALMONELLOSIS

The treatment of paratyphoid fever is the same as that for typhoid. Salmonella food-poisoning is self-limiting and does not require antibiotic therapy, unless the patient is severely ill or blood cultures indicate systemic infection. As with typhoid, third-generation cephalosporins or fluoroquinolones are the most reliable agents. Early trials showed that use of antibiotics prolonged salmonella carriage (Aserkoff & Bennet 1969). Recent trials have confirmed that antibiotics are not useful in non-typhoid *Salmonella* gastroenteritis. Sanchez et al (1993) randomized 65 patients to ciprofloxacin (500 mg), co-trimoxazole (960 mg) or placebo twice daily for 5 days.

There was no difference between the three groups in terms of duration of diarrhoea, time to defervescence, or rate of clearance from stools. Carlstedt et al (1990) found that norfloxacin (400 mg twice daily for 7 days) did not shorten the carrier state. Funke et al (1993) found that ciprofloxacin treatment was followed by relapse in 4 of 14 (30%) of cases, and relapse was confirmed by ribotyping. In children with severe invasive salmonellosis, pefloxacin has been found to be effective when other antibiotics have failed (Gendrel et al 1993).

ESCHERICHIA COLI INFECTIONS

Esch. coli infections with enterotoxigenic (ETEC), entero-pathogenic (EPEC), enteroinvasive (EIEC), enterohaemor-rhagic (EHEC) or enteroaggregative (EAggEC) strains cause human disease, but these pathogens are difficult to identify in most routine microbiological laboratories. Consequently, information about these infections is limited, and there are few therapeutic trials. ETEC is a common cause of acute self-limiting diarrhoea in children in the tropics (Echeverria et al 1993) and in travellers (Steffen 1986, Farthing 1994b). Many of these episodes require no antibiotic therapy. EPEC probably plays a similar role. EIEC causes dysentery probably in around 5% of cases (Echeverria et al 1993), and EHEC strain 0157:H7 cause a milder form of bloody diarrhoea which is sometimes complicated by haemolytic uraemic syndrome or thrombotic thrombocytopenic purpura. The role of EAggEC in persistent diarrhoea is as yet unclear.

One trial to our knowledge has examined the potential for treatment of large numbers of infections with ETEC (Bandres et al 1992): 220 ETEC isolates in Mexico were sensitive to aztreonam, fluoroquinolones, gentamicin and furazolidone; 7% of strains were resistant to co-trimoxazole.

CAMPYLOBACTER JEJUNI INFECTION

Like non-typhoid salmonellae, *Campylobacter* spp. can cause mild, self-limiting diarrhoea or dysentery; abdominal pain is present in 70%, and fever in 90%. The decision to treat with antibiotics will be determined by the severity of the illness, but is usually recommended if there are major systemic manifestations.

Treatment with erythromycin, while accelerating clearance of the organism, does not alter the clinical illness. Ciprofloxacin is effective, but less information is available on its efficacy in vivo. Reina et al (1992) found resistance in *C. jejuni* to erythromycin (3.5%) and ciprofloxacin (11%), and in *Campylobacter coli* to the same agents (33% and 26%, respectively). Resistance is not a major problem in all parts of the world, but indicates the need for current sensitivity information in different geographic locations.

YERSINIA ENTEROCOLITICA INFECTION

Yersiniosis is an illness of variable severity, but can run a prolonged course. Infection may be complicated by a non-suppurative seronegative polyarthritis. Where infection is severe with dysentery or septicaemia, antibiotic therapy is mandatory, but otherwise it is not clearly beneficial (Griffiths & Gorbach 1993). Third-generation cephalosporins and fluoroquinolones seem to be the most effective agents (Gayraud et al 1993). Pham et al (1991) found amoxycillin–clavulanate to be effective against most strains, and all were sensitive to ciprofloxacin, chloramphenicol, tetracycline and trimethoprim.

NON-CHOLERA VIBRIOS, *AEROMONAS* AND *PLESIOMONAS* SPP.

This group includes *Vibrio parahaemolyticus*, non-O1 or non-O139 *V. cholerae*, *Aeromonas* spp. and *Plesiomonas shigelloides*. Like non-typhoid salmonellae, the illness is variable, and diagnosis is probably frequently missed as laboratories do not routinely attempt to isolate these organisms. Where treatment is indicated on the basis of symptoms, third-generation cephalosporins, tetracycline, chloramphenicol or fluoroquinolones are usually effective (Rahim et al 1992, Griffiths & Gorbach 1993, Koehler & Ashdown 1993).

CLOSTRIDIUM DIFFICILE INFECTION

Cl. difficile causes watery diarrhoea or pseudomembranous colitis. The organism is normally present in most neonatal stools but decreases in frequency to around 3% in adults. The relationship between carriage of *Cl. difficile* toxin A production and the development of clinical disease is poorly understood. When a toxin-generating *Cl. difficile* is isolated from diarrhoeal stool then treatment is warranted, and measures to limit transmission in hospitalized patients is necessary.

Treatment is with oral metronidazole (400 mg three times daily for 10 days) or oral vancomycin (125 mg four times daily for 10 days), which is slightly more effective (Bartlett 1990). Patients unable to take oral medication can be given intravenous metronidazole in the same dose. The problem is with relapse, particularly in the elderly. On relapse, vancomycin should be given if metronidazole was given the first time, or vice versa. Repeated courses may be needed and both drugs can be given in combination. Probiosis has

been tried in recurrent infection (Griffiths & Gorbach 1993) using *Lactobacillus*, *Bifidobacterium* and administration of an enema of normal human faeces (Flotterod & Hopen 1991). The treatment of recurrent relapses can be difficult, and should when at all possible be accompanied by withdrawal of concurrent antibiotics.

WHIPPLE'S DISEASE

This unusual disease is caused by *Trophyrema whippelii*. Treatment should include an antibiotic which can cross the blood–brain barrier as the central nervous system is the most common site of relapse, but may occur even if this rule is observed (Cooper et al 1994). In this patient, standard treatment with co-trimoxazole was complicated by relapse after 14 months, but responded to cefixime 400 mg twice daily for 11 months. It is difficult to conduct clinical trials in such a rare disease. It is customary to treat for 1 year; beginning with penicillin and streptomycin for 2 weeks, followed by doxycycline 100 mg/day. This regimen has appreciable toxic potential, so the use of cefixime is of interest. One report in 19 patients indicated success following 2 months of treatment with demeclocycline with or without chloramphenicol or amoxycillin; 3 patients relapsed. Some physicians use steroids initially in severely debilitated patients. Careful attention to nutritional supple-mentation is necessary, and must include folic acid and vitamin replacement.

INTESTINAL TUBERCULOSIS AND OTHER MYCOBACTERIAL INFECTION

Intestinal tuberculosis should be treated with routine antituberculous therapy (Ch. 59). Infection with *Mycobacterium avium* complex is confined to patients with AIDS (Chs 46, 59).

SMALL BOWEL BACTERIAL OVERGROWTH

Overgrowth with bacteria occurs in patients with structural abnormalities of the small bowel such as in strictures, diverticula, or bypassed surgical loops or in conditions associated with hypomotility such as scleroderma and idiopathic intestinal pseudo-obstruction. Bacterial overgrowth may lead to diarrhoea and malabsorption. Clinical improve-ment is generally obtained with metronidazole, tetracycline or a fluoroquinolone, but repeated courses are usually required if the underlying structural or motor abnormality remains.

Viral gastro-intestinal infections

CYTOMEGALOVIRUS INFECTION

This infection causes dysentery and is often accompanied by severe abdominal pain in immunocompromised patients, either in the context of AIDS or the iatrogenic immuno-suppression following cancer chemotherapy or transplantation. Its treatment is discussed more fully in Chapter 46.

INFECTIONS WITH ROTAVIRUS, ENTERIC ADENOVIRUSES TYPES 40 AND 41, SMALL ROUND STRUCTURED VIRUSES

These viruses cause acute, self-limiting watery diarrhoea, and should receive supportive management by fluid and electrolyte replacement, usually by ORT. Specific antiviral therapy is not available. Limited success has been reported by the oral administration of antirotavirus hyperimmune bovine colostrum, but this has not entered routine clinical practice.

Protozoal gasto-intestinal infections

GIARDIA LAMBLIA

The treatment of giardiasis is sometimes difficult because of the adverse effects of most antigiardial drugs and because none can be regarded as safe in pregnancy. Treatment failures occur with all the standard drugs, but the development of sensitivity testing for *Giardia* has allowed investigation of some of the mechanisms of treatment failure, including drug resistance.

The three major classes of drugs used to treat giardiasis are the nitroimidazole derivatives, the acridine dyes such as mepacrine (quinacrine) and the nitrofurans such as furazolidone (Adam 1991, Davidson 1984). The recommended treatment regimens for adults and children and an estimate of efficacy are outlined in Table 50.3. Metronidazole and tinidazole are probably the drugs of choice, since the treatment period is brief and compliance is generally good. However, the latter agent is not approved for treatment of giardiasis in the USA. Mepacrine is of similar efficacy to the nitroimidazole derivatives, but some studies suggest that it is less well tolerated. Of particular concern is the reversible toxic psychosis in adults, and skin problems, particularly in patients with underlying skin disorders such as psoriasis. Furazolidone appears to be a less effective drug in giardiasis but is widely used in children in the USA, partly because it is available as a suspension (Mendelson 1980, Quiros-Buelna 1989). Paromomycin has some activity against *Giardia* and since it is poorly absorbed has been suggested as a possible drug for use in pregnancy.

Recent studies suggest that the benzoimidazoles, drugs with broad-spectrum antihelminthic activity, may also be useful in the treatment of giardiasis (Meloni et al 1990). Their antigiardial activity probably relates to their interaction with β-tubulin and their ability, at least in vitro, to inhibit attachment. Mebendazole has in vitro activity against *Giardia* and was effective in one clinical study, although these findings have not been confirmed in other reports. Albendazole also has in vitro activity against *Giardia*, and clinical trials have confirmed its efficacy in human infection. Albendazole may be particularly useful in children in the developing world since treatment for intestinal helminths and *Giardia* can be administered at the same time.

Although not routinely available it is possible to produce drug-sensitivity profiles of *Giardia* using quantitative growth

Table 50.3 *Drug treatment of giardiasis*

Drug	Treatment regimen		Efficacy (%)
	Adults	Children	
Metronidazole	2 g (single dose) daily for 3 days *or* 400 mg three times daily for 5 days	15 mg/kg daily (max. 750 mg for 10 days)	>90
Tinidazole	2 g single dose	50–75 mg/kg in a single dose	>90
Mepacrine (quinacrine)	100 mg three times daily for 5–7 days	2 mg/kg three times daily for 5–7 days	>90
Furazolidone	100 mg four times daily for 7–10 days	2 mg/kg three times daily for 7–10 days	>80

assays or evaluating inhibition of adherence of the parasite to biological or artificial substrata (Gillin & Diamond 1981, Boreham et al 1984, Gordts et al 1985, Hoyne et al 1989, Inge & Farthing 1987). These assays have clearly shown that *Giardia* isolates vary in their sensitivity to standard antigiardial drugs and that resistance may develop in vitro following long-term exposure to a nitroimidazole derivative. The development of resistance has also been described in vivo in a chronically infected individual who was treated repeatedly but unsuccessfully with a nitroimidazole derivative.

CRYPTOSPORIDIOSIS

There is no therapy of demonstrable efficacy for the eradication of *Cryptosporidium parvum*. The majority of infections occur in children, in waterborne epidemics, or in patients with AIDS. Most of the infections in immuno-competent individuals are self-limiting, but some of these individuals have persisting infection. For many AIDS patients, symptomatic therapy with anti-diarrhoeal agents and analgesics is all that is available, but some centres use paromomycin which may reduce the intensity of infection (Ch. 46). Interesting reports of eradication with hyper-immune bovine colostrum have yet to make any impact on clinical practice.

ENTAMOEBA HISTOLYTICA

Two classes of drugs are used in the treatment of amoebic infection. Luminal amoebicides such as diloxanide furoate and iodoquinol act on organisms in the intestinal lumen and are not effective against organisms in tissues. Tissue amoebicides, such as metronidazole, dehydroemetine and chloroquine, are effective in the treatment of invasive amoebiasis, but less effective in the treatment of organisms in the bowel lumen. Table 50.4 summarizes treatment protocols for asymptomatic carriers, patients with intestinal infection and those with amoebic liver abscess.

In non-endemic areas, asymptomatic patients may be treated with diloxanide furoate, paromomycin or iodoquinol. Iodoquinol and its analogue, iodochlorhydroxyquin are effective against intraluminal amoebae, but it causes myeloptic neuropathy after long-term use and is now contraindicated. The value of treatment of asymptomatic carriers in endemic areas is questionable because of the high rate of reinfection.

Metronidazole is the drug of choice for amoebic colitis as it is very effective against the trophozoite; however, it has little effect on the cyst and therefore treatment should be followed by a luminal agent such as diloxanide furoate. Tinidazole may be used as an alternative to metronidazole.

Metronidazole or tinidazole followed by diloxanide furoate is the treatment of choice for liver abscess. The potential

Table 50.4   *Treatment of amoebiasis*

	Adult dosage	Paediatric dosage
Asymptomatic intestinal carrier		
1st choice: diloxanide furoate	500 mg t.i.d. for 10 days	20 mg/kg daily divided in 3 doses for 10 days
2nd choice: paromomycin	25–30 mg/kg daily in 3 doses for 7–10 days	25–30 mg/kg daily divided in 3 doses for 7–10 days
or		
iodoquinol	650 mg t.i.d. for 20 days	20–40 mg/kg/day divided in 3 doses for 20 days
Intestinal infection		
1st choice: metronidazole followed by	750–800 mg t.i.d. for 10 days	35–50 mg/kg daily divided in 3 doses for 10 days
diloxanide furoate*	500 mg t.i.d. for 10 days	20 mg/kg daily divided in 3 doses for 10 days
tinidazole followed by	2 g/day for 2–3 days	50–60 mg/kg daily for 3 days
diloxanide furoate*	500 mg t.i.d. for 10 days	20 mg/kg daily divided in 3 doses for 10 days
2nd choice: paromomycin	25–30 mg/kg daily in 3 doses for 7–10 days	25–30 mg/kg daily divided in 3 doses for 7–10 days
Amoebic liver abscess		
1st choice: metronidazole followed by	750–800 mg t.i.d. for 10 days	35–50 mg/kg daily divided in 3 doses for 7–10 days
diloxanide furoate*	500 mg t.i.d. for 10 days	20 mg/kg daily divided in 3 doses for 10 days
or		
tinidazole followed by	2 g/day for 3–5 days	50–60 mg/kg daily for 5 days
diloxanide furoate*	500 mg t.i.d. for 10 days	20 mg/kg daily divided in 3 doses for 10 days
2nd choice: dehydroemetine followed	1–1.5 mg/kg daily (max 90 mg/day) i.m. for 5 days	
by diloxanide furoate*	500 mg t.i.d. for 10 days	20 mg/kg daily divided in 3 doses for 10 days

* Paromomycin or iodoquinol may be used as an alternative to diloxanide furoate.

cardiovascular and gastro-intestinal adverse effects of dihydroemetine and emetine limit their use and remain as second-line treatment. Higher relapse rates are associated with chloroquine than with other therapeutic agents. Aspiration of a liver abscess may be necessary in some cases, particularly in large abscesses where rupture appears to be imminent and for large lesions in the left lobe where the risk of rupture is increased. The need for open surgical drainage has decreased since the success of percutaneous drainage.

LESS COMMON INFECTIONS

Isospora belli and *Sarcocystis* spp. rarely cause disease in immunocompetent humans. Infection in the immunocompetent is treated with co-trimoxazole 960 mg twice daily for 14 days, but this may need to be increased to achieve reliable eradication. Diclazuril is also reported to be effective. The recently described protozoan, *Cyclospora cayatenensis* can also be treated effectively with co-trimoxazole 960 mg twice daily for 7–10 days. Other protozoa such as *Cheilomastix mesnili* or *Entamoeba coli*, do not cause disease and require no therapy.

Microsporidia are discussed in Chapter 63.

Intestinal helminthiases

See Chapter 64.

Helicobacter pylori infection

Since the discovery of this organism (previously referred to as *Campylobacter pylori*) by Marshall & Warren (1984), it has become clear that it is responsible for the vast majority of benign duodenal and gastric ulcers, and recent evidence implicates it in the pathogenesis of gastric MALT lymphoma and gastric adenocarcinoma.

Eradication of *H. pylori* allows healing of peptic ulcers and relapse is then very uncommon unless the infection recurs. Recurrence of infection in the industrialized world usually indicates failure of eradication rather than reinfection, as the yearly risk of acquiring *H. pylori* infection in adult life is less than 1%. Eradication is only known to be of benefit in the presence of gastroduodenal pathology. We do not yet have evidence of value in prevention of gastric carcinoma or risk reduction for this cancer. Several regimens are available for eradication of the infection, and choice between them is largely determined by local cost, efficacy and considerations of compliance. For a general review, see Dooley (1993).

The regimens in common use are outlined in Table 50.5. Following eradication, success or failure is best determined by [¹³C]urea breath test, but an acceptably sensitive alternative would be histological examination and culture of two antral biopsies and two corpus biopsies. Antibodies persist for at least 6 months following eradication, and serological examination is therefore not helpful. Urease testing or histological analysis of single gastric biopsies are insensitive, and unsuitable for confirmation of eradication.

Table 50.5 *Regimens available for eradication of* H. pylori*

Drug	Dose	Duration (days)	Efficacy (% eradication)	Reference
Bismuth subcitrate	120 mg ×4	7	91	Sung et al (1995)
Tetracycline	500 mg ×4	7		
Metronidazole	400 mg ×4	7		
Omeprazole	40 mg	14	96	Bell et al (1993)
Amoxycillin	500 mg ×3	14		
Metronidazole	400 mg ×3	14		
Omeprazole	20 mg	28	85	Collins et al (1991)
Tetracycline	500 mg ×3	7		
Metronidazole	400 mg ×3	7		
Omeprazole	20 mg ×2	14	85	Tytgat (1994)
Amoxycllin	1 g ×2	14		
Omeprazole	20 mg	7	95	Bazzoli et al (1994)
Clarithromycin	250 mg ×2	7		
Tinidazole	500 mg ×2	7		
Ranitidine	300 mg	56	88	Hentschel et al (1993)
Amoxycillin	750 mg ×3	12		
Metronidazole	500 mg ×3	12		

* Examples of popular regimens are given; the list is not exhaustive. For further details, consult Tytgat (1994).

It is also important to allow 1 month after completion of eradication therapy before attempting to confirm eradication, as the organism may still be present but undetectable in this period. In most centres it will be impossible to test every patient for persisting infection after attempted eradication. It is our policy to check whether eradication has been successful, either if symptoms recur or if the patient initially presented with a complicated ulcer such as with bleeding or perforation.

References

Adam R D 1991 The biology of *Giardia* spp. *Microbiological Reviews* 55: 706–732

Aleksic S, Katz A, Aleksic V, Bockemuhl J 1993 Antibiotic resistance of *Shigella* strains isolated in Germany 1989–1990. *International Journal of Medical Microbiology, Virology, Parasitology and Infectious Diseases* 279: 484–493

Al-Waili N S, Al-Waili B H, Saloom K Y 1988 Therapeutic use of mebendazole in giardial infections. *Transactions of the Royal Society for Tropical Medicine and Hygiene* 82: 438

Arnold K, Hong C S, Nelwan R et al 1993 Randomized comparative study of fleroxacin and chloramphenicol in typhoid fever. *American Journal of Medicine* 94: 195S–200S

Arora R K, Gupta A, Joshi N M, Kararia V K, Lall P, Anand A C 1992 Multidrug resistant typhoid fever: study of an outbreak in Calcutta. *Indian Journal of Paediatrics* 29: 61–66

Aserkoff B, Bennet J V 1969 Effect of antibiotic therapy in acute salmonellosis on the fecal excretion of salmonellae. *New England Journal of Medicine* 281: 636–640

Bandres J C, Mathewson J J, Ericsson C D, Dupont H L 1992 Trimethoprim/sulphamethoxazole remains active against ETEC and *Shigella* species in Guadalajara, Mexico. *American Journal of Medical Sciences* 303: 289–291

Bartlett J G 1990 *Clostridium difficile*: clinical considerations. *Reviews in Infectious Diseases* 12 (suppl 2): S243–S251

Bazzoli F, Zagari R M, Fossi S et al 1994 Short term low dose triple therapy for the eradication of *H. pylori*. *European Journal of Gastroenterology and Hepatology* 6: 773–777

Bell G D, Powell K U, Burridge S M et al 1993 *H. pylori* eradication: efficacy and side effect profile of a combination of omeprazole, amoxycillin and metronidazole compared with four alternative regimens. *Quarterly Journal of Medicine* 86: 743–750

Bennish M L, Salam M A, Haider R, Barza M 1990 Therapy for shigellosis II: randomized, double-blind comparison of ciprofloxacin and ampicillin. *Journal of Infectious Diseases* 162: 711–716

Bennish M L, Salam M A, Hossain M A et al 1992a Antimicrobial resistance of *Shigella* isolates in Bangladesh, 1983–1990. *Clinics in Infectious Diseases* 14: 1055–1060

Bennish M L, Salam M A, Khan W A, Khan A M 1992b Comparison of 1 or 2 day ciprofloxacin with five day therapy. *Annals of Internal Medicine* 117: 727–734

Bhattacharya M K, Nair G B, Sen D et al 1992 Efficacy of norfloxacin for shigellosis: a double-blind randomised clinical trial. *Journal of Diarrhoeal Diseases Research* 10: 146–150

Boehme C, Rodriguez G, Illesca V, Reydet P, Serra J 1992 Shigellosis in children of the IX region of Chile. *Revista Medica de Chile* 120: 1261–1266

Boreham P F, Phillips R E, Shepherd R W 1984 The sensitivity of *Giardia intestinalis* to drugs in vitro. *Journal of Antimicrobial Chemotherapy* 14: 449–461

Bratoeva M P, John J F Jr 1994 In vivo R-plasmid transfer in a patient with a mixed infection of shigella dysentery. *Epidemiology and Infection* 112: 247–252

Butler T, Rumans L, Arnold K 1982 Response of typhoid fever caused by chloramphenicol-susceptible and chloramphenicol-resistant *Salmonella typhi*. *Reviews of Infectious Diseases* 4: 551–561

Carlstedt G, Dahl P, Niklasson P M, Gullberg K, Banck G, Kahlmeter G 1990 Norfloxacin treatment of salmonellosis does not shorten the carrier stage. *Scandinavian Journal of Infectious Diseases* 22: 553–556

Cavallo J D, Bercion R, Baudet J M, Samson T, France M, Meyran M 1993 Antibiotic sensitivity of 140 strains of *Shigella* isolated in Djibouti. *Bulletin de la Societe de Pathologie Exotique et de ses Filiales* 86: 35–40

Chakravorty B, Jain N, Gupta B, Rajvansi P, Sen M K, Krishna A 1993 Chloramphenicol resistant typhoid fever. *Journal of the Indian Medical Association* 91: 10–13

Collins R, Keane C, O'Morain C 1991 Omeprazole and colloidal bismuth subcitrate with or without antibiotics in the treatment of *H. pylori* associated duodenal ulcer disease. *Gastroenterology* 100: A48

Cooper G S, Blades E W, Remler B F, Salata R A, Bennert K W, Jacobs G H 1994 Central nervous system Whipple's disease. *Gastroenterology* 106: 782–786

Davidson R A 1984 Issues in clinical parasitology: the treatment of giardiasis. *American Journal of Gastroenterology* 79: 256–261

Dooley C 1993 *Helicobacter pylori*. *Gastroenterology Clinics of North America* 22 (1)

Dutta P, Rasaily R, Saha M R et al 1993 Ciprofloxacin for treatment of severe typhoid fever in children. *Antimicrobial Agents and Chemotherapy* 37: 1197–1199

Echeverria P, Savarino S J, Yamamoto T 1993 *Escherichia coli* diarrhoea. *Baillières Clinical Gastroenterology* 7 (2): 243–262

Echeverria J, Seas C, Carillo C, Mosterino R, Ruiz R, Gotuzzo E 1995 Efficacy and tolerability of ciprofloxacin prophylaxis in adult household contacts of patients with cholera. *Clinical Infectious Diseases* 20: 1480–1484

Eidlitz-Marcus T, Cohen Y H, Nassinovitch M et al 1993 Comparative efficacy of 2 and 5 day courses of ceftriaxone for treatment of severe shigellosis in children. *Journal of Paediatrics* 123: 822–824

Eko F O, Utsalo S J 1991 Antimicrobial resistance trends of shigella isolates from Cakabar, Nigeria. *Journal of Tropical Medicine and Hygiene* 94: 407–410

Fallon R J, Mandal B K, Mayon-White R T, Scott A C 1988 Assessment of antimicrobial treatment of acute typhoid and paratyphoid fevers in Britain and the Netherlands. *Journal of Infection* 16: 129–134

Farthing M J G 1994a Oral rehydration therapy. *Pharmacology and Therapeutics* 64: 477–492

Farthing M J G 1994b Travellers' diarrhoea. *Gut* 35: 1–4

Ferrecio C, Morris J G, Valdirieso C et al 1988 Efficacy of ciprofloxacin in the treatment of chronic typhoid carriers. *Journal of Infectious Diseases* 157: 1235–1239

Flotterod O, Hopen G 1991 Refractory *C. difficile* infection: untraditional treatment of antibiotic-induced colitis. *Tidsstrift for Den Norske Laegeforeming* 11: 1364–1365

Funke G, Nemes P, Luthy-Hottenstein J, Altwegg M 1993 Effect of ciprofloxacin therapy in duration of bacterial excretion in acute salmonella gastroenteritis. *Schweizerische Medizinische Wochenschrift* 123: 1935–1940

Gayraud M, Scavizzi M R, Mollaret H H, Guillevin L, Hornstein M J 1993 Antibiotic treatment of *Yersinia enterocolitica* septicemia. *Clinics in Infectious Diseases* 17: 402–410

Gendrel D, Raymond J, Legall M A, Bergeret M, Badoual J 1993 Use of pefloxacin after failure of initial antibiotic treatment in children with severe salmonellosis. *European Journal of Clinical Microbiology and Infectious Diseases* 12: 209–211

Gillin F D, Diamond L S 1981 Inhibition of clonal growth of *Giardia lamblia* and *Entamoeba histolytica* by metronidazole, quinacrine and other anti-microbial agents. *Journal of Antimicrobial Chemotherapy* 8: 305–316

Girgis N I, Kilpatrick M E, Farid Z, Sultan Y, Podgore J K 1993 Cefixime in the treatment of enteric fever in children. *Drugs under Experimental and Clinical Research* 19: 47–49

Girgis N I, Kilpatrick M E, Farid Z, Mikhail I A, Bishay E 1990 Ceftriaxone versus chloramphenicol in treatment of enteric fever. *Drugs under Experimental and Clinical Research* 16: 607–609

Gordts B, Hemelhof W, Asselman C, Butzler J 1985 In vitro susceptibility of 25 *Giardia lamblia* isolates of human origin to six commonly used anti-protozoal agents. *Antimicrobial Agents and Chemotherapy* 28: 378–380

Gotuzzo E, Guerra J G, Benavente L et al 1988 Use of norfloxacin to treat chronic typhoid carriers. *Journal of Infectious Diseases* 157: 1221–1225

Gotuzzo E, Seas C, Echeverria J, Carillo C, Mosterino R, Ruiz R 1995 Ciprofloxacin for the treatment of cholera: a randomized, double-blind, controlled clinical trial of a single daily dose in Peruvian adults. *Clinical Infectious Diseases* 20: 1485–1490

Griffiths J K, Gorbach S L 1993 Other bacterial diarrhoeas. *Baillière's Clinical Gastroenterology* 7 (2): 263–305

Harnett N 1992 High level resistance to trimethoprim, co-trimoxazole and other antibacterial agents among clinical isolates of *Shigella* in Ontario, Canada. *Epidemiology and Infection* 109: 463–472

Hentschel E, Brandstatter G, Dragosics B et al 1993 Effect of ranitidine and amoxicillin plus metronidazole on the eradication of *H. pylori* and the recurrence of duodenal ulcer. *New England Journal of Medicine* 328: 308–312

Hoffman S L, Punjabi N H, Kumala S 1984 Reduction of mortality in chloramphenicol-treated severe typhoid fever by high-dose dexamethasone. *New England Journal of Medicine* 310: 82–88

Hoyne G F, Boreham P F L, Parsons P G, Ward C, Biggs B 1989 The effect of drugs on the cell cycle of *Giardia intestinalis*. *Parasitology* 99: 333–339

Hyams K C, Bourgeois A L, Merrell B R et al 1991 Diarrheal disease during Operation Desert Shield. *New England Journal of Medicine* 325: 1423–1428

Inge P M G, Farthing M J G 1987 A radiometric assay for anti-giardial drugs. *Transactions of the Royal Society for Tropical Medicine and Hygiene* 81: 345–347

International Study Group 1995 Multicentre evaluation of reduced-osmolality oral rehydration salts solution. *Lancet* 345: 282–285

Islam A, Butler T, Kabir I, Alam N H 1993 Treatment of typhoid fever with ceftriaxone for 5 days or chloramphenicol for 14 days: a randomised clinical trial. *Antimicrobial Agents and Chemotherapy* 37: 1572–1575

Kagalwalla A F, Khan S N, Kagalwalla Y A, Alola S, Yaish H 1992 Childhood shigellosis in Saudi Arabia. *The Pediatric Infectious Diseases Journal* 11: 215–219

Koehler J M, Ashdown L R 1993 In vitro susceptibilities of tropical strains of *Aeromonas* species from Queensland, to 22 antimicrobial agents. *Antimicrobial Agents and Chemotherapy* 37: 905–907

Kruse H, Kariuki S, Soli N, Olsvik O 1992 Multiresistant Shigella from African AIDS patients. *Scandinavian Journal of Infectious Diseases* 24: 733–739

Kubin R 1993 Safety and efficacy of ciprofloxacin in paediatric patients – a review. *Infection* 21: 413–421

Lasserre R, Sangalang R P, Santiago 1991 Three day treatment of typhoid fever with two different doses of ceftriaxone, compared to 14 day therapy with chloramphenicol. *Journal of Antimicrobial Chemotherapy* 28: 765–772

Mahoney F J, Farley T A, Burbank D F, Leslie N H, McFarland L M 1993 Evaluation of an intervention programme for the control of an outbreak of shigellosis among institutionalized persons. *Journal of Infectious Diseases* 168: 1177–1180

Marshall B J, Warren J R 1984 Unidentified curved bacilli in the stomach of patients with gastritis and peptic ulceration. *Lancet* i: 1311–1315

Mathai D, Kudva G C, Keystone J et al 1993 Short course ciprofloxacin for enteric fever. *Journal of the Association of Physicians of India* 41: 428–430

Meloni B P, Thompson R C A, Reynoldson J A, Seville P 1990 Albendazole: A more effective antigiardial agent in vitro than metronidazole or tinidazole. *Transactions of the Royal Society of Tropical Medicine and Hygiene* 84: 375–379

Mendelson R 1980 The treatment of giardiasis. *Transactions of the Royal Society of Tropical Medicine and Hygiene* 74: 438–439

Murphy G S, Bodhidatta L, Echeverria P 1993 Ciprofloxacin and loperamide in the treatment of bacillary dysentery. *Annals of Internal Medicine* 118: 582–586

Navqi S H, Bhutta Z A, Farooqui B J 1992 Therapy of multidrug resistant typhoid in 58 children. *Scandinavian Journal of Infectious Diseases* 24: 175–179

Pham J N, Bell S M, Lanzarone J Y 1991 Biotype and antibiotic sensitivity of 100 clinical isolates of *Yersinia enterocolitica. Journal of Antimicrobial Chemotherapy* 28: 13–18

Pillay N, Adams E B, Northo-Coombes D 1975 Comparative trial of amoxycillin and chloramphenicol in treatment of typhoid fever in adults. *Lancet* ii: 333–334

Prado D, Lopez E, Liu H et al 1992 Ceftibuten and trimethoprim–sulphamethoxazole for treatment of *Shigella* and EIEC disease. *The Pediatric Infectious Diseases Journal* 11: 644–647

Quiros-Buelna E 1989 Furazolidone and metronidazole for treatment of giardiasis in children. *Scandinavian Journal of Gastroenterology* 24 (suppl 159): 65–69

Rahim Z, Ali A, Kay B A Rahim Z 1992 Prevalence of *Plesiomonas shigelloides* among diarrhoea patients in Bangladesh. *European Journal of Epidemiology* 8: 753–756

Reina J, Borrell N, Serra A 1992 Emergence of resistance to erythromycin and fluoroquinolones in thermotolerant *Campylobacter* strains isolated from feces. *European Journal of Clinical Microbiology and Infectious Diseases* 11: 1163–1166

Rogerson S J, Spooner V J, Smith T A, Richens J 1991 Hydrocortisone in chloramphenicol-treated severe typhoid fever in Papua New Guinea. *Transactions of the Royal Society of Tropical Medicine and Hygiene* 85: 113–116

Salam I, Katelaris P H, Leigh-Smith S, Farthing M J G 1994 Randomised trial of single-dose ciprofloxacin for travellers' diarrhoea. *Lancet* 344: 1537–1539

Sanchez C, Garcia-Restoy E, Garau J et al 1993 Ciprofloxacin and trimethoprim–sulphamethoxazole versus placebo in acute uncomplicated salmonella enteritis. *Journal of Infectious Diseases* 168: 1304–1307

Steffen R 1986 Epidemiologic studies of traveler's diarrhea, severe gastrointestinal infections and cholera. *Reviews of Infectious Diseases* 8 (suppl 2): S122–S130

Sung J J Y, Chung S C S, Ling T K W et al 1995 Antibacterial treatment of gastric ulcers associated with *H. pylori. New England Journal of Medicine* 332: 139–142

Tanaka-Kido J, Ortega L, Santos J I 1990 Comparative efficacies of aztreonam and chloramphenicol in children with typhoid fever. *The Pediatric Infectious Diseases Journal* 9: 44–48

Thirunarayanan M A, Jesudason M V, John J 1993 Resistance of *Shigella* to nalidixic acid and fluorinated quinolones. *Indian Journal of Medical Research Section A* 97: 239–241

Tytgat G N J 1994 Review article: treatments that impact favourably upon the eradication of *H. pylori* and ulcer recurrence. *Alimentary Pharmacology and Therapeutics* 8: 359–368

Uwaydah A K, al Soub H, Matar I 1992 Randomised prospective study comparing two dosage regimens of ciprofloxacin for the treatment of typhoid fever. *Journal of Antimicrobial Chemotherapy* 30: 707–711

Voogd C E, Schot C S, van Leeuwen W J, van Klingeren B 1992 Monitoring of antibiotic resistance in Shigellae isolated in the Netherlands. *European Journal of Clinical Microbiology and Infectious Diseases* 11: 164–167

World Bank 1993 World development report. Oxford University Press, Oxford

51

CHAPTER

Hepatitis

J. Main and H. C. Thomas

Introduction

Acute and chronic viral hepatitis continue to cause major morbidity and mortality world-wide. While many viral infections can lead to acute hepatitis, this chapter concentrates on the hepatotropic viruses, particularly those associated with chronic hepatitis.

Hepatitis A

Hepatitis A virus (HAV) is a member of the picornaviridae group and causes acute, mostly subclinical hepatitis, without chronicity. More severe disease is seen in older patients, particularly those with underlying liver disease such as chronic viral hepatitis or alcoholic liver disease. Hepatic failure occurs in 0.35% of all cases. Interferon has been reported to eliminate hepatitis A infection of cell cultures and has been tried as therapy for severe acute hepatitis (Yoshiba et al 1994); three patients with fulminant hepatic failure and one with acute severe hepatitis A were treated 19–33 days after the onset of hepatitis with interferon-β, 3 MU daily for 13–81 days. Liver function tests improved on therapy and all patients survived. Liver transplantation may be required for patients with fulminant hepatitis A.

Prevention

A major advance in the prophylaxis of HAV infection has been the development and licensing of a safe and effective vaccine. Before this only passive prophylaxis was available with γ globulin derived from pooled plasma from blood donors. This gave only short-term protection or attenuation of the disease, while failures have been attributed to the

decreasing seroprevalence of anti-HAV immunoglobulin G (IgG) in the donor population.

Hepatitis B virus infection

Epidemiology

There are an estimated 300 million carriers of hepatitis B virus (HBV) world-wide. In South-East Asia the carriage rate is as high as 20% in some countries and, although national vaccination programmes have commenced, it is likely to be several years before their impact becomes apparent. In the Western world HBV disease is mainly seen in intravenous drug users and homosexual men.

Natural history

Acute disease is usually asymptomatic, although fulminant hepatitis can occur. The risk of chronicity depends on the timing of infection. In vertical transmission there is a 95% chance of chronic infection and a subsequent life-time risk of 40% of dying in later life from the complications of chronic HBV. Host factors such as the immaturity of the neonatal immune system and viral factors such as tolerance to HBe antigen are thought to be responsible for the high rate of chronicity in this group. In adults infected with HBV the risk of chronic infection is 5–10%. Certain major histocompatibility complex (MHC) subtypes have higher rates of chronicity and some carriers appear to have a reduced ability to produce interferon. Higher rates of chronicity are seen in immunocompromised individuals such as those infected with human immunodeficiency virus (HIV). The main complications of chronic HBV infection result from chronic inflammation with the development of cirrhosis and hepatocellular carcinoma.

Precore mutants

For some years it was recognized in Mediterranean countries that a subgroup of patients with chronic hepatitis B were HBeAg negative and anti-HBe positive, but with evidence of ongoing viral replication (HBV DNA in serum) and liver damage. The virus was sequenced and a mutation identified in the precore region of the genome (Carman et al 1989). The molecular variant is known as the anti-HBe or precore variant, and it is thought that it arises in HBeAg carriers as a result of immune pressure. De novo infections have also been reported and some studies have suggested that precore acute infections are associated with a high incidence of fulminant disease.

Animal models

Hepadna virus infection has also been noted in several animal species including woodchucks, ground squirrels and Peking ducks. These animals have been studied extensively and are useful models and sources of hepatocyte cell lines for assessing potential antiviral agents.

ACUTE HEPATITIS

Acute hepatitis B infection is generally subclinical. In those with symptomatic disease no intervention is generally required and there is only a small risk of fulminant disease. HBV does not appear cytopathic and the acute hepatitis coincides with the host immune response. The potential for antiviral therapy in acute hepatitis B remains unclear. Although fatigue is common for some months after acute HBV this does not appear to relate to ongoing viral replication. Interferon-α has been prescribed for patients with acute type B hepatitis, but the numbers of patients in the studies have been too small to determine whether interferon can reduce the chance of chronicity or influence the outcome.

CHRONIC HEPATITIS B

The aims of antiviral therapy are to clear the virus and reduce the risk of chronic liver disease including cirrhosis and hepatocellular carcinoma. Viral clearance also reduces the risks of viral transmission to others.

Candidates for therapy

Patients are deemed to have chronic wild-type hepatitis B if they have a 6-month history of biochemical or histological evidence of hepatic inflammation and viral replication with HBe antigen in the serum. Patients with precore mutant infection will be HBe-antigen negative but will generally have chronic hepatitis and evidence of ongoing replication with HBcAg in liver and HBV DNA in serum. There is less experience of antiviral therapy for patients with precore mutant infection and most of the experience with antiviral therapy has been for patients with chronic wild-type infection.

Assessing the response to antiviral therapy

A complete response to antiviral therapy is defined as complete clearance of infection with sustained loss of HBe antigen, circulating HBV DNA and the development of anti-HBe antibodies. Long-term follow-up of successfully treated patients has shown that most patients will eventually also lose HBsAg and develop anti-HBs antibodies (Korenman et al 1991). The time taken to clear HBsAg appears to depend on the chronicity of the infection and can immediately follow HBeAg clearance in those with a short history or occur many years later in those with more chronic disease. There is uncertainty as to whether the persistence of HBsAg carriage in these patients is because of ongoing low-level viral replication or production of HBsAg by host cells following integration of part of the viral genome. Patients treated successfully also have an improvement in the level of inflammation of the liver and it is hoped that they will, if treated early enough in the course of their disease, have a reduced chance of developing cirrhosis and hepatocellular carcinoma. The chance of disease relapse seems small and has been mainly reported following the development or introduction of an immunosuppressive state.

For the patient with established cirrhosis successful antiviral therapy may lead to a reduction in the level of inflammation and sustain liver function for some years. Antiviral therapy is also considered in this group before transplantation in attempt to reduce the viral load and risk of graft infection.

TREATMENT

Interferons

Interferon-α has been administered for chronic HBV infection since 1976 and is now licensed in many countries for chronic carriers. Interferon-α has both immunomodulatory and antiviral actions.

Interferon-α enhances MHC class 1 display which is thought to facilitate immune recognition of infected hepatocytes. Other immunomodulatory effects include increased natural killer cell activity.

Interferon-α induces intracellular enzymes which interfere with viral protein synthesis. Interferons stimulate the production of about 30 host proteins. One set of antiviral proteins is known as 2',5'-oligoadenylate synthetase (2',5'-OAS) which leads to activation of ribonuclease (RNase)

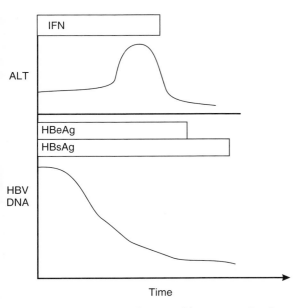

Fig. 51.1 *Chronic hepatitis B; successful response to interferon. IFN, interferon; ALT, alanine transaminase.*

enzymes which cleave mRNA. Interferon-α also induces protein kinases which inhibit the first step of protein synthesis. 2',5'-OAS and protein kinases are, however, fairly non-specific in their activity and can inhibit both the viral and host protein synthesis.

In patients treated with interferon-α a fall is seen in the levels of HBV DNA and in successfully treated cases this is sustained. The transaminase values remain stable until 6–8 weeks into the course of therapy when a rise in the transaminase value occurs (Fig. 51.1). This is thought to correspond to host recognition and immune lysis of infected hepatocytes. HBV DNA levels remain undetectable in serum and HBeAg is lost and anti-HBe antibodies are detected.

Patients may continue to be HBsAg positive for some time after successful therapy. It is thought that integration of viral genes occurs within the host genome, but with more prolonged follow-up it appears that eventually HBsAg is lost (Korenman et al 1991). Follow-up studies have demonstrated that following successful interferon therapy there is a reduction in the hepatic inflammation; the hope is that this will result in reduced risks of cirrhosis and hepatocellular carcinoma, but it may be several years before this is proven.

Interferon-α is administered by intramuscular or deep subcutaneous injection and the usual regimen is 5–10 MU three times weekly for 3–6 months, which most patients can be taught to self-administer. The response rate is about 40% in adult acquired disease (Table 51.1). Unfortunately, the response rate is very low in those with vertically acquired disease. Low response rates are also seen in immunocompromised patients such as those with HIV infection. Patients with low baseline serum HBV DNA values, who have high baseline transaminase values or active inflammation on liver biopsy are more likely to respond. It is therefore possible to target therapy to those most likely to respond, i.e. those with adult acquired disease, the HIV negative, those with low levels of HBV DNA and high baseline ALT, who on biopsy have evidence of active hepatitis without cirrhosis.

The main adverse effect with interferon is myelotoxicity; careful monitoring of the full blood count is required, particularly in those with severe liver disease and associated hypersplenism where the baseline blood counts tend to be low (Box 51.1). If significant leucopenia occurs, interferon should be discontinued and recommenced at a lower dose. Other side-effects include influenza-like symptoms with malaise, fever and myalgia. These side-effects are particularly seen with the first few doses of interferon and become less marked with time. Administration of the interferon at bedtime can help minimize these symptoms, as can paracetamol.

Table 51.1 *Treatment of chronic HBV: interferon monotherapy*

Dose (MU)	Schedule		Treated		Control		Study
	Frequency	Duration (weeks)	No. of patients	Loss of HBeAg (%)	No. of patients	Loss of HBeAg (%)	
2.5–7.5/m²	Daily	4	14	2 (14)	16	0 (0)	Anderson et al (1986)
5–10/m²	t.i.w.	12	37	12 (32)	24	1 (4)	Brook et al (1989)
10/m²	t.i.w.	24	23	6 (26)	23	0 (0)	Alexander et al (1987)
2.5–5/m²	t.i.w.	12	37	7 (19)	23	0 (0)	Dusheiko et al (1988)
5	t.i.w.	16	41	15 (37)	43	3 (7)	Perrillo et al (1990)
10	t.i.w.	16	39	6 (15)	36	3 (8)	Lok et al (1992)

t.i.w., Three times weekly.

Box 51.1 *Side-effects of interferon-α*

Fever and chills (less with subsequent doses)
Myalgia
Fatigue
Myelotoxicity (regular monitoring of full blood count required)
Impaired concentration
Altered mood (particularly depression)
Exacerbation or development of underlying autoimmune disease
Alopecia (usually reversible)
Arthralgia
Hypersensitivity reactions (rare)

Mild reversible hair loss has also been described. Depression can also occur, and patients with a background of major depressive disease require careful counselling and monitoring before embarking on a course of interferon. Interferon with its immunomodulatory effects can aggravate underlying autoimmune disease. Interferon antibodies can also occur, but their significance is unclear; the phenomenon is more commonly seen with prolonged courses prescribed for other types of chronic viral hepatitis or haematological conditions.

There are three main preparations of interferon-α. Lymphoblastoid interferon (Wellferon) is derived from lymphoblastoid cells infected with the Sendai virus. Interferon-α_{2a} (Roferon, Roche) and interferon-α_{2b} (Viraferon, Schering-Plough) are manufactured using recombinant DNA technology. Interferon-α_{2a} and -α_{2b} are derived from genetically engineered *Escherichia coli* containing DNA which codes for human interferon. The results of treatment with these types of interferon are very similar.

In one of the largest multicentre studies (Thomas et al 1994), 238 patients were randomized to receive no treatment, 2.5, 5 or 10 MU/m^2 three times weekly for 12–24 weeks. The clearance rate of HBeAg was 37% in the treatment group versus 13% in the group who received no treatment. There was no significant difference in the viral clearance rates in the different treatment groups, but a trend was seen with higher response rates seen in those treated with the higher dose.

Interferon-β. Interferon-β has also been prescribed for chronic HBV infection and so far the results appear similar to those seen with interferon-α.

Interferon-γ. Interferon as monotherapy or in combination with interferon-α has been tried in small studies of patients with chronic hepatitis B and found to confer no benefit to interferon-α as monotherapy.

Immunomodulatory

Corticosteroid. It is recognized that the withdrawal of corticosteroid therapy in patients who happen to be chronic HBV carriers can lead, on occasion, to viral clearance. Corticosteroid therapy is associated with a fall in the transaminase values, presumably because of immunosuppression. This is associated with increased viral replication and a rise in the HBV DNA levels. It has been postulated that the immune rebound which follows immunosuppressive therapy with corticosteroids could aid immune clearance. Small studies with corticosteroid treatment followed by adenine arabinoside (ara-AMP) have shown promise. Subsequent studies have evaluated the combination of corticosteroid treatment and withdrawal followed by interferon-α. Prednisolone has been prescribed in combination with interferon either as a pretreatment or given simultaneously, and generally appears to confer no benefit to interferon alone. It has been suggested that prednisolone pretreatment might benefit those with low baseline transaminase values and be helpful in treating those with vertically acquired infection, but this has not been confirmed in controlled trials (Lok et al 1992).

Thymic hormones. A number of thymic hormones have been investigated as potential agents for the treatment of chronic hepatitis B. One of the largest studies, using thymopentin, a synthetic pentapeptide, has been shown to stimulate maturation and function of T lymphocytes (Fattovich et al 1994). However, 30 patients randomized to receive no therapy or 6 months of thymopentin therapy demonstrated no benefit. A small pilot study (Farhat et al 1995) with thymosin fraction 5 (thymus derived) and thymosin-α_1 (synthetic) suggests that these agents are worth further investigation.

Levamisole. Levamisole has immunostimulatory effects, but these do not seem to be associated with an inhibitory effect on HBV. There have been reports (Fattovich et al 1992) of skin reactions following therapy.

Inosine pranobex. Inosine pranobex has also been tried, without convincing benefit.

Vaccines as therapy. Patients with chronic HBV infection generally have high levels of circulating HBsAg, so that administration of exogenous HBsAg would appear to confer little theoretical benefit. However, similar approaches have been tried as therapy for recurrent herpes simplex infection so that there is renewed interest in this approach. In a recent French study (Pol et al 1994), 32 patients were given three doses of hepatitis B vaccine (GenHevacB, 20 µg of HBsAg and pre-S2 protein) with aluminium hydroxide as adjuvant. During a 3-month follow-up period HBV DNA levels became undetectable in 10 (31%) patients and decreased in 4 (13%) patients. Six to nine months after the vaccine course interferon therapy was offered to all the patients in the study. Overall it was felt that vaccination alone inhibited viral replication in 44% of the patients in the study.

Nucleoside analogues. Nucleoside analogues have been studied as potential antiviral agents for chronic hepatitis B for many years. There has been renewed interest in this approach with the development of nucleoside analogues for treating HIV infection.

Adenine arabinoside and adenine arabinoside monophosphate. One of the first antiviral agents to be used in the treatment of chronic HBV was adenine arabinoside (ara-A), a nucleoside analogue (Bassendine et al 1981). A reduction in the serum levels of HBV DNA and transaminases followed the administration of ara-A. A few patients cleared hepatitis B. However, in most patients HBV DNA levels and transaminase values rose again immediately after cessation of treatment. It has been suggested that the rebound in alanine transaminase (ALT) values following cessation of ara-A may reflect immuno-suppressive activity of the drug. Only a few patients cleared HBe antigen.

ara-A is water insoluble and has to be given by intravenous infusion. The monophosphorylated derivative adenine arabinoside monophosphate (ara-AMP) is water soluble and can be given intramuscularly. A typical regimen is 10 mg/kg per 24 h for 5 days followed by 5 mg/kg per 24 h for a further 23 days. Although HBV DNA levels fell with therapy the rates of viral clearance were again low. In a US study (Perrillo et al 1985), very disappointing results were noted in contrast with more favourable response rates in a similar study from France. It is unclear whether host factors are important in determining response; for example, women had a good chance of responding in the French study.

Combining ara-AMP with immunomodulation has been tried. In small studies ara-A and ara-AMP have administered with corticosteroids. Another unsuccessful approach has been the combination of interferon and ara-AMP (Garcia et al 1987). Prolonged courses of ara-AMP have led to peripheral neuropathy, often painful and irreversible, and this concern has limited the drug's use. In an attempt to reduce the toxic side-effects, ara-AMP has been conjugated with human serum albumin which preferentially targets hepatocytes.

Acyclovir and famciclovir. HBV, unlike the herpes viruses, does not possess thymidine kinase necessary for the phosphorylation of acyclovir to its active triphosphate form, yet when given intravenously a transient inhibitory effect has been noted on HBV replication. This effect of acyclovir occurred only whilst on therapy, and no patient has achieved sustained viral loss. Famciclovir is the oral formulation of penciclovir (BRL 39123), a novel nucleoside analogue, which has efficacy against the herpes simplex and zoster viruses.

Famciclovir is better absorbed orally than is acyclovir, with absolute bioavailability in man of 77%. Penciclovir and famciclovir have been shown to inhibit duck hepatitis B viral replication in the Peking duck model. In addition, penciclovir has been shown to be a potent inhibitor of HBV replication in human hepatoma cells transfected with the HBV genome. A pilot study in patients with chronic hepatitis B virus infection has confirmed that the drug appears to have some inhibitory effects on HBV replication and further studies are

under way. Famciclovir is also being assessed for patients with end-stage hepatitis B undergoing assessment for liver transplantation. It has been suggested that maintenance therapy with famciclovir may prolong graft survival while the antiherpes effects may also be beneficial in protecting against reactivation of herpes simplex and varicella-zoster virus infection.

Reverse transcriptase inhibitors. Intensive research into reverse transcriptase inhibitors for therapy of HIV infection has led to renewed interest in nucleoside analogues as therapy for chronic HBV. HBV, like HIV, has a reverse transcriptase step in its replication cycle. Established anti-HIV agents such as zidovudine (azidothymdine (AZT)) didanosine (dideoxyinosine (DDI)) and zalcitabine (dideoxcytidine (DDC)) have all been shown to have inhibitory effects on hepadna viruses in cell culture. However, zidovudine alone or in combination with interferon-α appears to have no significant inhibitory effect on HBV replication when administered to patients.

Lamivudine. Lamivudine (3'-thiacytidine) is a deoxy-nucleoside analogue and reverse transcriptase inhibitor currently under trial as an anti-HIV agent. In vitro the drug is active against hepadna viruses. The low toxicity reported from the prolonged use of lamivudine in trials with HIV-infected patients has led to studies in patients with chronic HBV. Preliminary studies (Tyrrell et al 1993) with 4 weeks of therapy demonstrated a rapid fall in the HBV DNA levels but a rise on discontinuation. Studies with more prolonged monotherapy or in combination with interferon-α are under way.

Fialuridine. Fialuridine (FIAU) is a nucleoside analogue with inhibitory effects on HBV replication. Preliminary studies with short-term therapy demonstrated a fall in HBV DNA levels. In contrast with similar agents, this effect continued for some time after discontinuation of therapy. More prolonged therapy (67–90 days) regrettably led to fatal results in several patients. Some patients described symptoms suggestive of myopathy whilst on therapy, but they generally became ill after stopping therapy and their decline continued despite 'rescue' therapy with uridine and thymidine. The study was terminated when 2 of the 15 treated patients developed renal and liver failure. Lactic acidosis and pancreatitis were noted in other patients on the study. It has been postulated that fialuridine was toxic to host mitochondrial DNA. Similar effects have been reported following therapy of HIV-infected patients with other nucleoside analogues including zidovudine (Freiman et al 1993).

Ribavirin. Ribavirin (1-β-D-ribofuranosyl-1,2,4-triazole-3-carboxamide), a guanosine analogue, has broad-spectrum antiviral activity. Eighteen patients with chronic hepatitis B have been given ribavirin for 6 months (Fried et al 1994); a modest decrease in the HBV DNA levels and transaminase values occurred whilst on therapy.

TREATMENT OF SPECIFIC PATIENT GROUPS

Decompensated liver disease

In patients with HBV-associated cirrhosis and decompensated disease, interferon must be administered under close supervision. Such patients may have baseline leucopenia and thrombocytopenia and poorly tolerate high doses of interferon. There have also been reports of the immune lysis induced by interferon causing severe hepatitis and further hepatic decompensation. It has been noted when treating these patients that the rise in the transaminase values can occur within the first week of therapy and be associated with further hepatic decompensation (Kassianides et al 1988). A high rate of bacterial infection has also been noted when treating this group of patients which probably results from a combination of worsening liver function and interferon-induced neutropenia. Deaths have occurred following high-dose interferon and also following corticosteroid therapy. Studies of antiviral approaches continue in this group of patients and currently lower doses of interferon (0.5–1 MU/day three times weekly) followed by gradual escalation and careful monitoring are therefore recommended. These patients may be candidates for prolonged treatment with the newer nucleoside analogues in order to reduce viral replication and preserve liver function.

Transplantation

Liver transplantation is currently the only hope for patients with acute fulminant or end-stage hepatitis B liver disease. The graft reinfection rate with HBV is very high and graft failure occurs quickly in the setting of immunosuppression. One-year survival figures of 50% compare poorly with 80% for other types of liver disease. Cirrhosis has been described in transplanted livers within 200 days. High levels of viral replication are seen in the setting of antirejection immunosuppression and a pattern of 'fibrosing cholestatic hepatitis', rather than a hepatitic picture, is seen in many cases. Interestingly, the graft reinfection rate is lower in those with fulminant hepatitis B, perhaps as much of their liver damage relates to a strong host immune response and some of these patients are infected with the precore mutant form of the virus which may, because of the lack of production of tolerogenic HBeAg, provoke a stronger immune response than the wild-type virus. Hepatitis D virus (HDV) infection is also associated with a lower graft reinfection rate and has been attributed to the inhibitory effects of HDV on HBV replication.

Various strategies have been tried to reduce the graft reinfection rate including attempts to reduce the viral load prior to transplantation with interferon and other antiviral agents. Immune approaches have also been tried. Administration of high-dose hepatitis B immune globulin appears effective in preventing reinfection (Samuel et al 1993) but is very expensive and may need to be continued indefinitely. It may simply be delaying rather than eradicating reinfection. Monoclonal antibodies are also under development but both approaches have led to the development of mutations in the HBsAg gene of hepatitis B.

Interferon has theoretical problems for transplant patients in that the enhanced MHC display and immune activity can encourage rejection. Other strategies under trial include the administration of nucleoside analogues such as lamivudine and famciclovir. Such agents may need to be continued indefinitely as maintenance therapy.

Other immunocompromised patients (including HIV)

Immunosuppressed chronic HBV carriers are unlikely to respond to interferon as monotherapy and are another group where prolonged nucleoside therapy may be considered to limit viral replication.

Precore mutation infection

Interferon-α has been tried in patients with anti-HBe associated chronic hepatitis with variable results. In one of the larger studies (Hadziyannis et al 1990), 50 patients were randomized to receive either low-dose interferon (3 MU three times weekly) or no treatment. After 1 year 11 of the 17 (65%) evaluable patients in the treatment arm had normal transaminase values. Subsequent follow-up, however, detected a high relapse rate, and this has been seen in other studies. Brunetto and others (Brunetto et al 1991) analysed the results of interferon treatment of 90 patients with chronic anti-HBe-positive hepatitis included in four randomized controlled trials. Although transaminase values reduced to normal in about 70% of patients, there was a high relapse rate. Many of these patients had established cirrhosis, which may have reduced their chance of sustained response. Nucleoside analogues are now being tried in this group.

Extrahepatic manifestations. Interferon-α has also been used with some success in treating patients with HBV-associated glomerulonephritis. Significant reductions in proteinuria have been observed in some patients.

Hepatitis C virus

It was recognized by the 1970s that there were many cases of post transfusion hepatitis which resulted in chronic liver disease, although markers of infection for hepatitis A and hepatitis B were negative. Termed PT (post-transfusion or parenterally transmitted) non-A non-B hepatitis, it was only in 1989 that hepatitis C virus (HCV) was discovered and tests developed for blood-product screening and diagnosis.

Epidemiology

HCV accounts for more than 90% of post-transfusion hepatitis and is a common cause of liver disease in intravenous drug users and recipients of blood products. The seroprevalence is 0.07% in new UK blood donors and thought to be 1% in the general population. Seroprevalence rates of 25% have been described in Egypt, with higher levels in other African countries which remain unexplained and have led to theories regarding possible spread through mass immunization programmes or even possibly insect transmission. It is now also recognized that there are several major genotypes and subtypes of HCV. The pattern varies from country to country. In Egypt, for example, carriers of HCV are infected predominantly with type 4, whereas in the UK patients are infected with types 1, 2 and 3.

Natural history

The incubation period of HCV is 6–8 weeks, although shorter times have been reported following blood transfusion. The acute hepatitis is generally subclinical and HCV is not a major cause of acute fulminant hepatitis. Careful prospective and retrospective studies suggest that 60–80% of patients infected with HCV become chronic carriers. Generally, most carriers are asymptomatic. The chronic liver damage can range from mild hepatitis to cirrhosis and risk of hepatocellular carcinoma. The varying rate of progression is not understood. Host factors suggest that females are less likely to become chronic carriers after infection and that immunosuppressed patients are likely to develop more rapidly progressive disease. Viral factors also seem important and it seems that certain genotypes, for example type 1b, are associated with more severe disease. It has been estimated that 20% of carriers will develop cirrhosis. As yet there is no reliable clinical or other parameter which can help predict which patients will go on to develop more severe disease.

It is also recognized that there are a number of patients with chronic HCV infection who have normal liver biochemistry and yet significant liver disease on biopsy. A group of healthy carriers has also been demonstrated with ongoing HCV replication and yet normal liver biochemistry and histology.

ACUTE HEPATITIS

Despite the difficulties with diagnosing acute HCV infection, a number of small trials suggest that early antiviral therapy with interferon can reduce the risk of chronicity (Alberti et al 1991, Omata et al 1991, Viladomiu et al 1992). This is certainly worth considering when faced with a patient or health-care worker with a history of needlestick injury, a rising ALT value and positive HCV RNA. A suggested regimen would be similar to that used for chronic hepatitis C, i.e. interferon-α 3 MU three times weekly for 6 months.

CHRONIC HEPATITIS C

The aims of antiviral therapy are to clear the infection and to thereby reduce the chance of subsequent liver disease and risk of hepatocellular carcinoma. Treatment of the individual may also limit disease spread. It is likely to be several years before an effective anti-HCV vaccine can be developed.

TREATMENT

Acyclovir and corticosteroids have been shown to be of no benefit as therapy for chronic HCV. Interferon-α has been used since 1986 and is now licensed for chronic HCV infection in many countries. Pilot and subsequent studies have shown that with interferon a reduction was noted in the transaminase values within a few days of starting therapy, a very different pattern from that seen in the treatment of HBV infection. Although 50% of patients respond to therapy there is a very high relapse rate, and only about 20% of those treated with interferon have a sustained response (Table 51.2). In the early trials, assessing the response was confined to a reduction in the transaminase values and to improvement in the histopathological findings. Now with the availability of assays for hepatitis C viraemia there is increasing emphasis on virological rather than biochemical end-points, as it has been shown that those with the sustained response were generally those patients in whom HCV RNA became undetectable at the end of therapy. The response patterns are illustrated in Figure 51.2. A sustained response is currently defined as the sustained (at least 6 months) loss of HCV RNA and normalization of transaminase levels. A 6–12 month regimen of 3 MU interferon-α given three times weekly appears well tolerated. There is increasing evidence that more prolonged courses are associated with more sustained response rates. In a Scandinavian study, for example, interferon-α at a dose of 3 MU three times weekly was administered to 40 patients for 60 weeks. At the end of treatment ALT values had normalized in 24 (60%) patients, and after a follow-up period of up to 24 weeks after discontinuation of therapy remained normal in 15 patients. HCV RNA levels were negative in 17 of the responders in the follow-up period. In a controlled study comparing 6 with 12 months of interferon, better results followed the longer treatment period. This

Table 51.2 *Treatment of chronic HCV: interferon monotherapy*

| Dose (MU) | Schedule | | Treated | | Control | | Treated | Study |
	Frequency	Duration (weeks)	No. of patients	Normalization or near-normalization in ALT (%)	No. of patients	Normalization or near-normalization in ALT (%)	Sustained remission at follow-up (%)	
3	t.i.w.	24	58	26 (45)	51	4 (8)	38	Davis et al (1989)
2	t.i.w.	24	21	13 (62)	20	0 (0)	10	Di Bisceglie et al (1989)
3	t.i.w.	24	28	16 (56)	29	6 (20)	13	Causse et al (1991)
3	t.i.w.	24	26	18 (69)	25	1 (4)	30	Saracco et al (1990)
3	t.i.w.	24	18	13 (72)	18	3 (17)	29	Marcellin et al (1991)
3	t.i.w.	24	33	17 (52)	33	0 (0)	30	Cimino et al (1991)
6/3/6	t.i.w	48	35	31 (89)	31	0 (0)	44	Colombo et al (1991)

t.i.w., Three times weekly.

study also demonstrated that patients with cirrhosis were less likely to respond.

Other host factors have been studied and a complete response to interferon is more likely if the patient has a body weight less than 86 kg, has chronic persistent hepatitis, low levels of serum ferritin and a normal γ-glutamyl transpeptidase (Davis 1994).

The level of viraemia and genotype (Yoshioka et al 1992) may also be important in determining the response to treatment. In one Italian study (Chemello et al 1994a) of interferon therapy, 74% (of 19) patients with HCV type 3 infection had a long-term response (normal ALT values for at least 1 year after stopping therapy) compared with only 52% (of 23) of patients with type 2 and 29% (of 65) with type 1 infection. Genotype 1b is particularly associated with a poor response (Kanai et al 1992). Patients with type 1b infection tend to be older with more advanced disease, and it has been suggested that these factors may also influence outcome. The most recent studies on larger numbers of patients suggest that genotype may be an independent variable (Bellobuono et al 1994); it seems likely that determining the virus genotype will become more important in assessing the likelihood of response to therapy.

Compared to the 3 month treatment courses prescribed for chronic HBV infection, HCV regimens are generally longer and lower dose. Side-effects such as myalgia and myelotoxicity are therefore less, but prolonged administration of interferon can lead to the formation of interferon antibodies. Their clinical significance is unclear (Finter et al 1991): there are a few reports of patients who initially respond to interferon relapsing whilst on therapy and responding again when switched from recombinant to lymphoblastoid interferon.

For those patients who relapse following discontinuation of therapy there is currently no clearly defined strategy. Some studies have suggested that re-treating such patients is of no long-term benefit, while others have shown otherwise.

Ribavirin. Ribavirin (1-β-D-ribofuranosyl-1,2,4-triazole-3-carboxamide), a guanosine analogue, has also been used to treat chronic HCV. It is administered orally and is well tolerated. Mild haemolysis can occur and haemoglobin levels require monitoring. A pilot study (Reichard et al 1991) showed a drop in ALT on therapy and a fall in the HCV RNA values (Reichard et al 1993). The reductions in the ALT and HCV RNA levels occur much more gradually than is seen with interferon therapy, but in contrast to interferon therapy all patients have a biochemical relapse after therapy. It is unusual for patients, even with normal ALT values, to clear HCV RNA. This observation has been confirmed in a large randomized controlled study of ribavirin. Preliminary results suggest that the combination of interferon-α and ribavirin has a much greater chance of sustained virological and biochemical response than either therapy alone (Chemello et al 1994b, 1995). A further study suggests that this approach is also helpful for those who failed to respond to interferon as monotherapy (Brillanti et al 1994). These are very encouraging results and, if confirmed by larger studies, will make treatment more promising and cost-effective.

Decompensated disease. Compared with treatment for chronic HBV, lower doses of interferon are usually given for

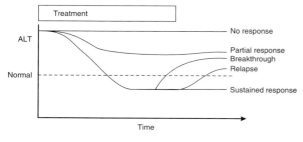

Fig. 51.2 *Chronic hepatitis C; treatment response criteria. ALT, alanine transaminase.*

longer periods and this is generally well tolerated by patients with severe disease. Those with hypersplenism may have low baseline white cell and platelet counts and dose reductions of interferon and careful monitoring may be required. There are anecdotal reports of patients on long-term maintenance regimens with either low-dose interferon or ribavirin used to palliate rather than cure the disease process.

HCV in transplant patients. Although there are reports of disease progression with immunosuppressive therapy, end-stage chronic HCV accounts for 20–40% of liver transplants in Europe and the USA. Although graft reinfection inevitably occurs, short-term survival is not impaired. Low-dose interferon and ribavirin are being assessed as potential maintenance therapy for transplant recipients.

Other immunocompromised patients (including HIV). Unlike patients with HIV and HBV infection, patients who are co-infected with HCV and HIV appear to have as much chance of responding to interferon-α as those who are HIV negative (Boyer et al 1992). However, there has been some concern regarding falls in CD4 count with interferon therapy when prescribed for chronic HCV in patients with HIV infection. The myelotoxic effects of interferon may limit its use if the patient is also taking other potentially myelotoxic drugs such as zidovudine or ganciclovir. Given the small chance of HCV clearance, most patients and physicians would wish to carefully review the potential benefit versus risk for the individual, depending on the severity of their liver disease and stage of HIV infection. Ribavirin as maintenance therapy would be a further option and appears well tolerated by this group.

Extrahepatic manifestations. HCV infection can be associated with glomerulonephritis and type II cryoglobulinaemia. There are reports of successful responses to interferon for both conditions.

Hepatitis D virus

Hepatitis D virus (HDV), or the delta agent, is the smallest virus known to infect man. It requires the presence of HBsAg in order to replicate, and in combination with HBV infection can cause rapidly progressive liver disease.

Epidemiology

There are three major epidemiological patterns of HDV infection. Epidemics are reported in the Amazon basin and other tropical areas. The second pattern is seen around the Mediterranean, where up to 10% of HBsAg carriers have evidence of HDV infection. The third pattern is a disease of high-risk individuals exposed to blood and blood products.

Natural history

There are two clinical patterns with HDV infection. Patients can become infected with HDV and HBV simultaneously; this 'co-infection' has high risks of serious acute hepatitis, but the risk of chronicity is only 10%. In patients who are already HBV carriers, 'superinfection' with HDV can also cause acute severe disease, but carries high risks of chronic HDV infection with often rapidly progressive disease. The development of cirrhosis has occurred within 2–3 years of infection, and hepatocellular carcinoma has also been reported.

Chronic HDV

Interferon-α appears to be of some benefit for patients with chronic HDV infection. Pilot studies have shown a reduction in the transaminase values and HDV RNA levels with therapy, but most patients relapse after cessation of treatment and prolonged treatment courses have been advocated (Rosina et al 1991). In one recent study (Farci et al 1994), 42 patients were randomized to receive no treatment or interferon-α (9 or 3 MU) three times weekly for 48 weeks; 10 of 14 patients treated with the higher dose, 4 of 14 patients on the lower dose and 1 of the 13 untreated patients had normalized transaminase values by the end of therapy. In 5 of the 10 responders the biochemical response persisted for up to 4 years.

Hepatitis E virus

Hepatitis E virus occurs in outbreaks in tropical countries and causes acute disease. It has a high mortality rate during pregnancy. Chronicity does not occur.

Hepatitis F

There is current debate about the existence of hepatitis F, which is thought to be another virus responsible for cases of acute, sporadic hepatitis in tropical zones.

Hepatitis G

Hepatitis G virus (HGV), like HCV, appears to be a flavivirus and may account for some of the cases of parenterally acquired non-A, non-B, non-C acute and chronic hepatitis.

With the availability of diagnostic tests for HGV antiviral trials are likely to be developed.

Summary

It is now possible to offer effective antiviral therapy for many patients with chronic hepatitis. Trials with new antiviral agents offer hope for many patients and are gradually increasing our knowledge and understanding of the pathogenesis and natural history of these diseases.

References

Alberti A, Chemello L, Benvegnu L et al 1991 Pilot study of interferon alpha-2a therapy in preventing chronic evolution of acute hepatitis C. In: Viral hepatitis and liver disease. Williams & Wilkins, Baltimore, p 656–658

Alexander G J M, Brahm J, Fagan E et al 1987 Loss of HBsAg with interferon therapy for chronic HBV. *Lancet* ii: 66–69

Anderson M G, Harrison T J, Alexander G J M et al 1986 Randomised controlled trial of lymphoblastoid interferon for chronic active hepatitis B. *Journal of Hepatology* 3 (suppl): S225–S227

Bassendine M F, Chadwick R G, Salmeron J et al 1981 Adenine arabinoside therapy in HBsAg-positive chronic liver disease: a controlled study. *Gastroenterology* 80: 1016–1021

Bellobuono A, Mondazzi L, Tempini S et al 1994 Efficacy of different regimens of alpha interferon in chronic hepatitis C and relationship between response and HCV genotype. *Journal of Hepatology* 21 (suppl): 35

Boyer N, Marcellin P, Degott C et al 1992 Recombinant interferon-alpha for chronic hepatitis C in patients positive for antibody to human immunodeficiency virus. Comite des Anti-Viraux. *Journal of Infectious Diseases* 165 (4): 723–726

Brillanti S, Garson J, Foli M et al 1994 A pilot study of combination therapy with ribavirin plus interferon alfa for interferon resistant chronic hepatitis C. *Gastroenterology* 107: 812–817

Brook M G, Chan G, Yap I et al 1989 Randomised controlled trial of lymphoblastoid interferon alfa in Europid men with chronic hepatitis B virus infection. *British Medical Journal* 299 (6700): 652–656

Brunetto M R, Oliveri F, Demartini A et al 1991 Treatment with interferon of chronic hepatitis B associated with antibody to hepatitis B e antigen. *Journal of Hepatology* 13 (suppl 1): S8–S11

Carman W F, Jacyna M R, Hadziyannis S et al 1989 Mutation preventing formation of hepatitis HB e antigen in chronic hepatitis B virus infection. *Lancet* ii: 588–591

Causse X, Godinot H, Chevallier M et al 1991 Comparison of 1 or 3 MU of interferon alfa-2b and placebo in patients with chronic non-A, non-B hepatitis. *Gastroenterology* 101: 497–502

Chemello L, Alberti A, Rose K et al 1994a Hepatitis C serotype and response to interferon therapy [letter]. *New England Journal of Medicine* 330: 143

Chemello L, Cavalletto L, Bernardinello E et al 1994b Response to ribavirin, to interferon and to a combination of both in patients with chronic hepatitis C and its relation to HCV genotypes. *Journal of Hepatology* 21 (suppl 1): S12

Chemello L, Cavalletto L, Bernardinello E et al 1995 The effect of interferon alfa and ribavirin combination therapy in naive patients with chronic hepatitis C. *Journal of Hepatology* 23 (suppl 2): 8–12

Cimino L, Nardone G, Citarella C et al 1991 Treatment of chronic hepatitis C with recombinant interferon alfa. *Ital J Gastroenterol* 23: 399–342

Colombo M, Rumi M G, Marcelli R et al 1991 Randomised controlled trial of recombinant interferon alfa in patients with chronic hepatitis C [abstract]. *Hepatology* 14: 101

Davis G L 1994 Prediction of response to interferon treatment of chronic hepatitis C. *Journal of Hepatology* 21: 1–3

Davis G L, Balart L A, Schiff E R et al 1989 Treatment of chronic hepatitis C with recombinant interferon alpha. *New England Journal of Medicine* 321: 1501–1506

Di Bisceglie A M, Martin P, Kassianides C et al 1989 Recombinant interferon alfa therapy for chronic hepatitis C: a randomized double blind placebo-controlled trial. *New England Journal of Medicine* 321: 1506–1510

Dusheiko G M, Kassianides C, Song E et al 1988 Loss of hepatitis B surface antigen in three controlled trials of recombinant interferon alpha-interferon for treatment of chronic hepatitis B. A R Liss, New York, p 844–847

Farci P, Mandas A, Coiana A et al 1994 Treatment of chronic hepatitis D with interferon alfa-2a. *New England Journal of Medicine* 330: 88–94

Fattovich G, Giustina G, Alberti A et al 1994 A randomised controlled trial of thymopentin therapy in patients with chronic hepatitis B. *Journal of Hepatology* 21: 361–366

Finter N B, Chapman S, Dowd P et al 1991 The use of interferon-alpha in virus infections. *Drugs* 42 (5): 749–765

Fried M W, Fong T-L, Swain M G et al 1994 Therapy of chronic hepatitis B with a 6 month course of ribavirin. *Journal of Hepatology* 21: 145–150

Garcia G, Smith C I, Weissberg J I et al 1987 Adenine arabinoside monophosphate (vidarabine phosphate) in combination with human leukocyte interferon in the treatment of chronic hepatitis B. *Annals of Internal Medicine* 107: 278–285

Hadziyannis S, Bramou T, Makris A et al 1990 Interferon alfa-2b treatment of HBeAg negative/serum HBV DNA positive chronic active hepatitis type B. *Journal of Hepatology* 11: S133–S136

Kanai K, Kato M, Okamato H et al 1992 HCV genotypes in chronic hepatitis C and response to interferon. *Lancet* 339: 1543

Kassianides C, Di Bisceglie A M, Hoofangle J H et al 1988 Alpha interferon therapy in patients with decompensated chronic type B hepatitis. In: Viral hepatitis and liver disease. A R Liss, London, p 840–843

Korenman J, Baker B, Waggoner J et al 1991 Long term remissions of chronic hepatitis B after alpha interferon. *Annals of Internal Medicine* 114: 629–634

Lok A S F, Wu P C, Lai C L et al 1992 A controlled trial of interferon with or without prednisolone priming for chronic hepatitis B. *Gastroenterology* 102: 2091–2097

Marcellin P, Boyer N, Giostra E et al 1991 Recombinant human alpha-interferon in patients with chronic non-A, non-B hepatitis. A multi-centre randomised controlled trial from France. *Hepatology* 13: 393–397

Omata M, Yokosuka O, Takano S et al 1991 Resolution of acute hepatitis C after therapy with natural beta interferon. *Lancet* 338: 914–915

Perrillo R, Regenstein F, Bodicky C et al 1985 Comparative efficacy of adenine arabinoside 5'-monophosphate and prednisone withdrawal followed by adenine arabinoside 5'-monophosphate in the treatment of chronic active hepatitis type B. *Gastroenterology* 88: 780–786

Perrillo R P, Schiff E R, Davis G L et al 1990 A randomised controlled trial of interferon alfa 2-b alone and after prednisone withdrawal for the treatment of chronic hepatitis B. *New England Journal of Medicine* 323: 295–301

Pol S, Driss F, Michel M-L et al 1994 Specific vaccine therapy in chronic hepatitis B infection. *Lancet* 344: 342

Reichard O, Andersson J, Schvarcz R et al 1991 Ribavirin treatment for chronic hepatitis C. *Lancet* 337: 1058–1061

Reichard O, Yun Z-B, Sonnersborg A et al 1993 Hepatitis C viral RNA titers in serum prior to, during and after oral treatment with ribavirin for chronic hepatitis C. *Journal of Medical Virology* 41: 99–102

Rosina F, Pintus C, Meschievitz C et al 1991 A randomised controlled trial of a 12 month course of recombinant human interferon alpha in chronic delta (type D) hepatitis: a multicenter Italian study. *Hepatology* 13: 1052–1056

Samuel D, Muller R, Alexander G et al 1993 Liver transplantation in European patients with the hepatitis B surface antigen. *New England Journal of Medicine* 329: 1842–1847

Saracco G, Rosina F, Torrani et al 1990 A randomised controlled trial of interferon alfa 2b as therapy for chronic non-A, non-B hepatitis. *Journal of Hepatology* 11: S34–S49

Thomas H C, Lok A S F, Carreno V et al 1994 Comparative study of three doses of interferon-α_{2a} in chronic active hepatitis B. *Journal of Viral Hepatology* 1: 139–148

Tyrrell D L J, Mitchell M C, De Man R A et al 1993 Phase II trial of lamivudine for chronic hepatitis B. *Hepatology* 18 (suppl): 112A

Viladomiu L, Genesca J, Estaban J I et al 1992 Interferon alpha in acute post-transfusion hepatitis C; a randomised controlled trial. *Hepatology* 16: 767–769

Yoshiba M, Inoue K, Sekiyama K et al 1994 Interferon for hepatitis A. *Lancet* 343: 288–289

Yoshioka K, Kakumu S, Wakita T et al 1992 Detection of hepatitis C virus by polymerase chain reaction and response to interferon alpha therapy: relationship to genotypes of hepatitis C virus. *Hepatology* 16: 293–299

Infections of the skin and soft tissues

S. Ash

Introduction

The skin and underlying soft tissues form a usually formidable defensive barrier against infection despite the fact that its surface is normally colonized by a variety of organisms. Disruption of the integrity of the integument, compromise of immune function, or spread of an organism via the circulation can lead to a wide spectrum of manifestations of dermatological infections.

Diagnosis may rely upon the appearance of the skin lesions alone. Isolation of the causative organism may be difficult, in many cases due to contamination by normal commensal skin flora.

Topical antimicrobial therapy can often result in the development of resistance, and also hypersensitivity; its success is often limited by the failure of adequate penetration into the skin and underlying tissue. However, one advantage of topical antimicrobial therapy is its lack of systemic complications and toxicity. Many of the topical agents in common use, either singly or in combination, are listed in Box 52.1.

Viral soft tissue infections

HERPES SIMPLEX VIRUS

Herpes simplex virus (HSV) types 1 and 2 cause herpes labialis and genital herpes. Many individuals suffer recurrent outbreaks of herpes labialis, often provoked by exposure to sunlight, coinciding with the premenstrual period, or precipitated by a bacterial lower respiratory tract infection. Early topical application of acyclovir cream may

Box 52.1 *Commonly used topical preparations*

Antibacterials	Disinfecting agents
Chloramphenicol	Benzalkonium chloride
Colistin	Cetrimide
Neomycin	Chlorhexidine
Mafenide	Hexachloraphane
Mupirocin	Chlorinated solutions
Nitrofurazone	Iodine compounds
Tetracyclines	Potassium permanganate
Fusidic acid	Troclosan
Gentamicin	Quinolones
Polymyxin	
Bacitracin	

There are also numerous commercial preparations of mixtures of these agents.

limit the severity and duration of the lesions. Systemic antivirals are rarely recommended for single attacks of herpes labialis, although prophylaxis with acyclovir for frequent recurrences has been shown effective (Rooney et al 1993). Genital herpes is dealt with in Chapter 58. Occasionally, in profoundly immunocompromised patients such as those with acquired immune deficiency syndrome (AIDS), severe and disseminated HSV may cause serious and life-threatening disease. In such instances, intravenous acyclovir is administered in a dose of 10 mg/kg i.v. every 8 h.

Some individuals may suffer from recurrent herpetic lesions, especially those with immunodeficiency. Long-term prophylaxis with an antiviral then becomes an option. Lower doses are generally recommended for such an indication, and acyclovir 200–400 mg orally 12-hourly are commonly used doses. The development of viral resistance is a potential risk in long-term use as a prophylactic.

Other antiherpetic agents such as famcyclovir and BVara-U may find a place in the therapy of herpes virus infections, but do not seem to hold any substantial advantage over acyclovir. Valiciclovir is a pro-drug offering better pharmacokinetics than acyclovir in that it is better absorbed and achieves comparatively higher plasma levels and a longer half-life, necessitating less frequent dosing. Its precise therapeutic place has yet to be established.

Foscarnet may be of value in treating acyclovir-resistant strains of herpes viruses. It is given intravenously in a dose of 20–200 mg/kg daily according to renal function after a 20 mg/kg priming dose over 30 min.

VARICELLA-ZOSTER VIRUS

Varicella-zoster virus (VZV) infects and establishes latency in most people by the time they reach adulthood. Childhood chickenpox is usually a benign self-limiting condition rarely complicated by a benign encephalitis with predominant cerebellar features. Treatment of primary cases in young patients is usually not warranted. However, some authorities recommend treating secondary cases acquired in family members of an index case, to be commenced within 24 h of the appearance of a rash in susceptible adults (acyclovir 800 mg five times daily for 5 days) and children (acyclovir 20 mg/kg four times daily for 5 days). Chickenpox in adults may be a more serious condition, complicated by viral pneumonia, particularly in cigarette smokers. Once again, therapy with acyclovir is indicated, starting as early as possible after the appearance of the rash. Antiviral therapy beginning more than 4 days into the illness, or certainly after lesions have scabbed and no new lesions are appearing, is of limited value. Acyclovir 800 mg five times daily orally for 7 days is recommended, with intravenous therapy a sensible option in cases of viral pneumonia at a dose of 5–10 mg/kg every 8 h. Chickenpox occurring in pregnant women or immunocompromised children, e.g. with AIDS, presents a special case probably best treated with intravenous acyclovir at a dose of 10 mg/kg every 8 h for 7–10 days. This group of patients may also benefit from the administration of zoster hyperimmune globulin, although shortages of this product at a particular time may affect indications and recommendations. Treatment of VZV infections has been reviewed recently by Whitley & Straus (1993).

Zoster (or shingles) may occur in anybody who bears latent infection with VZV. It is more frequent in those who are immunocompromised, in whom it may produce lesions in multiple dermatomes, and may also disseminate. Trials have indicated minor advantages to therapy with an antiviral if started in the first few days of an attack of shingles. It is claimed that the incidence of postherpetic neuralgia is reduced by antiviral treatment, although the data are not particularly convincing. Acyclovir, 800 mg five times daily for 5 days orally should be started as soon after the

appearance of the rash. Valiciclovir has just been licensed in the UK for the treatment of zoster, and is given orally in a dose of 1 g 8-hourly for 7 days. It is converted to acyclovir after absorption through the gut, but the pro-drug itself is much better absorbed than acyclovir. Valiciclovir may have possible therapeutic indications for other HSV and VZV infections in the future.

VZV may affect the eye if the dermatome affected in shingles is that of the first division of the trigeminal nerve. This is a painful condition that threatens eyesight. Systemic treatment should be supplemented with an ophthalmic preparation of acyclovir administered every 4 h. Cycloplegics administered topically may help prevent synechiae, and also relieve the discomfort of ciliary spasm. Topical chloramphenicol drops/ointment or fucidin ophthalmic ointment may also be used to prevent secondary bacterial infection.

HUMAN PAPILLOMA VIRUS

Human papilloma virus (HPV) causes warts in a variety of areas of the body, and those of the genital area are dealt with in Ch. 58. In immunocompromised patients, warts caused by HPV may be particularly severe and widespread. HPV lesions may, in many circumstances, be premalignant. Traditionally, treatment for warts has relied on ablative techniques such as freezing with liquid nitrogen, and the application of trichloracetic acid or podophyllin. Surgical removal may be necessary in some instances. Systemic and intralesional interferon-α has been used in trials of therapy for HPV-related warts, but the exact place of these remedies is yet to be established.

MOLLUSCUM CONTAGIOSUM

Molluscum contagiosum most commonly presents as a self-limiting disorder in childhood and usually requires no therapy. However, in patients with HIV-related immunodeficiency the lesions may persist, spread widely and enlarge. Therapy is generally unsatisfactory, but temporary relief may be obtained with the application of liquid nitrogen, 0.025% treretinoin cream, or even intralesional interferon-α.

HUMAN IMMUNODEFICIENCY VIRUS

Human immunodeficiency virus (HIV) infection may be associated with a vast array of dermatological infections; as summarized in Box 52.2. Full reference to these entities is made in Chapter 46 and also in an article by Ash & Hewitt (1994).

Box 52.2 *Dermatological conditions associated with HIV infection*

Infection

Bacterial: e.g. staphylococcal, streptococcal and mycobacterial infections, syphilis, donovanosis, lymphogranuloma venereum, chancroid, bacillary angiomatosis

Viral: e.g. herpes simplex virus, varicella-zoster virus, cytomegalovirus, human papilloma virus infections and molluscum contagiosum

Fungal: e.g. candida, sporotrichosis, dermatophytes, histoplasmosis, cryptococcus and pityriasis infections

Parasitic: e.g. scabies

Protozoal: e.g. toxoplasma, pneumocystis infections and leishmaniasis

Neoplastic

Kaposi's sarcoma
Lymphoma
Anorectal carcinoma
Squamous cell carcinoma

Inflammatory

Seroconversion illness
Vasculitis
Drug reactions
Aphthous ulcers
Seborrheic dermatitis, psoriasis, ichthyosis, porphyria cutanea tarda
Idiopathic generalized pruritus

Bacterial soft tissue infections

STAPHYLOCOCCAL INFECTIONS

Furunculosis and folliculitis

Furunculosis and folliculitis usually require no treatment or little more than treatment by lancing for the former condition. However, some individuals, despite their otherwise apparent health, may be subject to recurrent furunculosis or folliculitis and a regimen to reduce carriage of the causative staphylococcal organism may reduce the problem. Therapy with topical chlorhexidene 0.1% or 0.5% neomycin sulphate is recommended, with the nasal application of fucidic acid or a nasal preparation of chlorhexidene and neomycin. The problem of nasal carriage of family members of the patient may need addressing in order to increase the success of therapy. Systemic flucloxacillin 500 mg 6-hourly orally for 14 days has been used by some in addition to topical therapy in an effort to improve efficacy and prevent relapse.

Staphylococcal bullous impetigo

Staphylococcal bullous impetigo occurs more commonly around the mouth, and on the nose, ears and axillae. The staphylococci responsible are usually producers of exfoliatin, an enzyme causing cleavage of the upper epidermal layer. The lesions start as vesicles and progress to pus-filled bullae. Oral flucloxacillin, typically 500 mg 6-hourly for 5–7 days, with chlorhexidene topically to prevent spread is recommended.

Staphylococcal scalded skin syndrome

Staphylococcal scalded skin syndrome (SSSS, or toxic epidermal necrolysis) occurs mainly in children; the manifestations appear to be caused by an exaggerated response to the production of exfoliatin by the causative staphylococcal organism. It may affect large areas of skin, swabs from which characteristically fail to grow any significant organism. The syndrome may follow a primary impetigenous infection. Treatment consists of a β-lactamase resistant penicillin, supportive measures to combat losses of fluid, electrolytes, protein and heat, and a careful watch for secondary infections. Occasionally this syndrome may be seen in immunocompromised adults.

MULTIRESISTANT *STAPHYLOCOCCUS AUREUS*

Multiresistant *staphylococcus aureus* (MRSA) poses a particular problem for infection control in hospitals. This organism is now frequently found as a commensal colonizing the skin and nares of patients and staff within many hospitals in most countries around the world. Key measures to eradicate the organism include isolation of individual patients, or at least containment if many patients are involved. Topical therapy with nasal chlorhexidene/neomycin or muprirocin preparations plus chlorhexidene baths with application of mupirocin 2% ointment to colonized areas such as axillae and groin is often successful. Patients who then produce three successive negative swabs from multiple sites may then be released from isolation. Patients who acquire soft tissue infection with MRSA are usally treated with either vancomycin, 500 mg i.v. 6-hourly or 1 g 12-hourly as a slow infusion over 60 min with dose reduction in patients with renal insufficiency and plasma level monitoring; teicoplanin 400 mg i.v. daily is an alternative.

Staff colonized with MRSA should be given a period of leave during which they should apply the same measures detailed above, and be allowed to return to work only after negative swabs. Patients known to have had MRSA in the past should be isolated if they are readmitted, until proven free of contamination. It may be wise to adopt similar precautions for patients being transferred from one hospital to another where the former institution is known to have problems with MRSA.

Management of staphylococcal skin disorders has been reviewed by Williams & MacKie (1993).

STREPTOCOCCAL INFECTIONS

Group A streptococci

Group A streptococci (GAS) are a cause of many different types of soft tissue infections, ranging from superficial (e.g. impetigo) to deep (e.g. necrotizing fasciitis and myositis) and have enjoyed a resurgence of interest over the past few years as a result of its changing epidemiology (Todd 1993).

Streptococcal pyoderma

Streptococcal pyoderma is usually caused by *Streptococcus pyogenes* Lancefield group A. It is the commonest skin infection world-wide, especially in children, being more prevalent in tropical climates, and is associated with poor hygiene. It usually follows minor trauma, e.g. insect bites, and appears as a pustule surrounded by erythema. Systemic penicillin therapy is the treatment of first choice. However, the lesion may become secondarily infected (especially if a crust forms) with *Staph. aureus*. Response to antibiotics may then depend upon local resistance patterns of staphylococci, and flucloxacillin may be needed. An alternative is erythromycin.

Streptococcal cellulitis

Streptococcal cellulitis usually occurs on the extremities as a painful, hot, tense, red area with a poorly defined margin. It may be accompanied by lymphadenitis. Treatment consists of rest and elevation of the limb and parenteral penicillin. It is a common policy to cover the possibility of staphylococcal involvement (especially in diabetics) with the addition of flucloxacillin.

Erysipelas

Erysipelas is a more superficial form of streptococcal cellulitis that classically affects the face and also the abdomen of infants and the limbs in adults. It is again a hot, painful, red lesion, but with a well-defined margin, and vesicles may be present. Parenteral penicillin is the first choice for therapy (alternatives are erythromycin and first-generation cephalosporins).

With all these streptococcal infections of the skin, the causative organism may be one of the nephritogenic strains, and glomerulonephritis has been documented after these infections.

Cellulitis of the orbit and peri-orbital tissues

Cellulitis of the orbit and peri-orbital tissues deserve special mention. Bergin & Wright (1986) reviewed 49 cases, mean age 31 years, of whom 61% had abnormal sinus radiology. Few had a leucocytosis, and results from cultures of blood, conjunctiva, nose, antrum or abscess (where done) were disappointing. Blood cultures were positive in 30% of children under 5 years of age, but in only 12% of adults. The commonest organisms in adults were staphylococci and streptococci – including pneumococcus – and one may therefore recommend treatment with parenteral penicillin and flucloxacillin. In children, *Haemophilus influenzae* type b is more common and a third-generation cephalosporin is the first choice for therapy.

In a study of 166 children, Israele & Nelson (1987) made the distinction between orbital and peri-orbital cellulitis. Seventy-five per cent of cases of the less common orbital cellulitis are associated with pre-existing sinusitis, whereas predisposing causes of peri-orbital cellulitis are more commonly skin trauma/infection, upper respiratory tract infection, otitis media and, less often, sinusitis. The nature of the aetiological organism therefore reflects this difference. In peri-orbital cellulitis *H. influenzae* type b was most often implicated, whereas *Staph. aureus* and streptococci as well as *H. influenzae* type b and anaerobes were found to cause orbital cellulitis. Infection with *Haemophilus* is associated with sinusitis and an age below 5 years. Four per cent of patients were found to develop meningitis as a complication. For patients aged above 5 years with peri-orbital cellulitis secondary to skin trauma or infection, the authors recommend that antibiotic cover for Gram-positive cocci, e.g. erythromycin or ampicillin + flucloxacillin, is adequate (Israele & Nelson 1987). For those under 5 years of age, or with sinusitis, it is advisable to provide antibiotic cover for *Haemophilus* with a third-generation cephalosporin.

Cases of orbital cellulitis may need surgery to decompress the orbit in order to spare damage to the optic nerve.

Group B streptococci

Group B streptococci may cause a cellulitis/adenitis infection, typically in infancy, but also less commonly in older children. Occasionally, serious systemic infection and meninigitis may result. Parenteral penicillins or cephalosporins, e.g. 1.2 g 4-hourly i.v. benzylpenicillin are suitable antibiotics.

IMPETIGO CONTAGIOSA

Impetigo contagiosa is an infection of the superficial layers of the epidermis which occurs in two forms. The commoner is the vesicular, golden-crusted variety which is classically of streptococcal origin, but is commonly superinfected with staphylococci. Less common is the bullous variety, a pure staphylococcal infection, which may occur in hospital nurseries in the severe epidemic form called impetigo (or pemphigus) neonatorum. The streptococci and staphylococci are often of unusual types peculiar to skin infections. Distinct streptococcal types are involved in respiratory and skin infections, with a few uncommon types able to infect both sites. A review (Baltimore 1985) suggests that the majority of cases of impetigo (excluding the bullous form) are caused by streptococcus group A organisms, and only a minority by staphylococci, diphtheroids and Gram-negative bacilli. The most important complication was that of glomerulonephritis.

Comparison between therapeutic regimes is difficult, but topical antibiotics are less effective than systemic therapy (usually either penicillin or erythromycin). In cases where the lesions had both streptococci and staphylococci present, it appears that treating the streptococci alone is sufficient to clear the lesion. In contrast to this, another review article reporting on a study of 60 patients found *Staph. aureus* in all but one isolate, and of the 59 isolates with this organism, only one was sensitive to penicillin and ampicillin (Coskey & Coskey 1987). A further review (Blumer et al 1985) reports that staphylococci were more commonly found than streptococci in the lesions of impetigo. In fact, in hospitalized patients, *Staph. aureus* and *H. influenzae* type b were most common. These latter two articles recommend the use of a β-lactamase-resistant penicillin for outpatients (e.g. flucloxacillin), and parenteral cefuroxime or ceftriaxone for inpatient use.

The introduction of topical mupirocin for the treatment of impetigo has shown promising results (Eells et al 1986), and reports of an 88% success rate for staphylococcal lesions and 100% for group A β-haemolytic streptococci, compared to 47% and 0%, respectively, with the use of the polyethylene glycol base on its own (which itself has antibacterial properties). Additional local treatment for impetigo should still be included, with the gentle removal of crusts with either soap and water or 1% cetrimide solution.

Sycosis barbae may be considered as a form of impetigo, and may result from superficial injury to the skin incurred while shaving. In its mildest form, the condition will usually improve on stopping shaving for a few days. Otherwise it may benefit from one of the therapies used for the treatment of impetigo itself. Quinolone derivatives (e.g. Vioform) may be helpful in intractable cases.

Necrotizing infections and GAS gangrene

Necrotizing infections may occur in the deeper soft tissue elements, and generally have a polymicrobial cause,

although occasionally a single bacterial species is capable of causing disease (Lewis 1992). The most common isolates are β-haemolytic streptococci, α-haemolytic streptococci, *Staph. aureus*, combinations of anaerobes and other facultative anaerobes, and Gram-negative bacilli. Much publicity occurred in Europe and the USA during 1994 about group A streptococci (GAS) as a cause of necrotizing fasciitis. The so-called 'epidemic' appeared to represent little more then the usual incidence of serious GAS infections.

Necrotizing fasciitis is a rapidly progressive and often fatal infection of subcutaneous soft tissues, which goes by a variety of different names depending on the site and circumstance of disease. Allied conditions having sufficient similarity to be considered together include Meleney's synergistic gangrene and Fournier's gangrene of the scrotum. Division and categorization into subgroups is unnecessary and unhelpful as there are general principles of management applicable to all cases. Many cases occur in debilitated, diabetic, alcoholic and malnourished patients as well as those with intra-abdominal sepsis. Attention to these underlying problems may be necessary to achieve successful treatment.

The principles of treatment of necrotizing soft tissue infections (Box 52.3) involve urgent surgical debridement removing all non-viable tissue, intensive supportive care in terms of oxygen delivery to the area, and broad-spectrum antibiotic cover. An empirical choice of agent is based upon the likely need for the antibiotic to possess activity against Gram-positive and Gram-negative bacteria, including anaerobes. Various antibiotics, usually in combination, can be considered appropriate, and the following are typical examples:

- Ampicillin (1 g i.v. 6-hourly) + metronidazole (500 mg i.v. or rectally 6-hourly; or 400 mg p.o. 8-hourly) + ciprofloxacin (750 mg orally 12-hourly; or 400 mg i.v. 12-hourly)
  or
- Imipenem (500 mg i.v. 6-hourly)
  or
- Clindamycin (450 mg i.v. or p.o. 6-hourly) + ceftazidime (2 g i.v. 8-hourly if renal function normal)
  or
- Piperacillin/tazobactam (4.5 g i.v. 8-hourly).

Box 52.3 *Principles of management of patients with necrotizing fasciitis*

- Resuscitation, fluid replacement, etc.
- Supportive measures to improve oxygen delivery to tissues
- Surgical debridement of all non-viable tissue; second and third procedures may be necessary
- Broad-spectrum systemic antibiotic therapy (see text)
- Address any pre-existing or precipitating pathology
- Nutritional support

Although aminoglycosides are often recommended as part of an antibiotic cocktail, these drugs show poor activity in an anaerobic tissue environment.

Many cases will need repeated surgical procedures and require constant surgical review.

Nutritional support should also be considered in the management of each patient.

CLOSTRIDIAL INFECTIONS

Clostridial anaerobic cellulitis is a necrotizing infection of subcutaneous tissues, and by itself does not involve the deep fascia or muscle. Crepitus may be present due to gas formation. The causative organism is usually *Clostridium perfringens*; it follows surgery or trauma, especially when associated with the presence of a foreign body and necrotic tissue which provide an anaerobic environment in which the organism can thrive. Management is based on surgical debridement and drainage of pus with high parenteral doses of penicillin and another antibiotic if a second organism is isolated.

Clostridial myonecrosis is characterized by an acute, rapidly spreading myositis with gas formation, and severe systemic upset. About 80% of cases are caused by *C. perfringens*, with *Clostridium novyi*, *Clostridium septicum*, *Clostridium bifermentans* making up most of the remainder. Gas in the wound is frequently a late finding and reliance on its presence to confirm the diagnosis is dangerous. Avoidance of this infection is aided by surgical debridement of contaminated wounds. In elective surgical amputations through the thigh, and orthopaedic operations above the knee and below the waist, prophylactic penicillin should be given. Established infection has a high mortality, even with treatment. This consists of surgical debridement with a wide margin of excision, or sometimes amputation, and treatment with parenteral penicillin (6–12 g/day). The presence of other organisms may necessitate widening the spectrum of antibiotic cover. Exchange transfusions have been advocated for seriously ill patients with gross systemic upset. The benefits of hyperbaric oxygen remain difficult to assess as there are no well-controlled trials or comparisons of this mode of therapy with conventional management. It may itself have toxic effects on the lung and nervous system, and the transfer of a patient from one hospital to another possessing the facility carries its own morbidity.

Anaerobic streptococci may also cause myonecrosis and produce gas.

NON-CLOSTRIDIAL INFECTIONS

Non-clostridial anaerobic cellulitis can be caused by a variety of organisms such as peptostreptococci, peptococci and bacteroides. In addition, facultative species including coliforms, streptococci and staphylococci may be present. Some Enterobacteriaceae, pseudomonads, anaerobic streptococci, and bacteroides may all cause cellulitis and produce gas, and thus be confused with clostridial myonecrosis. The distinction is important because many Gram-negative organisms will not respond to penicillin treatment. Cefoxitin, or clindamycin and an aminoglycoside have been suggested as appropriate therapy for this condition.

OTHER CAUSES OF CELLULITIS

Other causes of cellulitis include that caused by *H. influenzae* (usually encapsulated type b strains), which is almost exclusively an infection of children, most often affecting the face, and giving rise to a well demarcated violet lesion. Because of the possibility of ampicillin resistance it has been the practice to treat with chloramphenicol, but reports of resistance to this agent now make a cephalosporin such as cefotaxime the drug of choice. Enterobacteriaceae (especially *Escherichia coli*, *Klebsiella* and *Enterobacter* spp.) may cause cellulitis in diabetics, in areas of ischaemia or trauma, or after surgery of the abdomen or perineum. The organisms may produce gas. Mixed infections of streptococci and anaerobes are not uncommon. Therapy consists of an aminoglycoside, or a third-generation cephalosporin, with metronidazole for anaerobe cover.

Erysipeloid

Erysipeloid is a cellulitis caused by the Gram-positive bacillus *Erysipelothrix rhusiopathiae*. It usually presents after minor injury to the fingers or hands of workers who carry raw fish, pork or poultry, and presents as a warm, tender, well-marginated lesion with a violet colour. The condition usually heals spontaneously after a few weeks, but will respond sooner to either penicillin or tetracycline.

CUTANEOUS ANTHRAX

This disease affects some 20 000–100 000 people per year world-wide. Its treatment was reviewed by Knudson (1986). Penicillin is still the drug of first choice. Where penicillin allergy is a problem, erythromycin or tetracycline are alternatives. Unlike the generally lethal pulmonary and intestinal forms, most cases of cutaneous anthrax respond well to penicillin therapy (2.4–3.6 g/day for 10–12 days). This usually reduces local inflammation and systemic symptoms, but does not affect the evolution of the typical local lesion and eschar. Despite treatment, some patients die of systemic disease at a time when response to therapy is apparently satisfactory. Excision of the lesion increases and prolongs both the local and systemic manifestations and has no place in treatment. In septicaemic illness, anti-anthrax serum is advisable to neutralize circulating toxin (Knudson 1986).

Some cases will have no history of occupational exposure to alert the physician to the diagnosis. In well patients who have been exposed, penicillin prophylaxis should be coupled with vaccination.

GRAM-NEGATIVE INFECTIONS

Pseudomonas aeruginosa is the most important of the Gram-negative organisms causing disease of the skin. It is an opportunist in diabetic, immunodeficient and burn patients. The features of infection often depend on the characteristics of the particular strain involved. The spectrum of soft tissue infections include infection of the toe web, finger and toe nails, and corneal ulceration. Nail infections may cause a greenish hue to the affected area, and are often associated with long periods of immersion in water during the course of the sufferer's occupation. The infection can usually be treated successfully by the application of a drying agent such as 10% aluminium chloride or alcohol. Surgical drainage may be required of an adjacent paronychia. General therapy of superficial pseudomonal infections includes drying of the area, the removal of any occlusions, and debridement where appropriate. Heavy infection can sometimes be detected by green fluorescence under an ultraviolet light.

Pseudomonas pyoderma may present as a primary infection, particularly in immunocompromised patients. Necrotic areas and haemorrhage are common, and it may also be accompanied by the typical vasculitic rash of ecthyma gangrenosum characteristic of septicaemic infections. 'Whirlpool-bath' folliculitis due to pseudomonal infection may occur some 24–48 h after a hot bath (which dilates ducts) in poorly chlorinated water. It presents as a maculopapular and pustular rash on the trunk, axillae and buttocks, and may be accompanied by malaise, low-grade fever, lymphadenopathy, tender breasts, vomiting and cramps. It is usually a self-limiting illness, but a few cases have been severe.

Erythrasma

Erythrasma is caused by *Corynebacterium minutissimum* which possesses keratolytic properties. The infected skin in erythrasma shows a striking pink fluoresence in ultraviolet light. Standard therapy consists of oral erythromycin, 250 mg 6-hourly for 2 weeks, but equally good results may be obtained with topical agents such as benzoic acid ointment, framycetin, and 2% sodium fucidate.

Burns

Initial therapy of severe burns patients with resuscitative measures, fluid replacement, etc., has led to an improvement in mortality figures during the early acute phase after injury. In the stages that follow in burns of an area greater than 30–40% body surface, however, the main cause of mortality is from infection. The principles of management are summarized in Box 52.4, and have been reviewed in excellent articles by Waymack & Pruitt (1990) and Deitch (1990).

Both Gram-positive and Gram-negative bacteria are commonly incriminated in burn sepsis as well as, occasionally, fungi. Infection with Gram-negative bacilli has been associated with a higher mortality rate. If there are clinical signs that the burns wound is infected (see below) empirical antibiotic therapy should be started before the results of bacteriology are known (see Box 52.4). Pseudomonal infections are particularly common, so much so that a few specialized burns units use intravenous immunoglobulins as a routine prophylactic. Gram-negative organisms infecting burn wounds may be either nosocomial in origin or may derive from endogenous contamination from the gut, especially in wounds located close to the perineum. Selective gut decontamination in this class of patient is still controversial (Ch. 44). Established infection with *Pseudomonas* requires treatment with an effective antipseudomonal regimen such as the combination of a parenteral aminoglycoside with ceftazidime or azlocillin. Ciprofloxacin may be a valuable drug in this situation, but as yet there are no results of large trials to prove its merit.

The particular organisms likely to be isolated from burn wounds (and their sensitivities) will vary from one burns unit to another. There is also likely to be a changing pattern

---

Box 52.4 *Principles of management of patients with burns*

- Immediate resuscitative measures; fluid replacement
- Wound toilet, e.g. irrigation with chlorhexidene 0.05%
- Surgical debridement of non-viable tissue
- Topical prophylactic antimicrobial agents (see Box 52.5), e.g. silver sulfadiazine
- Observation and microbial surveillance, wound biopsy and treatment of established infection with systemic antibiotics
- Empirical systemic antibiotic therapy of infected wounds, for example with:
  — piperacillin/tazobactam (4.5 g i.v. 8-hourly)
  or
  — ciprofloxacin (750 mg p.o. or 400 mg i.v. 12-hourly) + benzylpenicillin (1.2 g i.v. 4-hourly)
  or
  — clindamycin (450 mg i.v./p.o. 6-hourly) + ceftazidime (2 g i.v. 8-hourly)
- Surgical grafting
- General supportive measures, including nutrition.

of isolate identity with the passage of time within the same unit.

Prophylactic systemic antibiotics are not recommended as a routine.

Early recognition of infection in a burns wound requires frequent observation of the sites. Unfortunately, swabbing for microbiological culture may yield results that do not distinguish between infection and contamination, nor do they give any indication of the extent of infection. A change in the appearance of the lesion may signify infection. Haemorrhage, rapid eschar separation and a green discolouration are suspicious signs of bacterial invasion, and a black colour may indicate infection with fungi. Gram-positive infections generally, but not invariably, give rise to suppurative foci. Biopsy, with an ellipse of skin from the edge of a wound has been shown to give valuable information concerning the density of organisms in the tissue and also the extent of invasion into viable tissue.

Topical antimicrobials have been shown to lessen the progression of partial to full-thickness lesions. They may also prolong the sterility of established full thickness wounds, but it must be emphasized that there is still a need for adequate surgical removal of necrotic tissue, with or without grafting. Topical therapy for burns has recently been extensively reviewed by Manafo & West (1990). Agents commonly in use include those listed in Box 52.5. Topical prophylactic antimicrobial therapy is assumed to have played a large part in the improved outcome of patients with severe burn wounds, and has been shown to lessen the incidence of wound colonization which usually precedes infection, and which may eventually lead to delayed healing, and increased morbidity and mortality.

Actinomycosis

Actinomyces israeli is sensitive to penicillin, but therapy has to be prolonged because of poor penetration of antibiotic through the granulomatous and fibrotic structures that are a feature of the infected lesions in this condition; eradication may thus be difficult. Tetracyclines, erythromycin and clindamycin are also suitable drugs. For cervicofacial actinomycosis at least 6 weeks treatment is usually advisable with 1 g 6-hourly amoxycillin orally. Success has been reported with both tetracycline (3 g/day for 28 days; or 3 g/day for 10 days followed by 2 g/day for a further 18 days) and erythromycin (500 mg 6-hourly for 6 weeks), which may be useful in the penicillin-allergic patient.

Thoracic, abdominal, bone and disseminated actinomycosis may be difficult to eradicate. Penicillin is regarded as the drug of choice given in doses of 1.2 g i.v. 4-hourly. Therapy may be continued for between 2 and 3 months by changing to oral amoxycillin (1 g 6-hourly) after perhaps 3 weeks of parenteral penicillin. *A. israelii* is sensitive to both fucidin and clindamycin, and both these antibiotics may have an advantage in treating deep-seated infection because of their good penetrating ability. Surgical treatment to drain abscesses and excise sinus tracts is an important part of management, but on its own is not adequate treatment.

Actinomyces are often accompanied by small Gram-negative bacilli, *Actinobacillus actinomycetemcomitans*, and a *Haemophilus*-like organism *Haemophilus aphrophilus*. Both are relatively insensitive to penicillin, but sensitive to tetracycline, and this fact has supported the use of tetracycline in the therapy of this condition.

Box 52.5 *Topical therapy for burns*

Silver nitrate – has good antimicrobial activity, gives pain relief, has no effect on epithelial growth, but is difficult to apply, may cause electrolyte loss, is expensive, stains and does not penetrate eschar tissue well

Mafenide – is a good antimicrobial, is cheap, easy to apply and penetrates eschar well, but is painful, hampers epithelial growth, and may cause systemic acidosis

Silver sulphadiazine – is a good antimicrobial which is easy to apply, and provides pain relief without effect on epithelial growth, but which discolours and is expensive

Gentamicin – causes emergence of resistant strains and fungal growth

Povidone iodine – may be painful, and can be inactivated by proteins in the wound, has an inhibitory effect on phagocytosis and has been shown to cause systemic acidosis

Chlorhexidene – is innocuous, painless and easy to apply

Tetanus

This infection is caused by the anaerobic, spore-forming, Gram-positive bacillus, *Clostridium tetani*. Infection most commonly arises after penetrating trauma to the soft tissues and contamination with soil. However, in many cases the initial lesion and source of infection is never found. Classically, there is the retention of foreign material in the tissues, and tissue necrosis giving rise to an anaerobic environment which favours growth of the organism and toxin production. The incubation period of the illness is proportional to the distance of the lesion from the central nervous system, and generally falls between 3 and 21 days. A more severe and prolonged illness tends to follow a short incubation period.

Treatment consists of the administration of human antitetanus antiserum, surgical exploration of the lesion if identified, benzylpenicillin 1.2 g i.v. 4-hourly for 10 days, and management in a quiet, dimly lit environment. Muscular spasms may be reduced by using benzodiazepines such as diazepam. Heavy sedation, however, may compromise respiratory function which should be monitored closely. Dantrolene may be effective as a muscle relaxant, but without depressing respiration. Prolonged use of dantrolene may cause hepatic damage. Prognosis has been improved by the introduction of paralysis and ventilation when the disease appears to be progressing towards the development of convulsions. Periods of several weeks may be necessary, and if so H_2-antagonists and anticoagulation should be given.

Acne vulgaris

This is an inflammatory condition, probably caused by the accumulation of free fatty acids in the follicles of the skin produced by the action of bacterial lipolytic enzymes on triglycerides. The principal organism incriminated is usually *Propionibacterium acnes*. Antimicrobial treatment is therefore directed at reducing the bacterial population responsible, thereby decreasing the formation of free fatty acids. Therapy with antibiotics has been shown to improve the condition in many trials, but these have also shown a large placebo effect. Nevertheless, antibiotic therapy has an established place in the treatment of acne. The pathogenesis and treatment of acne vulgaris has recently been reviewed by Cunliffe & Eady (1992). Oral antimicrobials, namely tetracyclines, erythromycin and clindamycin, have been used for many years and recent studies have reported on the side-effects of such long-term therapy. Partly for this reason, topical antimicrobial therapy has enjoyed a resurgence of interest.

Topical antibiotics commonly used include tetracycline, clindamycin and erythromycin (with or without zinc), and are useful agents for treating mild to moderate acne. Systemic oral antibiotics e.g. tetracycline, doxycycline, minocycline and erythromycin, may be needed for more severe acne (Box 52.6). Minocycline is probably the best of these agents taken in a dose of 50 mg twice daily. Resistance of propionibacter to minocycline is rare, whereas it is much more common to the other tetracyclines and erythromycin.

Of equal, if not greater importance than antibiotic therapy are the many other strategies designed to affect the pathogenetic processes of acne advantageously. Benzoyl peroxide 10% has an antibacterial action thought to be due to the release of oxygen when the drug reacts with cysteine in the skin, and non-antimicrobial therapy for acne can be classified into groups of agents with sebostatic, comedolytic, exfoliant, anhydrotic and anti-inflammatory properties. Retinoic acid, which also has exfoliant actions, is the most commonly used comedolytic. Other exfoliants include resorcinol, and the use of cryotherapy and abrasives.

Box 52.6 *Systemic antibiotic therapy for moderate to severe acne*

- Minocycline 50 mg 12-hourly orally for a minimum of 6 weeks or
- Erythromycin 250 mg 8-hourly orally for 1–4 weeks and then 12-hourly until improvement occurs

Aluminium chloride hexahydrate 6.25% can be used as an anhydrotic, but is not particularly effective in most patients in reducing severity. The topical and systemic use of steroids as anti-inflammatory agents, is only likely to have a short-term beneficial effect, and may actually aggravate or induce acne. More recently, isoretinoin has been used as an oral systemic agent with remarkable success even in severe acne vulgaris. It is teratogenic and has a number of other side-effects, and is probably best reserved as second-line therapy. Antiandrogens such as cyproterone acetate, also have a place in the treatment of acne, and like oral isotretinoin, should be used with the guidance of a specialist with experience of their use.

Scabies and pediculosis

The usual manifestations of scabies and head lice are well known. Occasionally, particularly in patients with HIV, a very severe form of scabies – Norwegian scabies – may occur with widespread lesions covered in thick crusts and much inflammation. The treatment of choice for scabies remains either lindane, malathion or benzylbenzoate. Lindane should not be used in pregnancy or in children because of possible neurotoxicity, and benzylbenzoate is probably best avoided in children due to its irritant nature. Different districts operate a rotational policy for the use of these agents. An application is made to the whole body excluding the head and neck, and this is repeated the next day without bathing in the case of benzylbenzoate only, to be washed off finally 24 h later. The itch of the lesions may persist for some time until the dead 'skeleton' of the scabies mite has been disposed of by the host's immune defence mechanisms. Patients with AIDS and 'Norwegian-type' scabies may need to apply the medication to the neck and scalp area and repeat the whole procedure a second time 10–14 days after the first. Two newer agents are in use for the treatment of scabies and pediculosis: permethrin and phenothrin. These agents appear to have good efficacy and few side-effects, but have diminished activity against the eggs of lice. Molinari (1992) reviews these treatments and concludes that the treatment of choice in children with head lice is now a single application of permethrin 1% rinse and permethrin 5% cream for scabies. In areas of the world where economies dictate treatment regimens, sulphur ointment (6–10%) may be the only treatment available.

Malathion and carbaryl are also satisfactory treatments for head lice in adults. Aqueous lotions, left for 12 h on the scalp are preferred to shampoos. Lindane is not recommended for head lice due to a high rate of treatment failure. Systemic treatment with ivermectin has been reported to help treat the severe forms of scabies associated with HIV-infected individuals.

Fungal soft tissue infections

Fungal skin and soft tissue infections are discussed in Chapter 60.

References

Ash S, Hewitt C 1994 HIV-associated cutaneous disorders. *Current Opinion in Infectious Diseases* 7: 195–201

Baltimore R S 1985 Treatment of impetigo: a review. *Paediatric Infectious Diseases Journal* 4: 597–601

Bergin D J, Wright J E 1986 Orbital cellulitis. *British Journal of Opthalmology* 70: 174–178

Blumer J L, O'Brien C A, Lemon E, Capretta T M 1985 Skin and soft tissue infections: pharmacological approaches. *Paediatric Infectious Diseases Journal* 4: 336–341

Coskey R J, Coskey L A 1987 Diagnosis and treatment of impetigo. *Journal of the American Academy of Dermatology* 17: 62–63

Cunliffe W J, Eady E A 1992 A reappraisal and update on the pathogenesis and treatment of acne. *Current Opinion in Infectious Diseases* 5: 703–710

Deitch E A 1990 Review article: the management of burns. *New England Journal of Medicine* 323: 1249–1253

Eells L D, Mertz P M, Piovanetti D P et al 1986 Topical antibiotic treatment of impetigo with mupirocin. *Archives of Dermatology* 122: 1273–1277

Israele V, Nelson J 1987 Periorbital and orbital cellulitis. *Paediatric Infectious Diseases Journal* 6: 404–410

Knudson G B 1986 Treatment of anthrax in man: history and current concepts. *Military Medicine* 151: 71–77

Lewis R T 1992 Necrotising soft-tissue infections. *Infectious Diseases Clinics of North America* 6: 693–703

Molinari F 1992 Update on the treatment of pediculosis and scabies. *Pediatric Nursing* 8: 600–602

Monafo W W, West M A 1990 Current treatment recommendations for topical burn therapy. *Drugs* 40: 362–373

Rooney J F, Sraus S E, Nannix M L et al 1993 Oral acyclovir to suppress frequently recurrent herpes labialis: a double-blind, placebo-controlled trial. *Annals of Internal Medicine* 118: 268–272

Todd J K 1993 The resurgence of severe group A streptococcal disease. *Infectious Medicine* 10: 48–51

Waymack P J, Pruitt B A 1990 Burn wound care. *Advances in Surgery* 23: 261–289

Whitley R J, Straus S E 1993 Therapy for varicella-zoster virus infections: Where do we stand? *Infectious Disease Clinical Practice* 2: 100–108

Williams R E A, MacKie R M 1993 The staphylococci. Importance of their control in the management of skin disease. *Dermatologic Therapy* 11: 201–206

Infections of the central nervous system

H. P. Lambert

Meningitis

The likelihood of any particular cause varies greatly in different communities, and depends also on host factors which may or may not be evident when the patient is first seen.

The most common causes in community acquired meningitis, at all ages beyond the neonatal period, remain *Neisseria meningitidis, Haemophilus influenzae* and *Streptococcus pneumoniae.* Their frequency differs in different age groups; in early childhood all three organisms were found, with a predominance of *H. influenzae* and *N. meningitidis.* These two organisms were of approximately equal prevalence in Britain, but the inclusion of a conjugate vaccine against *H. influenzae* (HIB) has now greatly reduced the prevalence of this form of meningitis. *Haemophilus* meningitis becomes rare by school age, although it does occur in older children and in adults. At the older ages the pneumococcus becomes predominant, and is especially prominent in patients with various forms of immune suppression and in chronic alcoholics, and in meningitis associated with skull fractures.

Until recently, therefore, the meningococcus and the pneumococcus were responsible for virtually all pyogenic meningitis in school-aged children and adults. The increased number of patients with various forms of increased susceptibility in some communities has, however, somewhat altered this picture. In New York, for example, meningitis caused by various Gram-negative enteric bacilli and by *Listeria monocytogenes* have assumed prominence in renal transplant recipients, patients on renal dialysis programmes and those receiving immunosuppressive drugs for a variety of chronic disorders. The importance of alcoholism as a risk factor has been mentioned.

In the neonate, most cases are caused by enterobacteria, notably *Escherichia coli,* and by pseudomonads; most of the remaining cases are caused by streptococci and staphylococci. Group B streptococci have emerged into prominence in recent years, and are about as frequent as enterobacteria in the newborn, both in the USA and in the UK. An enormous variety of other organisms are capable of causing meningitis in the neonate, of which *L. monocytogenes* and *Salmonella* are especially notable, but the three species commonly found at older ages, are also occasionally responsible. The relative importance of different bacteria in the immediate post-neonatal period had been examined by Enzenauer et al (1983), who recorded several cases of group B streptococcal meningitis in the 1–2 month age group. Coliform meningitis was only encountered when neonatal complications had ensued, and *H. influenzae* was the most importance cause in this group.

When meningitis supervenes in chronic ear infection, in association with congenital defects of the central nervous system (CNS), or follows trauma, operation or lumbar puncture, the infecting organisms resemble those of neonatal meningitis, with a large proportion caused by staphylococci, streptococci, enterobacteria and pseudomonads, while the pneumococcus is also strongly represented in this group, especially in association with meningitis following fracture of the skull. Mixed infections, sometimes including anaerobic organisms, are also found.

DIAGNOSIS AND PRINCIPLES OF TREATMENT

Early diagnosis of bacterial meningitis is essential for successful treatment. The age of the patient is of some value in indicating which of the common bacteria is responsible, but the only sign commonly helpful on physical examination is the characteristic rash found in some patients with severe meningococcal infection. Because of this paucity of clinical evidence, early bacteriological diagnosis is of the utmost importance, and an expert opinion on a Gram-stained film of a specimen of cerebrospinal fluid (CSF) should be regarded as one of the few bacteriological emergencies. Other methods to supplement the Gram stain are now becoming more widely used. Rapid antigen-detection methods can be used to detect antigen in CSF, blood or urine, and suitably specific sera against the common causal pathogens are available. These methods enable a rapid causal diagnosis to be made in some patients, especially those who have received antibiotic treatment before lumbar puncture, in whom no bacteria can be seen in the Gram-stained CSF deposit. Countercurrent immune electro-phoresis (CIE) and other methods such as enzyme-linked immunosorbent assay (ELISA) have been supplanted by commercially prepared latex agglutination kits which are easy to use and give a result in a few minutes, but vary in their sensitivity and specificity. Polymerase chain reaction (PCR) tests are also available at reference centres.

No organism can be isolated from the CSF in some cases of purulent meningitis; the proportion varies between 12% and 25% in different series. One reason for this shortfall in causal diagnosis, which can be partly restored by rapid antigen-detection tests, is previous antibiotic treatment. This has the effect of reducing the number of positive CSF Gram-stained films and cultures, and occasionally the changes induced are so great that the CSF findings may simulate those of tuberculous or viral meningitis. The possibility of tuberculous meningitis particularly arises because, while the CSF cellular content may change greatly in number and character, the low glucose concentration normally found in pyogenic meningitis tends to persist.

PHARMACOKINETIC FACTORS

Antibiotic concentration in CSF

The factors affecting penetration of antibiotics into the CSF have been reviewed by Stone & Wise (1991) and by Ristuccia & Le Frock (1992). Chief among them are lipid solubility, ionization, the pH gradient between blood and CSF, protein binding, molecular size and configuration, the presence of active transport system and the degree of meningeal inflammation. The available data on CSF levels varies greatly from drug to drug, but it is possible to make a clinical classification (Box 53.1) into four groups:

- Therapeutic CSF concentrations may be reached by standard dosage and routes of administration
- A high therapeutic ratio allows adequate CSF concentrations to be achieved by high i.v. or i.m. doses; the CSF concentration is usually higher when the meninges are inflamed
- Drug toxicity disallows increase in dose, and CSF concentration may reach therapeutic levels only when the meninges are inflamed
- Little or no drug is found in the CSF with or without meningitis; intrathecal administration may be needed.

CSF penetration of the penicillins and the cephalosporins is poor. Low CSF/plasma ratios are found with uninflamed meninges and, although better penetration is achieved in meningitis, CSF concentrations still vary widely and unpredictably. The high therapeutic ratio of these compounds does, however, allow large doses to be given by the

---

Box 53.1 *Penetration of antimicrobial agents into CSF*

- Therapeutic CSF concentrations achieved by standard doses and routes of administration

  Chloramphenicol
  Sulphonamides
  Trimethoprim
  Fluoroquinolones[‡]
  Metronidazole
  Doxycycline*
  Isoniazid
  Rifampicin
  Pyrazinamide
  Ethionamide
  Amphotericin B

- Therapeutic CSF concentrations achieved by high i.v. or i.m. doses, especially in meningitis

  Penicillins[†]
  Cephalosporins

- Therapeutic CSF concentrations may be achieved by standard doses and routes in meningitis

  Clindamycin
  Vancomycin
  Tetracycline*
  Erythromycin
  Ethambutol
  Flucytosine

- Therapeutic CSF concentrations cannot be reliably achieved except where intrathecal route is possible

  Aminoglycosides[†]
  Polymyxin[†]
  Fusidate

* After repeated doses.
† Intrathecal preparations may be available.
‡ Varies with different agents of the group.

intravenous route, so that therapeutic levels can be achieved; suitable regimens are described later in this chapter. An extensive review of penetration of the newer cephalosporins into CSF has been made by Cherubin et al (1989), who conclude that they are more or less equivalent, with the exceptions of cefamandole and cefoperazone in which penetration was inadequate. With the other compounds, they feel choice should be based mainly on the appropriateness of the agent for the specific pathogen to be treated. Aminoglycosides penetrate into the CSF poorly or not at all; the problem of aminoglycoside therapy in coliform meningitis is discussed on page 751.

The evidence of erratic distribution within the CSF, and that antibiotics injected into the lumbar theca do not easily become distributed throughout the ventricular system, has led many physicians to a greatly diminished use of intrathecal therapy on the grounds that its risks outweigh the doubtful therapeutic advantage. There are, nevertheless, a few situations in which intrathecal treatment is indicated, when the ventricular route must be used. In some patients a ventricular reservoir may be needed when injections at this site are easily made. Doses and preparations for intrathecal injection should be very carefully checked.

Contribution of experimental studies

Although much information has been gathered about antibiotic concentrations in serum and CSF in human meningitis, ethical and practical limitations make it difficult to achieve a full picture of the conditions necessary for successful treatment. Many factors certainly contribute to the poor results of treatment in neonatal meningitis, and in Gram-negative bacillary meningitis in older age groups, but recent studies make it certain that failure to achieve appropriate concentration of the correct antibiotic at relevant sites is often related to these poor results. As elsewhere in the body, local foci of infection remain important and, in neonatal meningitis especially, persistent ventriculitis results in treatment failure. General principles apply here as elsewhere: the antibiotic regimen used must be active and, in this situation, bactericidal against the causal organism at concentrations regularly achieved in body fluids. Additional factors related to success or failure have been clarified by work on experimental animals, especially in a rabbit model of experimental meningitis, in which repeated estimations of bacterial counts and of antibiotic concentrations can be made. McCracken (1983) shows that, for some agents, the pharmacokinetic factors can be quite similar in the rabbit and the human infant. He concludes that measurement of the ratio of CSF area under curve to serum area under curve (CSF AUC/serum AUC × 100) after single doses and the mean relative concentrations after 9 h infusions give good predictions for CSF penetration in infants and children. Both in rabbits and children, best results are achieved if the bactericidal titre of the CSF for the relevant organism is at least 1 : 8, but the rate of decline in the bacterial population of the CSF is no greater even if this titre is much exceeded. Measurements of this type, both in experimental animals and in man, are helpful in the initial evaluation of new putative agents for treating meningitis, but are usually unnecessary in clinical practice once pharmacokinetic features of the drug have been well established.

Special features of antibiotics commonly used in the treatment of meningitis

Benzylpenicillin and ampicillin. In common with other β-lactam agents, these compounds penetrate the CSF poorly. Their low toxicity, however, enables this disadvantage to be overcome by high systemic dosage. These high doses normally necessitate intravenous therapy. Where conditions made this impracticable or hazardous, intramuscular injections can be used, but the large injection volumes are painful and not without danger of faulty siting. CSF concentrations appropriate for the treatment of penicillin-susceptible meningococcal or pneumococcal meningitis can be achieved with dosage of 150 mg/kg (250 000 units/kg) daily divided into 4-hourly intravenous doses (Hieber & Nelson 1977). The same general points apply to ampicillin and its congeners. The range of doses in controlled trials has varied from 150 to 400 mg/kg daily. It has been shown that the highest doses are unnecessary, and a standard dose regimen of 200 mg/kg daily is recommended. It needs to be emphasized that none of the oral forms of penicillin or ampicillin is suitable for treating meningitis. This means that the whole course of treatment must be given by injection – CSF penetration diminishing even further as meningeal inflammation begins to resolve. The short half-lives of these compounds makes it unwise to prolong the dose interval beyond 4–6 h.

Two specific unwanted effects have also to be considered. Neurological toxicity from penicillin (p. 265) presents a danger only when excessively high blood or CSF concentrations are reached. This sometimes occurs when very large doses are given intravenously in the presence of renal failure, but is especially associated with incorrectly high intrathecal dosage at a time when this form of administration was commonly used.

Cephalosporins. The spread of resistance to ampicillin, and to some extent to chloramphenicol, among strains of *H. influenzae* made it necessary to evaluate the use of cephalosporins in this and other forms of meningitis. The earlier compounds proved unsatisfactory, despite good in vitro activity, with a number of treatment failures; cefamandole also gave poor results. This situation changed with the introduction of extended-spectrum compounds such as cefotaxime. Their high intrinsic activity made it possible to achieve CSF concentrations many times greater than the minimum bactericidal concentrations (MBCs) of the common organisms causing meningitis, and their high degree of β-lactamase resistance made them suitable for treating ampicillin-resistant organisms. CSF concentrations and CSF/serum ratios for these and other agents used in treating meningitis are shown in Table 53.1. The wide variability and occasional low CSF concentrations are worth noting. During the 1980s many controlled trials (reviewed in the previous edition of this book) were made of different cephalosporins in meningitis. The largest groups studied were children with *H. meningitis*, and in most trials the compound under trial was compared with the ampicillin–chloramphenicol combination then prevailing as standard treatment for community-acquired childhood meningitis. These trials gave results generally similar, but not superior to, the standard regimen. Of the many compounds available, cefotaxime and ceftriaxone have been especially well studied. In addition to clinical comparisons with the standard regimens, many trials included measurements of rate of decline of bacterial counts in the CSF, and time to negative CSF cultures, which were again generally comparable in the two groups. In one trial (Barson et al 1985) comparing twice-daily ceftriaxone with chloramphenicol–ampicillin, repeat lumbar puncture 10–18 h after the start of treatment showed similar reductions of bacterial counts, but the median bactericidal titre in the CSF was 1 : 1024 in the ceftriaxone group compared with 1 : 4 in the conventional therapy group. Ceftriaxone concentrations in the CSF were 3–24% (mean 11.8%) of the serum concentration. These generally good results emboldened workers to study once-daily ceftriaxone dosage, allowing the possibility of largely outpatient treatment in patients who were well enough after the initial diagnostic assessment and initiation of treatment. Again, results were satisfactory; diarrhoea, the main unwanted effect, was not severe enough to necessitate a change of treatment. Duration of treatment has also been reduced, Lin

et al (1985) showing that the results with 7 days' treatment with ceftriaxone were as good as those after 10 days.

Ceftriaxone, like the other cephalosporins used in meningitis, is normally given intravenously, but sometimes this route is difficult to maintain through the entire course of therapy. A study involving CSF examination 4–6 h after intramuscular injection on the 3rd, 6th or 9th day of treatment (the normal intravenous route being used on the other days) showed satisfactory serum concentrations of ceftriaxone, and all CSF specimens showed bactericidal titres of a least 1 : 64 against the three common organisms (Bradley et al 1994).

Cefotaxime too has been extensively studied and shown effective in the common forms of bacterial meningitis, used mostly in a dose of 50 mg/kg daily. A large study of 85 infants and children prospectively randomized to receive cefotaxime or ampicillin and chloramphenicol (Odio et al 1986) showed similar progress in the two groups. The mean bactericidal titre in the CSF was 1 : 64 in the cefotaxime group and 1 : 8 in the ampicillin–chloramphenicol group. Other substantial studies by Wells et al (1984) and by Jacobs et al (1985) gave similar results, with useful data in the former study on serum and CSF concentrations of cefotaxime and its desacetyl derivative.

The increasing importance of drug resistance in *H. influenzae* infection, and the possible antagonism between ampicillin and chloramphenicol, led Finnish workers to conduct an important multicentre comparison in 220 children with meningitis (146 of them caused by *H. influenzae*) of chloramphenicol, ampicillin (initially with chloramphenicol), cefotaxime and ceftriaxone (Peltola et al 1989). Results were similar in the four treatment groups, but all four bacteriological failures were with chloramphenicol and treatment had to be changed more frequently in this group. Use of ampicillin was limited by the problem of resistance. These workers were unable to rank the other two agents. Cefotaxime has fewer adverse effects, but the high cost of both drugs greatly limits their potential in developing countries.

Although cefotaxime and ceftriaxone are perhaps the most widely used cephalosporins in meningitis, other β-lactam compounds have also been studied in *Haemophilus* meningitis, including ceftazidime, ceftizoxime and aztreonam, again usually in comparison with ampicillin and chloramphenicol. An earlier compound, latamoxef (moxalactam), no longer in common use, was also extensively evaluated in meningitis, and found a valid alternative to the standard regimen, with a reassuring follow-up report (Kaplan et al 1988) of the patient's status 2 years after therapy.

Cefuroxime, once used fairly widely in meningitis, proved inferior to ceftriaxone in a comparative trial (Schaad et al 1990) in 106 children with the common forms of bacterial meningitis. CSF cultures remained positive at 18–36 h in 1 of 52 in the ceftriaxone group compared with 6 of 52

Table 53.1 *Penetration of some agents into human CSF*

Agent	Conc. in lumbar CSF (mg)	CSF/serum (%)
Latamoxef	2.7 – 27	6.6 – 16.0
Ceftriaxone	2 – 42	1.1 – 31
Cefoperazone	<0.8 – 11.5	
Ceftazidime	2 – 56	1.6 – 46
Ceftizoxime	<0.5 – 29	23
Cefotaxime	3.7 ± 5.5	10
Desacetyl form	4.3 ± 7.1	55
Aztreonam	3.5 – 62	
Imipenem	0.5 – 11	
Cilastatin	0.1 – 10	
Ciprofloxacin	0.3 – 0.5	20 – 30

receiving cefuroxime, and substantial hearing loss was present at follow-up in two of the ceftriaxone and nine of the cefuroxime group. Although undoubtedly effective, this agent does now appear as somewhat inferior to many later compounds and is not now generally recommended for the treatment of meningitis. Lebel at al (1989), reviewing the results of four trials, noted positive CSF cultures 24 h into therapy in 9% of 174 patients given cefuroxime compared with none in 159 treated with ceftriaxone, and subsequent hearing impairment in 18% compared with 11% in the two groups.

Chloramphenicol. Although now little used in wealthier countries, chloramphenicol remains an important drug for meningitis in developing countries with low health budgets. It is highly effective in *H. influenzae* meningitis and its replacement by ampicillin in the USA and some other countries was partly reversed when ampicillin resistance emerged in this species in 1974. Unfortunately, strains resistant to chloramphenicol have also now appeared, although they are still rare in most countries. Chloramphenicol is also the drug of choice for meningococcal meningitis in the highly penicillin-allergic patient. The situation with pneumococcal meningitis is now becoming complicated by drug resistance and, although pneumococci are usually susceptible on disc testing, the efficacy of chloramphenicol is uncertain; this problem is discussed below, in the section on pneumococcal meningitis. Chloramphenicol is also frequently needed in neonatal meningitis, although now becoming superseded by newer agents. It is less effective against coliform organisms, against which its action is bacteriostatic, than against *H. influenzae* against which it is strongly bactericidal. In countries with low health budgets chloramphenicol provides an inexpensive drug, highly effective, and easy to administer, for most forms of meningitis. The risks of meningitis far exceed the small risk of aplastic anaemia from its administration.

The danger of excessive dosage of chloramphenicol in the neonate, with high blood concentrations causing the so-called 'grey syndrome' resulting from deficient hepatic glucuronidation, has long been known. It is now evident that wide variations of serum level may be attained by standard dosage, especially in the neonate, and there is a need to monitor serum levels, at any rate in infancy, in order to ensure adequate levels and to prevent toxicity. Assays are recommended every 48 h following the start of a standard regimen, the dose to be increased if peak concentrations are less than 20 mg and decreased if trough levels exceed 15 mg or peak levels exceed 30 mg. Unfortunately, some poor results are attributable to wrong dosage; the studies of Mulhall et al (1983) showed that only 20 of 70 neonates and infants treated in British paediatric units received the correct dose, and serious toxicity was always associated with a higher than recommended dose of 25 mg/kg in 24 h for preterm infants and for term infants in the first week of life, and 37.5–50 mg/kg for neonates over 7 days old. Infants beyond the neonatal period, and children, can be given 75 mg/kg. As to route of administration, oral administration often gives suboptimal levels in the neonate. Beyond this age, chloramphenicol can be given by mouth as soon as possible, often for the whole duration of treatment, since oral and intravenous routes are effective pharmacokinetically. The intravenous route does bear a disadvantage, at least potentially, over the oral one, since about one-third of the administered, intravenous, dose of chloramphenicol succinate is lost in the urine in unhydrolysed form and, whereas the oral dose of the palmitate correlates well with the AUC, the intravenous dose of succinate does not. Contrary to previous belief, however, the intravenous and intramuscular routes are equivalent in the extent of loss of unhydrolysed succinate, so that the choice between these routes, when oral administration is impossible, should be made on other grounds (Shann et al 1986). Dosage of antibiotics commonly used in the treatment of meningitis is summarized in Table 53.2.

Duration of treatment and assessment of response

The response to treatment in cases of acute meningitis is

Table 53.2 *Antibiotic dosage in meningitis*

	Dose in 24 h		Dose interval (h)	Route
	Adult (g)	Child (mg/kg)		
Benzylpenicillin	14.4	180–300	4	i.v. (i.m.)
Ampicillin	12	200	4	i.v. (i.m.)
Chloramphenicol*	3	50–100	6	i.v., oral
Cefotaxime	8	200	8	i.v. (i.m.)
Ceftriaxone	4	80	24	i.v. (i.m.)
Vancomycin*	2	40	6	i.v.

* Control by measurement of plasma concentrations desirable. Dose less in neonates.

usually extremely rapid. Except with coliform infections and tuberculous meningitis (Ch. 59), if uncomplicated cases are treated early, the cerebrospinal fluid is often sterile within 24 h of the onset of treatment and almost invariably within a week. Duration of treatment is discussed in relation to individual pathogens.

Difficulties are often encountered in judging the progress of treatment in meningitis. In particular, fever may be prolonged, and neurological signs or disturbance of consciousness may persist for a variable time during treatment. If progress is unsatisfactory, it is essential to review the evidence for the initial diagnosis, the basis on which the antibiotic regimen was chosen, and the dose and route of administration of the drug. However, prolonged fever seldom results from antibiotic failure, and it is rare to recover organism from the CSF within 48 h of starting treatment. Repeat lumbar punctures are therefore unnecessary if progress is satisfactory. The most common cause of prolonged fever in patients receiving intravenous treatment is phlebitis at injection sites, and similarly patients receiving intramuscular injections may have fever from muscle damage. Fever may be caused by metastatic foci of infection, such as arthritis in meningococcal septicaemia, while focal neurological complications such as subdural effusion, sinus thrombosis or brain abscess must be considered. The fever of infection may be supplanted by that of drug hypersensitivity, and very rarely a second organism may be introduced at lumbar puncture. Once antibiotic failure has been excluded, it is often best to stop treatment after 10–14 days, and to observe the patient's progress and temperature thereafter. Once therapy is established on a rational basis it is unnecessary and confusing to make frequent changes of treatment because fever persists. It is often found that the temperature returns to normal as soon as chemotherapy is discontinued. Other aspects of management not directly related to infection must, of course, always be taken into account. Among the most important are the prevention and management of shock, coma, fits, hyponatraemia and CSF block. The protection of family contacts in certain forms of meningitis will be discussed.

TREATMENT OF SPECIFIC INFECTIONS

Meningococcal meningitis

Although meningococcal meningitis is a serious illness and meningococcal shock syndrome one of the most rapidly fatal of all infections, the organism itself is easily eliminated by appropriate chemotherapy. The success of sulphonamides in meningococcal disease was an outstanding triumph of chemotherapy, but the rapid spread of resistant strains since their first appearance in 1963 rendered these agents unsuitable for first-choice treatment within a few years. The

mainstay of treatment is benzylpenicillin, administered as described on page 744. Susceptibility testing is necessary, since the appearance of strains of moderate resistance to penicillin, described especially in Spain (Saez-Nieto et al 1992). In the UK, the minimum inhibitory concentration (MIC) of penicillin for most strains is less than 0.1 mg/l, but in 1993 6% showed MICs of 0.16–1.28 mg/l. These levels are not clinically important if the correct dosage is used.

Ampicillin is as suitable as benzylpenicillin for meningococcal disease, and when the microbial diagnosis of pyogenic meningitis is uncertain, the cephalosporins discussed above, although mainly used in *Haemophilus* meningitis, are fully active also against meningococci. Patients who are allergic to the penicillins or whose illness is caused by a penicillin-resistant meningococcus are best treated with a cephalosporin or chloramphenicol, which are as effective as penicillin in meningococcal meningitis. If penicillin resistance in meningococci becomes widespread, it will again become important to consider the possible use of sulphonamides, especially in countries in which parenteral cephalosporins suitable for treating meningitis are prohibitively expensive for most patients. In this context it should be recalled that sulphonamides are highly effective if the infecting strains is a susceptible one. The compound chosen will depend on availability; for most suitable agents such as sulphadimidine or sulphadiazine, initial dosage is 50 mg/kg followed by 100 mg/kg daily in adults, or 200 mg/kg in children.

In sharp contrast to the situation with many other forms of meningitis, eradication of the organism can be achieved readily and unduly prolonged treatment is unnecessary. Treatment is often continued for 7 days, but 5 days suffices to eradicate infection fully and even shorter treatments have been effective. Viladrich et al (1986) treated 50 patients with meningococcal meningitis with intravenous penicillin for 4 days and even single-dose therapy with a parenteral preparation of long-acting chloramphenicol has been successfully used (Puddicombe et al 1984, Pecoul et al 1991).

Prophylaxis of meningococcal meningitis. Outbreaks of meningococcal meningitis in closed communities, especially of military recruits, are well recognized, but spread within family groups may also occur, especially in conditions of overcrowding. Sulphadiazine has been very effective for chemoprophylaxis, while many other agents successfully used for the treatment of meningitis are ineffective for this purpose. As a results, the emergence of sulphonamide-resistant strains posed a considerable problem. Rifampicin is much more effective than penicillin, ampicillin, tetracycline or erythromycin in controlling the carriage of sulphonamide-resistant strains and has therefore become the drug of first choice for chemoprophylaxis, unless the prevalent strain is known to be sulphonamide susceptible. A number of trials in the early 1970s established the degree of efficacy of rifampicin (85–90%) in immediate reduction of meningococcal carrier rate, but a substantial proportion of the residual strains isolated in the post-treatment period were rifampicin resistant; it is therefore possible that widespread use of rifampicin will be accompanied by an increase in strains resistant to this drug. Moderate success in controlling meningococcal carriage has also been achieved with a tetracycline, minocycline. Total clearance of carriers was achieved by using a combination of rifampicin and minocycline, but a third of the patients given both drugs experienced unpleasant side-effects. Sequential use of minocycline followed by rifampicin has also been employed. The dosage of drugs used in meningococcal prophylaxis is: rifampicin 600 mg twice daily for four doses (10 mg/kg body weight 12-hourly for four doses for children); sulphonamide 1.0 g twice daily for four doses, and minocycline 200 mg followed by 100 mg twice daily for 5 days. More recently, two useful additions to the range of drug available for clearing meningococcal carriers have been made. Single-dose oral ciprofloxacin in a dose of either 500 or 750 mg has proved notably effective, and is now the preferred agent for adult contacts. For example, Gaunt & Lambert (1988) reduced the prevalence of nasopharyngeal carriers from 19% to 1.5% in a naval training establishment using a single dose of 500 mg without, in this trial, the emergence of resistant strains. Similarly, Dworzack et al (1988) treated 46 persistent carriers with 750 mg in a single oral dose in a placebo-controlled double-blind trial. Twenty of the 22 placebo recipients remained positive, whereas 20 of 23 recipients of active drug showed negative results on swabbing 7 and 21 days later. Single-dose injection treatment with ceftriaxone has also been successful in clearing nasopharyngeal carriage (Schwartz et al 1988) and this is the agent of choice in pregnant contacts. The adult dose is 250 mg as a single intramuscular injection; children under 12 years should receive half this dose.

If meningococcal disease is suspected, the patient should be given parenteral penicillin and admitted to hospital immediately. All suspected cases should be notified to the relevant public health authority (in the UK the Consultant in Communicable Disease Control) and pernasal or throat swabs taken from all suspected cases. Within 24 h chemoprophylaxis should be offered to all household and mouth-kissing contacts, and to patients before discharge (CDR 1995). Contacts should be carefully advised about possible early symptoms and of the persisting risk, even if they have received prophylaxis. The use of vaccine should be considered if a group C (or A) strains is responsible.

Pneumococcal meningitis

Despite the extreme susceptibility of *Str. pneumoniae* to the agents commonly used in the treatment of meningitis, the mortality from pneumococcal meningitis remains disappointingly high, usually of the order of 20–30%. Penicillin

should be given in doses of 1.2 g 2–4-hourly; this is best achieved by injecting the doses into an intravenous infusion. After the first few days of treatment when the interval between doses can be increased to 4-hourly, it may become practical to change to the intramuscular route. Treatment should be continued for at least 14 days, since even fully susceptible pneumococci may be notably slow to clear from the CSF (Greenwood et al 1986).

Penicillin-resistant pneumococci are now widespread, and susceptibility testing of strains recovered from infected sites is essential. Infection at sites other than the CNS caused by strains with low-level penicillin resistance can often be successfully treated with high-dose ·penicillin, but CNS infections cannot be reliably controlled in this way, and penicillin is ineffective at any site in the presence of high-level resistance.

Experience of penicillin resistance in severe pneumococcal infections has been extensively reported from Barcelona, Spain. Viladrich et al (1988) note that 15 of 66 episodes of pneumococcal meningitis between 1981 and 1987 were caused by strains with MICs between 0.1 and 4.0 mg/l. Half of them were also chloramphenicol resistant. They achieved some success by using high-dose intravenous cefotaxime (about 300 mg/kg), but point out that infections caused by more highly resistant strains (>4 mg/l) may need another antibiotic such as vancomycin.

The treatment of penicillin-resistant pneumococcal meningitis presents a problem with no easy solutions. Chloramphenicol, the traditional alternative used in patients with penicillin allergy, and indeed the only practical alternative in places with limited health budgets, is sometimes successful, but may fail to control infection. Work from South Africa (Friedland & Klugman 1992) showed that many penicillin-resistant pneumococci, although susceptible to chloramphenicol on disc testing, had high MBC values associated with poor results of treatment. At present, high-dose cephalosporins such as cefotaxime or ceftriaxone are preferred for meningitis caused by penicillin-resistant pneumococci, although some cephalosporin-resistant strains are now being encountered. Vancomycin has also been used, but correct dosage is difficult to achieve and a number of failures have been recorded. It is suggested that vancomycin should be used (in penicillin/chloramphenicol-resistant pneumococcal meningitis) only when high-dose cephalosporins have failed (Viladrich et al 1991). Vancomycin may also have a place in combination with cephalosporins when diminished susceptibility to the cephalosporin has been demonstrated (Klugman 1994). Rifampicin, in combination with a cephalosporin or with vancomycin, and imipenem or meropenem, should also be considered in evaluating treatment options. Some of the newer fluoroquinolones (Ch. 32) with better activity against Gram-positive cocci than the earlier compounds, may come to have a role in this context.

In summary, meningitis caused by penicillin-resistant pneumococci should initially be treated with an extended-spectrum cephalosporin such as cefotaxime. Success, however, can by no means be guaranteed, and careful laboratory study of the isolate in relation to other possible antibiotic choices should be made.

Haemophilus meningitis

Changing methods of treatment for *Haemophilus* meningitis well illustrate the progressive limitation of treatment options which results from the spread of antibiotic resistance.

For many years chloramphenicol was unquestionably the drug of choice. It is bactericidal in concentrations which can readily be achieved in the CSF and is, indeed, superior to ampicillin in that respect. It then appeared that ampicillin was equally effective, and being free from the possible haematological toxicity of chloramphenicol, it became the drug most commonly used, especially in the USA.

As regards efficacy, there is little to choose between the two methods. Direct comparisons gave very similar results, except for a longer average duration of fever with ampicillin therapy and, in some reports, a higher relapse rate.

In 1974, the situation changed again when strains of *H. influenzae* type b, resistant to ampicillin by virtue of plasmid-mediated β-lactamase production, were described in meningitis and other systemic *Haemophilus* infections. These strains are now of such frequency as to preclude ampicillin as sole initial therapy for *Haemophilus* meningitis. The resistance is of a high order, and life-threatening infections, such as meningitis and acute epiglottitis caused by these strains, fail to respond to ampicillin even in large doses. A survey in the UK (Powell et al 1987), of 2434 strains, showed ampicillin resistance in 7.8%, resistance to chloramphenicol in 1.7%, to trimethoprim in 4.2% and to sulphamethoxazole in 3–5%. Of the 87 capsulated strains, 15 produced β-lactamase, but another nine, although β-lactamase negative, were also ampicillin resistant. At present about 15% of UK strains and 30% of American strains are β-lactamase producers.

These changing resistance patterns have led to the widespread use of cephalosporins as initial treatment in *Haemophilus* meningitis and in meningitis of uncertain aetiology. It is important to note that there is no evidence that cephalosporins give superior results; the sole reason for their use is the presence of antibiotic resistance. Treatment with chloramphenicol or ampicillin is entirely appropriate when isolates are susceptible, an especially important consideration in the many parts of the world with financial limitations on antibiotic budgets. US practice, before ampicillin resistance became common, favoured the initial use of chloramphenicol together with high dose ampicillin. The antagonism between ampicillin or penicillin and chloramphenicol makes it likely that this form of combined treatment effectively relies on the chloramphenicol component (Asmar & Dajani 1983), and it has been shown in a large study in Papua New Guinea that equivalent results are obtained whether chloramphenicol is used alone or in combination with penicillin (Shann et al 1985a). Another more recent trial has confirmed this finding (Kumar & Verma 1993).

A number of choices is available when cephalosporins are indicated for the treatment of *Haemophilus* meningitis, and the agent used will depend on availability and the prevalent antibiotic policy of the country or institution. After disappointing results with the earliest cephalosporins, the first notable success with these compounds was achieved with cefuroxime, but the possible limitations of this particular cephalosporin have been discussed in a preceding section of this chapter. In many countries cefotaxime or ceftriaxone are chiefly used; but, as indicated, many other extended spectrum cephalosporins are equally suitable for *Haemophilus* meningitis. It should be noted that cephalosporins are inactive against some of the less common Gram-negative organisms which may cause meningitis, against Listeria, and some of the compounds have relatively weak action against Gram-positive cocci. The generally low toxicity of β-lactam agents permits high parenteral dosage and this, together with the high intrinsic activity which these compounds show against common bacterial causes of meningitis, overcomes their other relevant general property of poor CSF penetration. CSF concentrations and CSF/serum ratios for these compounds in human studies are summarized in Table 53.1. The wide variability and occasional low concentrations in CSF are worth noting.

Protection of contacts. The risk of child contacts of patients with *Haemophilus* meningitis (and possibly other systemic *Haemophilus* infections) is of a similar order to that experienced by contacts of meningococcal disease. The overall risk is about 0.5% but about 2% in household contacts under 5 years of age. The high rate of nasopharyngeal carriage of the organism in contacts suggests the need for chemoprophylaxis. As with meningococcal infections, many agents effective in vitro, or even in the treatment of established infection, are ineffective in reducing carriage rates in the nasopharynx. Rifampicin, given in a dose of 20 mg/kg once daily for 4 days, has been shown to reduce carriage rates by 90% and the effect persists, to a lessening extent, for several weeks. Resistance to rifampicin has been seen, although most reisolates are still susceptible. These findings provided the basis for a number of trials, which showed a significant reduction of risk in contacts given rifampicin. The importance of correct dosage emerged clearly; in one study carriage was reduced by 97% in children given 20 mg/kg of rifampicin but only 63% in those given half that dose (and by 28% in the placebo group). Current recommendations have been influenced by the success of vaccination against invasive *Haemophilus* disease. Rifampicin chemoprophylaxis is now offered to all home contacts in households in which there are any unvaccinated or incompletely vaccinated children less than 4 years old. The index case should also be given rifampicin, since persistent nasopharyngeal carriage may re-emerge after the acute infection has been treated. Chemoprophylaxis is also given to adult and child contacts in pre-school-age groups if two or more cases of disease have occurred within 120 days.

It needs to be stressed that such a procedure does not obviate the need for careful observation of all contacts, since a workable policy for chemoprophylaxis cannot include all those at risk. Rifampicin does sometimes fail to eradicate carriage, and the risk of rifampicin resistance is as yet uncertain. Moreover, although the recolonization rate is reduced, this may still occur. Failure of rifampicin prophylaxis has been reported a number of times. Rifampicin chemoprophylaxis, although marginally effective, will have negligible effect on the total number of patients with invasive *H. influenzae* disease and is much less important than vaccination as a control measure. Current UK policy for the protection of contacts is discussed by Cartwright et al (1994).

Staphylococcal meningitis

This form of meningitis is usually encountered as a component of a generalized haematogenous infection, commonly in the elderly or in patients with serious underlying disease. In a series of 104 patients (Jensen et al 1993), 91% had bacteraemia, 21% endocarditis and 12% osteomyelitis. The mortality rate is high, and the course of the illness difficult to modify, even with appropriate therapy. The mainstay is a suitable penicillin, starting with flucloxacillin or an equivalent compound pending information from susceptibility tests. Results in the series quoted gave a suggestion that prognosis might be improved by the use of fusidic acid in conjunction with the penicillin. In the presence of antibiotic resistance other choices such as vancomycin and rifampicin will often be preferable. Staphylococcal meningitis also occurs as a postoperative infection, when the prognosis is generally more favourable than in the septicaemic form.

Streptococcus agalactiae meningitis

Group B streptococcal meningitis is chiefly of concern in neonates and is discussed in the section on neonatal meningitis. It is also occasionally encountered in adults. A review by Dunne & Quagliarello (1993) points out that nearly half the reported patients had no evident underlying disease; the others had urological or haematological disease or insulin-dependent diabetes mellitus. Bacteraemia was present in 83%. *Str. agalactiae* is susceptible to penicillin but the MIC is 5–8 times higher than that for *Streptococcus*

pyogenes. The most appropriate treatment options are high-dose benzylpenicillin or penicillin together with gentamicin, since the combination has been shown to be synergic in vitro.

Salmonella meningitis

Salmonella meningitis is most prevalent in neonates and is discussed in the section on neonatal meningitis.

Streptococcus suis meningitis

Streptococcus suis meningitis has a strong occupational association, with work involving pigs or pork. Meningitis may be associated with arthritis and other septicaemic manifestations, and deafness is a common sequel. Kay et al (1995), in a review including 25 of their own cases, note that isolates are susceptible to penicillin and ampicillin and to cephalosporins, co-trimoxazole and vancomycin. Although 2–3 weeks' treatment with penicillin or ampicillin is usually satisfactory, relapses sometimes occur requiring further treatment. Patients who also have endocarditis need longer periods of treatment.

Other Gram-negative bacillary meningitis

Meningitis caused by organisms such as *Esch. coli*, *Klebsiella* and *Proteus* spp. is mainly encountered in neonates, but has become less unusual at older ages, in patients with immunosuppression and other conditions such as chronic renal failure. As discussed on page 746, chloramphenicol is less effective in these infections than in *Haemophilus* meningitis. The value of ampicillin is vitiated by the high prevalence of resistance among these organisms, and effective use of aminoglycosides is difficult to achieve for the reasons discussed in the section on neonatal meningitis. For these reasons the cephalosporins have become of great importance here. One of these compounds, such as cefotaxime or ceftriaxone, can now be selected as agent of first choice for these forms of meningitis, but with several important caveats. First, although the MIC for most Gram-negative bacilli found in meningitis are low and greatly exceeded by attainable serum and CSF concentrations of these drugs, some organisms such as *Enterobacter cloacae* and *Acinetobacter* may have relatively high MICs and treatment may fail for this reason. Second, some of the newer agents are insufficiently active against pseudomonads to be used for meningitis of this cause; ceftazidime and aztreonam are probably best in this respect, but aminoglycoside treatment by intravenous and occasionally by the intraventricular route may be necessary. The possible use of aminoglycoside by the intrathecal route is to be especially borne in mind if an intraventricular reservoir needs to be inserted for neurosurgical reasons and is thus available.

Third, the foregoing recommendations apply only if Gram-negative rods are seen on the Gram-stained CSF film. Several of these agents, including ceftriaxone and aztreonam, have poor or no activity against Gram-positive cocci and cannot therefore be used as initial single-drug therapy for meningitis of unknown cause. The value of co-trimoxazole in some types of bacterial meningitis is discussed below. Fourth, resistance to cephalosporins is increasing.

Gram-negative organisms are also especially associated with nosocomial meningitis, especially associated with neurosurgical interventions and the presence of CSF fistulas or ventriculostomies. A variety of organisms may be involved and the serious potential of such episodes is illustrated by the report of 25 cases of *Acinetobacter* meningitis in a neurosurgical unit (Siegman-Igra et al 1993) over a 5-year period. Initial empirical antibiotic therapy was with a ureidopenicillin plus an aminoglycoside, and intrathecal administration of amikacin was given on a number of occasions.

Initial treatment of community-acquired meningitis when bacteriological diagnosis is unknown

In community-acquired meningitis, when no special risk factors have been identified, it is now usual to initiate treatment with a cephalosporin such as cefotaxime or ceftriaxone. Owing to the high prevalence of ampicillin resistance in *H. influenzae* (and in other Gram-negative pathogens), this has replaced the former practice of using a combination of ampicillin (or penicillin) and chloramphenicol. In the many parts of the developing world in which the three common organisms causing meningitis are still susceptible to chloramphenicol, this remains the agent of choice and, since it is clear that a chloramphenicol/penicillin combination is no better than chloramphenicol alone, we favour the use of chloramphenicol as sole agent in these circumstances. The low cost of this drug compared with that of cephalosporins, its good spectrum of activity against bacteria causing meningitis, and its good pharmacokinetic characteristics, combine to make it of continued value in developing countries and elsewhere.

NEONATAL MENINGITIS

Meningitis is a frequent accompaniment of neonatal septicaemia, and carries a high mortality and a high incidence of residual neurological damage. The variety of organisms which may be responsible has been described on page 811. Factors predisposing to neonatal meningitis are low birth weight, complications during labour and maternal puerperal infection, while other cases are associated with meningomyelocoele or other neurological defects. The Gram-negative organisms often responsible have a wide variety of

antibiotic susceptibility patterns, and it is particularly important in this group to obtain guidance from the laboratory as soon as possible, with CSF and blood cultures. The variety of possible causal organisms in neonatal meningitis led to the widespread use, pending bacteriological diagnosis, of a penicillin, usually ampicillin, and an aminoglycoside, usually gentamicin, as initial treatment. In view of the poor penetration of aminoglycosides into CSF, treatment was formerly supplemented by daily intrathecal injections of gentamicin.

The erratic distribution of drugs introduced into the lumbar theca has been recognized for some time; material injected into the lumbar theca becomes widely distributed through the ventricular system only if the injection volume is large, about 25% of the estimated CSF volume. Lumbar intrathecal injection does sometimes give adequate levels throughout the CSF, especially when hydrocephalus is present. The introduction of ventricular reservoirs allowing repeated CSF sampling enabled Kaiser & McGee (1975) to carry out a detailed series of studies which showed clearly that lumbar intrathecal injection gives high concentrations of gentamicin or tobramycin in the lumbar but not in the ventricular fluid, while intraventricular injection leads to high concentrations in both ventricular and lumbar fluids. To these doubts about the efficacy of lumbar intrathecal injections must be added the technical problems of repeated intrathecal injection in the neonate and the possibility that repeated injections can sometimes be shown to have been placed subdurally rather than into the subarachnoid space. Nor is the achievement of adequate ventricular concentrations of antibiotic merely a theoretical requirement, since ventriculitis is established as an important cause of treatment failure in neonatal meningitis, and addition of intraventricular treatment has sometimes been shown to sterilize the CSF when conventional treatment has failed. However, successive trials have shown that addition of gentamicin by the lumbar intrathecal route to a parenteral regimen of ampicillin and gentamicin did not improve the outlook, and that intraventricular administration carried a substantial risk (McCracken & Mize 1976, McCracken & Mize 1980).

The most appropriate initial regimen, if no organism is seen on the Gram stain of the CSF deposit, is a combination of ampicillin and an appropriate cephalosporin, usually cefotaxime or ceftriaxone. If Gram-negative bacilli are seen, the cephalosporin can be used as sole initial agent. The former regimen of ampicillin and gentamicin (or other aminoglycoside) is still widely employed, especially when health budgets are low. If must be accepted that the aminoglycoside component of this regimen may or may not achieve adequate concentrations in the CSF and its failure to do so may account for some treatment failures with persistent meningitis. An additional difficulty in devising rational schemes for neonatal meningitis is the increasing

Table 53.3 *Initial choices of antibiotic regimen for neonatal meningitis**

Early microbiological or epidemiological evidence	Provisional regimens
None	Ampicillin + cefotaxime *or* Ampicillin + gentamicin
Gram-negative bacilli	Cefotaxime
Ps. aeruginosa – possible	Ampicillin or antipseudomonal penicillin + ceftazidime
Staphylococcus – definite	Flucloxacillin *or* Vancomycin
Staphylococcus – possible	Flucloxacillin + cefotaxime *or* Vancomycin + cefotaxime
Str. agalactiae *L. monocytogenes*	Ampicillin + gentamicin Ampicillin + gentamicin

* Other suitable aminoglycosides or β-lactam agents may be chosen, depending on the antibiotic policy of the hospital.

prevalence of ampicillin resistance among the more common causal agents.

In many cases of neonatal meningitis suggestive but inconclusive evidence of the probable aetiology may be available; Table 53.3 gives guidance on initial regimens in various circumstances. Some other important causes of neonatal meningitis are discussed in the following pages.

Streptococcus agalactiae

Neonatal infections by this group of organisms have come to prominence in recent years, especially in the USA, and much is now known of their epidemiology and pathogenesis. Two syndromes are seen: an early septicaemic variety of rapid course and high mortality (50%) closely simulating the respiratory distress syndrome, and a meningitic syndrome developing somewhat later in the neonatal period. Group B streptococcal meningitis carries a high mortality (20%), as do other forms of neonatal meningitis. The median MICs of benzylpenicillin and ampicillin are 0.02 and 0.04 mg/l, respectively, with conventional inocula (10^5 colony forming units (CFU)), but rises appreciably with larger inocula. Since the CSF may contain 10^6–10^8 bacteria/ml, treatment by high doses of penicillin, in excess of 150 mg/kg daily by intravenous injection, is recommended.

In most patients treated with high-dose penicillin or ampicillin alone the CSF rapidly becomes and remains sterile. In some patients, however, a poor response or relapse has been noted. One reason for this may be failure to eradicate the organisms from focal sites such as the ventricles or cardiac valves. Another possibility is infection by a penicillin-tolerant strain, showing a high MBC/MIC

ratio. These difficulties, together with the demonstration of synergy in vitro and in animal models between penicillin and aminoglycosides against group B streptococci, suggest the initial use of benzylpenicillin in high dosage with an aminoglycoside. The latter drug may be withdrawn if clinical progress and further laboratory data on the causal organism are satisfactory. Some units, following the recommendation of the American Academy of Pediatrics, use penicillin or ampicillin as single agents.

Prophylaxis. Acquisition of these organisms by neonates is highly correlated with maternal carriage, although nosocomial transmission act as an additional source. Attempts have therefore been made to reduce the risk of neonatal group B streptococcal disease by a number of methods, which are discussed in Chapter 57.

Listeria meningitis

L. monocytogenes meningitis is probably less uncommon than was previously thought. When it occurs in the newborn, it appears to result from latent genital tract infection in the mother. It is also encountered in adults; some patients have no underlying disease, but *L. monocytogenes* meningitis is especially associated with lymphoreticular disease, immune suppression, as in transplant patients, and in pregnancy, diabetes and alcoholism. Strains of *Listeria* are in general susceptible to most of the main groups of antimicrobial drugs except the polymyxins, but variation among individual strains has been recorded, especially in relation to penicillins and sulphonamides, and it is important to establish the sensitivity pattern of the isolated strain. Lalloo et al (1992) found all their nine isolates susceptible to ampicillin, chloramphenicol, co-trimoxazole and gentamicin. A number of schemes of treatment have been used successfully, including tetracycline, co-trimoxazole and chloramphenicol. In recent years ampicillin in high dosage has become a popular method. Although tolerance or resistance to ampicillin has been shown in a number of strains, synergy has been demonstrated both in vivo and in animal models between ampicillin and aminoglycosides. A problem sometimes encountered in treating *Listeria* infections of the CNS is recurrence after apparent initial response. It is therefore important that isolates should be carefully studied to aid the selection of an optimal regimen.

A large number of reports of relatively small numbers of patients is available, but one of the larger studies (Bouvet et al 1982), dissented from the prevailing opinion which favours ampicillin or ampicillin with gentamicin for initial treatment. They report poor results from the combination in most patients with severe disease and favour the combination of chloramphenicol and an aminoglycoside despite the antagonism demonstrated in vitro for this combination against *L. monocytogenes*. Notwithstanding this report, we favour giving ampicillin with an aminoglycoside as initial therapy for known or suspected *Listeria* meningitis. This has the advantage of also providing one of the acceptable first-line treatments for meningitis of uncertain cause in neonate or immune-suppressed patients while more bacteriological information is being gathered. Co-trimoxazole is the main alternative. This combination has good in vitro activity and results in clinical practice have been very promising (Spitzer et al 1986). In adults the clinical syndrome may be that of meningoencephalitis or brain abscess rather than one of acute meningitis; treatment may need to be continued for a prolonged period. Other antibiotic schemes may be chosen on the basis of the resistance pattern of the isolated strain. Useful information about susceptibility and treatment regimens is given by Trautmann et al (1985), Tuazon et al (1982) and Kluge (1990).

Salmonella meningitis

This can occur at any age but is most prevalent in infancy. It is a major cause of neonatal meningitis in tropical countries and is also encountered as a nosocomial infection in infant nurseries. It carries a high fatality rate and neurological residua are common. Chloramphenicol was traditionally the mainstay of treatment but was relatively ineffective, the drug having a static effect only in contrast to its powerful bactericidal action on *H. influenzae*. Co-trimoxazole and the newer cephalosporins have had considerable success, but the rapid spread of antibiotic resistance in salmonellae has made many formerly appropriate agents ineffective. On this background there have been several favourable reports describing the value of quinolones in patients infected with highly resistant strains. Their success in many invasive salmonelloses and their ready penetration into the CSF, has led to their use in infant meningitis caused by Salmonellae and some other Gram-negative organisms in the belief that the life-threatening nature of these infections justifies their use in spite of some doubt about toxicity in infancy (p. 438). One report, for example, describes a good response in a baby with meningitis caused by a multiply resistant strain of *Salmonella paratyphi* A (Bhutta et al 1992). Ciprofloxacin has also been used successfully in other forms of Gram-negative bacillary meningitis in neonates (Green et al 1993). A useful summary of cephalosporins in salmonellosis is given by Bryan et al (1986).

The value of different agents has also been tested in experimental models. For example, in *Salmonella enteritidis* meningitis the rate of killing was better with ceftriaxone or imipenem than with chloramphenicol or co-trimoxazole; serum and CSF levels were very similar in this model to those found in man (Bryan & Sheld 1992).

Post-traumatic meningitis

This complication of CSF leak is most often pneumococcal in origin, although *H. influenzae* and *N. meningitidis* are occasionally responsible; rarely, post-traumatic meningitis is associated with other components of the respiratory tract flora such as streptococci. Antimicrobial prophylaxis is often administered as a preventive measure, especially in the initial period following head injury accompanied by CSF leak. There is, however, a dearth of well-controlled studies of this problem and such evidence as there is does not favour routine prophylaxis (British Society for Antimicrobial Chemotherapy 1994). If there is thought to be a real indication for chemoprophylaxis in an individual case, co-trimoxazole is probably the agent of choice, since it is easily administered, both components penetrate well into the CSF and the combination is appropriate for a high proportion of the relevant organisms.

Treatment for post-traumatic meningitis should assume a pneumococcal cause unless there is evidence to the contrary. The prognosis of this form of pneumococcal meningitis is more favourable than that of pneumococcal meningitis unassociated with previous head trauma.

Other candidate drugs in meningitis

The discussion in this chapter has centred around the roles of penicillin, ampicillin, chloramphenicol and the newer extended-spectrum β-lactam compounds. However, changing patterns of antibiotic resistance, and the possibility of very unusual causes of meningitis in immunosuppressed patients make it necessary to consider also reserve drugs which may sometimes be necessary. One such is co-trimoxazole. It has a wide antibacterial spectrum and favourable pharmacokinetic features in that both components penetrate the CSF freely. Resistance to this combination is increasing, however, in many bacterial species so that it could not properly be used as initial blind treatment for Gram-negative bacillary meningitis. The role of co-trimoxazole in bacterial meningitis is thoroughly reviewed by Levitz & Quintiliani (1984), who point to its potential value against organisms generally resistant to the newer cephalosporins, such as *Acinetobacter calcoaceticus*, *Burkholderia* (formerly *Pseudomonas*) *cepacia* and *Flavobacterium meningosepticum*, or only moderately susceptible to these agents, such as some *Serratia* and *Enterobacter* spp. Other possible indications are salmonella meningitis and listerial meningitis and success has been achieved with this combination in several patients with *Staphylococcus aureus* meningitis resistant to penicillin.

The newer quinolones penetrate well into the CSF; CSF/serum ratios are about 50% for enoxacin and pefloxacin and 20–30% for ciprofloxacin and ofloxacin (Scheld 1989, Wolff et al 1987). They may find a useful place in the treatment of Gram-negative bacillary meningitis, especially for organisms resistant to standard regimens (Seger et al 1990, Hooper & Wolfson 1991). CSF levels of the earlier compounds are marginal for control of Gram-positive cocci, but some newer compounds have a wider antibacterial spectrum and may prove effective (Ch. 32).

The emergence of difficult resistance patterns in staphylococci has led to a renewal of interest in vancomycin. This penetrates inflamed meninges, but Gump (1981) recommends additional intraventricular treatment if CSF culture is still positive after 48 h of intravenous treatment. He suggests intravenous dosage of 60 mg/kg daily for neonates and children, 2–3 g/day for adults, with intrathecal dosage ranging from 5 to 20 mg, to be repeated not more than five times. The increasing problems of antibiotic resistance, and very broad antibacterial spectrum of the carbapenems, led to studies of imipenem–cilastatin in meningitis. This proved unsatisfactory because of a high incidence of fits, and it remains to be seen whether meropenem retains its promise after favourable results in early trials (Scheld 1994).

NON-ANTIBIOTIC ASPECTS OF MANAGEMENT

The persistently high mortality and residual morbidity of bacterial meningitis make it especially important to consider other aspects of management which might diminish the impact of the disease. Fits must be controlled promptly and signs of increasing intracranial pressure treated with mannitol infusions. The widespread practice, in patients requiring artificial ventilation, of hyperventilation to low $P\mathrm{co_2}$, should not be employed, since it has been shown that this may reduce cerebral blood flow irregularly and perhaps to ischaemic levels in parts of the brain. Similarly, efforts should be made to avoid fluctuations in blood pressure which, in severe meningitis, may lead to changes in cerebral perfusion (Lambert 1994), and patients should be given correct fluid replacement rather than dehydrated in the often mistaken fear of inappropriate secretion of antidiuretic hormone.

The use of steroids in meningitis, attempted and abandoned 25 years ago, has now been reassessed and strongly argued in certain forms of meningitis. The rationale is to attempt to reduce the endogenously mediated inflammatory processes which lead to cerebral oedema and tissue damage, themselves possibly aggravated by rapid lysis of bacteria when antibacterial therapy is initiated. There is now good evidence in *H. influenzae* meningitis of childhood, with some evidence at other ages and in other aetiologies, that meningeal inflammation and, more importantly, neurological sequelae, are diminished when a short course of high-dose dexamethasone is given as early as possible, preferably 15–20 min before the first dose of antibiotic. Other measures to modulate the inflammatory process have been successful in experimental systems, but have not yet reached clinical practice.

Amoebic meningoencephalitis

The causative agent of the fulminant variety seen mainly in children and young adults after swimming in inland water in hot weather is usually of the genus *Naegleria*, which is sensitive in vitro to amphotericin and possibly to chloroquine, but not to the common antimicrobials, to emetine or to metronidazole. The syndrome caused by *Acanthamoeba/ Hartmanella* is more variable and sometimes subacute: although inactive in vitro, sulphonamides may possibly have a role in treatment. The biology of *Naegleria fowleri* is reviewed by John (1982). Miconazole appears active in vitro but not in mice. Tetracycline and rifampicin have a synergic effect with amphotericin in protecting mice, and have been employed together with amphotericin in some patients. Successful treatment was reported by Seidal et al (1982), who report only 3 survivors in about 100 cases recorded previously. The diagnosis was established early and their patient received amphotericin intravenously and intrathecally together with miconazole and, initially, a sulphonamide.

We make the suggestion that immediate treatment with amphotericin by intravenous and intrathecal routes should be used. An additional drug may be indicated if evidence in favour of this is available from local knowledge of the strain involved. The outlook in this form of meningitis is very grave.

Brain abscess

The mortality from brain abscess is high and has changed little in the antibiotic era. The reasons for this are certainly complex, but particularly important among them is the dangerously rapid rise of intracranial pressure which so often accompanies the development of brain abscess during the early stage of cerebritis. Discussion here is confined to antimicrobial aspects of treatment, but other aspects of management are of crucial importance, notably the control of raised intracranial pressure, and drainage (using stereotoxic computed tomography (CT) scanning) or excision of the abscess, as important in the brain as elsewhere. Surgical intervention may not be possible with multiple abscesses, and the advent of modern scanning has raised interest in the possibilities of non-surgical treatment if the condition can be recognized in the early stage of non-suppurative cerebritis. As in other forms of abscess, bacteria may be found in the abscess contents after many days of systemic chemotherapy.

The causal organisms differ to some extent in their order of frequency with the origins of the abscess, but several studies have amply confirmed the importance of anaerobic Gram-negative bacteria, especially *Bacteroides* and *Fusiformis* spp., and of aerobic and anaerobic streptococci.

Enterobacteria of various genera are commonly also found, and staphylococci are important in infection associated with trauma, and in spinal epidural abscess. Several species are often isolated from a single specimen when suitable selective technique are used, especially in abscesses of middle ear origin. De Louvois et al (1977a,b) stressed the strong association of *Bacteroides* spp. with temporal lobe abscess and the general importance of streptococci, especially *Streptococcus milleri*. Streptococci were the most prominent single pathogen in non-temporal lobe abscesses but, as Grace & Drake-Lee (1984) point out, *Bacteroides* spp. may also be found in abscesses of sinus origin. A similar distribution of causal organisms is found in cerebral abscess in childhood, common associations of which are cyanotic congenital heart disease, otitis, sinusitis, head injuries and cystic fibrosis (Fischer et al 1981). It has to be remembered that, although the dominant organism in cerebral abscesses are well documented, other less common agents are sometimes encountered, including species of actinomyces and nocardia and fungi.

An appropriate first-choice antimicrobial drug regimen must take into account not only this diverse flora, but also the characteristics of potentially effective drugs in penetrating brain tissue, CSF and abscess cavities. Data on these aspects may be found in the work of Black et al (1973), Picardi et al (1975), de Louvois et al (1983) and Stone & Wise (1991). Microbiological data may occasionally be available at the time chemotherapy is started, for example, when brain abscess is diagnosed during the course of a septicaemia of known aetiology. Generally, however, no such information is available and initial antibiotic policy must be based on the organisms known to be dominant in the aetiology of cerebral abscess, as described above, bearing in mind especially that the common forms of brain abscess are often polymicrobial. Some authors recommend variations of regimen based on the different frequency of various species found in cerebral abscess associated with different parameningeal or pulmonary sources. We do not think these differences are big enough to allow this sort of fine tuning and consider that a single unit policy for brain abscess associated with parameningeal or pulmonary sepsis is preferable.

These data indicate the basis of modern antibiotic treatment. High-dose ampicillin or penicillin retain an important role as effective against streptococci, including the microaerophilic species not susceptible to metronidazole, and against most of the relevant anaerobes. The recognition of anaerobes as an important component of the flora of many brain abscesses led to the use of metronidazole, especially relevant as *Bacteroides fragilis* and perhaps some strains of *Bacteroides melaninogenicus* (Mathisen et al 1984) are penicillin resistant but susceptible to metronidazole. This has led to the widespread use of metronidazole, together with ampicillin or penicillin, as

agents of first choice. Good results in otogenic abscess were reported by Ingham et al (1977), who found that metronidazole, given orally or intravenously, achieved high concentrations in pus or ventricular fluid. In addition to high-dose ampicillin or penicillin and metronidazole, it has been customary to include chloramphenicol in the regimen against the possibility that Gram-negative aerobes may also be involved. Now that extended spectrum cephalosporins of wide activity are available, and some of the limitations of chloramphenicol recognized, we now recommend that a cephalosporin be included as a component of the initial regimen.

Causal organisms in subdural empyema are generally similar to those in brain abscess and a similar antibiotic policy may be used. For staphylococcal brain abscess, pending detailed microbiological information, a combination of flucloxacillin (or similar isoxazolyl penicillin) and fusidic acid is suggested. Other abscesses of haematogenous origin may clearly need specific forms of chemotherapy different from those recommended for the common types associated with parameningeal sources in the ear or sinuses, and these must be tailored to the particular organism concern.

SPINAL EPIDURAL ABSCESS

The dominant organism is *Staph. aureus*, but all series of cases include an important minority caused by streptococci, and also a lesser number caused by Gram-negative bacilli of various species (Danner & Hartman 1987, Darouiche et al 1992). For this reason, we feel that initial antibiotic choice should consist of flucloxacillin together with an appropriate cephalosporin. Other choices may prove more suitable as more information becomes available. Instillation of penicillin into the abscess cavity is best avoided, since the procedure has potential dangers and failure to sterilize the abscess contents is not usually attributable to deficiency of antibiotic in the pus.

SHUNT INFECTIONS

These are discussed in Chapter 45.

Encephalitis

Although viral infections, some of them accessible to specific therapy, predominate as causes of encephalitis, it is important to remember other causes of these syndromes, since some of these are also amenable to treatment. The many viruses causing encephalitis for which no specific therapy is available are not considered here.

HERPES SIMPLEX ENCEPHALITIS

As nucleoside analogues were developed for antiviral chemotherapy, each was in turn used in the treatment of herpes simplex encephalitis, in the hope of reducing the impact of this devastating illness. Initial hopes for idoxuridine were disappointed by its toxicity and lack of benefit. Cytarabine too lacked efficacy, but evidence of modest benefit from systemic vidarabine was obtained. This agent was rapidly supplanted when acyclovir was introduced, when two notable trials established its value. The Swedish study of 51 confirmed cases (of 127 suspected) included 27 treated with acyclovir and 24 with vidarabine (Skoldenberg et al 1984). Of the acyclovir group, 9 (33%) were dead or severely disabled after 6 months and 15 (56%) had returned to normal life; the corresponding figures in the vidarabine group were 19 (76%) and 3 (13%). A comparative study in the USA of 208 patients with encephalitis, of whom 33% had biopsy-proven herpes simplex infection, revealed 43 early deaths in the vidarabine group and 13 deaths in those treated with acyclovir; the corresponding numbers after 18 months were 54 and 28, respectively. Functional assessment at 6 months recorded moderate disability in 22% and 9%, and functional normality in 14% and 38% in the two groups (Whitley et al 1986). Acyclovir is notably free of systemic toxicity (Ch. 40), but relapse has sometimes been seen after the completion of standard treatment, both with this agent and with vidarabine. It is possible that this risk would be diminished by using a combination of antiviral agents, but no firm evidence is available. The dose regimen for acyclovir is 10 mg/kg 8-hourly for 10–14 days for both adult and neonatal herpes encephalitis. Vidarabine is no longer used.

The role of brain biopsy before treatment has been much disputed. British centres have generally opted for using acyclovir in any patient who might have herpes simplex encephalitis, making appropriate changes as further evidence becomes available. This involves a large number of treatments in patients who, in the event, do not have herpes simplex encephalitis, but avoids the morbidity associated with brain biopsy from haemorrhage or cerebral oedema, which are encountered in 3% of subjects. The problem of early diagnosis will be greatly reduced by the use of PCR in specimens of CSF, when this technique becomes widely available.

VARICELLA-ZOSTER ENCEPHALITIS

Cases are too few for trials of substantial size to be achieved, and prognosis in the cerebellar form of the disease is usually good. Nevertheless, bearing in mind the activity of acyclovir against this virus and its low toxicity, we would recommend its use in this condition.

CREUTZFELDT–JAKOB DISEASE, PROGRESSIVE MULTIFOCAL LEUCOENCEPHALOPATHY AND SUBACUTE SCLEROSING PANENCEPHALITIS

Several forms of treatment, including antiviral drugs, interferon and transfer factor, have been tried in these commonly fatal conditions but no firm evidence to guide therapy is available, nor has any drug treatment of established value for rabies been established.

Some of the most important syndromes associated with encephalitic features and for which specific treatments are available are listed in Table 53.4, with reference to the relevant chapters in which they are discussed.

Table 53.4 *Some infections with major encephalitic components for which specific treatment is available*

Infection	Treatment	Page No.
Herpes simplex virus		
Neonatal herpes simplex virus	Acyclovir	732, 810
Varicella-zoster virus		
Influenza virus	Amantadine	692
Cytomegalovirus	Ganciclovir	668
Lyme borreliosis	Ceftriaxone, penicillin	778
Syphilis	Penicillin, etc.	815
Tuberculosis	Antimycobacterial drugs	833
Listeriosis	Ampicillin, co-trimoxazole	809
Rickettsial infections	Doxycycline	889
Malaria		Ch. 62
Trypanosomiasis		Ch. 63
Toxoplasmosis		Ch. 63

A number of infections of the central nervous system are discussed in other chapters, as follows:

- *Tuberculous meningitis*   Ch. 59
- *Neurosyphilis*   Ch. 58
- *Lyme disease*   Ch. 61
- *Neurobrucellosis*   Ch. 61
- *HIV disease*   Ch. 46.

References

Asmar B I, Dajani A S 1983 Ampicillin–chloramphenicol interactions against enteric Gram-negative organisms. *Pediatric Infectious Diseases* 2: 39–42

Barson W J, Miller M A, Brady M T, Powell D A 1985 Prospective comparative trial of ceftriaxone versus conventional therapy of bacterial meningitis in children. *Pediatric Infectious Diseases* 4: 362–368

Bhutta Z A, Farooqui B J, Sturm A W 1992 Eradication of a multiple drug resistant *Salmonella paratyphi*. A causing meningitis with ciprofloxacin. *Journal of Infection* 25: 215–219

Black P, Graybill J R, Charache P 1973 Penetration of brain abscess by systemically administered antibiotics. *Journal of Neurosurgery* 38: 705–709

Bouvet E, Suter F, Gilbert C, Witchitz J L, Bazinc Vachon F 1982 Severe meningitis due to *Listeria monocytogenes*. A review of 40 cases in adults. *Scandinavian Journal of Infectious Diseases* 14: 267–270

Bradley J S, Farhat C, Stamboulian D, Branchini O G, Debbag R 1994 Ceftriaxone therapy of bacterial meningitis; CSF concentrations and bactericidal activity after intramuscular injection in children treated with dexamethasone. *Pediatric Infectious Diseases Journal* 13: 724–728

British Society for Antimicrobial Chemotherapy. Infection in Neurosurgery Working Party 1994 Antimicrobial prophylaxis in neurosurgery and after head injury. *Lancet* 334: 1547–1551

Bryan J P, Rocha H, Scheld W M 1986 Problems in salmonellosis; rationale for clinical trials with newer beta-lactam agents and quinolones. *Reviews of Infectious Diseases* 8: 189–207

Bryan J P, Scheld W M 1992 Therapy of experimental meningitis due to Salmonella enteritidis. *Antimicrobial Agents and Chemotherapy* 36: 949–954

Cartwright K A V, Begg N T, Rudd P 1994 Use of vaccine and antibiotic prophylaxis in contacts and cases of *Haemophilus influenzae* type b (Hib) disease. *Communicable Disease Report* 4: R16–R17

Cherubin C E, Eng R H K, Norrby R, Modai J, Humpert G, Overturf G 1989 Penetration of newer cephalosporins into cerebrospinal fluid. *Review of Infectious Diseases* 11: 526–548

Communicable Disease Report 1995 Control of meningococcal disease: guidance for consultants in communicable disease control. 5: R189–200

Danner R L, Hartman B J 1987 Update of spinal epidural abscess. *Reviews Infectious Diseases* 9: 265–274

Darouiche R O, Hamill R J, Greenberg S B, Musher D M 1992 Bacterial spinal epidural abscess. *Medicine* 71: 369–385

de Louvois J, Gortvai P, Hurley R 1977a Antibiotic treatment of abscesses of the central nervous system: a multicentre prospective study. *British Medical Journal* 1: 958–967

de Louvois J, Gortvai P, Hurley R 1977b Bacteriology of abscesses of the central nervous system: a multicentre prospective study. *British Medical Journal* 2: 981–984

de Louvois J 1983 Antimicrobial chemotherapy in the treatment of brain abscess. *Journal of Antimicrobial Chemotherapy* 12: 205–207

Dunne D W, Quagliarello V 1993 Group B streptococcal meningitis in adults. *Medicine* 72: 1–10

Dworzack D L, Saunders C C, Horowitz E A et al 1988 Evaluation of single dose ciprofloxacin in the eradication of *N. meningitidis* from nasopharyngeal carriers. *Antimicrobial Agents and Chemotherapy* 32: 1740–1741

Enzenauer R W, Bass J W 1983 Initial antibiotic treatment of purulent meningitis in infants 1–2 months of age. *American Journal of Diseases of Childhood* 137: 1055–1056

Fischer E G, McLennan J E, Suzuki Y 1981 Cerebral abscess in children. *American Journal of Diseases of Childhood* 135: 746–749

Friedland I R, Klugman K P 1992 Failure of chloramphenicol therapy in penicillin-resistant pneumococcal meningitis. *Lancet* 339: 405–408

Gaunt P N, Lambert B E 1988 Single dose ciprofloxacin for the eradication of pharyngeal carriers of *N. meningitidis*. *Journal of Antimicrobial Chemotherapy* 21: 489–496

Grace A, Drake-Lee A 1984 Role of anaerobes in cerebral abscesses of sinus origin. *British Medical Journal* 288: 758–759

Green S D R, Ilong A, Cheesbrough J S, Tillotson G S, Hichens M, Felmingham D 1993 The treatment of neonatal meningitis due to Gram-negative bacilli with ciprofloxacin; evidence of satisfactory penetration into the CSF. *Journal of Infection* 26: 253–256

Greenwood B M, Hassan-King M, Cleland P G, McFarlane J T, Yahaya H N 1986 Sequential bacteriological findings in the CSF of Nigerian patients with pneumococcal meningitis. *Journal of Infection* 12: 49–56

Gump D W 1981 Vancomycin for treatment of bacterial meningitis. *Review of Infectious Diseases* 3: S289–S292

Hieber J P, Nelson J D 1977 A pharmacologic evaluation of penicillin in children with purulent meningitis. *New England Journal of Medicine* 297: 410–413

Hooper D C, Wolfson J S 1991 Fluoroquinolone antimicrobial agents. *New England Journal of Medicine* 324: 384–394

Ingham H R, Selkon J B, Roxby C M 1977 Bacteriological study of otogenic cerebral abscesses: chemotherapeutic role of metronidazole. *British Medical Journal* 2: 991–993

Jacobs R F, Wells T G, Steele R W, Yamauchi T 1985 A prospective randomized comparison of cefotaxime versus ampicillin and chloramphenicol for bacterial meningitis in children. *Journal of Pediatrics* 107: 129–133

Jensen A G, Espersen F, Skinhoj P, Roshdahl V T, Frimodt-Moller N 1993 *Staphylococcus aureus* meningitis. A review of 104 nationwide consecutive cases. *Archives of Internal Medicine* 153: 1902–1908

John D T 1982 Primary amebic meningo-encephalitis and the biology of *Naegleria fowleri*. *Annual Review of Microbiology* 36: 101–123

Kaiser A B, McGee Z A 1975 Aminoglycoside therapy of Gram-negative bacillary meningitis. *New England Journal of Medicine* 293: 1215–1220

Kaplan S L, Mason S K, Mason E D, Murphy M, Smith E O 1988 Follow-up of prospective randomized trial of ampicillin or chloramphenicol versus moxalactam treatment of *Haemophilus influenzae* type b meningitis. *Journal of Pediatrics* 112: 795–798

Kay R, Cheng A F, Tse C Y 1995 *Streptococcus suis* in Hong Kong. *Quarterly Journal of Medicine* 88: 39–47

Kluge R M 1990 Listerioses – problems and therapeutic options. *Journal of Antimicrobial Chemotherapy* 25: 887–890

Klugman K P 1994 Management of antibiotic-resistant pneumococcal infections. *Journal of Antimicrobial Chemotherapy* 34: 191–193

Kumar P, Verma I C 1993 Antibiotic therapy for bacterial meningitis in developing countries. *Bulletin of the World Health Organization* 71: 183–188

Lalloo U G, Coovadia Y M, Adhikari M, Poyiadji O 1992 *Listeria monocytogenes* meningitis at King Edward VII Hospital, Durban. A 10 year experience 1981–90. *South African Medical Journal* 81: 187–189

Lambert H P 1994 Neurological management. Meningitis. *Journal of Neurology, Neurosurgery and Psychiatry* 57: 405–415

Lebel M B, Hout M J, McCracken G H 1989 Comparative efficacy of ceftriaxone and cefuroxime for treatment of bacterial meningitis. *Journal of Pediatrics* 114: 1049–1054

Levitz R E, Quintiliani R 1984 Trimethoprim–sulphamethoxazole for bacterial meningitis. *Annals of Internal Medicine* 100: 881–890

Lin T-Y, Chrange D F, Nelson J D, McCracken G H 1985 Seven days of ceftriaxone therapy is as effective as ten days treatment for bacterial meningitis. *Journal of American Medical Association* 253: 3559–3563

Mathisen G E, Meyer R D, George W L, Citron D M, Finegold S M 1984 Brain abscess and cerebritis. *Review of Infectious Diseases* 6: S101–S106

McCraken G H 1983 Pharmacokinetic and bacteriological correlations between antimicrobial therapy of experimental meningitis in rabbits and meningitis in human; a review. *Journal of Antimicrobial Chemotherapy* 12 (suppl D): 97–108

McCracken G H, Mize S G 1976 A controlled study of intrathecal antibiotic therapy in Gram-negative enteric meningitis of infancy. *Journal of Pediatrics* 89: 66–72

McCracken G H, Mize S G, Therlkeld N 1980 Intraventricular gentamicin therapy in Gram-negative bacillary meningitis of infancy. Report of the second neonatal meningitis co-operative study group. *Lancet* i: 787–791

Mulhall A, de Louvois J, Hurley R 1983 Chloramphenicol toxicity in neonates; its incidence and prevention. *British Medical Journal* 287: 1424–1427

Odio C M, Faingezicht I, Salas J L, Guevera J, Mohs E, McCracken G H 1986 Cefotaxime versus conventional therapy for the treatment of bacterial meningitis of infants and children. *Pediatric Infectious Diseases* 5: 402–407

Pecoul B, Varaine F, Keita M et al 1991 Long-acting chloramphenicol versus intravenous ampicillin for treatment of bacterial meningitis. *Lancet* 338: 862–866

Peltola H, Anttila M, Rankonen O-V, Finnish Study Group 1989 Randomised comparison of chloramphenicol, ampicillin, cefotaxime and ceftriaxone for childhood bacterial meningitis. *Lancet* i: 1281–1287

Picardi J L, Lewis H P, Tan J S, Phair J P 1975 Clindamycin concentrations in the central nervous system of primates before and after head trauma. *Journal of Neurosurgery* 43: 717–720

Powell M, Koutsia-Carouzou C, Voutsinas D, Seymour A, William J D 1987 Resistance of clinical isolates of *Haemophilus influenzae* in United Kingdom 1986. *British Medical Journal* 295: 176–179

Puddicombe J B, Wali S S, Greenwood B M 1984 A field trial of a single intramuscular injection of long-acting chloramphenicol in the treatment of meningococcal meningitis. *Transactions of the Royal Society of Tropical Medicine and Hygiene* 78: 339–403

Ristuccia A M, Le Frock J L 1992 Cerebrospinal fluid penetration of antimicrobials. *Antibiotics and Chemotherapy* 45: 119–152

Saez-Nieto J A, Lujan R, Berron S et al 1992 Epidemiology and molecular basis of penicillin-resistant *Neisseria meningitidis* in Spain: a 5-year history. *Clinical Infectious Diseases* 14: 394–402

Schaad U B, Suter S, Gianella-Borradori A 1990 A comparison of ceftriaxone and cefotaxime for the treatment of bacterial meningitis in children. *New England Journal of Medicine* 322: 141–147

Scheld W M 1989 Quinolone therapy for infections of the central nervous system. *Reviews of Infectious Diseases* 11: S1194–S1202

Scheld W M 1994 Is there a place for carbapenems in the therapy of meningitis? *Current Opinion in Infectious Diseases* 7 (suppl 1): S33–S37

Schwartz B, Al-Tobaiqi A, Al-Ruwais A et al 1988 Comparative efficacy of ceftriaxone and rifampicin in eradicating pharyngeal carriage of Group A *Neisseria meningitidis*. *Lancet* i: 1239–1242

Seger S, Rosen N, Joseph G, Alpern E, Iran H, Rubinstein E 1990 Pefloxacin efficacy in Gram-negative bacillary meningitis. *Journal of Antibiotic Chemotherapy* 26 (suppl B): 187–192

Seidel J S, Harmatz P, Visvesvara G S, Cohen A, Edwards J, Turner J 1982 Successful treatment of primary amebic meningo-encephalitis. *New England Journal of Medicine* 306: 346–348

Shann F, Barker J, Poore P 1985a Chloramphenicol alone versus chloramphenicol plus penicillin for bacterial meningitis in children. *Lancet* ii: 681–684

Shann F, Linnemann V, Mackenzie A, Barker J, Gratten M, Crinis N 1985b Absorption of chloramphenicol sodium succinate after intramuscular administration in children. *New England Journal of Medicine* 313: 410–414

Siegmen-Igra Y, Bar-Yosef S, Gorea A, Avram J 1993 Nosocomial *Acinetobacter* meningitis secondary to invasive procedures: report of 25 cases and review. *Clinical Infectious Diseases* 17: 843–849

Skoldenberg B, Forsgren M, Alestig K et al 1984 Acyclovir versus vidarabine in herpes simplex encephalitis; rando-mised multicentre study in consecutive Swedish patients. *Lancet* ii: 707–711

Spitzer P G, Hammer S M, Karchmer A W 1986 Treatment of *Listeria monocytogenes* infection with trimethoprim–sulphamethoxazole; case report and review of the literature. *Review of Infectious Diseases* 8: 427–430

Stone J, Wise R 1991 Antimicrobial agents and the CNS. In: Lambert H P (ed) Infections of the central nervous system. B C Decker, Toronto

Trautmann M, Wagner J, Chahin M, Wein K E 1985 *Listeria* meningitis: report of 10 recent cases and review of current therapeutic recommendations. *Journal of Infection* 10: 107–114

Tuazon C U, Shamsuddin D, Miller H 1982 Antibiotic susceptibility and synergy of clinical isolates of *Listeria monocytogenes*. *Antimicrobial Agents and Chemotherapy* 21: 525–527

Valadrich P F, Pallares R, Ariza J, Rvfi G, Guidiol F 1986 Four days of penicillin therapy for meningococcal meningitis. *Archives of Internal Medicine* 146: 2380–2382

Valadrich P F, Guidiol F, Linares J, Rufi B, Ariza J, Parres R 1988 Characteristics and antibiotic therapy of adult meningitis due to penicillin-resistant pneumococci. *American Journal of Medicine* 84: 839–846

Viladrich P F, Guidiol F, Linares J et al 1991 Evaluation of vancomycin for therapy of adult pneumococcal meningitis. *Antimicrobial Agents and Chemotherapy* 35: 2467–2472

Wells T G, Tran J M, Brown A L, Marmer B C, Jacobs R F 1984 Cefotaxime therapy of bacterial meningitis in children. *Journal of Antimicrobial Chemotherapy* 14: 181–189

Whitley R J, Alford C A, Hirsch M S 1986 Vidarabine versus acyclovir therapy in herpes simplex encephalitis. *New England Journal of Medicine* 314: 144–149

Wolff M, Boutron L, Singlas E, Clair B, Decazes J M, Regnier B 1987 Penetration of ciprofloxacin into cerebrospinal fluid of patients with bacterial meningitis. *Antimicrobial Agents and Chemotherapy* 31: 899–902

Wong V K, Wright H T, Ross L A et al 1991 Imipenem/cilastatin treatment of bacterial meningitis in children. *Pediatric Infectious Diseases Journal* 10: 122–125

Bone and joint infections

R. J. Fass

Pathogenesis

Acute haematogenous osteomyelitis and septic arthritis are most common in infants, children and the elderly (Waldvogel et al 1970, Cooper & Cawley 1986, Gillespie 1990a). Skeletal involvement may be obvious during the acute bacteraemic phase or 1 or 2 weeks after a course of treatment for *Staphylococcus aureus* bacteraemia, when the patient may present with osteomyelitis of the femur, a spinal disk space infection or a septic hip. Occasionally, the bacteraemic episode is transient or inapparent.

In adults osteomyelitis is more usually a consequence of contiguous spread of infection from infected wounds, teeth, sinuses, ulcers, open fractures or after surgery (Waldvogel et al 1970). Host defenses and early, vigorous antimicrobial treatment of these infections frequently prevents spread to bone or aborts progression of early bone involvement. Joint involvement due to soft tissue infection is uncommon unless there is penetrating trauma, an overlying ulcer or spread from contiguous bone (Goldenberg & Reed 1985, Esterhai & Gelb 1991, Smith & Piercy 1995).

Early, aggressive treatment of acute bone and joint infections is important to achieve cure and prevent chronic infection when cure is more difficult (Waldvogel et al 1970, Goldenberg & Reed 1985, Cooper & Cawley 1986, Esterhai & Gelb 1991, Smith & Piercy 1995). Suboptimal or delayed treatment of skin or soft tissue infections when there is devitalized tissue due to trauma or vascular disease, as occurs with diabetic feet and pressure sores, are particularly common problems (Waldvogel et al 1970, Sugarman et al 1983, Gentry 1990, Lipsky et al 1990).

Nosocomial skeletal infections complicating total joint replacement or internal fixation of fractures are also important (Waldvogel & Vasey 1980, Inman et al 1984, Goldenberg & Reed 1985, Gillespie 1990a). They may occur early, due to contamination at the time of surgery, or from

infection in the postoperative period, or later, or as a recrudescence of a chronic, indolent infection or following bacteraemic seeding (Inman et al 1984, Gillespie 1990b).

Diagnosis

The diagnoses of osteomyelitis and septic arthritis require both clinical suspicion and reliable microbiological information (Waldvogel et al 1970, Goldenberg & Reed 1985, Cooper & Cawley 1986, Gentry 1990, Lipsky et al 1990, Esterhai & Gelb 1991, Smith & Piercy 1995). In addition to blood cultures, Gram stains and cultures of material obtained by aspiration or biopsy directly from the involved bone or joint are used to establish the aetiology. Material obtained from infected wounds, fistulae or ulcers may suffice when a single organism such as *Staph. aureus* is repeatedly isolated, but the results of such cultures are often misleading, leading to either undertreatment or overtreatment (Mackowiak et al 1978, Gentry 1990, Lipsky et al 1990).

To establish the diagnosis of osteomyelitis, visualization of the involved bone or bones using X-rays, radionuclide, magnetic resonance imaging (MRI) and/or computed tomography (CT) and, occasionally, radiolabelled white cell scans is necessary (Schauwecker et al 1990, Wegener & Alavi 1991). In acute disease, the initial X-rays are typically normal because abnormalities require time to evolve. They are still useful, however, to establish a baseline for subsequent comparisons. Scans and MRI are more sensitive for early disease and are often indicated for the diagnosis of acute haematogenous infection. Vigorous antimicrobial therapy of high-risk skin/soft tissue infections, which assumes that bone involvement is present, often resolves the issue regarding the presence or absence of bone involvement on clinical and X-ray follow-up.

Chronic osteomyelitis evolves over months or years and the resultant inflammatory bone destruction with sequestration of devascularized bone and reactive new bone formation cause obvious X-ray abnormalities. MRI and CT scans are helpful for defining the anatomical extent of disease, primarily for planning surgery (Schauwecker et al 1990, Wegener & Alavi 1991).

The interpretation of imaging studies may be confounded by neighbouring soft tissue infection, fractures, underlying skeletal, vascular or neuropathic disease, previous surgery or the presence of prostheses (Sugarman et al 1983, Lipsky et al 1990, Schauwecker et al 1990, Wegener & Alavi 1991).

For septic arthritis, joint aspiration to obtain material for Gram stain and culture should be accompanied by fluid analysis for cells, protein and glucose content to distinguish infectious from noninfectious arthritis. Imaging studies are not as important as with osteomyelitis, but may be helpful to detect joint destruction or define associated bone or soft tissue involvement (Goldenberg & Reed 1985, Esterhai & Gelb 1991, Wegener & Alavi 1991, Smith & Piercy, 1995)

Antimicrobial choice

The choice of antimicrobial regimen to treat a bone or joint infection is largely dependent on identifying the pathogen and determining its antimicrobial susceptibility. The bacterial species which commonly cause skeletal infections are shown in Box 54.1 (Waldvogel et al 1970, Nelson 1983, Sugarman et al 1983, Goldstein et al 1984, Inman et al 1984, Goldenberg & Reed 1985, Cooper & Cawley 1986, Brook 1987, Gentry 1990, Gillespie 1990b, Lipsky et al 1990, Nelson 1990, Esterhai & Gelb 1991, Goldstein &

Citron 1993, Smith & Piercy 1995). Drugs which have proven most effective in treating skeletal infections include the β-lactams (Nelson 1983, Gentry 1990, Nelson 1990, Smith & Piercy 1995), clindamycin (Feigin et al 1975, Kaplan et al 1982, Nelson 1983, Mader et al 1989, Nelson 1990) and the fluoroquinolones (Norrby 1989, Waldvogel 1989, Gentry 1990, Mader 1990, Gentry 1991). Vancomycin, teicoplanin, fusidic acid, co-trimoxazole, aminoglycosides and metronidazole have more limited indications. Macrolides and tetracyclines should be avoided.

Drug selection should not be based primarily on achievable bone and joint concentrations. Bone concentrations are quite variable and technically difficult to measure (Waldvogel & Vasey 1980), while concentrations in synovial fluid are more predictive of therapeutic response (Nelson 1971, Nelson et al 1978, Sattar et al 1983, Goldenberg & Reed 1985). Drug selection should generally also be independent of the site of infection, the route by which it was acquired, or the degree of chronicity.

STAPHYLOCOCCAL AND STREPTOCOCCAL INFECTIONS

β-Lactams, in high doses, are the preferred drugs for streptococcal and staphylococcal infections (Gentry 1990, Nelson 1990, Smith & Piercy 1995). Intravenous penicillin G is usually used for the former and flucloxacillin, nafcillin or oxacillin for the latter because most staphylococci produce penicillinase. In penicillin-allergic patients, cephalosporins (e.g. cefuroxime) may be substituted. For oral administration, drugs such as penicillin V, amoxycillin, cloxacillin, dicloxacillin, flucloxacillin and cephalexin may be used.

Clindamycin has been extensively used with excellent results for the treatment of staphylococcal osteomyelitis

Box 54.1 *Common pathogens in suppurative bone and joint infections.*

Haematogenous	Contiguous spread		
	Acute skin and soft tissue infections	Orofacial and dental infections	Diabetic foot and pressure sores
Staph. aureus	Staph. aureus	Streptococcus spp.	Staph. aureus
Streptococcus spp.	Str. agalactiae	Anaerobic cocci	Staph. epidermidis
H. influenzae[1]	Str. pyogenes	Fusobacterium spp.	Streptococcus spp.
Enterobacteriaceae[2]		Ps. melaninogenicus	Enterobacteriaceae
Staph. epidermidis[3,4]		Ps. multocida[7]	Ps. aeruginosa
Candida[4]		Eik. corrodens[8]	Ent. faecalis
N. gonorrhoeae[5]			Anaerobic cocci
Ps. aeruginosa[6]			Bacteroides spp.
			Clostridium spp.

[1] Infants and unimmunized children. [2] Elderly and neonates. [3] Bone and joint prostheses. [4] Intravenous devices.
[5] Young adults. [6] Injection drug use and foot puncture wounds. [7] Dog and cat bites. [8] Human bites.

(Feigin et al 1975, Kaplan et al 1982, Gentry 1990, Nelson 1990). For prolonged courses, oral clindamycin provides serum concentrations nearly comparable to those achieved intravenously (Fass 1980, Kaplan et al 1982). In an animal model of *Staph. aureus* osteomyelitis, clindamycin was more effective than cefazolin, presumably due to better bone penetration and possibly due to inhibition of glycocalyx formation (Mader et al 1989).

Fusidic acid is not available in the USA, but is used to treat staphylococcal skeletal infections in Europe, where it is combined with drugs such as penicillins, erythromycin or rifampicin (Coombs 1990, Drugeon et al 1994).

The glycopeptides, vancomycin and teicoplanin, are consistently active against methicillin-resistant staphylococci. They may not be as effective as β-lactams in treating serious infections caused by methicillin-susceptible *Staph. aureus* (Small & Chambers 1990, Fortún et al 1995) and should only be used to treat infections caused by multidrug-resistant Gram-positive organisms. In the USA, cotrimoxazole is probably the best alternate treatment for methicillin-resistant staphylococcal infections (Yeldandi et al 1988). In Europe, fusidic acid which is active against methicillin-resistant as well as methicillin-susceptible *Staph. aureus* may be used (Coombs 1990, Drugeon et al 1994).

HAEMOPHILUS INFLUENZAE INFECTIONS

Ampicillin or amoxycillin are preferred for β-lactamase negative *H. influenzae* infections; for resistant strains, expanded-spectrum cephalosporins are recommended (Nelson 1990). Ampicillin–sulbactam, amoxycillin–clavulanate and ciprofloxacin (in adults) are also satisfactory (Aronoff et al 1986).

ENTEROBACTERIACEAE AND *PSEUDOMONAS AERUGINOSA* INFECTIONS

A β-lactam plus an aminoglycoside has traditionally been recommended to treat infections caused by the Enterobacteriaceae and *Ps. aeruginosa*, but monotherapy with highly active expanded-spectrum β-lactams is satisfactory for many infections. Aminoglycoside toxicity, poor penetration and the necessity for prolonged parenteral administration has always been problematical, so that they should be avoided whenever possible (Gentry 1990, Smith & Piercy 1995).

There is now extensive experience using the fluoroquinolones, particularly ciprofloxacin, in treating aerobic Gram-negative skeletal infections (Norrby 1989, Gentry 1990, Mader 1990, Gentry 1991). It is highly active, available parenterally and orally, well tolerated during prolonged administration and has established efficacy.

GONOCOCCAL INFECTIONS

Skeletal involvement with the gonococcus is the result of haematogenous seeding and most commonly presents as tenosynovitis rather than as osteomyelitis or septic arthritis. Despite a high frequency of penicillin-G- and ampicillin-resistance among gonococci, strains that disseminate are usually susceptible (Goldenberg & Reed 1985, Smith & Piercy 1995). Because of the high prevalence of penicillin resistance among gonococci causing genital infections, however, expanded-spectrum cephalosporins such as ceftriaxone parenterally or cefixime orally are usually recommended (Smith & Piercy 1995). It is likely that the fluoroquinolones, ciprofloxacin and ofloxacin, would also be effective, but there is little clinical experience with these drugs in treating gonococcal skeletal infections.

OROFACIAL AND DENTAL INFECTIONS

Orofacial and dental infections are caused by oropharyngeal streptococci and anaerobes, and are appropriately treated with a penicillin or clindamycin (von Konow et al 1992). Human and animal bites may also include the Gram-positive skin flora of the victim as well as the mouth flora of the attacker (Goldstein et al 1984, Brook 1987, Goldstein & Citron 1993, Smith & Piercy 1995). Amoxycillin–clavulanate (or ampicillin–sulbactam) has an ideal spectrum against the organisms isolated from these infections; cephalosporins, macrolides, tetracyclines and fluoroquinolones are less consistently active (Brook 1987, Goldstein & Citron 1993, Smith & Piercy 1995). Clindamycin is also useful to treat infected bites but is not active against *Eikenella corrodens* (Robinson & James 1974), associated with human bites, or *Pasteurella multocida* (Goldstein et al 1988), associated with animal bites.

THE INFECTED DIABETIC FOOT AND PRESSURE SORES

Selecting the optimal antimicrobial regimen for treating these infections is difficult because infection may be caused by combinations of staphylococci, streptococci, enterococci, Enterobacteriaceae, *Ps. aeruginosa* and faecal anaerobes (Sugarman et al 1983, Lipsky et al 1990). The antimicrobial spectra of drugs potentially useful for treating these infections are shown in Table 54.1. Monotherapy may be appropriate, depending on the microbial aetiology. For example, a β-lactam–β-lactamase inhibitor may cover all the Gram-positive, Gram-negative and anaerobic pathogens present. Monotherapy with other drugs may not be adequate. Clindamycin covers staphylococci, streptococci and anaerobes, but not enterococci or aerobic Gram-negative

Table 54.1 *Clinically useful antimicrobials, by spectrum of activity, for treating aerobic–anaerobic bone and joint infections such as the diabetic foot and infected pressure sores*

Antimicrobial	Staphylococci*	Streptococci	Ent. faecalis	Enterobacteriaceae	Ps. aeruginosa	Anaerobes (oral)	Anaerobes (faecal)
Penicillin G, ampicillin, amoxycillin	+	+++	+++	±	0	++	+
Ampicillin–sulbactam, amoxycillin–clavulanate†	+++	+++	+++	+	0	+++	+++
Mezlocillin, piperacillin	±	+++	+++	++	++	+++	++
Piperacillin–tazobactam†	+++	+++	+++	+++	++	+++	+++
Cefotaxime, ceftizoxime, ceftriaxone	+++	+++	0	+++	±	+++	++
Ceftazidime	+++	±	0	+++	++	±	±
Cefoperazone	+++	+++	±	+++	++	+++	++
Imipenem	+++	+++	+++	+++	++	+++	+++
Ciprofloxacin	±	±	±	+++	++	±	±
Co-trimoxazole	+++	±	0	+++	0	0	0
Aminoglycosides	±	0	0	+++	+++	0	0
Clindamycin	+++	+++	0	0	0	+++	+++
Metronidazole	0	0	0	0	0	+++	+++
Vancomycin, teicoplanin	+++	+++	+++	0	0	±	±

0, Little or no clinical activity; ±, some in vitro activity, but not very useful clinically; +, good for a limited number of strains or organisms; ++, good for many strains or organisms; +++ good for most or all strains or organisms.
* Methicillin-susceptible strains; vancomycin or teicoplanin for resistant strains.
† Not necessary for non-β-lactamase-producing strains or for some β-lactamase-producing species such as *Ps. aeruginosa.*

bacilli. Metronidazole covers anaerobes but, unlike other anti-anaerobe drugs, has no activity against any aerobes. An aminoglycoside may be given in combination with a β-lactam for synergy against aerobic Gram-negative bacilli, but it should not be used as monotherapy. Co-trimoxazole covers staphylococci and Enterobacteriaceae but not enterococci or anaerobes. Ciprofloxacin covers Enterobacteriaceae and *Ps. aeruginosa* but it is suboptimal for Gram-positive cocci and inactive against anaerobic Gram-negative bacilli. Vancomycin or teicoplanin would be necessary to cover β-lactam-resistant Gram-positive organisms. On occasion, the diversity of pathogens present and their susceptibility patterns may justify the use of imipenem, despite its high cost.

Dose, route and duration of treatment

Skeletal infections have traditionally been treated with relatively high doses of intravenous antimicrobials – septic arthritis for 2–3 weeks and osteomyelitis for 4–6 weeks (Waldvogel et al 1970, Syrogiannopoulos & Nelson 1988,

Gentry 1990, Esterhai & Gelb 1991, Smith & Piercy 1995). In children, however, shorter courses of treatment were often adequate. Acute infections caused by *H. influenzae*, *Neisseria* spp. or streptococci should be treated for at least 10–14 days and those caused by *Staph. aureus*, Enterobacteriaceae or *Ps. aeruginosa* for at least 3 weeks (Nelson 1983, Syrogiannopoulos & Nelson 1988, Nelson 1990, Smith & Piercy 1995).

Acute infections in adults and chronic infections at any age need to be treated for longer (Waldvogel et al 1970, Goldenberg & Reed 1985, Esterhai & Gelb 1991). It is becoming increasingly popular to administer long-term, intravenous antibiotics at home using a surgically implanted central venous catheter and long half-life antibiotics in an attempt to reduce the length of hospital stay and associated costs (Gentry 1990). Complication rates of 20% have been reported (Couch et al 1987), however, and costs are still appreciable.

While prolonged intravenous treatment would certainly be appropriate when infection is associated with severe staphylococcal bacteraemia, it is probably unnecessary for most infections. The availability of highly active, predictably absorbed oral agents has obviated the need for prolonged intravenous antimicrobials with the attendant discomfort, complications and costs. Indeed, there is clear benefit from more prolonged treatment for some patients, such as those with chronic, recalcitrant osteomyelitis; treatment with an appropriate oral agent for 3–12 months should be considered in such cases (Waldvogel et al 1970, Feigin et al 1975, Nelson 1983, Lipsky et al 1990).

Oral penicillins, cephalosporins or clindamycin, after 5–10 days of initial intravenous therapy, have been effective in children (Feigin et al 1975, Tetzlaff et al 1978, Kaplan et al 1982, Nelson 1983). Similarly, treatment with intravenous, and then oral ampicillin–sulbactam has also been used successfully (Aronoff et al 1986).

Switching from intravenous to oral therapy has also been successful in adults (Black et al 1987); 21 adults with osteomyelitis or septic arthritis caused primarily by *Staph. aureus* and/or Enterobacteriaceae treated intravenously for a mean of 3.6 days followed by a mean of 43 days orally, had a satisfactory outcome. Cloxacillin, cephalexin (6–9 g/day plus probenecid) or co-trimoxazole (160/800 mg four times daily) were prescribed for the staphylococcal infected

and co-trimoxazole for those caused by the Enterobacteriaceae. Co-trimoxazole, at the same dose, was also used successfully to treat methicillin-resistant *Staph. aureus* osteomyelitis, usually after initial intravenous vancomycin (Yeldandi et al 1988).

Ciprofloxacin and, to a lesser extent, ofloxacin and pefloxacin, initially available only orally, have been extensively used to treat skeletal infections (Norrby 1989, Waldvogel 1989, Gentry 1990, Mader 1990, Gentry 1991). Borderline activity against streptococci and enterococci and the emergence of staphylococcal resistance (Fass et al 1995) indicates that the fluoroquinolones, when used to treat skeletal infections, should be restricted to aerobic Gram-negative infections. Our experience with oral ciprofloxacin to treat 21 patients with osteomyelitis was uniformly successful for those caused by Enterobacteriaceae and/or *Ps. aeruginosa*, but only 2/11 (18%) with concomitant Gram-positive and/or anaerobic pathogens had a satisfactory response.

Table 54.2   *Comparison of intravenous and oral antimicrobial regimens for treating skeletal infections in adults*

Drug	Dose	Approximate peak serum concentration (mg/l)	Usual MIC (mg/l) of appropriate pathogens
Intravenous			
β-Lactams			
Penicillin G	1–2 MU 4–6-hourly	10–20 U/ml	≤0.12
Ampicillin	1–2 g 4–6-hourly	20–50	≤0.25, 0.5–2*
Ampicillin–sulbactam	1.5–3 g 6-hourly	50–150	≤2, 2–8†
Nafcillin	1–2 g 4–6-hourly	40–80	≤0.5
Cefazolin	1–2 g 8-hourly	80–150	≤2
Ceftriaxone	1–2 g 24-hourly	100–250	≤4
Non-β-lactams			
Clindamycin	600 mg 8-hourly	8	≤0.5
Co-trimoxazole	160/800 mg 8-hourly	6/120	≤0.5/9.5
Ciprofloxacin	400 mg 8–12-hourly	4	≤0.25, 0.12–2**
Metronidazole	500 mg 6-hourly	15–25	≤4
Oral			
β-Lactams			
Penicillin V	500 mg q.i.d.	5	≤0.12
Amoxycillin	500 mg t.i.d.	5–10	≤0.25, 0.5–2*
Amoxycillin–clavulanate	500 mg t.i.d.	5–10	≤2, 2–8†
Dicloxacillin	0.5–1 g q.i.d.	10–25	≤2
Cephalexin	0.5–1 g q.i.d.	15–25	≤8
Cefixime§	400 mg q.d.	4	≤1
Non-β-lactams			
Clindamycin	300 mg q.i.d.	5	≤0.5
Co-trimoxazole‖	160/800 mg t.i.d.	4/100	≤0.5/9.5
Ciprofloxacin	500–750 mg b.i.d.	3–4	≤0.25, 0.12–2**
Metronidazole	500 mg q.i.d.	12	≤4

q.d., once daily; b.i.d., twice daily; t.i.d., three times daily; q.i.d., four times daily.
* MIC ≤0.12 mg/l for most susceptible organisms; 0.5–2 mg/l for *Ent. faecalis*.
† MIC ≤2 mg/l for β-lactamase-positive *H. influenzae*; 2–8 mg/l for susceptible Enterobacteriaceae.
§ Cefixime is indicated for Gram-negative organisms only.
‖ Peak serum concentrations at steady state are extrapolated from multiple studies.
** MIC ≤0.25 mg/l for Enterobacteriaceae; 0.12–2 mg/l for susceptible *Ps. aeruginosa*.

Oral therapy requires predictable absorption. Although β-lactams are often the preferred drugs for skeletal infections, oral derivatives can be unpredictably absorbed, even at high doses with probenecid (Prober & Yeager 1979, Nelson 1983, Aronoff et al 1986). Serum concentrations of intravenous and oral clindamycin far exceed those necessary to inhibit most staphylococci and streptococci (Feigin et al 1975, Fass 1980, Kaplan et al 1982). Likewise, serum concentrations of co-trimoxazole after intravenous and oral administration are virtually identical (data on file, Burroughs Welcome Co.) and are inhibitory to most staphylococci and Enterobacteriaceae. Oral and intravenous ciprofloxacin (Heller 1992) also results in serum concentrations in excess of those needed to inhibit most Enterobacteriaceae and *Ps. aeruginosa*. Serum concentrations of metronidazole after intravenous and oral administration are virtually identical (Houghton et al 1979) and exceed those needed to inhibit most anaerobes.

In Table 54.2, intravenous antimicrobials commonly used to treat skeletal infections are shown with recommended doses, observed peak serum concentrations and the usual minimum inhibitory concentrations (MICs) for pathogens appropriate for treatment. For each drug, doses of the oral preparation (or similar drug in the case of the β-lactams) with observed peak serum concentrations are provided for comparison. For the antipseudomonal β-lactams and glycopeptides, no oral equivalents are available and switching to oral therapy requires changing drug class.

Direct instillation or irrigation of infected bones or joints is no longer necessary with currently available antibiotics and thus the risks of secondary infection and chemical synovitis with a treatment of uncertain efficacy are avoided (Nelson 1983).

Monitoring antimicrobial therapy

Clinical and microbiological follow-up are important to ensure that resolution is progressing satisfactorily. This is particularly the case when the microbiological diagnosis has been equivocal or lacking. Serum bactericidal tests (SBTs) have been used to monitor the adequacy of treatment, but this is usually unnecessary. The tests suffer from poor standardization and validated guidelines for interpretation of results (Wolfson & Swartz 1985, Weinstein et al 1987). Infections due to gonococci and streptococci usually respond favourably, while staphylococcal and Gram-negative bacillary infections often do poorly (Cooper & Cawley 1986, Esterhai & Gelb 1991), regardless of the SBT test results.

Determining SBT titres (or, more simply, measuring drug levels) may be useful to confirm adequacy of drug

concentrations when treating with marginally active drugs or to assess the adequacy of concentrations with oral agents, particularly the penicillins and cephalosporins (Tetzlaff et al 1978, Prober & Yeager 1979, Kaplan et al 1982, Nelson 1983, Aronoff et al 1986, Black et al 1987, Syrogiannopoulos & Nelson 1988).

Surgery

Surgical procedures are indicated for a variety of reasons in the diagnosis and management of bone and joint infections (Waldvogel et al 1970, Waldvogel & Vasey 1980, Goldenberg & Reed 1985, Cooper & Cawley 1986, Gillespie 1990b, Lipsky et al 1990, Nelson 1990, Esterhai & Gelb 1991, Smith & Piercy 1995). Needle aspiration or biopsy may suffice for diagnosis or drainage. Arthroscopic drainage of joints may facilitate breaking up fibrinous joint material and removal of debris. More extensive procedures may be indicated to resect fistulae, debride ulcers or necrotic devascularized bone, remove foreign bodies, including joint prostheses, as well as improving locomotor stability, restoring vascular supply and joint reconstruction.

In some patients with diabetic foot ulcers, the vascular supply may be so poor or the infection so extensive that antimicrobial administration and debridement is insufficient to ensure eradication of infection and ultimate healing (Lipsky et al 1990). In such instances, prolonged chemotherapy may be futile and unnecessarily subject a patient to adverse drug effects, expenses and disability. Amputation may be advisable for cure and a return to baseline lifestyle (Waldvogel et al 1970). An analogous situation may occur with extensive decubitus ulcers. Early excision of the ulcer, aggressive debridement of involved bone and flap grafting to cover the wound may result in a satisfactory outcome (Mathes 1982). Risk factors predisposing to the initial infection should be reduced to avoid recurrence after this time-consuming and expensive procedure.

Internal fixation and prosthetic devices

It is particularly difficult to eradicate infection in the presence of foreign bodies, including prostheses (Gillespie 1990b). Overtly infected or unstable fixation devices and prosthetic joints should be removed. When it is not clear that they are infected or are required for stability, prolonged treatment may be tried, sometimes with removal at a later date. Alternately, one can remove the prostheses, use external fixation on a temporary basis, and then insert a new device at a later date when the infection has been eradicated (Waldvogel & Vasey 1980).

Joint replacement is now a commonly performed operative procedure. Initially, deep wound infection rates were about 10% but with greater experience, prophylactic antibiotics and unidirectional airflow systems, infection rates should be <2%. The use of gentamicin-impregnated cement and personnel isolator systems may also have contributed to reduced infection rates at some centres. The most commonly used prophylactic antimicrobial has been cefazolin or similar cephalosporin. Therapeutic agents should be selected, as for the treatment of other skeletal infections, based on microbial aetiology. Staphylococci are most common, but infections caused by streptococci, Gram-negative bacilli and, occasionally, anaerobes may be seen. Removal of the prosthesis, infected tissue and cement should be done with immediate (one-stage) or, preferably, delayed (two-stage) replacement of the prosthesis (Saravolatz 1993).

References

Aronoff S C, Scoles P V, Makley J T, Jacobs M R, Blumer J L, Kalamchi A 1986 Efficacy and safety of sequential treatment with parenteral sulbactam/ampicillin and oral sultamicillin for skeletal infections in children. *Reviews of Infectious Diseases* 8 (suppl 5): S639–S643

Black J, Hunt T L, Godley P J, Matthew E 1987 Oral antimicrobial therapy for adults with osteomyelitis or septic arthritis. *Journal of Infectious Diseases* 155: 968–972

Brook I 1987 Microbiology of human and animal bite wounds in children. *Journal of Pediatric Infectious Diseases* 6: 29–32

Coombs R R H 1990 Fusidic acid in staphylococcal bone and joint infection. *Journal of Antimicrobial Chemotherapy* 25 (suppl B): 53–60

Cooper C, Cawley M I D 1986 Bacterial arthritis in an English health district: a 10 year review. *Annals of the Rheumatic Diseases* 45: 458–463

Couch L, Cierny G, Mader J T 1987 Inpatient and outpatient use of the Hickman catheter for adults with osteomyelitis. *Clinical Orthopaedics and Related Research* 219: 226–235

Drugeon H B, Caillon J, Juvin M E 1994 In-vitro antibacterial activity of fusidic acid alone and in combination with other antibiotics against methicillin-sensitive and -resistant *Staphylococcus aureus. Journal of Antimicrobial Chemotherapy* 34: 899–907

Esterhai J L Jr, Gelb I 1991 Adult septic arthritis. *Orthopedic Clinics of North America* 22: 503–514

Fass R J 1980 Lincomycin and clindamycin. In: Kagan B M (ed) Antimicrobial therapy, 3rd edn. W B Saunders, Philadelphia, p 97–116

Fass R J, Barnishan J, Ayers L W 1995 Emergence of bacterial resistance to imipenem and ciprofloxacin in a university hospital. *Journal of Antimicrobial Chemotherapy* 36: 343–353

Feigin R D, Pickering L K, Anderson D, Keeney R E, Shackleford P G 1975 Clindamycin treatment of osteomyelitis and septic arthritis in children. *Pediatrics* 55: 213–223

Fortún J, Pérez-Molina J A, Añón M T, Martínez-Beltrán J, Loza E, Guerrero A 1995 Right-sided endocarditis caused by *Staphylococcus aureus* in drug abusers. *Antimicrobial Agents and Chemotherapy* 39: 525–528

Gentry L O 1990 Antibiotic therapy for osteomyelitis. *Infectious Disease Clinics of North America* 4: 485–499

Gentry L O 1991 Oral antimicrobial therapy for osteomyelitis. *Annals of Internal Medicine* 114: 986–987

Gillespie W J 1990a Epidemiology in bone and joint infection. *Infectious Disease Clinics of North America* 4: 361–376

Gillespie W J 1990b Infection in total joint replacement. *Infectious Disease Clinics of North America* 4: 465–484

Goldenberg D L, Reed J I 1985 Bacterial arthritis. *New England Journal of Medicine* 312: 764–771

Goldstein E J C, Citron D M 1993 Comparative susceptibilities of 173 aerobic and anaerobic bite wound isolates to sparfloxacin, temafloxacin, clarithromycin, and older agents. *Antimicrobial Agents and Chemotherapy* 37: 1150–1153

Goldstein E J C, Citron D M, Finegold S M 1984 Role of anaerobic bacteria in bite-wound infections. *Reviews of Infectious Diseases* 6 (suppl 1): S177–S183

Goldstein E J C, Citron D M, Richwald G A 1988 Lack of in vitro efficacy of oral forms of certain cephalosporins, erythromycin, and oxacillin against *Pasteurella multocida. Antimicrobial Agents and Chemotherapy* 32: 213–215

Heller A H 1992 Pharmacokinetic studies demonstrating equivalent doses of intravenous and oral ciprofloxacin. *Infections in Medicine* 9 (suppl B): 32–40

Houghton G W, Smith J, Thorne P S, Templeton R 1979 The pharmacokinetics of oral and intravenous metronidazole in man. *Journal of Antimicrobial Chemotherapy* 5: 621–623

Inman R D, Gallegos K V, Brause B D, Redecha P B, Christian C L 1984 Clinical and microbial features of prosthetic joint infection. *American Journal of Medicine* 77: 47–53

Kaplan S L, Mason E O Jr, Feigin R D 1982 Clindamycin versus nafcillin or methicillin in the treatment of *Staphylococcus aureus* osteomyelitis in children. *Southern Medical Journal* 75: 138–142

Lipsky B A, Pecoraro R E, Wheat L J 1990 The diabetic foot. Soft tissue and bone infection. *Infectious Disease Clinics of North America* 4: 409–432

Mackowiak P A, Jones S R, Smith J W 1978 Diagnostic value of sinus-tract cultures in chronic osteomyelitis. *Journal of the American Medical Association* 239: 2772–2775

Mader J T 1990 Fluoroquinolones in bone and joint infections. In: Sanders W E, Sanders C C (eds) Fluoroquinolones in the treatment of infectious diseases. Physicians & Scientists Publishing Co., Glenview, IL, p 71–86

Mader J T, Adams K, Morrison L 1989 Comparative evaluation of cefazolin and clindamycin in the treatment of experimental *Staphylococcus aureus* osteomyelitis in rabbits. *Antimicrobial Agents and Chemotherapy* 33: 1760–1764

Mathes S J 1982 The muscle flap for management of osteomyelitis. *New England Journal of Medicine* 306: 294–295

Nelson J D 1971 Antibiotic concentrations in septic joint effusions. *New England Journal of Medicine* 284: 349–353

Nelson J D 1983 A critical review of the role of oral antibiotics in the management of hematogenous osteomyelitis. In: Remington J S, Swartz M N (eds) Current clinical topics in infectious diseases. McGraw-Hill, New York, vol 4, p 64–74

Nelson J D 1990 Acute osteomyelitis in children. *Infectious Disease Clinics of North America* 4: 513–522

Nelson J D, Howard J B, Shelton S 1978 Oral antibiotic therapy for skeletal infections of children. I. Antibiotic concentrations in suppurative synovial fluid. *Journal of Pediatrics* 92: 131–134

Norrby S R 1989 Ciprofloxacin in the treatment of acute and chronic osteomyelitis: a review. *Scandinavian Journal of Infectious Diseases* 60 (suppl): 74–78

Prober C G, Yeager A S 1979 Use of the serum bactericidal titer to assess the adequacy of oral antibiotic therapy in the treatment of acute hematogenous osteomyelitis. *Journal of Pediatrics* 95: 131–135

Robinson J V A, James A L 1974 In vitro susceptibility of *Bacteroides corrodens* and *Eikenella corrodens* to ten chemotherapeutic agents. *Antimicrobial Agents and Chemotherapy* 6: 543–546

Saravolatz L D 1993 Infection in implantable prosthetic devices. In: Wenzel R P (ed) Prevention and control of nosocomial infections, 2nd edn. Williams & Wilkins, Baltimore, p 683–707

Sattar M A, Barrett S P, Cawley M I D 1983 Concentrations of some antibiotics in synovial fluid after oral administration, with special reference to antistaphylococcal activity. *Annals of the Rheumatic Diseases* 42: 67–74

Schauwecker D S, Braunstein E M, Wheat L J 1990 Diagnostic imaging of osteomyelitis. *Infectious Disease Clinics of North America* 4: 441–463

Small P M, Chambers H F 1990 Vancomycin for *Staphylococcus aureus* endocarditis in intravenous drug users. *Antimicrobial Agents and Chemotherapy* 34: 1227–1231

Smith J W, Piercy E A 1995 Infectious arthritis. *Clinical Infectious Diseases* 20: 225–231

Sugarman B, Hawes S, Musher D M, Klima M, Young E J, Pircher F 1983 Osteomyelitis beneath pressure sores. *Archives of Internal Medicine* 143: 683–688

Syrogiannopoulos G A, Nelson J D 1988 Duration of antimicrobial therapy for acute suppurative osteoarticular infections. *Lancet* i: 37–40

Tetzlaff T R, McCracken G H Jr, Nelson J D 1978 Oral antibiotic therapy for skeletal infections of children. II. Therapy of osteomyelitis and suppurative arthritis. *Journal of Pediatrics* 92: 485–490

von Konow L, Köndell P Å, Nord C E, Heimdahl A 1992 Clindamycin versus phenoxymethylpenicillin in the treatment of acute orofacial infections. *European Journal of Clinical Microbiology and Infectious Diseases* 11: 1129–1136

Waldvogel F A 1989 Use of quinolones for the treatment of osteomyelitis and septic arthritis. *Review of Infectious Diseases* 11 (suppl 5): S1259–S1263

Waldvogel F A, Medoff G, Swartz M N 1970 Osteomyelitis: a review of clinical features, therapeutic considerations and unusual aspects. *New England Journal of Medicine* 282: 198–206, 260–266, 316–322

Waldvogel F A, Vasey H 1980 Osteomyelitis: the past decade. *New England Journal of Medicine* 303: 360–370

Wegener W A, Alavi A 1991 Diagnostic imaging of musculoskeletal infection. *Orthopedic Clinics of North America* 22: 401–418

Weinstein M P, Stratton C W, Hawley H B, Ackley A, Reller L B 1987 Multicenter collaborative evaluation of a standardized serum bactericidal test as a predictor of therapeutic efficacy in acute and chronic osteomyelitis. *American Journal of Medicine* 83: 218–222

Wolfson J S, Swartz M N 1985 Serum bactericidal activity as a monitor of antibiotic therapy. *New England Journal of Medicine* 312: 968–975

Yeldandi V, Strodtman R, Lentino J R 1988 In-vitro and in-vivo studies of trimethoprim–sulphamethoxazole against multiple resistant *Staphylococcus aureus*. *Journal of Antimicrobial Chemotherapy* 22: 873–880

Infections of the eye

D. V. Seal and A. J. Bron

Introduction

This chapter gives an outline account of ocular infections and approaches to therapy. The eye presents special problems in relation to the delivery of drugs and the risks of local drug toxicity.

BARRIERS TO OCULAR PENETRATION

Surface epithelium

The normal conjunctiva and cornea are protected by a triple-layered tear film comprising an outer oily layer from the meibomian glands, an aqueous layer from lacrimal glands and an inner mucus layer, derived chiefly from conjunctival goblet cells. Repeated blinking maintains the spread and integrity of this protective layer. Tears have an antibacterial effect due to bacterial coating by tear immunoglobulin A (IgA), growth inhibition by lactoferrin iron chelation and cell wall lysis by a combination of IgG and complement, leaking through the conjunctiva from inflamed vessels.

Tear lysozyme acts on the bacterial cell membrane and has a direct antibacterial action on *Micrococcus lysodeikticus*, which is non-pathogenic in the eye. From the age of 40 years, tear volume and the concentration of tear components of lacrimal origin decrease due to reduced lacrimal gland function.

Pharmacokinetics

The bulbar conjunctival and corneal epithelia are relatively impermeable to water-soluble agents of small molecular size applied topically. Proprietary ophthalmic preparations, such as gentamicin sulphate, are available as eye drops or as ointments at high concentration (e.g. 0.3–1.0%) relative to

their effective antimicrobial concentration and are thus active in the treatment of surface ocular infections such as conjunctivitis. Agents with a relatively high lipid–water solubility coefficient (such as ciprofloxacine, chloramphenicol and the sulphonamides) can, in addition, penetrate the conjunctiva and cornea to enter deeper tissues.

Once the surface epithelium is breached, as with corneal ulceration, water-soluble drugs can diffuse into the anterior segment of the eye in high concentration. This can be enhanced by the use of fortified eye drops with drug concentrations exceeding those of commercially available preparations. However, this route is ineffective in providing concentrations in the posterior segment of the eye because a diffusion barrier exists across the lens–zonule compartment and anterior vitreous, and because drug is removed by diffusion across the anterior surface of the iris and across the posterior uvea. In addition, there is bulk movement of aqueous from the posterior chamber, through the pupil, and out through the conventional aqueous drainage pathway into the venous circulation.

The surface epithelial barrier can be circumvented therapeutically by delivering a bolus of drug under the conjunctiva (subconjunctival injection) or more deeply into the orbit (sub-Tenon's injection). These periocular routes will deliver effective antimicrobial concentrations into the anterior segment of the eye (e.g. cornea and anterior chamber) and to some extent into the posterior segment (e.g. the vitreous).

Blood–ocular barriers

In the uninflamed intact eye, barriers also exist to the transfer of antibiotic from the blood circulation into the ocular fluids. A blood–aqueous barrier inhibits the entry of water-soluble drugs across the epithelium of the ciliary body into newly formed aqueous, and there is also a blood–retinal barrier with similar properties. Although drugs may readily reach a high concentration within the extracellular space of the choroid via the fenestrated capillaries of the choriocapillaris, diffusion across the outer retina is obstructed by tight junctions between the cells of the retinal pigment epithelium (the outer blood–retinal barrier), and across the retinal capillaries by endothelial tight junctions (the inner blood–retinal barrier). Indeed, there is an active transport mechanism which removes anionic drugs from the aqueous across the pigment epithelium of the posterior iris, and from the cortical vitreous across the retinal capillary endothelial cells and the retinal pigment epithelium.

These barriers affect the ocular distribution of systemically administered drugs and their potential for entering the vitreous as well as the retention of drugs delivered directly into the vitreous space.

In the uninflamed eye, the highest aqueous concentration using the systemic route will be achieved by lipid-soluble drugs such as chloramphenicol, or lipophilic quinolones in lower concentration. Negligible concentrations will be achieved using water-soluble drugs, particularly those in anionic form (such as the penicillins and cephalosporins), which are actively transported out of the eye.

In the inflamed eye, the concentrations achieved in the ocular compartments are increased, owing to partial breakdown of the blood–aqueous barrier, so that effective antimicrobial concentrations may be produced in the

aqueous. However, concentrations reached in the vitreous with parenteral therapy are always much lower than those achieved in the aqueous, even in the inflamed eye with endophthalmitis. Vitreous concentrations after high-dose systemic therapy in such situations will be subtherapeutic and lower than those achievable by subconjunctival injection and, inevitably, than those produced by direct injection into the vitreous. The latter route is always favoured in the treatment of serious endophthalmitis.

The barriers referred to for the globe itself (Fig. 55.1) do not exist for other orbital structures and thus infections within the orbit or ocular adnexae (the eyelids, lacrimal gland and nasolacrimal system) are readily treatable with systemic antibiotics.

Bacterial infections of the eye

BLEPHARITIS

In 1946, Thygeson made the following distinction between blepharitis due to *Staphylococcus aureus* and that due to seborrhoea (Table 55.1).

McCulley et al (1982) has explored relationships between blepharitis, staphylococci and meibomianitis and, with Mathers et al (1991), has identified meibomianitis as a separate syndrome. It is characterized by excessive secretion of meibomian glands causing a gritty sensation and stickiness in the early morning. Later the glands may become blocked and secondarily infected causing a chalazia,

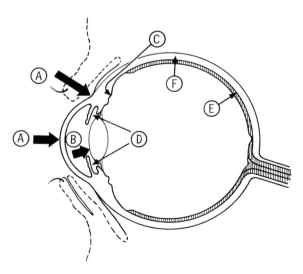

Fig. 55.1 *(A) Epithelial barrier (breached by an ulcer; negotiated by topical drops or subconjunctival injection). (B) Aqueous–vitreous barrier. (C) Blood–aqueous barrier limits entry into the aqueous from the blood. (D) Iris pigment epithelial pump removes anions from the aqueous. (E) Blood–retinal barrier; external, pigment–epithelial barrier. (F) Internal, capillary–endothelial barrier. There is an outward pumping of anions across the retina.*

Table 55.1 *Blepharitis due to* Staph. aureus *and seborrhoea*

	Staph. aureus	Seborrhoea
Seborrhoeic capitis	Occasionally present	Always present
Associated dermatoses	Acne, rosacea, impetigo, eczema	Seborrhoeic dermatitis
Unilateral or bilateral	Unilateral common	Always bilateral
Lid margin ulceration	Often	Absent
Associated conjunctivitis	Frequent, severe	Minimal or absent
Associated folliculitis	Common, acute	Absent
Associated keratitis	Marginal infiltrates and ulceration	Absent
Scales, crusting	Hard, tenacious, removal difficult	Greasy, easily removed
Microscopy, lid margin	Staphylococci	Pityrosporum ovale and leucocytes

or become deficient leading to an unstable tear film. This may be one cause of recurrent erosion syndrome.

Confusion exists over the role of coagulase-negative staphylococci (CoNS) in the above conditions. CoNS have been shown not to be involved in blepharitis per se (Wright et al 1994); in a rabbit model study (Mondino et al 1987) acute folliculitis and ulceration of the lid margin did not occur in a way similar to that caused by *Staph. aureus* (see below); in humans, no immune reaction could be demonstrated to CoNS. CoNS may have a secondary role in meibomianitis with production of lipases releasing toxic fatty acids from triglycerides and this may explain an apparent response to tetracycline (Dougherty et al 1991), but the pathogenesis is far from proven.

Ficker et al (1991b) investigated delayed hypersensitivity (DTH) to *Staph. aureus* in humans with chronic blepharitis of mixed aetiology and found that 40% of patients had enhanced cell-mediated immunity (CMI) to *Staph. aureus*; this did not occur in normals and was not found more frequently in atopes. This enhanced CMI to *Staph. aureus* was associated with folliculitis rather than meibomianitis. In addition, enhancement was more likely to be present with recurrent marginal ulceration that required steroid treatment.

Blepharitis is diagnosed by clinical examination. The lid margin is examined with a slit-lamp for evidence of folliculitis and collarettes (cuffing of infected secretion around the lashes). In the acute condition, there will be beads of pus and an ulcerated margin. When chronicity ensues, there is a loss or misdirection of lashes, telangiectasia and a swollen lid margin. There may be a history of recurrent marginal ulceration.

Culture of the lid margin requires 'scrubbing' with a swab soaked in sterile broth, and plating out directly on blood agar and a selective medium for *Staph. aureus*. If *Staph. aureus* is present, treatment should commence with Fucithalmic (topical 1% fusidic acid in gel). If laboratory cultures demonstrate resistance, tetracycline or Polytrim ointment can be used instead, if the isolate is sensitive. In acute blepharitis, flucloxacillin or erythromycin can also be given by mouth (500 mg four times a day for 4 days) and whole-body bathing commenced with chlorhexidine (Hibiscrub, Zeneca Pharmaceuticals).

CoNS may be cultured but should not be considered as pathogenic. They colonize 80% of normal and blepharitic lid margins; in the absence of meibomianitis, the presence of CoNS should be considered as part of the normal lid flora not requiring treatment with antibiotics.

In chronic blepharitis, regular lid hygiene should be performed with lid scrubs and baby lotion, and misdirected lashes removed. Intermittent therapy should be given with topical Fucithalmic (or less efficiently by Polytrim) to suppress the presence of *Staph. aureus* on the lids. Patients should be encouraged to wash with antiseptic soaps to suppress carriage of *Staph. aureus* at other skin sites, especially axillary and perineal; chlorhexidine (Hibiscrub) is the most efficacious product and gives a persistent antistaphylococcal effect on skin.

If no apparent response occurs, the blepharitic patient should be investigated in more detail. An algorithm has been published to assist with this (Ficker et al 1995). Patients are divided into those with and without enhanced CMI to *Staph. aureus*. This is determined by injecting intradermally 0.1 ml of killed *Staph. aureus* cells (10^8/ml preserved with 0.5% phenol) and 2.5 ng of protein A (Sigma Chemicals) into the forearm (Ficker et al 1995). An induration reaction is read at 48 h; enhancement is indicated by a positive result of >5 mm for killed *Staph. aureus* cells and >20 mm for protein A. The presence of *Staph. aureus* on the lid margin should be suppressed in enhanced patients; this situation occurs more commonly in association with rosacea.

Atopy

Atopic blepharitis should not be confused with staphylococcal blepharitis. The two may co-exist but atopic keratoconjunctivitis (AKC) is a separate disorder (Tuft et al 1991). Most normal, non-inflamed lids in patients with atopic dermatitis are colonized with *Staph. aureus* (Tuft et al 1992), as are the conjunctiva and nasal mucosa. The skin of patients with atopic dermatitis is also heavily colonized by *Staph. aureus*, but the reasons for this association are not understood. Management of concomitant *Staph. aureus* blepharitis in the atope follows the same procedures outlined above. While tear immunoglobulin E (IgE) levels are high, they are not directed against *Staph. aureus* antigens even in AKC patients.

Rosacea

Acne rosacea is also associated with blepharitis. The lids are often colonized by *Staph. aureus*, although it is not clear why the rosacea patient, like the atope, is more susceptible to this colonization than others. These patients also appear to have enhanced CMI to *Staph. aureus*, but it is not clear whether this is cause or effect. In a recent randomized, placebo-controlled cross-over trial (Seal et al 1995b), symptomatic improvement of blepharitis in mild rosacea occurred in 90% of patients receiving topical fusidic acid (Fucithalmic) compared to 50% in those on oral oxytetracycline. This response to tetracycline in rosacea has been found by others (Bartholomew et al 1982), but 25% responded to placebo. Such symptomatic improvement did not occur in non-rosacea blepharitis. There was no response to fusidic acid, and a 25% response to tetracycline. It is thus useful to distinguish rosacea-associated blepharitis as a separate group. Rosacea patients also develop a keratitis, which requires management with topical steroid.

CONJUNCTIVITIS

Conjunctivitis can be due to bacteria, chlamydia, viruses, helminths, fungi and protozoa. Non-infective forms due to allergy or toxicity also exist. Toxicity may be due to preservatives, such as thiomersal, associated with contact-lens wear or, occasionally, to circulating bacterial toxins, as in toxic shock syndrome due to *Staph. aureus* (TSST-1) and *Streptococcus pyogenes* (exotoxin A).

Clinical presentation

Bacterial conjunctivitis presents with an acute purulent discharge which frequently becomes bilateral. The presentation may be hyperacute with *Neisseria gonorrhoeae* with massive lid swelling and a characteristic, profuse yellow-green discharge. In the neonate this infection can progress rapidly to keratitis and perforation leading to blindness.

In viral and to a lesser degree chlamydial conjunctivitis, there is often a follicular conjunctival response, which is usually absent in bacterial infection. Bacterial conjunctivitis may also be watery and only mildly purulent. It is then often confused with viral or chlamydial disease, the latter beginning with a watery discharge that later becomes more purulent. Recent surveys have shown that both ophthalmologists and general practitioners often misdiagnose bacterial conjunctivitis. Enquiry should always be made of an associated urethritis or proctitis, which is the clue for chlamydial infection but need not be present.

Therapy

Therapy should include antibacterial drops or ointment for five days. If treatment fails, conjunctival specimens should be collected, together with specimens for chlamydia if thought appropriate. Empirical treatment for chlamydial infection with topical tetracycline ointment can be given while awaiting laboratory results, with systemic tetracycline or erythromycin 250 mg four times a day for 2 weeks to eradicate chlamydial carriage at other sites.

Adenovirus conjunctivitis may begin unilaterally, but commonly becomes bilateral and, depending on the causative type, may cause a disabling punctate keratitis. In its acute form it lasts up to 21 days; full recovery may take 28 days or longer. Management is palliative only, but culture should be undertaken if possible to confirm the diagnosis accurately. This is important in relation to potential epidemics.

Acute haemorrhagic conjunctivitis (AHC) may occur in epidemics and is due to enterovirus 70; mild paralysis occasionally ensues. In 1971, in the UK 76 cases occurred with enterovirus 70, but this was exceptional. AHC has occurred in pandemics in the tropics in 1969–1971 and 1980–1982. In Singapore, AHC was due to coxsackie A24 in

1970, but enterovirus 70 in 1971 and 1990. Diagnosis is usually clinical. Virus culture should be performed if possible. Treatment is symptomatic unless herpetic infection is present, when topical acyclovir can be used.

Microbial causes of conjunctivitis

Bacteria
- *Staph. aureus*, associated with blepharitis
- *Streptococcus pneumoniae*, associated with sinus disease
- *Str. pyogenes*, associated with throat infections
- *Listeria monocytogenes*, associated with rural and farmyard dust (Farmer's eye)
- *Corynebacterium diphtheriae*, associated with a pseudo-membrane
- *Neisseria meningitidis/gonorrhoeae*, associated with throat/genital infection
- *Pseudomonas aeruginosa*, associated with contact-lens wear
- *Klebsiella aerogenes* and *coliforms*, associated with contact-lens wear
- *Proteus* spp., associated with old age (more in men than women)
- *Moraxella* spp., associated with damaged ocular surface
- *Haemophilus influenzae*, associated with intrinsic throat flora.

Chlamydia
- *Chlamydia trachomatis*, associated with overcrowding in houses and flies (encouraged by cattle dung) in the Near and Middle East and tropics
- Trachoma/inclusion conjunctivitis (TRIC), associated with genital infection in Western countries (may be transmitted in swimming pools).

Viruses
- *Herpes simplex*, associated with corneal disease
- *Herpes zoster*, associated with shingles of the Vth nerve.
- Adenovirus, associated with epidemics from shipyards, close living quarters, and eye clinics (via tonometers and staff handling of patients); early diagnosis is required to bring outbreaks to a quick halt
- AHC: enterovirus 70, poliovirus and coxsackie A24 are associated with epidemics and occasional paralysis; it is associated with foreign travel, especially Singapore and Calcutta
- Conjunctivitis in measles, mumps and dengue is associated with systemic virus infection as with Epstein–Barr virus, associated with glandular fever, and hepatitis A, associated with systemic infection.

Helminths
- *Thellazia capillaris* and *californensis*, associated with birds in the Middle East and the USA
- Loa loa, subconjunctival worm occurring in tropical countries.

Protozoa include *Acanthamoeba* spp. associated with contact-lens wear, or rural corneal trauma and keratitis.

Fungi – fungal keratitis may be associated with an adjunctive conjunctivitis, but fungal conjunctivitis per se does not usually occur.

Microbial diagnosis and treatment

The patient's history and associated illness will often give a clue to the organism responsible.

Presumed bacterial conjunctivitis. Culture swabs should be collected and two smears prepared for Gram and acridine orange stains. Conjunctival swabs should be cultured on blood and chocolate agars (and a selected gonococcal agar if thought relevant). Culture should take place in CO_2 at 37°C for 48 h. Pathogens should be identified and sensitivity tests performed. Treatment should be given with preparations listed in Boxes 55.5 and 55.6.

Presumed chlamydial conjunctivitis. The diagnosis is confirmed by identifying the antigen using a monoclonal antibody test, e.g. 'Syvamicrotrak'. Conjunctival cells should be scraped using a spatula and placed on special slides provided in the kit test. This is much simpler and cheaper than specialist tissue culture.

The older and cheapest method involved staining the conjunctival cell smear with Giemsa stain and observing for intracytoplasmic (Bedson) bodies, within epithelial cells. (These are complete chlamydial cells lacking a traditional bacterial cell wall.) This method becomes more sensitive if the smear is observed under ultraviolet light, when the stained chlamydiae fluoresce yellow, non-specifically.

Presumed viral conjunctivitis. Swabs should be collected by rubbing the conjunctiva firmly and placing into viral transport medium to be sent fresh to the laboratory. These swabs will either be inoculated into tissue culture or used in immunofluorescent tests directed against viral antigen; a combination of both techniques can provide a rapid and sensitive result.

Other forms of conjunctivitis

If the conjunctiva contains a thellazia worm, it should be removed with forceps. Thellazia infection is a zoonosis from birds and occurs when fly-borne larvae from bird droppings are deposited on the conjunctival surface; it has been reported from California, the Middle East and India.

Acanthamoeba conjunctivitis and (epi)scleritis are secondary to the corneal infection and should be managed with it (p. 776).

Ophthalmia neonatorum

Ophthalmia neonatorum is defined as any purulent discharge from the eyes during the first 28 days of life. The prevalence

and treatment of this condition have been summarized by Ridgway (1986). Ophthalmia neonatorum in the UK occurs in 8.2–12% of live births, with gonococcal infection now rare. Elsewhere, the incidence of gonococcal conjunctivitis varies from 0.04% of live births in the West to 1.0% in parts of Africa. The incidence of neonatal chlamydial ophthalmia in London has been estimated to be less than 1%. Sandstrom et al (1984) isolated the following organisms in a case controlled study: *Haemophilus* (17%), *Staphylococcus* (17%), *Str. pneumoniae* (11%) and *Enterococcus* (8%). Positive cultures were obtained in 58% of cases with ophthalmia neonatorum and 5% in controls without conjunctivitis.

Neonatal prophylaxis against gonococcal infection is provided currently in the USA (and in the past in the UK), with one drop of silver nitrate 1% (Crede's solution) in each eye. Silver nitrate causes more ocular symptoms in the first week of treatment than an agent such as oxytetracycline hydrochloride.

Systemic treatment is essential for the treatment of gonococcal keratoconjunctivitis in neonates. Ridgway (1986) recommends 30 mg/kg of benzylpenicillin in two daily doses for 7 days. In recent years, however, the increasing frequency of isolation of penicillin-resistant strains has led to the use of β-lactamase-stable cephalosporins such as ceftriaxone 25–40 mg/kg intravenously every 12 h for 3 days combined with topical saline lavage and antibiotic ointment (e.g. Oc. gentamicin). Single-dose intramuscular therapy may be appropriate when there is no corneal involvement. As is the case with neonatal chlamydial ophthalmia, the infection must be treated systemically; topical therapy alone is not adequate.

TRACHOMA AND OTHER CHLAMYDIAL DISEASE

Ocular infection by *C. trachomatis* takes three forms: trachoma, adult chlamydial ophthalmia (ACO) and neonatal chlamydia ophthalmia (NCO). Trachoma affects 500 million people in developing countries and accounts for 5–10 million blind patients. It is caused by the serotypes A, B and C. In hyperendemic areas 30–50% of the population have active disease and 10% of the population exhibit blinding sequelae. Although infection may be encountered as early as the second month of life, active inflammatory disease is most common in the preschool age group. It is at this stage that the infection leads to the typical conjunctival scarring, which results in entropion and trichiasis and causes recurrent microbial keratitis from repeated corneal trauma. Blinding sequelae due to repeated corneal scarring from infection and trauma, occurs after the age of 40 years. Public health intervention is required to prevent spread of the infection at the childhood stage.

ACO, also known as inclusion conjunctivitis, and NCO, result from sexual transmission. They are caused by serotypes D-K. ACO has its greatest prevalence between the ages of 15 and 20 years. NCO may rarely occur immediately after birth, but presents most commonly in the first week or up to 6 weeks later.

Treatment

Chlamydia trachomatis is unresponsive to the aminoglycosides neomycin and gentamicin. It is partially sensitive to both chloramphenicol and penicillin, which adversely affect growth in subsequent cultures. For this reason, transport media suitable for chlamydial culture do not contain penicillin. *Chlamydia trachomatis* is fully sensitive to the tetracyclines, erythromycin and other macrolides including azithromycin, rifampicin and the quinolones, especially ofloxacin. It is also sensitive to chlorhexidine.

Topical treatment of trachoma with tetracycline or erythromycin ointment or quinolone drops can be effective locally but requires to be given three times daily for 5 weeks. In trachoma, treatment of other family members, or whole villages, is necessary to prevent reinfection. Treatment of the early active inflammatory stages is effective with a single dose of azithromycin.

Systemic therapy is necessary for the treatment or prophylaxis of the systemic manifestations of chlamydial disease such as cervicitis, uveitis, upper respiratory or ear disorders and Reiter's disease in ACO; pharyngitis, vaginitis and a potentially fatal pneumonitis associated with NCO.

For ACO, treatment with oral tetracycline, erythromycin or rifampicin for 2 weeks has been recommended; but long-acting tetracyclines, such as doxycycline and minocycline, offer convenience and improved compliance as fewer doses are required and dietary constraints are not necessary. Oral azithromycin therapy is effective with a single dose. The patient should be checked for genital carriage of chlamydia. In addition, in ACO, partner(s) should be checked for genital carriage and treated with erythromycin or azithromycin if positive.

A suitable treatment for NCO is oral erythromycin 50 mg/kg per 24 h in four divided doses for 2–3 weeks (Ridgway 1986). Topical therapy may be used adjunctively, but is inadequate on its own (see also Ch. 58).

CANALICULITIS

Recurrent unilateral conjunctivitis due to an antibiotic-sensitive bacterium such as *H. influenzae*, can be the presenting symptom of a canaliculitis due to *Actinomyces* spp. (formally *Streptothrix* or *Leptothrix*), or *Arachnia propionica*. The organism does not usually invade the canaliculus wall but forms a 'fungal' ball which obstructs the lumen. The canaliculus provides a micro-aerophilic environment which supports the growth of non-fastidious anaerobic bacteria, and becomes infected with endogenous flora.

Pus, massaged along the canaliculus to the punctum, can be Gram stained to show typical, branching Gram-positive bacilli. Prolonged anaerobic culture on blood agar plates is necessary to demonstrate actinomycetes. Thioglycollate broth should also be inoculated, since oxygen tension decreases with depth, so that the actinomycete ('breadcrumb') colonies grow and float at the appropriate level. Sensitivity tests should be performed.

Actinomycetes and *Arachnia* spp. are usually sensitive to penicillin, tetracycline and erythromycin but resistant to gentamicin and other aminoglycosides often used ineffectively to attempt cure. Initial treatment involves irrigating the canaliculus with penicillin. If this fails, surgery is needed. The canaliculus is opened and debrided. All material removed should be Gram-stained and cultured. The canaliculus should be treated with 5% povidone iodine for 5 min as an effective antiseptic. The canaliculus should be syringed daily for 7 days with penicillin and the patient reviewed at 3 months. Occasionally, repeat surgery and further povidone iodine and penicillin are required to effect a cure.

DACRYOCYSTITIS

Acute dacryocystitis is caused by stasis, due to distal obstruction of the nasolacrimal system. *Staph. aureus* or streptococci are the usual causes and infection may subside on systemic chemotherapy alone. However, drainage of a lacrimal sac abscess may occasionally be necessary, and ultimately the obstruction must be treated by dacryocysto-rhinostomy.

Chronic dacryocystitis commonly involves Gram-negative organisms as 'secondary' pathogens. It can only be effectively treated by relieving the nasolacrimal duct obstruction.

The postoperative infection rate in patients undergoing DCR is greatly reduced by intraoperative cefuroxime intravenously (750 mg), or a 5-day course of oral cefalexin 250 mg four times a day.

MICROBIAL KERATITIS

Suppurative bacterial keratitis presents clinically as a corneal stromal infiltrate or abscess with an overlying epithelial defect. Common causes of infection are given in Box 55.1. It is usually central, except in cases of trauma, but can be peripheral. Because the cornea is only about 0.5 mm thick, such an ulcer may rapidly progress to perforation within 24 h of onset. In the aphake or in the pseudophakic

Box 55.1   *Bacteria causing suppurative keratitis*

Gram-positive cocci
Staphylococcus aureus
Coagulase-negative staphylococci
Streptococcus pneumoniae
Streptococcus pyogenes
Streptococcus viridans
Anaerobic streptococci (rare)

Gram-negative diplobacilli
Moraxella spp.
Neisseria gonorrhoeae
Neisseria meningitidis

Gram-positive rods
Corynebacterium diphtheriae (rare)
Diphtheroids (rare)

Gram-negative rods
Pseudomonas aeruginosa
Proteus spp.
Klebsiella pneumoniae
Escherichia coli
Serratia marcescens
Acinetobacter spp.
Morganella morganii

Other enteric bacteria

Acid-fast bacteria
Mycobacterium chelonei
Nocardia asteroides

eye with a capsulotomy, access to the vitreous space is facilitated and a secondary endophthalmitis may supervene. There is an urgent need to treat bacterial keratitis with high doses of effective antibiotic. Supplementary corneal transplantation, or other reconstructive surgery, may be required at a later stage in the management of corneal scarring or perforation.

Bacteria account for over 80% of ulcerative keratitis occurring in northern climates and 60% in the south where fungal keratitis is more common. Mixed bacterial and fungal infection may also frequently occur in the tropics and occasionally as well in northern climates especially when associated with rural injuries.

In the past, suppurative keratitis was due chiefly to trauma, or occurred in compromised eyes with existing corneal disease. With the growth of contact-lens use in recent years, there has been a rapid increase in contact-lens-associated keratitis, most of which is bacterial (Erie et al 1993). In general, the risk is much less for hard- than soft-lens wearers and is greater with extended wear than daily wear. In a multicentre case-controlled study, the overall risk for ulcerative keratitis with extended-wear lenses was 4 times greater than that for daily wear. In addition, overnight wear of contact lenses increased the risk of keratitis to 10–15 times that occurring with daily wear alone (Schein et al 1989, Dart et al 1991). Soft-contact-lens

wear in corneal graft patients also increases the risk of microbial keratitis.

The incidence of contact-lens-associated microbial keratitis has been estimated to be 1 in 500 for extended-wear patients and 1 in 2500 in daily-wear patients (Poggio et al 1989). The bacteria responsible for contact-lens-associated keratitis include most of those usually associated with suppurative keratitis, but Gram-negative bacteria are more commonly encountered than Gram-positive and *Ps. aeruginosa* is more frequent than other Gram-negative bacteria (Poggio et al 1989, Stapleton et al 1995). Contamination of contact-lens care solutions is an important potential source of keratitis (Donzis et al 1987, Seal et al 1992); home-made solutions are a major risk factor.

Diagnosis

Diagnosis depends on smears and cultures from direct scrapes of the corneal ulcer. Detailed recommendations for the collection of specimens and the processing and interpretation of smears and cultures have been provided by Ficker et al (1991a).

One drop of unpreserved amethocaine or benoxinate is instilled to achieve anaesthesia. Preservatives must be avoided since they will inhibit bacterial replication. The surface material from the ulcer should be debrided using a swab. This may be plated on to blood or chocolate agar, but is less helpful than later scrapes since it usually contains only cellular debris and mucus. The base and edge of the ulcer are most likely to yield organisms. The second scrape should be taken for microscopy. Using a platinum Kimura spatula, a large-gauge sterile needle, or a surgical blade on a disposable handle, the base and edge of the ulcer is firmly scraped. A freshly sterilized instrument is used for each sample.

The material gathered should be firmly spread on a clean glass slide to create a thin film. This is air dried. The second scrape should be similarly used for a second slide film. The third scrape should be plated on to blood, chocolate and Sabouraud agars then a fluid medium, preferably brain–heart infusion, should be inoculated with the same blade. In addition, a Lowenstein–Jensen slope should be inoculated if the keratitis is chronic, although the atypical *Mycobacterium chelonae* will grow on blood agar incubated for 1 week at 37°C. For the chronic ulcer, blood agar should be incubated for one week in 4% CO_2 in order to culture *Nocardia* spp.

When *Acanthamoeba keratitis* is suspected an appropriate specimen for culture of this should also be taken (p. 776).

All media should be inoculated directly at the slit lamp or operating microscope. If possible, duplicate specimens should be taken to allow for culture at different temperatures. Transport medium should not be necessary. Culture of agar plates should always take place at 37°C for one week. The fluid media should be incubated at 30°C in 4%

CO_2 for at least 3 weeks. Anaerobic cultures should be considered when there is an unsatisfactory response to therapy.

Material collected should be stained for bacteria according to the clinical presentation (Ficker et al 1991a). Stains include: Gram stain and acridine orange for common bacteria; the modified Ziehl–Neelsen stain (decolourizing with 5% acetic acid only) for nocardia and mycobacteria; the full Ziehl–Neelsen stain for mycobacteria and the periodic acid Schiff (PAS) or methenamine silver (Grocott) stains for fungi and protozoal cysts. Selective stains include the use of labelled polyclonal or monoclonal antibodies. The acridine orange and Gram stain together will identify organisms in the majority (80%) of cases. It is also possible to maximize the available material and decolourize and restain the same slide with a further intermediate stain and finally an end stain; the choice of the stains involved should be governed by clinical suspicion.

Treatment of suppurative keratitis

A frequent approach is to use combination drop therapy with fortified preparations to cover the spectra of most infective possibilities. A common empirical combination is gentamicin forte 1.5% (15 mg/ml) with cefuroxime or cephazolin 5% (50 mg/ml).

Drops should be given hourly, day and night, for the first 3 days, then 2-hourly by day. Successful eradication of bacterial infection is reported in about 90% of patients treated in this way. Recently, equal success has been reported using commercial preparations of either ciprofloxacin 0.3% or ofloxacin 0.3% at the same frequency. Ofloxacin treatment may cause less irritation. Topical ciprofloxacin may leave microcrystalline deposits on the corneal surface which may have to be removed.

Subconjunctival injections are not necessary, provided an intensive fortified drop regimen is used, as the latter will produce therapeutic levels in the cornea which are sustained and without large fluctuation. If frequent topical applications are not possible, as in a child or a disturbed individual, subconjunctival injections of gentamicin 40 mg and cephazolin 100 mg can be used as an alternative, delivered under a general anaesthetic. Inclusion of adrenaline 0.3 ml (of 1 : 1000) in 1 ml of solution prolongs the effective concentration of antibiotic in the cornea and aqueous from about 6 to 24 h. Other potential regimens are given in Box 55.2.

The frequency of drop use varies from centre to centre. In the USA, it has been recommended that a regimen of fortified drops be given every 15–30 min day and night on an outpatient basis for 3 days. An outpatient approach is not feasible for all patients, and in the UK it is usual to admit patients to hospital. Antibiotic ointment may be given at night in the later stages of therapy once infection is under

Box 55.2 *Suppurative bacterial keratitis: specific antibiotic regimens for topical or periocular therapy*

Initial therapy
To treat unknown organism(s) (new case or no growth on presentation): cefuroxime (5%) + gentamicin (1.5%). This combination will treat the following organisms:

Staph. aureus
Coagulase-negative staphylococci
Streptococci
Haemophilus influenzae
Klebsiella spp.
Proteus spp.
Other enterobacteriaceae

***Pseudomonas aeruginosa* infection (culture-proven or suspected)** (Stapleton et al 1995): Ticarcillin or piperacillin (5%) + gentamicin (1.5%) and/or ceftazidime (5%) and/or ciprofloxacin (0.3%).

Note: Ticarcillin and piperacillin should not be used when penicillin allergy is suspected.
Cephalosporins should also be avoided when there is a history of an anaphylactic reaction to penicillin.

Nocardial and mycobacterial keratitis
See text.

Fungal keratitis (hyphae or yeasts seen on smear or fungus cultured)
Hyphal infection (*Aspergillus* spp., *Fusarium* spp.): Natamycin (5%) or amphotericin (0.15–0.3%).
Yeast infection (*Candida* spp.): clotrimazole (or other imidazole) at 1% in arachis oil eye drops or flucytosine 1% drops

control, but in the acute stages it may interfere with absorption from drop therapy. Systemic antibiotics have no place in the management of bacterial keratitis in the absence of limbal involvement or perforation.

Antibiotics are modified according to the results of cultures and the evaluation of the clinical response to initial therapy. If there is a clear clinical response, the same regime should be continued. Susceptibility tests may be misleading because they are performed on lower tissue antibiotic levels than can be achieved in the cornea during topical therapy. Therapy should be reduced by increasing the interval between drops every 3–4 days, not by reducing their concentration. The decision to terminate therapy is based on clinical response and the nature of the causative organism.

If there is no response, all topical therapy should be stopped in order to allow the drugs and preservatives to leach from the tissues. After 24 or 48 h the clinical condition is reappraised, and the cornea is scraped again. On this occasion a full search must be made for more exotic organisms which may have special culture requirements.

If no organism is identified, a second-line broad-spectrum empirical antibiotic regime should be started to include antimicrobial action against resistant streptococci, nocardia and mycobacteria. This may include drop therapy of topical vancomycin 50 mg/ml (5%) plus amikacin 50 mg/ml (5%)

and trimethoprim 0.1% (given as Polytrim) or ciprofloxacin (or ofloxacin) 3 mg/ml (0.3%). At night, use erythromycin 0.5% ointment or rifampicin 2.5% ointment instead.

Special cases. Treatment of *M. chelonae* infection requires topical amikacin or ciprofloxacin. This mycobacterium, which causes a chronic keratitis and may follow radial keratotomy, is resistant to the common antituberculous drugs.

Treatment of nocardial infection, presenting as a chronic refractory keratitis of several months' duration, is fraught with problems common with the disease at other sites (Godfrey Heathcote et al 1990). It usually requires a combination of surgery, to debulk the infectious load (partial or full keratoplasty), plus antibiotics. Antibiotics often fail on their own, despite apparent full sensitivity in vitro. A combination of topical amikacin (always) plus erythromycin and/or vancomycin and/or trimethoprim has been used successfully. Isolates are resistant to penicillin but may be sensitive to sulphonamides. The new generation of macrolides (azithromycin and clarithromycin) may prove useful in future.

Acanthamoeba infection

In the UK, this infection occurs in 1 in 10 000 contact lens wearers (7 per million population). In India it is much more commonly associated with rural, traumatic eye disease and presentation tends to be late (Sharma et al 1990); the role of co-existing trachoma remains to be elucidated. Early diagnosis greatly improves the outcome. A high index of suspicion must be maintained for all contact-lens-related keratopathies presenting with epithelial disturbances or infiltrations with a 'snowstorm' appearance on slit-lamp microscopy, multiple superficial abscesses or dendritiform ulcers. A keratoneuritis (corneal nerve infiltration) seen on slit-lamp microscopy is diagnostic for the condition. Similarly, persons who have been exposed to hot tubs or hot natural springs and have developed unusual corneal disease may have *Acanthamoeba* keratitis.

It is important to make an early diagnosis when the infection is limited to epithelial or anterior stromal invasion. As well as taking scrapes from the infiltrated epithelium, sheets of cells should be removed for both culture and microscopy. Positive diagnosis of *Acanthamoeba* keratitis can be made in vivo by confocal microscopy.

Wet mounts of epithelial scrapings have been found useful for identifying cysts, and establishing the diagnosis within 10 min of collection by simple light microscopy. A good epithelial scraping is collected by a sterile technique with a disposable sterile scalpel blade which is placed in a conical tube containing 2 ml saline (without potassium hydroxide). The tube is agitated on a vibrator, then centrifuged and the deposit inspected by wet-field microscopy at ×100.

If the diagnosis of *Acanthamoeba* keratitis has been missed and the disease has progressed significantly to the development of a stromal ring abscess, simple scrapes from the surface may not yield viable organisms. Cysts may be found in the midst of the abscess, but it can be difficult to encourage them to excyst and results may be delayed. In practice, time can be saved by proceeding directly to corneal biopsy, aiming to sample the deep infiltrate for viable trophozoites. Both culture and electron microscopy are useful here to demonstrate amoebae in the stromal tissue.

For culture, scrapes should be inoculated directly onto non-nutrient agar, ideally made up in Page's amoebal saline. If non-nutrient agar without Page's saline is used, then the plate should be inoculated again with a turbid suspension (on a swab) of heat-killed *K. aerogenes*, or other coliforms, as a nutrient source for the amoebae. The plate should be incubated at 32°C for 4 weeks; it should not be incubated at higher temperatures. Amoebae will usually, but not always, be visible by low power light microscopy after 1 week; after 2 weeks the whole plate is covered by the typical double-walled, star-shaped cysts. Each point of the star is the ostiole by which the internalized amoeba communicates with the outside world; it is normally plugged with mucopolysaccharide. For drugs to be effective, they have to penetrate the ostioles. Isolates should be sent to a reference laboratory for in vitro drug sensitivity testing. Where facilities for culture are not available, specimens may be mailed to a suitable laboratory.

Treatment. Treatment should start with 0.02% (200 mg/l) chlorhexidine in physiological saline (Hay et al 1994, Seal et al 1995a, Seal et al 1996) and Brolene (propamidine isethionate) 0.1% (1000 mg/l) in physiological saline. (If chlorhexidine is unavailable, polyhexamethylene biguanide (PHMB) (0.02%) can be used instead, but it is not licensed for use as a drug.)

These drugs are given every hour, day and night for the first 3 days, reducing to 2-hourly by day only. This requires the patient's admission to hospital. Adjunctive therapy includes oral flurbiprofen, for both non-steroidal anti-inflammatory and analgesic effects, and topical mydriatic. Thereafter, combination therapy is given 3-hourly by day for 2 months and then 4-hourly by day for 2 months more. Control is rapidly gained but treatment is needed for 2–6 months in some patients, partly because drop therapy is not an ideal vehicle with which to treat this infection.

If diagnosed early, cure is possible, with complete recovery of vision. One week after starting therapy however, there may be a corneal reaction to the lysis of dead amoebae, with localized stromal oedema and anterior chamber activity, which lasts up to 3 weeks (Seal et al 1996). Although this may be suppressed with steroids, their use is not encouraged. Cases presenting late, with considerable pain, ring abscess, inflammation and episcleritis, may need the introduction of steroids. This necessary measure will prolong the treatment period, but without it the patient may find the pain intolerable. Adjunctive immunosuppression has been advocated for the management of acanthamoeba scleritis.

Prevention. Contact-lens storage cases are contaminated with *Acanthamoeba* from the domestic water supply and airborne dust. Prevention involves use of acanthamoebacidal disinfectants in storage and cleaning solutions, of which the best is hydrogen peroxide at 3%; if PHMB is included as the disinfectant, then the minimum concentration for an acanthanmoebacidal effect is 5 mg/l or ppm (0.0005%). Chlorine is ineffective against cysts. Storage cases should never be washed in tap water, but with boiled water only, and they should be stored dry when not in use. This is important because coliform bacteria die quickly in dry conditions, and amoebae cannot then multiply.

ENDOPHTHALMITIS

Endophthalmitis implies infection of the vitreous compartment together with the retinal and uveal coats of the eye. It is most commonly encountered as a complication of intraocular surgery (such as cataract or glaucoma surgery) or following penetrating injury to the eye. In the former case, pathogens harboured in the lids and conjunctival sac may be responsible. For this reason, it is customary to administer prophylactic topical antibiotic preoperatively (e.g. G. chloramphenicol, gentamicin or fusidic acid). Preoperative lid or conjunctival sac culture is not practised because of the day-to-day variation in positive culture results. The formation of thin-walled drainage blebs after glaucoma operations using mitomycin C may predispose to late infections. Less commonly, endophthalmitis may arise endogenously in association with septicaemia (metastatic endophthalmitis).

Causes of acute endophthalmitis include *Str. pyogenes*, *Staph. aureus* and Enterobacteriaceae; when trauma occurs *Bacillus* spp. and clostridia are involved (Seal & Kirkness 1992). Causes of chronic endophthalmitis include CoNS, *Propioni acnes* and, occasionally, streptococci.

Whatever the basis of the infection, endophthalmitis is a potentially blinding disease with irreversible tissue damage occurring within 24–48 h. Early diagnosis and prompt treatment are essential. Bacterial endophthalmitis is treated by a combination of intravitreal and systemic antibiotic therapy. Subconjunctival therapy is a less satisfactory alternative to the intravitreal route. Management should always include a vitreous sample, with smears and cultures to identify the infecting organism and its sensitivities. A simultaneous injection of an antibiotic combination is given intravitreally and repeated at intervals (e.g. 48–72 h) depending on the intravitreal persistence of the drug selected and the clinical response. Intravitreal antibiotic doses are scaled down to avoid retinal toxicity (see Table 55.3).

Additional systemic therapy, which mirrors the intravitreal therapy, will maintain effective intravitreal levels for longer by reducing the diffusion gradient out of the eye. High doses are required and there is a need to be aware of the risks of systemic toxicity. After 24 h, if there is a clear clinical response, prednisolone is added to the systemic regimen to reduce the vitreous inflammatory response and subsequent vitreous organization (oral prednisolone 60 mg daily on a reducing scale). For the same reason, dexamethasone is added to the intravitreal injection. Antibiotic therapy is modified after 24–48 h according to the clinical response and the antibiotic-sensitivity profile of the cultured organism.

ORBITAL CELLULITIS

Orbital cellulitis is an infection of the extraocular orbital contents presenting with pain, proptosis and diplopia due to impaired extraocular muscle function. A few cases follow penetrating injury or are secondary to panophthalmitis, but the majority occur in association with sinusitis (Bergin & Wright 1986). The condition commonly affects children, where spread to the orbit across the thin orbital plate of the ethmoid bone occurs. Retroseptal infection requires multidisciplinary management because of the risk of extension to the eye or cranial cavity. Loculated pus must be drained. Delayed or inadequate treatment may lead to blindness or death.

Preseptal cellulitis may resemble orbital cellulitis when intense lid swelling is present, but the presence of normal ocular movements and absence of globe inflammation in preseptal disease helps to distinguish the two. The diagnosis can be resolved by magnetic resonance imaging (MRI). It is associated with sinusitis, ocular infection and infected wounds.

Parenteral therapy is designed to cover the common causative organisms: *H. influenzae*, *Staph. aureus*, *Str. pneumoniae* and *Str. pyogenes*. *H. influenzae* is the prominent cause of orbital cellulitis in young children and in this age group ampicillin–clavulanic acid (Augmentin) or cefuroxime are the drugs of choice. In view of the emergence of multiply-resistant strains of *H. influenzae*, consideration should be given to the use of a third-generation cephalosporin such as cefotaxime, particularly when the clinical response is poor or resistant organisms are isolated from nasal swabs. In adults, therapy is directed against streptococci and *Staph. aureus* with high-dose intravenous benzylpenicillin and flucloxacillin or, clindamycin or vancomycin, depending on local knowledge and the results of susceptibility tests.

LYME DISEASE (see also Ch. 61)

Although ocular manifestations are a rare feature of this

tick-borne disease, the spirochaete (*Borrelia burgdorferi*) invades the eye early and remains dormant, accounting for both early and late ocular manifestations. A non-specific follicular conjunctivitis occurs in approximately 10% of patients with early Lyme disease, while keratitis often occurs within a few months of onset, characterized by nummular, interstitial opacities. Inflammatory events include orbital myositis, episcleritis, vitritis, uveitis and retinal vasculitis. When serology is negative, a vitreous tap may be required for diagnosis. Neuro-ophthalmic manifestations include bilateral mydriasis, neuroretinitis, pigmentary retinopathy, involvement of multiple cranial nerves, optic atrophy, and disc oedema. Seventh nerve paresis can lead to neurotrophic keratitis. In endemic areas, Lyme disease may be responsible for approximately 25% of new-onset Bell's palsy.

Diagnosis is based on a history of exposure within an endemic area, positive serology and response to treatment (Lesser 1995). Antibodies may be measured by indirect enzyme-linked immunosorbent assay (ELISA) and western blot. Polymerase chain reaction (PCR) has been used successfully for vitreous and cerebrospinal fluid (CSF) (Karma et al 1995). Serum reagin tests are non-reactive in Lyme borreliosis, but false-positive specific tests for syphilis viz. FTA-ABS can occur.

Spirochaetes have been identified in the vitreous of a seronegative patient with vitritis and choroiditis and cultured from an iris biopsy in a treated patient. Therapy with doxycycline or amoxicillin is effective in the earliest stages, but serious late complications require high doses of intravenous penicillin or ceftriaxone.

WHIPPLE'S DISEASE

Whipple's disease is a rare systemic disorder with malaise, fever, migrating arthralgias, fatigue, abdominal discomfort, diarrhoea and weight loss. Ocular signs include uveitis, vitritis and retinal vasculitis. Small bowel biopsy shows characteristic, diastase-resistant, PAS-positive macrophages in the mucosal lamina propria. The aetiological agent has been identified as a Gram-positive actinomycete called *Tropheryma whipplii*. There is some evidence of a predisposing immunodeficiency (Schrenk et al 1994, Cerf et al 1995).

The condition, including its ocular features, may be treated successfully with antibiotics, but relapse is not uncommon and it is important to use antibiotics with good penetration of the blood–brain barrier to minimize central nervous system (CNS) complications. Combination therapy is therefore recommended, e.g. parenteral streptomycin and benzylpenicillin for 2 weeks followed by sulphamethoxazole (800 mg) and trimethoprim (160 mg) (co-trimoxazole) orally twice daily for 1 year.

TOXOPLASMA RETINOCHOROIDITIS (see also Ch. 61)

The intracellular protozoan parasite *Toxoplasma gondii* can enter the fetal retina during intra-uterine life, presenting as retinochoroiditis during the second and third decades, when it is the commonest cause of posterior uveitis. However, 1% of the population per year acquire toxoplasmosis as a primary infection which may be subclinical or cause a syndrome of lymph-node enlargement and fever. There is now evidence from various studies in children and adults that primary toxoplasmic infection can result in acute primary choroiditis more frequently than previously considered.

Small peripheral retinal lesions may be allowed to run their course, but lesions near the macula, optic disc or maculopapular nerve fibre bundle, or those associated with severe vitritis, should be treated. Therapy is directed against both the dividing organism and the inflammatory host response. The problem is complicated by the protozoan multiplying in 'tissue cysts' within cells which are impervious to drug penetration, so that recurrence can always be expected. *Toxoplasma* infection is encountered in immunocompromised patients (Ch. 46).

Treatment

Pyrimethamine and sulphadiazine act synergistically to interfere with folic acid synthesis. They should be commenced early in the course of the disease and continued for 4–6 weeks (Box 55.3). Pyrimethamine therapy should be avoided in early pregnancy and monitored closely due to the risk of bone marrow depression. Folinic acid supplements reduce this risk, but platelet and white cell counts should be performed weekly (Tabbara 1986).

Clindamycin has also been shown effective in the treatment of ocular toxoplasmosis (Lakhampal et al 1983) and has good ocular tissue absorption properties. It does,

---

Box 55.3 *Treatment of* Toxoplasma *retinochoroiditis (Tabbara 1986)*

Regimen	
Pyrimethamine*	100 mg stat then 25 mg/day orally for 4–6 weeks and
Sulphadiazine	2 g stat then 1 g orally four times daily for 4–6 weeks and
Folinic acid	3 mg orally or i.m. twice weekly
Alternative regimen	
Clindamycin†	300 mg orally four times daily for 4–6 weeks and
Sulphadiazine	2 g stat then 1 g orally four times daily for 4–6 weeks

* Pyrimethamine may cause bone marrow depression; leukocyte and platelet counts should be monitored weekly.
† Clindamycin may cause pseudomembranous colitis.

however, carry the risk of pseudomembranous colitis, although this is very small when used in outpatients.

Tetracycline and minocycline may also be effective, but have not yet been fully evaluated in clinical trials.

Oral corticosteroid therapy is indicated in vision-threatening disease, but should not be used without concurrent specific antiprotozoal therapy or in immunocompromised patients.

OCULAR *TOXOCARA* (LARVA MIGRANS) INFECTION

Toxocara canis is a worm whose natural host is the dog. Man is an accidental host, infected by ingesting the ova from dog-contaminated soil, in whom the larval stage develops causing visceral and ocular larva migrans, but adult worms are not found. These larvae migrate around the body and occasionally deposit themselves in the CNS, including the retina. Here, they can present as a possible tumour, for which eyes have been enucleated in the past.

Serological diagnosis only confirms previous exposure. Furthermore, the serological test may be negative when a choroidal lesion is present. Serological diagnosis is thus unreliable and should not be performed. Fine-needle biopsy in a reference centre with cytology for tumour cells and a test system for *toxocara* antigen is the best approach.

If the retinal lesion is peripheral, treatment is conservative or symptomatic, but if it is close to the macula, treatment is warranted. Oral diethylcarbamazine 3 mg/kg is given for 3 weeks. There may be symptoms of allergic reaction to the dying larvae, for which prednisolone is given. When blindness results it is usually unilateral, but bilateral blindness has been recorded.

Albendazole or a single dose of ivermectin are alternative therapies.

OCULAR ONCHOCERCIASIS

Ocular onchocerciasis, or 'river blindness', results from infection with the filarial parasite *Onchocerca volvulus*. The disease is endemic in areas of Africa and Central and South America where it is a major cause of blindness. The ocular manifestations include keratitis, anterior uveitis, glaucoma, chorioretinitis and optic neuritis.

For several decades diethylcarbamazine (DEC) and sumarin have been used systemically in the treatment of ocular onchocerciasis. Both are effective microfilaricidal drugs with a positive effect on keratitis and uveitis; they are, however, less beneficial in posterior segment disease. The use of DEC may be followed by a severe systemic reaction, which is largely prevented by the use of systemic corticosteroids. An appropriate therapeutic regimen has been provided by Taylor & Dax (1986).

Ivermectin (12 mg single dose) has also been shown to slowly eliminate microfilariae from the anterior chamber but with the advantages of producing minimal ocular inflammation and much less systemic reaction (Dadzie et al 1987). This drug represents an important advance in the mass therapy of onchocerciasis in endemic areas. It acts on the adult female worms to inhibit reproduction, and therefore no new microfilariae are produced for several months. It also kills microfilariae in tissue, including skin and the eye. It has to be given yearly so that the eradication programme is a continuous one. Ivermectin should not be given to children under 5 years, pregnant women or patients with other severe infections such as trypanosomiasis.

OCULOMYCOSIS (see also Ch. 60)

Fungal infections of the eye are invariably sight-threatening and include keratomycosis, exogenous or endogenous endophthalmitis and orbital mycosis. Although oculomycosis is rare in the UK, it may account for one third or more of infective corneal ulcers in some rural settings and in developing countries (Thomas 1994).

The fungi responsible for keratomycosis, with the exception of *Candida* spp. (common in the UK), are mainly filamentous. Those most frequently encountered are *Aspergillus*, *Fusarium* and *Curvularia*, but prevalence varies geographically. *Candida* is an important cause of endogenous endophthalmitis occurring preferentially in drug addicts and immunocompromised individuals.

Because of the toxicity of the most effective antifungal agents, the relatively narrow activity spectrum of some and the difficulties of clinical diagnosis, treatment is rarely instituted in the absence of direct evidence of fungal aetiology, based at least on the results of smears. Culture techniques are discussed on page 774. Some filamentous fungi such as *Fusarium* have been detected in the cornea in vivo by confocal microscopy.

Effective therapy requires mycological identification and, preferably, information about drug sensitivity. The number of drugs available for local ocular use is limited, not only by problems of local and systemic toxicity, but also by poor solubility or ocular penetration. Because of the infrequency of oculomycosis, no commercial antifungal preparations are available in the UK for local ocular use; eye drops are usually formulated from parenteral preparations as required.

Available drugs include the polyene antibiotics (amphotericin B, nystatin, natamycin), the cytostatic 5-fluorocytosine (flucytosine (5-FC)), and the imidazoles (clotrimazole, econazole, fluconazole, ketoconazole, itraconazole, miconazole, thiabendazole) (see Box 55.5 and Table 55.3).

Amphotericin B is active against a wide range of fungal organisms causing oculomycosis, including A*spergillus* spp., *Fusarium* spp. and *Candida* spp. It may be given topically as drops (0.05–0.5%), subconjunctivally or intravitreally. It is toxic by any of these routes but the use of topical preparations at concentrations of 0.15% or less will minimize toxicity, which relates in part to the presence of deoxycholate in the parenteral preparation. Amphotericin B is given parenterally by slow intravenous infusion in the management of endophthalmitis, often on a background of more widespread systemic infection, in addition to intravitreal therapy. Renal and haematological status must be kept under surveillance and drug levels monitored (Ch. 10).

Natamycin (Pimaricin) is a tetraene antifungal agent which has been used in the topical treatment of a wide range of fungi causing keratitis, including *Fusarium* spp. A 5% suspension (Natacyn) is available commercially in the USA. It has some topical toxicity.

Imidazoles have also been used effectively in the topical treatment of keratomycosis: clotrimazole, miconazole and econazole are effective against *Candida* spp. and *Aspergillus* spp. but not against the majority of *Fusarium* spp. They can be locally toxic. Ketoconazole is well absorbed after oral administration and is generally well tolerated, although hepatotoxicity is problematical. It has been used effectively in oculomycosis caused by *Fusarium* (Ishibashi 1983), combined with another antifungal agent to prevent the emergence of resistance. *Candida endophthalmitis* can be effectively treated with oral fluconazole combined with intravitreal amphotericin B, but vitrectomy and fluconazole alone have also been reported to be successful. Aqueous levels of fluconazole over 2 h after oral treatment with 200 mg were 2.7–5.4 mg/ml and vitreous levels up to 1.7 mg/ml. Corneal levels were low (0.031 mg/ml).

5-FC is only active against *Candida* spp. It is well absorbed by the oral route and achieves high blood and tissue levels. It has been used effectively in the treatment of *Candida endophthalmitis*, in combination with systemic or intravitreal amphotericin to prevent the otherwise rapid emergence of resistant strains. 5-FC has also been used topically (1% suspension) in the treatment of *Candida albicans* keratomycosis.

Virus infection of the eye

(See also Ch. 40)

Herpes simplex virus (HSV) and adenovirus may account for 1% of all acute conjunctivitis in an ophthalmic casualty department. Antiviral agents are available for the treatment of HSV and herpes zoster virus (HZV) infections, but not for adenovirus infection. A number of other ocular viral infections occur for which there is no specific antiviral therapy but topical antibiotics are often prescribed to reduce the risk of secondary bacterial infection.

HERPES SIMPLEX VIRUS EYE DISEASE

Primary HSV infection of the eye is a self-limiting disease which may be expressed as blepharitis, conjunctivitis or punctate keratitis. It may be followed by zosteriform spread along the axons of the Vth cranial nerve with the establishment of latency in the trigeminal ganglion. This may also follow asymptomatic infections. All subsequent ocular disease results from reactivation of virus, associated with peripheral shedding, and is termed 'recurrent' disease. Recurrent eye disease includes epithelial keratitis (dendritic and geographic ulcers), stromal keratitis (disciform and necrotizing), limbitis, keratouveitis, secondary glaucoma and, rarely, acute retinal necrosis (Holland 1994). Antiviral therapy is effective in the treatment of epithelial keratitis, but its role in the management of other forms of recurrent disease is less clear. No form of therapy affects the incidence of recurrences.

Ocular disease may be caused by HSV type 1 or 2. Type 1 usually produces non-genital infections and is transmitted by direct or indirect non-sexual contact. Type 2 is chiefly transmitted sexually. Consequently, most neonatal eye disease is caused by HSV-2 with transmission during transit through the birth canal. The majority of non-infantile ocular disease is caused by the type 1 virus. Of HSV keratoconjunctivitis, 1% is caused by type 2. Type 1 virus is generally more sensitive to antivirals than type 2 (Rotkis & Chandler 1985) and drug resistance does not appear to be a significant problem. Trifluorothymidine (F3T) may be more effective against type 2 virus which can produce a clinically more severe form of keratouveitis. Not all primary eye disease is followed by recurrent eye disease.

The first-generation antivirals, available for the topical treatment of superficial ocular infection with HSV, were idoxuridine (IDU), adenine arabinoside (ARA-A), and F3T. The latter is available commercially in the USA but not in the UK. However, a 1.0% solution in normal saline can be prepared from the dry powder in many hospital pharmacies. All three agents are extremely effective in blocking herpes virus replication; but, as they are incorporated into DNA of both infected and uninfected cells, they show significant toxicity with prolonged use.

The second-generation antivirals are those which are activated by virus-induced enzymes (e.g. thymidine kinase) and which therefore exert their action chiefly in infected cells. These drugs are more inhibitory to herpetic DNA polymerase than cellular polymerase, and preferentially inhibit viral DNA synthesis. They are less toxic than the first-generation agents and include acyclovir, bromovinyl-deoxyuridine (BVDU) and ethyldeoxyuridine (EDU). The topical regimens advocated for these compounds are listed in Table 55.2. In addition to these agents, human interferon has also been used clinically.

HSV has been found in human corneal stroma and in the aqueous of patients with uveitis, so the penetration of antiviral agents into these regions after topical application is of interest. IDU does not penetrate intact corneal epithelium, and aqueous entry is poor even in the presence of an epithelial defect.

ARA-A is found in the aqueous of an intact eye after frequent topical administration in low concentration; its less active metabolite hypoxanthine arabinoside is also present.

F3T does not penetrate intact epithelium, but effective concentrations may penetrate in the presence of an epithelial lesion. Acyclovir reaches effective aqueous levels in the intact eye after topical use (Poirier 1984) and has therefore been recommended for the treatment of uveitis, limbitis and secondary glaucoma.

Acyclovir is highly effective against the dendritic ulcer, in some studies appearing to be more effective than IDU and in others equally effective as ARA-A (Laibson et al 1982). Since acyclovir is less toxic than any of the first-generation antivirals, it would appear to be the treatment of choice for dendritic ulcer, with F3T and ARA-A as alternatives. BVDU and EDU also appear to be highly effective agents.

Dendritic keratitis may be self-limiting, with about 26% of placebo-treated cases resolving within 2–3 weeks. Antiviral therapy will produce a clinical cure in 76–100% and shorten the median healing time to as little as 3 days.

Simple wiping of infected epithelium from the cornea in dendritic keratitis promotes healing and prognosis is further improved with thermomechanical debridement (Sundmacher 1984), though neither treatment alone is as effective as the combination of debridement and antiviral therapy. Thermo-mechanical debridement in combination with high dose human interferon (HuIFN-β 3–10 × 10^6 units/ml) increases the rate of healing in comparison to a standard F3T regimen, while Sundmacher et al (1984) demonstrated the fastest healing of all using F3T plus HuIFN-β (30 × 10^6 units/ml), with a median healing time of 3 days, and 100% healing by 4 days. Clinical success has also been achieved using recombinant material (r-HuIFN-α_2 arg). Interferon appears to produce little toxicity topically apart from a mild reversible punctate keratitis.

Steroid use predisposes the conversion of untreated dendritic ulcer into the more aggressive, geographic ulcer. F3T is claimed to be the most effective treatment for this form of epithelial keratitis. Acyclovir and ARA-A were found to be equally effective in the study by Collum et al (1985). Where prolonged use occurs, acyclovir would be preferable because of its lower level of toxicity.

Antiviral agents have been used in prophylaxis against epithelial recurrence in two situations. The intensive use of topical corticosteroids in the management of rejection

Table 55.2 *Antiviral drugs for ocular therapy (modified from Pavan-Langston & Greene 1984)*

Drug	Form	Concentration	Frequency	Available in UK
Idoxuridine (IDU)	Ointment Drops	0.5% 0.1%	5 times daily for 14 days 1-hourly by day, 2-hourly by night for 14 days	Yes Yes
Vidarabine (ARA-A)	Ointment i.v.	3.0%	5 times daily for 14 days 1 mg in 2 ml 5% dextrose up to 1 mg/kg per 24 h	Yes Yes
Trifluorothymidine (F3T)	Drops	1.0%	Hourly by day, 2-hourly by night for 14 days	No*
Acyclovir (ACV)	Ointment Tablets i.v.	3.0% 200 mg	5 times daily for 14 days 400–800 mg 4-hourly for 5 days 5 mg/kg over 1 h every 8 h	Yes Yes Yes
Bromovinyldeoxyuridine (BVDU)	Drops Ointment	0.1% 0.5%	1–2-hourly by day 5 times daily for 14 days	No No
Ethyldeoxyuridine (EDU)	Drops Gel		1–2-hourly by day nocte	No No
Penciclovir	Tablet	125/250 mg	8-hourly for 5 days	Yes
Valciclovir	Tablet	125/250 mg	8-hourly for 5 days	Yes

* Not commercially available; can be produced in a hospital pharmacy.

episodes in corneal allografts, performed for herpetic corneal disease, should always be accompanied by antiviral prophylaxis. It was discovered early that the first-generation antivirals, such as IDU, would cause severe epithelial and even stromal toxicity confined to the graft, within weeks of prophylactic antiviral therapy on moderate dosage. Reduced-dose regimens have a better record in this respect (e.g. ARA-A once daily) but a careful watch for epithelial haze, oedema or punctate keratitis must be maintained. It would appear that second generation antivirals (e.g. acyclovir) have a major advantage in this area. The routine use long-term of postoperative antiviral prophylaxis, however, would seem not to be justified in view of the low incidence of spontaneous epithelial recurrence during the first postoperative year and the risks of the long-term exposure of the graft to a toxic agent (Ficker et al 1988).

Prophylactic antivirals are also used in patients receiving topical steroids to suppress the inflammatory features of herpetic keratouveitis. Similar considerations to those in corneal graft prophylaxis apply and risks of antiviral drug toxicity again arise because of the prolonged nature (weeks or months) of the immunosuppressive therapy.

Some experimental and clinical studies have implied that antiviral therapy will suppress stromal keratitis and uveitis. However, such studies are difficult to confirm, in part because the end-point of recovery is less clear than in epithelial disease. Most authors recommend the use of antivirals with good penetration characteristics (e.g. acyclovir) in the management of such disease in view of the presence of virus in these situations. A controlled trial of oral acyclovir in stromal keratitis in patients receiving topical steroids and trifluridine (Barron et al 1994), has shown no beneficial effect for this additional antiviral therapy. Another controlled trial in this group (Wilhelmus et al 1994), showed that topical steroid was significantly better than placebo in reducing persistent or progressive stromal inflammation but had no detrimental effect as assessed by visual outcome at 6 months.

No form of treatment will reduce the frequency of clinical recurrence.

Resistant strains of virus have been identified to IDU, ARA-A and F3T and have been responsible for clinical disease. Culture of HSV with acyclovir has permitted the emergence of acyclovir-resistant TK strains within 10 days, and this has raised some concerns as to the long-term expectation of clinical resistance to acyclovir and related drugs. ARA-A may be effective in the treatment of keratitis resistant to IDU, F3T and acyclovir in disease resistant to ARA-A and IDU and BVDU in cases resistant to IDU, ARA-A and F3T.

Penciclovir (Famvir) has recently been introduced to treat HSV-1 and HSV-2 and HZV; it is converted in vivo to the triphosphate by virus-induced thymidine kinase and has been shown to be active against acyclovir-resistant HSV.

Box 55.4 *Ocular toxicity of first-generation antiviral agents*

Allergic reactions
Contact dermatitis
Punctal stenosis
Epiphora
Meibomian gland change
Lid thickening
Ptosis
Follicular conjunctivitis
Epithelial keratopathy
Graft keratopathy
'Ghost' dendrites
Reduced epithelial healing
Filamentary keratitis
Stromal oedema
Reduced wound strength

Both first- and second-generation antivirals may cause hypersensitivity reactions, such as contact dermatitis (Box 55.4). This is uncommon, however, and there is usually no cross-hypersensitivity, allowing antivirals of either group to be substituted.

Corticosteroids may provoke the appearance of dendritic ulcers in some subjects, convert dendritic ulcers to geographic ulcers and worsen the overall prognosis of HSV keratitis. It has been suggested that the use of cortico-steroids in stromal keratitis may predispose to recurrences and that the use of antivirals alone may be preferable in mild disease (McGill 1987). Corneal perforation due to HSV rarely occurred before the steroid era. For these reasons, the use of steroids in the treatment of herpetic disease is controversial. Their use, however, is indicated in selected cases and always requires ophthalmic supervision. Steroids are capable of suppressing the inflammatory response in disciform and other forms of stromal keratitis and in uveitis, but rebound inflammation may occur on weaning therapy. It is important to give prophylactic antiviral therapy to patients receiving steroids in all but very low dosages due to the risk of activation of epithelial HSV keratitis. Regimens for steroid use are discussed by Cohen & Laibson (1984).

HERPES-ZOSTER VIRUS (HZV) OPHTHALMICUS

Involvement of the first division of the Vth cranial nerve by HZV is associated with a vast array of ocular complications ranging from involvement of the lids in the primary infection, to persistent conjunctivitis, keratouveitis, glaucoma, papillitis, ocular nerve palsy and deep ocular pain. Although the use of topical ocular steroids to suppress the inflammation does not have the dire consequences seen with HSV eye disease (e.g. induction of dendritic or geographic ulceration), studies by McGill & Chapman (1983) suggested that outcome in those treated with acyclovir alone was better than in those receiving steroids alone (acyclovir 3% ointment versus betamethasone 0.1% ointment, five times daily). No recurrence occurred in the acyclovir-treated group, whereas the recurrence rate was 63% in the steroid-only group. Such recurrences were more difficult to suppress than the initial disease features. Corneal epithelial disease healed significantly more quickly in the acyclovir patients. Acyclovir has been used intravenously in doses of 5 mg/kg 8-hourly or greater, and has been shown in some studies to be effective in improving the healing time of the rash and diminishing the pain associated with the early phase of the disease. Placebo-treated patients in a trial of intravenous acyclovir therapy suffered progression until topical acyclovir was started (McGill et al 1983). The studies of Van den Broek et al (1984) using intravenous acyclovir showed an effect on acute pain only.

There have been a number of reports of clinical benefit from oral administration of acyclovir (Cobo et al 1986), given at 600 mg five times daily. It was well tolerated and reduced the incidence and severity of dendritiform keratopathy, stromal keratitis and uveitis. Treatment within 72 h of the onset of skin lesions reduced pain in the acute phase of the disease but not postherpetic neuralgia. Other studies have indicated that doses of 800 mg five times daily are well tolerated and produce higher serum levels (McKendrick et al 1986). Pencyclovir is a new alternative, as discussed above, and is being marketed for its better effect in treating HZV.

ADENOVIRUS KERATOCONJUNCTIVITIS

Adenovirus is a common cause of acute conjunctivitis, presenting either in association with an upper respiratory tract infection, fever and malaise (pharyngoconjunctival fever), or as part of an outbreak of moderate or severe keratoconjunctivitis (epidemic keratoconjunctivitis).

Although antiviral agents, interferon and antibiotics have not been shown to affect the course of adenoviral kerato-conjunctivitis, some amelioration of symptoms has been observed in patients treated with trifluorothymidine.

Topical corticosteroids can suppress the symptoms and signs in adenovirus keratoconjunctivitis, but their use may be followed by a rebound keratitis and they must therefore be used judiciously. The effect of steroid therapy on the duration and outcome of the keratitis, however, has yet to be established.

OTHER VIRAL INFECTIONS

Most cases of measles are associated with conjunctivitis. Keratitis is a major cause of blindness in developing nations where secondary infection and vitamin A deficiency may be compounding factors. Although there is no specific antiviral agent available, topical antibiotics and systemic vitamin A

supplements will help prevent secondary bacterial infection.

Acute haemorrhagic conjunctivitis is usually caused by enterovirus 70 and occurs in epidemics in densely populated tropical and subtropical areas. The condition is self-limiting and without serious sequelae to the eye, although occasionally paralysis at other sites can ensue. Apart from the use of prophylactic antibiotics, management is directed toward curbing transmission of the disease.

ACQUIRED IMMUNE DEFICIENCY SYNDROME

Human immunodeficiency virus (HIV) has been identified in tear fluid, conjunctiva, corneal epithelium and retina, but the principal ophthalmic manifestations of acquired immune deficiency syndrome (AIDS) relate to florid opportunistic infections and to conjunctival and orbital involvement with Kaposi's sarcoma and other neoplasms. Therapy is directed against the relevant organism and is generally more intense and prolonged than is required in immunocompetent individuals (Ch. 46).

Cytomegalovirus (CMV) is the most common of the ocular opportunists and produces a haemorrhagic necrotizing retinitis (Schuman et al 1987).

During the first 7 years after infection, less than 1% of HIV-infected persons present with CMV retinopathy as the initial manifestation of AIDS, but CMV retinitis is found in about 16–19% of terminal AIDS patients and is bilateral in about 17%. The delay from presentation with HIV infection is shorter in bilateral cases. HSV, Epstein–Barr virus (EBV), and toxoplasma, may occasionally cause a clinically similar retinitis.

In a study of CMV retinitis in AIDS patients, 58% presented with unilateral disease and 15% of these developed contralateral infection, despite treatment with ganciclovir. 'Smoldering retinitis' was a clinical sign seen in 33% of the patients whose retinitis progressed while receiving ganciclovir. Response to therapy is partly related to immune status. At presentation, CMV retinitis does not frequently pose an immediate threat to vision, but it may do so with development of retinal detachment, in association with peripapillary disease or by affecting the central retina. Retinal detachment, an important cause of blindness from CMV retinitis, can be treated successfully by vitrectomy, silicone oil, and endolaser.

CMV retinitis occurring in AIDS patients implies a high risk for the development of CMV encephalitis, particularly when the retinitis involves the peripapillary region. On the other hand, in patients with AIDS without CMV retinitis, CNS symptoms are unlikely to be attributable to CMV encephalitis (Bylsma et al 1995).

Therapy. Progression of CMV retinitis may be delayed in the short-term by intravenous therapy with either ganciclovir or foscarnet. Repeated, local intravitreal therapy is more effective, and particularly valuable when there are no signs of disseminated CMV disease. The development of slow-release, intraocular implant systems promises to provide further improvements in management.

Dihydroxypropoxymethylguanine (DHPG; ganciclovir) (Ch. 40), a virostatic drug similar in structure to acyclovir, and trisodium phosphonoformate (foscarnet), improve or temporarily stabilize the retinitis in the majority of patients receiving long-term maintenance therapy (Orellana et al 1987, Le Huang et al 1989). Ganciclovir and foscarnet are equally effective in controlling CMV retinitis, but foscarnet is less well tolerated. Repeated therapy is indicated because of the high relapse rate. Ganciclovir is given by intravenous infusion over 1 h in a dose of 5 mg/kg every 12 h.

In a randomized trial of CMV retinitis therapy in AIDS, patients were either immediately treated with intravenous ganciclovir (5 mg/kg twice daily for 14 days and then once daily for 14 weeks), or treatment was deferred. Deferred patients whose retinitis progressed were offered ganciclovir. The median time to progression in the deferred treatment group was 13.5 days compared with 49.5 days in the immediate treatment group (Spector et al 1993). Intravenous administration of ganciclovir results in intravitreal concentrations which are subtherapeutic (0.93 ± 0.39 mg/ml) for many CMV isolates, which explains the difficulty of long-term complete suppression of CMV retinitis by this route.

Combined daily therapy with ganciclovir and foscarnet has recently been shown to be beneficial (Weinberg et al 1994), with prolonged intervals between progression without increased toxicity. Such therapy may halt the progress of peripheral outer retinal necrosis in AIDS patients.

Improved results have been achieved with cidofovir (CDV–HPMPC) treatment with 5 mg/kg once weekly for 2 weeks, then 5 mg/kg every other week, which delayed the progression of retinitis in AIDS patients compared to delayed therapy. Proteinuria (23%) and neutropenia (15%) are possibly related to therapy and may lead to discontinuation of the drug.

Intraocular delivery. Intravitreal injection of antiviral agents is an effective treatment of CMV retinitis, which avoids the risk of systemic toxicity. Intravitreal ganciclovir or foscarnet have been given on a weekly basis with little local ocular complication. An intravitreal dose of ganciclovir (200–400 µg) is as effective as intravenous therapy; a dose of 2 mg in 0.05–0.1 ml probably provides adequate intravitreal levels (0.25–1.22 µg/l) for up to 7 days. Levels at 24 h have been recorded as 143.4 µg/l and at 72 h as 23.4 µg/ l. The intravitreal dose of foscarnet is 2.4 mg in 0.1 ml. A lower dose of these agents has been given in patients whose eyes contain silicone oil in relation to retinal surgery.

Intravitreal cidofovir together with oral probenecid, has also been effective in halting progression of CMV retinitis.

More recently, the development of intraocular sustained-release devices have provided the opportunity to deliver controlled amounts of drugs for prolonged periods with minimum local toxicity.

Toxoplasmosis

Ocular involvement by toxoplasmosis is less common than CNS involvement. It may cause the presenting symptom, with blurred vision and floaters or pronounced visual loss from macular, papillomacular bundle or optic nerve head involvement (Holland et al 1988).

The retinochoroiditis is unassociated with a pre-existing retinochoroidal scar, suggesting that the lesions are a manifestation of acquired rather than congenital disease.

Lesions may be single or multifocal, in one or both eyes, or consist of massive areas of retinal necrosis. They may resemble those of CMV retinitis and may occur concurrently in the same eye. In comparison, toxoplasmic lesions tend to be thick and opaque, with smooth borders and a relative lack of haemorrhage.

Treatment of the toxoplasmic ocular infection with pyrimethamine, clindamycin and sulfadiazine is effective in over 75% of patients. Once resolution is observed, maintenance therapy is continued, as relapses occur in the absence of treatment. Corticosteroid treatment is unnecessary and its use has been associated with the development of CMV retinitis.

Pneum. carinii can cause a choroidopathy in patients with systemic spread from primary lung infections. Multiple yellow placoid fundus lesions are seen (Freeman et al 1989).

Candida albicans and *Cryptococcus neoformans* can also produce retinal lesions or endophthalmitis, particularly in AIDS patients who are intravenous drug users. A bilateral epithelial keratopathy caused by Encephalitozoon, has been described in an HIV-positive patient with cryptococcal meningitis, which responded to itraconazole given for the meningitis.

HZV ophthalmicus occurs in a more severe and chronic form in AIDS and may require prolonged systemic penciclovir therapy.

Microsporidial keratoconjunctivitis in a patient with AIDS responded to treatment with dibromopropamidine isethionate ointment.

Prophylaxis against post-operative infection

Postoperative infection is the most common form of exogenous bacterial endophthalmitis. Sources of organisms include the surgeon (hands, gloves, nose, technique), contaminated instruments, implants, drugs, irrigations and infusions, and also environmental and patient sources. Endophthalmitis also occurs after intravenous infusions and blood transfusion.

The bacterial flora indigenous to the conjunctival sac and eyelids are probably important. The lid margins exhibit transient pathogens delivered to them by the hands; and pathogenic organisms may populate the lash follicles.

The lid margins may also be colonized with *Staph. aureus*, especially in atopes. Although similar cultures may be obtained from the two eyes, cultural findings from normal lids vary over a 24–48 h period. For this reason, it is no longer customary to perform preoperative cultures, even before intraocular surgery, and reliance is usually placed on 24 h of antibiotic prophylaxis, preoperative antiseptic preparation and aseptic technique.

Topical antibiotic drops given one day preoperatively are effective in reducing the bacterial flora of the eye. Various preparations are commercially available; gentamicin sulphate (0.3%) decreases both lid and conjunctival staphylococcal cultures but is ineffective against streptococci and *Propionibacterium acnes*. Broad-spectrum cover is advisable, but chloramphenicol should be used with caution because of its known toxicity for bone marrow – its advantage is penetration of the surface epithelium.

Apt et al (1985) showed that saline irrigation of the conjunctival sac increased the variety of flora present on culture of the conjunctiva, whereas application of two drops of povidone iodine 5% in balanced salt solution reduced both the number and variety of organisms present; this latter preparation is still in favour and should be instilled into the conjunctival sac for at least 5 min before surgery.

CATARACT SURGERY

The expected rate of endophthalmitis following modern cataract surgery with lens implantation is in the region of 0.1 to 0.7%. While this rate is low, the risk of blindness in the affected eye presents a challenge to reduce the infection rate further.

Surgical technique reflects the skill of the operator. In cataract surgery, some bacteria (predominantly CoNS or *P. acnes*) will enter the wound or gain access during irrigation. To combat this, some surgeons add an antibiotic, such as gentamicin 5 mg/l or vancomycin, to the irrigant fluid, but endophthalmitis may still occur despite such measures. Contamination also occurs when the sterile intra-ocular lens is opened and held in the air around the eye before placement. This could be reduced by carrying out surgery in ultraclean air conditions. In addition, if the intra-ocular lens (IOL) touches the conjunctival surface it can become contaminated with CoNS or *P. acnes*, because the conjunctival surface is not sterile, even after prophylactic antibiotics and antiseptics. Repeated entry of the anterior

chamber by instruments carries the same risk. A study of DNA typing by restriction fragment length polymorphism between postoperative CoNS cultures from lids and those causing endophthalmitis has shown similarity in 85% of cases (Speaker et al 1991), suggesting that most patients become infected by their own bacterial flora.

Careful closure of the wound is important. Loose sutures carry bacteria and may cause a stitch abscess directly or on suture removal. This is often due to *Staph. aureus*, which may arise from contamination with lid flora, particularly in atopes of whom 70% have lid colonization with *Staph. aureus*. This can be a particular problem in diabetics or those with rheumatoid arthritis, both of whom are particularly susceptible to *Staph. aureus* infection. The infection can progress from a stitch abscess to a sclerokeratitis, which may be refractory to the usual combination of topical gentamicin forte and cefuroxime and require debridement and a lamellar keratectomy.

Fungi (*Candida* spp. and *Aspergillus* spp.) may cause endophthalmitis following cataract surgery, the source being lid and, rarely, aerial contamination with spores. Studies have shown that 4% of blepharitic lids are contaminated with *Aspergillus* spores, possibly because the inflamed surface is 'sticky'.

Subconjunctival antibiotics are routinely given in relation to surgery. There is debate whether to give them immediately prior to surgery, at the onset of anaesthesia (as currently practised in other surgical disciplines), during surgery or immediately after surgery. The most established practice is to give one subconjunctival injection of cefuroxime 125 mg, or gentamicin 20 mg, at the end of surgery, and this practice is encouraged. It will provide good antibiotic prophylaxis against *Staph. aureus*, *Str. pyogenes*, CoNS and *P. acnes*. Gentamicin as an alternative gives poor streptococcal coverage and has no effect on *P. acnes*. If intra-operative prophylaxis is favoured, then adding cefuroxime or gentamicin to the irrigation fluid is practical, but antibiotic irrigation fluids have only a small effect on bacterial numbers in the limited period of exposure. Vancomycin should be reserved for therapy and *not* used for prophylaxis.

Many surgeons favour giving topical antibiotic drops for one week after cataract surgery to prevent postoperative infection; chloramphenicol is often used, but the cautions noted above should be observed (Kirkness et al 1995).

REMOVAL OF AN INTRAOCULAR FOREIGN BODY

Intraocular penetration of a projectile into the posterior segment of the eye is a medical emergency, especially when involving metal splinters arising from hammering farmyard equipment, dirty or soil-contaminated items and machinery. A review of 20 years experience found that 8% of patients developed endophthalmitis, of whom half lost all light perception (Seal & Kirkness 1992). While Brinton et al (1984) advocated antibiotic prophylaxis for intraocular foreign body (IOFB) removal, this is not universally practised. We consider that all patients with an IOFB require antibiotic prophylaxis.

Bacillus spp. are the most virulent pathogens carried by an IOFB, and infection usually results in visual loss. *Staph. aureus*, coliforms, streptococci and, occasionally, *Clostridium perfringens*, are equally likely to cause sight-threatening endophthalmitis. Because magnet removal is crude, a track of necrotic tissue is left behind which is seeded with bacteria. For this reason antibiotic prophylaxis should be used for all IOFB removals. The following regimen is suggested:

- Intravitreal gentamicin 200 μg + vancomycin 1000 μg (or clindamycin 600 μg)
- Subconjunctival gentamicin 40 mg + clindamycin 34 mg
- Topical gentamicin (forte) 15 mg/ml + clindamycin 20 mg/ml
- Intravenous therapy – give adequate dosage for weight, with similar antibiotics injected intravitreally.

MANAGEMENT OF SURGERY IN ATOPY

The atopic individual has a special relationship with *Staph. aureus*, which colonizes the skin, including that of the eyelids and nasal mucosa to a high degree (Tuft et al 1992). *Staph. aureus* also colonizes, and may infect, eczematous skin. Care is therefore needed when planning surgery, particularly if the patient has an associated blepharitis. The following regimen is suggested, in addition to others given above.

- Whole-body bathing, including shampooing hair, with chlorhexidine 4% impregnated soap (Hibiscrub) for 72 h prior to surgery
- Topical antistaphylococcal prophylaxis for 72 h prior to surgery with fusidic acid (Fucithalmic)
- Povidone iodine 5% in balanced salt solution to the conjunctivae for 8 min before operating
- Postoperative fusidic acid 750 mg three times a day (enteric coated capsules) or trimethoprim for 5 days (together with subconjunctival cefuroxime 125 mg immediately postoperatively as listed above, if having cataract surgery).

Modes of delivery of antibiotics

Many modes of delivery discussed here are outside the specifications of the product licence for the agent and are therefore used at the clinician's responsibility.

TOPICAL PREPARATIONS

Drops and ointments are the standard means of administering antibiotics to the surface of the eye, either for prophylaxis or treatment (Boxes 55.5 and 55.6). Ointments prolong contact time and therefore permit less frequent

Box 55.5 *Selected topical antimicrobial drops: commercially available and fortified extemporaneous preparations*

Antibacterial eye drops	Fortified*	Commercial preparation
Amikacin	25/50 mg/ml	
Bacitracin	10 000 U/ml	Not in UK
Cefazolin	50 mg/ml	
Ceftazidime	50 mg/ml	
Cefuroxime	50 mg/ml	
Cephalothin	50 mg/ml	
Chloramphenicol[†]		5 mg/ml
Ciprofloxacin		3 mg/ml
Gentamicin	15 mg/ml	3 mg/ml
Framycetin		5 mg/ml
Fusidic acid		10 mg/ml, gel basis (Fucithalmic)
Neomycin		5 mg/ml
Ofloxacin		3 mg/ml
Oxacillin	66 mg/ml	
Penicillin G	5000 U/ml (0.3%)	
Piperacillin	50 mg/ml	
Propamidine isethionate		1 mg/ml
Sulphacetamide		100–300 mg/ml
Tetracycline		10 mg/ml, oil vehicle
Ticarcillin	50 mg/ml	
Tobramycin	15 mg/ml	3 mg/ml
Teicoplanin	25 mg/ml	
Vancomycin	50 mg/ml	

Combinations

Neosporin +		
Polymyxin B		5000 U/ml
Gramicidin		25 U/ml
Neomycin		2.5 mg/ml
Polytrim +		
Polymyxin B		10 000 U/ml
Trimethoprim		1 mg/ml

Antifungal eye drops

Amphotericin[‡]	1.5–3.0 mg/ml
Clotrimazole	1% in arachis oil
Econazole	1% in arachis oil
Fluconazole	1% in arachis oil
Flucytosine	1%
Itraconazole	1% in arachis oil
Miconazole	1% in arachis oil
Natamycin[‡]	50 mg/ml

Antiprotozoal eye drops[§]

Propamidine isethionate (Brolene)	0.1% (1 mg/ml)
Chlorhexidine digluconate	0.02% (200 mg/l)

* Produced in hospital pharmacy.
† Use with caution because of known risk of bone marrow aplasia and *never* prescribe for more than 8 weeks (Kirkness et al 1995).
‡ Aqueous suspension.
§ For the treatment of *Acanthamoeba* keratitis (Hay et al 1994, Seal et al 1995a).

Box 55.6 *Antimicrobial   eye   ointments   (commercial preparations)*

Antibacterial eye ointments
Chloramphenicol*	1%
Chlortetracycline	1%
Erythromycin	0.5% (not commercially available)
Framycetin	0.5%
Gentamicin	0.3%
Neomycin	0.5%
Rifampicin	2.5% (not commercially available)
Sulphacetamide	2.5–10%
Tetracycline	1%

Antibacterial ointment combinations
Graneodin +	
Neomycin	0.25%
Gramicidin	0.025%
Polyfax +	
Bacitracin	500 U/g
Polymyxin B	10 000 U/g
Polytrim +	
Trimethoprim	0.5%
Polymyxin B	10 000 U/g

Antiamoebal eye ointment
Nystatin	3.3% (not commercially available)

Antiprotozoal eye ointment
Dibromopropamidine	0.15%
(Brolene)	

* Use with caution because of known risk of bone marrow aplasia and *never* prescribe for more than 8 weeks.

instillation and are less likely to be washed out of the eye. In recent years, the preparation of fortified antibiotic eye drops has been advocated for the successful treatment of suppurative keratitis. Fortified drops are prepared by combining commercially available parenteral preparations with artificial tear preparations or sterile water to widen the range and concentration of agents used.

To achieve high levels of chemotherapeutic agents in the posterior segment of the eye, local delivery of antibiotic by periocular or intravitreal injection is employed. Recently, iontophoresis has been re-explored as a means of driving ionized agents into the posterior segment in high concentration, but has not yet gained general use in practice. Systemic administration of a drug achieves far lower levels in the tissues of the globe than these techniques, but is used as an adjunct to other routes in the treatment of endophthalmitis. It is effective alone in the treatment of adnexal disease. Some of these techniques are considered in more detail below.

PERIOCULAR INJECTION

Subconjunctival delivery involves the injection of 0.25–1.0 ml of antibiotic solution deep to the conjunctiva. There is some leakage of antibiotic back into the conjunctival sac, but the bolus chiefly acts as a depot for diffusion which will produce transient high levels of antibiotic in cornea, sclera, choroid and aqueous and, to a lesser and variable extent, the vitreous. Vitreous levels are lower because of the absorption of drug into the choroidal and retinal circulations, and because of the natural barriers to penetration into the vitreous across the retina (see above). Appropriate doses for subconjunctival injection are given in Table 55.3.

Table 55.3 *Selected intravitreal and periocular antibiotics*

Agent	Intravitreal injection*		Periocular injection, dose (mg)	Intravenous injection, dose
	Dose (µg)	Effective duration (h)		
Amikacin	400	24–48		15 mg/kg every 24 h[†]
Ampicillin	500	24	100–125	1 g 4-hourly
Amphotericin	5–10	24–48	Not used	0.1–1.0 mg/kg every 24 h[†]
Carbenicillin	2000	16–24	100	3 g 4-hourly
Cefazolin	2000	16	100	1 g 4-hourly
Cefuroxime	2000		125	1.5 g 6-hourly
Chloramphenicol[†]			24	0.75 g 6-hourly
Clindamycin	1000	16–24	150	0.75 g 8-hourly
Erythromycin	500	24	50	0.5 g 6-hourly
Flucloxacillin			100	1 g 6-hourly
Gentamicin	100–200	48	72–96	5 mg/kg every 24 h[†]
Methicillin	2000	40	100	1 g 4-hourly
Oxacillin	500	24	100	2 g 4-hourly
Penicillin			300–600	3 MU 4-hourly
Vancomycin	1000	72	25	1 g 12-hourly

* Maximum intravitreal injection volume is usually 0.2 ml, i.e. 0.1 ml of each agent used in combination.
† Chloramphenicol given systemically penetrates to the vitreous to treat acute bacterial endophthalmitis satisfactorily providing the organism is sensitive to it; it should be reserved for therapy when intravitreal antibiotics cannot be given, but must be used within 48 h of the start of endophthalmitis if useful vision is to be saved.
‡ Administered in three divided doses.

Peak aqueous levels are achieved in the first hour and effective levels are maintained for about 6 h. Inclusion of adrenaline in the subconjunctival injection prolongs antibiotic activity for 24 h or more, so that injections may be repeated less frequently. This is contraindicated in patients with cardiac disease, and caution must be exercised in the aged, or when patients are receiving general anaesthesia with halothane. Where possible, the injection is delivered close to the site of infection, since tissue levels are highest near the site of the injection.

A sub-Tenon's injection is delivered in a similar volume but more deeply into the orbit, beneath Tenon's capsule and close to the sclera. Care must be taken to avoid penetration of the globe. It is said to achieve higher levels in the posterior eye than the more anterior subconjunctival route.

Ofloxacin and ciprofloxacin have not yet been used routinely by the intravitreal route to treat endophthalmitis, although ciprofloxacin has been shown to be relatively non-toxic intravitreally in rabbits and to be removed by the active transport route similarly to cephalosporins. Recent studies by other routes (von Gunten et al 1994, El Baba et al 1994) have shown that insufficient intravitreal levels are achieved to treat serious infective endophthalmitis.

Periocular injections require local anaesthesia, and are not without complications. Conjunctival ischaemia and necrosis may occur locally and orbital haemorrhage and penetration of the globe have been reported. Although high aqueous levels can be achieved, they are not sustained, and the use of frequent topical application of fortified antibiotic preparations is generally preferred to repeated periocular injections in the treatment of microbial keratitis.

ANTERIOR CHAMBER AND INTRAVITREAL INJECTION

Lavage of the anterior chamber with antibiotic solutions has been employed in the past in the treatment of serious ocular infections, but has limited value since aqueous levels will quickly be reduced by diffusion and by bulk removal of aqueous from the anterior chamber as part of its normal circulation.

Intravitreal injection of antibiotic has a much more important role to play in the treatment of endophthalmitis. Antibiotic may persist in the vitreous space in effective concentrations for up to 96 h. Only a small volume is injected (up to 0.2 ml). To avoid excessive elevation of ocular pressure an equal volume of vitreous fluid is removed prior to injection. Amounts injected are based on studies of toxicity in animals (including primates), since the retina is very sensitive in this respect.

The technique involves entering the vitreous via the pars plana to avoid retinal injury. This approach is also used to collect a vitreous sample and may be combined with a total vitrectomy to reduce the infective load and facilitate diffusion of injected drugs. The intravitreal injection is given through the same entry site and can be repeated at intervals depending on the drug(s) selected.

Antibiotic injected into the vitreous is removed by the anterior and posterior routes. The anterior route involves diffusion into the posterior chamber and removal by bulk flow in the aqueous humour and (for anionic drugs) by transport across the pigment epithelium of the iris and into the circulation. The posterior route involves diffusion across the retina, and (for anionic drugs) active transport by the retinal vessels or retinal pigment epithelium.

For these reasons, cationic drugs such as gentamicin have longer half-lives in the vitreous than anionic drugs such as penicillin, which are actively transported out of the vitreous space. This effect persists, though in lesser degree, in the inflamed eye. Persistence of drug in the vitreous can be prolonged if the same drug is given systemically at the same time, since the outward diffusion gradient is decreased. In the case of certain anionic drugs, such as the penicillins, cephalosporins and ciprofloxacin, levels can be further increased by systemic administration of probenecid. This raises plasma levels by inhibiting renal tubular excretion, and will also block active transport of antibiotic out of the eye.

THE SYSTEMIC ROUTE

Systemic medication may be used to treat preseptal and orbital cellulitis, dacryoadenitis, acute dacryocystitis and the rare condition of ocular erysipelas (necrotizing fasciitis of the eyelids, which may need surgical debridement). In the management of chronic blepharitis, tetracyclines used in low dose (e.g. oxytetracycline 250 mg twice daily) may act by an effect on meibomian oil composition through inhibition of bacterial lipase (Dougherty et al 1991). In rosacea-associated blepharitis, oral tetracycline 250 mg twice daily or doxycycline 100 mg once daily, will be effective in 50% of patients (Seal et al 1995b).

Systemic medication may be combined with local therapy in the treatment of ophthalmia neonatorum due to *Gonococcus, Chlamydia* or, rarely, *Pseudomonas* spp. It will also be used in the treatment of adult patients with chlamydial or gonococcal eye disease.

Systemic chemotherapy has no place in the management of uncomplicated bacterial keratitis. It is usually employed in high dosage in the treatment of bacterial endophthalmitis or CMV retinitis and is mandatory in the management of metastatic endophthalmitis associated with septicaemia when the systemic disease must also be treated. Because of the risks of systemic toxicity, high-dose regimens should be closely monitored.

References

Apt L, Isenberg S, Yoshimori R 1985 Antimicrobial preparation of the eye for surgery. *Journal of Hospital Infection* 6 (suppl A): 163–172

Barron B A, Gee L, Hauck W W et al 1994 Herpetic eye disease study – a controlled study of oral acyclovir for Herpes simplex stromal keratitis. *Ophthalmology* 101: 1871–1882

Bartholomew R S, Reid B J, Chessborough M J, Macdonald M, Galloway N R 1982 Oxytetracycline in the treatment of ocular rosacea: a double-blind trial. *British Journal of Ophthalmology* 66: 386–388

Bergin D J, Wright J E 1986 Orbital cellulitis. *British Journal of Ophthalmology* 70: 174–178

Brinton G S, Topping T M, Hyndiuk R A 1984 Post-traumatic endophthalmitis. *Archives of Ophthalmology* 102: 547–550

Bylsma S S, Achim C L, Wiley C A et al 1995 The predictive value of cytomegalovirus retinitis for cytomegalovirus encephalitis in acquired immunodeficiency syndrome. *Archives of Ophthalmology* 113: 89–95

Cerf M, Marche C, Ciribilli J M 1995 Whipple's disease: a single or multiple origin. *Presse Medicale* 24: 119–128

Cobo L M, Foulks G N, Liesegang T et al 1986 Oral acyclovir in the treatment of acute herpes zoster ophthalmicus. *Ophthalmology* 93 (6): 763–770

Cohen E J, Laibson P R 1984 The use of corticosteroids in herpes simplex keratitis. In: Blodi F C (ed) Herpes simplex infections of the eye. Churchill Livingstone, New York, p 109–116

Collum L M T, Logan P, McAutiffe-Curtin D, Hung S O, Patterson A , Rees P J 1985 Randomised double-blind trial of acyclovir (Zovirax) and adenine arabinoside in herpes simplex amoeboid corneal ulceration. *British Journal of Ophthalmology* 69: 847–850

Dadzie K Y, Bird A C, Awadzi K, Schulz-Key H, Gilles H M, Aziz M A 1987 Ocular findings in a double-blind study of ivermectin versus diethylcarbamazine versus placebo in the treatment of onchocerciasis. *British Journal of Ophthalmology* 71: 78–85

Dart J, Stapleton F, Minassian D 1991 Contact lenses and other risk factors in microbial keratitis. *Lancet* 338: 650–653

Donzis P B, Mondino B J, Weissman B A et al 1987 Microbial contamination of contact lens care systems. *American Journal of Ophthalmology* 104: 325–333

Dougherty J M, McCulley J P, Silvany M E, Meyer D R 1991 The role of tetracycline in chronic blepharitis. *Investigative Ophthalmology and Vision Science* 32: 2970–2975

El Baba F, Trousdale M, Gauderman J et al 1992 Intravitreal penetration of oral ciprofloxacin in humans. *Ophthalmology* 99: 483–486

Erie J C, Nevitt M P, Hodge D O, Ballard D J 1993 Incidence of ulcerative keratitis in a defined population from 1950 to 1988. *Archives of Ophthalmology* 111: 1665–1671

Elkins B S, Holland G N, Opremcak E M et al 1994 Ocular toxoplasmosis misdiagnosed as cytomegalovirus retinopathy in immunocompromised patients. *Ophthalmology* 101 (3): 499–507

Ficker L A, Kirkness C M, Rice N S C, Steele A D McG 1988 Longterm prognosis for corneal grafting in herpes simplex keratitis. *Eye* 2: 400–408

Ficker L, Kirkness C M, McCartney A, Seal D V 1991a Microbial keratitis – the false negative. *Eye* 5: 549–559

Ficker L, Ramakrishnan M, Seal D V, Wright P 1991b Role of cell-mediated immunity to staphylococci in blepharitis. *American Journal of Ophthalmology* 111: 473–479

Ficker L, Seal D V, Wright P 1996 Staphylococcal blepharitis. In: Wilhelmus K, Pepose G, Holland G (eds) Ocular infection and immunity. Mosby, Chicago, ch 61

Freeman W R, Gross J G, Labelle J et al 1989 Pneumocystis carinii choroidopathy. A new clinical entity. *Archives of Ophthalmology* 107: 863–867

Godfrey Heathcote J, McCartney A, Rice N, Peacock J, Seal D V 1990 Endophthalmitis caused by exogenous nocardial infection in a patient with Sjögren's syndrome. *Canadian Journal of Ophthalmology* 25: 29–33

Hay J, Kirkness C M, Seal D V, Wright P 1994 Drug resistance and *Acanthamoeba* keratitis: the quest for alternative antiprotozoal chemotherapy. *Eye* 8: 555–563

Holland G 1994 Standard diagnostic criteria for the acute retinal necrosis syndrome. *American Journal of Ophthalmology* 117: 663–666

Holland G N, Rao N A, Sidikaro Y et al 1988 Ocular toxoplasmosis in patients with the acquired immunodeficiency syndrome. *American Journal of Ophthalmology* 106: 653–667

Ishibashi Y 1983 Oral ketoconazole therapy for keratomycosis. *American Journal of Ophthalmology* 95 (3): 342–345

Karma A, Seppala I, Mikkila H, Kaakkola S, Viljanen M, Tarkkanen A 1995 Diagnosis and clinical characteristics of ocular Lyme borreliosis. *American Journal of Ophthalmology* 119 (2): 127–135

Kirkness C M, Seal D V, Hay J 1995 Topical chloramphenicol: use or abuse. *Eye* 9: vii–viii

Laibson P R, Pavan-Langston D, Yeakley W R, Lass J 1982 Acyclovir and vidarabine for the treatment of herpes simplex keratitis. *American Journal of Medicine* 73 (1A): 281–285

Lakhampal V, Schocket S S, Nirankari V S 1983 Clindamycin in the treatment of toxoplasmic chorioretinitis. *American Journal of Ophthalmology* 95: 605–613

Le Huang P, Girard B, Robinet M et al 1989 Foscarnet in the treatment of cytomegalovirus in the acquired immune deficiency syndrome. *Ophthalmology* 96: 865–874

Lesser R L 1995 Ocular manifestations of Lyme disease. *American Journal of Medicine* 98 (4A): 60S–62S

Mathers W D, Shields W J, Sachdev M S, Petroll W M, Jester J V 1991 Meibomian gland dysfunction in chronic blepharitis. *Cornea* 10 (4): 277–285

McCulley J P, Dougherty J M, Deneau D G 1982 Classification of chronic blepharitis. *Ophthalmology* 89: 1173–1179

McGill J 1987 The enigma of herpes stromal disease. *British Journal of Ophthalmology* 71 (2): 118–125

McGill J, Chapman C 1983 A comparison of topical acyclovir with steroids in the treatment of herpes zoster kerato-uveitis. *British Journal of Ophthalmology* 67 (11): 746–750

McGill J, MacDonald D R, Fall C, McKendrick G D 1983 Intravenous acyclovir in acute herpes zoster infection. *Journal of Infection* 6 (2): 157–161

McKendrick M W, McGill J I, White J E, Wood M J 1986 Oral acyclovir in acute herpes zoster. *British Medical Journal* 293: 1529–1532

Mondino B J, Caster A I, Dethlefs B 1987 A rabbit model of staphylococcal blepharitis. *Archives of Ophthalmology* 105: 409–412

Orellana J, Teich S A, Friedman A H, Lerebours F, Winterkorn J, Mildvan D 1987 Combined short- and long-term therapy for the treatment of cytomegalovirus retinitis using ganciclovir (BWB759U). *Ophthalmology* 94 (7): 831–838

Pavan-Langston D, Greene B 1984 Antiviral therapy of herpes simplex virus ocular disease. In: Blodi F C (ed) Herpes simplex infections of the eye. Churchill Livingstone, New York, p 91–99

Poggio E C, Glynn R J, Schein O D et al 1989 The incidence of ulcerative keratitis among users of daily wear and extended wear soft contact lenses. *New England Journal of Medicine* 321: 779–783

Poirier R H 1984 Intraocular penetration of vidarabine monophosphate, trifluridine, and acyclovir. In: Blodi F C (ed) Herpes simplex infections of the eye. Churchill Livingstone, New York, p 101–108

Ridgway G L 1986 A fresh look at ophthalmia neonatorum. *Transactions of the Ophthalmological Society of the UK* 105: 41–42

Rotkis W M, Chandler J W 1985 Antiviral agents. In: Easty D I,

Smolin G (eds) External eye disease. Butterworths, London, p 154–185

Sandstrom K I, Bell T A, Chandler J W et al 1984 Microbiological causes of neonatal conjunctivitis. *Journal of Pediatrics* 105: 706–711

Schein O D, Glynn A G, Poggio E C et al 1989 The relative risk of ulcerative keratitis among users of daily-wear and extended-wear soft contact lenses. *New England Journal of Medicine* 321: 773–778

Schrenk M, Metz K, Heiligenhaus A, Layer P, Bornfleld N, Wessing A 1994 Ocular involvement in Whipple's disease. *Klinische Monatsblatter fur Augenheilkunde* 204 (6): 538–541

Schuman J S, Orellana J, Friedman A H, Teich S A 1987 Acquired immunodeficiency syndrome (AIDS). *Survey of Ophthalmology* 31 (6): 384–410

Seal D V, Kirkness C M 1992 Criteria for intravitreal antibiotics during surgical removal of intraocular foreign bodies. *Eye* 6: 465–468

Seal D V, Hay J, Kirkness C M 1995a Chlorhexidine or polyhexamethylene biguanide for *Acanthamoeba* keratitis. *Lancet* 345: 136

Seal D V, Hay J, Kirkness C M et al 1996 Successful medical therapy of *Acanthamoeba* keratitis with chlorhexidine and propamidine. *Eye* 10 (4): in press

Seal D V, Wright P, Ficker L, Hagan K, Troski M, Menday P 1995b Placebo controlled trial of fusidic acid gel and oxytetracycline for recurrent blepharitis and rosacea. *British Journal of Ophthalmology* 79: 42–45

Seal D V, Stapleton F, Dart J 1992 Possible environmental sources of *Acanthamoeba* sp. in contact lens wearers. *British Journal of Ophthalmology* 76: 424–427

Sharma S, Srinivasan M, George C 1990 Diagnosis of *Acanthamoeba* keratitis. *Indian Journal of Ophthalmology* 38: 50–56

Speaker M G, Milch F A, Shah M K, Eisner W, Kreiswirth B N 1991 Role of external bacterial flora in the pathogenesis of acute postoperative endophthalmitis. *Ophthalmology* 98: 639–649

Spector S A, Weingeist T, Pollard R B et al 1993 A randomized, controlled study of intravenous ganciclovir therapy for cytomegalovirus peripheral retinitis in patients with AIDS. AIDS Clinical Trials Group and Cytomegalovirus Cooperative Study Group. *Journal of Infectious Diseases* 168 (3): 557–563

Stapleton F, Dart J K G, Seal D V, Matheson M 1995 Epidemiology of *Pseudomonas aeruginosa* in contact lens wearers. *Epidemiology and Infection* 114: 395–402

Sundmacher R 1984 The role of interferon in prophylaxis and treatment of dendritic keratitis. In: Blodi F C (ed) Herpes simplex infections of the eye. Churchill Livingstone, New York, p 129–146

Tabbara K F 1986 Ocular toxoplasmosis. In: Tabbara K F, Hyndiuk R A (eds) Infections of the eye. Little Brown and Co., Boston, p 635–652

Taylor H R, Dax E M 1986 Ocular onchocerciasis. In: Tabbara K F, Hyndiuk R A (eds) Infections of the eye. Little Brown and Co., Boston, p 653–664

Thomas P A 1994 Mycotic keratitis – an underestimated mycosis. *Journal of Medical and Veterinary Mycology* 32: 235–256

Tuft S J, Kemeny D M, Dart J K G, Buckley R J 1991 Clinical features of atopic keratoconjunctivitis. *Ophthalmology* 98: 150–158

Tuft S J, Ramakrishnan M, Seal D V, Kemeney D M, Buckley R J 1992 Role of *Staphylococcus aureus* in chronic allergic conjunctivitis. *Ophthalmology* 99: 180–184

van den Broek P J, van der Meer J W M, Mulderj D, Versteegj M, Mattie H 1984 Limited value of acyclovir in the treatment of uncomplicated herpes zoster: a placebo-controlled study. *Infection* 12 (5): 338–341

von Gunten S, Lew D, Paccolat F et al 1994 Aqueous humor penetration of ofloxacin given by various routes. *American Journal of Ophthalmology* 117: 87–89

Weinberg D V, Murphy R, Naughton K 1994 Combined daily therapy with intravenous ganciclovir and foscarnet for patients with recurrent cytomegalovirus retinitis. *American Journal of Ophthalmology* 117: 776–782

Wilhelmus K R, Gee L, Hauck W W et al 1994 Herpetic eye disease study – a controlled trial of topical corticosteroids for H. simplex stromal keratitis. *Ophthalmology* 101: 1883–1896

Wright P, Ficker L, Seal D V 1994 Staphylococci and the outer eye: relationship of colonisation and immunity to disease. In: Bialasiewicz A, Schaal K (eds) Infectious diseases of the eye. Aeolus Press, Buren, p 65–74

Urinary tract infections

S. R. Norrby

Introduction

This chapter deals with cystitis, pyelonephritis, prostatitis and urethritis caused by pathogens other than sexually transmitted ones like Neisseria gonorrhoeae, Chlamydia trachomatis, Trichomonas vaginalis and Ureaplasma urealyticum.

Cystitis and pyelonephritis are characterized by significant bacteriuria, which was originally defined by Kass as 10^5 colony forming units (cfu) or more per millilitre of a voided urine sample, or any bacterial count in urine obtained by catheterization or bladder puncture. This concept has now been redefined (Table 56.1) based on studies showing that by lowering the bacterial counts the diagnostic sensitivity can be increased without marked loss of specificity.

Both cystitis and pyelonephritis can be classified as symptomatic or asymptomatic, complicated or uncomplicated, and sporadic or recurrent. This classification is

Table 56.1 *Definitions of bacteriuria in midstream urine samples. Note that in all patients with symptomatic infections, pyuria must also be present**

Type of infection	Definition
Acute uncomplicated cystitis in women	
Infections caused by GNB	$\geq 10^3$ cfu/ml
Infections caused by staphylococci	$\geq 10^2$ cfu/ml
Acute uncomplicated pyelonephritis	
Infections caused by GNB	$\geq 10^4$ cfu/ml
Infections caused by staphylococci	$\geq 10^3$ cfu/ml
Complicated infections and infections in men	$\geq 10^4$ cfu/ml
Patients with asymptomatic bacteriuria	$\geq 10^5$ cfu/ml in 2 samples

GNB, Gram-negative bacteria.
* Modified from Rubin et al (1992).

meaningful since aetiology, choice of antibiotics and treatment times differ considerably between various types of infection.

Asymptomatic bacteriuria is common in girls and occurs in 1–7% of adult women, depending on age. All patients with long-term urinary catheters have significant bacteriuria which in most patients is asymptomatic. Many patients with cystitis who do not respond bacteriologically to antibiotic treatment but have persistent bacteriuria are asymptomatic.

Complicated cystitis or pyelonephritis is defined as infection in patients with anatomical or functional defects which facilitate establishment of bacteriuria. Examples of such defects are congenital anomalies of the urethra, ureters or kidneys, foreign bodies (stones, catheters), residual bladder urine due to obstructions or neurological diseases, tumours and obstructions of the urethra by strictures, prostatic hyperplasia, prostatic cancer or prostatitis. Diseases which may aggravate the course of a pyelonephritis, e.g. diabetes mellitus with nephropathy and malignant hypertension, are sometimes considered complicating factors, but these conditions do not increase the risk of establishment of bacteriuria. Significant bacteriuria in a man should always be considered a complicated urinary tract infection. The length of the male urethra prevents ascending infections and establishment of bacteriuria in a healthy man.

Cystitis and pyelonephritis are often recurrent infections. Recurrences occur both in patients with uncomplicated and complicated infections but are more common in the latter. Recurrent urinary tract infections can be subclassified into relapse, when the same bacterial strain causing the previous episode is isolated, or reinfection, when the causative pathogen is a new strain. There is no internationally accepted definition of a recurrent urinary tract infection. In clinical trials it is often defined as more than one episode in 6 months or more than two episodes in a year. Thus sporadic infections occur less than twice in 6 months or less than *three times in a year. It should be noted that this classification does not include chronic infections; chronic pyelonephritis and chronic glomerulonephritis are inflammatory diseases, albeit often aggravated by infections.*

Urethritis is an inflammation of the urethra without concomitant significant bacteriuria. In patients with sexually transmitted diseases urethritis is a well-defined concept (Ch. 58). However, when such organisms are not identified and significant bacteriuria is not present the urethral syndrome becomes a microbiologically poorly defined disease without identified aetiology.

Prostatitis is an inflammation of the prostate gland which often also involves the seminal vesicles. When prostatitis is caused by bacterial pathogens it is subdivided into acute and chronic bacterial prostatitis which may or may not be associated with significant bacteriuria.

EPIDEMIOLOGY AND PATHOGENESIS

Urinary tract infections occur in all ages and are most common in sexually active women. Below the age of 3 years, symptomatic cystitis or pyelonephritis is somewhat more common in boys than in girls due the higher frequency of congenital defects of the male urethra. In the very old, bacteriuria is more common in men than in women due to the high frequency of prostate disease.

Cystitis and pyelonephritis are infections caused by the aerobic faecal flora. The pathogenesis of these infections can be considered from two aspects: host factors and virulence factors of the infecting organisms.

Host factors

Host factors of importance for establishment of bacteriuria are those mentioned above defining a complicated cystitis or pyelonephritis. In addition, the short length of the female urethra explains the higher frequency of bacteriuria in adult women than in adult men. In women without urinary tract defects, bacteria can ascend the urethra and reach the bladder, something which is impossible in men. In postmenopausal women atrophy of the vaginal mucosa is an important and treatable (with oestrogen) complicating factor which is surprisingly often overlooked.

Establishment of significant bacteriuria in a woman is facilitated by a high number of bacteria in the periurethral area. This is achieved during sexual intercourse, which often leads to bacteriuria if the bladder is not emptied postcoitus.

In men, especially those who are sexually active, the source of a bacteriuria may be a prostatitis. Otherwise a prerequisite for bacteria to reach the bladder in sufficient amounts to establish bacteriuria is a turbulent urine flow which may result from strictures or obstruction of the urethra. Irrespective of age and gender pyelonephritis almost invariably results from bacteria ascending the ureters. This is facilitated by defects in the ureteral bladder sphincters causing ureteral reflux during micturition. Such defects may be congenital but are also common in pregnant women during the latter half of pregnancy due to the pressure of the uterus on the bladder. Pyelonephritis is also common in patients with ureteral stones or stones in the renal pelvis. Pyelonephritis and renal abscesses resulting from haematogenous dissemination of bacteria from other infectious foci is extremely rare, but may be seen in patients with endocarditis.

Virulence factors

Virulence factors of the organisms causing cystitis and pyelonephritis have been extensively studied. With the most common aetiologic agent, *Escherichia coli*, it has been demonstrated that an important virulence factor is the ability of the bacterial cells to adhere to epithelial cells in the urinary tract mucosa. This is achieved by antigens located in the fimbriae of the bacteria which adhere to glycosphingolipid receptors on the epithelial cells. As a result of adherence, transportation of bacteria in the urethra and the ureters is facilitated. Another consequence of adherence is that cytokines, e.g. interleukin-1, -6 and -8, are released and that invasive infections are facilitated. Adherence is important in patients without complicating factors, but seems less important when such factors are present. Other defined bacterial virulence factors are the antigenic structures of Enterobacteriaceae, the O, H and K antigens and the polysaccharide capsules. Virulence factors in Gram-positive organisms of importance in urinary tract infections are less extensively studied.

AETIOLOGY

Bacteriuria is acquired by the faecal–genital route, often via periurethral colonization in women. With the exception of patients who have rectovesical fistulas or other abnormal communications between the bladder and the intestines or vagina, anaerobic bacteria do not cause bacteriuria. The most common organisms causing bacteriuria are listed in Table 56.2.

In women with sporadic uncomplicated cystitis or pyelonephritis, the aetiology is quite predictable. About 85% of these patients will have infections caused by *Esch. coli*. The second most common organism is *Staphylococcus saprophyticus* which accounts for about 10% of the infections. However, in North Europe *Staph. saprophyticus* has a seasonal pattern. It is normally not found between November and March and reaches a peak in July and August when it causes up to 40% of all uncomplicated infections. The reason for this variation is unknown.

Table 56.2 Aetiology of cystitis and pyelonephritis

Species	Dominant type of infection
Escherichia coli	All types
Staphylococcus saprophyticus	Uncomplicated cystitis and pyelonephritis in women during April to September
Klebsiella spp.	Recurrent/complicated infections
Enterobacter spp.	Recurrent/complicated infections
Enterococcus spp.	Recurrent/complicated infections
Proteus spp.	Tumours or stones
Morganella morganii	Recurrent/complicated infections
Pseudomonas spp.	Recurrent/complicated infections, bladder catheters
Other organisms	Recurrent infections

Esch. coli is also the most common aetiology in recurrent and/or complicated cystitis and pyelonephritis, but other Gram-negative organisms as well as enterococci become increasingly frequent. Of importance in these patients is the antibiotic treatment given for the preceding episode. That treatment is likely to have selected resistant organisms. Organisms such as Enterobacter spp., Pseudomonas aeruginosa, Pseudomonas spp., Acinetobacter spp. and Citrobacter spp. typically appear in patients who have received repeated antibiotic courses or who have acquired their bacteriuria in hospital.

Proteus spp., Morganella morganii and Providencia spp., which all grow in alkaline pH are common in patients with kidney or bladder stones or tumours. Since Proteus spp. are also common in the praeputial flora, they are often a contaminant in urine samples from young boys.

Fungal growth in the urine is in most cases seen with Candida albicans or other Candida spp. The clinical importance of funguria is uncertain or doubtful in patients with bladder catheters. In patients without catheters growth of candida may reflect a renal infection resulting from haematological dissemination of the organisms. In rare cases candiduria is also seen as a result of the formation of a mycelial ball in the bladder, a mycetoma.

DIAGNOSIS

Clinical diagnosis

Patients with cystitis are afebrile and the dominating symptoms are dysuria, frequent micturition and/or suprapubic pain. Sometimes macroscopic haematuria is present, especially in infections caused by Staph. saprophyticus. With the exception of haematuria these symptoms are difficult or impossible to differentiate from those of urethritis unless the patient has a urethral discharge.

Pyelonephritis is a systemic infection and patients develop fever and may also have signs of septicaemia, which occurs in up to 30% of patients with this infection. Other symptoms are chills and flank pain. Differential diagnoses are urinary stones, cholecystitis, appendicitis and basal pneumonia. The clinical symptoms of pyelonephritis are often masked by patients taking drugs with analgesic and/or antipyretic activity.

In children, urinary tract infections often present with few clinical symptoms and fever may be the only symptom of pyelonephritis.

Acute prostatitis is characterized by symptoms similar to those of cystitis, but patients also have tenderness and enlargement of the prostate on rectal palpation. In chronic prostatitis the symptoms may be more diffuse and the prostate is often normal on rectal examination.

Radiological diagnosis

Radiological examinations are rarely indicated in the acute phase of a urinary tract infection. An exception is when an obstruction of a ureter is suspected in a patient with signs of pyelonephritis or with recurrent cystitis, radiological examinations for identification of congenital anatomical defects and/or ureteral reflux should be performed.

In adults who have recovered from pyelonephritis radiological examination is recommended to exclude renal scars from childhood episodes of pyelonephritis.

Laboratory diagnosis

The keystone in the diagnosis of cystitis and pyelonephritis is demonstration of significant bacteriuria. The reference technique is the quantitative urine culture. The sample can be obtained as a clean-catch (midstream) urine or by bladder puncture or catheterization. Bladder puncture is the preferred technique in small children, especially boys. After sampling the urine must be kept chilled (but not frozen) until analysed. In situations where the samples must be transported over long periods of time to a laboratory, a dip-slide culture can be used. With this technique an agar covered slide is dipped in urine and incubated overnight at room temperature or in a small incubator. It provides results in terms of quantity of bacteria and differentiation of Gram-negative and Gram-positive organisms. The slide can subsequently be sent to a microbiological laboratory for determination of species and antibiotic susceptibility.

In patients with infections caused by Gram-negative bacteria other than Pseudomonas spp. bacteriuria can also be demonstrated by the nitrite test, a rapid paper strip test. Nitrite is formed by bacterial metabolism of nitrate and is not normally present in urine. A positive nitrite test has a very high specificity. The sensitivity, however, is low since the method requires bacteria to have multiplied in the bladder, and since Gram-positive bacteria and pseudomonas do not form nitrite.

Urine cultures should always be obtained in patients with complicated infections, recurrent infections or pyelonephritis. In patients with sporadic uncomplicated cystitis aetiological diagnosis is optional.

Pyuria is a marker for significant bacteriuria. Demonstration of pyuria is best achieved by microscopy of unspun urine using a Bürker chamber and defining pyuria as $>10 \times 10^6$ leucocytes per litre of urine. The second-best method is to use a leucocyte esterase paper strip test. Sediment microscopy has a low reliability since it is a technique which cannot be standardized. Marked pyuria in a patient with negative bacteriological cultures should lead to a suspicion of renal tuberculosis (Ch. 59).

There is no specific laboratory test for differentiation of cystitis and pyelonephritis. Patients with pyelonephritis normally have increased serum concentrations of C-reactive protein (CRP) and peripheral white blood cells (WBCs) may be increased. Erythrocyte sedimentation rate is not always increased when the patient is first seen but is likely to rise during the following days. A regular finding in patients with acute pyelonephritis is that the concentrating ability of the kidneys is reduced. This can be measured as urine osmolality after 12 h of no fluid intake or, more easily, by a subcutaneous (not nasal) challenge with antidiuretic hormone. This test cannot be used when the patient is febrile and it is therefore a confirmatory test which can be done when the patient has improved.

Bacteria causing pyelonephritis form complexes with antibodies, and detection of antibody-coated bacteria by immunofluorescence has been used as a method to differentiate cystitis and pyelonephritis. However, this test has tended to show a high frequency of false-positive results if a reasonable sensitivity is sought, or too many false-negative results if the specificity of the test is high.

The aetiological diagnosis of prostatitis is difficult. The most ambitious technique is to culture four samples: (i) the first portion of a voided urine sample; (ii) a midstream urine portion; (iii) prostate secretion obtained by rectal massage of the prostate; and (iv) the first portion of new voided urine sample. Patients with acute or chronic bacterial prostatitis should be culture positive in all four of these samples.

Antibiotic treatment

Antibiotic treatment of cystitis and pyelonephritis is normally empirical. Women with acute cystitis are rarely prepared to wait 24 h for treatment and patients with acute pyelonephritis should be treated as soon as possible to avoid damage to the kidneys and to reduce the risk of serious systemic manifestations of the infection.

PHARMACOKINETIC REQUIREMENTS

All antibiotics used for treatment of urinary tract infections with significant bacteriuria should be excreted via the kidneys. This makes drugs like chloramphenicol and the tetracyclines less suitable since they are lipid soluble, with elimination mainly via liver metabolism resulting in very low urine concentrations. In patients with pyelonephritis it is also important that the antibiotic achieves serum concentrations sufficiently high to eliminate bacteraemia. With renally excreted antibiotics therapeutic concentrations are normally achieved in the renal parenchyma.

In patients with prostatitis special pharmacokinetic requirements apply. The prostate tissue is difficult to penetrate and the pH of prostatic and vesicular fluid varies and is often altered by infection. Hence, the drugs used must be active at a wide range of pH values. Finally, in chronic prostatitis calculi may be present which reduce the efficacy of antibiotic treatment.

Safety considerations

Uncomplicated cystitis is an infection which constitutes no threat to the patient if adequately treated. When such infections are treated it is a prerequisite that the antibiotics used have the highest possible degree of safety; serious or life-threatening adverse effects cannot be accepted even if they appear in very low frequencies. On the other hand, in patients with pyelonephritis, the infection per se constitutes a considerable risk to the patient, which makes adverse effects to the treatment given more acceptable if a high degree of efficacy can be expected.

CHOICE OF ANTIBIOTICS

Of paramount importance in this respect is the local antibiotic resistance pattern. It is not possible to extrapolate susceptibility data generated in one country to another. There may be marked differences between hospitals in the same country in the frequency of resistance to commonly used antibiotics. The local microbiological laboratories must provide data from regular resistance surveillance studies performed on clinically relevant collections of bacterial strains. Results obtained in outpatients should be considered separately from hospital-generated data.

Documentation of antibiotic efficacy

Treatment of urinary tract infections with antibiotics aims at eliminating the symptoms and, most importantly in patients with cystitis or pyelonephritis, the bacteriuria. Systematic evaluations of antibiotic efficacy are made in clinical trials. Table 56.3 lists minimal requirements on clinical trials of antibiotic treatment of cystitis and

Table 56.3 *Requirements for clinical trials of antibiotic treatment of urinary tract infections*

Criterion	Requirements
Type of infection	A single type only e.g. uncomplicated cystitis in women or complicated infections in either sex
Sample size	For trials in cystitis, at least 200 patients with confirmed bacteriuria per treatment group; smaller samples for complicated infections and pyelonephritis
Entry criteria	Verified pyuria and/or positive nitrite test, typical symptoms, urine for culture
Control	Well-documented regimen
Design	Always prospective, controlled and randomized. Preferably double-blind
End-points	Bacteriological efficacy, clinical efficacy and safety. Efficacy to be analysed 5–9 days and 4–6 weeks after treatment
Analyses	Both intention-to-treat analysis of outcome in all patients randomized and per-protocol analysis of patients fulfilling defined criteria, e.g. minimum treatment time, bacteriuria pretreatment and at least one follow-up visit

pyelonephritis. Most trials initiated by pharmaceutical companies today fulfill these criteria. However, before the mid-1980s many clinical trials included too few patients to allow valid conclusions to be drawn.

TREATMENT OF CYSTITIS

Cystitis accounts for approximately 85% of all infections with significant bacteriuria. Typically, about 75% of women with cystitis have sporadic infections and 25% recurrent infections. Complicated infections are found in only about 2% of unselected patients. Most patients with cystitis are women aged 15–50 years.

In addition to antibiotic treatment, it is important to provide advice to the patients on how to prevent recurrences. Sexually active women should be told that emptying the bladder after intercourse will reduce the risk of recurrence.

As mentioned above, cystitis in older women is often due to atrophic changes of the vaginal mucosa, increasing the periurethral bacterial inoculum. Elderly women should therefore be examined for vaginal atrophy and, if present, such atrophy should be treated with oestrogen to prevent recurrences.

Although cystitis is a self-limiting benign infection in most patients, antibiotic treatment is recommended. The most important reason for using antibiotic treatment in this

condition is to prevent ascending infections and pyelo-nephritis.

A large number of antibiotics are used for treatment of uncomplicated cystitis. A general rule is that oral β-lactam antibiotics (ampicillin, amoxycillin, carbacephems, cephalosporins, co-amoxiclav and other β-lactam–β-lactamase inhibitor combinations and mecillinam) seem to be considerably less efficacious in eradicating bacteriuria than trimethoprim–sulphonamide combinations, trimethoprim or fluoroquinolones (Table 56.4). This is not due to more frequent resistance to β-lactams than to other antibiotics in bacteria causing bacteriuria. A possible explanation is that β-lactam antibiotics are rapidly eliminated, i.e. the urine becomes free from antibacterial drug within about 12 h after the last treatment dose. With trimethoprim, co-trimoxazole and fluoroquinolones, on the other hand, high concentrations in the urine are maintained for 24 h or more after the end of treatment. Another possibility is that the latter drugs reduce the periurethral inoculum more effectively than β-lactams, thereby reducing the risk of recurrences.

There are no major differences in clinical efficacy between antibiotics used for treatment of uncomplicated cystitis. Irrespective of whether the bacteriuria is eliminated or not, symptoms tend to disappear after 3 days. Thus, there is a poor correlation between clinical and bacteriological efficacy.

The duration of treatment in uncomplicated cystitis is a controversial issue. Recommendations range from a large single dose to 10 days or more. A short treatment course offers better patient compliance, reduced costs and minimized risks of adverse effects. However, all antibiotics tested in sufficiently large trials have been found to be less effective if used as a single dose than when longer treatment

Table 56.4 *Bacteriological efficacy in a study comparing a β-lactam (ritipenem axetil) with a fluoroquinolone (norfloxacin) for 5 days' treatment of uncomplicated cystitis in women* *

Follow-up and outcome	Treatment	
	Ritipenem axetil	Norfloxacin
5–9 days post-treatment		
No bacteriuria	51/122 (42%)	77/114[†] (68%)
Superinfection	22/122 (18%)	20/114 (18%)
Persistence	41/122 (34%)	12/114[†] (11%)
Not assessable	8/122 (7%)	5/114 (4%)
3–4 weeks post-treatment		
No bacteriuria	31/59 (53%)	52/82 (63%)
Recurrence	17/59 (29%)	16/82 (20%)
Reinfection	11/59 (19%)	8/82 (10%)
Not assessable	0/59	6/82 (7%)

* Modified from The Swedish Urinary Tract Infection Study Group (1995).
[†] p <0.001.

Table 56.5 *Comparative efficacy of trimethoprim–sulphonamide combinations and β-lactam antibiotics when used for different treatment times in patients with uncomplicated cystitis**

Treatment time	Rate of eradication of bacteriuria	
	Trimethoprim + sulphonamide	β-Lactam
Single dose	267/300 (89%)	58/ 60 (66%)
3 days	139/147 (95%)	282/343 (82%)
>5 days	294/308 (96%)	370/423 (88%)

* Modified from Norrby (1990).

times have been employed (Table 56.5). Differences exist between antibiotics. For co-trimoxazole and other combinations of trimethoprim and sulphonamides, e.g. trimethoprim plus sulphadiazine (co-trimazin), high cure rates could be demonstrated after administration of a single dose. Treatment for 3 days improved the efficacy, but no further benefits were achieved with longer treatment times. However, with prolonged treatment the frequencies of adverse events increased drastically in patients receiving trimethoprim–sulphonamide combinations, while the safety of β-lactam antibiotics was far less affected by the treatment time (Table 56.6).

Fluoroquinolones seem also to be relatively effective if used for 3 days or less, and probably little is gained by increasing the treatment time to 5 days or more.

It is recommended that a short (3 days or less) course of co-trimoxazole or another trimethoprim–sulphonamide combination, or of trimethoprim only is used as first-line treatment of sporadic uncomplicated cystitis when the local susceptibility pattern so allows. When safety is considered, trimethoprim is to be preferred over co-trimoxazole or other trimethoprim–sulphonamide combinations. However, the documentation of efficacy is less comprehensive for trimethoprim since for many years co-trimoxazole was the gold standard in clinical trials. In pregnant women nitrofurantoin or a β-lactam antibiotic for 5–7 days should be the drugs of choice. β-Lactam antibiotics should otherwise generally be used restrictively due to their poor bacteriological efficacy. Older, non-fluorinated quinolones should not be used for the treatment of any type of urinary

tract infection. They are considerably less active than the fluorinated quinolones and resistance emerges in high frequency with these antibiotics. Moreover, resistance to older quinolones increases the risk of resistance to fluoroquinolones. Resistance to these antibiotics is chromosomal. With the non-fluorinated derivatives, a single mutation of one of the bacterial genes coding for the DNA-gyrase (topoisomerase I), which is the target for quinolones, will result in resistance. Such mutations occur in a frequency of about 10^{-8}. The new fluoroquinolones are 100–1000 times more active and two consecutive mutations are required in species such as *Esch. coli* before the organisms become resistant. This is likely to occur at a frequency of 10^{-16}. If an older quinolone is used the first mutation is often initiated. The risk for mutation to resistance against the fluoroquinolones if they are used then increases from 10^{-16} to 10^{-8}.

Patients with recurrent uncomplicated cystitis are more likely to have bacteriuria caused by organisms other than *Esch. coli* or *Staph. saprophyticus*. Pathogens which should be covered are enterococci and *Klebsiella* spp. The choice of antibiotic will depend on the treatment used for the preceding episode. Fluoroquinolones are antibiotics which, if not used in the same patient recently, are very likely to be effective. To preserve their value in the treatment of these more serious infections as well as patients with pyelonephritis, these antibiotics are not recommended as first-line drugs for treatment of uncomplicated sporadic cystitis.

Following treatment of uncomplicated sporadic cystitis, no follow-up procedures are warranted. Patients should be told to come back if they again experience clinical symptoms.

Antibiotics for treatment of uncomplicated sporadic cystitis can often be chosen without urine cultures, based on knowledge of the local antibiotic susceptibility pattern. In patients with complicated infections, which are typically recurrent, and in patients with uncomplicated infections which recur, urine cultures should be performed routinely.

Antibiotics used for treatment of complicated and recurrent cystitis are the same as those used in sporadic uncomplicated infections. However, β-lactams tend to perform even less well than in sporadic cases and treatment should continue for 5 days or longer. In these patients urine should be cultured after treatment. The goal should be to identify and eliminate the complicating factor, if present.

Table 56.6 *Frequencies of adverse events reported after treatment of uncomplicated cystitis**

Treatment time	No. of patients with adverse events	
	Trimethoprim + sulphonamide	β-Lactam
Single dose	30/404 (7%)	23/212 (11%)
3 days	13/195 (7%)	55/630 (9%)
≥5 days	101/406 (25%)	126/934 (14%)

* Modified from Norrby (1990).

TREATMENT OF PYELONEPHRITIS

Pyelonephritis may be a life-threatening infection. In adults, septicaemia may lead to septic shock. In children there is a marked risk of development of renal scars, which in turn may lead to permanent renal damage if the patient develops recurrent urinary tract infections involving the affected kidney. Correct choice of empirical antibiotic treatment is therefore essential. The first therapeutic decision to be taken is whether or not the patient needs parenteral treatment. If an injectable antibiotic is needed, there are several alternatives for empirical treatment. In patients with sporadic infections which are community acquired, a second-generation cephalosporin (e.g. cefuroxime), an aminoglycoside or, in some countries, co-trimoxazole are likely to be effective. Ampicillin, amoxicillin and first-generation cephalosporins (cephalothin, cefazolin, cephradine and others) against which more than 10% of *Esch. coli* strains are resistant, are not recommended. In patients with hospital-acquired infections a third-generation cephalosporin (e.g. ceftazidime, cefotaxime or ceftriaxone), a carbapenem (imipenem or meropenem), an aminoglycoside or a fluoroquinolone (e.g. ciprofloxacin or ofloxacin) are effective in most countries.

Renal function is always reduced in the acute phase of pyelonephritis. This, together with the fact that β-lactams, aminoglycosides and quinolones all achieve high concentrations in urine, blood and renal tissues, allows the use of low doses, e.g. cefuroxime 750 mg three times daily, 3 mg/kg body weight per day of gentamicin, netilmicin or tobramycin and intravenous ciprofloxacin 200 mg twice daily.

Some patients with pyelonephritis can be given oral antibiotics throughout the course of treatment. Antibiotics to be preferred are the fluoroquinolones which are more efficacious than oral β-lactam antibiotics. Since quinolones are not recommended for pregnant women and since the therapeutic efficacy of oral (but not parenteral) β-lactams must be questioned, it is recommended that oral treatment is not used initially in pregnant women with signs of pyelonephritis.

An insufficiently studied problem is what drug to use when a patient started on parenteral treatment is to be switched to an oral regimen. Clinical trials of antibiotics have traditionally not been directed towards this problem, and few studies have evaluated the normal clinical situation, i.e. that a patient is treated parenterally for 24–48 h and then continued on an oral antibiotic. At present the best choice for oral follow-up to an injectable antibiotic in a patient with pyelonephritis seems to be a fluoroquinolone.

Treatment should be continued for 2 weeks in pyelonephritis. Longer treatment times seem not to increase the cure rates but are likely to result in higher frequencies of adverse reactions to the antibiotics used. The efficacy of treatment given for pyelonephritis should be followed up with urine cultures at least once after treatment.

ASYMPTOMATIC BACTERIURIA

Most patients with asymptomatic bacteriuria should not be treated. This is certainly true for patients with bladder catheters. Treatment will in such cases only result in the selection of increasingly resistant bacterial strains and, if the patients should develop a systemic infection, it may be difficult to find an active antibiotic. Early studies indicated that asymptomatic bacteriuria in the elderly was correlated with an increased mortality. However, more recent investigations have failed to show that bacteriuria per se is an independent risk factor for increased mortality. In one such study antimicrobial treatment of asymptomatic bacteriuria did not affect mortality. Exceptions from this rule are pregnant women and patients who are to undergo urogenital tract surgery. Both these groups should be screened for bacteriuria and treated if found positive. Antibiotics recommended are those used for treatment of uncomplicated cystitis. In other categories of patients, e.g. the elderly and those with diabetes mellitus, screening for bacteriuria is not recommended since treatment of asymptomatic bacteriuria has not been proven to have beneficial effects.

PROPHYLAXIS AND LONG-TERM TREATMENT

Antibiotic prophylaxis of cystitis and pyelonephritis should be used very restrictively. Patients with frequent recurrences of these infections should be investigated in order to find and eradicate the complicating factors leading to the recurrences. In some patients episodes of cystitis or pyelonephritis may require long periods of treatment to prevent recurrences before surgery is performed. An important group in which such prophylaxis is indicated is children with congenital anatomical defects. Several studies have indicated that reflux and pyelonephritis in young children is correlated with renal cortical damage and scarring.

In a small fraction of patients with recurrent cystitis or pyelonephritis, mainly young girls, no complicating factor can be identified. Such patients benefit from prophylaxis and should be given nitrofurantoin or trimethoprim once daily before going to bed. The treatment is normally continued for 6 months, but several years of treatment may be required.

TREATMENT OF PROSTATITIS

Antibiotic treatment of prostatitis differ from those of cystitis and pyelonephritis, with respect to both choice of antibiotics and treatment times. In patients in whom gonorrhoea and chlamydial infection have been excluded, identification of the aetiology can be tried using the method described with segmented urine culture. However, in most cases this procedure is too cumbersome and treatment is started without aetiological verification. Drugs frequently used and well documented are co-trimoxazole, tetracyclines such as doxycycline, and fluoroquinolones. Treatment times are 3 weeks or longer.

TREATMENT OF FUNGURIA

When a *Candida* spp. is isolated in the urine and considered a clinically relevant finding, treatment should be given. Amphotericin is generally active against candida and resistance has never been reported. However, the drug is difficult to administer and has considerable nephrotoxicity. The azole derivatives, e.g. fluconazole and itraconazole, are metabolized in the liver and achieve low urine concentrations. Resistance to these drugs may occur, and *Candida krusei* is normally resistant. A good choice for treatment of candiduria, if the isolated organisms are susceptible is flucytosine, which is excreted by the kidneys and achieves high concentrations in renal tissue. However, if flucytosine is used, caution should be taken not to use too high doses which may lead to adverse reactions. Optimally, serum concentrations of flucytosine should be monitored and kept between 25 and 100 mg/l during the entire dose interval.

References

Norrby S R 1990 Short-term treatment of uncomplicated urinary tract infections in women. *Reviews of Infectious Diseases* 12: 458–467

Rubin E H, Shapiro E D, Andriole V T, Davis R J, Stamm W E 1992 Evaluation of new anti-infective drugs for the treatment of urinary tract infections. *Clinical Infectious Diseases* 15 (suppl 1): S216–S217

The Swedish Urinary Tract Infection Study Group 1995 Interpretation of the bacteriological outcome of antibiotic treatment for uncomplicated cystitis: impact of the definition of significant bacteriuria in a comparison of ritipenem axetil with norfloxacin. *Clinical Infectious Diseases* 20: 507–513

Further information

Abrutyn E, Mossey J, Berlin J A, Levison M, Pitsakis P, Kaye D 1994 Does asymptomatic bacteriuria predict mortality and does antimicrobial treatment reduce mortality in elderly ambulatory women? *Annals of Internal Medicine* 120: 827–833

Ditchfield M R, Decampo J F, Nolan T M et al 1994 Risk factors in the development of early renal cortical defects in children with urinary tract infections. *American Journal of Roentgenology* 162: 1393–1397

Jonsson M, Englund G, Nörgård K 1990 Norfloxacin vs. pivmecillinam in the treatment of uncomplicated lower urinary tract infections in hospitalized elderly patients. *Scandinavian Journal of Infectious Diseases* 22: 339–344

Kass E H 1957 Bacteriuria and diagnosis of infections of the urinary tract: with observations on the use of methionine as a urinary antiseptic. *Archives of Internal Medicine* 100: 709–714

Kraft J K, Stamey T A 1977 The natural history of symptomatic recurrent bacteriuria in women. *Medicine (Baltimore)* 56: 55–60

Kunin C M 1992 Guidelines for the evaluation of new anti-infective drugs for the treatment of urinary tract infection: additional considerations. *Clinical Infectious Diseases* 15: 1041–1044

Naber K G 1989 Use of quinolones in urinary tract infections and prostatitis. *Reviews of Infectious Diseases* 11: S1321–S1337

Otto G, Sandberg T, Marklund B I, Ulleryd P, Svanborg C 1993 Virulence factors and *pap* genotype in *Escherichia coli* isolates from women with acute pyelonephritis, with or without bacteremia. *Clinical Infectious Diseases* 17: 448–456

Sandberg T, Englund K, Lincolm K, Nilsson L G 1990 Randomised double-blind study of norfloxacin and cefadroxil in the treatment of acute pyelonephritis. *European Journal of Clinical Microbiology and Infectious Diseases* 9: 317–322

Smellie J M, Poulton A, Prescod N P 1994 Retrospective study of children with renal scarring associated with reflux and urinary infection. *British Medical Journal* 308: 1193–1196

Stamm W E 1983 Measurement of pyuria and its relation to bacteriuria. *American Journal of Medicine* 75: 53–58

Stamm W E, Counts G W, Running K R, Fihn S, Turck M, Holmes K K 1982 Diagnosis of coliform infection in acutely dysuric women. *New England Journal of Medicine* 307: 463–468

Urinary Tract Infection Study Group 1987 Coordinated multicenter study of norfloxacin versus trimethoprim-sulfamethoxazole treatment of symptomatic urinary tract infections. *Journal of Infectious Diseases* 155: 170–177

Infections in obstetrics

F. Smaill

Introduction

Infection in pregnancy has consequences for the mother and her unborn child. Decisions regarding therapy need to be made carefully, balancing the risks and benefits to mother and fetus. While most infection that occurs in pregnancy is without serious consequence, it is important to recognize the unique vulnerability of the developing fetus to infection and the potential for significant maternal disease.

General principles of drug use in pregnancy and the puerperium

The pharmacokinetics of drugs in pregnancy

The physiological changes in pregnancy, that primarily serve to increase the delivery of blood and nutrients to the fetus, may modify the pharmacokinetics of many drugs, with potential therapeutic implications (Table 57.1). Body fat and red cell volume are increased. However, no overall trend in pharmacokinetic parameters has been observed, nor have generally applicable principles for the disposition of drugs in pregnancy been established (Cummings 1983). For drugs with rapid rates of excretion, minimal metabolism and direct renal clearance, e.g. some β-lactam antibiotics and the aminoglycosides, lower serum levels have been documented during pregnancy (Philipson 1979). The clearance of ampicillin, which is excreted largely unchanged by the kidney, is increased over the non-pregnant state (330 vs 238 ml/min) but, because the apparent volume of distribution is increased, the half-life is only slightly shorter (39

vs 44 min). Peak concentrations achieved after each dose are, however, reduced. Serum levels of gentamicin are lower, but the half-life of gentamicin is usually within the range found in non-pregnant individuals.

The consequences of the altered pharmacokinetics of antibiotics in pregnancy on the treatment of infection have not been systematically reviewed. It seems reasonable, however, with most β-lactam antibiotics to give the maximum recommended dose for serious infections. For aminoglycosides and other drugs with a narrow toxic/therapeutic ratio, where the clearance of the drug is difficult to predict and where fetal toxicity is of concern, frequent serum assays are advised. A critical review of aminoglycoside monitoring in pregnancy, however, is lacking.

Placental transfer of drugs

Most drugs are transported across the placenta passively by simple diffusion from a high to a low concentration. The transfer rate across the placenta is related to the surface area of the placenta, the membrane thickness, physico-chemical properties of the drug, and the concentration gradient. As pregnancy progresses functional and structural changes take place in the placenta. The surface area of the placenta increases from 5 m^2 at 28 weeks to 11 m^2 at term. In early pregnancy the fetal blood may be separated from maternal blood by a distance of 20–40 μm, while at term the effective membrane thickness is reduced to 2 μm, facilitating the passage of drugs.

The concentration gradient across the placenta is a function of the amount of drug administered to the mother, the volume of drug distribution (V_d) in the maternal and fetal extracellular space, uterine blood flow, and maternal and fetal drug excretion. Both the amplitude and duration of maternal serum levels affect the amount of drug transmitted. Higher concentrations of antimicrobial agents are generally attained in fetal serum and amniotic fluid by bolus rather

Table 57.1   *Pregnancy-associated physiological changes and their potential influence on antimicrobial pharmacokinetic parameters (Chow & Jewesson 1985, Mucklow 1986)*

Physiological change (estimate of increase)	Pharmacokinetic parameter(s)	Therapeutic implication(s)
Increased total body water (up to 8 l) and intravascular volume (by 40%)	Increased apparent volume of distribution (decreased peak plasma concentrations, increased half-life)	Possible need for larger loading doses
	Reduced concentration of albumin and other plasma proteins (larger fraction of unbound drug, increased tissue/plasma distribution, increased drug clearance)	Possible underestimation of serum concentrations of free or active drug; Possible need for more frequent dosing
Increased cardiac output (by 30–50%), renal blood flow (by 50–80%) and glomerular filtration rate (by 40–50%)	Increased drug clearance	Subtherapeutic drug concentrations; Possible need for increased dose and/or decreased dosing interval
Increased progesterone-activated hepatic metabolism	Increased rate of biotransformation to either active or inactive metabolites	Possible need for increased dose and/or decreased dosing interval

Decreased gastro-intestinal motility
    Delayed gastric emptying
    Delayed transit time
	Reduced rate of absorption from small bowel Increased rate of absorption from gastro-intestinal tract	Unpredictable absorption of orally administered drugs

than by continuous infusion. Transfer of drug to the fetus will also affect the effective concentration of drug in the mother.

During pregnancy, uterine blood flow is increased as a consequence of increased cardiac output and decreased uterine vascular resistance. Flow may be diminished by pressure on the great arteries by the uterus or it may be altered by pathological changes in the vasculature, as can occur in hypertension or diabetes. In hypertension of pregnancy, changes in the configuration of the spiral arteries opening into the placental bed can reduce blood flow by as much as 40%. During parturition, alterations in intrauterine pressure due to myometrial activity will modify maternal blood flow into the intervillous space.

A drug with a molecular weight of <500 Da, high lipid solubility, a low degree of ionization and a low affinity for protein binding is able to traverse the placenta readily. As a result of the reduction in albumin and serum protein concentrations during pregnancy more free drug is available although the clinical consequences of this are not well understood. Only free drug can pass into tissues and inhibit bacterial growth. Protein binding, however, is rarely the rate-limiting step in drug transfer because the dissociation of bound drug occurs more rapidly than transfer across the placenta. The contribution of drug metabolism by the placenta to fetal pharmacokinetics is probably minimal.

For some antibiotics, such as ampicillin, cefotaxime, and sulfonamides, fetal concentrations approach or exceed those in maternal serum (Table 57.2). Antibiotics with low transplacental transfer include cephalothin, dicloxacillin,

Table 57.2   *Transplacental passage of selected antimicrobial agents (Sáez-Llorens & McCracken 1995, Briggs et al 1995)*

Antimicrobial agent	Trimester	Fetal serum levels (% of maternal)	Adverse effects to fetus or infant	Risk category*
Acyclovir	3	125 – 140	None known	C
Amikacin	1, 2	8 – 16	Potential ototoxicity	C
	3	30 – 50		
Amoxicillin	3	30	None	B
Ampicillin	1, 2	50 – 250	None	B
	3	20 – 200		
Azithromycin	–	–	None known	B
Carbenicillin	2, 3	60 – 100	None	B
Cefazolin	1, 2	2 – 27	None	B
	3	36 – 69		
Cefotaxime	2	80 – 150	None	B
Cefoxitin	3	11 – 133	None	B
Ceftriaxone	3	9 – 120	None	B

Table 57.2 *Cont'd*

Antimicrobial agent	Trimester	Fetal serum levels (% of maternal)	Adverse effects to fetus or infant	Risk category*
Cefuroxime	3	18–108	None	B
Cephalexin	3	33	None	B
Cephalothin	3	10–40	None	B
Chloramphenicol	3	30–106	Potential circulatory collapse	C
Ciprofloxacin	–	–	Arthropathy in immature animals	C
Clarithromycin	–	–	None known	C
Clindamycin	2	10–25	None	B
	3	30–50		
Cloxacillin	3	20–97	None	B
Dicloxacillin	3	7–12	None	B
Erythromycin	2, 3	1–20	None	B
Fluconazole	–	–	None known	C
Gentamicin	2, 3	21–44	Potential ototoxicity; potentiation of $MgSO_4$ neuromuscular weakness	C
Imipenem	3	14–52	Potential seizure activity	C
Metronidazole	3	100	Mutagenic in bacteria; carcinogenic in rodents; not teratogenic in animals	B
Nafcillin	3	16	None	B
Nitrofurantoin	3	38–92	Haemolysis in G-6-PD deficiency	B
Penicillin G	1, 2	26–70	None	B
	3	15–100		
Sulfonamides	3	13–275	Haemolysis in G-6-PD deficiency; jaundice and potential kernicterus.	B
Tetracyclines	3	10–90	Adverse effects on bone and teeth, possible inguinal hernia	D
Tobramycin	1, 2	20	Potential ototoxicity	D
Trimethoprim	1, 2	27–131	Folate antagonist; teratogenic in animals	C
Vancomycin	–	–	Potential ototoxicity	B

G-6-PD, glucose-6-phosphate dehydrogenase.
* Definition of FDA pregnancy categories:
A Controlled studies in women fail to demonstrate a risk to the fetus in the first trimester and the possibility of fetal harm appears remote.
B Either animal-reproduction studies have not demonstrated a fetal risk but there are no controlled studies in pregnant women or animal-reproduction studies have shown an adverse effect that was not confirmed in controlled studies in the first trimester.
C Either studies in animals have revealed adverse effects on the fetus and there are no controlled studies in women or studies in women and animals are not available. Drugs should only be given if the potential benefit justifies the potential risk to the fetus.
D There is positive evidence of human fetal risk, but the benefits from use in pregnant women may be acceptable despite the risk.

erythromycin, and tobramycin. Erythromycin crosses the placenta but in concentrations too low to treat most pathogens. Data are not available on placental transfer of the new macrolides. Many of the studies on which values for placental transfer of drugs are derived were performed on cord blood, involve very small numbers and did not control for gestational age or time of administration, explaining in part the wide variation seen. Drug levels within umbilical cord blood may not represent the true levels in either the fetal vascular nor extravascular compartments.

Differences in fetal drug concentrations of certain antibiotics may in part be explained by differences in protein binding. Levels of highly protein bound antibiotics tend to be considerably lower in fetal serum that in maternal serum. Dicloxacillin (96% protein bound) crosses poorly, while ampicillin (20% protein bound) reaches high levels in the fetus.

Predicting with any accuracy the pharmacokinetics of a drug within the fetus is difficult because of the multiple variables involved (Mucklow 1986). Only unionized drug can traverse the lipid biological membrane. The degree of drug ionization is determined by the intrinsic properties of the drug (pK_a) and the pH of the medium. Fetal blood is relatively acidic (pH 7.25, compared with 7.45 in maternal blood), resulting in more unionized drug in the fetal circulation. There are more red cells per unit volume in fetal blood to take up drug and there are differences in serum proteins which affect drug binding. Fetal albumin concentrations rise as pregnancy progresses. Before 30 weeks of gestation, very little adipose tissue is available to take up lipid-soluble drugs. In the fetal circulation, up to 40% of the umbilical blood bypasses the fetal liver via the ductus venosus and, as a result, drug may not be metabolized by hepatic enzymes before it reaches fetal tissues. While the fetal liver probably does possess many of the metabolic capabilities of the adult liver, certain enzyme pathways are immature. The excretion of drugs by the fetal kidney is decreased; aminoglycoside antibiotics and penicillins are cleared slowly, and potentially may accumulate after repeated doses.

The major route for drug transfer to the amniotic fluid is via the living fetus. Water-soluble drugs are excreted in the fetal urine. Lipid-soluble compounds may diffuse directly across the fetal membranes. Peak fetal serum levels occur 1 to 3 h later than the maternal peak. Peak levels in amniotic fluid are reached later still, reflecting delays in fetal excretion. For ampicillin, amniotic fluid concentrations reach 20% of the maternal serum and peak in about 8 h, but for gentamicin, levels in the amniotic fluid may exceed maternal serum concentration. Drug molecules in the amniotic fluid may be ingested by the fetus and reabsorbed from the gastro-intestinal tract, further complicating the estimate of fetal drug exposure.

The placental transmission of antimicrobial agents has been thoroughly reviewed by Charles (1993a).

Excretion into breast milk

Adverse effects associated with maternal antibiotic use while breast feeding are uncommon, although the evidence for the safety of drugs in this setting has been determined by anecdotal evidence rather than by carefully controlled long-term studies. As a general rule, the concentration of antimicrobial agents in breast milk is so low that harmful effects are unlikely to occur.

Most drugs are transferred into breast milk by simple diffusion; active secretion is uncommon (Wilson et al 1980). Factors influencing the concentration of antibiotics in breast milk include maternal serum concentration of unbound drug, water and lipid solubility, degree of ionization, serum- and milk-binding capability and molecular weight of the antibiotic (Rivera–Calimlim 1987).

Rather than being produced and stored in the breast between feedings, milk is formed as the infant suckles. The fat content of milk is affected by the maternal diet and varies with the infant feeding pattern and time of day. Drugs with a high lipid solubility tend to accumulate in milk, but the concentration of drugs with low lipid solubility, e.g. penicillin, is low.

The protein content of milk falls rapidly during the first week postpartum, but mature milk shows little diurnal or feed-to-feed variation in protein content. Drugs that are highly serum protein bound do not achieve high concentrations in milk. Milk has a lower protein content than plasma and milk protein binds drug less avidly that does plasma protein. There are no data pertaining to antibiotic concentrations in the colostrum. Because blood flow and permeability are increased during the colostral phase, drug concentrations may be increased.

Only the non-ionized fraction of the unbound antibiotic will diffuse across the lipid membrane to enter the alveolar membrane where milk is formed. The pH of breast milk is generally lower than maternal plasma; a range of 6.35–7.65 (average 7.08) is cited. Drugs that are weak bases, such as erythromycin, trimethoprim and tetracyclines, ionize and concentrate in milk, whereas weak acids, such as ampicillin, do not. In general, the concentrations of metronidazole, sulfonamides and trimethoprim in breast milk are similar to those in maternal serum, whereas those of chloramphenicol, erythromycin and tetracycline are approximately 50–75%. Available data suggest that the β-lactam antibiotics and aminoglycosides achieve a low maximum concentration in milk (Sáez-Llorens & McCracken 1995).

Recommendations on the use of drugs in breast feeding are provided (Committee on Drugs 1994) and summarized in Table 57.3. For most antibiotics breast feeding is safe. As a general guideline, if an antibiotic is safe to administer to an infant, it is safe to administer to a lactating women. Chloramphenicol should be avoided and drugs metabolized by glucose-6-phosphate dehydrogenase (G-6-PD) should be used with caution where a possibility of enzyme deficiency exists. Ciprofloxacin and ofloxacin are excreted into breast milk in concentrations similar to those found in plasma, and the drug is likely to be well absorbed from the neonatal gastro-intestinal tract. Because the quinolones have been shown to cause permanent lesions of the cartilage of weight-bearing joints, as well as other signs of arthropathy in immature animals, breast-feeding during quinolone therapy is not recommended.

The oral availability of gentamicin and vancomycin is poor and any drug that is excreted into breast milk is unlikely to be absorbed. Neonatal serum levels of gentamicin can, however, be detected but are too low to be either therapeutically useful or toxic.

In theory, an infant could develop bacterial resistance to an antimicrobial agent by receiving subtherapeutic dose in maternal milk, but in practice no known cases of therapeutic failure caused by lactational exposure have occurred. There are case reports of antibiotic-associated colitis developing in an infant as a consequence of exposure to antibiotics in breast milk, but a causal effect has not always been convincingly demonstrated.

Safety of antibiotics used in pregnancy

No antimicrobial agent currently available has been positively implicated as a human teratogen. Some drugs are clearly associated with serious fetal abnormalities. The precise stage of embryonic development when the fetus is exposed to a drug is important in determining the extent

Table 57.3 *Antibiotic use and breast feeding*

Drug	Recommendation	Comments
Aminoglycosides and vancomycin	Compatible with breast feeding	Poorly absorbed through infant's gastro-intestinal mucosa; theoretical potential for ototoxicity
Chloramphenicol	Not recommended	Possible idiosyncratic bone marrow suppression
Isoniazid	Compatible with breast feeding	Toxic effects have not been reported. Potential for hepatotoxicity. Because pyridoxine deficiency in the neonate can cause seizures and breast milk has relatively low levels of pyridoxine, infants should probably receive supplemental pyridoxine
Metronidazole	Effect on nursing infant unknown, but may be of concern	Some experts recommend that because the drug is mutagenic in vitro breast feeding be discontinued when therapy is given to the mother
Quinolones (ciprofloxacin, norfloxacin, ofloxacin)	Not recommended	Theoretically may affect cartilage development of weight-bearing joints
Tetracycline	Usually compatible with breast feeding, since absorption of drug is negligible	Some recommend that its use be avoided, if possible, because of the potential for dental staining in the infant's unerupted teeth
Sulfonamides (including dapsone)	Usually compatible with breast feeding	Risk of kernicterus if the infant is premature, ill or jaundiced; haemolysis with G-6-PD deficiency
Nalidixic acid, nitrofurantoin,	Usually compatible with breast feeding	Haemolysis in infant with G-6-PD deficiency
Penicillins and cephalosporins	Compatible with breast feeding	Development of hypersensitivity though exposure to the minute quantities of penicillin ingested by a neonate is probably more theoretical than actual concern

G-6-PD, glucose-6-phosphate dehydrogenase.

and nature of the teratogenic effect. The time of maximum susceptibility of the human fetus extends from implantation to the completion of organogenesis by 12 weeks of pregnancy, but the potential for causing defects in limb formation extends to the end of the first trimester.

An estimate of the risk to the fetus assigned to various antibiotics is included in Table 57.2, using the definitions provided by the US Food and Drug Administration (see the footnote to the table for explanation). Briggs et al (1995) provide a thorough description of the available evidence for the safety of individual drugs.

There are no known or suspected teratogenic effects associated with the use of the penicillins and cephalosporins. Although for many of the newer penicillins and cephalosporins there are no data on their use in pregnancy, animal studies have not demonstrated any developmental toxicity and these agents are expected to be safe. Erythromycin base has been safely used in pregnancy; erythromycin estolate, however, has been associated with subclinical but reversible hepatotoxictiy in 10–15% of women given the drug in late pregnancy and its use is not recommended.

Available data have produced conflicting conclusions on the safety of metronidazole in pregnancy. Although the drug is mutagenic in bacteria and carcinogenic in rodents, these properties have never been shown in humans. The drug is not an animal teratogen. Several studies, case reports and reviews have described the safe use of metronidazole during pregnancy. Overall, no association with congenital malfor-

mations, abortions or stillbirths was found although some investigators have suggested that the risk of an adverse outcome is increased when the agent is used in early pregnancy.

Tetracyclines are contraindicated in pregnancy. Tetracycline forms a complex with calcium orthophosphate and is incorporated into growing bones and teeth undergoing calcification. It is this complex which is responsible for the brown discolouration observed in deciduous teeth if tetracycline is given in the second half of pregnancy. Tetracycline has been shown to cause inhibition of fibula growth in premature infants but is not known to be teratogenic. Large doses of intravenous tetracycline have resulted in fatal hepatotoxicity in a pregnancy.

Ototoxicity has been described in infants whose mothers were treated with streptomycin. Kanamycin use has also been reported to have caused ototoxicity in infants exposed to the drug in utero. No cases have been reported in association with gentamicin, tobramycin or amikacin, although, because all the aminoglycosides are ototoxic drugs, a theoretical potential for side-effects exists. There is no evidence that in utero exposure to vancomycin is associated with auditory nerve damage, although again this is possible. It is prudent to monitor maternal serum levels of these potentially ototoxic drugs and ensure that levels remain in the therapeutic range.

Although a lack of dietary folate has been associated with neural tube defect and supplementation is recommended before conception and during early pregnancy, no congenital abnormalities have been observed in association with antibiotics whose mechanism of action is by interfering with bacterial folate synthesis, e.g. trimethoprim and pyrimethamine. Supplemental folic acid should be administered when these drugs are used but will not interfere with the antibacterial activity of the drug.

The greatest concern with sulfonamide use during pregnancy is when the drug is given close to delivery. Particularly with the long-acting agents, significant levels may persist in the newborn for the first several days of life. The sulfonamides compete with bilirubin for binding to plasma albumin. Unbound bilirubin can diffuse across the blood–brain barrier and may result in kernicterus. Because sulfonamides are teratogenic in some species of animals, human teratogenicity has been suspected, but not confirmed. With the sulfonamides and most antimalarials, haemolytic anaemia may occur with glucose-6-phosphate deficiency.

Chloramphenicol is now rarely the drug of choice for the treatment of infection. Its use during pregnancy is usually avoided because of potential haematological toxicity. The drug is not known to cause congenital defects. Although there are no reports of an increased risk of malformations or musculoskeletal problems associated with the use of the quinolones during the first trimester of pregnancy, these agents are relatively contraindicated in pregnancy, but probably could be safely used where they were clearly the drug of choice (Berkovitch et al 1994).

Our limited knowledge of the behaviour of antimicrobial agents in the pregnant woman and the fetus makes it difficult to provide evidence-based guidelines on the use and safety of drugs in pregnancy. As general principles, however, unnecessary drug use should always be avoided, particularly in the first trimester of pregnancy. Presumptive therapy for a possible infection is rarely indicated and for some infections treatment may be safely delayed. Where there is clinical or microbiological evidence of infection and effective treatment is indicated, the safest but most appropriate antibiotic regimen should be chosen. The route of administration and dose will be determined by the severity of the infectious process; levels of potentially toxic drugs, e.g. aminoglycosides, should be monitored. In any decision to use antimicrobial agents during pregnancy it must be assumed that serious, uncontrolled infection will always be a greater threat to mother and child than the possibility of an adverse drug event.

Specific therapeutic problems in pregnancy and childbirth

Comprehensive reviews of the epidemiology, pathogenesis,

diagnosis and treatment of infections in pregnancy and childbirth can be found in texts such as Charles (1993b) and Pastorek (1994). Infections in the fetus and newborn infant are dealt with exhaustively by Remington & Klein (1995).

CHORIOAMNIONITIS AND INTRA-AMNIOTIC INFECTION

Clinically evident intra-amniotic infection is associated with maternal fever and tachycardia, fetal tachycardia, uterine tenderness, foul odour of the amniotic fluid and maternal leucocytosis, although few patients show all these signs and symptoms. The number of vaginal examinations, internal fetal monitoring and duration of ruptured membranes and labour have been identified as risk factors for infection. An increased caesarean section rate, increased perinatal mortality and increased risk of neonatal sepsis occur as complications. Subclinical chorioamnionitis is much more common. The frequent finding of histological chorioamnionitis and recovery of microorganisms from amniotic fluid in association with preterm labour and preterm rupture of membranes provide evidence of a role for infection in preterm birth.

Most intra-amniotic infection occurs by the ascending route when organisms colonizing the lower genital tract cross either intact or ruptured membranes. Less commonly, infection can be haematogenous, e.g. *Listeria*, or bacteria may be introduced during an invasive procedure. While some of the organisms present in the lower genital tract are clearly recognized as pathogens, e.g. *Neisseria gonorrhoeae* and *Chlamydia trachomatis*, infection is most commonly polymicrobial and involves the indigenous cervicovaginal flora. Anaerobes, mycoplasmas, *Gardnerella vaginalis*, group B streptococci and aerobic Gram-negative rods are the most common organisms associated with intra-amniotic infection.

While Gram stain and culture of amniotic fluid can confirm the diagnosis of clinically evident intra-amniotic infection, most antibiotic decisions are made empirically. A combination of ampicillin and gentamicin has been proven safe and effective. While an argument can be made for including an agent with anaerobic activity, e.g. clindamycin or metronidazole, comparative studies have yet to show this is associated with an improved outcome. Antibiotic treatment should be initiated as soon as the diagnosis is made; delaying therapy until after delivery is associated with an increased rate of neonatal sepsis (Gibbs et al 1988).

There is evidence from randomized trials that antibiotic treatment of preterm labour with ruptured membranes delays delivery and reduces maternal and neonatal infection, although no reduction in perinatal mortality has been demonstrated (Mercer & Arheart 1995). No single regimen seems preferable. Amoxicillin, ampicillin and erythromycin have been most often studied; a broad-spectrum regimen of ampicillin, gentamicin and clindamycin has also been evaluated. Despite the association of subclinical intra-amniotic infection with preterm birth, studies have shown an inconsistent effect of antibiotics for preterm labour with intact membranes (Romero 1993, Norman 1994) and at present a general recommendation about their use in this setting cannot be made. Antibiotic therapy is not ordinarily indicated for prolonged ruptured membranes at term unless maternal fever supervenes.

C. trachomatis, N. gonorrhoeae, Trichomonas vaginalis, Mycoplasma hominis, Ureaplasma urealyticum and group B streptococci have been implicated in preterm birth, but because of the difficulty controlling for sociodemographic variables and multiple infections, the association of a specific infection with an adverse pregnancy outcome is unclear. Certain of these microorganisms, however, are transmitted to the infant during delivery. Neonatal conjunctivitis is a consequence of maternal infection with *N. gonorrhoeae* or *C. trachomatis* and maternal colonization is a risk factor for group B streptococcal infection (see below for treatment recommendations).

Vaginal colonization with the genital mycoplasmas *U. urealyticum* and *M. hominis* is common, but the pathogenic potential of these organisms is unclear. There is an association between chorioamnionitis and the isolation of *M. hominis* but most amniotic fluids that are positive for *M. hominis* also contain more virulent bacteria. Endometritis with isolation of *M. hominis* from the bloodstream is recognized as a cause of postpartum fever; treatment with tetracycline, erythromycin or clindamycin is sometimes indicated, although most infections settle without therapy. *U. urealyticum* is associated with preterm labour and low birth-weight; erythromycin treatment of maternal infection, however, does not influence neonatal outcomes (Eschenbach et al 1991). Antibiotic therapy for infertility or to prevent spontaneous abortion associated with mycoplasma infections is not justified. *U. urealyticum* can cause pneumonia in newborn infants, particularly those born prior to 34 weeks gestation, and is associated with an increased risk of chronic lung disease of prematurity. Therapy with erythromycin is indicated in clinically ill neonates (Cassell et al 1993).

In bacterial vaginosis, a common vaginal infection in women of child-bearing age, there is an alteration in the normal flora of the genital tract, characterized by replacement of lactobacilli with anaerobes and *G. vaginalis*. Evidence is accumulating that bacterial vaginosis is associated with chorioamnionitis and preterm birth. In the non-pregnant patient, oral metronidazole is the drug of choice. Oral clindamycin, intravaginal clindamycin cream and intravaginal metronidazole preparations are safe and effective alternatives in pregnancy. Asymptomatic bacterial vaginosis is common, but currently there is no evidence to support screening of pregnant patients for this infection.

ANTIBIOTIC PROPHYLAXIS AND CAESAREAN SECTION

The risk of infection after both emergency and elective caesarean section is substantial. The risk of infection after caesarean section is increased with prolonged rupture of the membranes and length of labour. Although serious complications are uncommon in women undergoing elective caesarean section, up to 10% may develop a wound infection and the incidence of fever or endometritis is similar to that in the group undergoing emergency caesarean section. There is strong evidence from randomized trials (Smaill 1994a) that antibiotic prophylaxis will reduce the incidence of fever or endometritis (odds ratio 0.30; CI 0.27–0.34), wound infection (odds ratio 0.38; CI 0.31–0.45) and serious infection, e.g. pelvic abscess, peritonitis or septicaemia (odds ratio 0.24; CI 0.19–0.30). Data from trials of antibiotic prophylaxis for elective caesarean sections confirm that prophylaxis is also of benefit in this population, albeit at lower risk of infectious complications (Smaill 1992).

Infections following caesarean section are either wound infections, from which *Staphylococcus aureus* may be isolated, or associated with endometritis, when Gram-negative aerobes and anaerobes predominate. Any antibiotic with activity against at least some of the potential pathogens has been shown to be better than placebo in reducing infection. No particular regimen is clearly superior; a cephalosporin such as cefazolin is cheap and effective and appropriate as a standard regimen. My own policy is to administer a single dose of intravenous cefazolin 1 g. Unless treating infection already present at the time of caesarean section, no more than one dose is required. There is some evidence that antibiotics with a broader spectrum of activity may be more efficacious. The results of a meta-analysis have shown a trend towards an improved outcome with a second- or third-generation cephalosporin compared with cefazolin (odds ratio for fever or endometritis 0.82; CI 0.67–1.02), but the available evidence does not warrant the routine use of these more expensive, broad-spectrum agents.

Principles of surgical prophylaxis have established that the maximum concentration of antibiotic should be present in the tissues when the incision is made. It is my recommendation that antimicrobial prophylaxis for caesarean section, as with all other surgical procedures, be given in a timely fashion prior to or with the induction of anaesthesia. A theoretical argument is often made for delaying administration until after the cord has been clamped to avoid exposure of the baby to antibiotics, but there is no good evidence to support this widespread practice.

POSTPARTUM INFECTIONS

Caesarean section is the major risk factor for the

development of postpartum endometritis. With prolonged labour and ruptured membranes, large numbers of bacteria are introduced into the endometrial cavity. Following caesarean section, these bacteria in surgically traumatized and devitalized tissue can overwhelm local host defences and infection may become established.

Infection is usually caused by organisms that are indigenous to the cervicovaginal flora. Changes in the vaginal flora, with an increase in the concentration of anaerobes (in particular *Bacteroides* spp. and *Prevotella* spp.) occur in the puerperium. Most postpartum endometritis is associated with group B streptococci, enterococci, other aerobic streptococci, *G. vaginalis*, *Escherichia coli*, *Prevotella bivia*, other *Bacteroides* spp. and peptostreptococci. Infection occurring within the first 24 h is more likely to be due to aerobic organisms; after 3 days a mixed anaerobic infection is more common. *Clostridium perfringens* is rarely isolated from endocervical cultures and is infrequently responsible for postpartum endometritis. Fulminant infections with this organism are rare, but the signs of clostridial myonecrosis (gas gangrene, hyperbilirubinaemia, disseminated intravascular coagulation, hypotension and oliguria) must alert the physician to prompt surgical intervention.

The presence of fever, lower abdominal pain, uterine tenderness and leucocytosis suggest the diagnosis of endometritis. There may be signs of a wound infection. Genital tract cultures are rarely of value in confirming infection in patients with endometritis because obtaining a satisfactory specimen without contamination from the lower genital tract is difficult. Unless blood cultures are positive or a fluid collection can be aspirated under sterile conditions, decisions regarding antibiotic therapy need to be made empirically. Most cases are polymicrobial. Although there is evidence that the initial regimen should include anti-anaerobic activity, evidence from randomized trials has not established the most effective regimen. Appropriate initial regimens include clindamycin and gentamicin, a combination of ampicillin, gentamicin and metronidazole, or cefotetan. In this patient population, there is generally no contraindication to the safe and effective use of an aminoglycoside. Studies of single-agent therapy, e.g. pipericillin, cefotaxime, imipenem and ticarcillin–clavulanic acid, have not demonstrated an advantage of these broad-spectrum agents over standard regimens, although many of the studies have lacked the power to detect small differences in outcome. Knowledge of local bacterial resistance patterns, the usual infecting organisms and cost of the alternative regimens should be used to establish guidelines for the appropriate initial therapy of postpartum endometritis.

A rapid clinical response is usual; intravenous therapy continued for 24–48 h after the patient becomes afebrile is adequate and in most cases further treatment with oral antibiotics is not necessary. Failure of the initial antimicrobial therapy may be due to failure to treat a significant pathogen, e.g. *Enterococcus* spp. or *Staph. aureus* or the presence of a focal collection, e.g. wound or pelvic abscess, that requires formal drainage.

Although infection with group A streptococci is an uncommon cause of maternal morbidity, there are reports that serious infections with a virulent strain of *Streptococcus pyogenes*, associated with a toxic-shock-like syndrome, are increasing in frequency (Ch. 41). These strains retain their susceptibility to penicillin, although for serious infections clindamycin is advocated and there is some evidence that intravenous immunoglobulin may be beneficial. The organism occasionally is cultured from the lower genital tract of asymptomatic women, but strains that cause severe infections are usually acquired nosocomially.

Other infectious causes of puerperal fever include mastitis, urinary tract infection and septic pelvic thrombophlebitis. Septic pelvic thrombophlebitis rarely occurs as a complication of puerperal endometritis. Bacteria introduced into the endometrial cavity gain access to the vascular system and injure the vascular endothelium. Thrombogenesis is accentuated by the hypercoagulable state in pregnancy and the marked venous stasis that occurs in the pelvic vasculature after delivery. Infection presents either with the acute onset of spiking fevers and severe, localized abdominal pain or subacutely with persisting fever despite appropriate antibiotic therapy. Sometimes an ultrasound scan will demonstrate the thrombus, but usually investigations help exclude an alternative cause, e.g. abscess on computer tomography. Empirical anticoagulation with defervescence within 24–48 h may be the only way to establish the diagnosis.

Puerperal mastitis presents with breast tenderness, chills and fever. *Staph. aureus* is the most common causative organism, although infection with coagulase-negative staphylococci, group A and group B streptococci and *Haemophilus influenzae* is recognized. Antibiotic therapy, guided by the results of Gram stain and culture of expressed milk, should be promptly initiated. A penicillinase-resistant penicillin or first-generation cephalosporin is usually appropriate initial therapy and safe with continued breast feeding. If an abscess is confirmed, incision and drainage are necessary.

The management of abortion-related infection has been reviewed by Stubblefield & Grimes (1994). Infection is usually polymicrobial and derived from the normal flora of the genital tract with the important addition of sexually transmitted organisms including *N. gonorrhoeae* and *C. trachomatis*. Choosing the best empirical regimen may be difficult. An antibiotic regimen suitable for treating postpartum endometritis, e.g. ampicillin, gentamicin and metronidazole, is in general adequate, but the addition of doxycycline or use of a regimen that includes a drug with some activity against *C. trachomatis*, e.g. clindamycin, may be necessary. If penicillinase-producing *N. gonorrhoeae* is suspected, the regimen should be modified to include a third-generation cephalosporin, e.g. ceftriaxone, or a quinolone.

Group B streptococcal infections

Group B streptococci (GBS) are part of the normal vaginal flora and colonize the lower genital tract of up to 30% of women. The rate of vertical transmission from a colonized mother to her infant during delivery is approximately 50%. Rates for neonatal group B streptococcal disease are approximately 2/1000 to 3/1000 live births, but show considerable geographic variation, making the establishment of universal guidelines for the prevention of disease difficult. The risk of early-onset streptococcal disease is increased in premature and low-birth-weight babies, and in those pregnancies complicated by prolonged rupture of membranes, fever or chorioamnionitis. These groups have been targeted for prophylaxis (Box 57.1).

Attempting to eradicate maternal colonization with GBS antenatally is unsuccessful. The effect of antibiotics is transient and by the time of delivery most women are again culture positive. The lower gastro-intestinal tract is the likely reservoir for GBS. Evidence from randomized trials has, however, confirmed that intrapartum administration of antibiotics to pregnant women colonized with GBS is effective and will reduce infant colonization and infection (Smaill 1994b).

Intravenous ampicillin (2 g initially followed by 1–2 g every 4–6 h) or penicillin G (5 million units every 6 h) until delivery is recommended. Amstey & Gibbs (1994) suggest that the pharmacokinetics and spectrum of activity of penicillin may make it the better choice. Intravenous clindamycin (300–600 mg 8-hourly) or erythromycin (500 mg to 1 g 6-hourly) are alternatives in penicillin-allergic women. Chlorhexidine disinfection of the vagina during labour has been studied and warrants further evaluation (Burman et al 1992).

Despite the publication of guidelines from august bodies for the prevention of GBS infections in the newborn, the optimum strategy for maternal chemoprophylaxis is unknown. Three alternative strategies have been recommended:

Box 57.1 *Obstetric risk factors for which intrapartum chemoprophylaxis for group B streptococci is recommended*

- Preterm labour (<37 weeks gestation)
- Term labour (≥37 weeks gestation)
  - Prolonged rupture of membranes. Chemoprophylaxis should be given if labour is likely to continue beyond 18 h (neonatal benefits are optimally achieved if antibiotics are given at least 4 h prior to delivery)
  - Maternal fever during labour (>38°C orally)
- Previous delivery of a newborn with GBS, regardless of current GBS colonization status
- Previously documented GBS bacteriuria

1. Universal screening of all pregnant women at 26–28 weeks gestation and intrapartum chemoprophylaxis of GBS colonized women with identified risk factors (Box 57.1)
2. No universal screening but intrapartum chemoprophylaxis for all women with identified risk factors (Box 57.1)
3. Performance of a rapid antigen test and culture for GBS during labour in women with identified risk factors and chemoprophylaxis for women whose rapid test or culture is positive.

There are difficulties with each one of these options. Maternal colonization can be intermittent, raising concerns about the value of culture early in pregnancy, and unfortunately the sensitivity of rapid antigen tests to detect maternal colonization during labour continues to be disappointing. Whether chemoprophylaxis should only be given to women with identified risk factors has not yet been established. While the risk of neonatal disease is increased in 'at risk' pregnancies, 70% of early onset group B streptococcal disease occurs in term infants, many of whom have no identifiable risk factors. Carefully performed cost-effective analyses have not resolved the issue.

Despite inadequate data on the prevalence of GBS disease in my community, I currently recommend intrapartum chemoprophylaxis to all women with identified risk factors (option 2 above). Neither in my laboratory nor on the labour ward is any rapid screening test performed; the sensitivity of these tests remains too low to justify their use and their cost. Until more information about the best way to collect, transport and process 'screening' cultures done at 26–28 weeks is available, and we can ensure that the results of these cultures are available in a timely fashion at the onset of labour, I do not advocate the option of universal screening.

URINARY TRACT INFECTIONS (Ch. 56)

Asymptomatic bacteriuria complicates 5–8% of all pregnancies. The incidence of asymptomatic bacteriuria in pregnancy is not significantly different from that in non-pregnant women, but without treatment one-third of pregnant women will develop acute pyelonephritis. *Esch. coli* accounts for most urinary tract infections, with other Gram-negative organisms, *Enterococcus faecalis* and GBS making up the rest. Urinary tract infection is associated with premature delivery and low birth weight; effective treatment of asymptomatic bacteriuria reduces these adverse outcomes (Smaill 1994c).

Evidence from randomized trials has confirmed that any one of several antimicrobial agents, e.g. trimethoprim, co-trimoxazole, amoxicillin, nitrofurantoin and cephalexin, is safe and effective for treating urinary tract infection in pregnancy. Although the most appropriate duration of therapy has not been determined, short-course regimens are advocated. For asymptomatic bacteriuria and cystitis, a 3-day course of therapy is adequate in most instances. For women with recurrent infections, continuous prophylaxis with nitrofurantoin 100 mg and regular surveillance cultures are equally effective alternative management strategies.

For the treatment of pyelonephritis, the initial choice of an antimicrobial regimen is usually empirical. Despite the potential toxicity of the aminoglycosides, a combination of gentamicin with ampicillin or a first-generation cephalosporin remains an effective and safe regimen, providing coverage against the most common urinary pathogens. Because of the inherent difficulties of using the aminoglycosides in pregnancy, it is reasonable to modify this regimen when the susceptibility of the organism is known. The second- or third-generation cephalosporins, e.g. cefuroxime or cefotaxime, and the extended-spectrum penicillins, e.g. pipericillin, may be appropriate choices. Parenteral therapy need only be continued until there has been a clinical response. There is limited evidence that for women with pyelonephritis who are perceived as being at low risk of bacteraemia, initiating treatment with oral antibiotics is safe and effective (Angel et al 1990).

LISTERIOSIS

The changes in cell-mediated immunity that occur in pregnancy result in decreased resistance to infection with intracellular organisms, such as *Listeria monocytogenes*. Maternal listeriosis usually presents as an influenza-like illness, but infection may not be recognized until preterm labour ensues. When fever and chills predominate, pyelonephritis may be suspected. Maternal symptoms usually subside quickly, with or without treatment. Listeriosis should be considered when a premature infant develops a septicaemic illness or a full-term infant presents with meningitis.

Listeria spp. are ubiquitous in nature and transient gastro-intestinal carriage is common. While most listeriosis is sporadic, food-borne outbreaks and clusters of perinatal cases have been reported. Most fetal infection occurs by transplacental spread following maternal bacteraemia. Early diagnosis and treatment of *Listeria* sepsis may reduce fetal morbidity and mortality. Maternal blood cultures are often positive. Gram stain and culture of amniotic fluid, if chorioamnionitis is suspected, may quickly confirm the diagnosis.

Although there are no controlled studies of treatment for *L. monocytogenes* infections, a combination of ampicillin and gentamicin is the recommended regimen. *In vitro* studies and an animal model have shown that the aminoglycoside enhances the bactericidal activity of the penicillin, which alone is only bacteriostatic. The cephalosporins have no activity and should never be administered as sole agent if

Listeria infection is suspected. Treatment options for the penicillin allergic pregnant patient are limited. Trimethoprim–sulfamethoxazole is effective but its use is relatively contraindicated as delivery of a preterm infant is a likely consequence of infection. The organism is usually sensitive to erythromycin *in vitro* and use of this drug is an option.

TUBERCULOSIS IN PREGNANCY

This topic is discussed in Ch. 59. It is worth emphasizing that untreated tuberculosis presents a greater threat to the mother and her infant than any antituberculous therapeutic regimen and that none of the first-line drugs are known to be teratogenic. Streptomycin should be avoided because of fetal ototoxicity. Because isoniazid interferes with pyridoxine metabolism and there are increased requirements for this vitamin in pregnant women, pyridoxine supplementation (50 mg/day) should be given. Women taking antituberculous medications can safely breast feed.

Routine isoniazid prophylaxis during pregnancy is controversial. While some physicians prefer to wait until after delivery, others will begin treatment immediately or delay therapy until after the first trimester. Women in the postpartum period may be at increased risk of isoniazid hepatotoxicity and should be closely monitored (Snider & Caras 1992).

SEXUALLY TRANSMITTED DISEASES IN PREGNANCY (Ch. 58)

Erythromycin is used most often to treat chlamydial cervicitis in pregnancy, but some women are unable to complete a therapeutic course because of gastro-intestinal side-effects, specifically nausea and vomiting. Amoxicillin has been recommended as an alternative (Magat et al 1993) but, because of failures with both this regimen and erythromycin, a test of cure is indicated when treating chlamydial infections in pregnancy. Single-dose azithromycin, approved for the treatment of chlamydia cervicitis, has been shown in a small study to be effective for the treatment of chlamydial infections in pregnant patients who cannot tolerate erythromycin (Bush & Rosa 1994), although data on its safety in pregnancy are lacking.

Current treatment regimens for penicillinase-producing strains of *N. gonorrhoeae*, that include ceftriaxone, cefixime and spectinomycin, are safe and effective in pregnancy. Ciprofloxacin, ofloxacin and the tetracyclines, however, should not be administered.

Therapy of syphilis in pregnancy should be with doses of penicillin appropriate to the stage of disease and does not differ from standard treatment regimens. Infection of the fetus may occur at any stage of maternal disease, although it is more likely during primary or secondary infection than in latent or tertiary disease when spirochaetaemia is less. Erythromycin is a second-line drug but, because it is less effective in preventing intrauterine infections, consideration should be given to desensitizing pregnant women with syphilis and penicillin allergy (Wendel at al 1985). Following treatment, maternal non-treponemal serology should be followed monthly for the remainder of the pregnancy; evidence of a rise in titre or absence of a four-fold decline after 3 months requires retreatment. Stoll (1994) comprehensively reviews the management of an infant born to a mother with reactive serological tests for syphilis.

TOXOPLASMOSIS

Acute toxoplasma infection is usually asymptomatic and, without an efficient screening programme, establishing a diagnosis of primary infection during pregnancy is difficult. A rise in maternal immunoglobulin G (IgG) titre or the presence of specific IgM antibody usually indicates acute infection but fetal infection can only be confirmed by the recovery of the parasite from fetal blood or amniotic tissue or, more recently, with a polymerase chain reaction test on amniotic fluid. In the first trimester, although infection is rare, fetal damage is severe. If acute toxoplasmosis is acquired later in pregnancy, there is a greater possibility that the parasite will affect the placenta and spread to the fetus. Treatment of women who acquire toxoplasma infection during pregnancy can reduce the incidence and severity of fetal infection. Although spiramycin will reduce the frequency of maternal transmission, pyrimethamine–sulfadiazine is more effective in treating fetal infection and the use of this combination, with folinic acid supplementation, is recommended if primary maternal infection is confirmed. Alternating the two regimens for the duration of pregnancy has also been advocated. Toxoplasmosis is discussed in more detail in Chapter 63 in which the issue of pregnancy is also discussed, and is reviewed extensively by Wong & Remington (1994).

Although evidence from controlled trials is lacking, it is recommended that infected infants be treated for the first year of life, and there is some support for the concept of routine neonatal screening for subclinical infections with treatment to reduce long-term sequelae (Guerina et al 1994).

VIRAL INFECTIONS

Treatment of primary genital herpes simplex virus (HSV) infections with acyclovir will reduce the severity of symptoms and shorten the duration of viral shedding; prophylaxis with acyclovir will reduce symptomatic recurrences. Although acyclovir has been safely used in pregnancy, experience during the first trimester is very limited. For women with disabling symptoms related to frequent and severe recurrences during pregnancy, prophylactic acyclovir is probably indicated. Viral shedding from the genital tract may occur without visible lesions and despite acyclovir therapy. Infants born to a mother with a history of genital herpes should be observed closely and empirical therapy with acyclovir started if symptoms suggestive of HSV develop. Delivery by caesarean section is only warranted if clinically obvious herpetic lesions are present in labour.

Adults who develop chicken pox may develop severe disease, particularly pneumonia, and in pregnancy the morbidity and mortality from varicella is probably increased. Transplacental transmission of varicella can result in the congenital varicella syndrome, estimated at about 2% following maternal varicella in the first 20 weeks of pregnancy. Oral acyclovir, if started within 24 h of the onset of rash, is recommended for the treatment of adults who develop chicken pox, and pregnant women at any stage of gestation who develop chicken pox should also be offered acyclovir. The adverse effects of acyclovir on fetal development are theoretical, while the maternal morbidity from chicken pox is real. Oral therapy with acyclovir 800 mg five times daily started as soon as possible after the onset of the rash should be adequate, with intravenous treatment reserved for complicated chicken pox or zoster infections. The benefit of therapy begun after 24 h has not been demonstrated and I do not routinely recommend treatment if 3–4 days have elapsed since the onset of rash. For the individual patient the cost of therapy is also a valid factor in the decision to treat.

Congenital cytomegalovirus (CMV) usually occurs after an asymptomatic primary maternal infection which, unless serial antibody levels are obtained, goes undiagnosed. Although the antiviral drugs, ganciclovir and foscarnet have activity against CMV, there is no experience with these agents in pregnancy. Without safe and effective therapies, routine screening for primary maternal CMV infection or fetal infection during pregnancy is not recommended.

Zidovudine is a dideoxynucleoside analogue, with potent inhibitory activity against the HIV reverse transcriptase enzyme. Despite initial concerns about the use of this class of drug in pregnancy, there is good evidence that the use of zidovudine in pregnant women with HIV infection is safe and will reduce perinatal transmission of infection (Connor et al 1994). The most appropriate regimen still has to be determined, but maternal treatment with zidovudine 500 mg/day after the 14th week of pregnancy, intravenous zidovudine during labour and treatment of the newborn infant for the first 6 weeks of life is currently advised. Recommendations advocating routine screening for HIV infection during pregnancy are strengthened by these results.

NEONATAL SEPSIS

The incidence of neonatal sepsis is significantly associated with low birth weight. Mortality is several times higher in infants weighing <1500 g. As a consequence of advances in neonatal care which have resulted in improved survival of low-birth-weight infants, bacterial sepsis and meningitis are frequently encountered clinical problems. The management of these infections is discussed by Klein & Marcy (1995).

Epidemiology

Two patterns of infection, early onset and late onset, are described. Early onset disease presents within the first few days of life as a fulminant, multisystem illness. It is often associated with maternal risk factors, e.g. premature rupture of membranes, chorioamnionitis or maternal fever. Many of the infants are preterm and of low birth weight and mortality is high. Late onset infections are more likely to progress slowly and be associated with focal signs, with meningitis being the most common.

Most of the infecting bacteria associated with neonatal sepsis, both early and late onset, are acquired from the maternal genital tract during delivery. Group B streptococci, *Esch. coli* and *L. monocytogenes* are the likely organisms. Late-onset infection is also associated with organisms that the infant is exposed to in the nursery, neonatal intensive care unit or household. *Staph. aureus*, coagulase-negative staphylococci, enterococci and Gram-negative enteric bacteria may be encountered when infection is acquired in the hospital.

Diagnosis

It is difficult to make the diagnosis of neonatal sepsis from history or clinical findings. The most reliable clinical signs include diminished responsiveness, poor feeding, respiratory distress and changes in peripheral perfusion. If *in utero* infection has occurred, signs may be present at birth. Up to a quarter of infants with bacteraemia will have concurrent meningitis, more in low-birth-weight infants. Infants who present with septicaemia caused by coagulase-negative staphylococci may present with a subacute picture, although some will have symptoms not unlike those with more virulent organisms. The septic work-up should include culture of peripheral venous blood and urine and lumbar puncture with examination of cerebrospinal fluid (CSF). Cultures from superficial sites are unhelpful and do not establish the presence of systemic infection.

Pharmacology of antibiotics in the neonate

The physiological immaturity of enzyme systems in the neonate, the relatively large extracellular fluid volume and rapidly changing renal function affect the pharmacokinetic properties of drugs in the neonate. Deficiency of hepatic glucuronyl transferase in newborns leads to diminished conjugation of chloramphenicol, increasing the accumulation of free drug in serum. The peak serum concentration of aminoglycosides is lower and it takes longer for these drugs to be excreted in neonates than in older infants, thus affecting dosing regimens. Some antibiotics, e.g. sulfonamides and ceftriaxone, can displace bilirubin from albumin-binding sites and potentially increase the risk of kernicterus. Renal function dramatically increases during the first 2 weeks of life, but in the sick neonate is decreased by any condition that reduces renal blood flow, e.g. dehydration, hypoxia or hypotension. Because of these rapid changes in renal function, drug levels may need to be closely monitored in the neonatal period.

Selection of antibiotics

Because of the subtle clinical signs, the rapidity with which infection progresses and the high mortality rate, presumptive antibiotic therapy needs to be started early. Suggested regimens are outlined in Table 57.4. Modification of the initial regimen should be made when culture results are available.

Newborn infants in intensive care units have a high rate of sepsis. Infants can become colonized with resistant organisms, e.g. *Enterobacter cloacae*, and nosocomial transmission of infection can occur. Local knowledge of the likely nosocomial pathogens and their susceptibility patterns will influence the initial empirical regimen. In many units, coagulase-negative staphylococci have assumed a prominent role as nosocomial pathogens. Because coagulase-negative staphylococci are frequent skin contaminants, managing an infant with suspected sepsis whose blood culture is positive for coagulase-negative staphylococci can be difficult.

The duration of therapy is determined by culture results and the response to treatment. If the infant was treated for presumed sepsis but the results of cultures are negative, the infant is well and an ongoing infectious process is not suspected, antibiotics can be stopped. If the mother received intrapartum antibiotics and cultures are negative and the infant remains asymptomatic, antibiotics need not be continued. Otherwise, empirical treatment probably should be continued for 7–14 days, depending on the initial response to therapy. Treatment for focal infection should be longer, e.g. for osteomyelitis a 4-week course is recommended. The minimum duration of treatment for meningitis caused by group B streptococci or Gram-negative enteric bacilli is 21 days.

The relative toxicity of the aminoglycosides and their poor penetration into the CSF make the third-generation cephalosporins attractive for the empirical management of neonatal sepsis. However, the rapid emergence of resistant Gram-negative bacteria when cefotaxime was used has led to

Table 57.4 *Choice of antimicrobial agents for neonatal infection*

Clinical setting	Infecting organisms	Suggested regimen	Comment
Initial therapy for presumed sepsis	Group B streptococcus, *Esch. coli, L. monocytogenes*	Ampicillin and gentamicin	In most circumstances, appropriate for early and late onset disease
	Group B streptococcus	Penicillin or ampicillin (with or without gentamicin)	For meningitis, both ampicillin and gentamicin should probably be continued for 7–10 days (or until CSF is sterile). Routine in vitro testing for penicillin tolerance is not recommended
	L. monocytogenes	Ampicillin and gentamicin	Resistant to cephalosporins
Initial therapy for hospital-acquired sepsis	*Staph. aureus,* coagulase-negative staphylococci, enterococci, Gram-negative enteric bacteria	Cloxacillin or first-generation cephalosporin or vancomycin and gentamicin.	Increased risk of staphylococcal infection with indwelling vascular catheters. Nurseries with MRSA should use vancomycin.
	Coagulase-negative staphylococci e.g. *Staph. epidermidis*	Vancomycin	Some strains (<20%) will be sensitive to cloxacillin; removal of a colonized line may be necessary
	Enterococcal infections (*Ent. faecalis, Ent. faecium*)	Ampicillin or penicillin and aminoglycoside, or vancomycin	Increasingly resistant isolates including vancomycin resistance
Gram-negative meningitis	*Esch. coli, Klebsiella* spp. other Gram-negative enteric bacteria	Third-generation cephalosporin (e.g. cefotaxime), usually combined with an aminoglycoside for first 7–10 days of treatment	The combination of ampicillin and gentamicin remains an acceptable alternative if the isolate is susceptible; ceftazidime or pipericillin with an aminoglycoside for *Pseudomonas* infections
Necrotizing enterocolitis	Gram-negative enteric bacteria, anaerobes, coagulase-negative staphylococci	Ampicillin and gentamicin	Clindamycin or vancomycin may be indicated
Other infections	*Gardnerella vaginalis*	Ampicillin and gentamicin	Susceptibility testing of isolates not standardized
	H. influenzae	Third-generation cephalosporin (ampicillin if β-lactamase negative)	Most strains causing neonatal sepsis are not-typable

CSF, cerebrospinal fluid; MRSA, methicillin-resistant *Staph. aureus.*

recommendations that the use of the third-generation cephalosporins be restricted to proven Gram-negative meningitis and cases where renal failure precludes the use of an aminoglycoside. Although ceftriaxone has been used for the treatment of neonatal infections, limited experience with the drug in this population and concerns about protein binding mean it cannot be recommended for routine therapy in neonatal sepsis (Sáez-Llorens & McCracken 1995).

Vancomycin is well tolerated and can be safely administered to the neonate. Although vancomycin has not clearly been shown to be nephrotoxic, serum levels should be monitored regularly, especially if the drug is administered in

conjunction with an aminoglycoside. With the minimal inflammation seen in ventriculoperitoneal shunt infections, vancomycin concentrations within the CSF are generally low. The management of shunt infections caused by coagulase-negative staphylococci may include direct instillation of vancomycin into the ventricle.

The importance of anaerobic bacteria as a cause of serious neonatal infection is unclear. *Bacteroides fragilis*, resistant to penicillin, seems to be an uncommon pathogen, although clindamycin will be included if an anaerobic infection is suspected, e.g. necrotizing enterocolitis with perforation. Metronidazole has been inadequately evaluated in the neonatal period, in part because of fears of teratogenicity and mutagenicity, and its use probably should be reserved for situations where it is clearly the drug of choice, e.g. in *B. fragilis* meningitis.

In an attempt to overcome the antibody deficiency in newborns, intravenous immunoglobulin (IVIG) has been advocated in the treatment of neonatal sepsis (Hill 1993) although its use has not been uniformly endorsed. There is no evidence that the use of prophylactic IVIG will prevent nosocomial infection in low-birth-weight infants. The use of steroids, granulocyte transfusions or haematopoietic growth factors remains experimental in the management of neonatal sepsis.

OTHER INFECTIONS

Infants with disseminated candida infections may appear clinically identical to those with bacterial sepsis, but the diagnosis is often difficult because blood cultures are frequently negative. In utero infection may result in disseminated pulmonary or mucocutaneous infection, while infection acquired from the infected vagina during birth usually only results in mucocutaneous disease. Risk factors for nosocomial acquisition of systemic fungal infection include prior antibiotic use, indwelling lines and total parenteral nutrition. Amphotericin remains the standard therapy for systemic infection, often combined with 5-flucytosine if there is evidence of central nervous system involvement. Experience with the use of fluconazole in the neonate is limited, but it has been used successfully to treat disseminated *Candida albicans* infections.

Neonatal enteroviral infections may present with a sepsis-like illness, most often noted with coxsackieviruses B2 to B5 and echovirus types 5, 11 and 16. Bacterial infections of the newborn can mimic neonatal HSV infections and presumptive therapy with acyclovir is often initiated pending the outcome of viral cultures.

References

Amstey M S, Gibbs R S 1994 Is penicillin G a better choice than ampicillin for prophylaxis of neonatal group B streptococcal infections? *Obstetrics and Gynecology* 84: 1058

Angel J L, O'Brien W F, Finan M A, Morales W J, Lake M, Knuppel R A 1990 Acute pyelonephritis in pregnancy: a prospective study of oral versus intravenous antibiotic therapy. *Obstetrics and Gynecology* 76: 28–32

Berkovitch M, Pastuszak A, Gazarian M, Lewis M, Koren G 1994 Safety of the new quinolones in pregnancy. *Obstetrics and Gynecology* 84: 535–538

Briggs G G, Freeman R K, Yaffe S J 1995 Drugs in pregnancy and lactation, 4th edn. Williams & Wilkins, Baltimore

Burman L G, Christensen P, Christensen K et al 1992 Prevention of excess neonatal morbidity associated with group B streptococci by vaginal chlorhexidine disinfection during labour. *Lancet* 340: 65–69

Bush M R, Rosa C 1994 Azithromycin and erythromycin in the treatment of cervical chlamydial infection during pregnancy. *Obstetrics and Gynecology* 84: 61–63

Cassell G H, Waites K B, Watson H L et al 1993 *Ureaplasma urealyticum* intrauterine infection: role in prematurity and disease in newborns. *Clinical Microbiology Reviews* 6: 69–87

Charles D 1993a Placental transmission of antimicrobial agents. In Charles D (ed) Obstetric and perinatal infections. Mosby Year Book, St Louis, p 314–324

Charles D (ed) 1993b Obstetric and perinatal infections. Mosby Year Book, St Louis

Chow A W, Jewesson P J 1985 Pharmacokinetics and safety of antimicrobial agents during pregnancy. *Reviews of Infectious Diseases* 7: 287–313

Committee on Drugs 1994 The transfer of drugs and other chemicals into human milk. *Pediatrics* 93: 137–150

Connor E M, Sperling R S, Gelber R et al 1994 Reduction of maternal-infant transmission of human immunodeficiency virus type 1 with zidovudine treatment. *New England Journal of Medicine* 331: 1173–1180

Cummings A J 1983 A survey of pharmacokinetic data from pregnant women. *Clinical Pharmacokinetics* 8: 344–354

Eschenbach D A, Nugent R P, Rao A V et al 1991 A randomized placebo-controlled trial of erythromycin for the treatment of *Ureaplasma urealyticum* to prevent premature delivery. *American Journal of Obstetrics and Gynecology* 164: 734–742

Gibbs R S, Dinsmoor M J, Newton E R, Ramamurthy R S 1988 A randomized trial of intrapartum versus immediate postpartum treatment of women with intra-amniotic infection. *Obstetrics and Gynecology* 72: 823–828

Guerina N G, Hsu H-W, Meissner H C et al 1994 Neonatal serological screening and early treatment for congenital *Toxoplasma gondii* infection. *New England Journal of Medicine* 330: 1858–1863

Hill H R 1993 Intravenous immunoglobulin use in the neonate: role in prophylaxis and therapy of infection. *Pediatric Infectious Disease Journal* 12: 549–558

Klein J O, Marcy S M 1995 Bacterial sepsis and meningitis. In: Remington J S, Klein J O (eds) Infectious diseases of the fetus and newborn infant, 4th edn. W B Saunders, Philadelphia, p 835–890

Ledward R S, Hawkins D F, Stern L 1991 Drug Treatment in Obstetrics, 2nd edn. Chapman & Hall, London

Magat A H, Alger L S, Nagey D A, Hatch V, Lovchik J C 1993 Double-blind randomized study comparing amoxycillin and erythromycin for the treatment of *Chlamydia trachomatis* in pregnancy. *Obstetrics and Gynecology* 81: 745–749

Mercer B M, Arheart K L 1995 Antimicrobial therapy in expectant management of preterm premature rupture of membranes. *Lancet* 346: 1271–1279

Mucklow J C 1986 The fate of drugs in pregnancy. *Clinics in Obstetrics and Gynecology* 13: 161–175

Norman K, Pattinson R C, de Souza J, de Jong P, Moller G, Kirsten G 1994 Ampicillin and metronidazole in preterm labour: a multicentre, randomized controlled trial. *British Journal of Obstetrics and Gynaecology* 101: 404–408

Owen J, Groome L J, Hauth J C 1993 Randomized trial of prophylactic antibiotic therapy after preterm amnion rupture. *American Journal of Obstetrics and Gynecology* 169: 976–981

Pastorek J G II (ed) 1994 Obstetric and gynecologic infectious diseases. Raven, New York

Philipson A 1979 Pharmacokinetics of antibiotics in pregnancy and labour. *Clinical Pharmacokinetics* 4: 297–309

Remington J S, Klein J O (eds) 1995 Infectious diseases of the fetus and newborn infant. W B Saunders, Philadelphia

Rivera-Calimlim L 1987 The significance of drugs in breast milk. *Clinics in Perinatalogy* 14: 51–70

Romero R, Sibai B, Caritis S et al 1993 antibiotic treatment of preterm labor with intact membranes: A multicenter, randomized, double-blinded, placebo-controlled trial. *American Journal of Obstetrics and Gynecology* 169: 764–774

Sáez-Llorens X, McCracken G H 1995 Clinical pharmacology of antibacterial agents. In: Remington J S, Klein J O (eds) Infectious diseases of the fetus and newborn infant, 4th edn. W B Saunders, Philadelphia, p 1287–1336

Smaill F 1992 Antibiotic prophylaxis and caesarean section. *British Journal of Obstetrics and Gynaecology* 99: 789–790

Smaill F 1994a. Prophylactic antibiotics in caesarean section (all trials). In: Enkin M W, Keirse M J N C, Renfrew M J, Neilson J P (ed) Pregnancy and childbirth module. Cochrane database of systematic reviews. 'Cochrane Updates on Disk', Oxford, Update Software, 1994, Disk Issue 1, Review No. 03690, 3 August 1994

Smaill F 1994b Intrapartum antibiotics for group B streptococcal colonization. In: Enkin M W, Keirse M J N C, Renfrew M J, Neilson J P (ed) Pregnancy and childbirth module. Cochrane database of systematic reviews. 'Cochrane Updates on Disk', Oxford, Update Software, 1994, Disk Issue 1, Review No. 03006, 5 October 1994

Smaill F 1994c Antibiotic vs no treatment for asymptomatic bacteriuria. In: Enkin M W, Keirse M J N C, Renfrew M J, Neilson J P (ed) Pregnancy and childbirth module. Cochrane database of systematic reviews. 'Cochrane Updates on Disk', Oxford, Update Software, 1994, Disk Issue 1, Review No. 03170, 22 April 1993

Snider D E Jr, Caras G J 1992 Isoniazid-associated hepatitis deaths: a review of available information. *American Review of Respiratory Disease* 145: 494–497

Stoll B J 1994 Congenital syphilis: evaluation and management of neonates born to mothers with reactive serologic tests for syphilis. *Pediatric Infectious Diseases Journal* 13: 845–853

Stubblefield P G, Grimes D A 1994 Septic abortion. *New England Journal of Medicine* 331: 310–314

Wendel G D, Stark B J, Jamison R B et al 1985 Penicillin allergy and desensitization in serious infections during pregnancy. *New England Journal of Medicine* 312: 1229–1232

Wilson J T, Brown R D, Cherek D R 1980 Drug excretion in human breast milk. *Clinical Pharmacokinetics* 5: 1–66

Wong S-Y, Remington J S 1994 Toxoplasmosis in pregnancy. *Clinical Infectious Diseases* 18: 853–862

Sexually transmitted infections

A. R. O. Miller

Introduction

The sexually transmitted diseases (STDs) are a heterogeneous collection of infectious conditions where the principal (although not exclusive) mode of spread is by sexual contact. Antimicrobial agents play a major part in their treatment and control (Box 58.1), although additional measures such as screening, contact tracing and health education are equally vital. Health education and modification of sexual behaviour play a fundamental role in controlling the spread of the sexually transmitted infections for which chemo-

therapeutic options remain limited (such as human immuno-deficiency virus (HIV) infection). When the last edition of this book was prepared, the use of quinolones and the new macrolides for the treatment of STDs was just beginning and the rapid development of these agents since then has altered practice in many STD clinics.

In the USA, the Centers for Disease Control, Atlanta (CDC) from time to time issues a policy document on the management of STDs and its most recent guidelines were published in 1993 (CDC 1993). No such consensus has ever been established in the UK and individual STD clinics continue to develop their own regimens.

Box 58.1 *Recommended treatments for STDs*

Syphilis
Early syphilis
• Bicillin 2 ml/day i.m. for 10 days (equivalent to procaine penicillin 600 mg/day)
• Doxycycline 300 mg/day orally for 15 days (in penicillin-allergic patients)

Late syphilis with normal lumbar puncture
• Bicillin 2 ml/day i.m. for 15 days
• Doxycycline 300 mg/day orally for 30 days (in penicillin-allergic patients)

Neurosyphilis
• Aqueous benzylpenicillin G 2.4 g i.v. 6-hourly for 15 days
• Ceftriaxone 500 mg/day i.v. for 15 days (in penicillin-allergic patients)

Careful follow-up is mandatory for all patients but is even more important in those who did not receive penicillin or in those who are infected with HIV.

Gonorrhoea
Uncomplicated urethritis, pharyngitis or proctitis
• Azithromycin 1 g orally as a single (supervised) dose
• Cefotaxime 500 mg i.m. as a single dose (followed by doxycycline to eradicate *Chlamydia*)

Disseminated gonococcal infection
• Ceftriaxone 1 g/day i.v. for a few days followed by cefixime 400 mg orally twice daily to complete 7 days treatment (or longer if there was joint involvement)

Non-specific genital infection (and/or confirmed chlamydia urethritis, cervicitis)
• Azithromycin 1 g orally as a single dose
• Doxycycline 100 mg twice daily for 7 days

Box 58.1 *Cont'd*

Pelvic inflammatory disease
- Co-amoxiclav 1.2 g i.v./orally 8-hourly and doxycycline 100 mg orally twice daily for 7–10 days
- Clindamycin 300 mg i.v./orally 6-hourly and doxycycline 100 mg twice daily for 7–10 days

Genital herpes
Acute primary attack
- Acyclovir 200 mg orally five times daily for 5 days

Recurrent attacks
- Acyclovir 400 mg orally twice daily with prodromal symptoms
- Acyclovir 400 mg orally twice daily for long-term suppression

Chancroid
- Azithromycin 1 g orally as a single dose

Vulvovaginitis
Candida
- Fluconazole 150 mg orally as a single dose
- Miconazole 200-mg pessary at night for 3 days

Trichomonas
- Metronidazole 2 g orally as a single dose

Bacterial vaginosis
- Metronidazole 2 g orally as a single dose

Syphilis

Syphilis remains an important STD because of its long term consequences. Recent reports from the USA and UK suggest that the incidence may be falling in the 1990s after a sharp rise seen in the late 1980s (Catchpole 1992, Webster & Rolfs 1993), but there is no room for complacency.

Penicillin remains the drug of choice for all stages of infection and the only indication for alternative therapy is in the patient who is genuinely penicillin allergic. *Treponema pallidum*, the cause of syphilis, cannot be cultured in the laboratory and therefore conventional sensitivity testing cannot be done. However, clinical experience has produced well-validated treatment regimens that are generally effective. Long-term follow-up with serological testing is mandatory to ensure complete cure. There may be slight individual variations between centres depending on the availability of drugs and expertise.

It is appropriate to review the various preparations that are of relevance to the treatment of STDs because considerable confusion continues to surround them. The US literature continues to recommend the use of the long-acting penicillins for the treatment of syphilis, but neither benzathine penicillin nor even benethamine penicillin are now available in UK and the only long-acting preparation still obtainable is bicillin. This is a combination of procaine penicillin 1.8 g and benzylpenicillin 360 mg.

Some references continue to express penicillin doses in units rather than milligrams. One million units (1 mega unit) of aqueous benzylpenicillin G is equivalent to 600 mg.

EARLY SYPHILIS

This is empirically defined as primary or secondary syphilis or latent disease of less than 1 year's duration. The classic work by Idsoe (1972) has shown that *T. pallidum* will be killed by maintaining a serum level of 0.03 μg/l of penicillin for at least 7 days. The level of penicillin must not fall below this for more than 24 h or treponemes will regenerate. This is achieved by a single injection of 2.4 MU of benzathine penicillin, which will provide adequate levels of penicillin for 3–4 weeks (Idsoe 1972). Occasional relapses have been reported with this regimen but are not necessarily indications for changing – they merely emphasize the requirement for scrupulous follow-up (Jorgensen et al 1986, Markovitz et al 1986). This remains the treatment favoured by the CDC, although other US authorities suggest additional dosages (Musher 1988, Tramont 1994).

As discussed above, the long acting penicillins are no longer available in the UK and most clinics would use intramuscular bicillin 2 ml/day for 10 days. This will give a daily dose of 600 mg of procaine penicillin (with a small dose of benzylpenicillin, 120 mg/day). Petersen et al (1984) have shown 600 mg/day of procaine penicillin to be effective, and Dunlop (1985) has argued that this should be the treatment of choice in early syphilis.

This regimen does not produce treponemicidal levels of penicillin in the cerebrospinal fluid (CSF) even with the addition of probenecid (Goh et al 1984) and Lukehart et al's work (1988) has suggested that treponemes penetrate the CSF in early syphilis. They isolated virulent *T. pallidum* (by rabbit inoculation) from the CSF of 12 out of 40 patients with primary or secondary syphilis and found positive CSF serology in four more. This was irrespective of HIV status. These findings question the arbitrary distinction of syphilis into early and late disease and would argue that all patients with syphilis should have a lumbar puncture to exclude neurological involvement.

LATE SYPHILIS

Certainly any patient with syphilis of longer than a year's duration, any evidence of neurological disease or who is HIV seropositive (see below) must have a lumbar puncture. If there is evidence of neurosyphilis then high-dose penicillin therapy is mandatory. The best way to ensure this is to admit the patient to hospital and treat with intravenous benzylpenicillin 2.4 g every 6 h for 2 weeks, but this is an expensive option. It may be acceptable to give a few days of intravenous treatment and then follow up with daily intramuscular therapy (procaine penicillin 2.4 g/day) to complete 2 weeks of treatment. Few trial data are available, although Philcox et al (1987) showed that 1.2 g of procaine penicillin for 20 days was adequate treatment for neurosyphilis. These results have been questioned by Van der Walke et al (1988) following their work on penicillin concentrations in the CSF.

If there is no evidence of neurological infection it seems appropriate to treat late syphilis with procaine penicillin 600 mg/day for a slightly longer period than for early syphilis. Trial data are lacking, but Thin (1989) recommends 15 days and this seems entirely reasonable.

SYPHILIS IN THE PRESENCE OF HIV INFECTION

It seems possible that the immune suppression produced by infection with HIV could alter the natural history and clinical features of infection with *T. pallidum*, and anecdotal case reports would suggest that this may be the case (Johns et al 1987, Hutchinson et al 1991, Katz et al 1993). The CDC (1993) continues to recommend no change in the regimen for individuals co-infected with HIV and syphilis and this approach has been supported by at least one study (Gourevitch et al 1993) but has been questioned by other authors (Corcoran & Ridgeway 1994, Musher & Baughin 1994). Horowitz et al (1994) have described a patient who, despite 10 days of intravenous high-dose penicillin, had clinical (and post mortem) evidence of neurosyphilis 3 years later. Gordon et al (1994) have reported 11 HIV-infected patients with symptomatic neurosyphilis. Five had previously received 2–5 g of benzathine penicillin for treatment of early syphilis. All were treated with high-dose intravenous benzylpenicillin G for 10 days. One patient developed a clinical relapse of neurosyphilis and three others had laboratory evidence of ongoing CSF infection. In the accompanying editorial, Musher & Baughin (1994) comment that these results are not unexpected as penicillin will produce a clinical cure of syphilis rather than complete eradication of infection, and therefore, clinical relapse is prevented by an intact immune system. Once again the answer must lie with determined follow-up and early retreatment for symptomatic or laboratory indication of relapse. Extending the initial treatment is not recommended on present evidence.

SYPHILIS IN THE PENICILLIN ALLERGIC

Penicillin is the preferred therapy for all stages of syphilis and is the only agent with which there is substantial experience. Therefore, any history of penicillin allergy requires careful evaluation. The CDC recommends skin testing and desensitization. The traditional alternative has been tetracycline in divided doses of 2 g/day for 15 or 30 days depending on whether the infection is considered 'early' or 'late'. Doxycycline in a single daily dose of 300 mg may produce better rates of compliance, and Fiumara (1982) has demonstrated its clinical efficacy in early syphilis, although Zenilman et al (1993) have described treatment failure in a 50-year-old HIV-negative female who was allergic to penicillin and who was diagnosed with early latent syphilis. She was treated with oral doxycycline 100 mg twice daily for 2 weeks. Six months later she received a further 30 days of the same treatment because of a persisting positive serological evaluation. After a further month her serology remained positive and a lumbar puncture showed evidence of asymptomatic neurosyphilis. She was desensitized to her penicillin allergy and successfully treated with intravenous penicillin (14.4 g/day for 14 days). Although an anecdotal case report, this does indicate that extreme care should be taken with the use of doxycycline for syphilis.

If tetracycline is contraindicated (e.g. in pregnancy) then erythromycin is usually considered an alternative, although it does not penetrate the blood–brain barrier or cross the placenta well and may be ineffective in treating neurosyphilis.

Third-generation cephalosporins are accepted treatment for bacterial meningitis and it seems reasonable to use them for treating syphilis in the genuinely penicillin allergic. Hook et al (1988) showed that ceftriaxone will cure asymptomatic neurosyphilis, but there remains a paucity of data.

SYPHILIS IN PREGNANCY AND CONGENITAL SYPHILIS

Throughout the developed world it is standard practice that a pregnant woman has a serological test for syphilis as part of her antenatal evaluation. If positive she should be treated with penicillin in a regimen appropriate to her suspected clinical stage. If there is any doubt about the duration of infection then she should have a lumbar puncture. A mother who is penicillin allergic should receive erythromycin but, as noted above, this drug does not cross the placenta effectively. El Tabbakh et al (1994) have described an infant who was congenitally infected despite erythromycin therapy and Pickering (1985) has stressed that infants born to mothers whose syphilis has been treated with erythromycin should receive penicillin soon after birth.

Infection of the fetus in utero is especially likely in the early stages of maternal infection and in the later stages of pregnancy. It is unlikely to occur if the mother receives adequate penicillin therapy during pregnancy, but it has been reported (Mascola et al 1984). If the mother has not received penicillin then the neonate should be treated either with daily intravenous benzylpenicillin 30 mg/kg in two divided doses or daily intramuscular procaine penicillin 50 mg/kg for 10 days (Pickering 1985) (see also Ch. 57).

FOLLOW-UP

Patients who have been treated for early syphilis should have follow-up non-treponemal serology (e.g. Venereal Disease Reference Laboratory) performed at 3, 6 and 12 months after treatment. Retreatment should be considered if the VDRL titre shows a four-fold increase or, having been high, fails to show a four-fold decrease within 12 months. For late syphilis follow-up should be extended for 2 years, and for neurosyphilis the patient should be kept under review for at least 3 years with CSF examinations at 6-month intervals.

EPIDEMIOLOGICAL TREATMENT

Sexual contacts of patients with infectious syphilis have a high chance of developing the disease within 3 months of contact and therefore should receive prophylactic treatment with a regimen appropriate for early syphilis.

JARISCH–HERXHEIMER REACTION

Following antibiotic treatment of syphilis (especially with penicillin which is rapidly treponemicidal) the patient often develops an unpleasant reaction of fever, myalgia, headache and malaise. This reaction is most likely to take place with the treatment of early syphilis, when it may be alarming and unpleasant but not dangerous. In late syphilis it might cause a lesion to enlarge and produce more organ damage, so attempts are often made to reduce the incidence and severity of the reaction with steroids. However, there is little good evidence that they do modify the reaction.

Gonorrhoea

Infection caused by *Neisseria gonorrhoeae* is readily transmitted by sexual contact and may produce disease in several anatomical sites. Its usual presentation is as either urethritis or cervicitis, but it may also infect the rectum and pharynx or become disseminated to cause septicaemia (with or without arthritis).

Although penicillin has traditionally been used to treat gonorrhoea, there has been increasing concern about penicillin resistance. *N. gonorrhoeae* can become resistant to penicillin by a number of mechanisms. Genetic mutation can alter the ribosomes, the envelope proteins or the penicillin binding proteins in the so-called chromosomally mediated resistant organisms (CMRNG). Alternatively, a plasmid transmitted gene can code for the production of a β-lactamase and give rise to penicillinase-producing *N. gonorrhoeae* (PPNG). These were first described by Phillips in 1976 and their mechanisms further defined by Easmon in 1985. There is little evidence that PPNG is becoming endemic in the UK (Sherrard & Barlow 1993). Warren & Phillips (1993) reviewing PPNG at St Thomas' Hospital from 1976 until 1990 concluded that its prevalence had remained stable at about 5% since 1982. Nevertheless, it is no longer common practice to use penicillin preparations for treating gonorrhoea in the UK or the USA. In Australia, the prevalence of penicillin resistance is higher: the Australian Gonococcal Surveillance Programme reported (1993) an 8% prevalence of intrinsic resistance and a 13% incidence of PPNG in 1993. Like Sherrard & Barlow they related PPNG acquisition to overseas travel.

DUAL INFECTION

Many of those infected with *N. gonorrhoeae* will also have acquired infection with *Chlamydia trachomatis* or other infective causes of non-specific genital infection (NSGI). Richmond et al (1980) showed that chlamydia can be recovered from nearly 50% of women with endocervical gonorrhoea and Bradley et al (1980) demonstrated their presence in more than 30% of men with gonococcal urethritis.

The ideal antimicrobial agent would consistently eradicate both *N. gonorrhoeae* and *C. trachomatis* from any anatomical site with a single oral dose, with no side-effects and without being or becoming susceptible to resistance mechanisms. It would also eradicate incubating syphilis, be safe in pregnancy and cheap. Such an agent does not exist, and treatment remains a compromise. It is usual to give single-dose therapy to treat the gonorrhoea, followed by a more prolonged course of an antichlamydial agent. Although the agent used to treat the chlamydia would probably be effective against gonorrhoea as well, it may not be as reliable as the specific antigonococcal agent and there is always concern about patient compliance with a multidosage regimen.

The general trend in the evolution of treatment regimens for gonorrhoea is for a new agent to be used in a high dose (often multidosage) regimen initially; the dosage is then reduced in subsequent trials until the lowest possible dose demonstrating clinical efficacy is derived. Cure rates of less than 95% are not regarded as acceptable.

CHOICE OF AGENT

Many agents are effective in treating *N. gonorrhoeae* in either single or multiple doses and the choice of agent often depends on local habit, availability and cost. The groups of drugs most commonly used are quinolones, cephalosporins and macrolides.

Quinolones

Ciprofloxacin in a single oral dose has been well studied and, although the CDC recommends 500 mg, there are good data to support the use of 250 mg which would produce significant financial savings (Balachandran et al 1992, Otubu et al 1992, Hook et al 1993). These studies have confirmed cure rates in excess of 97%, irrespective of the site of infection and production of penicillinase. Norfloxacin 800 mg (Bogaerts et al 1993), enoxacin 400 mg (Covino et al 1993a), ofloxacin 400 mg (Maiti et al 1991) and fleroxacin 400 mg (Lassus et al 1992) have all demonstrated similar single dose efficacy. Quinolones remain expensive compounds and recently there has been some concern about decreased sensitivity of *N. gonorrhoeae* in vitro (Bogaerts et al 1993, CDC 1994).

Injectable cephalosporins

Ceftriaxone (Ch. 14) has recently been introduced into the UK. The CDC was recommending its use for treating gonorrhoea in 1989 and it remained top of the CDC list in 1993. Hansfield & Hook had shown its efficacy in a single dose of 125 mg i.m. in 1987. Unfortunately, as ceftriaxone is only available in vials of 250 mg, most experience is with

this dosage, but recent studies confirm that its high level of efficacy is maintained at the lower dose (Hook et al 1993, Handsfield et al 1994).

Cefotaxime has very similar activity to ceftriaxone, but lacks the long half-life. Nevertheless, single-dose efficacy was demonstrated by De Konig et al in 1983 (1 g) and by Boakes et al in 1981 (500 mg). Mogabgab & Lutz (1994) have also shown that 500 mg intramuscular cefotaxime is as effective as 250 mg ceftriaxone in treating uncomplicated gonorrhoea and have drawn attention to a 31% cost saving using this regimen. McCormack et al (1993) obtained similar results in a multicentre study of 613 patients comparing 500 mg of cefotaxime with 250 mg ceftriaxone.

It is probable that most of the third-generation injectable cephalosporins would show similar clinical efficacy. Second-generation agents such as cefoxitin and cefuroxime have shown efficacy, but this is usually achieved in combination with probenecid (Miller 1992), an additional complication which we would not now recommend.

Oral cephalosporins

Some clinics prefer to administer intramuscular treatment because compliance is assured and there is no chance of vomiting or incomplete absorption. However, many clinics and patients prefer oral treatment and there is considerable experience with oral cephalosporins. Oral cefuroxime axetil 1 g is certainly effective, and in a recent trial produced a 98% cure rate (Kinghorn et al 1992). Third-generation oral cephalosporins are also useful. Oral cefixime 400 mg as single dose is recommended by the CDC (1993). Large studies of its use in a single dose of 400 or 800 mg support this recommendation (Handsfield et al 1991, Portilla et al 1992, Dunnett & Moyer 1992). Verdon et al (1993) showed 95% efficacy in eradicating rectal or urethral gonorrhoea in 125 subjects (mainly men) with a single dose of 200 mg cefixime, although they remain reluctant to recommend this dosage for routine use. Cefpodoxime proxetil is equally effective and is recommended by the CDC in a dose of 200 mg, although a recent dose ranging study demonstrated equal clinical efficacy with a single dose of 50 mg (Novak et al 1992). All these oral cephalosporin regimens have been very well tolerated and can be used in pregnancy. There are few data on their effect on incubating syphilis and they would not be expected to have a significant effect on chlamydia.

Macrolides

Erythromycin has long been used as a second-line treatment for non-specific genital infection (NSGI) but has not been reliably effective against gonorrhoea since the mid-1970s and is no longer regarded as appropriate therapy. However, the new macrolides (and closely related azalide compounds) do have useful activity against chlamydia and gonorrhoea.

Azithromycin (Ch. 27) has been particularly well studied (Steingrimsson et al 1992). Waugh (1993) treated 118 patients who had culture-proven *N. gonorrhoeae* infection with a single dose of azithromycin 1 g. Bacteriological eradication was confirmed in 93% of those with urethritis and all those (small numbers) with cervical, pharyngeal or rectal infection. Proven co-existing chlamydial infection in 22 subjects was eradicated by this regimen. Handsfield et al (1994), unhappy with the results of the single 1 g dosage, have recently evaluated a 2 g dose, with 98.9% eradication of *N. gonorrhoeae*, irrespective of anatomical site or penicillinase production. However, they reported a 35.5% incidence of gastro-intestinal side-effects, much higher than the incidence previously reported with the 1 g dosage.

Steingrimsson et al (1994) have subsequently shown that 1 g of azithromycin in a single dose is as effective as 7 days of doxycycline in treating gonorrhoea or NSGI. Side-effects were reported as negligible and they achieved a 96% success rate in eradicating *N. gonorrhoeae*. Similar results (95% cure) were achieved in West Africa by Odugbemi et al (1993).

There are no data on the use of azithromycin in pregnancy. There is no evidence of animal teratogenicity, and it is likely to be safe for mother and fetus, but its efficacy may be reduced and therefore follow-up should be even more scrupulous (Handsfield et al 1994).

It would be reasonable to recommend 1 g azithromycin in a single dose as the treatment of choice for uncomplicated gonorrhoea infections, irrespective of the anatomical site. The drug could be taken under supervision to ensure compliance. Any of the quinolone or cephalosporin treatments must be followed by a course of doxycycline.

Disseminated gonococcal infection is relatively rare and no centre has major experience. It seems sensible to follow the CDC guidelines, and we recommend treatment with an injectable third-generation cephalosporin (cefotaxime 1 g every 8 h or ceftriaxone 1 g every 24 h). Once the patient is improving clinically, therapy is continued with an oral third-generation cephalosporin (e.g. cefixime 400 mg every 12 h) or a quinolone (ciprofloxacin 500 mg every 12 h) to complete a week's total course.

Non-specific genital infection

Non-specific genital infection (NSGI) includes urethritis, mucopurulent cervicitis and proctitis not caused by *N. gonorrhoeae*. The majority of cases are caused by *C. trachomatis*. The next most commonly associated organism is *Ureaplasma urealyticum* (previously known as 'genital mycoplasma'). Some of the remaining cases are caused by herpes simplex virus or *Trichomonas vaginalis*, and in a

significant proportion of cases no initiating organism is identified. *C. trachomatis* (and possibly some of the other listed organisms) can also cause pelvic inflammatory disease (PID), urethral syndrome and perihepatitis (Miller 1992). Chlamydial infection is often acquired simultaneously with gonorrhoea.

A definitive microbiological diagnosis of *C. trachomatis* infection is becoming increasingly available in STD clinics, but rarely alters the clinical management. A diagnosis of NSGI is made by demonstrating inflammation of the appropriate area (e.g. more than five pus cells per oil immersion field on a urethral swab) and excluding gonorrhoea. It is then usual to treat the patient presumptively for chlamydia. Positively identifying or excluding the presence of *C. trachomatis* may be helpful if the condition does not settle or relapses early after apparently appropriate treatment.

ANTIBIOTIC SUSCEPTIBILITY OF *C. TRACHOMATIS*

C. trachomatis is generally very sensitive in cell culture to tetracyclines, macrolides and rifampicin. Quinolones, sulphonamides and some β-lactams show moderate antichlamydial activity, and aminoglycosides, trimethoprim and other β-lactams show less activity (Sanders et al 1986). Occasional clinical isolates resistant to erythromycin and tetracycline have now been reported by Jones et al (1990). Agacfidan et al (1993) have shown that azithromycin in vitro is cidal for chlamydia.

TETRACYCLINE TREATMENT

Until recently, most STD clinics used a tetracycline preparation as first choice for treating NSGI and advised erythromycin for those patients in whom tetracycline preparations were inappropriate. Oral tetracycline in a dose of 500 mg or 250 mg four times a day is clinically effective although many clinics give a dose of 500 mg twice a day to improve patient compliance. Katz et al (1992) recently showed that compliance with a 7-day course of four times a day agents (tetracycline or erythromycin) was very poor, irrespective of whether the patient was symptomatic.

Doxycycline in a dose of 100 mg twice a day has become the accepted gold standard for the treatment of NSGI and is recommended by the CDC (1993). In 1981 Jordan showed that this resulted in much better compliance, although it is of course more expensive than tetracycline and causes gastro-intestinal side-effects. Many studies confirm the clinical efficacy of this regimen (Romanowski et al 1993, Lister et al 1993, Lauharanta et al 1993). Single-dose doxycycline has an unacceptably low rate of eradication

(Arya et al 1978). Minocycline developed a reputation for producing dizziness, but in a direct comparison with twice daily doxycycline Romanowski et al (1993) showed that if given in a single nightly dose of 100 mg it had equivalent efficacy and a similar rate of adverse side-effects.

AZITHROMYCIN

The use of single-dose azithromycin to treat gonorrhoea has been discussed above and there are numerous studies now available to show that a single dose of 1 g is effective in treating NSGI and/or chlamydial infection. Martin et al (1992) compared single-dose azithromycin 1 g with the standard 7 days of doxycycline (100 mg twice a day) in 457 patients with uncomplicated NSGI and a positive antigen test for *C. trachomatis*. The 266 subjects available for evaluation showed bacteriological and clinical cure rates in excess of 95% for both regimens. There was no significant difference between regimens in terms of efficacy or side-effects. Other studies have confirmed this level of efficacy for azithromycin and have shown it to be as effective as the standard 7 days of doxycycline (Lauharanta et al 1993, Nilsen et al 1992, Lister et al 1993, Steingrimsson et al 1994).

Nilsen et al (1992) showed that the clinical cure rate with single-dose azithromycin was equivalent to 7 days of doxycycline, even when *C. trachomatis* could not be identified, although there are few data on the use of azithromycin specifically against *Ureaplasma*.

QUINOLONES

Quinolones show moderate antichlamydial activity in the laboratory. Kitchen et al (1990) showed clinical efficacy with 400 mg of ofloxacin once daily for 7 days, and Maiti et al (1991) showed clinical and microbiological cure with 200 mg twice daily for 7 days. The CDC (1993) recommend 300 mg of ofloxacin twice daily for 7 days. Conflicting claims for the action of ciprofloxacin have been made (Miller 1992), but a recent study by Hooton et al (1990) has suggested that even in dosages as high as 2 g/day it gives an inadequate cure rate. This raises a question about its use as a monotherapy for treating pelvic inflammatory disease (see below).

Our current recommendation for the treatment of NSGI therefore is azithromycin in a single dose of 1 g. This should improve compliance and give an acceptably high rate of eradication, although patients should still be encouraged to return for a test of cure. It will also have the advantage of treating gonorrhoea effectively (see above). Standard doxycycline therapy of 100 mg twice daily for 7 days would be second-line therapy.

Pelvic inflammatory disease

The term 'pelvic inflammatory disease' (PID) refers to infective inflammation of the female upper genital tract. It usually presents with lower abdominal pain and there may be associated fever, dyspareunia and vaginal discharge. The clinical severity may vary from mild pelvic discomfort, when out-patient treatment is obviously appropriate, to a severe acute abdomen and toxaemia requiring emergency admission, parenteral antibiotics and, possibly, surgical intervention. Infection may be confined to the uterine lining (endometritis) and/or the fallopian tubes (salpingitis), or it may spread to produce peritonitis. The infection may become walled off to form an abscess and any attack of PID may produce long-term pelvic pain and have serious consequences for future fertility (Westrom 1975, Westrom et al 1992). Many episodes of PID probably occur without symptoms and are diagnosed retrospectively at subsequent investigations for infertility. Acute PID is usually a spontaneous event in a sexually active female, but occasionally it may be related to a procedure such as dilatation and curettage or the insertion of an intrauterine contraceptive device (Westrom 1980, Farley et al 1992).

The pathogenesis of PID remains ill understood, and clinical diagnosis remains imprecise. Organisms such as enterococci, *Clostridia*, *Bacteroides* or *Gardnerella* spp. may be isolated as part of normal vaginal flora, and isolation of organisms from vagina or cervix of a patient with PID does not necessarily denote that they are the cause of the clinical syndrome. Numerous studies have drawn attention to the polymicrobial basis of the condition, and it is generally accepted that the gold standard for microbiological diagnosis remains laparoscopic sampling of endometrial or fallopian secretions (Miller 1992). Stacey et al (1992) have recently emphasized the important role of both *N. gonorrhoeae* and *C. trachomatis* in producing PID. Antibiotic therapy needs to be directed against these two sexually transmitted pathogens as well as against other aerobic and anaerobic organisms that may have a secondary role, or may in some cases be the principal pathogen.

Many studies have shown the efficacy of a large number of antibiotic combinations in achieving clinical resolution of symptoms. However, less is known about their effectiveness in eradicating low-grade persistent endometrial infection or reducing the incidence of long-term problems (such as infertility, tubal pregnancy or chronic pelvic pain).

The CDC (1993) continues to recommend intravenous cefoxitin (2.0 g 6-hourly) and doxycycline (intravenously or orally, 100 mg 12-hourly). Cefoxitin has the advantage over other cephalosporins of having useful activity against Gram-negative anaerobic organisms such as *Bacteroides fragilis*, a potential pathogen. (An alternative would be cefotetan, but other third-generation cephalosporins require the addition of metronidazole or clindamycin to cover anaerobes.) The alternative regimen for inpatients is clindamycin 900 mg i.v. 8-hourly and gentamicin in a standard dosage. This is followed with oral doxycycline or clindamycin to complete 14 days of therapy. Campbell & Dodson (1990) have previously demonstrated good efficacy of clindamycin in eradicating *C. trachomatis*, although it is not conventionally regarded as an antichlamydial agent for the treatment of NSGI. In a recent study clindamycin/gentamicin produced a satisfactory clinical outcome in 87% and eradicated *C. trachomatis* in 100% (European Study Group 1992). Landers et al (1991) compared cefoxitin–doxycycline with tobramycin–clindamycin and demonstrated a 98.5% response in uncomplicated PID and a 81% response in patients with a tubovarian abscess for both regimens. *C. trachomatis* was eradicated from all patients.

Because the literature on antibiotic treatment of PID is so complex and many studies are not directly comparable, several large meta-analyses have been carried out (Walker et al 1993, Dodson 1994). Dodson reviewed 101 clinical trials involving over 4000 patients and concluded that there was no statistically significant difference in cure rates between single-agent and combination therapy or between those regimens which specifically treated chlamydia and those which did not. However, good anaerobic cover was beneficial. Walker et al (1993) reviewed 34 studies using rigorous criteria to exclude trials where the methodology or clinical and microbiological data were inadequate. Again clinical cure was equivalent with combinations or single agents and specific antichlamydial activity did not seem to be of benefit. Several of the studies reviewed showed ciprofloxacin or ofloxacin to be highly effective despite their lack of major activity against anaerobic organisms or chlamydia. More recent studies have again displayed good efficacy with either ciprofloxacin and ofloxacin in both in- and outpatients (Thadepalli et al 1991, Soper et al 1992, Martens et al 1993). In contrast to Dodson, Martens et al (1993) questioned whether anti-anaerobic activity is of importance.

Despite its demonstrated efficacy against both *N. gonorrhoeae* and *C. trachomatis* (see above), azithromycin has not been studied in the treatment of PID, and although it seems logical to use it in this context we must await evidence from good clinical trials. An attractive combination would be co-amoxiclav, to treat aerobic and anaerobic agents together with azithromycin, to give additional antigonococcal activity and treat chlamydia. Co-amoxiclav alone was reported over 90% effective in Jordanian women with PID although, as none of them had gonococci or chlamydia isolated, the microbiological results of this study seem rather unusual (Uri et al 1992). In Nairobi, Kosseim et al (1991) showed ampicillin–sulbactam to be as effective as cefoxitin–doxycycline in 101 women. However, the clinical response in both groups was disappointing (70%), as was

the high incidence of post-PID tubal obstruction. McGregor et al (1994) achieved a much better cure rate (86–91%) with ampicillin–sulbactam and showed this regimen to be comparable with cefoxitin–doxycycline for PID and with clindamycin–gentamicin for postpartum endometritis. If chlamydia were detected in the ampicillin–sulbactam group with PID, then doxycycline was added.

Thus, despite extensive study and review, the situation remains complex and there continues to be controversy over how important antichlamydial and antigonococcal activity are, how important anaerobic cover is and how important other aerobic Gram-positive and Gram-negative organisms are. It seems likely that rapidity of antibiotic administration is more crucial than the actual choice of agent (Witkin & Ledger 1993). Hillis et al (1993) have reported that a 48-h delay in seeking care after the onset of pain in salpingitis trebles the probability of subsequent infertility or ectopic pregnancy.

We recommend co-amoxiclav (1.2 g 8-hourly) which can be started intravenously and subsequently be given orally in reduced dosage) together with doxycycline 100 mg twice daily. Treatment should be given for at least 10 days and for 14 days if there is slow clinical resolution. An alternative combination is doxycycline and clindamycin which would give excellent cover against gonorrhoea, chlamydia and anaerobic infection.

Genital herpes infection

Genital herpes can be a painful, distressing and embarrassing condition that may recur and lead to considerable anxiety and psychosexual morbidity. However, there is little evidence of serious long-term organic sequelae. The condition is caused by infection with herpes simplex virus (HSV). There are two recognized serotypes: HSV-1 and HSV-2. HSV-1 tends to cause peri-oral cold sores and HSV-2 tends to cause genital lesions, but the clinical presentations are interchangeable. Like all herpes virus infections, infection with HSV is life-long. The primary infection usually produces the most serious clinical problems and is a self-limiting condition (except in those with impaired immunity). The virus then usually remains latent indefinitely, but in some cases it will produce recurrent clinical attacks (which are generally milder than the primary episode but may still cause significant distress). Non-infected individuals may acquire their infection from someone who is latently infected and symptom-free, but who is still shedding live virus.

Antiviral therapy is aimed at reducing viral shedding and symptomatology of the primary (and recurrent) attacks and suppressing or aborting recurrent attacks. As with all STDs it is important to make a definitive diagnosis, exclude other causes for genital ulceration (syphilis or chancroid) and exclude other co-existing STDs such as urethritis.

ACYCLOVIR IN THE PRIMARY ATTACK

Acyclovir (Ch. 40) is highly active against HSV and is now well established as the treatment of choice for primary attacks (Nilsen et al 1982). The CDC (1993) recommends 200 mg orally five times daily for 10 days or until clinical resolution is achieved. Most clinics in UK would limit treatment to 5 days. Wald et al (1994) have recently compared 4 g/day of acyclovir with the standard dose of 1 g/day and found no statistically significant difference in the duration of symptoms or viral shedding between the two groups. Adverse gastro-intestinal events were more common with the higher dose. They did demonstrate that starting treatment (with either dose) within the first 3 days of the symptoms developing shortened the duration of the first episode. Treating a primary infection does not eliminate the virus, nor will it reduce the risk of subsequent recurrences.

TREATMENT OF RECURRENT ATTACKS

It is less clear that acyclovir is of value in shortening the duration or severity of a secondary episode of genital herpes. The CDC (1993) states that there may be limited benefit provided that treatment is given within the prodromal period or within 2 days of the onset of lesions, but it is not generally recommended. Mindel, in his 1991 review, would agree with this conclusion. However, Whatley & Thin (1991) showed that if patients had frequent recurrences with a well-recognized prodrome and could be taught to start treatment early then acyclovir in a dose of either 400 mg twice daily or 200 mg five times daily for 5 days was effective in shortening or aborting attacks. A dose of 200 mg acyclovir twice daily was ineffective. It would seem that patient selection and education is crucial if this strategy is to work.

SUPPRESSION OF RECURRENT ATTACKS

There is less dispute over the use of long term acyclovir to suppress frequent recurrences, although the definition of 'frequent' will vary between individuals and physicians. Certainly attacks recurring more than once every 1–2 months should make the clinician consider some form of modifying strategy – either patient-initiated treatment (as above) or long-term suppressive therapy. There is now considerable experience with the latter and the consensus view is that acyclovir 400 mg twice daily is the appropriate dosing regimen. Many of the long-term studies are now

reporting 5-year results that continue to show efficacy and safety. Goldberg et al (1993) have reported a multicentre trial started in 1984 using acyclovir 400 mg twice daily. Patients who had 12 or more annual recurrences before starting treatment were having a mean recurrence rate of less than one per year after 5 years, and more than 20% of the study population have been recurrence free for the whole 5 years. There is no evidence of any serious side-effects or cumulative toxicity from acyclovir. Kaplowitz et al (1991) report similar results from their 3-year study. Isoprinosine 500 mg twice daily was much less effective than acyclovir 400 mg twice daily and in fact showed no significant benefit over placebo (Kinghorn et al 1992).

In summary, acute primary episodes of genital HSV infection should be treated with acyclovir 200 mg five times daily for 5 days. Recurrent attacks should not receive acute treatment but if they become frequent then initially the patient should be offered self-treatment, and if that strategy fails the use of long-term suppressive therapy should be considered. If recurrences are completely suppressed treatment should be withdrawn at 1 year to see if it is still required.

ACYCLOVIR IN PREGNANCY

Although acyclovir is not recommended in pregnancy for the treatment of genital HSV there is no evidence of an increase over expected number of birth defects or a consistent pattern of birth defects in mothers who have used it (Andrews et al 1992). Haddad et al (1993) have treated five pregnant women with a history of recurrent genital herpes in whom HSV was isolated after 37 weeks' gestation. Although appropriate plasma levels of acyclovir were obtained, asymptomatic shedding of HSV was not reduced and one of the neonates became infected, so it seems that acyclovir is ineffective in preventing neonatal infection. (See also Ch. 57.)

Chancroid

Chancroid is a cause of genital ulceration accompanied by painful and often suppurative inguinal lymphadenopathy. It is caused by the sexually transmitted organism *Haemophilus ducreyi* and until recently was not regarded as a major problem in Western STD practice as it was relatively uncommon and has no long-term sequelae. However, interest in chancroid has increased with the implication that genital ulceration facilitates HIV heterosexual transmission, particularly in the developing world (Plourde et al 1992a). A recent outbreak amongst San Francisco prostitutes has heightened this interest (Flood et al 1993).

THERAPY OF CHANCROID

H. ducreyi can be cultured (with difficulty) in the laboratory, and therefore in vitro sensitivity testing is available and generally correlates well with clinical results. Most strains remain sensitive to erythromycin and this continues to be recommended by the CDC (1993) although, since the dose is 500 mg orally four times daily for 7 days, there are likely to be significant compliance problems (see above). Knapp et al (1993) have reviewed in vitro susceptibilities of isolates from Thailand and the USA, and have documented resistance to tetracycline, co-trimoxazole and, possibly, amoxicillin–clavulanic acid. However, all isolates were sensitive to ceftriaxone, ciprofloxacin, ofloxacin, erythromycin and azithromycin. Azithromycin is proving to be highly effective and is recommended by the CDC (1993) in a single oral dose of 1 g.

Ceftriaxone was shown to be effective in a single dose of 250 mg i.m. by Bower et al (1987) in Kenya and this remains a CDC recommendation. However, in a study of 133 men in Nairobi, Tyndall et al (1993) have recently shown that this regimen was no longer effective. The outcome was worse in those who were infected with HIV, but there was still a significant clinical failure rate in HIV-negative subjects and therefore the use of this regimen, at least in Kenya, must be questioned.

There is increasing resistance of *H. ducreyi* to both trimethoprim and sulphonamides, and co-trimoxazole is no longer reliably effective (Plourde et al 1992b). However, a single intramuscular dose of spectinomycin 2 g still seems to be safe and effective (Guzman et al 1992). Ciprofloxacin remains effective and Plourde and colleagues (1992b) have shown good efficacy for a single dose of fleroxacin 400 mg.

Lymphogranuloma venereum

Lymphogranuloma venereum (LGV) is caused by C. *trachomatis*, but the strains appear more invasive than those which produce urethritis and produce a painful adenopathy. It is not clear why this is a rare condition when NSGI and *C. trachomatis* are so common. Antimicrobial therapy is not of proven benefit, but it is common to treat with a tetracycline preparation. The good antichlamydial activity of azithromycin might suggest it as an appropriate agent to consider, but there are currently no clinical data available. The Centers for Disease Control (1993) recommend doxycycline 100 mg twice daily for 21 days, with erythromycin as an alternative.

Granuloma inguinale

This is another uncommon condition in the UK. It is a granulomatous destruction of skin and subcutaneous tissues of the genital region caused by the bacterial agent *Calymmatobacterium granulomatis*. Suggested treatment is with quinolones, co-trimoxazole or ceftriaxone. Single-dose ceftriaxone is known to be ineffective, but repeated dosing in chronic lesions may be very effective (Merianos et al 1994).

Vulvovaginitis

Abnormal vaginal discharge and/or vulval pruritis are common causes of presentation to STD clinics and to primary care physicians and gynaecologists. Although these symptoms may suggest mucopurulent cervicitis caused by *N. gonorrhoeae* or *C. trachomatis*, they are more often presentations of vulvovaginitis and may be precipitated by three major conditions: fungal vaginitis caused by candida species (usually *Candida albicans)*; trichomonas vaginitis caused by the protozoan *Trichomonas vaginalis*; and bacterial vaginitis (BV). This last condition was first described by Gardner & Dukes in 1955 and, as it lacks some features of true inflammation, it is often called 'bacterial vaginosis' rather than vaginitis. Vulvovaginitis is not usually caused by a sexually transmitted infection but it usually presents to STD clinics and clearly it is essential to exclude and/or treat potentially sexually transmitted pathogens. In recognition of this shift away from concentration purely on sexually transmitted infection and disease, many STD clinics in the UK have now changed their title to clinics of Genitourinary Medicine (GUM).

The diagnosis of vaginitis/vaginosis can be made by examination of the discharge. In trichomonas and BV the vaginal pH will be greater than 4.5. Addition of 10% potassium hydroxide solution to the slide will produce the characteristic fishy odour of amines with both trichomonas and BV (positive whiff test). Slides are then examined under the microscope. *Candida* pseudohyphae may be readily identified in the potassium hydroxide slide, whereas motile *Trich. vaginalis* is more easily spotted in a saline mounted slide. In BV the saline slide often reveals 'clue cells', i.e. squamous epithelial cells that have their borders obscured with bacteria.

VULVOVAGINAL CANDIDIASIS

The CDC (1993) estimate that 75% of women will have one or more episodes of vulvovaginal candidiasis (VVC) in their lifetime. Predisposing factors include pregnancy, diabetes mellitus, the oral contraceptive pill, steroids and HIV infection. It is not usually a sexually transmitted condition and there is no indication for routine epidemiological treatment of male sexual partners. However, men infected with *Candida* may occasionally develop a balanitis which can be helped by topical anticandidal preparations.

Treatment

VVC is treated with agents active against species of *Candida* and these can be applied topically or given orally for their systemic effect. Topical preparations usually come in the form of cream or pessary for intravaginal and vulval application. Two topical treatments widely used in the UK and USA are the imidazole agents miconazole or clotrimazole. Nystatin is now less commonly used as it is felt to be less effective. Clotrimazole pessaries are given in doses of: a single 500 mg dose; 200 mg/day for 3 days; or 100 mg/day for 6 days. Forssman & Milsom (1985) showed an equivalent cure (80–95%) and relapse rate with each of these strategies. Miconazole is given in a 3-day course of 200 mg/day or a 7-day course of 100 mg/day with similar efficacy. Oral agents for the treatment of acute VVC are not recommended in the USA (CDC 1993), but there is an increasing literature on their use which is becoming more widespread. Most importantly, patients prefer it. Osser et al (1991) found that 75% of women preferred oral therapy, and Merkus (1990) found that only 5% preferred local treatment. Osser showed that a single dose of fluconazole 150 mg had a significantly higher clinical and mycological cure rate than local econazole. He concluded that oral and topical agents show equivalent results for the treatment of acute VVC. A meta-analysis by Patel et al (1992) came to similar conclusions and suggested that single-dose oral fluconazole was cost-effective. Itraconazole 200 mg for 3 days is also effective (Silva-Cruz et al 1991). Itraconazole 200 mg once monthly for 6 months proved to be a successful and well-tolerated suppressive therapy for women with chronic recurrent VVC (Creatsas et al 1993).

It would therefore seem reasonable to offer oral fluconazole (150-mg capsule, single dose) as standard therapy for acute VVC, unless there are compelling reasons for using local therapy.

TRICHOMONAS VAGINITIS

This is caused by a sexually transmitted pathogen, although the male is usually asymptomatic. The drug of choice remains metronidazole. Lossick (1982) reviewed the various studies using this drug and concluded that the single 2-g dose had a median cure rate of 96%, minimized noncompliance and used less drug than multiple-dosage regimens. This regimen is recommended by the CDC and it is felt that male sexual partners should be treated with a similar course. If there is clinical failure then a more prolonged course of metronidazole should be given. Single-dose tinidazole 2 g has similar efficacy (Gabriel et al 1982).

BACTERIAL VAGINOSIS

This is a clinical syndrome resulting from the overgrowth of anaerobic bacteria to replace the lactobacillus species predominating in the normal vaginal flora. The main organism is *Gardnerella vaginalis* but *Bacteroides* spp. and other anaerobic organisms are also implicated. *G. vaginalis* is part of the normal vaginal flora in up to 50% of women, and so only women who are symptomatic should be treated, although some clinicians maintain that if this condition is identified at a screening clinic it should be treated. As the aim is to reduce the anaerobic flora it is appropriate to use antibiotics known to be active against anaerobes, and therefore clindamycin and metronidazole are the usual agents. Metronidazole has been extensively studied and employed in clinical practice (Lossick 1990). There has been dispute over whether single-dose metronidazole therapy (2 g) is as effective as the other standard regimen of 500 mg twice daily for 7 days. Svedberg et al (1985) found a lower cure rate and a higher relapse rate with single-dose therapy, and the CDC (1993) favours the multidosage regimen. However, a recent review by Sweet (1993) suggested that single-dose metronidazole was equally effective. Livengood et al (1994) have shown that intravaginal metronidazole gel 5 g twice daily is an effective, safe and well-tolerated treatment for BV, so the choice of regimen depends on the individual preference of the patient or clinician.

Clindamycin cream was shown to be effective by Dhar et al (1994), and Greaves et al (1988) found that oral clindamycin 300 mg twice daily for 7 days was effective and well tolerated.

Quinolones have proved less effective for the treatment of BV and these clinical findings are consistent with their relative lack of anaerobic activity (Covino et al 1993b, Carmona et al 1987).

Single-dose metronidazole is therefore the preferred option for treatment of this condition, with oral clindamycin as an option for those in whom metronidazole is contraindicated or not tolerated.

References

Agacfidan A, Moncada J, Schachter J 1993 In vitro activity of azithromycin (CP-62993) against *Chlamydia trachomatis* and *Chlamydia pneumoniae*. *Antimicrobial Agents and Chemotherapy* 37 (9): 1746–1748

Andrews E B, Yankaskas B C, Cordero J F, Schoeffler K, Hampp S 1992 Acyclovir in pregnancy register: six years' experience. *Obstetrics and Gynecology* 79: 7–13

Arya O P, Alergant C D, Annels E H, Carey P B, Glosk A K, Goddard A D 1978 Management of non-specific urethritis in man. *British Journal of Venereal Disease* 54: 414–421

Australian Gonococcal Surveillance Programme 1993 The incidence of gonorrhoea and the antibiotic-sensitivity of gonococci in Australia, 1981–1991. *Genitourinary Medicine* 69: 364–369

Balachandran T, Roberts A P, Evans B A, Azadian B S 1992 Single dose therapy of anogenital and pharyngeal gonorrhoea with ciprofloxacin. *International Journal of STD and AIDS* 3 (1): 49–51

Boakes A J, Barrow J, Eykyn S, Phillips I 1981 Cefotaxime for spectinomycin resistant *Neisseriae gonorrhoeae*. *Lancet* ii: 96

Bogaerts J, Tello W M, Akingeneye J, Mukantabana V, Van Dyck E, Piot P 1993 Effectiveness of norfloxacin and ofloxacin for treatment of gonorrhoea and decrease of in vitro susceptibility to quinolones over time in Rwanda. *Genitourinary Medicine* 69: 196–200

Bowmer M I, Nsanze H, D'Costa L J et al 1982 Single-dose ceftriaxone for chancroid. *Antimicrobial Agents and Chemotherapy* 31: 67–69

Bradley S B, Fisher L M, Dalton H P 1980 Recovery of *Chlamydia trachomatis* from patients of a south-eastern venereal disease clinic. *American Journal of Clinical Pathology* 73: 774–781

Campbell W F, Dodson M G 1990 Clindamycin therapy for *Chlamydia trachomatis* in women. *American Journal of Obstetrics and Gynecology* 162 (2): 343–347

Carmona O, Hernandez-Gonzalez S, Kobelt R 1987 Ciprofloxacin in the treatment of nonspecific vaginitis. *American Journal of Medicine* 82 (suppl 4A): 321–323

Catchpole M A 1992 Sexually transmitted diseases in England and Wales: 1981–1990. *Communicable Disease Review* 2 (1): R1–R7

Centers for Disease Control 1993 Sexually transmitted diseases treatment guidelines. *Morbidity and Mortality Weekly Report* 42 (suppl RR-14): 1–99

Centers for Disease Control 1994 Decreased-susceptibility of *Neisseria gonorrhoeae* to fluoroquinolones – Ohio and Hawaii 1992–1994. *Morbidity and Mortality Weekly Report* 43 (18) 325–327

Corcoran G D, Ridgeway G L 1994 Antibiotic chemotherapy of bacterial sexually transmitted diseases in adults: a review. *International Journal of STD and AIDS* 5 (3): 165–171

Covino J M, Smith B L, Cummings M C, Benes S, Draft K, McCormack W M 1993a Comparison of enoxacin and ceftriaxone in the treatment of uncomplicated gonorrhoea. *Sexually Transmitted Diseases* 20 (4): 227–229

Covino J M, Black J R, Cummings M, Zwahl B, McCormack W M 1993b Comparative evaluation of ofloxacin and metronidazole in the treatment of bacterial vaginosis. *Sexually Transmitted Diseases* 20 (5): 262–264

Creatsas G C, Charalambidis V M, Zagotzidou E H, Anthopoulou H N, Michailidis D C, Aravantinos D I 1993 Chronic or recurrent vaginal candidosis: short term treatment and prophylaxis with itraconazole. *Clinical Therapeutics* 15 (4): 662–671

De Konig, G A, Tio D, van den Hoek J A et al 1983 Single 1 gram dose of cefotaxime in the treatment of infection due to penicillinase-producing strains of *Neisseria gonorrhoeae*. *British Journal of Venereal Disease* 59: 100–102

Dhar J, Arya O P, Timmins D J et al 1994 Treatment of bacterial vaginosis with a three day course of clindamycin vaginal cream: a pilot study. *Genitourinary Medicine* 70 (2): 121–130

Dodson M G 1994 Antibiotic regimens for treating acute pelvic inflammatory disease. An evaluation. *Journal of Reproductive Medicine* 39 (4): 285–296

Dunlop E M C 1985 Survival of treponemes after treatment: comments, clinical conclusions and recommendations. *Genitourinary Medicine* 61: 293–301

Dunnett D M, Moyer M A 1992 Cefixime in the treatment of uncomplicated gonorrhoea. *Sexually Transmitted Diseases* 19 (2): 92–93

Easmon C S F 1985 Gonococcal resistance to antibiotics. *Journal of Antimicrobial Chemotherapy* 16: 409–417

El Tabbakh G H, Elejalde B R, Broekhuizen F F 1994 Primary syphilis and nonimmune fetal hydrops in a penicillin-allergic woman. A case report. *Journal of Reproductive Medicine* 39 (5): 412–414

European Study Group 1992 Comparative evaluation of clindamycin/gentamicin and cefoxitin/doxycycline for treatment of pelvic inflammatory disease: a multi centre trial. *Acta Obstetrica et Gynecologica Scandinavica* 71 (2): 129–134

Farley T M M, Rosenburg M J, Rowe P J, Chen J H, Meirik O 1992 Intrauterine devices and pelvic inflammatory disease: an international perspective. *Lancet* 339: 785–788

Fiumara N J 1982 Treating syphilis with tetracycline. *American Family Physician* 26: 131–133

Flood J M, Saraffian S K, Bolan G A et al 1993 Multistrain outbreak of chancroid in San Francisco. *Journal of Infectious Disease* 167: 1106–1111

Forssman L, Milsom I 1985 Treatment of recurrent vaginal candidiasis. *American Journal of Obstetrics and Gynecology* 152: 959–961

Gabriel G, Robertson E, Thin R N 1982 Single dose treatment of trichomonas. *Journal of International Medical Research* 10: 129–130

Gardner H L, Dukes C D 1955 *Haemophilus vaginalis* vaginitis. A newly defined species infection previously classified 'nonspecific' vaginitis. *American Journal of Obstetrics and Gynecology* 69: 962–976

Goh B T, Smith G W, Samarasinghe L, Singh V, Lim K S 1984 Penicillin concentrations in serum and cerebrospinal fluid after intramuscular injection of aqueous procaine penicillin 0.6 MU with and without probenicid. *British Journal of Venereal Disease* 60: 371–373

Goldberg L H, Kaufman R, Kurtz T O et al 1993 Long term suppression of recurrent genital herpes with acyclovir. A 5-year benchmark study. *Archives of Dermatology* 129 (5): 582–587

Gordon S M, Eaton M E, George R et al 1994 The response of symptomatic neurosyphilis to high-dose intravenous penicillin G in patients with human immunodeficiency virus infection. *New England Journal of Medicine* 331 (22): 1469–1473

Gourevitch M N, Selwyn P A, Davenny K et al 1993 Effects of HIV infection on the serologic manifestations and response to treatment of syphilis in intravenous drug users. *Annals of Internal Medicine* 118 (5): 350–355

Greaves W L, Chungafung J, Morris B, Haile A, Townsend J L 1988 Clindamycin versus metronidazole in the treatment of bacterial vaginosis. *Obstetrics and Gynecology* 72: 799–802

Guzman M, Guzman J, Bernal M 1992 Treatment of chancroid with a single dose of spectinomycin. *Sexually Transmitted Diseases* 19 (5): 291–294

Haddad J, Langer B, Astruc D, Messer J, Lokiec F 1993 Oral acyclovir and recurrent genital herpes during late pregnancy. *Obstetrics and Gynecology* 82 (1): 102–104

Handsfield H H, Hook E W 1987 Ceftriaxone for treatment of uncomplicated gonorrhoea: routine use of a single 125 mg dose in a sexually transmitted diseases clinic. *Sexually Transmitted Diseases* 14: 227–230

Handsfield H H, McCormack W M, Hook E W et al 1991 A comparison of single dose cefixime with ceftriaxone as treatment for uncomplicated gonorrhoea. *New England Journal of Medicine* 325 (19): 1337–1341

Handsfield H H, Dalu Z A, Martin D H, Douglas J M, McCarty J M, Schlossberg D 1994 Multicenter trial of single-dose azithromycin vs. ceftriaxone in the treatment of uncomplicated gonorrhoea. *Sexually Transmitted Diseases* 20: 107–111

Hillis S D, Joesoef R, Marchbanks P A, Wasserheit J N, Cates W, Westrom L 1993 Delayed care of pelvic inflammatory disease as a risk factor for impaired fertility. *American Journal of Obstetrics and Gynecology* 168: 1503–1509

Hook E W, Roddy R E, Handsfield H H 1988 Ceftriaxone therapy for incubating and early syphilis. *Journal of Infectious Diseases* 158: 891–894

Hook E W, Jones R B, Martin D H et al 1993 Comparison of ciprofloxacin and ceftriaxone as a single-dose therapy for uncomplicated gonorrhoea in women. *Antimicrobial Agents and Chemotherapy* 37 (8): 1670–1673

Hooton T M, Rogers M E, Medina T G et al 1990 Ciprofloxacin compared with doxycycline for nongonococcal urethritis. Ineffectiveness against *Chlamydia trachomatis* due to relapsing infections. *Journal of the American Medical Association* 264 (11): 1418–1421

Horowitz H W, Valsamis M P, Wicher V et al 1994 Cerebral syphilitic gumma confirmed by the polymerase chain reaction in a man with human-immunodeficiency virus infection. *New England Journal of Medicine* 331 (22): 1488–1491

Hutchinson C M, Rompalo A M, Reochart C A 1991 Characteristics of syphilis in patients attending Baltimore STD clinics: multiple bugle risk subgroups and interactions with HIV infection. *Archives of Internal Medicine* 151: 511–516

Johns D R, Tierny M, Felenstein D 1987 Alteration in the natural history of neurosyphilis by concurrent infection with human immunodeficiency virus. *New England Journal of Medicine* 316: 1569–1572

Jones R B, Van der Pol B, Martin D H, Shepard M K 1990 Partial characterization of *Chlamydia trachomatis* isolates resistant to multiple antibiotics. *Journal of Infectious Diseases* 162: 1309–1315

Jordan W C 1981 Doxycycline vs. tetracycline in the treatment of men with gonorrhoea: the compliance factor. *Sexually Transmitted Disease* 8 (suppl): 105–109

Jorgensen J, Tikjob G, Weismann K 1986 Neurosyphilis after treatment of latent syphilis with benzathine penicillin. *Genitourinary Medicine* 62: 129–131

Kaplowitz L G, Baker D, Gelb L et al 1991 Prolonged continuous acyclovir treatment of normal adults with frequently recurring genital herpes simplex virus infection. *Journal of the American Medical Association* 265 (6): 747–751

Katz B P, Zwickl B W, Caine V A, Jones R B 1992 Compliance with antibiotic therapy for *Chlamydia trachomatis* and *Neisseria gonorrhoeae*. *Sexually Transmitted Diseases* 19: 351–354

Katz D A, Berger J R, Duncan R C 1993 Neurosyphilis: a comparative study of the effects of infection with human immunodeficiency virus. *Archives of Neurology* 50: 243–249

Kinghorn G R, Woolley P D, Thin R N, DeMaubeuge J, Foidart J M, Engst R 1992 Acyclovir vs isoprinosine (immunovir) for suppression of recurrent genital herpes simplex infection. *Genitourinary Medicine* 68 (5): 312–316

Kitchen V S, Donegan C, Ward H, Thomas B, Harris J R W, Taylor-Robinson D 1990 Comparison of ofloxacin with doxycycline in the treatment of-nongonococcal urethritis and cervical chlamydial infection. *Journal of Antimicrobial Chemotherapy* 26 (suppl D): 99–105

Knapp J S, Back A F, Babst A F, Taylor D, Rice D J 1993 In vitro susceptibility of isolates of *Haemophilus ducreyi* from Thailand and the USA to currently recommended and newer agents for the treatment of chancroid. *Antimicrobial Agents and Chemotherapy* 37 (7): 1552–1555

Kosseim M, Ronald A, Plummer F A, D'Costa L, Brunham R C 1991 Treatment of acute pelvic inflammatory disease in the ambulatory setting: trial of cefoxitin and doxycycline versus ampicillin–sulbactam. *Antimicrobial Agents and Chemotherapy* 35 (8): 1651–1656

Landers D V, Wolner-Hanssen P, Paavonen J et al 1991 Combination antimicrobial chemotherapy in the treatment of acute pelvic inflammatory disease. *American Journal of Obstetrics and Gynecology* 164 (3): 849–858

Lassus A, Abath Filho L, Santos Junior M F, Belli L 1992 Comparison of fleroxacin and penicillin G plus probenicid in the treatment of acute uncomplicated gonococcal infections. *Genitourinary Medicine* 68 (5): 317–320

Lauharanta J, Saarinen K, Mustonen M T, Happonen H P 1993 Single dose azithromycin versus seven-day doxycycline in the treatment of non-gonococcal urethritis in males. *Journal of Antimicrobial Chemotherapy* 31 (suppl E): 177–183

Lister P J, Balachandran T, Ridgway G L, Robinson A J 1993 Comparison of azithromycin and doxycycline in the treatment of non-gonococcal urethritis in men. *Journal of Antimicrobial Chemotherapy* 31 (suppl E): 185–192

Livengood C H, McGregor J A, Soper D E, Newton E, Thomason J L 1994 Bacterial vaginosis: efficacy and safety of intravaginal metronidazole treatment. *American Journal of Obstetrics and Gynecology* 170 (3): 759–764

Lossick J G 1982 Treatment of *Trichomonas vaginalis* infections. *Review of Infectious Diseases* 4 (suppl) S801–S808

Lossick J G 1990 Treatment of sexually transmitted vaginosis/vaginitis. *Reviews of Infectious Diseases* 12 (suppl 6): S665–S681

Lukehart S A, Hook E W, Baker-Zander S A et al 1988 Invasion of the central nervous system by Treponema pallidum: implications for diagnosis and treatment. *Annals of Internal Medicine* 109: 855–862

Maiti H, Chowdhury F H, Richmond S J, Stirland R M, Tooth J A, Bhattacharyya M N, Stock J K 1991 Ofloxacin in the treatment of uncomplicated gonorrhoea and chlamydial genital infection. *Clinical Therapeutics* 13 (4): 441–447

Markovitz D M, Beutner K R, Maggio R P, Reichmann R C 1986 Failure of recommended treatment for secondary syphilis. *Journal of the American Medical Association* 225: 1767–1768

Martens M G, Gordon S, Yarborough D R, Faro S, Binder D, Berkeley A 1993 Multicentre randomized trial of ofloxacin versus cefoxitin and doxycycline in outpatient treatment of pelvic inflammatory disease. *Southern Medical Journal* 86 (6): 604–610

Martin D H, Mroczkowski T F, Dalu Z A et al 1992 A controlled trial of a single dose of azithromycin for the treatment of chlamydial urethritis and cervicitis. *New England Journal of Medicine* 327 (13): 921–925

Mascola L, Pelosi R, Blount J H et al 1984 Congenital syphilis: why is it still occurring? *Journal of the American Medical Association* 252: 1719–1722

McCormack W M, Mogabgab W J, Jones R B, Hook E W, Handsfield H H 1993 Multicentre comparative study of cefotaxime and ceftriaxone for treatment of uncomplicated gonorrhoea. *Sexually Transmitted Diseases* 20 (5): 269–273

McGregor J A, Crombleholme W R, Newton E, Sweet R L, Tuomala R, Gibbs R S 1994 Randomised comparison of ampicillin-sulbactam to cefoxitin and doxycycline or clindamycin and gentamicin in the treatment of pelvic inflammatory disease or endometritis. *Obstetrics and Gynaecology* 83(6): 998–1004

Merianos A, Gilles M, Chuah J 1994 Ceftriaxone in the treatment of chronic donovanosis in central Australia. *Genitourinary Medicine* 70 (2): 84–89

Merkus J M 1990 Treatment of vaginal candidiasis: orally or vaginally? *Journal of the American Academy of Dermatology* 23: 568–572

Miller A R O 1992 Sexually transmitted disease. In: Lambert H P, O'Grady F W (eds) Antibiotic and chemotherapy, 6th edn. Churchill Livingstone, New York: 428–438

Mindel A 1991 Is it meaningful to treat patients with recurrent herpetic infections? *Scandinavian Journal of Infectious Diseases* 80 (suppl) S27–S32

Mogabgab W J, Lutz F B 1994 Randomised study of cefotaxime versus ceftriaxone for uncomplicated gonorrhea. *Southern Medical Journal* 87 (4): 461–464

Musher D M 1988 How much penicillin cures early syphilis? *Annals of Internal Medicine* 109: 849–851

Musher DM 1991 Syphilis, neurosyphilis, penicillin and AIDS. *Journal of Infectious Diseases* 163 (6): 1201–1206

Musher D M, Baughin R E 1994 Neurosyphilis in HIV infected persons. *New England Journal of Medicine* 331 (22): 1516–1517

Nilsen A E, Aasen T, Halsos A M et al 1982 Efficacy of oral acyclovir in the treatment of initial and recurrent genital herpes. *Lancet* ii: 571–573

Nilsen A, Halsos A, Johansen A, Torud E, Moseng D, Anestad G, Storvold G 1992 A double blind study of single dose azithromycin and doxycycline in the treatment of chlamydial urethritis in males. *Genitourinary Medicine* 68 (5): 325–327

Odugbemi T, Oyewolw F, Isichei C S, Onwukeme K E, Adeyemi-Doro F A 1993 Single dose of azithromycin for therapy of susceptible sexually transmitted diseases: a multicentre open evaluation. *West African Journal of Medicine* 12 (3): 136–140

Osser S, Haglund A, Westrom L 1991 Treatment of candidal vaginitis. A prospective randomized investigator-blind multicenter study comparing topically applied econazole with oral fluconazole. *Acta Obstetrica and Gynecologica Scandinavica* 70 (1): 73–78

Otubu J A, Imade G E, Sagay A S, Towobola O A 1992 Resistance of recent *Neisseria gonorrhoeae* isolates in Nigeria and outcome of single-dose treatment with ciprofloxacin. *Infection* 20 (6): 339–341

Patel H S, Peters M D, Smith C L 1992 Is there a role for fluconazole in the treatment of vulvovaginal candidiasis? *Annals of Pharmacotherapy* 26 (3): 350–353

Petersen C S, Jorgensen B B, Pedersen NS 1984 Treatment of early infectious syphilis in Denmark. A retrospective serological study. *Danish Medical Bulletin* 31: 70–72

Philcox D V, Callanan J J, Forder A A 1987 Treatment of neurosyphilis. *South African Medical Journal* 72: 110–113

Phillips I 1976 Beta-lactamase producing penicillin resistant gonococcus. *Lancet* ii: 656–657

Pickering L K 1985 Diagnosis and therapy of patients with congenital and primary syphilis. *Pediatric Infectious Diseases* 4: 602–605

Plourde P J, Plummer F A, Pepin J et al 1992a Human immunodeficiency virus type I infection in women attending a sexually transmitted diseases clinic in Kenya. *Journal of Infectious Disease* 166: 86–92

Plourde P J, D'Costa L J, Agoki E et al 1992b A randomized double-blind study of the efficacy of fleroxacin versus trimethoprim–sulfamethoxazole in men with culture-proven chancroid. *Journal of Infectious Diseases* 165 (5): 949–952

Portilla I, Lutz B, Montalvo M, Mogabgab W J 1992 Oral cefixime versus intramuscular ceftriaxone in patients with uncomplicated gonococcal infections. *Sexually Transmitted Diseases* 19 (2): 94–98

Richmond S J, Paul I D, Taylor P K 1980 Value and feasibility of screening women attending STD clinics for cervical chlamydial infection. *British Journal of Venereal Disease* 56: 92–96

Romanowski B, Talbot H, Stadnyk M, Kowalchuk P, Bowie W R 1993 Minocycline compared with doxycycline in the treatment of nongonococcal urethritis and mucopurulent cervicitis. *Annals of Internal Medicine* 119 (1): 16–22

Sanders L L, Harrison R, Washington A E 1986 Treatment of sexually transmitted chlamydial infection. *Journal of the American Medical Association* 225: 1750–1756

Sherrard J, Barlow D 1993 PPNG at St Thomas' Hospital – a changing provenance. *International Journal of STD and AIDS* 4 (6): 330–332

Silva-Cruz A, Andrade L, Sobral L, Francisca A 1991 Itraconazole versus placebo in the management of vaginal candidiasis. *International Journal of Gynaecology and Obstetrics* 36 (3): 229–232

Soper D E, Brockwell N J, Dalton H P 1992 Microbial aetiology of urban emergency department acute salpingitis: treatment with ofloxacin. *American Journal of Obstetrics and Gynecology* 167 (3): 553–660

Stacey C M, Munday P E, Taylor-Robinson D et al 1992 A longitudinal study of pelvic inflammatory disease. *British Journal of Obstetrics and Gynaecology* 99: 994–999

Steingrimsson O, Olaffson J H, Thorarinsson H, Ryan R W, Johnson R B, Tilton R C 1992 Azithromycin in the treatment of sexually transmitted disease. *Journal of Antimicrobial Chemotherapy* 25 (suppl A): 109–114

Steingrimsson O, Olaffson J H, Thorarinsson H, Ryan R W, Johnson R B, Tilton R C 1994 Single dose azithromycin treatment of gonorrhoea and infections caused by *C. trachomatis* and *U. urealyticum* in men. *Sexually Transmitted Diseases* 21(1): 43–46

Svedberg J, Steiner J F, Deiss F, Steiner S, Driggers D A 1985 Comparison of single dose vs. one week course of metronidazole for symptomatic bacterial vaginosis. *Journal of the American Medical Association* 254: 1046–1049

Sweet R L 1993 New approaches to the treatment of bacterial vaginosis. *American Journal of Obstetrics and Gynecology* 169 (2): 479–482

Sweet R L, Bartlett J G, Hemsell D L, Solomkin J S, Tally F 1992 Evaluation of new anti-infective drugs for the treatment of acute pelvic inflammatory disease. *Clinical Infectious Disease* 15 (suppl 1): S53–S61

Thadepalli H, Mathai D, Scotti R, Bansal M B, Savage E 1991 Ciprofloxacin monotherapy for acute pelvic infections: a comparison with clindamycin plus gentamicin. *Obstetrics and Gynecology* 78 (4): 696–702

Thin R N 1989 Treatment of venereal syphilis. *Journal of Antimicrobial Chemotherapy* 24: 481–483

Tramont E C 1994 *Treponema pallidum* (*syphilis*). In: Mandell G L, Bennet J E, Dolin R (eds) Principles and practice of infectious diseases, 4th edn. Churchill Livingstone, New York

Tyndall M, Malisa M, Plummer F A, Ombetti J, Ndinya-Achola J O, Ronald A R 1993 Ceftriaxone no longer predictably cures chancroid in Kenya. *Journal of Infectious Diseases* 167 (2): 469–471

Uri F I, Sartawi S A, Dajani Y F, Masoud A A, Barakat H F 1992 Amoxycillin/clavulanic acid (augmentin) compared with triple drug therapy for pelvic inflammatory disease. *International Journal of Gynaecology and Obstetrics* 38 (1): 41–43

Van der Walke P G M, Kraai E J, Van Voorst Vader P C, Haaxma-Reiche H, Snide J A M 1988 Penicillin concentrations in cerebrospinal fluid during repository treatment regimen for syphilis. *Genitourinary Medicine* 64: 223–225

Verdon M S, Douglas J M, Wiggins S D, Habdsfield H H 1993 Treatment of uncomplicated gonorrhoea with single doses of 200 mg cefixime. *Sexually Transmitted Diseases* 20 (5): 290–293

Wald A, Benedetti J, Davis G, Remington M, Winter C, Corey L 1994 A randomized double-blind, comparative trial comparing high and standard dose oral acyclovir for first episode genital herpes. *Antimicrobial Agents and Chemotherapy* 38 (2): 174–176

Walker C K, Kahn J G, Washington A E, Peterson H B, Sweet R L 1993 Pelvic inflammatory disease: meta-analysis of antimicrobial regimen efficacy. *Journal of Infectious Diseases* 168: 969–978

Warren C, Phillips I 1993 Penicillinase producing *Neisseria gonorrhoeae* from St Thomas' Hospital 1976–1990 – the first fifteen years. *Genitourinary Medicine* 69: 201–207

Waugh MA 1993 Open study of the safety and efficacy of a single dose of azithromycin for the treatment of uncomplicated gonorrhoea in men and women. *Journal of Antimicrobial Chemotherapy* 31 (suppl E): S193–S198

Webster L A, Rolfs R T 1993 Surveillance for primary and secondary syphilis – United States, 1991. *Morbidity and Mortality Weekly Report* 42 (SS–3): 12–19

Westrom L 1975 Effect of acute pelvic inflammatory disease on fertility. *American Journal of Obstetrics and Gynaecology* 121: 707–713

Westrom L 1980 Incidence, prevalence and trends of acute pelvic inflammatory disease and its consequences in industrialized countries. *American Journal of Obstetrics and Gynaecology* 128: 880–892

Westrom L, Joesoff R, Reynolds G, Hagdu A, Thompson S E 1992 Pelvic inflammatory disease and fertility. *Sexually Transmitted Diseases* 19: 185–192

Whatley J D, Thin R N 1991 Episodic acyclovir therapy to abort recurrent attacks of genital herpes simplex infection. *Journal of Antimicrobial Chemotherapy* 27 (5): 677–681

Witkin S S, Ledger W J 1993 New directions in the diagnosis and treatment of pelvic inflammatory disease. *Journal of Antimicrobial Chemotherapy* 31: 197–199

Zenilman J M, Rand S, Barditch P, Rompalo A M 1993 Asymptomatic neurosyphilis after doxycycline therapy for early latent syphilis. *Sexually Transmitted Diseases* 20 (6): 346–347

Mycobacterial infections

A. M. Elliot and H. P. Lambert

The resurgence of tuberculosis

The resurgence of tuberculosis, on an international scale, has been one of the most alarming developments in infectious diseases over the last decade and has overturned the complacency engendered by the antibiotic era. The World Health Organization (WHO) predict that between 1990 and 2000 there will be a global increase in the annual number of new tuberculosis cases from 7.5 million to 10.2 million, and in the annual number of deaths from tuberculosis from 2.5 million to 3.5 million (Editorial 1994). *Mycobacterium tuberculosis* causes more adult deaths than any other single pathogen, a quarter of all preventable adult deaths (Bloom & Murray 1992).

Yet the disease is curable. Effective antituberculous drugs were among the earliest antibiotics to be discovered and used, and the elegant studies which elucidated the principles of their action are a paradigm of clinical research. There are several reasons for this paradox.

First, tuberculosis is a disease associated with poverty, social disruption, crowded living conditions and poor nutrition. Case rates declined in industrialized countries as living conditions improved, even before effective treatment became available. As a consequence of the continuing decline, the impetus for research and for investment in control measures weakened in these countries. However, a similar decline in case rates did not occur in many developing countries, where widespread economic hardship and changes in social structure (such as the migration of rural populations to new cities, often to live in crowded shanty towns) provided conditions which favoured the disease. In these countries the requirements for an effective tuberculosis treatment programme were hard to fulfil. These include identification of infectious cases, purchase of drugs and maintenance of the chain of supply to the patient, and keeping patients in

the programme to complete the long course of treatment. The result was that case rates often, at best, remained stable, and the prevalence of infection in the adult population remained well over 50%. Against this background, the global epidemic of human immunodeficiency virus (HIV) infection has had a grave impact, because the virus renders individuals profoundly susceptible to the development of active tuberculosis, both following new infection (Alland et al 1994, Small et al 1994) and through reactivation of latent disease (Selwyn et al. 1989). The association between tuberculosis and HIV was first reported in the USA (Pitchenik et al 1984). A rise in case rates, concurrent with the epidemic of HIV, was noted particularly in New York City, where the problem was compounded by a lack of treatment facilities, many having been closed as tuberculosis case rates had declined (Brudney & Dobkin 1991). Inadequate treatment programmes had also allowed drug-resistant tuberculosis to develop in a significant group of patients (Iseman 1993), and such patients became sources for outbreaks of multidrug-resistant primary disease, especially among HIV-positive contacts, facilitated by inadequate precautions for isolation of infectious cases in hospital (Edlin et al 1992). However, the impact of the association between tuberculosis and HIV has been incomparably greater in sub-Saharan Africa where the prevalence of latent disease among adults had remained high. Tuberculosis case rates have risen in many countries in parallel with the HIV epidemic, for example, more than doubling between 1985 and 1991 in Malawi and Zambia (Nunn et al 1994). In this setting the combined impact of the two infections is focused on young adults, at the height of their social and economic importance, and crucial to the development of their countries. While Africa currently bears the greatest burden, with approximately 4 million dually infected people (Snider et al 1994), an even greater number of cases is predicted for countries in Asia, with the denser populations and higher, prior prevalence of infection with *M. tuberculosis*, as the HIV epidemic expands there (WHO 1994a).

In this chapter we describe the principles by which current regimens for the treatment of tuberculosis were developed, indicating how these regimens should be used for the individual patient, together with appropriate adjuncts to therapy. The implications of co-infection with HIV for the approach to therapy for individual patients are also discussed. The implementation of therapy within a tuberculosis control programme is then addressed.

The development of treatment regimens

Current regimens of chemotherapy must be viewed against a background of 45 years of development during which the scope and limitations of antituberculous drugs have been explored and their usage refined by a combination of experimental studies and international clinical trials, in which the work of the British Medical Research Council has played a central role. The earlier regimens using streptomycin, isoniazid and para-amino salicylic acid (PAS) required long periods of daily treatment, of the order of 1–2 years, in order to achieve success. They were highly successful when operated by enthusiastic and well-trained chest clinic staff, but results were much inferior in the conditions which more usually prevail both in wealthy and in developing countries.

Major changes followed the introduction of rifampicin and the re-discovery of pyrazinamide (Fox 1985). These included the introduction of new regimens involving short-course chemotherapy, intermittent chemotherapy, and a combination of the two, and the abandonment of sanatorium treatment and of surgery, although there has now been a limited return of surgical treatment in some cases of resistant disease.

The many controlled trials conducted during the decades of antituberculous therapy which preceded the HIV era and the emergence of multiple resistance established a number of important principles. Predominant was the need to use more than one agent to prevent the emergence of bacterial resistance. Since single-drug resistance emerged early, this meant that, in practice, three drugs were used initially, so that it was likely, pending results of susceptibility tests, that at least two effective agents were being administered. Another crucial result of these trials was to define the duration of treatment necessary to achieve success with different regimens, that is, clinical and radiographic quiescence and an acceptably low relapse rate following treatment. It is clear that no easily applicable drug regimen is satisfactory in smear-positive disease if given for less

than 6 months, although 4-month regimens (described later), are effective in smear- and culture-negative tuberculosis. Reduction of treatment courses to 6 months has been made possible by the use of pyrazinamide during the first phase of treatment, usually for 2 months. Evidence from a number of trials, however, suggests that results are not improved by continuing pyrazinamide for the whole period of therapy, suggesting that the eradicative action of this drug is mainly exerted during the early phase of treatment. By contrast, the benefit of rifampicin is exerted throughout, probably by eliminating small numbers of bacilli as they enter a metabolically active phase. In regimens not including pyrazinamide, the minimum effective duration of treatment with regimens including isoniazid and rifampicin is 9 months.

A major impact resulting from the chemotherapy trials has been to provide validated regimens suitable for a variety of different social, medical and financial conditions. In this context the results of trials of intermittent therapy are especially important, since it is evident that treatment programmes, however well based, are often difficult to implement (p. 842) and one effective way of doing so is direct observation of every dose as it is taken. Most intermittent regimens rely on isoniazid and rifampicin, given two or three times weekly, following an intensive phase of daily treatment, but in some trials intensive phases as short as 2 weeks have been used. Schemes involving three times weekly administration of various four- or five-drug regimens without an initial daily phase have also been used with success. These regimens not including an initial intensive phase confirmed the importance of pyrazinamide in achieving eradication since the relapse rate was 3–4% in patients with initially drug-susceptible organisms treated with combinations including this agent, but 10.3% with the non-pyrazinamide containing regimen (Hong Kong Chest Service/British MRC 1987).

Isoniazid metabolism shows genetic polymorphism, 40% of Europeans and 70% of Chinese being rapid acetylators, and there was some apprehension that intermittent therapy might be less effective in rapid acetylators. Trials in Singapore and Hong Kong, however, showed that higher relapse rates were seen in rapid acetylators only when isoniazid was given (with rifampicin) once weekly after an initial intensive phase, and even this defect could be overcome by a more intensive initial phase. Twice weekly continuation regimens showed no disadvantage to the rapid inactivators (Hong Kong Chest Service/British MRC 1984).

The great preponderance of clinical trials has involved adults with smear-positive pulmonary tuberculosis, the most serious, and infectious, form of the disease. It could reasonably be asked whether shorter and less demanding treatments might be effective in less florid pulmonary disease. This was explored in large studies in Chinese patients in Hong Kong. These showed that 2- or 3-month courses of treatment were inadequate in smear-negative patients whose pretreatment sputum cultures proved positive, but that 4-month schemes using isoniazid, rifampicin, pyrazinamide and streptomycin daily or three times weekly gave good results (Hong Kong Chest Service/ Tuberculosis Research Centre Madras/British MRC 1989). The evidence that pyrazinamide acts mainly during the first 2 months, together with evidence that streptomycin is probably an unnecessary component of this regimen, makes it likely that a simpler 4-month scheme consisting of isoniazid and rifampicin throughout, with pyrazinamide for the first 2 months, should be entirely adequate for smear-negative disease in areas with a low prevalence of drug-resistant organisms. An even simpler regimen was used in a trial in the USA (Dutt et al 1989) involving 452 smear-negative, culture-negative patients who were treated with isoniazid and rifampicin alone for 4 months. Five patients relapsed during a follow-up of 6–78 months.

REGIMENS CURRENTLY WIDELY USED IN THE UK, THE USA AND MANY OTHER COUNTRIES

Antituberculous therapy in the UK and in many other countries with well-developed chest clinic services has followed the principles outlined, reinforced by the results of nationally based studies. In the UK, The British Thoracic and Tuberculosis Association (now the British Thoracic Society) established, before the reintroduction of pyrazinamide, that a daily regimen of isoniazid and rifampicin for 6 months supplemented in the first 2 months by ethambutol or streptomycin was followed by a high relapse rate of 5%,

but if continued for 9, 12 or 18 months the results were excellent. Later follow-up showed only 11 relapses among the 493 patients available for study. The 9-month scheme was then compared with two 6-month regimens of daily isoniazid and rifampicin, supplemented during the first 2 months by pyrazinamide together with either ethambutol or streptomycin. Both gave excellent results and follow-up for at least 3 years after completion of chemotherapy revealed relapse in only 2 of 119 patients, one during the first and the other during the fourth year after completion of treatment (British Thoracic Society 1984). It is now considered that streptomycin or ethambutol are not needed in the intensive phase if the prevalence of resistance in the population concerned is low. Some of the widely used schemes of daily and intermittent chemotherapy are summarized in Table 59.1 which also describes the widely used conventions for abbreviating drug names in antituberculous therapy.

It is clear that many available regimens of proved efficacy are available from which a choice suitable to local needs and policies can be made. The problems of compliance and the organizational difficulties in establishing good tuberculosis control services, however, remain formidable; these, and the problem of management of drug resistance, are discussed elsewhere in this chapter.

Tuberculosis in children and pregnant and lactating women

Although earlier trials of antituberculous therapy generally excluded children and pregnant women, there is now abundant evidence that treatment of children should follow the proven regimens used in adult tuberculosis, with suitable

Table 59.1 *Short-course regimens for the treatment of tuberculosis*

Intensive phase	Continuation phase	Comments
Daily throughout		
2 months H R Z	4 months H R	Used if frequency of primary resistance is low
E H R Z S H R Z	H R H R	E and S are interchangeable in the intensive phase. Used if frequency of primary isoniazid resistance likely to be significant (>4%)
2 months (E) H R	7 months H R	Longer duration but suitable when administration of pyrazinamide is undesirable
2 months H R Z	2 months H R	Suitable for sputum-smear-negative cases in areas of low primary resistance.
Intermittent		
2 months S H R Z E H R Z } daily	4 months H R H R } two or three times weekly	
6 months S H R Z E H R Z } three times weekly		These two schemes are especially valuable in the presence of primary resistance to H or S, or H and S

E, ethambutol; H, isoniazid; R, rifampicin; S, streptomycin; Z, pyrazinamide.

dose adjustments and precautions about the detection of drug toxicity. Numerous studies of 9-month regimens in children, summarized by the American Academy of Pediatrics (1992), have shown comparable results to those achieved in adults, both in wealthy countries and under difficult conditions in developing countries. For example, Biddulph (1990), working in Papua New Guinea, gave isoniazid, rifampicin, pyrazinamide and streptomycin daily to 639 children for the first 2 months, followed by isoniazid and rifampicin twice weekly for 4 months, observing a generally rapid favourable response and only seven relapses in those in whom follow-up was achieved, mostly during the first 3 months. Adverse drug reactions were few (2%), mostly to streptomycin.

There are, however, some problems specific to childhood tuberculosis. Sputum samples are rarely available, because cavitary disease is much less common than in adults, and because children are usually unable to provide sputum specimens. Ethambutol is included in several schemes which have been recommended for childhood tuberculosis, but we think it unwise to give it to any child too young to understand the normal caveats about, or to report visual symptoms, or in whom visual acuity cannot be tested. Directly observed treatment, to be promoted at all ages, is especially to be encouraged in children.

Drug dosages are given in Part II of this book, and should be adhered to, although drug toxicity is not especially notable in children. Problems of extrapulmonary tuberculosis common to children and adults are discussed in the relevant sections below, and the problem of neonatal contacts is discussed in the section on chemoprophylaxis.

Antituberculous treatment may be necessary during pregnancy, and naturally most concern relates to the use of drugs during the first trimester. Snider et al (1980) consider that the only real hazard is potential ototoxicity from streptomycin and that none of the other agents has proved teratogenic for the human fetus when given in normal doses. Nevertheless, some experimental evidence of teratogenicity from rifampicin and the lack of information about pyrazinamide makes for some anxiety in deciding on a suitable regimen in early pregnancy. We think that, since treatment will only be administered during the first trimester for pressing indications such as open cavitary disease, it would be best then to give full therapy with isoniazid, rifampicin and pyrazinamide, with additional pyridoxine supplements. Davidson (1995) reports that pyrazinamide has been included in the regimen for treating tuberculosis in pregnancy in Los Angeles for many years, with no reported adverse effects.

NON-PULMONARY TUBERCULOSIS

Tuberculous meningitis

Tuberculosis of the central nervous system, although now rare in wealthier countries, remains an important cause of illness, disability and death, especially in children, in many developing countries. Prognosis is broadly related to the stage of the disease when treatment is begun. Unfortunately, the underlying and devastating pathology of tuberculous meningitis, with basal arachnoiditis, vascular occlusion, cerebrospinal fluid (CSF) block and tuberculomas, is often well established at the time of diagnosis and the patient's neurological grade may change rapidly for the worse before chemotherapy could be expected to influence the outcome. It is very important to start treatment as early as possible, and suspicion of tuberculous meningitis fully justifies a policy of immediate whole-hearted treatment. If an alternative diagnosis is established treatment can be changed, and the probability of establishing a bacteriological diagnosis of tuberculous meningitis is, in any case, little diminished during the first week or two of treatment. To summarize the evidence on CSF penetration of antituberculous drugs (Ch. 37), isoniazid penetrates well into the CSF. It has been customary to use larger than conventional doses in tuberculous meningitis, but this is probably unnecessary and increases the risk of isoniazid toxicity. Pyrazinamide shows very good CSF penetration. Ellard et al (1987) found that in Chinese patients with tuberculous meningitis CSF concentrations 2 h after the dose were about 75% of serum concentration. Five and 8 h after dosing they were about 10% higher than the corresponding serum concentrations. Rifampicin concentrations in CSF are about 10% of the corresponding serum concentrations, probably representing efficient penetration of the non-protein-bound fraction of the drug. Isoniazid penetrates the CSF rapidly, achieving peak concentrations of about 30 times the minimum inhibitory concentration (MIC) for *M. tuberculosis*. By contrast, rifampicin and streptomycin penetrate slowly, achieving CSF concentrations only slightly in excess of the MIC (Ellard et al 1993). Both streptomycin and ethambutol cross the CSF barrier relatively poorly and only when the meninges are inflamed. Ethionamide shows good penetration, even in the absence of meningitis.

In contrast to the position with pulmonary and some other forms of tuberculosis, the wide variations in the course of the disease and the difficulties in its diagnosis (now lessening with new molecular techniques) has meant that few controlled trials of substantial size are available. Treatment policies have thus been based on the results of older trials, on the known pharmacokinetics of the agents, and on such evidence as is available from more recent clinical studies. Initial treatment should certainly include isoniazid (adults 300 mg and children 10 mg/kg), rifampicin (600 mg in adults weighing >50 kg, 450 mg in adults weighing <50 kg, and 10 mg/kg in children) and pyrazinamide (adults 1.5–2.0 g daily, children 35 mg/kg daily), all as single daily doses. Workers in Hong Kong (Teoh & Humphries 1991) recommend the inclusion of daily streptomycin for the first 2 or 3 months, and it should certainly be included if rifampicin is unavailable because of its cost. Most authorities, including the American Academy of Pediatrics (1992), who also include streptomycin in the regimen during the first 2 months, recommend that treatment is continued for 1 year, but several studies have discontinued treatment at 9 months with no evident difference in results (Phuapradit & Vejjajiva 1987), and Jacobs et al (1992) used a 6-month regimen including streptomycin as well as the three principal agents in the 2-month initial phase, continuing with rifampicin and isoniazid only during the remaining 4 months. Intrathecal streptomycin is no longer used, although there was evidence of benefit in older regimens before the newer antituberculous drugs were introduced.

Non-antibiotic aspects of treatment are important. Whether steroids are beneficial in tuberculous meningitis has long been controversial, but the balance of evidence now favours their use (Girgis et al 1991) in the initial stage of treatment. One specific indication for their use is to reduce rising intracranial pressure associated with tuberculomas, which may enlarge in the early weeks and months of therapy. By contrast, raised intracranial pressure caused by CSF block leading to hydrocephalus should be treated by shunting as soon as possible. Physicians working in areas with a high prevalence of tuberculous meningitis consider that early establishment of ventriculoperitoneal shunt for hydrocephalus is important in improving the long-term neurological outlook.

All studies of tuberculous meningitis have confirmed that the most important prognostic determinants are the neurological grade at presentation, and the patient's age, the prognosis being notably worse in young children (Teoh & Humphries 1991). A study of three different regimens, all of 12 months' duration, in 180 children with tuberculous meningitis (Ramachandran et al 1986), revealed a mortality of 27%, perhaps associated with their young age (50% were less than 3 years old) and their advanced neurological grade, only 13% being fully conscious and without focal neurological signs.

Lymph-node tuberculosis

Tuberculosis of lymph nodes tends to run an indolent course. Nodes may be slow to diminish in size, and may appear, enlarge and even break down to form sinuses during or after appropriate chemotherapy. Radiographic enlargement of the hilar nodes may take 2 or 3 years to resolve completely. Physicians should not be deterred by events like these from continuing treatment by established regimens, which have been shown effective in controlled trials. The British Thoracic and Tuberculosis Association conducted a series of trials of treatment of lymph node disease. These included 9-month regimens of rifampicin and isoniazid supplemented with either ethambutol or pyrazinamide for the first 2

months, and a 6-month regimen of rifampicin and isoniazid supplemented with pyrazinamide for the first 2 months. A 6- to 30-month follow-up of 157 patients who completed therapy (Campbell et al 1993) showed no significant differences in these regimens with respect to enlargement of nodes, the development of new nodes or sinuses, or in the need for operations. There were nine clinical relapses, but these were unconfirmed by culture in the five in which material was obtained. A 6-month regimen including pyrazinamide has also been shown successful in lymph node tuberculosis in children (Jawahar et al 1990).

Bone and joint tuberculosis

The extensive studies of spinal tuberculosis carried out by the British Medical Research Council over a period of 20 years in Hong Kong, Korea and East Africa have served as a model for the treatment of bone and joint tuberculosis generally. In particular, they have defined the role of treatments additional to chemotherapy. The 18-month regimens prevalent during the 1970s were shown to be highly successful, and the good results were not improved by bed rest, by a plaster jacket, or by surgical debridement – results of great importance for countries with limited medical resources. A more radical operation used in Hong Kong with bone grafting and anterior spinal fusion gave improved results compared with simple debridement, but this is a major procedure requiring sophisticated resources. In terms of functional result, the radical operation was no better than ambulatory chemotherapy, although it was superior in producing complete bony fusion with less subsequent deformity.

Later trials, following the introduction of short-course chemotherapy, gave equally satisfactory results, and it now seems certain that short-course chemotherapy by one of the established regimens is very effective and can be used as the mainstay of treatment in patients without substantial neurological impairment. An excellent detailed account of these studies has been provided by Girling et al (1988). It should be emphasized that appreciable impairment of spinal cord function was an exclusion criterion in these trials, and it should not be supposed that chemotherapy obviates the need for urgent intervention in developing spinal cord compression.

Other forms of extrapulmonary tuberculosis

There have been few formal studies of chemotherapy for tuberculous pleural effusion, but there seems no reason to think that the standard short-course regimens already discussed would be any less effective in this than in other forms of the disease. In effusions unaccompanied by evident parenchymal disease, the bacillary load is presumably small. This may have formed the rationale, together with the known low rate of drug resistance in their region, for the regimen of 6 months' treatment with isoniazid and rifampicin used by Canete et al (1994) in 130 patients with tuberculous pleural effusion. There were no relapses in a follow-up of 6–96 months, and residual pleural thickening was seen in only nine patients. Despite these good results, we think it would be best to use one of the regimens established for pulmonary disease.

The remarkably high prevalence of tuberculous pericarditis in the Transkei has enabled extensive studies of this dangerous form of tuberculosis. The benefit conferred by corticosteroids in conjunction with antituberculous chemotherapy in this condition, and in tuberculous pleural effusion, is discussed later in this chapter. The chemotherapeutic regimen employed in the pericarditis trial was intensive, comprising isoniazid, rifampicin, pyrazinamide and streptomycin daily for 14 weeks followed by continued daily treatment with isoniazid and rifampicin to a total of 6 months (Strang et al 1988).

There have been few systematic studies of urological tuberculosis, but again there seems no special reason to depart from the standard schemes, although here too shorter schemes have been used on the grounds that the bacillary load is probably small. Repeated ultrasound examinations and occasional urograms are used to monitor the integrity of the urinary tract. Close collaboration between urologist and physician are valuable; stents may be employed, and nephrectomy is occasionally indicated. Steroids are sometimes used in the hope of diminishing the likelihood of ureteric stricture. A large group of patients with various forms of non-pulmonary tuberculosis has been treated with one of the regimens of short-course chemotherapy used in the USA, consisting of rifampicin and isoniazid daily for 1 month and twice weekly for another 8 months (Dutt et al 1986). Of the 305 patients treated, 205 were followed for 1 year after completion of therapy, and no microbiological relapses were recorded.

Drug-resistant tuberculosis

Drug-resistant tuberculosis in the USA has brought this issue to the recent attention of the international press. But the problem is not new, and was known to occur as the result of inadequate tuberculosis treatment programmes. No geographical area is immune, and current events re-emphasize the importance of vigilance and of the maintenance of rigorous tuberculosis control programmes (Crofton 1994).

Recent molecular analyses have identified the genetic mechanisms of drug resistance in *M. tuberculosis*. In general, the results so far have shown that resistance arises, for each drug studied, through mutations at a small number of sites in one or two chromosomal genes. Thus, for isoniazid, resistance has been linked to mutations in either the catalase peroxidase (katG) gene (Zhang et al 1992) or in the inhA gene, the latter apparently encoding an enzyme involved in mycolic acid synthesis for the cell wall (Banerjee et al 1994). For rifampicin, resistance has been correlated with point mutations in the gene encoding the RNA polymerase β subunit (rpoB) (Telenti et al 1993); for streptomycin, the genes for ribosomal S12 protein (rpsL) and for 16S ribosomal RNA (rrs) (Finken et al 1993); and for fluoroquinolones, the DNA gyrase A gene (gyrA) (Takiff et al 1994). In an international study, 37 clinical isolates from patients with a wide array of countries of origin were examined (Heym et al 1994). It was shown that these known mutations were associated with resistance in 78% of strains with isoniazid resistance, all the strains with rifampicin resistance and 60% of strains with streptomycin resistance; the same chromosomal mutations occurred in single- and multidrug-resistant strains and in primary resistance (present in the initial isolate, before treatment) and acquired resistance (developing during treatment). Most reassuringly, there was no evidence for a single new mutation conferring resistance simultaneously to many drugs, nor for transposable genetic material (such as a plasmid) which might transmit drug resistance between populations of mycobacteria. Furthermore, the findings were in keeping with existing hypotheses about the development of drug resistant disease, on which the approach to the prevention and management of drug resistant tuberculosis are based: namely that, in an untreated patient with drug-susceptible disease, mutant organisms which are resistant to single drugs occur spontaneously in the mycobacterial population at a predictable frequency (about one in 10^6 for isoniazid, one in 10^8 for rifampicin); and that the frequency of bacilli resistant to more than one drug in such a population is vanishingly small. The use of a single drug in the treatment of such a patient applies selective pressure, favouring resistant organisms, so that the patient initially improves, but then relapses as the organisms resistant to the single drug multiply. This was clearly seen in the early trials of streptomycin. In the new population of mycobacteria, with all organisms resistant to the first drug, there will now be a low frequency of organisms spontaneously resistant to other drugs also. The addition of a second drug to the failing regimen then applies selective pressure in favour of organisms resistant to two drugs. Because of the very low frequency of organisms in the original population which were spontaneously resistant to both drugs, the emergence of resistance could have been prevented entirely by the use of two drugs from the outset. The essential principles in the prevention and management of drug-resistant tuberculosis are, therefore: first, that patients should always be treated with at least two drugs to which their infecting organism is sensitive; and, second, that a single drug should never be added to a failing regimen.

MANAGEMENT OF DRUG-RESISTANT TUBERCULOSIS

The management of disease caused by organisms resistant to a single drug presents little difficulty in programmes using the established short-course regimens (Table 59.1). This was demonstrated by an analysis of the pooled results of treatment for patients with initial resistance to isoniazid or streptomycin in the British Medical Research Council (BMRC) studies (Mitchison & Nunn 1986). It was found that, using 6-month regimens which included rifampicin throughout the treatment, the outcome was nearly as good for patients with organisms resistant to either streptomycin or isoniazid alone as for patients with fully drug-sensitive strains. In patients with organisms resistant to both isoniazid and streptomycin there were more failures and relapses, and emergence of additional resistance to rifampicin was seen with some regimens. However, other schemes were still very effective; for example, the 6-month regimens in which isoniazid, rifampicin, pyrazinamide, and either ethambutol or streptomycin, were used throughout treatment (Table 59.1) (Mitchison & Nunn 1986, Hong Kong Chest Service/BMRC 1987). In the combined BMRC studies rifampicin resistance was rare, and (as in the current outbreaks in the USA) was seldom seen in isolation. The outcome in patients with organisms resistant to both isoniazid and rifampicin (and in some cases also streptomycin) was especially poor: 5 of 8 patients failed therapy, and 2 more relapsed after completion of treatment. This disastrous combination, of resistance to both isoniazid and rifampicin (with or without resistance to other drugs), is now used to define 'multidrug resistant' *M. tuberculosis*.

In some circumstances, resistance can arise rapidly. This has been seen, for example, in the emergence of fluoroquinolone resistance in *M. tuberculosis* in New York City (Sullivan et al 1995): 22 patients were identified in less than 2 years, at least 18 of them HIV positive. Five of the infections were nosocomial, and six patients had primary infection with fluoroquinolone-resistant organisms.

The successful management of a patient with multidrug-resistant tuberculosis is difficult and costly, and this is why prevention of such cases is paramount. The second-line drugs currently in use are summarized in Table 59.2. Confronted by such a patient the first steps are to obtain as accurate a drug history as possible (both from the patient and from records), and to obtain material for renewed culture and sensitivity testing; this should be conducted in an experienced reference laboratory. Any drug which has previously been used in such a patient must be regarded as suspect, and the drug history may be a better predictor of the likely efficacy of a regimen than laboratory sensitivity studies (Goble et al 1993). Common patterns of cross-resistance (for example between isoniazid and ethionamide, and between rifampicin and the new rifamycins, such as rifabutin) should also be taken into account. A regimen should then be devised, ideally comprising at least two, and preferably three, drugs to which the patient has not been exposed and to which the organism is known to be sensitive. Given the limited number of available medications, compromises may be necessary, but a regimen should be chosen as close as possible to this ideal. To avoid inadvertently giving a single effective drug it may be advisable to delay the new regimen until information is complete, if the patient is not too ill. The second-line drugs are much more likely than first-line drugs to produce undesirable side-effects. Patients require much encouragement, with palliation of

Table 59.2 *Second-line drugs for the management of tuberculosis**

Drug	Comments
Injectable drugs	
Amikacin	One of these is selected. VIIIth nerve toxicity important
Kanamycin	Require audiometry monthly, and examination of vestibular function.
Capreomycin	
Oral drugs	
Ofloxacin	Quinolones are associated with gastro-intestinal upsets, anxiety, thrush. Efficacy is probably good. One of these is
Ciprofloxacin	selected. Ofloxacin is suggested as first choice because of its higher achievable serum concentration/minimal inhibitory concentration ratio
Ethionamide	Some cross-resistance with isoniazid. Gastro-intestinal upset, hepatitis, arthralgia
p-Aminosalicylic acid	Gastro-intestinal upset, rash, salt retention and oedema
Cycloserine	Mood disturbance, psychosis, seizures. Should be given with pyridoxine[†]
Clofazimine	Efficacy uncertain. Causes skin pigmentation
New rifamycins (e.g. rifabutin)	Often show cross-resistance with rifampicin

* Based on material from Iseman (1993) and Goble (1994).
† Recommended adult dose of pyridoxine, 50–200 mg/day (Goble 1994).

drug-induced symptoms, to enable them to tolerate 'minor' adverse effects, and because of the seriousness of the disease it may even be necessary for the patient to endure serious adverse effects (such as hearing loss) if no alternative treatments are available. Supervision of therapy is therefore a very important component of the management of these cases. Even with optimum care the success rate in multidrug-resistant tuberculosis is poor: analysis of 171 cases treated at the National Jewish Center in Denver between 1976 and 1983 revealed initial success with conversion to negative cultures in only 65% of cases, and relapse-free long-term survival in only 56% (Goble et al 1993). It is possible that the outlook may be improved, for patients with localized pulmonary disease, by resection of the worst affected areas (Iseman 1993). The surgical procedures are difficult, because of adhesions and fibrosis with anatomical distortion and should be undertaken only by an experienced surgeon. Surgery must be accompanied by continuing drug therapy. Because of the relatively poor sterilizing activity of second-line drugs it is recommended that therapy for these cases (with or without surgery) should be continued for at least 2 years after conversion to negative culture. A valuable and detailed practical account of the management of these difficult cases has been provided by the work of Goble (1986, 1994).

The approach described above can only be used where resources are plentiful. Where resources for health care are constrained we suggest the following approach to the patient with suspected drug-resistant tuberculosis. Such a patient will have had active disease despite therapy for several months, and may have been non-compliant with treatment, or may be known to have drug-resistant disease. Full supervision of therapy is therefore advocated, which may lead to cure and the prevention of emergence of additional resistance. If possible, a specimen is sent to a reference laboratory for culture and sensitivity testing, because even a result obtained months later may assist in decisions on therapy. A regimen is then chosen empirically, for example employing all available first-line drugs, such as streptomycin, isoniazid, rifampicin, pyrazinamide and ethambutol, perhaps given thrice weekly for 6 months under supervision. This regimen will allow cure in the vast majority of cases resistant to a single drug other than rifampicin, and also in combined resistance to streptomycin and isoniazid, as described earlier. Treatment beyond 6 months is considered if sensitivity results became available indicating resistance to rifampicin, and the patient is responding well. An alternative 're-treatment' regimen, based on similar principles, is recommended by the WHO, and comprises 2 months of daily isoniazid, rifampicin, pyrazinamide, ethambutol and streptomycin, followed by 1-month of the same drugs without streptomycin, and then by isoniazid, rifampicin and ethambutol either daily, or three times weekly, for 5 months ($2\ HRZES/1\ HRZE/5H_3R_3E_3$ or $5\ HRE$).

If the patient fails on one of these regimens they must, unfortunately, be considered incurable, and treatment should be discontinued to avoid diverting scarce resources from treatable patients. The WHO suggests that continued monotherapy with isoniazid may be considered for such cases, with the hope that it will suppress the disease to a small extent (WHO 1991).

The long-term isolation of unfortunate individuals who suffer from untreatable, persistently smear-positive multi-drug-resistant tuberculosis is a social problem which is hard to resolve and must be addressed in the context of their particular society.

Tuberculosis in the HIV-positive patient

The interaction between M. tuberculosis and HIV is a reciprocal one. It is well established that infection with HIV promotes the development of active tuberculosis in individuals infected with M. tuberculosis. Adult HIV-positive patients may present with classical, upper lobe, cavitary tuberculosis, especially in the early stages of HIV infection with a relatively intact immune response (Mukadi et al 1993). In these cases the diagnosis may usually be readily confirmed by examination of the sputum smear. However, with more advanced immunosuppression unusual pulmonary presentations occur, such as non-cavitating, middle or lower lobe pneumonia, and the sputum smear may be negative, so that diagnosis may be delayed (Elliott et al 1993). Disseminated disease, lymph node, pleural and pericardial disease are also common (Elliott et al 1990, De Cock et al 1992).

More recently, evidence has accrued to suggest that the reciprocal effect is also important, namely that active tuberculosis accelerates the progression of HIV disease. In Haiti, Pape et al (1993) carried out a placebo-controlled study of prophylaxis with isoniazid in asymptomatic HIV-positive individuals and found that isoniazid not only afforded protection against the development of active tuberculosis, but also reduced the rate of progression to symptomatic HIV disease. Whalen et al (1995) report that survival is shortened in HIV-positive patients with tuberculosis compared with HIV-positive controls, matched for CD4+ T-cell count. Studies in vitro also provide evidence that M. tuberculosis has the capacity to promote the proliferation of HIV in lymphocytes and macrophages (Wallis et al 1992).

It follows that rapid diagnosis of tuberculosis, and implementation of therapy to reduce the activity of the disease as quickly as possible, are likely to be crucial in the management of tuberculosis in HIV-infected individuals.

Fortunately, there is considerable evidence that tuberculosis itself responds well to conventional regimens in the HIV-positive patient, with improvement in symptoms, weight gain, resolution of radiological abnormalities (Elliott et al 1995a), and reduction in bacillary load in sputum (Brindle et al 1993) comparable to that seen in HIV-negative patients. The high mortality is seldom attributable to tuberculosis itself, once treatment is established (Nunn et al 1992) unless compliance with treatment is poor (Elliott et al 1995b). There is evidence that the inexpensive regimen with strepto-mycin, isoniazid and thiacetazone in the intensive phase which has been widely used in developing countries may be inferior to regimens with rifampicin, pyrazinamide and isoniazid in the intensive phase, the former being associated with less efficient sterilization of sputum after 2 months of treatment (Okwera et al 1994) and a higher mortality (Nunn et al 1992, Okwera et al 1994, Elliott et al 1995b). This is in keeping with the concept that rapid elimination of bacilli and suppression of active tuberculosis may be important in limiting the progression of HIV-associated disease.

Sometimes, rapid confirmation of the diagnosis of tuberculosis may be difficult and, where clinical suspicion is high and other diagnoses have been excluded as far as possible, a trial of antituberculous therapy may be necessary to avoid delay (Anglaret et al 1994). Failure to respond within 2–4 weeks (in a patient known to be compliant with therapy) suggests that the diagnosis is unlikely and that the patient should be re-evaluated.

A number of additional issues arise in the management of an HIV-positive patient with tuberculosis. First, there is a higher incidence of adverse drug reactions, especially rashes, than in the HIV-negative patient, and patients sometimes show adverse reactions to several drugs (Pozniak et al 1992). This applies to most antituberculous drugs, but especially to thiacetazone, with which there has been a high incidence of Stevens–Johnson syndrome, with significant mortality (Nunn et al 1991): this drug should therefore be avoided in patients known to be HIV-positive, and should, if possible, be eliminated from treatment policies in areas where HIV is highly prevalent.

A second issue is that antituberculous drugs, especially rifampicin and the quinolones, may be poorly absorbed in HIV-positive individuals, even in the absence of a significant history of diarrhoea and this may be relevant in a patient whose response to treatment is unexpectedly poor (Berning et al 1992). However, isoniazid apparently remains well absorbed, and evidence from a small number of patients suggests that in general the early outcome of treatment (measured by sputum conversion) may not be greatly affected by the lower serum drug levels which occur (C A Peloquin, personal communication). The effects on long term outcome and emergence of drug resistance remain to be assessed.

Drug interactions should be given special consideration in HIV-positive patients, because they frequently receive a large number of medications. Of note is the interaction between rifampicin and ketoconazole, in which serum levels of both drugs may be reduced (Engelhard et al 1984). Fortunately, no important adverse interaction between antituberculous therapy and zidovudine has been reported, although the anaemia associated with tuberculosis may be exacerbated (Antoniskis et al 1992).

The necessary duration of therapy in the HIV-positive patient is another difficult issue. Studies in Africa have shown increased recurrence rates in HIV-positive patients who received regimens without rifampicin in the continuation phase (which usually comprised isoniazid with thiacetazone or ethambutol or streptomycin) (Perriens et al 1991, Hawken et al 1993, Elliott et al 1995a). To some extent, the poor outcome in these studies may have been associated with incomplete adherence with therapy. In addition, some cases of recurrent disease may have resulted from reinfection with a new strain, rather than relapse of the original infection (Godfrey-Faussett et al 1994), an event particularly likely to occur in areas where tuberculosis is endemic. A more recent study from Zaire in which daily isoniazid, rifampicin, pyrazinamide and ethambutol for 2 months was followed by twice weekly isoniazid and rifampicin found that a total course of 12 months in HIV-positive patients was associated with a lower relapse rate (1.9%) than a course of 6 months (9%), but the relapse rate among HIV-negative patients treated for 6 months (5.3%) was not statistically significantly different from the HIV-positive group treated for 6 months, suggesting that factors other than HIV status may have contributed to the outcome in this study (Perriens et al 1995). In contrast, a study in Spain using a 6-month (presumably daily) regimen with isoniazid and rifampicin throughout, supplemented by pyrazinamide and ethambutol for the first 2 months, achieved good results with only one relapse over a median follow-up of 55 months (Soriano et al 1988). In response to this uncertainty, and accumulating data, the recommendations of the American Thoracic Society have changed from their earlier suggestion that at least 9 months' therapy should be given, or 6 months from conversion to negative culture status, whichever longer. Currently, routine extension of therapy beyond standard duration is not suggested, but careful monitoring of the patient is emphasized (American Thoracic Society 1994). Studies which should help to resolve this issue are in progress. At present, we favour the use of standard duration of therapy with a regimen containing rifampicin throughout, with attention to careful follow-up of patients after completion of therapy, if possible. If close follow-up is not possible, HIV-positive patients should be strongly advised to seek attention promptly should symptoms recur, given the risk of both reinfection and relapse.

The outcome of treatment of HIV-positive patients with multidrug-resistant tuberculosis is frequently poor (Fischl et al 1992, Busillo et al 1992). This is not surprising, since the diagnosis of drug resistance is often delayed. In addition, the weaker bactericidal effect of the second-line drugs presumably means that such patients are inevitably exposed to the deleterious effects of active tuberculosis for a longer period than are those with fully drug-sensitive disease, even when an appropriate regimen has been started. The addition of second-line drugs to the initial regimen may, therefore, be considered in HIV-positive patients with active tuberculosis and known exposure to a drug-resistant patient, pending their own sensitivity results.

Mycobacterium bovis infections

Mycobacterium bovis causes disease in man and in domestic and wild animals. In countries such as the UK and the USA where pasteurization of milk and tuberculin testing of cattle are now routinely performed, disease caused by *M. bovis* has become rare, although not eliminated. For example, in the UK infection of cattle still occurs, and wild animals, especially badgers, are thought to be important reservoirs of infection. Elsewhere the infection is seen in deer (Fanning & Edwards 1991) and in game animals (Clancey 1977), and this may present an increasing problem with more widespread farming and ranching of these animals for venison. In the UK, continued surveillance of cattle herds means that the chain to human disease is now seldom complete. Most recent cases in the indigenous UK population have been in patients aged 60 years or more, suggesting reactivation of latent disease, while younger patients with the disease are more often of southern European origin, or from the Indian subcontinent (Hardie & Watson 1992). Similarly, in the USA, disease due to *M. bovis* is seen particularly in patients of Hispanic origin (Dankner et al 1993).

M. bovis is capable of causing a spectrum of disease in humans similar to that caused by *M. tuberculosis*, but with a preponderance of cervical lymph node and gastrointestinal disease; about 30–50% of patients have pulmonary disease (Hardie & Watson 1992, Dankner et al 1993).

M. bovis is naturally resistant to pyrazinamide. A 9-month regimen of isoniazid and rifampicin, supplemented by ethambutol or streptomycin in the first 2 months, is suitable (Table 59.1).

BCG-RELATED DISEASE

Bacille Calmette–Guerin (BCG) is an attenuated strain of *M. bovis* and shares its characteristic resistance to pyrazinamide. BCG has been observed to cause disease in a number of settings. Following vaccination with BCG, the commonest complications are chronic abscess formation and ulceration at the site of inoculation, often associated with incorrect injection technique, and disease in the local lymph nodes (Lotte et al 1984). The best approach to the management of these complications remains controversial. Spontaneous resolution is usual, but may take many months. The options for intervention are antibiotic therapy and surgery. Some authors suggest that antibiotic therapy with isoniazid (de Souza et al 1983) or erythromycin (Murphy et al 1989) may be helpful for abscesses or ulcers at the site of injection, but it is uncertain whether any benefit over the natural course of resolution is obtained. Studies from Turkey have suggested that neither isoniazid, isoniazid plus rifampicin, nor erythromycin alter the outcome of regional lymphadenitis (Caglayan et al 1987), but surgical removal of the affected gland was clearly successful (Oguz et al 1992). The evidence suggests that specific intervention is unnecessary unless the nodes are very large, or rapidly enlarging (when spontaneous drainage is frequent): in such patients surgical excision of the gland is recommended.

Rare cases of disseminated mycobacterial disease have been reported after BCG vaccination, and this has become of greater concern in the context of HIV infection, with several case reports of disseminated disease due to BCG in AIDS patients, even as long as 30 years after vaccination (Reynes et al 1989). However, prospective studies have so far failed to show any overall increase in complications of BCG when given to asymptomatic HIV-positive neonates (Ryder et al 1993, Weltman & Rose 1993). Vigilance is necessary, since disease due to BCG in these infants may be delayed (Besnard et al 1993).

Controlled trials of BCG vaccination in children with HIV have not yet been carried out, but are needed to determine whether BCG has any protective effect against tuberculosis in this group and whether BCG itself has any adverse effect on the rate of progression of HIV infection, as postulated for patients with active tuberculosis. In view of the difficulty in identifying truly HIV-infected infants at birth, and the importance of protecting infants against serious forms of tuberculosis in the context of increasing numbers of adult cases in the community, the WHO recommendation to vaccinate all infants except those with clinical evidence of AIDS is at present still appropriate in developing countries.

Over the last few years, instillation of BCG into the bladder has been shown to be a very effective form of immunotherapy for transitional cell carcinoma. Widespread application of this technique has led to the recognition of a number of adverse consequences, especially if the procedure involves traumatic catheterization or the patient has concurrent cystitis (Lamm et al 1992). Complications have included fatal mycobacterial sepsis, and many forms of focal mycobacterial disease due to BCG, including pulmonary disease, vertebral osteomyelitis, mycobacterial aneurysm formation and psoas abscess. Local disease in the urinary tract, with cystitis and epididymo-orchitis, also occurs, and the symptoms of frequency, urgency and spasmodic pain may continue for months in cystitis, despite good treatment with control of the infection. Treatment of established disease caused by BCG should be conducted as for tuberculosis at the same site, with a regimen suitable for *M. bovis* (that is, not requiring pyrazinamide). It has been suggested that corticosteroids may be a useful adjunct to therapy in patients with life-threatening mycobacterial sepsis following bladder instillation of BCG (de Haven et al 1992).

CORTICOSTEROIDS AS AN ADJUNCT TO THERAPY

The use of corticosteroids as an adjunct to antituberculous therapy has been considered in a number of situations and has shown definite benefit for specific indications in controlled trials (Box 59.1). In general, the benefit is produced by a reduction, first, in the active inflammatory response and, second, in the severity of subsequent fibrosis, presumably by interference with the production of the chain of cytokines which leads to fibrosis. The beneficial effects of corticosteroids in tuberculous pericarditis (Strang et al 1988) have already been described (p. 836). Similarly, in patients with tuberculous pleural effusion, Lee et al (1988) showed that the use of prednisolone was associated with more rapid resolution of symptoms and resorption of pleural fluid. In Lee's study, pleural adhesions persisted in 1 of 21 patients who received prednisolone and 3 of 19 who received placebo. This difference was slight, but the earlier literature supported the suggestion that corticosteroid therapy can reduce the frequency of persistent pleural adhesions. It was of note that the addition of corticosteroids after adhesions were established appeared to have no beneficial effect. The use of corticosteroids in tuberculous meningitis has been

Box 59.1 *Indications in which the use of corticosteroids may be considered as an adjunct to antibiotic therapy in patients with tuberculosis*

Indications validated by controlled trials
- Pericarditis (Strang et al 1988)
- Pleural effusion (Lee et al 1988)
- Meningitis (Girgis et al 1991)

Additional possible indications related to tuberculosis
- Ocular infection
- Genito-urinary infection (especially involving the ureter)
- Peritonitis
- Mediastinal lymph node disease (with obstruction of the bronchi)

Absolute indication
- Addison's disease (replacement therapy)

Indication not directly related to tuberculosis
- Severe cutaneous drug reaction

controversial but, as discussed above, in their study including both children and adults, Girgis et al (1991) showed significant reductions both in mortality and in the frequency of late complications of tuberculous meningitis in patients who received corticosteroids.

A number of additional possible indications for adjunctive therapy with corticosteroids are listed in Box 59.1: most are rare, and therefore difficult to study. In general, corticosteroids are considered in situations where fibrosis and scarring are likely to have a particularly deleterious effect, for example in the eye, in iridocyclitis, with the potential sequel of glaucoma.

Corticosteroids should not, of course, be used without a firm diagnosis and concurrent adequate antituberculous therapy.

Presentations of tuberculosis (such as pleural and pericardial disease) in which adjunctive therapy with corticosteroids might be considered are common in HIV-infected patients, and the balance of risks and benefits may be different in this group. The adverse effects of iatrogenic immunosuppression may be greater, for example with the possible exacerbation of Kaposi's sarcoma (Gill et al 1989), reactivation of herpes zoster (Elliott et al 1992) and cytomegalovirus (Nelson et al 1993). The benefits of reduced scarring and contraction may be less important, since this process may be less prominent in HIV-positive cases (Elliott et al 1995a). On the other hand, suppression of the inflammatory response may, theoretically, produce additional benefits in the HIV-positive individual, by reducing the stimulus to proliferation of HIV associated with activation of the immune response by *M. tuberculosis*. However, until further information is available, we consider that the use of corticosteroids should usually be avoided in HIV-positive tuberculosis patients, especially in those with advanced HIV infection.

IMMUNOTHERAPY

Immunotherapy has been attempted at intervals during the history of tuberculosis and has recently attracted renewed attention. It is hoped that ways may be found to enhance the immune response to the organism, thereby allowing the required duration of chemotherapy to be reduced, and improving the outcome of treatment when marginal drug regimens are employed against drug-resistant disease.

Koch treated patients suffering from cutaneous tuberculosis (lupus vulgaris) with tuberculin injections (at a site remote from the disease) and noted that an inflammatory response in the diseased skin occurred, which was followed by healing. A similar response was seen when vitamin D was used in the treatment of lupus vulgaris in the 1940s. However, both these forms of therapy had to be abandoned because the simultaneous inflammatory response at sites of disease in deep tissues, such as the lungs or the vertebrae, had disastrous consequences.

More recently, cytokine therapy has been used experimentally in patients with lepromatous leprosy and with intractable non-tuberculous mycobacterial disease. In the case of leprosy, there is evidence that treatment with either interleukin-2 or γ-interferon may lead to a reduction in the bacillary load in the skin, but treatment with γ-interferon has been complicated by a high frequency of the severe reversal reaction erythema nodosum leprosum (Kaplan 1993). In contrast, a good response has been achieved using γ-interferon in a small number of HIV-negative patients with severe disease caused by non-tuberculous mycobacteria, without any such adverse effect (Holland et al 1994). γ-Interferon therapy is now under investigation in the USA as an adjunct to therapy in patients with multidrug-resistant tuberculosis. In view of the role of the immune response in the pathogenesis of tuberculosis there is considerable concern that immunostimulation may, once again, have deleterious effects in these patients, and the outcome of preliminary investigations is awaited with interest.

Grange et al (1994) have suggested that it may be possible to switch the balance of the immune response in tuberculosis from a destructive to a protective process; in particular, that it may be possible to achieve this by vaccination of patients with a preparation of killed *Mycobacterium vaccae*, as an adjunct to tuberculosis treatment. Again, clinical studies designed to test this hypothesis are in progress.

Another area in which immunological intervention may prove useful is in modulating the interaction between tuberculosis and HIV. It has been suggested that this process may be mediated by the production of high levels of the cytokine tumour necrosis factor α (TNF-α) during active tuberculosis (Wallis et al 1992), and that it may be possible to control this response by using the drug thalidomide, which specifically inhibits the production of TNF-α by activated macrophages in a dose-dependent manner (Kaplan 1993). If this intervention proves beneficial in preliminary trials it will clearly be necessary to seek an alternative drug or analogue of thalidomide without the current drug's teratogenic potential before the intervention can be widely implemented.

Implementation of therapy

Successful tuberculosis control requires political and financial commitment, and a well-planned and efficiently run programme. A review of many of the practical issues involved in programme application has been written by Fox (1985) on the basis of his extensive experience in India and other countries. It should be borne in mind that, in contrast to many other diseases, the cure of tuberculosis is important not only for the individuals concerned, but also, by diminishing spread of the organism, for the general public health. For this reason many countries provide tuberculosis treatment free of charge to the patient.

Choice of a regimen

National tuberculosis control programmes select treatment regimens and provide guidelines for their use. This is essential for the ordering of drugs and to ensure delivery of supplies in proportion to case-detection rates. The regimen and guidelines can be kept very simple, since, as we have seen, short-course regimens (Table 59.1) are suitable for the majority of new patients, including those who are HIV positive. It is of note that the apparently cheap 'standard' regimen of thiacetazone plus isoniazid, supplemented by streptomycin for the first 2 months, has been calculated to be less cost-effective than short-course regimens, because the 'standard' regimen is associated with a higher rate of incomplete treatment and relapse, and therefore carries the costs of retreatment and of treatment of additional secondary cases (Murray et al 1991).

Combined preparations

A number of combined preparations of drugs for tuberculosis have been formulated, and are routinely used in the UK; for example, the dual combination of isoniazid plus rifampicin, and the triple combination of isoniazid plus rifampicin plus pyrazinamide. Combinations have the great advantage that they prevent monotherapy, and they are therefore especially useful for unsupervised therapy. There have, however, been some problems with the bioavailability of component drugs in combinations (Acocella 1989), and these preparations should therefore be purchased only from reputable companies where proper quality control is assured (Fox 1990).

Supervision of therapy

It is notoriously difficult to persuade patients to complete a long course of therapy. Styblo (1989) has advocated admission of all cases to hospital for the first 2 months (the intensive phase) of treatment, and achieved good success with this policy in Tanzania. However, there are many countries in which this is impossible, not least with the rapidly increasing case loads of tuberculosis associated with the HIV epidemic. Intermittent regimens, which allow supervised outpatient therapy (Fox 1983) have been shown effective in HIV-negative patients and are likely also to be effective in HIV-positive patients, although this has yet to be formally demonstrated. They can also greatly reduce drug costs (Iseman et al 1993). A programme of directly observed, intermittent, outpatient therapy was shown to be successful in Denver, USA, with less than 10% loss to follow up (Cohn et al 1990). More recently, the implementation of directly observed therapy elsewhere in the USA has been associated with reduced relapse rates and reduced rates of drug-resistant disease (Weis et al 1994). The benefits of a programme of supervised, intermittent, ambulatory therapy (SIAT) are compelling, but the question remains whether such a programme can be implemented where case loads are very high, resources and health workers few, and travel difficult. Wilkinson (1994) has demonstrated that a programme of SIAT can be introduced in this type of setting by recruiting community members, such as store keepers, to supervise therapy: 89% of surviving patients in his study completed treatment.

Convenience of the patient

A crucial aspect of the success of Wilkinson's programme was that the convenience of the patient was considered in the choice of treatment supervisor. In situations where supervised therapy is currently impossible, the minimum requirement for a treatment programme is that drugs should be reliably supplied and accessible to the patient.

Chemoprophylaxis of tuberculosis

Antituberculous drugs may be used to prevent disease in two different ways. Most commonly, they may be given to people known to be infected, as judged by positive tuberculin skin tests, but without clinical or radiographic evidence of disease. They are also sometimes used, as in a neonate whose mother has active tuberculosis and in other circumstances of high risk of infection, to prevent or delay primary infection. In recent years the special problem of chemoprophylaxis in HIV-infected subjects has assumed major importance. We consider the topic under two main headings corresponding to HIV status.

CHEMOPROPHYLAXIS IN THE ABSENCE OF HIV INFECTION

Accepted indications for chemoprophylaxis vary a good deal from country to country, depending on the local risks of tuberculosis and on economic and organizational factors. They can, however, be categorized in a way which allows for effective local policies to be developed.

1. Contacts of newly diagnosed cases of tuberculosis. Contacts should have a tuberculin skin test and a chest radiograph. Those with positive skin tests and an abnormal radiograph should be investigated and treated on the usual principles as presumed cases of tuberculosis. Healthy contacts with a normal chest radiograph and positive skin tests should receive chemoprophylaxis. The scheme for the management of close contacts of pulmonary tuberculosis in the UK is shown in Fig. 59.1

2. Subjects with known recent tuberculin conversion (not due to BCG), should also be given chemoprophylaxis. These will be mostly identified in contact groups.

Chemoprophylaxis is also recommended in children in whom positive (grades 3 and 4) skin tests are found, even if they are not known as recent contacts of an infectious case. The upper age limit for prophylactic chemotherapy will vary with the prevalence of infection in the community, and in many parts of the world this type of preventive management is impossible to implement. At present in the UK, chemo-prophylaxis is recommended (Ormerod et al 1994, Joint Tuberculosis Committee of the British Thoracic Association 1994) in children under 16 years, and possibly in young adults, especially if they are known to have recently converted. Two regimens at present suggested by the British Thoracic Society are isoniazid alone daily for 6 months, or isoniazid and rifampicin both daily for 3 months.

3. Patients with illnesses thought to increase their likelihood of developing tuberculosis. These indications are generally much more contentious and tend to be applied more widely in the USA than they are in the UK. The American Thoracic Society (1994) suggests chemoprophy-laxis in tuberculin-positive patients with:

- Diabetes mellitus
- Prolonged steroid therapy
- Immunosuppressive therapy
- Some haematological and reticulo-endothial diseases
- Injected-drug users, even if HIV negative
- End-stage renal disease.
- Severe weight loss or chronic undernutrition
- Other adults less than 35 years old coming from high prevalence areas, or from underprivileged populations, or in long-term care.

We feel that the possible benefits of chemoprophylaxis on as wide a scale as this may well be outweighed by the risks of isoniazid toxicity, increasing as they do with age, and that the necessary precautions and close follow-up recommended in the hope of lessening the risks will often fail to be achieved. A sensible compromise is suggested by Bateman (1993) in the particular case of patients receiving steroids. Noting that review of the literature gives little evidence of increased risk of tuberculosis in these patients, but that there are uncertainties about the influence of dose and of underlying lung disease, he suggests the use of chemo-prophylaxis in patients on steroids who have 'healed' or previously treated tuberculosis, and in tuberculin-positive subjects with small parenchymal lesions. Such a compro-mise approach might well be applied, together with consideration of other individual risk factors, in other patients in vulnerable groups.

The benefits of chemoprophylaxis have been well documented in patients with silicosis in Hong Kong. Three regimens, isoniazid alone for 24 weeks, isoniazid and rifampicin for 12 weeks, and rifampicin alone for 12 weeks,

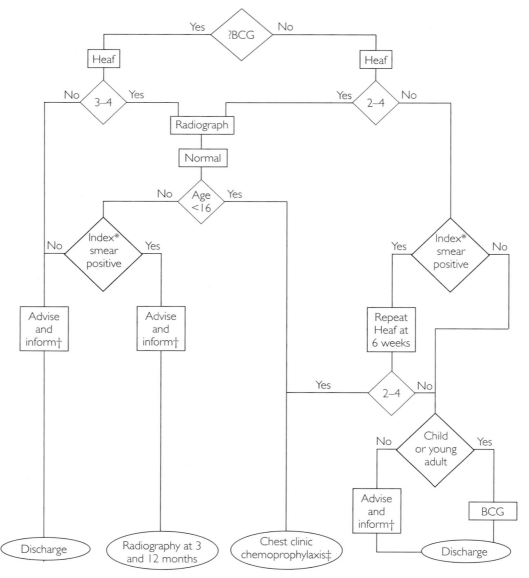

Fig. 59.1 *Examination of close contacts of pulmonary tuberculosis. Contacts of non-pulmonary tuberculosis need not usually be examined (see text). Note: Children under 2 years who have not had BCG vaccination and who are close contacts of a smear-positive adult index patient should receive chemoprophylaxis irrespective of tuberculin status (plus BCG vaccination later if applicable). *Negative test in immunosuppressed subjects does not exclude tuberculous infection. †Advise patient of tuberculosis symptoms, inform GP of contact. ‡Persons eligible for, but not given, chemoprophylaxis should have a chest radiograph at 3 and 12 months. (Reproduced with permission from Joint Tuberculosis Committee of the British Thoracic Association 1994, Control and prevention of tuberculosis in the UK, Thorax 49: 1193–1200.)*

were shown to diminish, but by no means abolish, the very high incidence of tuberculosis in patients with silicosis. At 5-year follow-up, the rate in the treated groups was 13% and that in the placebo group 27%. There was no significant difference between the treated groups and an important

additional finding was the lack of hepatotoxicity in those receiving rifampicin for 3 months (Hong Kong Chest Service/ TB Research Centre Madras/British MRC 1992).

4. The use of chemoprophylaxis on a larger scale. The above limited indications must be distinguished from the use of chemoprophylaxis on a much larger scale. The early trials of the US Public Health Service were concerned with groups at very high risk: Alaskan villages in which 'the disease was so widespread that for practical purposes everyone could be regarded as a close contact of an active case of tuberculosis'; patients in mental institutions; and people with inactive tuberculous lesions. The trials greatly reduced morbidity in compliant subjects during the year in which isoniazid was given, with lesser but significant reduction continued into a 5- to 10-year follow-up. The International Union against Tuberculosis (IUAT 1982), in a trial involving 28 000 adults with fibrotic pulmonary lesions in various European countries, achieved a reduction in culture-positive tuberculosis in a 5-year follow-up which increased from 31% in those who had received 12 weeks of isoniazid, to 69% in those given 24 weeks' chemoprophylaxis, to 93% in those receiving isoniazid for 1 year. The 24-week scheme was recommended because this gave the best ratio of cases of tuberculosis prevented per case of hepatitis attributed to isoniazid.

These results led to enthusiasm for even more widespread application of the method, which could in theory be extended to the whole tuberculin-positive component of a population. It is evident, however, that such schemes entail much isoniazid toxicity for little benefit, together with serious administrative difficulties, and that chemoprophylaxis is best restricted to particular groups along the lines of the foregoing discussion.

5. Infants of mothers with tuberculosis. A special and important problem is presented by the infant of a mother with tuberculosis, because of their intimate contact and the infant's high degree of susceptibility to disease. If the disease has been diagnosed and treated satisfactorily during pregnancy and is quiescent at term, the infant is given BCG and followed appropriately. A serious problem arises if the diagnosis is made late in pregnancy or even after delivery. If the infant is vaccinated with BCG at birth, segregation is necessary until the tuberculin test has converted, but separation from the mother is undesirable and in many countries discontinuation of breast feeding is very hazardous to the infant. In such circumstances the infant should be given oral isoniazid (preferably under supervision) until the mother is non-infectious; in practice, it is usually more practical to continue for 4–6 months, after which BCG can be given. If isoniazid-resistant BCG is available, vaccination need not be deferred until after the period of chemoprophylaxis.

CHEMOPROPHYLAXIS IN HIV-POSITIVE PATIENTS

It is evident from the foregoing discussion of the interaction between tuberculosis and HIV, and in particular from the study by Pape et al (1993) in Haiti, that isoniazid chemoprophylaxis can be expected to play a valuable role in the reduction of morbidity in HIV-positive patients, both from tuberculosis and from HIV. In countries with good resources and a low overall incidence of tuberculosis, the first step is tuberculin testing of all newly identified HIV-positive individuals. It is of note that the tuberculin test may be positive in some cases, even when patients have become anergic to standard control antigens (Markowitz et al 1993), so that tuberculin testing is helpful even in patients with advanced HIV disease when the result is positive; however, a negative tuberculin test in an HIV-positive individual who is anergic to control antigens does not exclude infection with *M. tuberculosis*. There is now considerable evidence that chemoprophylaxis reduces the incidence of active tuberculosis in tuberculin-positive, HIV-positive individuals and these patients should be considered for isoniazid prophylaxis for 1 year, after active tuberculosis has been excluded (Selwyn et al 1992, Pape et al 1993).

HIV-positive patients with advanced immunosuppression and cutaneous anergy are also at high risk of developing active tuberculosis when they come from populations with a high prevalence of infection. This was clearly demonstrated by Selwyn et al (1992) among HIV-positive drug users in New Jersey, USA, where the incidence of tuberculosis among anergic individuals (none of whom received isoniazid) was almost as high as that among tuberculin-positive individuals who did not receive isoniazid (6.6 and 9.7 cases per 100 person-years of follow-up, respectively). In this study none of the tuberculin-positive patients who received isoniazid developed tuberculosis during the follow-up period. HIV-positive individuals who are anergic to control antigens should therefore receive chemoprophylaxis regardless of their tuberculin status if they come from a group at high risk of infection. In addition to drug users, this includes HIV-positive immigrants from countries where tuberculosis is endemic.

The countries most severely affected by HIV and tuberculosis are also those in which resources for chemoprophylaxis are least likely to be available. Population screening for HIV and active tuberculosis and the implementation of chemoprophylaxis as a public-health measure are clearly impossible. However, HIV-infected individuals are frequently identified in the context of current programmes, for example in antenatal screening, sexually transmitted disease clinics, voluntary HIV testing centres and pre-employment medical examinations. Since antiviral therapy is seldom available there has been little to offer the individuals so identified, but the provision of tuberculosis chemoprophylaxis is now being considered (Mwinga 1994). One of the greatest difficulties encountered so far has been the exclusion of active tuberculosis among candidates for prophylaxis, since this may greatly increase screening costs and delay decisions on therapy: in a pilot study in Uganda, nearly 6% of candidates screened were found to have sputum-smear-positive tuberculosis (Aisu et al 1992).

Adherence with therapy may also be incomplete, and in a preliminary study in Zambia only 54% of participants completed therapy (Mwinga et al 1992). An outstanding question is for how long chemoprophylaxis should be continued. Wadhawan et al (1992), in Zambia, reported isoniazid given for 6 months conferred protection, but that the effect declined after treatment was discontinued; and in the study in Haiti, two cases of active tuberculosis occurred after the end of treatment in the group who had received isoniazid. This suggests that either the elimination of endogenous organisms was incomplete or the patients succumbed to new, exogenous infection. The latter is likely to occur in countries where tuberculosis is highly endemic, and further data are needed to determine whether limited courses of chemoprophylaxis are useful, or whether life-long chemoprophylaxis is required in this setting. Despite these difficulties and uncertainties, this method of prevention does offer some potential as a useful intervention for selected groups in developing countries (Walley & Porter 1995).

Atypical mycobacterial disease

Infections caused by atypical mycobacterial species form a large and varied group. An association of immunosuppression with infection by these organisms was recognized long before the advent of AIDS, but the link with HIV now predominates in this context and is discussed in Chapter 46. Atypical mycobacterial infection not associated with overt immunosuppression principally affects three main systems, causing pulmonary disease, often in association with predisposing lung conditions, lymphadenitis, predominantly in children, and skin and soft tissue infection (Wolinsky 1992).

Treatment regimens are often difficult to establish because of the varied antibiotic susceptibility of different species and isolates, and the treatment chosen should be determined by careful susceptibility testing of the isolate. Guidance is given in Table 59.3, but in general *Mycobacterium kansasii* is susceptible to ethambutol and rifampicin, and mostly resistant to isoniazid and pyrazinamide. Treatment regimens for *Mycobacterium avium/intracellulare* are based on various combinations involving rifabutin, ethambutol, aminoglycosides and the newer macrolides such as clarithromycin and azithromycin; fluoroquinolones, cycloserine and ethionamide have also been included. The rapidly growing species are generally resistant to the standard antituberculous agents; a large number of individual case reports describing the treatment of particular

infections is available, and individual testing is especially important. Few studies on any substantial scale other than those of the *M. avium/M. intracellulare* complex in AIDS (Ch. 46) have been made; one exception is a substantial multicentre trial of treatment of *M. kansasii* pulmonary infection (Research Committee, British Thoracic Society, 1994). This concerned 173 patients treated with rifampicin and ethambutol for 9 months. All the isolates were susceptible to these agents but resistant to isoniazid and pyrazinamide. In a follow-up period of 51 months 15 relapses were recorded, 3 of them possibly reinfections. A notable feature was the high mortality from other causes, emphasizing the strong association of *M. kansasii* infection with other serious pulmonary disease. Many authorities prefer to include isoniazid in the regimen, since the relapse rate was lower, although over a shorter follow-up period, in a study in which isoniazid was given in addition to the other two drugs.

Leprosy

The treatment and control of leprosy is a specialized topic and only the main features of its chemotherapy can be discussed here. Dapsone remained the mainstay of chemotherapy for many years after its introduction in 1947. Its high activity and encouraging pharmacokinetic features led to hopes that, although treatment had to be continued for many years, drug resistance might not prove a problem, and dapsone monotherapy was widely used in mass campaigns for leprosy control during the 1950s and 1960s. This optimism proved unjustified and, as with tuberculosis but over a longer time-scale, monotherapy was followed by an important problem of drug resistance. Primary dapsone resistance, that is, resistance in previously untreated patients, also appeared.

Relapse was not always associated with dapsone resistance, but with recrudescence of a population of persisters remaining dormant during chemotherapy, even when this had been continued for many years, a situation again comparable with that found in tuberculosis. By about 1977 it was recognized that mass treatment using dapsone alone could no longer be justified. Combination therapy was introduced, involving the addition of several other agents with anti-*Mycobacterium leprae* activity. Rifampicin is very rapidly bactericidal for the leprosy bacillus, and the slow generation time of the organism allows for infrequent administration, at monthly intervals. Persisters are, however, found after rifampicin treatment and, as with dapsone, may survive over many years of chemotherapy as a potential source of relapse. Clofazimine is also an effective agent which can be used in daily or intermittent dosage, with the

Table 59.3 *Medical treatment of disease caused by atypical mycobacteria. (*after Mahmoudi & Iseman 1993)*

Species	Recommended treatment[†]	Duration (months)	Anticipated response (%)	Comments
M. avium complex	**Rifampin, ethambutol, clarithromycin ± streptomycin.** Others: ciprofloxacin, amikacin, ethionamide, cycloserine, clofazimine	18–36	50–75	Use more drugs if extensive or life-threatening infection. Surgery may be useful for localized pulmonary disease
M. kansasii	**Rifampin, ethambutol, isonicotinic acid hydrazide ± streptomycin**	15–18	90	Previously untreated cases respond well to this regimen. But acquired resistance may compromise outcome in treated patients
M. chelonae	**Cefoxitin, amikacin ± clarithromycin.** Others: ciprofloxacin, imipenem, minocycline, doxycycline	?	10–20	Typically, improve on therapy, but relapse when drugs are stopped or resistance evolves to agents being used
M. fortuitum	**Clarithromycin, doxycycline, minocycline.** Others: ciprofloxacin, sulphonamide, imipenem	?	50–75	More responsive to therapy than *M. chelonae*. Less likely to involve lungs than *M. chelonae*
M. marinum	**Clarithromycin, doxycycline, minocycline.** Others: sulphonamide, rifampin, ethambutol,	2–6	80–100	
M. xenopi, M. szulgai, M. malmoense, M. scrofulaceum, M. simiae	**Rifampin, ethambutol, clarithromycin ± streptomycin.** Others: amikacin, ciprofloxacin, ethionamide, cycloserine, clofazimine	18–36	Variable but poor	Similar to *Mycobacterium avium* complex in resistance and response to therapy. No good studies, due to rarity

* Reproduced by permission from A Mahmoudi & M D Iseman 1993 *Chest Surgery Clinics of North America* 3: 729–736.
† Drugs in bold type are primary agents; others may prove useful.

additional advantage of an anti-inflammatory effect of some value in the control of erythema nodosum leprosum (ENL) reactions. Its main drawback is the red-brown pigmentation which it induces in the skin and conjunctiva, with darkening of the lesions themselves. Its other unwanted effects are abdominal discomfort and diarrhoea, which is usually mild but may be severe when a high dosage is given over a prolonged period. Ofloxacin or minocycline can be used as alternatives to clofazimine. Prothionamide and ethionamide, formerly used for this purpose, are no longer recommended because of their toxicity.

Combination chemotherapy for leprosy might be expected to have advantages similar to those found with tuberculosis, i.e. prevention of drug resistance, killing of persisters, rapid reduction of infectivity and a shortened duration of treatment. These arguments resulted in an important initiative

by the WHO in promulgating standard chemotherapeutic programmes for field use, employing multidrug treatment (MDT) for all forms of the disease, and using supervised treatment whenever possible (WHO Study Group 1982). The two main regimens recommended are:

● *Multibacillary leprosy* (including lepromatous and borderline cases)
  — Rifampicin   600 mg monthly,   supervised
  — Dapsone   100 mg daily,   unsupervised
  — Clofazimine   300 mg monthly,   supervised;
                +50 mg daily,   unsupervised
The regimen to be continued for at least 2 years and, if possible, as long as skin smears are positive; the patient is then kept under supervision for 5 years after completion of chemotherapy

- *Paucibacillary leprosy* (including tuberculoid and indeterminate cases; smear-positive cases in these clinical classifications should, however, be treated as multibacillary)
  - Rifampicin   600 mg monthly,   supervised
  - Dapsone   100 mg daily,   unsupervised

Treatment is continued for 6 months and patients are then kept under observation for another 2 years. More recent guidelines (WHO 1994b) have confirmed these recommendations.

These regimens have been generally successful and have enabled the duration of treatment to be much shortened with resulting improved compliance. Nevertheless, a number of problems are encountered in MDT (Waters 1993), especially the long duration of treatment required for multibacillary leprosy. A particular concern is the risk of relapse in this form of the disease, and this has recently been reviewed by the WHO. Rates were generally low, only 0.77% in groups with a long follow-up of 9 years. The WHO Leprosy Unit also found that 50% of the relapses occurred in the first 3 years, and 75% in the first 6 years, after stopping MDT, but Jakeman (1995) considers the results may be less good with treatment and control programmes of varied quality. Moreover, although MDT has become the preferred form of chemotherapy, its superiority is not always evident, as in the international trial by Dietrich et al (1994), in which dapsone alone, dapsone and rifampicin, and a four-drug regimen with additional prothionamide and isoniazid were compared in 307 patients with 3 years of treatment and 5 years of follow-up. The main effect of combination treatment was to accelerate regression of active disease, and there were only three relapses.

A major issue in leprosy treatment is whether the duration of treatment can be reduced, with resulting benefits in improved compliance and achieving effective control programmes. A number of claims for shorter courses of treatment with various combinations of the conventional agents have been made (Pattyn 1993), but Waters (1993) considers the best hope lies with new regimens which combine some of the newer bactericidal antileprosy drugs with rifampicin. The newer agents now under trial include the fluoroquinolones sparfloxacin, ofloxacin and pefloxacin, the macrolide clarithromycin, and minocycline, all of which have shown promising results in experimental systems and in pilot clinical studies. A WHO trial has been initiated including a regimen of ofloxacin and rifampicin, both given daily for only 30 days, and other possible methods include fully supervised monthly regimens.

Lepra reactions

The treatment of leprosy is punctuated by reactions. These are of two main types and chemotherapy should be continued unaltered in either case. Reactions in borderline disease are associated with downgrading or upgrading of lesions, and are caused by increased cellular hypersensitivity. Neuropathy may worsen and new skin lesions appear. These are treated with prednisolone, starting with 30–40 mg/day and reducing the dose over several weeks or months. ENL in lepromatous leprosy is caused by an Arthus reaction, and may be treated similarly with steroids. They should be given in short courses only since the sometimes prolonged or episodic character of ENL may lead to excessive steroid use and consequent toxicity. Clofazimine in increased dosage is useful in suppressing ENL, but its action is relatively slow. Mild or moderate ENL can often be controlled by thalidomide 100–400 mg at night in men and post-menopausal women (Wheate 1988). In mild reactions aspirin may suffice. Other possible interventions are discussed in the section in this chapter on immunological control.

Chemoprophylaxis of leprosy

The success of MDT has also encouraged a more optimistic attitude to chemoprophylaxis, which was hitherto applied sporadically or not at all. The evidence of protection of contacts by BCG vaccine is now strong and contacts of lepromatous leprosy should, where possible, be offered chemoprophylaxis with rifampicin. An optimal regimen has not been defined but Waters (1993) suggests six doses of rifampicin at monthly intervals.

References

Acocella G 1989 Human bioavailability studies. *Bulletin of the International Union Against Tuberculosis and Lung Disease* 64: 38–40

Aisu T, Raviglione M C, Van Praag E et al 1992 Feasibility of isoniazid preventive chemotherapy for HIV-associated tuberculosis (TB) in Uganda: preliminary results. *World Congress on Tuberculosis*. Washington, November 1992, Abstract 36A

Alland D, Kalkut G E, Moss A R et al 1994 Transmission of tuberculosis in New York City. An analysis by DNA fingerprinting and conventional epidemiologic methods. *New England Journal of Medicine* 330: 1710–1716

American Academy of Pediatrics 1992 Chemotherapy for tuberculosis in infants and children. *Pediatrics* 89: 161–165

American Thoracic Society 1994 Treatment of tuberculosis and tuberculosis infection in adults and children. *American Review of Respiratory and Critical Care Medicine* 149: 1359–1374

Anglaret X, Saba J, Peronne C et al 1994 Empiric antituberculosis treatment: benefits for earlier diagnosis and treatment of tuberculosis. *Tubercle and Lung Disease* 75: 334–340

Antoniskis D, Easley A C, Espina B M, Davidson P T, Barnes P F 1992 Combined toxicity of zidovudine and antituberculosis chemotherapy. *American Review of Respiratory Disease* 145: 430–434

Banerjee A, Dubnau E, Quemard A et al 1994 inhA, a gene encoding a target for isoniazid and ethionamide in *Mycobacterium tuberculosis. Science* 263: 227–230

Bateman E D 1993 Editorial. Is tuberculosis chemoprophylaxis necessary for patients receiving corticosteroids for respiratory disease? *Respiratory Medicine* 87: 485–487

Berning S E, Huitt G A, Iseman M D, Peloquin C A 1992 Malabsorption of antituberculous medications by a patients with AIDS. *New England Journal of Medicine* 327: 1817–1818

Besnard M, Sauvion S, Offredo C et al 1993 Bacille Calmette–Guerin infection after vaccination of human immunodeficiency virus-infected children. *Pediatric Infectious Diseases Journal* 12: 993–997

Biddulph J 1990 Short course treatment for childhood tuberculosis. *Pediatric Infectious Diseases Journal* 9: 794–801

Bloom B R, Murray C J L 1992 Tuberculosis: commentary on a reemergent killer. *Science* 257: 1055–1064

Brindle R J, Nunn P P, Githui W, Allen B W, Gathua S, Waiyaki P 1993 Quantitative bacillary response to treatment in HIV-associated pulmonary tuberculosis. *American Review of Respiratory Disease* 147: 958–961

British Thoracic Society 1984 A controlled trial of 6 months chemotherapy in pulmonary tuberculosis. Final report; results during the 36 months after the end of chemotherapy and beyond. *British Journal of Diseases of the Chest* 78: 330–336

Brudney K, Dobkin J 1991 Resurgent tuberculosis in New York City: human immunodeficiency virus, homelessness, and the decline of tuberculosis programs. *American Review of Respiratory Disease* 144: 745–749

Busillo C P, Lessnau K-D, Sanjana V et al 1992 Multidrug resistant *Mycobacterium tuberculosis* in patients with human immunodeficiency virus infection. *Chest* 102: 797–801

Caglayan S, Yegin O, Kayran K, Timocin N, Kasirga E, Gun M 1987 Is medical therapy effective for regional lymphadenitis following BCG vaccination? *American Journal of Diseases of Children* 141: 1213–1214

Campbell I A, Ormerod L P, Friend J A R, Jenkins P A, Prescott R J 1993 Six months versus 9 months chemotherapy for tuberculosis of lymph nodes: final results. *Respiratory Medicine* 87: 621–623

Canete C, Galarza I, Granados A, Farrero E, Estopa R, Manresa F 1994 Tuberculous pleural effusion; experience with 6 months treatment with isoniazid and rifampicin. *Thorax* 49: 1160–1161

Clancey J K 1977 The incidence of tuberculosis in lechwe (marsh antelope). *Tubercle* 58: 151–156

Cohn D L, Catlin B J, Peterson K L, Judson F N, Sbarbaro J A 1990 A 62-dose, 6-month therapy for pulmonary and extrapulmonary tuberculosis. A twice-weekly, directly observed, and cost-effective regimen. *Annals of Internal Medicine* 112: 407–415

Crofton J 1994 Multidrug resistance: danger for the Third World. In: Porter J D H, McAdam K P W J (eds) Tuberculosis: back to the future. Wiley, Chichester

Dankner W M, Waecker N J, Essey M A, Moser K, Thompson M, Davis C E 1993 *Mycobacterium bovis* infections in San Diego: a clinicoepidemiologic study of 73 patients and a historical review of a forgotten pathogen. *Medicine* 72: 11–37

Davidson P T 1995 Managing tuberculosis during pregnancy. *Lancet* 346: 199–200

De Cock K M, Soro B, Coulibaly I M, Lucas S B 1992 Tuberculosis and HIV infection in sub-Saharan Africa. *Journal of the American Medical Association* 268: 1581–1587

De Haven J I, Traynellis C, Riggs D R, Ting E, Lamm D L 1992 Antibiotic and steroid therapy of massive systemic bacille Calmette–Guerin toxicity. *Journal of Urology* 147: 738–742

De Souza G R M, Sant'Anna C C, Silva J R L, Mano D B, Bethlem N M 1983 Intradermal BCG vaccination complications – analysis of 51 cases. *Tubercle* 64: 23–27

Dietrich M, Gaus W, Kern P, Meyers W M 1994 An international randomized study with long term follow-up of single versus combination chemotherapy of multibacillary leprosy. *Antimicrobial Agents and Chemotherapy* 38: 2249–2257

Dutt A K, Moers D, Stead W W 1986 Short course therapy for extrapulmonary tuberculosis. *Annals of Internal Medicine* 104: 7–12

Dutt A K, Moers D, Stead W W 1989 Smear and culture-negative pulmonary tuberculosis. Four month short course chemotherapy. *American Review of Respiratory Disease* 139: 867–870

Editorial 1994 The global challenge of tuberculosis. *Lancet* 344: 277–279

Edlin B R, Tokars J I, Grieco M H et al 1992 An outbreak of multidrug-resistant tuberculosis among hospitalized patients with the acquired immunodeficiency syndrome. *New England Journal of Medicine* 326: 1514–1521

Ellard G A, Humphries M J, Gabriel M, Teoh R 1987 Penetration of pyrazinamide into cerebrospinal fluid in tuberculous meningitis. *British Medical Journal* 294: 284–285

Ellard G A, Humphries M J, Allen B W 1993 CSF drug concentration and the treatment of tuberculous meningitis. *American Review of Respiratory Disease* 148: 650–655

Elliott A M, Luo N, Tembo G, Halwiindi B et al 1990 The impact of human immunodeficiency virus on tuberculosis in Zambia: a cross-sectional study. *British Medical Journal* 301: 412–415

Elliott A M, Halwiindi B, Bagshawe A et al 1992 Use of prednisolone in the treatment of HIV positive tuberculosis patients. *Quarterly Journal of Medicine, New Series* 85: 307–308, 855–860

Elliott A M, Namaambo K, Allen B et al 1993 Negative sputum smear results in HIV positive patients with pulmonary tuberculosis in Lusaka, Zambia. *Tubercle and Lung Disease* 74: 191–194

Elliott A M, Halwiindi B, Hayes R J et al 1995a The impact of human immunodeficiency virus on response to treatment and recurrence rate in patients treated for tuberculosis: two-year follow-up of a cohort in Lusaka, Zambia. *Journal of Tropical Medicine and Hygiene* 98: 9–21

Elliott A M, Halwiindi B, Hayes R J et al 1995b The impact of human immunodeficiency virus on mortality in patients treated for tuberculosis in a cohort study in Lusaka, Zambia. *Transactions of the Royal Society of Tropical Medicine and Hygiene* 89: 78–82

Engelhard D, Stutman H R, Marks M I 1984 Interaction of ketoconazole with rifampin and isoniazid. *New England Journal of Medicine* 311: 1681–1683

Fanning A, Edwards S 1991 *Mycobacterium bovis* infection in human beings in contact with elk (*Cervus elaphus*) in Alberta, Canada. *Lancet* 338: 1253–1255

Finken M, Kirschner P, Meier A, Wrede A, Bottger E C 1993 Molecular basis of streptomycin resistance in *Mycobacterium tuberculosis*: alterations in the ribosomal protein S12 gene and point mutations within a functional 16S ribosomal RNA pseudoknot. *Molecular Microbiology* 9: 1239–1246

Fischl M A, Daikos G L, Uttamchandi R B et al 1992 Clinical presentation and outcome of patients with HIV infection and tuberculosis caused by multiple-drug-resistant bacilli. *Annals of Internal Medicine* 117: 184–190

Fox W 1983 Compliance of patients and physicians: experience and lessons from tuberculosis – II. *British Medical Journal* 287: 101–105

Fox W 1985 Short-course chemotherapy for pulmonary tuberculosis and some problems of its programme applica-

tion with particular reference to India. *Bulletin of the International Union against Tuberculosis* 60: 40–49

Fox W 1990 Drug combinations and the bioavailability of rifampicin. *Tubercle* 71: 241–245

Gill P S, Loureiro C, Bernstein-Singer M, Rarick M U, Sattler F, Levine A M 1989 Clinical effect of glucocorticoids on Kaposi sarcoma related to the acquired immunodeficiency syndrome (AIDS). *Annals of Internal Medicine* 110: 937–940

Girgis N I, Farid Z, Kilpatrick M E, Sultan Y, Mikhail I A 1991 Dexamethasone adjunctive treatment for tuberculous meningitis. *Pediatric Infectious Disease Journal* 10: 179–183

Girling D J, Darbyshire J H, Humphries M J, O'Mahoney G 1988 Extrapulmonary tuberculosis. *British Medical Bulletin* 44: 738–756

Goble M 1986 Drug-resistant tuberculosis. *Seminars in Respiratory Infections* 1: 220–229

Goble M 1994 Drug resistance. In: Friedman L N (ed) Tuberculosis, current concepts and treatment. C R C Press, Boca Raton, FL

Goble M, Iseman M D, Madsen L A, Waite D, Ackerson L, Horsburgh C R 1993 Treatment of 171 patients with pulmonary tuberculosis resistant to isoniazid and rifampin. *New England Journal of Medicine* 328: 527–532

Godfrey-Faussett P, Githui W, Batchelor B et al 1994 Recurrence of HIV-related tuberculosis in an endemic area may be due to relapse or reinfection. *Tubercle and Lung Disease* 75: 199–202

Grange J M, Stanford J L, Rook G W, Onyebujoh P, Bretscher P A 1994 Tuberculosis and HIV: light after darkness. *Thorax* 49: 537–539

Hardie R M, Watson J M 1992 *Mycobacterium bovis* in England and Wales: past, present and future. *Epidemiology and Infection* 109: 23–33

Hawken M, Nunn P, Gathua S et al 1993 Increased recurrence of tuberculosis in HIV-1-infected patients in Kenya. *Lancet* 342: 332–337

Heym B, Honore N, Truffot-Pernot C et al 1994 Implications of multidrug resistance for the future of short-course chemotherapy of tuberculosis: a molecular study. *Lancet* 344: 293–298

Holland S M, Eisenstein E M, Kuhns D B et al 1994 Treatment of refractory disseminated nontuberculous mycobacterial infection with interferon gamma. *New England Journal of Medicine* 330: 1348–1355

Hong Kong Chest Service/British Medical Research Council 1984 Study of a fully supervised programme of chemotherapy for pulmonary tuberculosis given once weekly in the continuation phase in the rural areas of Hong Kong. *Tubercle* 65: 5–15

Hong Kong Chest Service/British Medical Research Council 1987 Five year follow-up of a controlled trial of five 6-month regimens of chemotherapy for pulmonary tuberculosis. *American Review of Respiratory Disease* 136: 1339–1342

Hong Kong Chest Service/Tuberculosis Research Centre, Madras/British MRC 1989 A controlled trial of 3-month, 4-month and 6-month regimens of chemotherapy for sputum smear-negative pulmonary tuberculosis. *American Review of Respiratory Disease* 139: 871–876

Hong Kong Chest Service/Tuberculosis Research Centre, Madras/British Medical Research Council 1992. A double blind placebo-controlled trial of three chemoprophylactic regimens in patients with silicosis in Hong Kong. *American Review of Respiratory Disease* 145: 36–41

International Union against Tuberculosis Committee on Prophylaxis 1982 Efficacy of various durations of isoniazid preventive therapy for tuberculosis; 5 years of follow-up in the IUAT trial. *Bulletin of the World Health Organization* 60: 555–564

Iseman M D 1993 Treatment of multidrug-resistant tuberculosis. *New England Journal of Medicine* 329: 784–791

Iseman M D, Cohn D L, Sbarbaro J A 1993 Directly observed treatment of tuberculosis. We can't afford not to try it. *New England Journal of Medicine* 328: 576–578

Jacobs R F, Sunakorn P, Chotpitayasunonah T, Pope S, Kelleher K 1992 Intensive short course chemotherapy for tuberculous meningitis. *Pediatric Infectious Diseases Journal* 11: 194–198

Jakeman P 1995 Risk of relapse in multibacillary leprosy. *Lancet* 345: 4–5

Jawahar M S, Sivasubramanian S, Vijayan V K et al 1990 Short course chemotherapy for tuberculous lymphadenitis in children. *British Medical Journal* 301: 359–362

Joint Tuberculosis Committee of the British Thoracic Association 1994 Control and prevention of tuberculosis in the UK. *Thorax* 49: 1193–1200

Kaplan G 1993 Recent advances in cytokine therapy in leprosy. *Journal of Infectious Diseases* 167 (suppl 1): S18–S22

Lamm D L, van der Meijden P M, Morales A et al 1992 Incidence and treatment of complications of bacillus Calmette–Guerin intravesical therapy in superficial bladder cancer. *Journal of Urology* 147: 596–600

Lee C H, Wang W J, Lan R S, Tsai Y H, Chiang Y C 1988 Corticosteroids in the treatment of tuberculous pleurisy. A double-blind, placebo-controlled, randomised study. *Chest* 94: 1256–1259

Lotte A, Wasz-Hockert O, Poisson N, Dumitrescu N, Verron M, Couvet E 1984 BCG complications. *Advances in Tuberculosis Research* 21: 107–193

Mahmoudi A, Iseman M D 1993 Medical management of mycobacteria other than tuberculosis. *Chest Surgery Clinics of North America* 3: 729–736

Markowitz N, Hansen N I, Wilcosky T C et al 1993 Tuberculin and anergy testing in HIV-seropositive and HIV-seronegative persons. *Annals of Internal Medicine* 119: 185–193

Mitchison D A, Nunn A J 1986 Influence of initial drug resistance on the response to short-course chemotherapy of pulmonary tuberculosis. *American Review of Respiratory Disease* 133: 423–430

Mukadi Y, Perriens J H, St Louis M E et al 1993 Spectrum of immunodeficiency in HIV-1-infected patients with pulmonary tuberculosis in Zaire. *Lancet* 342: 143–146

Murphy P M, Maters D L, Brock N F, Wagner K F 1989 Cure of bacille Calmette–Guerin vaccination abscesses with erythromycin. *Reviews of Infectious Diseases* 11: 335–337

Murray C J L, DeJonghe E, Chum H J, Nyangulu D S, Salomao A, Styblo K 1991 Cost effectiveness of chemotherapy for pulmonary tuberculosis in three sub-Saharan African countries. *Lancet* 388: 1305–1308

Mwinga A, Elliott A, Halwiindi B et al 1992 One year follow up on patients in a pilot study to determine efficacy of chemoprophylaxis in the prevention of HIV-related tuberculosis in Zambia. *World Congress on Tuberculosis*, Washington, November 1992, Abstract 35A

Mwinga A G 1994 Preventive therapy for tuberculosis. Discussion. In: Porter J D H, McAdam K P W J (eds) Tuberculosis, back to the future. Wiley, Chichester

Nelson M R, Erskine D, Hawkins D A, Gazzard B G 1993 Treatment with corticosteroids – a risk factor for the development of clinical cytomegalovirus disease in AIDS. *AIDS* 7: 375–378

Nunn P, Kibuga D, Gathua S et al 1991 Cutaneous hypersensitivity reactions due to thiacetazone in HIV-1 seropositive patients treated for tuberculosis. *Lancet* 337: 627–630

Nunn P, Brindle R, Carpenter L et al 1992 Cohort study of human immunodeficiency virus infection in patients with tuberculosis in Nairobi, Kenya: analysis of early (6-month) mortality. *American Review of Respiratory Disease* 146: 849–854

Nunn P P, Elliott A M, McAdam K P W J 1994 The impact of human immunodeficiency virus on tuberculosis in developing countries. *Thorax* 49: 511–518

Oguz F, Mujgan S, Alper G, Alev F, Neyzi O 1992 Treatment of bacillus Calmette–Guerin associated lymphadenitis. *Pediatric Infectious Disease Journal* 11: 887–888

Okwera A, Whalen C, Byekwaso F et al 1994 Randomised trial of thiacetazone and rifampicin-containing regimens for pulmonary tuberculosis in HIV-infected Ugandans. *Lancet* 344: 1323–1328

Ormerod L P, Shaw R J, Mitchell D M 1994 Tuberculosis in the UK: current issues and future trends. *Thorax* 49: 1085–1089

Pape J W, Jean S S, Ho J L, Hafner A, Johnson W D 1993 Effect of isoniazid prophylaxis on incidence of active tuberculosis and progression of HIV infection. *Lancet* 342: 268–272

Pattyn S R 1993 Search for effective short course regimens for the treatment of leprosy. *International Journal of Leprosy* 61: 76–81

Peloquin C A, personal communication. National Jewish Center for Immunology and Respiratory Medicine, 1400 Jackson Street, Denver, CO 80206, USA

Perriens J H, Colebunders R L, Karahunga C et al 1991 Increased mortality and tuberculosis treatment failure rate among human immunodeficiency virus (HIV) seropositive compared with HIV seronegative patients with pulmonary tuberculosis treated with 'standard' chemotherapy in Kinshasa, Zaire. *American Review of Respiratory Disease* 144: 750–755

Perriens J H, St Louis M E, Mukadi Y B et al 1995 Pulmonary tuberculosis in HIV-infected patients in Zaire. A controlled trial of treatment for either 6 or 12 months. *New England Journal of Medicine* 332: 779–784

Phuapradit P, Vejjajiva A 1987 Treatment of tuberculous meningitis; role of short course chemotherapy. *Quarterly Journal of Medicine, New Series* 62: 249–258

Pitchenik A E, Cole C, Russell B W, Fischl M A, Spira T J, Snider D E 1984 Tuberculosis, atypical mycobacteriosis, and the acquired immunodeficiency syndrome among Haitian and non-Haitian patients in South Florida. *Annals of Internal Medicine* 101: 641–645

Pozniak A L, MacLeod G A, Maxwell M, Legg W, Weinberg J 1992 The influence of HIV status on single and multiple drug reactions to antituberculous therapy in Africa. *AIDS* 6: 809–814

Ramachandran P, Duraipandian M, Nagarajan M, Prabhakar R, Ramakrishnan C V, Trpathy S P 1986 Three chemotherapy studies of tuberculous meningitis. *Tubercle* 67: 17–29

Research Committee, British Thoracic Society 1994 *M. kansasii* pulmonary infection: a prospective study of the results of 9 months treatment with rifampicin and ethambutol. *Thorax* 49: 442–445

Reynes J, Perez C, Lamaury I, Janbon F, Bertrand A 1989 Bacille Calmette–Guerin adenitis 30 years after immuni-

sation in a patient with AIDS. *Journal of Infectious Diseases* 160: 727

Ryder R W, Oxtoby M J, Batter V et al 1993 Safety and immunogenicity of bacille Calmette–Guerin, diphtheria–tetanus–pertussis, and oral polio vaccines in newborn children in Zaire infected with human immunodeficiency virus type 1. *Journal of Pediatrics* 122: 697–702

Selwyn P A, Hartel D, Lewis V A et al 1989 A prospective study of the risk of tuberculosis among intravenous drug users with human immunodeficiency virus infection. *New England Journal of Medicine* 320: 545–550

Selwyn P A, Sckell B M, Alcabes P et al 1992 High risk of active tuberculosis in HIV-infected drug users with cutaneous anergy. *Journal of the American Medical Association* 268: 504–509

Small P M, Hopewell P C, Singh S P et al 1994 The epidemiology of tuberculosis in San Francisco. A population-based study using conventional and molecular methods. *New England Journal of Medicine* 330: 1703–1709

Snider D E, Layde P M, Johnson M W, Lyle M A 1980 Treatment of tuberculosis during pregnancy. *American Review of Respiratory Disease* 122: 65–79

Snider D E, Raviglione M C, Kochi A 1994 Global burden of tuberculosis. In: Bloom B R (ed) Tuberculosis: pathogenesis, protection, and control. *American Society for Microbiology*, Washington, DC

Soriano E, Mallolas J, Gatell J M et al 1988 Characteristics of tuberculosis in HIV-infected patients: a case control study. *AIDS* 2: 429–432

Strang J I G, Kakaza H H S, Gibson D G et al 1988 Controlled clinical trial of complete open surgical drainage and of prednisolone in treatment of tuberculous pericardial effusion in Transkei. *Lancet* ii: 759–764

Styblo K 1989 Overview and epidemiologic assessment of the current global tuberculosis situation with an emphasis on control in developing countries. *Reviews of Infectious Diseases* 11 (suppl 2): S339–S346

Sullivan E A, Kreiswirth B N, Palumbo L et al 1995 Emergence of fluoroquinolone-resistant tuberculosis in New York City. *Lancet* 345: 1148–1150

Takiff H E, Salazar L, Guerrero C et al 1994 Cloning and nucleotide sequence of the *Mycobacterium tuberculosis* gyrA and gyrB genes, and detection of quinolone resistance mutations. *Antimicrobial Agents and Chemotherapy* 38: 773–780

Telenti A, Imboden P, Marchesi F et al 1993 Detection of rifampicin-resistance mutations in *Mycobacterium tuberculosis*. *Lancet* 341: 647–650

Teoh R, Humphries M J 1991 Tuberculous meningitis. In: Lambert H P (ed) Infections of the central nervous system. Edward Arnold, London

Wadhawan D, Hira S, Mwansa N, Perine P 1992 Preventive tuberculosis chemotherapy with isoniazid among persons infected with HIV-1. International Conference on AIDS, Amsterdam, Abstract No. TuB 0536

Walley J, Porter J 1995 Chemoprophylaxis in tuberculosis and HIV infection. British Medical Journal 310: 1621–1622

Wallis R S, Ellner J J, Shiratsuchi H 1992 Macrophages, mycobacteria and HIV: the role of cytokines in determining mycobacterial virulence and regulating viral replication. Research in Microbiology 143: 398–405

Waters M F R 1993 Chemotherapy of leprosy – current status and future prospects. Transactions of the Royal Society of Tropical Medicine and Hygiene 87: 500–503

Weis S E, Slocum P C, Blais F X et al 1994 The effect of directly observed therapy on the rates of drug resistance and relapse in tuberculosis. New England Journal of Medicine 330: 1179–1184

Weltman A C, Rose D N 1993 The safety of bacille Calmette–Guerin vaccination in HIV infection and AIDS. AIDS 7: 149–157

Whalen C, Horsburgh C R, Hom D, Lahart C, Simberkoff M,

Ellner J 1995 Accelerated course of human immunodeficiency virus infection after tuberculosis. American Journal of Respiratory and Critical Care Medicine 151: 129–135

Wheate H W 1988 Management of leprosy. British Medical Bulletin 44: 791–800

Wilkinson D 1994 High-compliance tuberculosis treatment programme in a rural community. Lancet 343: 647–648

Wolinsky E 1992 Mycobacterial diseases other than tuberculosis. Clinical Infectious Diseases 15: 1–10

World Health Organization 1991 Guidelines for tuberculosis treatment in adults and children in national treatment programmes. WHO/TUB/91.161. WHO, Geneva

World Health Organization 1994a Tuberculosis, HIV on collision course in Asia. Press Release WHO/63. WHO, Geneva

World Health Organization 1994b Chemotherapy of leprosy. Technical Report Series 847

World Health Organization Study Group 1982 Chemotherapy of leprosy for control programmes. WHO Technical Report Series No. 675. WHO, Geneva

Zhang Y, Heym B, Allen B, Young D, Cole S 1992 The catalase–peroxidase gene of Mycobacterium tuberculosis. Nature 358: 591–593

60

Fungal infections

D. W. Denning

The treatment of most fungal infections has become considerably more complex over recent years for several reasons. Firstly, the increasing number of patients with acquired immune deficiency syndrome (AIDS) and human immunodeficiency virus (HIV) infection has yielded a new spectrum of fungal disease for which different therapeutic strategies have had to be devised or are being studied in clinical trials. Secondly, several new antifungals have been licensed or are under investigation, giving clinicians much greater choice but generating new questions such as the appropriate dose, and issues related to combination or sequential therapy. Thirdly, a much greater range of fungal pathogens are now

observed clinically due to changes in prophylaxis, international travel and changing medical care. Fourthly, resistance, especially in *Candida* spp. in HIV infection, is an increasing problem.

This chapter aims to give clinicians up-to-date recommendations for the treatment of all forms of fungal disease. This classification, summarized in Table 60.1, will form the structure of this chapter. *Pneumocystis carinii*, although now classified as a fungus taxonomically, is covered in Chapter 46. Developments in antifungal therapy are occurring rapidly in the mid-1990s and new data are likely to modify some recommendations in the future.

Table 60.1 *Classification of fungal infections*

	Normal host	Compromised host
Allergic	Allergic bronchopulmonary aspergillosis Allergic aspergillus sinusitis	
Saprophytic	Fungal sinusitis Aspergilloma	
Superficial	Tinea capitis, corporis, cruris and pedis Seborrhoeic dermatitis Pityriasis versicolor Paronychia Onychomycosis Otomycosis	Tinea Seborrhoeic dermatitis Onychomycosis
Subcutaneous and submucosal	Chromoblastomycosis Subcutaneous zygomycosis Sporotrichosis Rhinosporidiosis Lobomycosis Mycetoma Mycotic keratitis	 Sporotrichosis
Mucosal	Oropharyngeal candidosis Genital candidosis	Oropharyngeal candidosis Oesophageal candidosis

Table 60.1 *Cont'd*

	Normal host	Compromised host
Deep invasive	Urinary candidosis	Candidaemia
		Focal candidosis
		Pulmonary aspergillosis
		Focal aspergillosis
	Cryptococcosis	Cryptococcosis
	Coccidioidomycosis	Coccidioidomycosis
	Histoplasmosis	Histoplasmosis
	Blastomycosis	Blastomycosis
	Paracoccidioidomycosis	Sporotrichosis
		Mucormycosis
		Fusarium spp.
		Pseudallescheria boydii
		Trichosporon spp.
		Blastoschizomyces spp.
		Penicillium marneffei
		Other rare mycoses

THE ROLE OF SUSCEPTIBILITY TESTING OF FUNGI IN GUIDING TREATMENT

Susceptibility testing of antifungal agents has, until recently, had little application, but is useful when there is variability within a species to an antifungal agent. Certain fungi are intrinsically resistant to some antifungals (Table 60.2) and testing is inappropriate. In contradistinction, some fungi are apparently uniformly susceptible to certain antifungals, e.g. *Histoplasma capsulata* to itraconazole and amphotericin B. In these instances, susceptibility testing is only required if patients fail to respond, although non-compliance, drug interactions or failure of absorption leading to low antifungal concentrations are more likely explanations.

The reasons for doing susceptibility tests are given in Table 60.3. At present these are done in reference laboratories. It is not clear whether susceptibility testing to different amphotericin B preparations is appropriate. Delivery to the fungal cell may be important and differences (sometimes major) have been seen between different amphotericin B preparations, but these data are not yet correlated with clinical response.

Selected antifungal combinations are useful clinically. In experimental murine models, combinations have shown both synergy and antagonism which are isolate dependent. In vitro synergy studies are complex, but are occasionally useful clinically. The combination of amphotericin B and flucytosine in vitro against *Aspergillus* spp. is equally synergistic and antagonistic against tested isolates. If this finding is validated clinically, routine synergy testing would become desirable. Likewise, amphotericin B and rifampicin are often synergistic in vitro, but the worth of this combination has yet to be proven clinically.

Table 60.2 *Intrinsically resistant fungi*

Species	Antifungal agents
Candida krusei	Fluconazole
	Ketoconazole
*Candida glabrata**	Fluconazole
	Ketoconazole
	Itraconazole
*Candida tropicalis**	Fluconazole
	Flucytosine
*Candida lusitaniae**	Amphotericin B
Candida inconspicua	Fluconazole
Candida norvegenisis	Fluconazole
Malassezia spp.	Amphotericin B
Trichosporon spp.	Amphotericin B
Aspergillus spp.	Ketoconazole
	Fluconazole
Mucorales	Azoles
	Flucytosine
Scedosporium apiospermum (*Pseudallescheria boydii*)	Amphotericin B
Scedosporium prolificans	Amphotericin B
	Azoles
	Flucytosine
Paecilomyces	Amphotericin B
Fusarium spp.	Azoles
	Flucytosine
Penicillium spp.	Ketoconazole
Sporothrix schenkii	Amphotericin B
Madurella spp.	Amphotericin B
	Flucytosine

*A substantial proportion or majority of isolates.

Table 60.3 Indications for susceptibility testing in antifungal therapy

Fungus	Clinical setting	Antifungal
Candida spp.	Oral or oesophageal candidosis in AIDS (when unresponsive to treatment)	Fluconazole Ketoconazole Flucytosine
	Candidaemia Focal deep infections	Flucytosine Amphotericin B Fluconazole
Candida tropicalis	All infections	Fluconazole Flucytosine
Candida glabrata	Urinary tract infections	Flucytosine Fluconazole
	All other infections	Fluconazole Itraconazole
Candida lusitaniae	All infections	Amphotericin B
Rare fungi	All	Fluconazole Itraconazole Flucytosine Amphotericin B
All	When unresponsive to treatment or prophylaxis breaththrough	Fluconazole Itraconazole Amphotericin B Flucytosine
All	When in vitro resistance documented and first-line susceptibility testing shows resistance or tolerance	Synergy tests including rifampicin and amphotericin B or fluconazole and flucytosine

Allergic fungal disease

ALLERGIC BRONCHOPULMONARY ASPERGILLOSIS

First reported in 1952 from the London Chest Hospital, allergic bronchopulmonary aspergillosis (ABPA) is classified in five stages: acute remission, exacerbation, corticosteroid-dependent, asthma and fibrotic (Hinson et al 1952, Patterson et al 1982). ABPA also complicates asthma and cystic fibrosis.

Patients in remission require no therapy. Acute exacerbations are best treated with systemic corticosteroid therapy; usually a daily dose of 40–60 mg prednisolone for 7–10 days. Response is gauged both clinically and serologically; serum immunoglobulin E (IgE) levels should fall and radiological infiltrates should clear.

Many patients, however, require continuous corticosteroid therapy to sustain remission. For these a number of different antifungal strategies have been tried. Oral ketoconazole is ineffective (Shale et al 1987, Fournier 1987). In the only controlled trial of antifungal therapy, inhaled natamycin twice daily was also ineffective (Currie et al 1990). There have been anecdotal reports of amphotericin B by inhalation showing some benefit. The new azole itraconazole in a dose of 200–400 mg/day has shown benefit in two open studies. In one study, five of six patients who were corticosteroid dependent responded (Denning et al 1991a), the one who failed had low serum itraconazole concentrations. In another study, several patients responded, but the stage of disease and measurement of response were not well characterized (de Beule et al 1988). One of the difficulties in the management of ABPA in cystic fibrosis patients is the relatively poor bioavailability of itraconazole which, together with the tendency of the disease to wax and wane, justifies a controlled study to determine benefit.

In summary, the role of antifungal therapy in the management of ABPA remains contentious. For those who are corticosteroid dependent or severely disabled, a trial of itraconazole 400 mg/day is warranted, and if there is no improvement measurement of serum concentrations may be useful as a guide to appropriate dosing. It is thought that corticosteroids slow the progression of ABPA to pulmonary fibrosis which otherwise generally occurs between 5 and 11 years after the diagnosis.

Occasionally, ABPA is not caused by *Aspergillus* spp. but by *Candida* or *Trichophyton* spp. In these circumstances, if antifungal therapy is considered appropriate, this should be guided by known activity of the agent against the fungus in question.

ALLERGIC ASPERGILLUS SINUSITIS

This condition is associated with the presence of eosinophils and Charcot-Leyden crystals histologically in the context of *Aspergillus* sinusitis, which together establish the diagnosis of allergic aspergillus sinusitis (Jonathan et al 1989, Kutzenstein 1983, Manning et al 1991). Most cases are treated by surgical debridement. The use of corticosteroids or antifungal therapy is controversial. A treatment strategy similar to that in ABPA would be appropriate.

Saprophytic fungal disease

FUNGAL SINUSITIS

Aspergillus spp. are the commonest cause of fungal sinusitis although numerous other agents have been implicated. In the majority, the fungus is not truly invasive and surgical aeration of the sinus is usually curative. An algorithm is helpful in distinguishing saprophytic from invasive disease (de Carpentier et al 1994). Antifungal therapy is only required for those with histologically demonstrated mucosal invasion by fungal hyphae or if destruction is present on computed tomography (CT) scan.

The next most common cause of sinusitis are the dematiaceous fungi such as *Bipolaris*, *Dreschlera* and *Exserohilum* spp. and others. These occur in normal hosts, often young patients, and tend to be subacute in presentation. These infections tend to be highly resistant to therapy and are slowly progressive leading to ocular palsy and cerebral invasion. Some success has been reported with very large doses of itraconazole (e.g. 800–1200 mg/day).

ASPERGILLOMA

The vast majority of fungus balls of the lungs are due to *Aspergillus* spp. with rare cases due to *Pseudallescheria boydii* or Mucorales. This discussion will focus on aspergillomas. Approximately 10% of aspergillomas resolve spontaneously, making uncontrolled observations in small numbers of patients difficult to interpret. In addition, *Aspergillus* antibody titres vary considerably over time.

Several therapeutic strategies have been used in treating aspergillomas. Systemic antifungal therapy with ketoco-nazole is ineffective. Itraconazole 200 mg/day is of marginal symptomatic and little radiological benefit (Campbell et al 1991). This probably reflects, at least in part, the lack of delivery of drug to the fungus ball and the chronic fibrotic/inflammatory changes in the surrounding lung. A dose of 400 mg/day may have been more appropriate.

Instillation of the aspergilloma with nystatin and amphotericin B has been tried with some benefit, especially with amphotericin B. Repeated instillations are usually necessary (in one study daily for 15 days (Lee et al 1993)). Communication between the cavity and the airways is usual, so the instilled agent usually leaks into the airways. Repeated instillations are not very effective for complex and/or bilateral aspergillomas. The incorporation of amphotericin B in gelatin or glycerin that solidifies at 37°C (Giron et al 1993, Munk et al 1993) deserves further evaluation.

Many patients with aspergillomas are corticosteroid dependent, because of other pulmonary or systemic disease, which carries a slightly greater risk of invasive aspergillosis. Whether systemic antifungal therapy would prevent this is unclear.

Surgery may be necessary for patients with recurrent haemoptyses, but is fraught with difficulty particularly for complex aspergilloma, because of the vascular adherent pleura, while the remaining chest cavity may become infected with *Aspergillus* (Daly et al 1986). In those patients with major haemoptysis and simple aspergillomas, surgery offers an 84% 5-year survival compared with a 41% survival with conservative therapy (Jewkes et al 1983). Surgical removal of pleural aspergillomas and thoracoplasty is prone to many complications and is best avoided (Massard et al 1992).

In most instances of haemoptysis, abnormal and novel vascular connections to the systemic circulation are implicated, e.g. internal mammary or other arteries. Aspergillomas may also lead to an extensive network of small vessels. In patients unfit for surgery, with recurrent haemoptyses, embolization may be appropriate in order to occlude these vessels permanently. The patient must lie still for 3–4 h during the procedure, which may be a major limiting factor. Approximately 50–70% of embolization procedures are successful (Rémy & Jardin 1990), although 50% will relapse.

Superficial mycoses

Tinea capitis, cruris, corporis and pedis are widespread in the normal population and particularly common in HIV-positive patients. They are caused by a variety of dermatophytes of *Trichophyton*, *Microsporum* and *Epidermophyton* spp.

TINEA CAPITIS

Tinea capitis may manifest as alopecia with little apparent inflammation to a kerion which is an inflammatory mass of hair, exudate, fungus and granulation tissue that can mimic a squamous cell carcinoma, and is more common in children. A Wood's light examination and mycological sampling make the diagnosis. The mycological cause of tinea capitis varies geographically. In the UK, *Trichophyton tonsurans* predominates over *Microsporum*. In other parts of the world, *Trichophyton violaceum* and *Trichophyton soudananse* are more common.

Topical therapy is usually ineffective. Oral griseofulvin (500–1000 mg/day after food for 2–3 months) has the disadvantage of being protracted and requiring repeat mycological testing after 1 month. In adults, terbinafine 250 mg/day or itraconazole 200 mg/day are appropriate but must be continued for 4 weeks (Table 60.4). In children with tinea capitis caused by *M. canis*, a 6-week course of either itraconazole 100 mg or griseofulvin 500 mg/day exhibited equivalent efficacy of 88%, but itraconazole was better tolerated (Lopez-Gomez et al 1994).

TINEA CRURIS

Tinea cruris is more common in young men than women, producing a confluent, red, scaly rash covering the groin, scrotum and thighs. It is caused by various dermatophytes but *Candida* spp. can be involved if the skin is wet and macerated (intertrigo). Topical imidazoles such as clotrimazole, miconazole or sulconazole twice daily for at least 2 weeks are usually effective (Table 60.4). Oral itraconazole (200 mg/day for 1 week) (Parent et al 1994) or terbinafine 250 mg/day for 7 days (Farag et al 1994) are highly effective if topical agents fail.

TINEA CORPORIS

Tinea corporis tends to affect exposed areas of the extremities and may be treated systemically, as for tinea cruris (Table 60.4).

TINEA PEDIS

Tinea pedis (athlete's foot) affects about 30% of the population, and often recurs. Terbinafine cream 1% twice daily for 1 week compares well with 1% clotrimazole cream twice daily for 4 weeks (97% versus 84% response) (Evans 1994) (Table 60.4). It does not seem to be a major problem in HIV infection; *Trichophyton rubrum* can be grown from foot-skin scrapings in about 40% of HIV-positive patients, more commonly in late-stage disease, though with little symptomatic infection (Korting et al 1993). Moccasin-type tinea pedis affecting the soles is invariably due to *T. rubrum* and is often recalcitrant to therapy. Three weeks therapy with either terbinafine 250 mg/day or itraconazole 200 mg/day are the best options.

SEBORRHOEIC DERMATITIS, PITYRIASIS VERSICOLOR AND DANDRUFF

There is a range of superficial diseases related to superficial colonization with *Malassezia furfur* (*Pityrosprum ovale*). Pityriasis versicolor is a superficial skin infection of the upper trunk, primarily without an inflammatory component or scaling. Seborrhoeic dermatitis causes excess scaling of the edge of the scalp, face and anterior chest associated with an inflammatory component.

Dandruff (or its equivalent in babies – cradle cap) is characterized by excessive scaling but minimal inflam-

Table 60.4 *Treatment of tinea infections*

Condition	Agent	Daily dose	Duration
Tinea capitis	Griseofulvin	1000 mg	2–3 months
	Itraconazole	200 mg	4–6 weeks
Tinea cruris	Clotrimazole	Topical b.i.d.	2–3 weeks
	Miconazole	Topical b.i.d.	2–3 weeks
	Sulconazole	Topical b.i.d.	2–3 weeks
	Itraconazole	200 mg	1 week
	Terbinafine	250 mg	1 week
Tinea corporis	Itraconazole	200 mg	1 week
	Terbinafine	250 mg	1 week
Tinea pedis	Terbinafine, 1% cream	Topical b.i.d.	1 week
	Clotrimazole, 1% cream	Topical b.i.d.	1 week
Moccasin-type tinea pedis	Itraconazole	200 mg	3 weeks
	Terbinafine	250 mg	3 weeks

b.i.d., twice daily.

mation, and is largely a cosmetic problem. Use of medicated shampoo containing ketoconazole is effective if used frequently, but relapse is common. Alternatives include topical selenium sulphide shampoo or zinc pyrithione solutions. Cradle cap in babies requires no therapy but can be treated with olive oil, which is inoffensive and safe.

Pityriasis versicolor can be treated with 2.5% selenium sulphide shampoo applied nightly for at least 7 days (80% response) (Del Palacio Hernandez et al 1987). Topical griseofulvin cream 1% and terbinafine cream are also effective. Many patients do not like topical applications; oral itraconazole 200 mg/day for 7 days is 85% effective (Delescluse, 1990).

Seborrhoeic dermatitis is a common problem. Some authors have stated a lifetime incidence of 10% for the normal population with an incidence in HIV-infected patients of 50% (Staughton 1990). Seborrhoeic dermatitis frequently accompanies symptomatic HIV infection and tends to worsen as the immune deficit progresses. It may also be associated with folliculitis. *M. furfur*, a polymorphic yeast, is the aetiological agent (Ingham & Cunningham 1993). The relative contribution of a cell-mediated response or hypersensitivity to yeast colonization compared with a simple infection are poorly understood.

Seborrhoeic dermatitis is a chronic disease that relapses rapidly after treatment. It may also be difficult to effect improvement despite good antifungal therapy and anti-inflammatory agents. Topical corticosteroids have largely been supplanted by the use of topical ketoconazole with or without a steroid component. Lithium succinate 8% ointment is also effective. These treatments compare favourably with alternatives such as selenium sulphide and zinc pyrithione containing preparations. Patients with very inflammatory lesions benefit from combined hydrocortisone 1% and antifungals applied locally. Oral itraconazole 200 mg/day is also effective (Ingham & Cunningham 1993) and has useful in vitro activity against *M. furfur* (Delescluse 1990). Fluconazole is not very effective, especially in those with AIDS. Maintenance therapy is not recommended for seborrhoeic dermatitis, unless it is very severe.

FUNGAL NAIL DISEASE (PARONYCHIA AND ONYCHOMYCOSIS)

Fungi may affect the nail fold (paronychia) or the nail itself (onychomycosis). Paronychia is usually caused by *Candida albicans* and occasionally other *Candida* species. Confirmation by culture is desirable because there are more cases of paronychia due to bacteria, especially *Staphylococcus aureus*, than *Candida* spp. Onychomycosis is caused by a variety of fungi; the commonest are *T. rubrum* and *Trichophyton interdigitale* (*mentagrophytes*), which cause about 80% of cases in the UK; uncommon causes include *Trichophyton erinacea*, *T. soudanense*, *T. tonsurans*, *T.*

violaceum, *Epidermophyton floccosum* and *M. canis*. Non-dermatophyte moulds that occasionally cause onychomycosis, usually of the toenail, include *Fusarium* spp., *Aspergillus* spp., *Acremonium* spp., *Scytalidium dimidiatum*, *Scytalidium hyalinium* and *Scopulariopsis brevicaulis*. Some causes of onychomycosis are due to *C. albicans* and *Candida parapsilosis*.

Candida paronychia

Candida paronychia will usually respond, if it is mild and localized, to imidazole or terbinafine cream or nystatin ointment applied topically for 1–3 weeks. In addition, patients should refrain from excessive washing, which is the usual primary reason for the development of paronychia. This will often mean a period off work. For patients with extensive *Candida* paronychia or an immunodeficiency state, including chronic mucocutaneous candidosis, itraconazole 200 mg/day for 3–6 weeks is usually adequate, although some patients require longer term maintenance therapy to prevent recurrence. Patients who also have *Candida* onychomycosis together with paronychia require longer therapy. Fluconazole is also active against *Candida*, doses of 50–200 mg/day are effective depending on the severity of disease and how immunocompromised the patient is. Terbinafine may be an inferior choice in immunocompromised patients because it is not fungicidal against *C. albicans* although it is against other *Candida* species.

Onychomycosis

The treatment of onychomycosis depends on the nature of the infecting fungus, whether finger nails or toenails are involved, how many nails are involved, the pattern of nail involvement, the age of the patient and whether the patient is immunocompromised (British Society for Medical Mycology 1995). In localized distal finger nail disease, in the non-immunocompromised patients topical therapy is appropriate (Box 60.1). The combination of tioconazole with undecylenic acid applied twice a day for 4–6 weeks is one option. Alternatively, amorolfine nail paint applied weekly for the same duration has an equivalent efficacy rate (40%) (Zang & Bergstaesser 1992). A more radical solution is dissolution of the nail with 40% urea paste, a procedure

---

Box 60.1   *Options for treatment of onychomycosis*

Topical therapy	
40% Urea paste	once daily
Tioconazole + undecylenic acid (Trosyl)	twice daily
Amorolfine	weekly
Systemic therapy	
Griseofulvin	500–1000 mg/day
Itraconazole	200 mg/day
Terbinafine	250 mg/day

usually undertaken by a chiropodist. The above options may also be appropriate for non-dermatophyte onychomycosis of one or two toenails involving less than 80% of the nail. However, the cure rate of topical therapy is only about 40% and many months of treatment are required, thus dissolution of the nail with urea paste may be a preferred option for these patients.

For patients with proximal nail involvement or extensive nail disease, which may also include skin around the nails, systemic therapy is appropriate (Box 60.1). Griseofulvin (≥500 mg/day) was the standard therapy for these infections until recently. The response rates after 4–8 months of therapy for finger nails is 90% and for toenails treated for 12–18 months is 40% (Roberts 1991). Both itraconazole 200 mg/day (Hay et al 1990) or terbinafine 250 mg daily (Goodfield et al 1992) yields responses in excess of 75% for toenail involvement with dermatophytes. Itraconazole 100 mg/day is no more effective than griseofulvin. Itraconazole accumulates in the nail and nail plate and many dermatologists treat for 1 week in every month until cure is obtained (usually 3 months for finger nails and 6–12 months for toenails). Relapse may occur after discontinuation of therapy. Another strategy is alternating months of treatment. These intermittent regimens yield slightly lower efficacy but at substantially lower cost. Terbinafine should be administered daily for 3 months for finger nails and 6–12 months for toenails and has been shown to be cost-effective (Arikian et al 1994).

In patients with non-dermatophyte onychomycosis of the toenails, itraconazole may be appropriate for those caused by *Aspergillus* and possibly *Acremonium* spp. However, it will not be effective therapy for *Fusarium* onychomycosis and the data supporting its use for *Scopulariopsis* and *Scytalidium* infections are limited.

In leukaemic patients with onychomycosis it is important to ascertain whether it is due to *Fusarium*. Removal of the nail may prevent disseminated *Fusarium* infection, which carries a high mortality (Nelson et al 1994).

Onychomycosis is common in those with AIDS and includes a superficial white onychomycosis caused by *Candida* or dermatophytes or a more destructive generalized disease. Systemic therapy with itraconazole 200–400 mg/ day for 3 months for finger nails and 6–12 months for toenails is recommended. Terbinafine 250 mg/day is another option, although the response rate in AIDS patients is not known (Elmets 1994). Treatment is primarily for cosmetic reasons rather than to prevent dissemination, which is rare.

Onychomycosis in children is usually a dermatophyte infection and fluconazole syrup 2–3 mg/kg is appropriate in very small children.

OTOMYCOSIS (OTITIS EXTERNA)

Otomycosis is a relatively common problem in non-immunocompromised patients. It may be caused by bacteria or fungi. The latter are more likely in humid climates and in those with poor hygiene. The causative fungi include *Aspergillus niger* and *C. albicans* among others. However, the diagnosis can be elusive and superficial white patches may be all that is seen in the ear canal.

The vast majority of cases of otomycosis respond to a combination of thorough cleaning of the ear canal and local antifungal therapy. Clotrimazole powder or cream applied at least twice daily for a minimum of a week is probably the best primary therapy. Alternatives include cresyl acetate solution, gentian violet (1%), or topical ketoconazole, econazole or amphotericin B (Patow 1995). Care should be taken in the application of any of these compounds if the tympanic membrane is perforated, as hearing loss has been reported.

Occasionally, invasive otomycosis of the bone, in particular of the mastoid, occurs when there is perforation of the tympanic membrane. It is usually caused by *Aspergillus fumigatus*, but occasionally other organisms such as *Pseudallescheria boydii* are implicated. Many, but not all, patients are immunocompromised. These patients require systemic antifungal therapy according to the nature of the organism; surgical debridement is often necessary in addition.

Subcutaneous mycoses

There is a wide range of fungi that cause subcutaneous mycoses. The clinical hallmark is chronic deep induration usually with sinuses which extrude pus or fungal material. Management requires isolation of the fungus as many different species can be involved; the clinical picture alone is not sufficiently distinct to differentiate one from another.

CHROMOBLASTOMYCOSIS (CHROMOMYCOSIS)

Chromoblastomycosis is a chronic infection of the skin and subcutaneous tissue of non-immunocompromised individuals caused by several dematiaceous fungi, including *Fonsecaea pedrosi*, *Fonsecaea compacta*, *Phialophora verrucosa*, *Cladosporium carrionii*, *Rhinocladiella aquaspersa* and *Botryomyces caespitosus*. It is world-wide in distribution, but more common in tropical and subtropical areas.

Therapy is unsatisfactory. Small lesions can be surgically excised. Treatment with locally applied heat is sometimes efficacious, either alone or in combination with antifungal therapy (Randhawa et al 1994). Cryotherapy is also effective, especially for localized disease (Pimentel, 1989).

Response rates differ depending on the species of fungus implicated. Reasonable results have been obtained with oral itraconazole (200 mg/day) with or without flucytosine (100 mg/kg daily) (Restrepo et al 1988, Bayles 1992, Queiroz-Telles et al 1992). Thiabendazole (2 g/day) is also effective with or without flucytosine (Bayles 1989). Fluconazole appears to be ineffective even at doses of 400 mg/day (Diaz et al 1992).

SUBCUTANEOUS ZYGOMYCOSIS

Subcutaneous zygomycosis is distinct from invasive zygomycosis and mucormycosis (p. 874). *Basidiobolus ranarum* causes an indolent, painless, slowly progressive disease in children and adolescents in tropical countries, particularly Uganda. It is best treated with a saturated solution of potassium iodide 1.5–2 g/day for at least 3 months (Randhawa et al 1994). Ketoconazole 400 mg/day and itraconazole 100–200 mg/day have also been effective in small numbers of patients.

Conidiobolomycosis is a nasal and facial disease of adults seen primarily in central and western Africa. It causes gross nasal and facial distortion. Unfortunately, nothing has been shown to cure the disease, although it may be arrested by trimethoprim–sulphamethoxazole (960 mg three times daily for at least 6 months) (Randhawa et al 1994, Restrepo 1994). Surgery should be limited because it may spread the disease.

SPOROTRICHOSIS

Sporotrichosis is caused by *Sporothrix schenckii* and usually manifests as lymphocutaneous disease. A small proportion of non-immunocompromised patients have other sites of disease including osteoarticular forms, pneumonia and meningitis.

Lymphocutaneous disease responds well to potassium iodide (15–120 drops/day of saturated solution). However, although inexpensive, it is unpleasant to take and treatment has to continue for 3–6 months. The response rate exceeds 90%. Local application of heat or infrared treatment is also useful (Randhawa et al 1994). Ketoconazole and systemic amphotericin B are ineffective. Itraconazole 100–200 mg/day appears to be superior to fluconazole 200–400 mg/day (Hiruma et al 1991, Bayles 1992, Diaz et al 1992) in that response rates in uncontrolled studies are higher and tissue sterilization occurs earlier. If itraconazole is used a 3–6 month course provides cure in excess of 90%.

Osteoarticular and other deep forms of sporotrichosis are a major therapeutic challenge. Response rates to intravenous amphotericin B are mediocre to poor, particularly in pulmonary disease in which almost all patients have died.

Itraconazole 200–400 mg/day is effective for most cases of osteoarticular disease, but so far has not been very effective for pulmonary disease. Probably larger doses or a new more effective antifungal agent is required. Data on the response of *Sporothrix* meningitis are lacking.

In immunocompromised patients, particularly AIDS patients, sporotrichosis may be much more aggressive, invasive and destructive and less responsive to therapy. Itraconazole 400 mg/day after a loading dose is recommended. Repeated cultures and clinical assessment guide the response. Treatment should extend for many months, and in AIDS patients, probably for life.

RHINOSPORIDIOSIS

Rhinosporidiosis is a relatively rare disease caused by *Rhinosporidium seeberi*. It occurs in India, Sri Lanka, South America and Africa. Most cases are submucosal, causing polypoid masses in the nose and conjunctiva. However, it may involve subcutaneous tissues, other parts of the respiratory or urogenital tracts or anal canal. The organism does not grow in conventional media, but is quite distinctive in histological sections.

The only known effective therapy is surgical excision with electrocoagulation of the base of the lesion (Randhawa et al 1994). Recurrence is common. One report indicates that dapsone 100 mg/day may prevent recurrence (Nair 1979).

LOBOMYCOSIS

This is a rare, slowly progressive subcutaneous disease reported mostly from Latin and South America. It is caused by an uncultured fungus tentatively called *Loboa loboi*. The disease does not disseminate. Antifungal therapy is usually unsuccessful. Surgical excision of lesions is the only effective remedy (Rios-Fabra et al 1994).

MYCETOMA (MADUROMYCOSIS)

Mycetoma is a chronic, progressive destructive infection of the distal limbs involving all tissues. Numerous different organisms may be implicated and the appropriate treatment depends on the causative organism (Welsh 1993). There are three broad groups of infecting organisms: the true fungi; the higher bacteria, such as *Actinomyces*, *Nocardia* and *Streptomyces*; and bacteria including *Staphylococcus* species. This discussion concerns only the fungi causing mycetoma, but distinguishing between the various causes is essential for successful therapy.

The causative agent varies with the locality so that *P. boydii* is the most common cause in Europe and the USA.

Madurella grisea is more common in South America and *Madurella mycetomatis* in India. Sinuses form in the affected area and spore grains are often extruded through the sinus which provide a diagnostic sample. Sometimes the colour of the grain, if it is not available for culture and microscopy, can indicate a particular organism.

The agents of mycetoma are almost always resistant to amphotericin B and flucytosine. They may be sensitive to one of the azoles; for example, *P. boydii* may respond to miconazole, ketoconazole or, more likely, itraconazole. Ketoconazole or itraconazole are often effective if administered for several months or years (Venugopal & Venugopal 1993, Restrepo 1994). Doses should not be less than 400 mg/day. Amputation is frequently required if the disease is extensive and progressive or bone pain becomes unrelenting (Welsh 1993). However, many mycetomas remain relatively localized for long periods of time, with or without therapy.

FUNGAL KERATITIS

Fungal keratitis is a relatively common problem in subtropical and tropical areas. *Fusarium* and *Aspergillus* spp. are the most important causes. Mycotic keratitis may also be caused by *Candida* spp. and, in particular, *C. albicans*, but also *Candida guilliermondii*, *Candida kefyr* and *C. parapsilosis*. Over 70 species of fungi have been reported to cause this disease, including a number of dematiacious organisms (Ishibashi et al 1987).

The principles involved in the management of mycotic keratitis include rapid specialist assessment to evaluate any threat of corneal perforation or malignant glaucoma, correction of predisposing factors, appropriate antifungal and judicious surgical therapy (Thomas 1994).

Fusarium keratitis should be treated with topical amphotericin B deoxycholate 0.15%. Natamycin 5% ophthalmic solution may be superior to amphotericin B, although local bioavailability in corneal tissue is only 2% and therefore topical natamycin is inappropriate for infection involving the aqueous humour or other deep sites.

Aspergillus keratitis is treated with amphotericin B, clotrimazole or econazole local solution; 1% solutions are commercially available, but the azoles can be prepared in arachis oil at the same concentration. Oral itraconazole 200–400 mg/day is also effective in 75% of cases of *Aspergillus* keratitis (Thomas et al 1988).

Candida keratitis is treated with local nystatin, clotrimazole or ketoconazole 2% suspension (Torres et al 1985). Mycotic keratitis caused by unusual organisms should be treated with the most appropriate agent, although empirical therapy with either oral ketoconazole or oral itraconazole may be necessary.

Surgery is sometimes required for cases which fail to respond to medical therapy or where there is a threat of ocular perforation or the formation of a descemetocoele. Surgical procedures include debridement or lamella keratectomy, and formation of a conjunctival flap over a severely ulcerated area of the cornea or penetrating keratoplasty if a donor cornea is available. If possible surgery should be preceded by medical therapy for as long as possible.

Mucosal candidosis

Mucosal fungal infections are extremely common. The vast majority are caused by *C. albicans* and occasionally by other yeasts, especially *Candida glabrata*, and rarely by filamentous moulds such as *Aspergillus* spp.

OROPHARYNGEAL CANDIDOSIS

Before the AIDS epidemic, oropharyngeal candidosis (OPC) was largely seen in patients at the extremes of age, those receiving inhaled steroids or antibiotic therapy, following oral cavity radiotherapy and after cytotoxic chemotherapy. *C. albicans* is the primary pathogen and rarely *C. glabrata* and *Candida krusei*. The commonest pattern of OPC is the pseudomembranous form, but an exanthematous type is also found. Occasionally, denture-related candidosis or angular cheilitis are the primary manifestations. In AIDS, the pseudomembranous form predominates.

Topical agents such as nystatin or amphotericin B oral suspension (1 ml 6-hourly for 2–3 weeks) are effective in non-immunocompromised patients. Clotrimazole troches available in the USA are also effective. Miconazole oral gel in a dose of 10 ml 6-hourly is particularly useful for denture-related candidosis. In patients taking inhaled steroids with oropharyngeal candidosis, the use of a large-volume spacer will minimize the problem.

In immunocompromised patients, fluconazole 50–100 mg/day is more effective than topical therapy and is the agent of first choice, with response rates in excess of 90%. Ketoconazole and itraconazole are also effective at doses of 200–400 mg/day but are less well absorbed in conditions of hypochlorhydria which complicate AIDS and bone marrow transplantation. Improved serum of levels of both itraconazole and ketoconazole are achieved by acid drinks such as orange juice or cola and food.

OESOPHAGEAL CANDIDOSIS

Oesophageal candidosis usually co-exists with oropharyngeal disease, although in 30% of cases, no oral lesions are visible. Before AIDS, most cases occurred in cancer patients, typically also on corticosteroids or neutropenic. Oesophageal infection is confined to HIV-positive patients with more advanced disease, typically when the CD4 count is below $100 \times 10^6/l$, and is itself an AIDS-defining condition. There are rare reports of oesophageal candidosis in immunocompetent individuals and recently after omeprazole therapy, suggesting that hypochlorhydria favours colonization as well as reducing ketoconazole absorption.

For treatment, ketoconazole 200–400 mg/day is slightly inferior but less expensive than fluconazole 100 mg/day (Hernandez-Sampelayo 1994). Treatment duration should be 10–14 days. If the diagnosis was not proven by endoscopy and symptoms persist, endoscopy is then indicated to rule out other (usually viral) causes of oesophagitis. Resistance or drug interactions may account for the failure to respond; if available, serum drug concentrations can be measured. Relapse is common.

Azole resistance

The incidence of fluconazole resistance and azole cross-resistance has risen with the widespread use of azoles in the context of AIDS (Law et al 1994). Estimates of the incidence of azole resistance vary from 5% to 20%, depending on the definition and the CD4 count of the cohort of patients. Baily et al (1994) identified a group of patients with persistent oropharyngeal or oesophageal candidosis despite a dose of ≥100 mg fluconazole for at least 10 days. Isolates from these patients were less susceptible in vitro to fluconazole (minimum inhibitory concentration (MIC) ≥ 12.5 mg/l). Several other studies have also shown a good correlation between susceptibility testing and failure in OPC in AIDS (Ghannoum et al 1996).

The management of azole resistant oropharyngeal or oesophageal candidosis is not well studied and is somewhat empirical (Box 60.2). Higher doses of fluconazole (400 mg/day) are usually effective, as are other oral azoles such as ketoconazole 400–800 mg/day or itraconazole 400–600 mg/day. Isolates with only slightly elevated MIC values to either ketoconazole or itraconazole are more likely to respond. Itraconazole solution has been studied for this indication and is moderately successful. Oral amphotericin B and nystatin are relatively ineffective.

Box 60.2 *Options for treatment of azole resistant oropharyngeal and oesophageal candidosis in AIDS*

- Fluconazole 400–800 mg/day
- Ketoconazole 400–800 mg/day
- Itraconazole capsules 400–600 mg/day
- Itraconazole oral solution 200 mg/day
- Combination therapy: azole + flucytosine 75 mg/kg daily
- Amphotericin B 0.5–1 mg/kg i.v. daily
- Experimental antifungal therapy

When oral therapy fails, intravenous amphotericin B is the best, and usually only option. However, even this often fails. The dose should be a minimum of 0.7 mg/kg daily initially. It may be combined with flucytosine. Improvement should be assessed primarily by symptomatology, not by the visual appearance of the mouth. Complete clearance of oral plaques of *Candida* is hard to achieve with any of the above regimens, although symptoms usually improve.

VULVOVAGINAL CANDIDOSIS

Vulvovaginal candidosis is common. By a mean age of 24 years, 60% of 76 women had suffered at least one episode of vulvovaginal candidosis (Sawyer et al 1994). Among these women, 36% had at least one episode a year and 3% had it 'almost all the time'. Certain conditions increase the incidence and possibly the severity of vulvovaginal candidosis. These include pregnancy, antibiotic use, diabetes mellitus, cystic fibrosis and probably advanced HIV infection (Sawyer et al 1994, BSMM 1995). One study in HIV-seropositive women showed an increased prevalence of 2.5 times that found in controls, which correlated with the CD4 cell count (Spinillo et al 1994). In these patients there is often a worse response to initial treatment and a shorter time to relapse. Over 90% of cases are caused by *C. albicans* and about 5% by *C. glabrata*; various other species such as *Candida tropicalis* comprise the remainder.

Treatment may be local or systemic (Table 60.5). There is a spontaneous resolution rate over 7 days of up to 50%. Local treatment regimens with azoles yield response rates

---

Table 60.5 *Treatment regimens for vulvovaginal candidosis*

Antifungal agent	Formulation	Dose	Duration
Local therapy			
Clotrimazole	Vaginal tablet	200 mg	3 daily doses
Clotrimazole	Vaginal tablet	500 mg	1 dose
Econazole	Vaginal tablet	150 mg	3 daily doses
Miconazole	Pessary	100 mg	7 daily doses
Miconazole	Pessary	200 mg	3 daily doses
Miconazole	Pessary	1200 mg	1 dose
Nystatin	Vaginal tablet	100 000 U	14 daily doses
Terconazole	2% cream	5 g	3 daily doses
Clotrimazole	1% cream	5 g	7–14 daily doses
Clotrimazole	10% cream	5 g	1 dose
Butoconazole	2% cream	5 g	3 daily doses
Miconazole	2% cream	5 g	7 daily doses
Fenticonazole	2% cream	5 g	7 daily doses
Tioconazole	2% cream	5 g	3 daily doses
Tioconazole	6.5% cream	5 g	1 dose
Systemic therapy			
Fluconazole	Capsule	150 mg	1 dose
Itraconazole	Capsule	200 mg	2 dose
Ketoconazole	Tablet	400 mg	5 daily doses

of 80–90%. Many different regimens are available which vary primarily in cost. Women without predisposing factors such as pregnancy will usually prefer single-dose or 3-day treatments. Responses are slower in those with predisposing factors and 5- to 14-day treatment regimens are generally preferable, if topical therapy is preferred. Nystatin, one to two pessaries inserted high into the vaginal vault nightly for 14 nights, has a slightly lower response rate (80%) than the azoles, but is most useful for azole-resistant organisms such as *C. glabrata*. Oral therapy is preferred by many women. Fluconazole as a single dose of 150 mg or itraconazole two 200 mg doses 8 h apart are effective in over 90% of patients. Itraconazole may be preferable for *C. glabrata* infections.

In pregnancy, local therapy with a clotrimazole 500 mg vaginal tablet is usually effective and does not expose the fetus to an antifungal (Lindeque & Van Niekerk 1984). This is probably desirable in the first trimester, although there is no evidence that azoles are teratogenic in humans. Later in pregnancy, systemic therapy with fluconazole or itraconazole are accepted alternatives (Inman et al 1994).

Suppressive treatment may be indicated for very frequent episodes. The therapeutic options include local treatment with single-dose clotrimazole 500 mg fortnightly which, whilst not achieving a mycological cure, suppresses symptoms, and intermittent single-dose oral treatment with fluconazole 150 mg. Alternatively continuous therapy for a few months sometimes reduces the subsequent frequency of relapse (BSMM 1995). There is no evidence to date of resistance resulting from such a regimen.

Deep invasive mycoses

SYSTEMIC *CANDIDA* INFECTION

Most cases of systemic candidosis arise from the gastro-intestinal tract. In leukaemic patients, mucosal involvement of the stomach, small bowel and colon are frequently demonstrable at autopsy without dissemination to other organs, indicating local invasion. Candidaemia follows mucosal invasion. Candidaemia may be detected by blood cultures (50–75% of autopsy proven cases of *Candida* infection) or may be manifest subsequently by specific organ involvement, e.g. endophthalmitis and osteomyelitis.

Until recently, the majority of candida infections have been caused by *C. albicans* (85–90%). However, currently a higher proportion (30–60%) of non-*albicans* species now cause candidaemia (Price et al 1994). Most *C. albicans* isolates are susceptible to fluconazole, flucytosine and amphotericin B. *C. glabrata* is less susceptible to all antifungal agents, but particularly the azoles (Table 60.2).

Box 60.3 *Indications for flucytosine in* Candida *infections*

Superficial infection
Mucosal infections failing azole therapy (combined with an azole or polyene)

Urinary tract infection (without disseminated disease)
Candiduria due to fluconazole-resistant *Candida* spp.

Candidaemia
Extremely ill patient*
C. glabrata, C. lusitaniae infection*
Neonates*

Focal *Candida* infection
Endophthalmitis*
Endocarditis or other vascular involvement*
Meningitis*

* Always in combination with amphotericin B or fluconazole.

C. krusei is intrinsically resistant to fluconazole and less susceptible to amphotericin B (Table 60.2). About 50% of *C. tropicalis* isolates are resistant to fluconazole in vitro. *C. lusitaniae* may be intrinsically resistant to amphotericin B or may develop resistance during therapy (Table 60.2).

Amphotericin B or, increasingly, one of the lipid-associated preparations is commonly used for the treatment of systemic *Candida* infection. The appropriate doses are given in the sections below for conventional amphotericin B. If a lipid-associated preparation (e.g. AmBisome, Amphocil or Abelcet) is selected, then it is recommended that at least three times the dose of conventional amphotericin B should be used.

Fluconazole is a useful, well-tolerated agent for susceptible systemic *Candida* infections. Doses in adults should not be less than 400 mg/day for very ill patients, while some data support using 800 mg/day for candidaemia in intensive-care-unit patients (Grainger et al 1992). Details are given in the sections below.

There are very few data supporting the use of either ketoconazole or itraconazole for systemic *Candida* infection. The lack of an intravenous preparation has hampered the study of both agents. They may have a role in long-term suppressive therapy for infections due to fluconazole-resistant isolates.

The present indications for flucytosine are shown in Box 60.3; usually it is given in combination with amphotericin B or fluconazole. If the organism is later found to be resistant to flucytosine the drug should be discontinued. Appropriate dosing depends on renal function, haemofiltration and dialysis, but in a patient with normal renal function should be 100–150 mg/kg daily in 3 or 4 divided doses. Serum concentrations must be monitored (BSAC 1991).

Candidaemia

Candidaemia is the most common life-threatening form of invasive candidiasis and all patients require therapy.

Neonates. Therapy should be started if the neonate is

clinically unstable or deteriorating with any skin breaks from which *Candida* has been grown, or positive urine microscopy or culture for yeast. A single positive blood culture is an absolute indication for treatment.

The combination of flucytosine and amphotericin B remains the treatment of choice for babies with candidal infection (Butler & Baker 1988, Leibovitz et al 1992). If the platelet count allows, a lumbar puncture to exclude *Candida* meningitis should be done. It is beneficial to remove any risk factors if possible, e.g. broad-spectrum antibiotics and corticosteroids. Umbilical catheters should be changed (Dato & Dajani 1990). Neonates appear to tolerate amphotericin B and flucytosine well, although the monitoring of flucytosine concentrations should be commenced within 48 h of initiating therapy and carried out 2–3 times a week. Flucytosine should be administered twice daily initially. Complications besides meningitis include renal outflow obstruction, osteomyelitis or arthritis, cutaneous abscesses and myocarditis/endocarditis. With aggressive therapy the mortality rate in neonates (10%) is lower than in adults.

Fluconazole is also effective in neonates with candidaemia at a minimum dose of 5 mg/kg daily. As the mortality of neonatal candidaemia is low with amphotericin B and flucytosine, and there are few published data on the efficacy of fluconazole as primary therapy, fluconazole should be reserved for follow-on therapy which should be continued for at least 4 weeks, or longer if significant immunocompromissing factors are still present.

Neutropenia and bone-marrow-transplant patients. Neutropenic patients require a minimum of 1 mg/kg daily of amphotericin B, and if there is a poor or no response the dose of amphotericin B should be increased or a lipid associated preparation used. Fluconazole is not presently recommended for patients who are profoundly neutropenic, although some data suggesting equal efficacy are now available (De Pauw et al 1995).

Non-neutropenic adults and children. Empirical therapy for candidaemia should be started if candiduria or heavy colonization at other sites is documented together with deteriorating clinical status or signs of infection. A single positive blood culture is an absolute indication for treatment. There is a wide spectrum of severity of illness in candidaemia. Some patients are ambulant and essentially well, while others are critically ill. The intensity and duration of therapy will differ between these two groups, but all patients should receive amphotericin B or fluconazole.

The first randomized trial of candidaemia in non-neutropenic adults (Rex et al 1994) has shown that fluconazole 400 mg/day is equivalent to amphotericin B 0.5–0.6 mg/kg daily. The response rates were 70% and 79%, respectively. However, uncertainty remains about the optimal dose for fluconazole. For example, 30 surgical or intensive care unit patients with candidaemia treated with 5 mg/kg had a 60% response rate, whereas the next 30

patients in the same unit treated with 10 mg/kg had an 83% response rate (Presterl et al 1993). The dose of fluconazole should be doubled in patients undergoing haemofiltration as the drug is rapidly cleared by this route. Patients who present in septic shock due to candidaemia have a poor outlook and should be treated with either amphotericin B (at least 0.6 mg/kg daily) and flucytosine or fluconazole and flucytosine.

Patients with candidaemia should ideally have their central venous catheters changed, without the use of a guide wire. Arterial catheters, in general, do not require changing.

Controversy exists over the necessity to remove Hickman catheters in cancer patients with candidaemia. Quantitative cultures of blood taken from the line and from a peripheral vein before treatment should indicate if the Hickman catheter is infected; colony counts ≥ 25 colony forming units (cfu)/culture or ≥ 2.5 cfu/ml are a positive indicator for an intravascular source of infection (Talenti & Roberts 1989). The additional work of quantitative cultures by the microbiology laboratory is well worth the effort, given the implications of changing a Hickman catheter.

Duration of therapy. The most appropriate duration of therapy for candidaemia is unclear. Short courses of amphotericin B (e.g. <500 mg) are inadequate in terms of preventing death and the late complications of candidaemia. Doses ranging from 0.5–1.5 g amphotericin B are appropriate depending in part on the severity of the illness, the weight of the patient and the convenience of continued administration of intravenous amphotericin B. A reasonable approach now that fluconazole is available is the initial use of intravenous amphotericin B or fluconazole (with or without flucytosine) in hospital followed by continued oral fluconazole for 2–8 weeks depending on the type of patient, provided the organism is fluconazole susceptible.

Some implanted devices such as Dacron grafts, ventricular pacemakers and prosthetic joints are surgically impossible to remove. If they are infected these patients are best placed on long-term fluconazole therapy if the isolate is susceptible (British Society for Antimicrobial Chemotherapy 1994).

Candida meningitis

Candida meningitis is relatively uncommon and occurs in: neonates (see above); as part of disseminated candidosis in other patients; and as a complication of ventriculoatrial or ventriculoperitoneal shunts. In the treatment of *Candida* meningitis unrelated to a shunt, flucytosine should be used because of its excellent cerebrospinal fluid (CSF) penetration. In patients with infected shunts, removal of the shunt is of critical importance. If the isolate is susceptible to fluconazole, this would be an appropriate first-line agent in combination therapy with flucytosine if the patient is critically ill.

Candida peritonitis or wound drainage in surgical patients

Candida peritonitis following extensive abdominal surgery can be insidious in onset and is often associated with bacterial peritonitis or mixed yeast and bacterial cultures in wound drainage. Therapy is appropriate when *Candida* is the only isolate from a deep collection or as a heavy growth from a drain with clinical features of sepsis. A combination of peritoneal lavage without further laparotomy and either fluconazole or amphotericin B with or without flucytosine is usually appropriate.

Chronic ambulatory peritoneal dialysis

Candida peritonitis related to chronic ambulatory peritoneal dialysis (CAPD) usually responds to fluconazole or amphotericin B if the peritoneal catheter is removed. The nephrotoxicity of amphotericin B is not of concern in these patients but fluconazole is a reasonable alternative choice.

Hepatosplenic candidosis (chronic disseminated candidosis)

Hepatosplenic candidosis is a distinctive clinical entity in leukaemic patients. Following recovery from neutropenia, patients complain of abdominal pain, have an enlarged liver, and sometimes spleen, have a rising plasma alkaline phosphatase, and on scanning there are small defects in the substance of the liver, spleen and kidneys. Directed biopsy or splenectomy show small or large granulomata surrounding yeasts and hyphae. Cultures are usually negative.

Management consists of prolonged high-dose antifungal therapy. The choice of initial antifungal depends on what prophylactic antifungal was used (if any) and, if cultures are positive, the antifungal susceptibility of the organism. If the patients received fluconazole prophylaxis then amphotericin B and flucytosine would be an appropriate choice (Blade et al 1992). If the patient did not receive prophylaxis, but did receive empirical amphotericin B, then fluconazole 400–800 mg/day would be appropriate (Anaissie et al 1991, Kauffman et al 1991), probably with flucytosine. The lipid-associated amphotericin B preparations accumulate in the liver and spleen, but there is very little data supporting their use. Treatment should continue for several weeks. Delay in further cytotoxic chemotherapy is appropriate until clear improvement has been obtained. Subsequent bone-marrow transplantation is not precluded (Bjerke et al 1994).

Urinary tract candidosis and candiduria

From 1% to 9% of hospitalized patients have *Candida* grown from their urine. Typically this occurs in patients who have been catheterized, have received antibiotics or who are diabetic (Storfer et al 1994, Occhipinti et al 1994). For those in the intensive care unit candiduria is a good marker for candidaemia, and systemic treatment is appropriate if the patient manifests features of systemic sepsis (British Society for Antimicrobial Chemotherapy 1994). Urinary tract candidosis implies candiduria and evidence of outflow obstruction with fungal balls, a parenchymal abscess or other evidence of urinary tract disease. These patients require therapy, as 10% develop candidaemia (Storfer et al 1994). However, no criteria exist to distinguish colonization from infection (Wong-Beringer et al 1992) and a decision to treat is based on the likelihood of candidaemia, local symptomatology and demonstration of obstruction or fungal balls.

The penetration of amphotericin B into the urine is poor if given intravenously. However, a 10-day course of 1 mg/kg daily is effective for candiduria without obstruction (Kohn et al 1987). Fluconazole is an alternative first-line therapy if the species of *Candida* isolated is susceptible (Voss et al 1994). For patients with *C. glabrata* infections, fluconazole and flucytosine susceptibility testing will help guide therapy. Fluconazole is unlikely to sterilize the urinary tract if a catheter, ureteric stent or nephrostomy tube remains in place. Obstructive nephropathy due to pelvic fungal balls usually requires surgical exploration for removal.

Patients with persistent candiduria related to long-term indwelling urinary catheters may respond (50% response) to amphotericin B bladder washouts and catheter change. If used, amphotericin B 5–10 mg with an intravesical dwell time of 2 h is appropriate once or twice daily for no longer than 2 days (Sanford 1993).

Asymptomatic patients, without structural abnormalities of the urinary tract, do not require therapy, although follow-up is desirable.

Candida endocarditis

Candida primarily causes prosthetic-valve endocarditis, but occasionally causes native valve endocarditis as a complication of candidaemia in non-neutropenic patients (1%). Intravenous drug abuse and total parenteral nutrition are risk factors. Amphotericin B 1 mg/kg daily or fluconazole (≥400 mg/day) both with flucytosine is recommended. Virtually all patients, except neonates, will require valve replacement. It is not known if the timing of surgery is important in response. Relapse may occur many months after apparently successful therapy.

Candida suppurative thrombophlebitis

Resection of the affected vein or artery in accessible sites in addition to systemic antifungal therapy is appropriate. If the great veins in the chest are involved, resection is impossible. Prolonged high dose amphotericin B and flucytosine followed by fluconazole are usually necessary to eradicate the infection.

Candida **ophthalmitis**

Candida ophthalmitis manifests as a chorioretinitis or endophthalmitis and complicates about 10% of episodes of candidaemia. It rarely occurs in neutropenic patients. Most species of *Candida* have been implicated. Endophthalmitis may not be manifest until several days or weeks after treatment has commenced. Large, progressive or symptomatic lesions will usually require a partial vitrectomy. Microscopy of the vitreous fluid while the patient is still anaesthetized can guide the need for intravitreal dosing of amphotericin B (5 mg). Systemic amphotericin B and flucytosine is indicated in all cases as combination therapy, since amphotericin B penetrates into the vitreous poorly. Fluconazole is a preferred agent if the *Candida* species is susceptible, since vitreous penetration is good.

Candida **arthritis**

Candida arthritis is usually a complication of candidaemia (particularly in intravenous drug abusers) or follows prosthetic joint replacement. Fluconazole ≥200 mg/day may be successful, but in patients with infected non-prosthetic joints systemic amphotericin B is more appropriate initially. Flucytosine should be added if there is no improvement within 5–7 days, or fluconazole substituted. In those with infected prosthetic joints, replacement of the joint together with the removal of all cement and necrotic bone should be undertaken when technically feasible. When this is difficult to achieve, long-term suppressive therapy may be necessary.

Candida **osteomyelitis**

Candida osteomyelitis requires debridement of necrotic bone if extensive disease is present. Bone grafting may be done simultaneously if necessary in the case of vertebral osteomyelitis. Systemic amphotericin B with or without flucytosine is appropriate therapy, with fluconazole a useful alternative. Therapy should continue for several months until radiological improvement and inflammatory markers have settled.

INVASIVE ASPERGILLOSIS

Most patients with invasive aspergillosis are immunocompromised. Untreated invasive aspergillosis carries a nearly 100% mortality. At present, outcome depends as much on immune status and the speed of progression of disease as on the treatment administered. The speed of progression varies; it is most rapid in liver- and bone-marrow-transplant patients and those with profound neutropenia. Death typically occurs in 5–14 days from the first clinical features which are often non-specific. A successful outcome requires at least 14 days' therapy, and therefore early empirical therapy is critically important in these highly immunocompromised patients. In contrast, in less immunocompromised patients such as AIDS patients, disease progression is often slower, allowing a diagnosis before treatment.

Neutropenia

Standard criteria for the initiation of therapy for invasive aspergillosis in the neutropenic patient are shown in Box 60.4 (Denning 1994). Empirical conventional amphotericin B for neutropenic fever in a dose of 1–1.25 mg/kg daily is necessary for successful therapy. One of the lipid-associated amphotericin B preparations may be substituted for conventional amphotericin B if infusion-related or renal toxicity is a problem – using a dose of 3–5 mg/kg daily. If presumed invasive aspergillosis is progressing despite amphotericin B 1 mg/kg daily, alternative regimens include itraconazole (see below), a lipid-associated amphotericin B and, occasionally, surgery (see below).

Box 60.4 *Criteria for initiation of antifungal therapy for invasive aspergillosis*

Neutropenia (<500 × 10^6/l) including aplastic anaemia
- Isolation of *Aspergillus* from any site including nose swab, blood, broncho-alveolar lavage or positive microscopy/cytology for hyphae, etc.
- New pulmonary infiltrates on chest X-ray
- Infiltrates on CT scan of chest showing characteristic features, e.g.
  — halo or crescent sign
  — pleural based sharply angulated lesion
  — pleural based lesion with pneumothorax
- Persistent fevers (>7 days) with any localizing clinical features, e.g.
  — chest pain
  — dry cough
  — facial/ sinus pain
  — epistaxis
  — hoarseness
  — new skin lesions consistent with aspergillosis
- Any sudden intracranial event including stroke or fit with or without fever

Solid organ transplantation or allogeneic bone-marrow transplantation
- Radiological infiltrate with isolation of *Aspergillus* from respiratory secretions, broncho-alveolar lavage or blood
- Evidence of ulcers/bronchitis on bronchoscopy with hyphae visualized in broncho-alveolar lavage
- Histological or cytological evidence of hyphae from any tissue
- Any sudden intracranial event including stroke or fit with or without fever.

AIDS
- Respiratory symptoms, abnormal chest X-ray or bronchoscopy and isolation of *Aspergillus* or visualization of hyphae
- Cerebral lesions unresponsive to therapy for toxoplasmosis or a single enhancing lesion consistent with aspergillosis
- Histological or cytological evidence of hyphae from any site (culture not obtained or pending)

Persistent profound neutropenia is often associated with a fatal outcome in invasive aspergillosis. In these patients G-CSF or GM-CSF may be administered, although its effect is unproven. While there is a substantial shortening of the period of neutropenia which reduces the period at risk, it has yet to be shown that cytokine adjunctive therapy is beneficial for an established fungal infection. Patients whose leukaemia has relapsed also respond less well (Ribrag et al 1993).

Secondary prophylaxis is indicated in those with persistent *Aspergillus* disease who require further cytotoxic chemotherapy or bone marrow transplantation (Robertson & Larson 1988). Typically, amphotericin B (1 mg/kg daily) is co-administered with the cytotoxic regimen (Karp et al 1988). Secondary prophylaxis is particularly indicated for patients with *Aspergillus* sinusitis, as these patients have a 50% relapse rate. Surgery may also be appropriate (see below).

Bone-marrow transplantation

Following allogeneic bone-marrow transplantation, invasive aspergillosis occurs during or immediately after the short period of aplasia or with graft-versus-host disease, weeks or months after transplantation. Disease progression may be extremely rapid, and treatment should be administered at first suspicion of disease and discontinued if the suspicion proves groundless. Lipid-associated amphotericin B is widely used to avoid nephrotoxicity, although oral itraconazole should also be considered (Denning et al 1992, Denning et al 1994b). Absorption of itraconazole in bone-marrow transplant patients is often poor, but if the patient is eating and has limited gastro-intestinal disease it is a potentially useful option given the very poor response to amphotericin B in this patient group.

Solid organ transplantation

In solid organ transplant recipients with suspected fungal infection the criteria for initiation of therapy differ to those with neutropenia (Box 60.4) (Denning, 1994). The differential diagnosis of pneumonitis is wider and there is a higher frequency of *Aspergillus* tracheobronchitis. In addition, solid organ transplantation patients are more prone to *Aspergillus* mediastinitis, sternal osteomyelitis and wound infections, which are clear indications for therapy. Late infections, often presenting as pulmonary nodules, are also typical of solid organ transplant recipients (Haramati et al 1993). In transplant recipients on cyclosporin, a lipid-associated amphotericin B preparation is preferred if intravenous therapy is required, to prevent synergistic nephrotoxicity. The dose is uncertain, but 3–5 mg/kg daily is probably appropriate. Once intravenous therapy is no longer required, oral itraconazole may be administered if appropriate (see below) (Denning et al 1994b).

AIDS

In AIDS, invasive aspergillosis tends to be a relatively subacute disease evolving over 3–12 weeks. It is possible to make a positive diagnosis before therapy (Box 60.4) (Khoo & Denning 1994). The major exception to this is intracranial disease. Neither itraconazole nor amphotericin B are very effective, and most patients with AIDS and invasive aspergillosis succumb although some have responded to oral itraconazole, preceded by amphotericin B (Denning 1991b, Denning et al 1994b). Aspergillosis in these patients is often complicated by haemoptysis which is frequently fatal.

Relatively non-immunocompromised patients

There are a small number of patients with mild or no immunocompromising factors. Typically these are patients with chronic pulmonary disease on corticosteroids, diabetes mellitus, alcohol abuse or other corticosteroid-treated diseases. These patients usually respond slowly to amphotericin B or itraconazole (Denning et al 1994).

Therapeutic choice. The standard therapeutic agent for the treatment of invasive aspergillosis is amphotericin B deoxycholate. The overall response rate in amphotericin B treated patients is 35%. However this varies substantially from patient group to patient group (Denning 1996). Among the azoles, itraconazole has reasonable activity against *Aspergillus* spp., whereas ketoconazole and fluconazole have none. The success rate for itraconazole varies substantially between different host groups (Denning et al 1994). The two major considerations in the initial choice of therapy are whether the patient can take oral medication and absorb it, and whether the patient is taking cyclosporin or renal dysfunction is present.

If the patient is eating and is not taking drugs that induce the metabolism of P450 enzyme (e.g. rifampicin, phenytoin, carbamazepine, phenobarbitone), itraconazole is a reasonable therapeutic choice (Tucker et al 1992). Absorption is impaired by H_2 antagonists and intestinal problems, such as graft-versus-host disease, and HIV infection. The dose of itraconazole is 200 mg thrice daily for 4 days followed by 200 mg twice daily; higher doses (e.g. 800 mg/day) may be appropriate for cerebral aspergillosis. Itraconazole should be taken with food or an acidic carbonated drink. Serum concentrations of itraconazole should ideally be measured after 5–10 days, since reasonable response rates have been achieved if serum concentrations exceed 1 mg/l (high-performance liquid chromatography (HPLC)) or 5 mg/l (bioassay (Denning et al 1994)).

If oral therapy is contraindicated, conventional amphotericin B intravenously should be used in a dose of 0.8–1.0 mg/kg daily, regardless of renal dysfunction, except in neutropenic patients in whom 1–1.25 mg/kg daily is more appropriate (Table 60.6). If renal dysfunction occurs or is likely to be a problem because of concurrent cyclosporin,

Table 60.6 *Treatment regimens for invasive aspergillosis*

Drug	Route	Daily dose	
		Neutropenia Bone-marrow transplant Cerebral aspergillosis Endocarditis	Other patient groups or sites
Amphotericin B deoxycholate	i.v.	1–1.25 mg/kg	0.8–1.0 mg/kg
AmBisome (Liposomal)	i.v.	5 mg/kg	? 4 mg/kg
Amphocil (ABCD)	i.v.	6 mg/kg	? 4 mg/kg
Abelcet (ABLC)	i.v.	5 mg/kg	5 mg/kg
Itraconazole:			
Loading dose	Orally	600–800 mg	600 mg
Continuation	Orally	400–600 mg	400 mg

then one of the lipid-associated amphotericin B preparations may be appropriate (Table 60.6). There is currently no scientific data to choose between these compounds on grounds of efficacy. These high dosages should be continued for a minimum of 2 weeks until a therapeutic response has been obtained, and continued for 4–6 weeks in total.

The clinical state of the patient is not necessarily a guide as to whether to give oral itraconazole or intravenous amphotericin B. Responses have been obtained in profoundly neutropenic patients with extensive disease using oral itraconazole alone, where amphotericin B therapy has been ineffective, while the converse is also true. Drug absorption, bioavailability and toxicity are the key determinants of drug choice.

Combination therapy. The place of amphotericin B and itraconazole in combination is uncertain. Theoretically, antagonism is more likely than synergy, as itraconazole inhibits the synthesis of ergosterol to which amphotericin B binds. Limited animal data suggest that antagonism is a real phenomenon, although the magnitude of the effect may be concentration and time dependent. It is therefore recommended that treatment be with one or other drug alone.

The role of adjunctive therapy with either rifampicin or flucytosine is unclear. Amphotericin B with flucytosine improves clinical response rates marginally (Denning & Stevens 1990) and is indicated for certain sites of disease (e.g. brain, meninges, heart valve, eye) to which amphotericin B penetrates poorly. Antagonism is well documented in vitro for amphotericin B and flucytosine (Denning et al 1992).

Rifampicin and amphotericin B are often synergistic in vitro (Denning et al 1992). However, rifampicin induces the metabolism of immunosuppressants, particularly corticosteroids, and thus rejection or graft-versus-host disease could develop in transplant recipients. Rifampicin is also a powerful inducer of P450 enzymes, so its use for more than 3 days precludes the subsequent use of itraconazole (Tucker et al 1992). As itraconazole is useful as salvage or follow-on therapy, the use of rifampicin is not advised.

Treatment of invasive aspergillosis should continue for as long as the patient is immunocompromised and until there has been either complete or near complete resolution of disease. Aspergillosis characteristically causes vascular invasion and infarction of tissue so that drug delivery is poor, the response slow and relapse common if therapy is terminated early (Denning et al 1994). In the neutropenic patient treatment should continue until the neutrophil count exceeds $1.0 \times 10^9/l$ and there has been regression of disease radiologically. Eradication of the disease may require surgery (see below). In solid organ transplant patients therapy should be continued until there is a complete or near complete clinical response. Few AIDS patients and allogeneic bone marrow transplant recipients survive with aspergillosis, but here long term itraconazole is appropriate (Denning 1994).

Surgical excision. There are several indications for surgery in invasive aspergillosis (Denning & Stevens 1990) (Box 60.5). These include life-threatening haemoptysis (Kibbler et al 1988), where lesions impinge on the great vessels or major airways early surgical resection may prevent fatal haemoptysis or tracheal perforation. In patients awaiting bone-marrow transplantation, resection of a persistent lesion despite antifungal therapy will prevent recrudescence.

Box 60.5 *Indications for surgery in invasive aspergillosis*

Absolute indication
Endocarditis
Endophthalmitis
Major haemoptysis
Epidural abscess

Possible indication
Bone aspergillosis
Invasive external otitis
Invasive sinusitis
Localized unresolved pulmonary aspergillosis

Biopsy of the nasal mucosa is necessary for diagnosis in patients with invasive sinus aspergillosis. Surgery is also an essential part of the management of patients with *Aspergillus* endophthalmitis, endocarditis and, probably, osteomyelitis (Box 60.5).

CRYPTOCOCCAL INFECTIONS

Pulmonary cryptococcosis

Pulmonary cryptococcosis is uncommon but presents subacutely. The diagnosis is made by sputum culture, bronchoscopy, transbronchial, or open or percutaneous lung biopsy. It is essential to exclude meningeal disease in these patients. If the disease is confined to the lungs, the agents of choice are fluconazole or itraconazole, with ketoconazole or amphotericin B as alternatives, for 2–3 months.

In AIDS and other immunocompromised patients, pulmonary cryptococcosis may precede or reflect disseminated disease. Isolated pulmonary cryptococcosis requires therapy for 4–6 months initially. Maintenance therapy may be required, but should be individualized depending on resolution of disease and the immune status of the patient.

Cryptococcal meningitis

Cryptococcal meningitis may manifest few symptoms and is diagnosed by a positive CSF culture or cryptococcal antigen. Those with altered mental status should be classified as high risk (Saag et al 1992). Untreated the disease is uniformly fatal. This can be reduced to 10% with therapy.

AIDS. Those with high-risk disease should be treated with amphotericin B ≥0.7 mg/kg daily and flucytosine 75–150 mg/kg daily (Larsen et al 1990) for at least 2 weeks. Amphotericin B therapy should continue at high dosage if the response is suboptimal. Rarely is more than 6 weeks amphotericin B required, as long as follow-on azole therapy is given.

The various preparations of amphotericin B show comparable efficacy (40–65% in AIDS without flucytosine). AmBisome 3 mg/kg (Coker et al 1993), Amphocil 3 mg/kg and ABLC 5 mg/kg have yielded comparable response rates to deoxycholate amphotericin B in small numbers of patients.

Early death and blindness in cryptococcal meningitis reflects a markedly elevated CSF pressure (Denning et al 1991c, Rex et al 1993), which can exceed 500 mmH$_2$O. CT and magnetic resonance imaging (MRI) scans can be normal. Where pressures exceed 350 mmH$_2$O, pressure-reducing measures such as oral acetazolamide, insertion of lumbar or ventricular drains or repeated lumbar punctures are indicated. Steroids are less useful.

Those with normal mental status and AIDS may be treated with fluconazole 400 mg/day (Saag et al 1992) or itraconazole 400 mg/day (Denning et al 1989b). However, the response rates are lower compared with amphotericin B (Larsen et al 1990, de Gans et al 1992). As life-long maintenance therapy will be required with an azole, an initial 10–14 day course of amphotericin B with flucytosine is recommended in all patients. This can then be followed by fluconazole. Flucytosine slightly improves the outcome in the first 2 weeks of therapy, but has a major effect in preventing relapse over the next year of therapy. The prostate and meninges act as nidi of infection despite successful therapy (Larsen et al 1989). Fluconazole 200 mg/day is superior to placebo and also weekly amphotericin B (Bozzette et al 1991 Powderly et al 1992) and itraconazole 200 mg/day (Nelson et al 1994). The dose of fluconazole may need to be increased in those receiving rifampicin or other enzyme inducers.

Non-AIDS patients. In non-AIDS but immunocompromised patients, fluconazole in doses of 200 or 400 mg/day has a response rate of about 85% and is an agent of choice unless the patient is severely obtunded or the CSF pressure is moderately elevated (see above). *C. neoformans* var. *gattii* produces a higher mortality; amphotericin B with flucytosine may be the best treatment for such patients.

The duration of therapy in immunocompromised or other patients should be for many months or even years until the cryptococcal antigen titre in the CSF has fallen to zero or nearly zero. A post-treatment CSF cryptococcal titre of >8 is predictive of relapse (Diamond and Bennett 1974). It is probably appropriate to overtreat than stop and have to retreat which is often less successful.

HISTOPLASMOSIS

Histoplasmosis presents in several forms, including acute pulmonary histoplasmosis shortly after exposure, chronic cavitary, nodular or mediastinal disease, localized extrapulmonary and disseminated histoplasmosis. In AIDS and other immunocompromised patients disseminated histoplasmosis is most common and life-threatening.

Acute pulmonary histoplasmosis

In the normal host, acute pulmonary histoplasmosis does not require therapy unless it is severe with high, prolonged fever, significant hypoxaemia and major systemic disturbance (Box 60.6). Oral itraconazole 200 mg/day is the treatment of choice. Patients with acute pulmonary histoplasmosis who are immunocompromised should always be treated.

Chronic pulmonary histoplasmosis

Chronic cavitary, other intrathoracic forms of histoplasmosis and localized extrapulmonary forms (e.g. oral or gastro-

Box 60.6   *Treatment of histoplasmosis*

Acute pulmonary histoplasmosis
- None
- Itraconazole

Chronic pulmonary or localized histoplasmosis
- Itraconazole
- Ketoconazole
- Fluconazole
- Amphotericin B

Disseminated histoplasmosis
- Amphotericin B
- Itraconazole

Maintenance therapy in AIDS
- Itraconazole
- Weekly amphotericin B
- Fluconazole

intestinal ulcers or adrenal disease) require therapy. The response to intravenous amphotericin B 0.3–0.5 mg/kg daily for 3–4 weeks to a total of 1.5 g (Saag & Dismukes 1988) gives high response and cure rates. Because of the inconvenience and toxicity of this regimen, certain forms of histoplasmosis were deemed inappropriate for therapy. These included those with few symptoms, thin-walled cavities and early pulmonary lesions. However, oral therapy with the imidazoles and triazoles (see below) now favours treatment of almost all culture-positive cases (Box 60.6).

Ketoconazole therapy (400 mg/day) has a similar response rate (84%) to amphotericin B (Dismukes et al 1985) but in high dose is toxic (Sugar et al 1987). Itraconazole 200–400 mg/day appears to be slightly more efficacious than ketoconazole (85–97% response rates) (Negroni et al 1987, Dismukes et al 1992). The duration of therapy is uncertain but ranges from 6 to 12 months depending on response. Fluconazole is less active than itraconazole (Diaz et al 1992). Central nervous system disease should be treated with intravenous amphotericin B initially and with itraconazole 400 mg/day as follow-on therapy (Wheat et al 1990a).

Medical therapy for mediastinal fibrosis due to *H. capsulatum* is ineffective (Loyd et al 1988) and surgical treatment carries a high complication rate. This emphasizes the importance of early effective therapy for milder forms of the disease.

Disseminated histoplasmosis

In the immunocompromised patient with disseminated histoplasmosis (usually AIDS) the clinical condition of the patient determines first-line therapy (Box 60.6). In those in whom the diagnosis is made early and do not have features of severe systemic toxicity, confusion or poor oxygenation should be treated with itraconazole initially at 400 mg/day

reducing to 200 mg/day when a response has been noted. Itraconazole levels should be measured. In the very ill, intravenous amphotericin B 0.8–1 mg/kg daily is appropriate. Defervescence of fever may be slightly more rapid in patients treated with amphotericin B than itraconazole, but the response to both agents exceeds 90% in patients with disseminated histoplasmosis. Fluconazole 400 mg/day is slightly less effective than itraconazole 200 mg/day. Ketoconazole is not recommended.

Maintenance therapy of histoplasmosis is indicated as the relapse rate is extremely high. Itraconazole 200 mg/day is the preferred agent (Box 60.6) (Wheat et al 1993). In patients in whom itraconazole is contraindicated, fluconazole 200–400 mg/day is reasonably effective (Norris et al 1994). Both these regimens are preferable to long-term weekly amphotericin B (McKinsey et al 1989).

Histoplasma capsulata var. *dubosii* infection

A relatively rare form of histoplasmosis is caused by *H. capsulata* var. *dubosii* and occurs in central and Southern Africa. It is primarily a cutaneous disease, but thin-walled pulmonary cavities are well recognized. Disseminated forms may rarely complicate AIDS. Cutaneous disease responds to itraconazole, but pulmonary disease has a high relapse rate. Amphotericin B followed by itraconazole is recommended.

COCCIDIOIDOMYCOSIS

Coccidioidomycosis is endemic to North, Central and South America and is caused by *Coccidioides immitis* acquired by inhalation.

Primary coccidioidomycosis (valley fever)

Approximately 60% of infected persons suffer a primary illness which ranges from a mild flu-like illness to severe, progressive pneumonia. Treatment is only indicated for primary coccidioidomycosis if the patient is particularly ill with persistent high fever or hypoxia, or if the patient is immunocompromised. The latter include solid organ transplant recipients and HIV-positive patients with CD4 counts $<250 \times 10^6/l$. Patients with severe disease should receive intravenous amphotericin B 1 mg/kg daily. Those not quite so ill should receive itraconazole 400 mg/day. Treatment should be given for 4–8 weeks only.

Chronic pulmonary coccidioidomycosis

Less than 10% of patients develop chronic coccidioido-mycosis. This may be confined to the lung (50–70% of cases) or involve other organs. Therapy is indicated for virtually all these cases. The later pulmonary manifestations include asymptomatic nodules, small thin- or thick-walled cavities

Table 60.7 *Response of pulmonary coccidioidomycosis to azoles*

Agent	Dose (mg)	% response	% relapse	Response rate 1 year post-Rx
Ketoconazole	400	23	9	21
	800	32	44	18
Itraconazole	400	57	16	49
Fluconazole	200	34	39	21
	400	61	36	39

and progressive consolidation. The nodules are often mistaken for a malignant process and are removed surgically only to discover their nature histologically. Patients usually have serological evidence of infection or a positive skin test for *Coccidioides*. Therapy is not indicated for asymptomatic patients with nodular disease, although continued observation is appropriate.

Patients with cavitary disease and cough usually have positive sputum cultures and serological evidence of coccidioidomycosis. Therapy is indicated to control symptoms and prevent progression of disease. The results of therapy for chronic pulmonary coccidioidomycosis are summarized in Table 60.7. No agent yields better than a 60% response rate, but either itraconazole 400 mg/day or fluconazole 400 mg/day are appropriate. The initial response may take up to 9 months. Treatment should continue for 6 months beyond the last symptom or maximal improvement, which typically means 1–2 years of therapy. Even so, relapse is common, as indicated in Table 60.7. Those with a negative coccidioidin skin test during therapy and a peak complement fixation titre of ≥1/256 are approximately five times more likely to relapse, regardless of which therapy is used.

Severely ill patients with pneumonia high fever and hypoxaemia should be treated with systemic amphotericin B. If they are immunocompromised the response is poor. Patients with diffuse lung disease fare worse than those with focal disease. This has been well evaluated in AIDS, where the respective mortality rates are 70% and 30% (Fish et al 1990).

Extrapulmonary coccidioidomycosis

Other forms of coccidioidomycosis, including lymphoreticular, cutaneous, osteoarticular and genitourinary, respond to antifungal therapy better than does pulmonary disease. Itraconazole 400 mg/day for several months or years has response rates of approximately 90% (Tucker et al 1990a). In patients with osteoarticular disease, stabilization of the bone may be important to prevent pathological fractures. It may take many years for bone remodelling to occur. Surgical resection of easily accessible draining lymph nodes may be appropriate if the response to antifungal therapy is slow.

Coccidioidal meningitis. Meningitis due to *Cocc. immitis* is a slowly progressive lymphocytic meningitis with a 100% mortality if untreated. Some patients are extremely ill and die within weeks of presentation, others have a more indolent course over a period of up to 2 years. Coccidioidal meningitis does not respond to systemic ketoconazole or amphotericin B, and for this reason intrathecal amphotericin B was the mainstay of therapy until the triazoles were introduced. Intrathecal amphotericin B is administered daily initially in slowly ascending doses together with narcotic premedication. The dose of intrathecal amphotericin B is prepared in 5 ml of 5% dextrose. Cerebrospinal fluid (5 ml) is removed at lumbar puncture. A cisternal puncture is preferable in patients with spinal block or in whom lumbar puncture is difficult. The 5 ml of amphotericin B in 5% dextrose is given slowly intrathecally over a period of about 3–5 min with the patient in a head-down position. The lumbar-puncture needle is then removed and the patient remains head-down for 2 h. The initial dose of amphotericin B is 0.05 mg, which is increased by 0.05 mg each day until the level of tolerance is reached, up to a maximum of 1.2 mg. In general, few patients can tolerate more than 0.5 mg/day during the acute phase. During the maintenance phase higher doses can be given weekly or alternate weekly. In patients unable to tolerate a therapeutic dose, 25 mg hydrocortisone should also be given intrathecally with some amelioration of adverse effects. The response to therapy is judged by following the CSF glucose, white cell count and antibody titres. Unfortunately, intrathecal amphotericin B often causes a rise in the CSF white cell count.

Communicating hydrocephalus and other rather complex alterations of CSF flow are common in patients with coccidioidal meningitis. CSF pressures should be measured intermittently and ventriculoperitoneal shunts inserted for those with hydrocephalus. Such shunts clearly alter CSF flow and may create additional difficulties in delivering intrathecal amphotericin B to the sites of disease. Sometimes an Ommaya reservoir is necessary. CSF flow studies are important to determine how amphotericin B is delivered in and around the brain in this context. Vasculitic and encephalitic complications are also occasional complications of coccidioidal meningitis (Williams et al 1992).

Itraconazole 400 mg/day and fluconazole ≥400 mg/day are also effective in patients with coccidioidal meningitis (Tucker et al 1990a). Fluconazole has the theoretical advantage of better CSF penetration, but this has not been clearly translated into a better response rate. In general, the fluconazole response rate in coccidioidal meningitis is 70–90%, which contrasts with the intrathecal amphotericin B response rate of 40–100% depending on the series.

The treatment of coccidioidal meningitis is for life. No regimen is curative, and relapse is virtually universal in all patients.

Coccidioidomycosis in immunocompromised patients

A question that arises for patients in endemic areas of coccidioidomycosis who require a solid organ transplant is whether or not a prior history of coccidioidomycosis is a contraindication to transplantation. One study of six such patients showed that none treated with long-term ketoconazole reactivated (Hall et al 1993). In those who develop coccidioidomycosis post-transplantation, life-long therapy is recommended. Coccidioidomycosis complicating AIDS carries a poor outlook when disseminated or of a diffuse pulmonary pattern (Fish et al 1990). Such patients should be treated with intravenous amphotericin 1 mg/kg daily and followed, if successful, by an oral azole for life.

BLASTOMYCOSIS

Blastomycosis is endemic to North America and Africa (Baily et al 1991). It causes primary pulmonary infection. Cutaneous and osseous lesions indicate dissemination. Meningitis occurs in 3–10% of patients. The disease is usually relatively indolent. A few present with rapidly progressive pneumonia leading to the adult respiratory distress syndrome (Meyer et al 1993) and, although life-threatening, a successful outcome is possible. There are rare reports of blastomycosis in AIDS (Pappas et al 1993).

In patients who are acutely unwell or immunocompromised (Pappas et al 1993) amphotericin B 1 mg/kg daily is appropriate. This should be continued until the patient is improved and stable. In less acutely ill patients itraconazole 200 mg/day is the treatment of choice (Dismukes et al 1992). It is slightly superior to ketoconazole (Dismukes et al 1985). Treatment should be for 6–12 months in non-immunocompromised patients and longer in the immunocompromised. In patients with pulmonary disease and osseous disease more prolonged treatment may be necessary.

PARACOCCIDIOIDOMYCOSIS

Paracoccidioidomycosis is caused by *Paracoccidioides brasiliensis* and is endemic to Latin America. Males are affected more frequently than females, although a similar sex frequency is seen in pre-pubertal girls and post-menopausal women. Chronic pulmonary or disseminated disease is common and may mimic malignancy or tuberculosis which co-exist in 30% of those with pulmonary involvement. Mucosal and cervical node involvement is relatively common. A few cases have been reported in AIDS with low CD4 counts (Cunliffe & Denning 1995).

Sulphadiazine 4–6 g/day (adults) or 60–100 mg/kg daily (children) in divided doses is reasonably effective for mild and moderately disseminated disease or as follow-on therapy after initial amphotericin B treatment. The dose of sulphadiazine can be reduced when clear evidence of improvement has occurred. Therapy should be continued for 2 years to avoid relapse, but the development of resistance during treatment is relatively common. In severe or disseminated cases amphotericin B 0.5–1 mg/kg daily to a total of 1.5–2 g is appropriate. In mild cases in whom sulphonamides are contraindicated, itraconazole 100–200 mg/day for 6 months is curative (Vargas Flores 1992, Rios-Fabra et al 1994). The relapse rate is only 3–5%. Ketoconazole 200–400 mg/day for 12 months is an alternative and yields a 90% response rate (Rios-Fabra et al 1994). Fluconazole is also effective (Diaz et al 1992).

PENICILLIUM INFECTIONS

Penicillium species are ubiquitous airborne fungi which rarely cause infection. The exception is *Penicillium marneffei* localized to south-east China, Burma, northern Thailand, Vietnam and Indonesia (Deng et al 1988, Supparatpinyo et al 1991). *P. marneffei* is a primary pathogen and may cause focal or fatal progressive disseminated disease. It is a major problem in AIDS in northern Thailand where approximately a third of such patients develop disseminated *P. marneffei* infections with CD4 counts $<100 \times 10^6/l$ (Supparatpinyo 1994).

P. marneffei is highly susceptible in vitro to miconazole, itraconazole, ketoconazole and flucytosine, but is less susceptible to amphotericin B and fluconazole (Supparatpinyo 1994). The response of disseminated disease in those with AIDS parallels these in vitro responses, thus mild to moderately severe *P. marneffei* infections should be treated with itraconazole 400 mg/day or ketoconazole 400 mg/day. Seriously ill patients should be treated with amphotericin B 1 mg/kg daily, but there is a substantial failure rate, possibly attributable at least in part to the seriousness of the infection.

Relapse is common when therapy is stopped. In those with AIDS oral maintenance therapy with itraconazole is appropriate.

MUCORMYCOSIS (ZYGOMYCOSIS)

Several clinical patterns of mucormycosis are described in varying patient populations; rhinocerebral and pulmonary disease are most common. There are a large number of different causal genera and species described. Subcutaneous zygomycosis affects a small subgroup (p. 861). Diagnosis is often difficult, partly because cultures are frequently negative, for reasons that are not clear. Histology is required for early diagnosis, which is critical for a more favourable outcome. The clinical features of zygomycosis are similar to those of invasive aspergillosis, although the histological appearances of the hyphae are distinct. Azoles are ineffective; the organism is resistant to flucytosine in vitro.

Treatment requires large doses of amphotericin B (≥ 1 mg/kg daily) (Table 60.8). The evidence for synergy between amphotericin B and rifampicin is anecdotal. Limited data indicate that AmBisome and Amphocil are efficacious in mucormycosis in doses of 3–10 mg/kg daily (Ng & Denning 1995). Correction of an underlying immune defect such as diabetic ketoacidosis or neutropenia is also desirable.

Surgery is critically important in the management of localized mucormycosis, as antifungal therapy is relatively ineffective alone. In particular, the rhinocerebral form, localized pulmonary disease (Tedder et al 1994) and cutaneous varieties (Vainrub et al 1988) require surgery for a successful outcome. In general, the surgery needs to be radical and may need to be repeated depending on disease progression. Disseminated disease is usually fatal, regardless of therapy.

FUSARIUM INFECTIONS

Most disseminated *Fusarium* infections complicate leukaemia, other haematological malignancies, or bone marrow transplantation. Most are due to *Fusarium solani*, but other species have been implicated. Disseminated disease with fungaemia is usual; 75% of patients have skin lesions. Pneumonia and sinusitis also occur. Sometimes infection arises from an affected toenail.

Treatment is often ineffective and restricted to amphotericin B in doses of at least 1 mg/kg daily together with a granulocyte/macrophage colony-stimulating factor if the patient is still profoundly neutropenic. No patient with persistent neutropenia has survived this infection (Rabodonirina et al 1994, Nelson et al 1994, Martino et al 1994).

PSEUDALLESCHERIA BOYDII INFECTIONS

Pseudallescheria boydii is the anamorph of *Scedosporium apiospermum* and causes superficial skin disease, mycetoma, sinusitis, cerebral abscess in leukaemia and rare systemic infections such as endocarditis in immunocompromised patients. Disease expression is similar to that of *Aspergillus*, but is much less common. Rarely it causes a fungal ball in the lung. *Pseudall. boydii* is resistant to amphotericin B in vitro (Walsh et al 1995) and in vivo (Walsh et al 1992). Intravenous miconazole and oral itraconazole are the agents of choice (Dworzack et al 1989, Goldberg et al 1993).

Patients with a cerebral abscess due to *Pseudall. boydii* require large doses of intravenous miconazole (45 mg/kg daily) (Dworzack et al 1989). A serum concentration of 1 mg/l is desirable and should be measured by drug assay when this is available. Treatment is continued for months and oral itraconazole (at least 400 mg/kg daily) may be substituted for intravenous miconazole. The treatment of

Table 60.8 *Treatment of mucormycosis*

	Medical therapy	Surgery*
Subcutaneous		
Conidiobolomycosis	Yes, various, high relapse rate,	No
Basidiobolomycosis	potassium iodide 30 mg/kg	No
Wound or burn associated	Amphotericin B† 1.0–1.5 mg/kg ± rifampicin	Resections of affected areas (multiple if necessary)
Rhinocerebral	Amphotericin B† 1.0–1.5 mg/kg ± rifampicin	Resection to margins of affected tissue on CT scan
Pulmonary	Amphotericin B† 1.0–1.5 mg/kg ± rifampicin	Lobectomy or pneumonectomy if exclusively or predominantly unilateral
Gastro-intestinal	Amphotericin B† 1.0–1.5 mg/kg ± rifampicin	
Cerebral	Amphotericin B† 1.0–1.5 mg/kg ± rifampicin	Resection of lesion
Renal	Amphotericin B† 1.0–1.5 mg/kg ± rifampicin	Nephrectomy
Disseminated	Amphotericin B† 1.0–1.5 mg/kg ± rifampicin	Not feasible

* Other than diagnostic biopsy.
† Also consider new lipid-associated amphotericin B preparations in doses exceeding 3 mg/kg for life-threatening disease.

other forms of *Pseudall. boydii* infection are essentially along the same lines as described for invasive aspergillosis using itraconazole rather than amphotericin B.

TRICHOSPORON INFECTIONS

The taxonomy of the genus *Trichosporon* has been revised recently and it has become difficult to correlate the old literature with the new nomenclature. *Trichosporon capitatum* is now classified as *Blastoschizomyces capitatus* but causes a similar disease process in leukaemia to *Trichosporon beigelii* (Martino et al 1990). Other than this, most infections are caused by *Trichosporon beigelli* or closely related species. The term *Trichosporon* spp. will be used here, although for the most part this relates to *Trichosporon beigelii*.

Trichosporon spp. cause three forms of disease: white piedra, a superficial infection of hair shafts found in the Tropics; endocarditis; and disseminated infection in neutropenic patients (Tashiro et al 1994). Data suggest that although isolates may be inhibited by amphotericin B they are not killed (Walsh et al 1990) and that the preferred agents for life-threatening *Trichosporon* infections are the azoles (Anaissie et al 1992). Large doses of fluconazole (e.g. 400–800 mg/day) should be used for the control of this rapidly lethal infection, with subsequent tailoring depending on response. The majority of isolates are also resistant to flucytosine.

For patients with *Trichosporon* endocarditis surgery is essential, particularly in those with an infected prosthetic heart valve (Keay et al 1991); large and prolonged doses of fluconazole or another azole should be given.

OTHER RARE FUNGAL DISEASES

There are other rare fungal infections too numerous to discuss here. The reader is referred to authoritative texts and recent literature (Warnock & Richardson 1991, Cunliffe & Denning 1995).

Prophylactic and pre-emptive therapy of fungal disease

PROPHYLAXIS

Prophylaxis is here defined as the use of an antimicrobial agent for all patients with the same condition prior to the development of an infection and regardless of individual markers of risk. Pre-emptive therapy is defined as the selective use of an antimicrobial agent in patients at particularly high risk before disease is apparent, e.g. those colonized with *Aspergillus* before cytoreductive chemotherapy. Empirical therapy is defined as the early treatment of a suspected infectious disease because of clinical or radiological abnormalities, but without laboratory confirmation. An example of the latter is treatment with amphotericin B in a profoundly neutropenic patient who has developed a cough. Secondary prophylaxis is the retreatment of a proven or probable infectious disease during another period of high risk, e.g. further chemotherapy or bone marrow transplantation. Clearly the use of prophylaxis, pre-emptive and empirical therapy are interrelated in a given patient population and must be considered together.

Some populations are at such high risk of fungal disease that all such patients should receive prophylaxis; the best examples are bone marrow transplant recipients and the use of pneumocystis prophylaxis in advanced HIV disease. The latter is covered in Chapter 46. In most other settings the benefits of prophylaxis are less clearly defined. At present, antifungal prophylaxis is not indicated for intensive-care-unit patients, surgical patients, neonates, patients with burns, inherited immune deficiency states or those with solid tumours.

Neutropenia and bone marrow transplantation

Remission induction therapy for leukaemia involves multiple courses of intensive cytoreductive chemotherapy with discrete episodes of neutropenia; corticosteroids may also be used. Patients whose leukaemia does not go into remission or who relapse have a very high incidence of invasive fungal infections at autopsy (Ribrag et al 1993). Even the majority of those who go into remission will develop an invasive fungal infection during neutropenia (Robertson & Larson 1988). The important fungi to protect against are various species of *Candida* and *Aspergillus*, while any given choice may also protect against several other rare fungi (Walsh & Lee 1993).

Prophylaxis may be appropriate for patients who will have at least 7 days of profound neutropenia, to prevent invasive fungal infections. Prophylaxis is not indicated for shorter periods of neutropenia. Any benefit of prophylaxis increases with the duration of profound neutropenia. Prophylaxis may also protect against mucosal candidosis which is common in acute leukaemia. Table 60.9 shows the more common prophylactic choices. Clearly neither topical oral regimens nor fluconazole protect against invasive aspergillosis. Likewise, aerosolized or a nasal spray of amphotericin B will not protect against mucosal or invasive candidosis, although it may protect against rare other airborne fungi such as the Mucorales. Ketoconazole is not sufficiently effective for prophylaxis against *Candida* and has no activity against *Aspergillus*.

Table 60.9 *Prophylaxis of invasive fungal infection during neutropenia and bone marrow transplantation*

Regimen	Neutropenia		Bone marrow transplantation*	
	Candida	Aspergillus	Candida	Aspergillus
Fluconazole 50–150 mg/day	?	NA	?	NA
Fluconazole 400 mg/day	?	NA	P	NA
Itraconazole 200–400 mg/day	?	?	?	?
Amphotericin B i.v. 0.15–1 mg/kg	?	?	?	?
Amphotericin B oral ≤200 mg/day	NA	NA	NA	NA
Amphotericin B orally >200 mg/day	?	NA	?	NA
Amphotericin B, intranasal/nebulized	NA	?	NA	?
Nystatin, orally	NA	NA	NA	NA

P, proven; ?, of possible value but unproven; NA, not appropriate or not efficacious.
* The term bone marrow transplantation (BMT) refers to those at greatest risk, e.g. allogeneic BMT (especially mismatched or unrelated), autologous BMT without use of growth promoters, second BMT, etc.

Fluconazole probably has some efficacy in protecting against invasive candidosis in acute leukaemia, but this was not shown in a study of 257 patients (Winston et al 1993). One likely reason for the failure to show a difference was the high (70%) incidence of empirical amphotericin B usage usually started on day 3 or 4 of neutropenic fever. In other studies of similar populations of patients, lower doses of fluconazole and less frequent use of empirical amphotericin B had similar incidences of invasive fungal infection (Philpott-Howard et al 1993, Menichetti et al 1994). Thus lower doses of fluconazole (e.g. 50–150 mg/day) are probably appropriate (British Society for Antimicrobial Chemotherapy 1993). Breakthrough *C. krusei* or *C. glabrata* fungaemia or invasive aspergillosis may be problematic.

Itraconazole has not yet been well evaluated for antifungal prophylaxis. It has the potential to prevent invasive aspergillosis and *C. krusei* infections. However, the capsule formulation is not always uniformly well absorbed and low serum concentrations have been associated with failure, both in therapy and prophylaxis. A new liquid preparation of itraconazole is currently under evaluation for prophylaxis.

The prophylaxis of fungal infections during and after bone-marrow transplantation has been the subject of some recent controlled trials. Fluconazole 400 mg/day was highly effective compared with placebo in preventing *Candida* infections and reduced mortality due to *Candida* (Goodman et al 1992). In one study 40% of the doses of fluconazole were given intravenously (Goodman et al 1992). The optimal duration of prophylaxis is not yet clear, but may extend beyond the end of neutropenia in allogeneic bone-marrow-transplant patients. Many studies in leukaemia patients, some of which have included some bone-marrow-transplant patients have shown that 50–150 mg/day of fluconazole is as effective as oral amphotericin B prophylaxis. There is some debate about whether the high daily dose of fluconazole (400 mg) is necessary for prophylaxis in the bone-marrow-transplant setting.

Secondary prophylaxis is indicated for patients with prior or current invasive aspergillosis, candidaemia, hepato-splenic candidosis, mucormycosis and other rarer fungal infections. Management may involve surgery and will also require individualization of the antifungal regimen depending on the infecting organism and response to therapy. A typical regimen is amphotericin B 1 mg/kg daily starting on the day chemotherapy is given (Karp et al 1988).

AIDS

Two studies have shown the benefit of fluconazole 100 mg/day for the prevention of cryptococcal disease and mucosal candidosis in patients with AIDS, although this regimen was ineffective in preventing histoplasmosis (Nightingale et al 1992, Powderley et al 1995). However, the cost of preventing each case of cryptococcal meningitis is high. Long-term primary fluconazole may also carry a risk of the development of fluconazole resistance. Primary prophylaxis is not warranted to prevent oral candidosis in patients with HIV infection.

Solid organ transplantation

Very few studies have addressed antifungal prophylaxis in the solid organ transplant patient. The frequency of disseminated or life-threatening fungal infections is low in the renal transplant recipient unless there are major problems with rejection, and prophylaxis is not indicated for these patients. There are higher risks associated with heart transplantation, of invasive candidosis, aspergillosis and *Pneumocystis carinii* pneumonia, but it is not possible to recommend routine prophylaxis in these patients (British Society for Antimicrobial Chemotherapy 1993). Similarly, no data support the use of prophylaxis in the lung transplant recipient, although this group is worthy of study. The frequency of deep candidosis in liver transplant patients is high and therefore prophylaxis may be appropriate in the first month after transplantation for these patients. An amphotericin B preparation is probably most appropriate given the diversity of fungi causing disease in these patients.

References

Anaissie E, Bodey G P, Kantarjian H et al 1991 Fluconazole therapy for chronic disseminated candidiasis in patients with leukaemia and prior amphotericin B therapy. *American Journal of Medicine* 91: 142–150

Anaissie E, Gokaslan A, Hachem R et al 1992 Azole therapy for trichosporonosis: clinical evaluation of eight patients, experimental therapy for murine infection, and review. *Clinical Infectious Diseases* 15: 781–787

Arikian S R, Einarson T R, Kobelt-Nguyen G, Schubert F 1994 A multinational pharmacoeconomic analysis of oral therapies for onychomycosis. The Onychomycosis Study Group. *British Journal of Dermatology* 130: 35–44

Baily G G, Robertson V J, Neill P, Garrido P, Levy L F 1991 Blastomycosis in Africa: clinical features, diagnosis, and treatment. *Reviews of Infectious Diseases* 13: 1005–1008

Baily G G, Perry F M, Denning D W, Mandal B K 1994 Management of candidiasis after failure of fluconazole in an HIV cohort. *AIDS* 8: 787–792

Bayles M A H 1989 Chromomycosis. *Baillières Clin Med Commun Dis* 4: 45–70

Bayles M A H 1992 Tropical mycoses. *Chemotherapy* 38 (suppl 1): 37–44

Bennett J E, Dismukes W E, Dumar R J et al 1979. A comparison of amphotericin B alone and combined until flucytosine in the treatment of cryptococcal meningitis. *New England Journal of Medicine* 301: 126–131

Berenguer J, Diaz-Mediavilla J, Urra D, Munoz P 1989 Central nervous system infection caused by *Pseudalleschria boydii*: case report and review. *Reviews of Infectious Diseases* 11: 890–896

Bjerke J W, Meyers J D, Bowden R A 1994 Hepatosplenic candidiasis – a contraindication to marrow transplantation? *Blood* 84: 2811–2814

Blade J, Lopez-Guillermo A, Rozman C et al 1992 Chronic systemic candidiasis in acute leukemia. *Annals of Hematology* 64: 240–244

Bozzette S A, Larsen R A, Chiu J et al 1991 A placebo-controlled trial of maintenance therapy with fluconazole after treatment of cryptococcal meningitis in the acquired immunodeficiency syndrome. *New England Journal of Medicine* 324: 580–584

British Society for Antimicrobial Chemotherapy Working Party on Fungal Infection 1991 Laboratory monitoring of antifungal chemotherapy. *Lancet* 357: 1577–1580

British Society for Antimicrobial Chemotherapy Working Party on Fungal Infection 1992 Treatment of fungal infections in AIDS. *Lancet* 340: 648–651

British Society for Antimicrobial Chemotherapy Working Party on Fungal Infection 1993 Chemoprophylaxis for candidiasis and aspergillosis in neutropenia and transplantation: a review and recommendations. *Journal of Antimicrobial Chemotherapy* 32: 5–21

British Society for Antimicrobial Chemotherapy Working Party on Fungal Infection 1994 Management of deep *Candida* infection in the surgical and intensive care unit patient. *Intensive Care Medicine* 20: 522–528

British Society for Medical Mycology Group on Diagnostic Mycology 1995 Management of genital candidosis. *British Medical Journal* 310: 1241–1244

Butler K M, Baker C J 1988 *Candida*: an increasingly important pathogen in the nursery. *Pediatric Clinics of North America* 35: 543–563

Campbell J H, Winter J H, Richardson M S, Shankland G S, Banham S W 1991 Treatment of pulmonary aspergilloma with itraconazole. *Thorax* 46: 839–841

Coker R J, Viviani M, Gazzard B G et al 1993 Treatment of cryptococcosis with liposomal amphotericin B (AmBisome) in 23 patients with AIDS. *AIDS* 7: 829–835

Cunliffe N A, Denning D W 1995 Uncommon invasive mycoses in AIDS. *AIDS* 9: 411–420

Currie D C, Lueck C, Milburn H J et al 1990 Controlled trial of natamycin in the treatment of allergic bronchopulmonary aspergillosis. *Thorax* 45: 447–450

Daly R C, Pairolero P C, Piehler J M, Trastek V F, Spencer Payne W, Bernatz P E 1986 Pulmonary aspergilloma: Results of surgical treatment. *Journal of Thoracic Cardiovascular Surgery* 92: 981–988

Dato V M, Dajani A S 1990 Candidaemia in children with central venous catheters: role of catheter removal and amphotericin B therapy. *Pediatric Infectious Diseases Journal* 9: 309–314

de Beule K, de Doncker P, Cauwenbergh G et al 1988 The treatment of aspergillosis and aspergilloma with itraconazole, clinical results of an open international study (1982–1987). *Mycoses* 31: 476–485

de Carpentier J, Ramamurthy M, Taylor P, Denning D W 1994 An algorithmic approach to aspergillus sinusitis. *Journal of Otolaryngology and Laryngology* 108: 314–318

De Gans J, Portegies P, Tiessens G et al 1992 Itraconazole compared with amphotericin B plus flucytosine in AIDS patients with cryptococcal meningitis. *AIDS* 6: 185–190

Delescluse J 1990 Itraconazole in tinea versicolor: a review. *Journal of the American Academy of Dermatology* 23: 551–554

Del Palacio Hernandez A, Delgado Vincent S, Menendez Romos F, Rodriguez-Noriega Belaustegui A 1987 Randomized comparative clinical trial of itraconazole and selenium sulfide shampoo for the treatment of pityriasis versicolor. *Reviews of Infectious Diseases* 9 (suppl 1): 121–127

Deng Z, Ribas J L, Gibson D W, Connor D H 1988 Infections caused by *Penicillium marneffei* in China and Southeast Asia: review of eighteen published cases and report of four more Chinese cases. *Reviews of Infectious Diseases* 10: 640–652

Denning D W 1994 The treatment of invasive aspergillosis. *Journal of Infection* 28 (suppl 1): 25–33

Denning D W 1996 Therapeutic response in invasive aspergillosis. *Clinical Infectious Diseases* In press

Denning D W, Stevens D A 1990 Antifungal and surgical treatment of invasive aspergillosis: review of 2121 published cases. *Reviews of Infectious Diseases* 12: 1147–1201

Denning D W, Tucker R M, Hanson L H, Stevens D A 1989a Treatment of invasive aspergillosis with itraconazole. *American Journal of Medicine* 86: 791–800

Denning D W, Tucker R M, Hanson L H, Hamilton J R, Stevens D A 1989b Itraconazole therapy of cryptococcal meningitis and cryptococcosis. *Archives of Internal Medicine* 149: 2301–2308

Denning D W, Van Wye J, Lewiston N J, Stevens D A 1991a Adjunctive therapy of allergic bronchopulmonary aspergillosis with itraconazole. *Chest* 100: 813–819

Denning D W, Armstrong R W, Lewis B H, Stevens D A 1991b Elevated cerebrospinal fluid pressure in patients with cryptococcal meningitis and acquired immunodeficiency syndrome. *American Journal of Medicine* 91: 267–272

Denning D W, Follansbee S, Scolaro M, Norris S, Edelstein D, Stevens D A 1991c Pulmonary aspergillosis in AIDS. *New England Journal of Medicine* 324: 654–662

Denning D W, Hanson L H, Perlman A M, Stevens D A 1992 In vitro susceptibility and synergy studies of *Aspergillus* species to conventional and new agents. *Diagnostic Microbiology and Infectious Diseases* 15: 21–34

Denning D W, Stepan D E, Blume K G, Stevens D A 1992 Control of invasive pulmonary aspergillosis in a bone marrow transplant patient with oral itraconazole. *Journal of Infection* 24: 73–79

Denning D W, Lee J Y, Hostetler J S et al 1994 NIAID Mycoses Study Group multicenter trial of oral itraconazole therapy of invasive aspergillosis. *American Journal of Medicine* 97: 135–144

de Pauw B E, Raemaekers J M M, Donnelly J P, Kullberg B-J, Meis J F G M 1995 An open study on the safety and efficacy of fluconazole in the treatment of disseminated *Candida* infections in patients treated for hematological malignancy. *Annals of Hematology* 70: 83–87

Diamond R D, Bennett J E 1974 Prognostic factors in crytococcal meningitis. A study in 111 cases. *Annals of Internal Medicine* 80: 176–181

Diaz M, Negroni R, Montero-Gei F et al 1992 A Pan-American 5-year study of fluconazole therapy for deep mycoses in the immunocompetent host. *Clinical Infectious Diseases* 14 (suppl 1): S68–S76

Dismukes W E, Cloud G, Bowles C et al 1985 Treatment of blastomycosis and histoplasmosis with ketoconazole: results of a prospective randomized clinical trial. *Annals of Internal Medicine* 103: 861–872

Dismukes W E, Bradsher R W, Cloud G C et al 1992 Itraconazole therapy for blastomycosis and histoplasmosis. *American Journal of Medicine* 93: 489–497

Dworzack D L, Clark R B, Borkowski W J et al 1989 *Pseudallescheria boydii* brain abscess: association with near-drowning and efficacy of high-dose, prolonged miconazole therapy in patients with multiple abscesses. *Medicine* 68: 218–224

Elmets C A 1994 Management of common superficial fungal infections in patients with AIDS. *Journal of the American Academy of Dermatology* 31: S60–S63

Evans E G V 1994 A comparison of terbinafine (Lamisil) 1% cream given for one week with clotrimazole (Canesten) 1% cream given for four weeks, in the treatment of tinea pedis. *British Journal of Dermatology* 130 (Suppl 43): 12–14

Farag A, Taha M, Halim S 1994 One-week therapy with oral terbinafine in cases of tinea cruris/corporis. *British Journal of Dermatology* 131: 684–686

Fish D G, Ampel N M, Galgiani J N et al 1990 Coccidioidomycosis during human immunodeficiency virus infection. A review of 77 patients. *Medicine* 69: 384–391

Fournier E C 1987 Trial of ketoconazole in allergic broncho-pulmonary aspergillosis. *Thorax* 42: 831

Galgiani J M, Stevens D A, Graybill J R et al 1988 Ketoconazole therapy of progressive coccidioidomycosis. Comparison of 400- and 800-mg doses and observations at higher doses. *American Journal of Medicine* 84: 603–610

Ghannoum M A, Rex J H, Galgiani J N 1996 Susceptibility testing of fungi: current status of correlation of in vitro data with clinical outcome. *Journal of Clinical Microbilogy* 34: 489–495

Giron J M, Poey C G, Fajadet P P, Balagner G B et al 1993 Inoperable pulmonary aspergilloma: Percutaneous CT-guided injection with glycerin and amphotericin B paste in 15 cases. *Radiology* 188: 825–827

Goldberg S L, Geha D J, Marshall W F, Inwards D J, Hoagland H C 1993 Successful treatment of simultaneous pulmonary

Pseudallescheria boydii and *Aspergillus terreus* infection with oral itraconazole. *Clinical Infectious Diseases* 16: 803–805

Goodfield M J D, Andrew L, Evans E G V 1992 Short term treatment of dermatophyte onychomycosis with terbenafine. *British Medical Journal* 304: 1151–1154

Goodman J L, Winston D J, Greenfield R A et al 1992 A controlled trial of fluconazole to prevent fungal infections in patients undergoing bone marrow transplantation. *New England Journal of Medicine* 326: 845–851

Graninger W, Presterl E, Schneeweiss B, Teleky B, Georgopoulos A 1993 Treatment of *candida albicans* fungaemia with fluconazole. *Journal of Infection* 26: 133–146

Hall K A, Sethi G K, Rosado L J, Martinez J D, Huston C L, Copeland J G 1993 Coccidioidomycosis and heart transplantation. *Journal of Heart and Lung Transplantation* 12: 525–526

Haramati L B, Schulman L L, Austin J H M 1993 Lung nodules and masses after cardiac transplantation. *Radiology* 188: 491–497

Hay R J, Clayton R M, Moore M K, Midgely G 1990 Itraconazole in the management of chronic dermatophytosis. *Journal of the American Academy of Dermatology* 23: 561–564

Hernandez-Sampelayo T, Multicentre Study Group 1994 Fluconazole versus ketoconazole in the treatment of oropharyngeal candidiasis in HIV-infected children. *European Journal of Clinical Microbiology and Infectious Diseases* 13: P340–P344

Hinson K F W, Moon A J, Plummer N S 1952 Bronchopulmonary aspergillosis. A review and a report of eight new cases. *Thorax* 7: 317–333

Hiruma M, Kawada A, Ohata H, Noda T, Takahashi H, Ishibashi A 1991 Clinical experience with itraconazole in cutaneous mycoses. *Clinical Reports* 25: 571–577

Ingham E, Cunningham A C 1993 *Malassezia furfur*. *Journal of Medical and Veterinary Mycology* 31: 265–288

Inman W, Pearce G, Wilton L 1994 Safety of fluconazole in the treatment of vaginal candidiasis. A prescription-event monitoring study, with special reference to the outcome of pregnancy. *European Journal of Clinical Pharmacology* 46: 115–118

Ishibashi Y, Hommura S, Matsumoto Y 1987 Direct examination vs culture of biopsy specimens for the diagnosis of keratomycosis. *American Journal of Ophthalmology* 103: 636–640

Jewkes J, Kay P H, Paneth M, Citron K M 1983 Pulmonary aspergilloma: analysis of prognosis in relation to haemoptysis and survey of treatment. *Thorax* 38: 572–578

Jonathan D, Lund V, Milroy C 1989 Allergic aspergillus sinusitis – an overlooked diagnosis? *Journal of Laryngology and Otology* 103: 1181–1183

Karp J E, Burch P A, Merz W G 1988 An approach to intensive antileukemia therapy in patients with previous invasive aspergillosis. *American Journal of Medicine* 85: 203–206

Katzenstein A-L A, Sale S R, Greenberg P A 1983 Allergic *Aspergillus* sinusitis: a newly recognised form of sinusitis. *Journal of Allergy and Clinical Immunology* 72: 89–93

Kauffman C A, Bradley S F, Ross S C, Weber D R 1991 Hepatosplenic candidiasis: successful treatment with fluconazole. *American Journal of Medicine* 91: 137–141

Keay S, Denning D W, Stevens D A 1991 Endocarditis due to *Trichosporon beigelii*: In vitro susceptibility of isolates and review. *Reviews of Infectious Diseases* 13: 383–386

Khoo S, Denning D W 1994 *Aspergillus* infection in the acquired immune deficiency syndrome. *Clinical Infectious Diseases* 19 (suppl 1): 541–548

Kibbler C C, Milkins S R, Bhamra A, Spiteri M A, Noone P, Prentice H G 1988 Apparent pulmonary mycetoma following intensive aspergillosis in neutropenic patients. *Thorax* 43: 108–112

Kohn D B, Uehling D T, Peters M E, Fellows K W, Chesney P J 1987 Short-course amphotericin B therapy for isolated candiduria in children. *Journal of Pediatrics* 110: 310–313

Korting H C, Blecher P, Stallman D, Hamm G 1993 Dermatophytes on the feet of HIV infected patients: and frequency species distribution, localization and antimicrobial susceptibility. *Mycoses* 36: 271–274

Larsen R A, Bozette S, McCutchan A et al 1989 Persistent *Cryptococcus neoformans* infection of the prostate after successful treatment of meningitis. *Annals of Internal Medicine* 11: 125–128

Larsen R A, Leal M A, Chan L S 1990 Fluconazole compared with amphotericin plus flucytosine for cryptococcal meningitis in AIDS. *Annals of Internal Medicine* 113: 183–187

Law D, Moore C B, Wardle H M, Ganguli L A, Keaney M G L, Denning D W 1994 High prevalence of antifungal resistance in *Candida* spp. from patients with AIDS. *Journal of Antimicrobial Chemotherapy* 34: 659–668

Lee K S, Kim H T, Kim Y H, Choe K O 1993 Treatment of haemoptysis in patients with cavitary aspergilloma of the lung: value of percutaneous instillation of amphotericin B. *American Journal of Radiology* 161: 727–731

Leibovitz E, Iuster-Reicher A, Amitai M, Mogilner B 1992 Systemic candidal infections associated with use of peripheral venous catheters in neonates: a 9-year experience. *Clinical Infectious Diseases* 14: 485–491

Lindeque B G, Van Niekerk W G 1984 Treatment of vaginal candidiasis in pregnancy with a single clotrimazole 500 mg vaginal pessary. *South African Medical Journal* 65: 123–124

Lopez-Gomez S, Del Palacio A, Van Cutsem J, Soledad Cuetara M, Iglesias L, Rodriguez-Noriega A 1994 Itraconazole versus griseofulvin in the treatment of tinea capitis: a double-blind randomized study in children. *International Journal of Dermatology* 33: 743–747

Loyd J E, Tillman B F, Atkinson J B, Des Prez R M 1988 Mediastinal fibrosis complicating histoplasmosis. *Medicine* 67: 295–310

McKinsey D S, Gupta M R, Riddler S A, Driks M R, Smith D L, Kurtin P J 1989 Long-term amphotericin B therapy for disseminated histoplasmosis in patients with acquired immunodeficiency syndrome (AIDS). *Annals of Internal Medicine* 111: 655–659

Manning S C, Schaefer S D, Close L G, Vuitch F 1991 Culture-positive allergic fungal sinusitis. *Archives of Otolaryngology and Head & Neck Surgery* 117: 174–178

Martino P, Venditti M, Micozzi A et al 1990 *Blastoschizomyces capitatus*: an emerging cause of invasive fungal disease in leukemia patients. *Reviews of Infectious Diseases* 12: 570–582

Martino P, Gastaldi R, Raccah R, Girmenia C 1994 Clinical patterns of *Fusarium* infections in immunocompromised patients. *Journal of Infection* 28 (suppl 1): 7–15

Massard G, Roeslin N, Wihlm J-M, Dumont P, Witz J-P, Morand G 1992 Pleuropulmonary aspergilloma: clinical spectrum and results of surgical treatment. *Annals of Thoracic Surgery* 54: 1159–1164

Menichetti F, Del Favero A, Martino P et al 1994 Preventing fungal infection in neutropenic patients with acute leukemia: Fluconazole compared with oral amphotericin B. *Annals of Internal Medicine* 120: 913–918

Meyer K C, McManus E J, Maki D G 1993 Overwhelming pulmonary blastomycosis associated with the adult respiratory distress syndrome. *New England Journal of Medicine* 329: 1231–1236

Munk P L, Vellet A D, Rankin R N, Müller N L, Ahmad D 1993 Intracavitary aspergilloma: transthoracic percutaneous injection of amphotericin gelatin solution. *Radiology* 188: 821–823

Nair K K 1979 Clinical trial of diaminodiphenylsulfone (DDS) in nasal and nasopharyngeal rhinosporidiosis. *Laryngoscope* 89: 291–295

Negroni R, Palmieri O, Koren F, Tiraboschi I N, Galimberti R L 1987 Oral treatment of paracoccidioidomycosis and histoplasmosis with itraconazole in humans. *Reviews in Infectious Diseases* 9 (suppl 1): S47–S50

Nelson M R, Fisher M, Cartledge J, Rogers T, Gazzard B G 1994 The role of azoles in the treatment and prophylaxis of cryptococcal disease in HIV infection. *AIDS* 8: 651–654

Nelson P E, Dignani M C, Anaissie E J 1994 Taxonomy, biology and clinical aspects of *Fusarium* species. *Clinical Microbiology Reviews* 7: 479–504

Ng T T C, Denning D W 1995 Liposomal amphotericin B (AmBisome) therapy of systemic fungal infections – evaluation of UK compassionate use data. *Archives of Internal Medicine* 155: 1093–1098

Nightingale S D, Cal S X, Peterson D M et al 1992 Primary prophylaxis with fluconazole against systemic fungal infections in HIV-positive patients. *AIDS* 6: 191–194

Norris S, Wheat J, McKinsey D et al 1994 Prevention of relapse of histoplasmosis with fluconazole in patients with the acquired immunodeficiency syndrome. *American Journal of Medicine* 96: 504–508

Occhipinti D J, Gubbins P O, Schreckenberger P, Danziger L H 1994 Frequency, pathogenicity and microbiologic outcome of non-*Candida albicans* candiduria. *European Journal of Clinical and Microbiological Infectious Diseases* 13: 459–467

Pappas P G, Threlkeld M G, Bedsole G D, Cleveland K O, Gelfand M S, Dismukes W E 1993 Blastomycosis in immunocompromised patients. *Medicine* 72: 311–325

Parent D, Decroix J, Heenen M 1994 Clinical experience with short schedules of itraconazole in the treatment of tinea corporis and/or tinea cruris. *Dermatology* 189: 378–381

Patow C A 1995 Fungi as a cause of otitis. *Journal of the American Medical Association* 273: 25

Patterson R, Greenberger P A, Radin R C, Roberts M 1982 Allergic bronchopulmonary aspergillosis: staging as an aid to management. *Annals of Internal Medicine* 96: 286–291

Philpott-Howard J N, Wade J J, Mutfi G J, Brammer K W, Ehninger G, Multicentre Study Group 1993 Randomized comparison of oral fluconazole versus oral polyenes for the prevention of fungal infection in patients at risk of neutropenia. *Journal of Antimicrobial Chemotherapy* 31: 973–984

Pimentel E R A, Castro L G M, Cuce L C, Sampaio S A P 1989 Treatment of chromomycosis by cryosurgery with liquid nitrogen: a report on eleven cases. *Journal of Dermatology, Surgery and Oncology* 15: 72–77

Powderly W G, Saag M S, Cloud G A et al 1992 A controlled trial of fluconazole or amphotericin B to prevent relapse of cryptococcal meningitis in patients with the acquired immunodeficiency syndrome. *New England Journal of Medicine* 326: 793–798

Powderley W G, Finkelstein D, Feinberg J et al 1995 A randomised trial comparing fluconazole with clotrimazole traches for the prevention of fungal infections in patients with advanced human immunodeficiency virus infection. *New England Journal of Medicine* 332: 700–705

Price M F, LaRocco M T, Gentry L O 1994 Fluconazole susceptibilities of *Candida* species and distribution of species recovered from blood cultures over a 5-year period. *Antimicrobial Agents and Chemotherapy* 38: 1422–1424

Queiroz-Telles F, Purim K S, Fillus J N et al 1992 Itraconazole in the treatment of chromoblastomycosis due to *Fonsecaea pedrosoi*. *International Journal of Dermatology* 31: 805–812

Rabodonirina M, Piens M A, Monier M F, Gueho E, Fiere D, Mojon M 1994 *Fusarium* infections in immunocompromised patients: case reports and literature review. *European Journal of Clinical Microbiology and Infectious Diseases* 13: 152–161

Randhawa H S, Budimulja U, Bazaz-Malik G et al 1994 Recent developments in the diagnosis and treatment of subcutaneous mycoses. *Journal of Medical and Veterinary Mycology* 32 (suppl 1): 299–307

Rémy J, Jardin M 1990 Angiographic management of bleeding: bronchial bleeding. In: Dondelinger R F, Rossi P, Kurdziel J C, Wallace S (eds) Interventional radiology. Thieme, New York, p 325–341

Restrepo A 1994 Treatment of tropical mycoses. *Journal of the American Academy of Dermatology* 31: S91–S102

Restrepo A, Gonzalez A, Gomez I, Arango M, De Bedout C 1988 Treatment of chromoblastomycosis with itraconazole. *Annals of the New York Academy of Sciences* 544: 504–516

Rex J H, Larsen R A, Dismukes W E, Cloud G A, Bennett J E 1993 Catastrophic visual loss due to *Cryptococcus neoformans* meningitis. *Medicine (Baltimore)* 72: 207–224

Rex J H, Bennett J E, Sugar A M et al 1994 A randomized trial comparing fluconazole with amphotericin B for the treatment of candidemia in patients without neutropenia. *New England Journal of Medicine* 331: 1325–1330

Ribrag V, Dreyfus F, Venot A, Leblong V, Lanore J J, Varet B 1993 Prognostic factors of invasive pulmonary aspergillosis in leukemic patients. *Leukaemia and Lymphoma* 10: 317–321

Rios-Fabra A, Restrepo Moreno A, Isturiz R E 1994 Fungal infection in Latin American countries. *Infectious Disease Clinics of North America* 8: 129–154

Roberts M M 1991 Developments in the management of superficial fungal infections. *Journal of Antimicrobial Chemotherapy* 28 (suppl A): 47–58

Robertson M J, Larson R A 1988 Recurrent fungal pneumonias in patients with acute nonlymphocytic leukemia undergoing multiple courses of intensive chemotherapy. *American Journal of Medicine* 84: 233–239

Saag M S, Dismukes W E 1988 Treatment of histoplasmosis and blastomycosis. *Chest* 93: 848–851

Saag M S, Powderly W G, Cloud G A et al 1992 Comparison of amphotericin B with fluconazole in the treatment of acute AIDS-associated cryptococcal meningitis. *New England Journal of Medicine* 326: 83–89

Sanford J P 1993 The enigma of candiduria: evolution of bladder irrigation with amphotericin B for management – from anecdote to dogma and a lesion from Machiavelli. *Clinical Infectious Diseases* 16: 145–147

Sawyer S M, Bowes G, Phelan P D 1994 Vulvovaginal candidiasis in young women with cystic fibrosis. *British Medical Journal* 308: 1609

Shale D J, Faux J A, Lane D J 1987 Trial of ketoconazole in non-invasive pulmonary aspergillosis. *Thorax* 42: 26–31

Sharkey P K, Rinaldi M G, Dunn J F, Hardin T C, Fetchick R J, Graybill J R 1991 High-dose itraconazole in the treatment of severe mycoses. *Antimicrobial Agents and Chemotherapy* 35: 707–713

Spinillo A, Michelone G, Cavanna C, Colonna L 1994 Clinical and microbiological characteristics of symptomatic vulvovaginal candidiasis in HIV seropositive women. *Genitourinary Medicine* 70: 268–272

Staughton R 1990 Skin manifestations in AIDS patients. *British Journal of Clinical Practice* 71 (suppl): 109–113

Storfer S P, Medoff G, Fraser V J, Powderly W G, Dunagan W C 1994 Candiduria: retrospective review in hospitalized patients. *Infectious Diseases Clinical Practice* 3: 23–29

Sugar A M, Alsip S, Galgiani J N et al 1987 Pharmacology and toxicity of high dose ketoconazole. *Antimicrobial Agents and Chemotherapy* 31: 1874–1878

Supparatpinyo K, Nelson K E, Merz W G et al 1993 Response to antifungal therapy by human immunodeficiency virus-infected patients with disseminated *Penicillium marneffei* infections and in vitro susceptibilities of isolates from clinical specimens. *Antimicrobial Agents and Chemotherapy* 37: 2407–2411

Supparatpinyo K, Khamwan C, Baosoung V, Nelson K E, Sirisanthana T 1994 Disseminated *Penicillium marneffei* infection in southeast Asia. *Lancet* 344: 110–113

Talenti A, Roberts G D 1989 Fungal blood cultures. *European Journal of Clinical Microbiology and Infectious Diseases* 8: 825–831

Tashiro T, Nagai H, Kamberi P, Goto Y, Kikuchi H, Nasu M, Akizuki S 1994 Disseminated *Trichosporon beigelii* infection in patients with malignant diseases: immunohistochemical study and review. *European Journal of Clinical and Microbiological Infectious Diseases* 13: 218–224

Tedder M, Spratt J A, Anstadt M P, Hedge S S, Tedder S D, Lowe J E 1994 Pulmonary mucormycosis: results of medical and surgical therapy. *Annals of Thoracic Surgery* 57: 1044–1050

Thomas P A 1994 Mycotic keratitis – an underestimated mycosis. *Journal of Medical and Veterinary Mycology* 32: 235–256

Thomas P A, Abraham D J, Kalavathy C M, Rajasekaran J 1988 Oral itraconazole therapy for mycotic keratitis. *Mycoses* 31: 271–279

Torres M A, Mohamed J, Cavazos-Adame H, Martinez L A 1985 Topical ketoconazole for fungal keratitis. *American Journal of Ophthalmology* 100: 293–298

Tucker R M, Denning D W, Arathoon E G, Rinaldi M G, Stevens D A 1990a Itraconazole therapy of non-meningeal coccidioidomycosis: clinical and laboratory observations. *Journal of the American Academy of Dermatology* 23: 593–601

Tucker R M, Denning D W, Dupont B, Stevens D A 1990b Itraconazole therapy for chronic coccidioidal meningitis. *Annals of Internal Medicine* 112: 108–112

Tucker R M, Galgiani J N, Denning D W et al 1990c Treatment of coccidioidal meningitis with fluconazole. *Reviews of Infectious Diseases* 12 (suppl 3): S380–S389

Tucker R M, Hanson L H, Denning D W et al 1992 Interaction of azoles with rifampin, phenytoin and carbamazepine: in vitro and clinical observations. *Clinical Infectious Diseases* 14: 165–174

Vainrub B, Macareno A, Mandel S, Musher D M 1988 Wound zygomycosis (mucormycosis) in otherwise healthy adults. *American Journal of Medicine* 84: 546–548

Vargas Flores J 1992 El itraconazol en la paracoccidioidomicosis (experiencia en 40 casos bolivianos). *Revista Argentina de Micologia* XV. T-4/P.84.

Venugopal P V, Venugopal T V 1993 Treatment of eumycetoma with ketoconazole. *Australasian Journal of Dermatology* 34: 27–29

Voss A, Meis J F G M, Hoogkamp-Korstanje J A A 1994 Fluconazole in the management of fungal urinary tract infections. *Infection* 22: 247–251

Walsh M, White L, Atkinson K, Enno A 1992 Fungal *Pseudallescheria boydii* lung infiltrates unresponsive to amphotericin B in leukaemic patients. *Australian and New Zealand Journal of Medicine* 22: 265–268

Walsh T J, Lee J W 1993 Prevention of invasive fungal infections in patients with neoplastic diseases. *Clinical Infectious Diseases* 17 (suppl 2): S486–S480

Walsh T J, Melcher G P, Rinaldi M G et al 1990 *Trichosporon beigelli*, and emerging pathogen resistant to amphotericin B. *Journal of Clinical Microbiology* 28: 1616–1622

Walsh T J, Peter J, McGough D A, Fothergill A W, Rinaldi M G, Pizzo P A 1995 Activities of amphotericin B and antifungal azoles alone and in combination against *Pseudallescheria boydii*. *Antimicrobial Agents and Chemotherapy* 39: 1361–1364

Warnock D W, Richardson M D (eds) 1991 Fungal infections in the compromised patient, 2nd edn. Wiley, Chichester

Welsh O 1993 Mycetoma. *Seminars in Dermatology* 12: 290–295

Wheat L J, Batteiger B E, Sathapatayavongs B 1990a *Histoplasma capsulatum* infections of the central nervous system. A clinical review. *Medicine* 69: 244–260

Wheat L J, Connolly-Stringfield P A, Baker R L et al 1990b Disseminated histoplasmosis in the acquired immune deficiency syndrome: clinical findings, diagnosis and treatment and review of the literature. *Medicine* 69: 361–364

Wheat L J, Hafner R, Wulfsohn M et al 1993 Prevention of relapse of histoplasmosis with itraconazole in patients with the acquired immunodeficiency syndrome. *Annals of Internal Medicine* 118: 610–616

Wheat L J, Hafner R, Korzun A H et al 1995 Itraconazole treatment of disseminated histoplasmosis in patients with the acquired immunodeficiency syndrome. *American Journal of Medicine* 98: 336–342

Williams P L, Johnson R, Pappagianis D et al 1992 Vasculitic and encephalitic complications associated with *Coccidioides immitis* infection of the central nervous system in humans: report of 10 cases and review. *Clinical Infectious Diseases* 14: 673–682

Winston D J, Chandrasekar P H, Lazarus H M et al 1993 Fluconazole prophylaxis of fungal infections in patients with acute leukemia. *Annals of Internal Medicine* 118: 495–503

Wong-Beringer A, Jacobs R A, Guglielmo B J 1992 Treatment of funguria. *Journal of the American Medical Association* 267: 2780–2785

Zang M, Bergstraesser M 1992 Amorolfine in the treatment of onychomycosis and dermatomycoses (an overview). *Clinical and Experimental Dermatology* 17 (suppl 1): 61–70

Zoonoses

R. N. Davidson

Brucellosis

About 230 000 human cases of brucellosis occur annually (Sturchler 1988). The responsible species are, in order of importance: *Brucella melitensis* (the animal hosts are goat, sheep and camels), *Brucella abortus* (cattle, buffalo, camels), *Brucella suis* (pig and reindeer), *Brucella ovis* (sheep) and *Brucella canis* (dogs). Brucellae are shed in large numbers in milk, urine and products of conception of infected animals, and man is infected by direct contact with infected animals or, more commonly, by ingestion of unpasteurized milk or milk products. In man the disease may be acute or chronic, though it is no longer a fashionable aetiology of chronic fatigue syndromes.

Therapy of brucellosis is complicated by the intracellular location of the organism in reticulo-endothelial cells, where optimal concentrations of antibiotics are difficult to achieve. Central nervous system brucellosis and brucella endocarditis are rare, but particularly difficult to treat (McLean et al 1992).

ANTIBIOTIC THERAPY

Therapy with single drugs such as tetracycline, doxycycline or rifampicin has a relapse rate of 5–40%, and thus combination therapy is generally recommended (Acocella et al 1989, Hall 1990). The combination of trimethoprim–sulfamethoxazole alone is unsatisfactory: Ariza et al (1985a) reported relapses in 13 of 28 patients treated with co-trimoxazole for 45 days. Quinolones as single agents also appear inadequate: 4 of 15 uncomplicated adult cases treated with ciprofloxacin relapsed (al Sibai 1992). Ceftriaxone is even less effective: although it has good in vitro activity against *Brucella*, a dose of 2 g/day produced an initial clinical response in only 2 of 8 patients, and one of these relapsed (Lang et al 1992).

Drug combinations

It is unclear whether drug combinations provide synergy, prevent resistance, or act against different subpopulations of brucellae; nonetheless, combinations are far more effective than single agents. Most trials compare one combination against another, but leave important questions unaddressed. In the case of aminoglycosides, for example, it is unclear whether streptomycin is better than gentamicin; whether multiple daily doses of aminoglycosides are better than single daily doses; or whether adding streptomycin for 2 weeks is as good as 6 weeks. For all regimens initial response rates are higher than long-term cure rates, since relapses occur with all regimens usually within the first 6 months.

The World Health Organization (WHO) recommends doxycycline 200 mg/day plus rifampicin 600–900 mg/day for ≥6 weeks (WHO 1986). Although initial response rates are identical, streptomycin + doxycycline has been shown to have lower relapse rates than rifampicin + doxycycline (Ariza 1985b, Montejo et al 1993). A meta-analysis of six trials (a total of 544 patients) found that 5% of patients treated with streptomycin + doxycycline relapsed, versus 16% of rifampicin + doxycycline recipients (Solera et al 1994). Ariza et al (1992) suggested that the lower relapse rates of doxycycline + streptomycin may be confined to a subgroup of patients with brucella spondylitis. In their study of 95 patients, the overall relapse rate of doxycycline + streptomycin was 14.4% vs 5.9% for rifampicin + doxycycline in unselected cases; however, for those without spondylitis the relapse rates were 4.9% vs 4.3%. In other studies, rifampicin + doxycycline has had relapse rates as low as 3% (Akova et al 1993). It is not clear whether courses of rifampicin + doxycycline longer than 6 weeks would be superior, or if the relapse rate of any two agents combined could be reduced if a third agent is added.

Combinations of other oral agents are also promising. In a study of 61 patients, rifampicin + ofloxacin was better tolerated than rifampicin + doxycycline, and the relapse rate was identical: only 3% of each group relapsed (Akova et al 1993).

In children, the combination of trimethoprim–sulfamethoxazole (10–12 mg/kg daily trimethoprim, 50–60 mg/kg daily sulfamethoxazole) plus rifampicin (15–20 mg/kg daily) for 6 weeks has been highly effective: only 4 of 113 children relapsed, and all the relapsed patients responded to repeat therapy with the same agents (Khuri Bulos et al 1993). Co-trimoxazole plus rifampicin has also been recommended for pregnant women (Janbon 1993), with an alternative being trimethoprim–sulfamethoxazole plus an aminoglycoside (Young 1995).

Complicated brucellosis

As with other bacterial infections, abscesses due to *Brucella* should be surgically drained if possible. In cases of *Brucella* endocarditis, therapy with streptomycin plus doxycycline may be improved by the addition of rifampicin (Pratt et al 1978), but surgical removal of the valve may be necessary (Jacobs et al 1990).

Central nervous system involvement is best treated with a combination of three or more drugs. Of note, doxycycline crosses the blood–brain barrier better than generic tetracycline, but it is only available in an oral formulation. Neurobrucellosis has been treated with combinations of streptomycin, doxycycline, rifampicin and trimethoprim–sulfamethoxazole, but, despite this, the clinical sequelae may be severe (McLean et al 1992). It may be logical to add a third-generation cephalosporin in neurobrucellosis (Lang et al 1992), but this has not been tested in clinical practice.

Animal bites

About 85% of dog, cat and other animal bites will become infected with either animal oral flora or human skin flora. As well as wound cleaning and debridement, and tetanus and rabies prophylaxis, antimicrobial prophylaxis should be considered (Weber & Hansen 1991, Goldstein 1995). The following bite wounds warrant antimicrobial prophylaxis: moderate/severe injuries <8 h old (most infections present clinically >8 h after the bite); possible bone or joint penetration; face, genital and hand wounds; and bites suffered by patients with underlying illness such as liver disease or local conditions such as limb oedema or prosthetic joints. The organisms commonly isolated are: *Staphylococcus aureus*, *Staphylococcus intermedius*, *Pasteurella multocida*, *Capnocytophaga canimorsus* (formerly called 'dysgonic fermenter 2' (DF2)), anaerobes and *Eikenella corrodens*. Amoxycillin–clavulanic acid has good activity against these organisms, and is the best choice both for prophylaxis of infection-prone bites and for empirical treatment of infected bites prior to the results of cultures from the wound being available. Infected bites may be polymicrobial, even if a single species is cultured. Co-trimoxazole may substitute for amoxycillin–clavulanic acid if the patient is allergic to amoxycillin, although clinical efficacy data are lacking. Prophylaxis for 3–5 days should suffice; treatment of established infections should be more prolonged, and punctures over or near a joint observed carefully for osteomyelitis or septic arthritis. Prophylaxis with amoxycillin–clavulinic acid will, incidentally, prevent rat-bite fever, though co-trimoxazole will not.

Tularaemia

Tularaemia is a plague-like zoonosis occurring occasionally in Europe (excluding the UK), North America and the former USSR, where it is enzootic in a large number of animal species (Sturchler 1988). The causative organism, *Francisella tularensis*, a Gram-negative coccobacillus, infects man either by direct animal contact or when bitten by ticks or biting flies which have fed on infected animals. Six clinical syndromes of tularaemia are recognized: ulceroglandular, glandular, oculoglandular, oropharyngeal, typhoidal and pulmonary (Penn 1995).

TREATMENT

Streptomycin is the antibiotic of choice (Penn et al 1987, 1995), at a dose of 7.5–15 mg/kg i.m. 12-hourly for 7–14 days, the higher doses being used for more severe illness. A case of tularaemic meningitis has been treated successfully with the combination of streptomycin and tetracycline given for 1 week, followed by tetracycline alone for an additional 2 weeks (Hutton & Everett 1985).

Gentamicin has been used to treat 10 patients with pulmonary, typhoidal or ulceroglandular tularaemia, with uniform success and no relapses. The recommended dose is 3–5 mg/kg daily in divided doses, and a peak gentamicin concentration of at least 5 mg/l is desirable (Mason et al 1980).

A single case of unsuspected tularaemia with multisystem failure was cured with imipenem–cilastatin (Lee et al 1991).

Ciprofloxacin and, to a lesser extent, norfloxacin, ofloxacin, and pefloxacin, have good in vitro activity against *F. tularensis*. Patients have been successfully treated with ciprofloxacin 750 mg 12-hourly, and norfloxacin 400 mg 12-hourly (Syrjala et al 1991).

Tetracycline or chloramphenicol are bacteriostatic for *F. tularensis* and have unacceptable relapse rates (Penn 1995). Although ceftriaxone has excellent in vitro activity against *F. tularensis*, it fails in clinical practice (Cross & Jacobs 1993).

Anthrax

Bacillus anthracis, a Gram-positive spore-forming rod, causes acute infection in wild and domestic herbivores, and about 4000–8000 human cases annually (Sturchler 1988), with occasional epidemics. Human cutaneous infections follow contact with anthrax spores on animal hair or hides, either in an industrial or agricultural setting. More rarely, spores may be inhaled or ingested, causing respiratory and gastro-intestinal anthrax: both are usually lethal (Lew 1995).

In vitro, 44 isolates of *B. anthracis* isolated from wild game were highly susceptible to ampicillin, streptomycin, chloramphenicol, erythromycin, tetracycline, methicillin and netilmicin. More than 90% of the isolates were sensitive to clindamycin, gentamicin and cefoxitin. Only 84.1% of the isolates were highly sensitive to penicillin G, the remainder being moderately sensitive. There was complete resistance to co-trimoxazole (Odendaal et al 1991).

Cutaneous anthrax is rarely fatal if treated with intravenous penicillin G 12 g/day for 10–12 days. Patients who are allergic to penicillin should be treated with erythromycin, tetracycline or chloramphenicol (Knudson 1986, Singh et al 1992). Surgical debridement of the black, necrotic eschar is contraindicated. Systemic steroids have been used for the extensive oedema, but their efficacy is unproven.

Plague

Plague is caused by a bipolar staining Gram-negative bacillus, *Yersinia pestis*. A disease of world-wide distribution, plague is epizootic and enzootic in many urban and rural areas. In the bubonic form, man is infected by the bite of an infected flea. From the infected lymph nodes the infection may spread, and death is by overwhelming septicaemia. Patients with pulmonary involvement may transmit the disease, as pneumonic plague; rare forms such as plague meningitis or pharyngitis may also occur (Butler et al 1976, Butler 1995).

The true frequency of human plague is uncertain, because underreporting is likely, as well as wrong attribution of outbreaks of pneumonic or septicaemic illness to plague without confirmation by culture (John 1994). Official estimates are of about 1000 human cases annually (Sturchler 1988, Butler 1995). Untreated bubonic plague has a case fatality rate of >50%, whilst pneumonic and septicaemic forms are invariably fatal without treatment (John 1994). Treatment reduces this dramatically, the critical factor being early initiation of antibiotic treatment. When 28 patients were treated in a well-equipped hospital, 6 deaths occurred: 3 of 8 cases of pneumonic plague and 3 of 19 cases of bubonic plague died. All the fatalities were attributed to a failure to treat initially with an antibiotic appropriate for plague (Crook & Tempest 1992). Plague has an incubation period of 2–8 days, and has been reported in travellers who have recently returned from a plague-endemic area. This includes both tropical and temperate zones (Mann 1982).

Nearly all strains of *Y. pestis* are susceptible to streptomycin, tetracycline, chloramphenicol, ampicillin, cephalothin and trimethoprim–sulphamethoxazole. Drug resistance seems to be rare; Marshall et al (1967) found only 2 of 156 strains resistant to streptomycin, and none resistant to tetracycline or chloramphenicol. There is thus no rationale for the use of multiple antibiotics to treat plague (Butler 1995).

Streptomycin, at a dose of 30 mg/kg daily in two divided doses, intramuscularly for 10 days, is still probably the therapy of choice for most forms of plague (Butler et al 1976, 1977, Butler 1995). Meyer (1950) observed a case-fatality rate in India of only 10% in patients treated with streptomycin, compared with 21% in those treated with sulphonamides. Although combined treatment with strepto-mycin and tetracycline is often recommended, there is little evidence that these two drugs are more effective than streptomycin alone. Alternative regimens are tetracycline, 2–4 g/day in four doses for 10 days, or chloramphenicol, 4 g/day (60 mg/kg daily) in divided doses for 10 days, following an initial loading dose of 25 mg/kg (Butler et al 1977). Plague meningitis should be treated with either chloramphenicol or ampicillin.

In addition to antibiotics, patients with plague will often require intensive care for septicaemic shock. There is no evidence that corticosteroids are beneficial. Patients with any form of plague should be maintained in strict isolation for the first 48 h after initiation of treatment. Relapses after treatment are very uncommon.

Household contacts of patients with bubonic plague, and casual or close contacts of a patient with pneumonic plague, should receive chemoprophylaxis for 7 days after their last exposure with either tetracycline 250 mg 6-hourly, doxycycline 100 mg/day or co-trimoxazole 480 mg 12-hourly. Babies and pregnant women in the first trimester should take amoxycillin, and older children should take co-tri-moxazole. Stand-by or prophylactic 7 day courses of the same drugs are recommended for travellers visiting areas where a plague outbreak is confirmed or suspected.

Bartonellosis (Carrion's disease)

Though not a zoonosis, bartonellosis is transmitted by the bite of infected sandflies of the genus *Phlebotomus (Lutzomyia)*. The aetiological agent is *Bartonella bacilliformis*, a Gram-negative obligate aerobic organism (Roberts 1995). It is found only in the Andean river valleys of Peru, Ecuador and Colombia, and in endemic foci 5–10% of the population may be asymptomatic carriers, or have chronic haemangiomatous lesions called verrugas. Acute infection is known as Oroya fever, and is characterized by a malaria-like illness with severe haemolytic anaemia. In blood films bartonellae may be seen adherent to erythrocytes or within macrophages. The illness may be fatal, particularly if complicated by salmonellosis, tuberculosis or other infections; or it may gradually resolve spontaneously, with the development of a chronic cutaneous phase (verruga peruviana). Oroya fever responds well to penicillin, streptomycin or chloramphenicol (Schultz 1968). Chloramphenicol is a logical choice if secondary infection with *Salmonella* is suspected (Urteaga & Payne 1955, Cuadra 1956).

Treatment of verruga peruviana is symptomatic. Lesions may respond to antibiotics or require surgical excision.

Rat-bite fever

The term 'rat-bite fever' comprises two distinct diseases caused by two very different organisms, *Streptobacillus moniliformis* (a pleomorphic Gram-negative bacillus) and *Spirillum minus* (a short, thick Gram-negative spirochaete with darting motility). Both organisms are common inhabitants of the pharynx of both wild, pet, and laboratory rats in all parts of the world. Both organisms are susceptible to penicillin.

Humans usually acquire the disease through the bite of a rat, though a history of a bite is sometimes absent in *Strep. moniliformis* infections, which may be acquired by oral ingestion (Rygg & Bruun 1992). Sometimes *Strep. moniliformis* is seen in food- or milk-borne outbreaks, known as Haverhill fever (McEvoy et al 1987).

SPIRILLUM MINUS

The initial bite heals promptly, but becomes inflamed 1–4 weeks later, with regional lymphadenitis, fever and constitutional symptoms. *Spir. minus* may be demonstrated in dark-field illumination of exudate from the chancre-like bite or in thick blood films (Bhatt & Mirza 1992).

Spir. minus is highly sensitive to phenoxymethylpenicillin 500 mg orally every 6 h, for 10 days. Initiation of treatment may be followed by the Jarisch–Herxheimer reaction. Endocarditis due to *Strep. moniliformis* requires more prolonged therapy with higher doses of penicillin (Washburn 1995).

STREPTOBACILLUS MONILIFORMIS

The illness is that of fever, with minimal lymphadenopathy or reaction at the site of the bite; a rash and arthritis often occur after a few days. Uncomplicated *Strep. moniliformis* infection may be treated with intramuscular or intravenous benzylpenicillin 600 mg 12-hourly for 7–10 days, but when patients have responded promptly to treatment, oral phenoxymethylpenicillin, tetracycline or ampicillin, each for 10 days, may be used. Limited experience with oral erythromycin, clindamycin or chloramphenicol suggests that these are effective. Complications such as septic arthritis, meningitis and pneumonia require more intensive treatment with intravenous penicillin. For endocarditis due to *Strep. moniliformis*, McCormack et al (1967) recommended 4.8 million units (approximately 3 g) of procaine penicillin per day intramuscularly for 4 weeks if the organism is very susceptible to penicillin (minimum inhibitory concentrations (MIC) <0.1 mg/l) and 20 million units (12 g) of benzylpenicillin intravenously per day for 6 weeks in infections due to more resistant strains.

Prophylaxis against rat-bite fever

Infections due to both *Spir. minus* and *Strep. moniliformis* should, in theory, be adequately prevented by a 3-day course of penicillin 500 mg 6-hourly, or doxycycline 100 mg/day; however, the efficacy of prophylaxis has not been assessed in clinical practice.

Cat-scratch disease, bacillary angiomatosis and other infections due to *Rochalimea*

Rochalimea are small Gram-negative rods which cause several syndromes that sometimes overlap. The clinical features of these syndromes have recently been reviewed

(Adal et al 1994, Cotell & Noskin 1994, Slater & Welch 1995, Fischer 1995).

Rochalimea henselae and *Rochalimea quintana* (renamed *Bartonella henselae* and *Bartonella quintana*) may cause cutaneous bacillary angiomatosis, with or without systemic dissemination. This syndrome is seen mainly, but not exclusively in human immunodeficiency virus (HIV) positive or immunocompromised patients; if involving liver and spleen, the syndrome is called bacillary peliosis hepatis. Fever and bacteraemia are other common features.

R. henselae (and, more rarely and controversially, an unrelated organism named *Afipia felis*) are the cause of cat-scratch disease.

R. quintana is the cause of trench fever, which is not a zoonosis, but spread by the human body louse.

Rochalimea elizabethae has been isolated from the blood of an immunocompetent patient with endocarditis (Daly 1993).

Rochalimea henselae causes asymptomatic bacteraemia in as many as 41% of asymptomatic domestic cats (Koehler et al 1994). Infection is linked to ownership of cats and particularly kittens less than a year old. Though the mode of transmission is unproven, cat scratches and bites, as well as flea or tick bites, are implicated.

TREATMENT

There have been no systematic studies of antimicrobials in any of the syndromes due to *Rochalimea*. The organisms are sensitive in vitro to most antimicrobials, except amino-glycosides, but treatment failures with β-lactams, co-trimoxazole and quinolones have occurred in severely immunocompromised patients.

Cat-scratch disease. The benign lymphadenitis will resolve spontaneously (average duration 3 months) (Fischer 1995). Antimicrobials do not dramatically hasten resolution and are not generally recommended.

In immunocompetent patients with systemic symptoms, a 2–4 week course of erythromycin or doxycycline is recommended (Adal et al 1994), but occasional cases of unresponsiveness and relapse, requiring several combinations of antimicrobials, have been documented (Lucey et al 1992).

In immunocompromised patients, untreated bacillary angiomatosis with or without dissemination will be progressive and potentially fatal. Doxycycline 100 mg 12-hourly or erythromycin 500 mg 6-hourly are the drugs of choice. Cutaneous lesions should begin to resolve in 4–7 days, and have resolved after 4 weeks of treatment. Treatment should continue for 3 months or for as long as the underlying immunosuppressive condition lasts (Cotell & Noskin 1994, Adal et al 1994).

Leptospirosis

Pathogenic leptospires all belong to the species *Leptospira interrogans*; serovar *canicola* is most frequent in the USA and Europe, and *icterohaemorrhagiae* most commonly causes the severe form (Weil's disease).

It is primarily a disease of wild and domestic animals, who may asymptomatically pass large numbers of leptospires in their urine. Humans are infected mainly due to occupational or recreational contact with contaminated surface water, commonly during the summer. In endemic areas seroprevalence is 5–10% (Sturchler 1988), and travel-associated leptospirosis can often be diagnosed in febrile travellers when serology is performed. Rats are the most common source of human infection in developing countries, and dogs and livestock in industrialized countries (Farrar 1995).

Prophylaxis

Doxycycline 200 mg once weekly was tested against placebo in 940 US soldiers undergoing 3 weeks of jungle training in Panama (Takafuji et al 1984). One of 469 men (0.2%) receiving doxycycline and 20 of 471 (4.2%) receiving placebo developed leptospirosis, a prophylactic efficacy of 95%. Leptospirosis developed after a prolonged incubation period of 40 days in a laboratory technician who received a dose of penicillin (including benzathine penicillin, procaine penicillin and benzylpenicillin) within 1 h after exposure in a laboratory accident (Gilks et al 1988), suggesting that amoxycillin or ampicillin might be ineffective as prophylaxis. Physicians may be asked to advise on prophylaxis for cave explorers, canoeists, etc., who have ingested potentially infected water, as many clubs issue their members with cards warning about leptospirosis. Although only 29–48 cases were reported annually in England and Wales during the period 1990–1992 (Ferguson 1993), physicians may yet feel obliged to prescribe a prophylactic drug: doxycycline 200 mg/day for 3 days should be effective, though this schedule has not been assessed in clinical practice.

TREATMENT

Doxycycline 100 mg 12-hourly for 7 days, begun within 3 days of the onset of symptoms, was superior to placebo in 29 US soldiers (McClain et al 1984). The illness was shortened by 2 days, and leptospiruria did not develop. In moderately or severely ill patients, intravenous penicillin 1.2 g for 5–7 days should be used, even if the patient has been ill for several days. Watt et al (1988) evaluated the effect of a 7-day course of intravenous penicillin on severe advanced leptospirosis in a randomized placebo-controlled double-blind trial involving 42 patients. All but one patient had been ill for at least 5 days. Duration of fever, duration of renal impairment, hospital stay and duration of leptospiruria were all decreased by treatment with penicillin. Thus treatment with penicillin is effective in leptospirosis, even when therapy is begun late in the course of the disease. Intravenous ampicillin 1 g 6-hourly or cefotaxime are alternatives to penicillin, though clinical data are lacking (Farrar 1995). Chloramphenicol is ineffective in both experimental and human infections. The Jarisch–Herxheimer reaction may occur 4–6 h after initiation of penicillin therapy in some patients (Vaughan et al 1994).

Lyme disease

Lyme disease is a multisystem disorder caused by the spirochaete *Borrelia burgdorferi* (Burgdorfer et al 1982). The vectors are ticks of the *Ixodes ricinus* complex, namely *I. ricinus* in Europe, *Ixodes dammini* (also called *I. scapularis*) and *I. pacificus* in the USA. About 50 000 cases of Lyme disease have been reported from 47 states of the USA, since its description in 1975 (Steere et al 1977). It has subsequently been reported from Europe, Scandinavia, the former USSR, China, Japan and Australia. The transmission season is summer.

Lyme disease is characterized in a third of cases by erythema chronicum migrans, spreading from the site of a tick bite 3–22 days earlier. A febrile illness follows, when *Borr. burgdorferi* disseminates throughout the body. Late complications, including arthritis, neurologic abnormalities and myocardial conduction defects, occur fairly frequently (Steere 1989).

Prophylaxis

Amoxycillin 500 mg 6-hourly or doxycycline 100 mg 12-hourly for 10 days will prevent Lyme disease (Shapiro et al 1992). However, this is unlikely to be cost-effective, as the risk of infection after a bite in an endemic area is estimated as 1% or less (Magid et al 1992, Volkman et al 1993). In cases of penicillin allergy, erythromycin 250 mg 6-hourly or 30 mg/kg daily in divided doses (Steere 1989) or cefuroxime axetil (Nadelman et al 1992) are recommended. *Borr. burgdorferi* is resistant in vitro to rifampicin, ciprofloxacin and aminoglycosides.

A physician may nonetheless prescribe prophylaxis for patients with a history of tick bite if follow-up of the patient cannot be assured, or to satisfy patients' expectations, as many patients are aware that chronic joint and neurological involvement does not respond consistently to antimicrobials.

TREATMENT

The drugs of choice are doxycycline 100 mg 12-hourly or amoxycillin 500 mg 6-hourly. Those allergic to penicillins may be treated with erythromycin 250–500 mg 6-hourly or cefuroxime axetil 500 mg 12-hourly.

For patients with erythema chronicum migrans, 10 days of oral therapy is sufficient. Patients with disseminated disease should receive 20–30 days of therapy, and those with arthritis should receive 30 days. Amoxycillin can usefully be combined with probenecid 500 mg 8-hourly in patients with chronic arthritis: these patients are more difficult to treat successfully, and repeat courses may be necessary.

Patients with objective neurological abnormalities (neuroborreliosis) should receive 3–4 weeks of intravenous antimicrobials. Most experience is with ceftriaxone 2 g/day, though cefotaxime 2 g 8-hourly and benzylpenicillin 3 g 6-hourly have all been recommended as alternatives (Pfister et al 1991). Ceftriaxone i.v. 2 g/day for 14 days is significantly more effective than penicillin in the treatment of both Lyme arthritis and neurological manifestations of this infection. Characteristics of ceftriaxone, which may contribute to its effectiveness, are its long half-life, greater activity against *Borr. burgdorferi* in vitro and the high microbicidal concentrations achieved in the brain and cerebrospinal fluid (Dattwyler et al 1988). Patients with chronic fatigue do not generally improve with antimicrobial treatment, even when given repeated courses. A standard recommendation is not to treat chronic fatigue with antimicrobials, even if serology for *Borr. burgdorferi* is positive; yet many physicians do so, being aware of the subtlety of abnormalities which neuroborreliosis can produce (Kaplan et al 1992).

Although occasional patients may relapse or become reinfected after treatment for Lyme disease, the main cause of failure to respond to antimicrobials is misdiagnosis, due to false-positive Lyme serology or for other reasons (Steere 1989, Steere et al 1993).

Relapsing fever

Relapsing fever is characterized by recurrent episodes of fever and spirochaetaemia, separated by afebrile intervals during which spirochaetes are rarely found in the blood. Louse-borne relapsing fever, transmitted by the human body louse, is caused by *Borrelia recurrentis*; epidemics and pandemics have affected approximately 50 million people this century, with millions of deaths (Johnson 1985, Teklu et al 1983).

Tick-borne relapsing fever, transmitted by ticks, is caused by many different species of *Borrelia*, and is milder.

TREATMENT

Tetracyclines, erythromycin, penicillin and chloramphenicol have been used successfully. Treatment with any effective antibiotic typically induces the Jarisch–Herxheimer reaction within 2 h of initiating therapy, and coincides with the clearing of spirochaetaemia (Warrell et al 1983). It is not prevented by prior treatment with prednisolone, but may be diminished with meptazinol (Teklu et al 1983).

Louse-borne relapsing fever responds to a single oral dose of tetracycline 500 mg, doxycycline 100 mg or erythromycin 500 mg (Perine et al 1974, Perine & Teklu 1983). Duration of fever is longer in patients treated with penicillin, and there are more frequent failures and relapses (Butler et al 1978, Warrell et al 1983). Patients who cannot be treated with an oral agent may be given a single dose of tetracycline 250 mg intravenously.

Tick-borne relapsing fever has a higher rate of treatment failures or relapses. Treatment should therefore be with 5–10 days of tetracycline 500 mg 6-hourly, doxycycline 100 mg 12-hourly, or erythromycin 500 mg 6-hourly (Horton & Blaser 1985).

Rickettsioses

These are due to *Rickettsia rickettsii, Rickettsia conorii, Rickettsia australis, Rickettsia sibirica, Rickettsia akari, Rickettsia prowazeki, Rickettsia typhi, Rickettsia tsutsugamushi* and *Coxiella burnetii*.

Rickettsiae are small, fastidious, obligate intracellular coccobacilli. With the exception of *Rick. prowazeki* (epidemic typhus), all are zoonoses, and with the exception of *Coxiella burnetii* (Q fever), all are unable to survive outside a mammalian host or vector (Woodward & Hornick 1985).

The spotted fever rickettsiae mainly circulate in hard ticks, rodents and domestic animals in rural and peri-domestic habitats. They produce fever, malaise and, often, a vasculitic rash. The most familiar is *Rick. rickettsii* (Rocky Mountain spotted fever). This occurs only in the Western hemisphere and is the most severe, with a case-fatality rate of 20% if untreated. *Rick. conorii* (African tick-bite fever, fievre boutonneuse or Mediterranean spotted fever) may itself have some subspecies: the strain in Zimbabwe seems particularly mild, as almost all adults in parts of Zimbabwe have antibodies to *Rick. conorii*, despite few clinical cases (Kelly & Mason 1991). In Israel, by contrast, *Rick. conorii* was isolated from the blood of three previously healthy children with fatal infections (Yagupsky & Wolach 1993). *Rick. australis* and *Rick. sibirica* are similar clinically, but occur in Australia and Siberia.

Rick. akari (rickettsialpox) differs: it occurs in cities, has a mouse host and mite vector, and causes a papulovesicular rash.

The typhus group comprises *Rick. prowazeki*, responsible for epidemics among refugees (hosts, human; vectors, lice); *Rick. typhi*, also called *Rick. mooseri*, responsible for sporadic cases in slums and on farms (hosts, rodents; vectors, fleas); and *Rick. tsutsugamushi*, responsible for scrub typhus in Asia (hosts, wild rodents; vectors, mites).

Prophylaxis

In a large placebo-controlled study involving more than 1000 military personnel on the Pescadores Islands, a weekly dose of 200 mg doxycycline, continued throughout the period of residence in the endemic area, reduced the incidence of scrub typhus by approximately 80% (Olson et al 1980).

TREATMENT

For all the rickettsioses, tetracycline 0.5–1 g 6-hourly orally or 0.5 g 6-hourly intravenously, or doxycycline 100 mg 12-hourly are both highly effective. The duration of treatment is 5–7 days, or 2–3 days after the temperature returns to normal.

In a small series of cases of louse-borne relapsing fever and typhus in Ethiopia, a single 100 mg dose of doxycycline by mouth cured all patients, and there were no relapses (Perine et al 1974). In patients with scrub typhus, a single dose of doxycycline 200 mg orally was as effective as a 7-day course of tetracycline, and no relapses occurred among the patients given single-dose doxycycline (Brown et al 1978). In a retrospective series of Thai patients with murine typhus, a single dose of doxycycline 200 mg (52 patients) was as effective as 5–10 day course of chloramphenicol (9 patients) and significantly shortened the duration of fever compared to placebo (Silpapojakul et al 1993).

Children who are moderately or severely ill can be treated with a 2-day course of tetracycline or doxycycline without appreciable risk of deposition of drug in bones and teeth; alternatively, chloramphenicol may be used for children.

Chloramphenicol appears to be highly effective against rickettsioses in a dose of 2–4 g/day orally or intravenously in divided doses for 7 days.

Ruiz & Merrero (1992) compared ciprofloxacin 750 mg versus doxycycline 100 mg, each 12-hourly for 7 days, in 70 Spanish patients with Mediterranean spotted fever (*Rick. conorii*), and found the two drugs to be equally effective.

The fluoroquinolones are highly active against *Rickettsia* in vitro, and limited clinical experience suggests that they are effective in the treatment of all rickettsial syndromes (Eaton et al 1989, Gudiol et al 1989).

Brill–Zinsser disease is a recrudescence of illness in an individual who has had epidemic typhus previously, for example among immigrants from Eastern Europe whose initial infection occurred during World War II. It responds to treatment with tetracycline (Green et al 1990).

Q FEVER

Q fever is a world-wide zoonosis caused by *Coxiella burnetii*, which differs from other rickettsia in its high resistance to desiccation and its ability to survive for long periods in the environment. Human infection is usually acquired by inhalation of small numbers of airborne organisms when in proximity to infected domestic animals, hides, manure, dust, milk and, especially, placentae (Langley et al 1988). In endemic areas, over 10% of individuals may have antibodies to *Coxiella burnetii*, and most recall no characteristic illness.

Acute Q fever is characterized by fever and chills, severe headache and myalgia. The syndrome may be that of atypical pneumonia, and hepatitis is commonly present. Chronic Q fever usually involves the cardiac valves and presents as subacute bacterial endocarditis with negative blood cultures, and a vasculitic rash is present in 20%. It occurs months to as many as 20 years after initial infection with *C. burnetii*.

Treatment

Untreated, acute Q fever lasts from a few days to 2 weeks. Treatment with either tetracycline 500 mg four times daily or doxycycline 100 mg twice daily usually results in defervescence within 48 h (Spelman 1982). Treatment should be continued for 2 weeks. Since acute Q fever is usually a mild self-limiting disease, it is difficult to ascertain with certainty whether or not antimicrobial therapy substantially alters the course of the illness. In one large series, the duration of fever was 2 days in patients receiving tetracycline, 1.7 days in those receiving doxycycline, and 3.3 days in those who received no treatment (Spelman 1982). Q fever pneumonia is usually an undiagnosed 'atypical pneumonia', and thus erythromycin is often the antimicrobial chosen. In a double-blind comparison, doxycycline 100 mg 12-hourly or erythromycin 500 mg 6-hourly, both for 10 days, were administered to 48 patients with acute Q fever pneumonia. Doxycycline produced a more rapid reduction in fever, and fewer side-effects than erythromycin. There were no differences in any other clinical or radiological measures, and by day 40 the chest radiograph was normal in 47 of the patients (Sobradillo et al 1992). In a small series, patients with Q fever pneumonia did not respond to erythromycin at doses as high as 4 g/day, whereas the addition of rifampicin 600 mg/day resulted in cure (Marrie 1995).

Prophylactic administration of tetracycline was found ineffective when given soon after infection of human volunteers (Tigertt & Benenson 1956).

Therapy for Q fever endocarditis is controversial, because combinations of antimicrobials are necessary, and relapses may follow discontinuation of therapy, even after prolonged courses (Levy et al 1991, Fernandez Guerrero 1993). A logical choice is doxycycline plus co-trimoxazole, or doxycycline plus rifampicin, continued for 2 years (Marrie 1995).

Ehrlichiosis

Ehrlichia sennetsu has been known to cause an acute febrile illness in Japan and the Far East since 1953, and in 1986 another human pathogen, *Ehrlichia chaffeensis* (originally misidentified as *Ehrlichia canis*), was found in the USA (Maeda et al 1987). *E. chaffeensis* has an unknown, probably canine, reservoir host, and is transmitted to man by the bite of a tick. About 1 week later there is an abrupt onset of fever, headache and myalgia; rash and oedema may occur (particularly in children), and leukopenia, thrombocytopenia and hepatitis are common (Fishbein et al 1994). The organism may rarely be seen in vacuoles within circulating monocytes, or the diagnosis made by a four-fold rise or fall in antibodies to *E. chaffeensis* or to the antigenically related *E. canis*.

Many cases are asymptomatic, and serological surveys of febrile patients have shown ehrlichiosis to be as common as rickettsial infections in parts of the USA (Walker & Dumler 1995). Fatal cases have been reported.

TREATMENT

In vitro, *E. chaffeensis* is susceptible to doxycycline and rifampicin, but resistant to chloramphenicol, ciprofloxacin, erythromycin, co-trimoxazole, penicillin and gentamicin (Brouqui & Raoult 1992).

Doxycycline 200 mg/day or tetracycline 500 mg 6-hourly for 7 days appear to be highly effective (Everett et al 1994, Walker & Dumler 1995). When a tetracycline was given to outpatients with nonspecific febrile symptoms, only 3 of 49 were subsequently hospitalized, whereas 35 of 38 patients who received antimicrobials other than tetracyclines required hospitalization. Among hospitalized patients, those not receiving tetracyclines or chloramphenicol had a more protracted course, and severe illness was seen more commonly among patients who were over 60 years old, or who did not receive a tetracycline or chloramphenicol within the first week of symptoms (Fishbein et al 1994).

E. chaffeensis has produced a persistent, eventually fatal, infection in an immunocompromised patient, which did not respond to tetracycline plus chloramphenicol (Dumler et al 1993).

Viral zoonoses

No specific treatment is established for: yellow fever; dengue; rabies; Japanese encephalitis; St Louis encephalitis; picornaviruses (swine vesicular, foot-and-mouth); alphaviruses (Western equine encephalitis, Eastern equine encephalitis, Venezuelan equine encephalitis); Rift Valley fever, Californian virus, phleboviruses; tick-borne viruses (tick-borne encephalitis (Central Europe and Far East, Omsk haemorrhagic fever, etc.); arenaviruses (lymphocytic choriomeningitis, Marburg); pox/parapox (monkeypox); Ross River fever; or Chikungunya fever.

Lassa fever

Tribavirin (ribavirin), a guanosine analogue, has broad-spectrum antiviral activity. It is contraindicated in pregnant women.

Prophylaxis

For needle stick or other high-risk contact, oral tribavirin 5 mg/kg 8-hourly for 2–3 weeks would be a logical step (Peters & Johnson 1995), although of unproven efficacy.

TREATMENT

Tribavirin should be given intravenously as a loading dose of 30 mg/kg, followed by 15 mg/kg 6-hourly for 4 days, then 7.5 mg/kg 8-hourly for 6 days. In a study in Sierra Leone, tribavirin reduced mortality from 55% to 5%, if begun within 6 days of the onset of symptoms (McCormick et al 1986).

Tribavirin has proved beneficial in Argentine haemorrhagic fever (Enria & Maiztegui 1994) and, although unproven, may be useful in Bolivian, Venezuelan and Brazilian haemorrhagic fevers, all of which are caused by arenaviruses (Peters & Johnson 1995).

Tribavirin is of established benefit in Hantavirus infections (Huggins et al 1991), and has also been used in Hantavirus pulmonary syndrome.

References

Acocella G, Bertrand A, Beytout J et al 1989 Comparison of three different regimens in the treatment of acute brucellosis: a multicentre multinational study. *Journal of Antimicrobial Agents and Chemotherapy* 23: 433–439

Adal K A, Cockerel C J, Petri W A 1994 Cat scratch disease, bacillary angiomatosis, and other infections due to Rochalimea. *New England Journal of Medicine* 330: 1509–1515

Akova M, Uzun O, Akalin H E, Hayran M, Unal S, Gur D 1993 Quinolones in treatment of human brucellosis: comparative trial of ofloxacin rifampin versus doxycycline rifampin. *Antimicrobial Agents and Chemotherapy* 37: 1831–1834

al Sibai M B, Halim M A, el Shaker M M, Khan B A, Qadri S M 1992 Efficacy of ciprofloxacin for treatment of *Brucella melitensis* infections. *Antimicrobial Agents and Chemotherapy* 36: 150–152

Ariza J, Gudiol F, Pallares R, Rufi G, Fernandez Viladrich P 1985a Comparative trial of co-trimoxazole versus tetracycline streptomycin in treating human brucellosis. *Journal of Infectious Diseases* 152: 1358–1359

Ariza J, Gudiol F, Pallares R, Rufi G, Fernandez Viladrich P 1985b Comparative trial of rifampin doxycycline versus tetracycline streptomycin in the therapy of human brucellosis. *Antimicrobial Agents and Chemotherapy* 28: 548–551

Ariza J, Gudiol F, Pallares R et al 1992 Treatment of human brucellosis with doxycycline plus rifampin or doxycycline plus streptomycin. A randomized, double blind study. *Annals of Internal Medicine* 117: 25–30

Bhatt K M, Mirza N B 1992 Rat bite fever: a case report of a Kenyan. *East African Medical Journal* 69: 542–543

Brouqui P, Raoult D 1992 In vitro antibiotic susceptibility of the newly recognized agent of ehrlichiosis in humans, *Ehrlichia chaffeensis. Antimicrobial Agents and Chemotherapy* 36: 2799–2803

Brown G W, Saunders J P, Singh S, Huxsoll D L, Shirai A 1978 Single dose doxycycline therapy for scrub typhus. *Transactions of the Royal Society of Tropical Medicine and Hygiene* 72: 412–416

Burgdorfer W, Barbour A G, Hayes S F, Benach J L, Grunwaldt E, Davis J P 1982 Lyme disease a tick borne spirochaetosis? *Science* 216: 1317–1319

Butler T 1995 *Yersinia* spp. including plague. In: Mandell G L, Bennett J E, Dolin R (eds) Mandell, Douglas and Bennett's principles and practice of infectious diseases, 4th edn. Churchill Livingstone, New York, p 2070–2078

Butler T, Levin J, Linh N N, Chau D M, Adickman M, Arnold K 1976 *Yersinia pestis* infection in Vietnam. II. Quantitative blood cultures and detection of endotoxin in the cerebrospinal fluid of patients with meningitis. *Journal of Infectious Diseases* 133: 493–499

Butler T, Mahmoud A A F, Warren K S 1977 Algorithms in the diagnosis and management of exotic diseases. XXV. Plague. *Journal of Infectious Diseases* 136: 317–320

Butler T, Jones P K, Wallace C K 1978 *Borrelia recurrentis* infection: single dose antibiotic regimens and management of the Jarisch–Herxheimer reaction. *Journal of Infectious Diseases* 137: 573–577

Cotell S L, Noskin G A 1994 Bacillary angiomatosis. Clinical and histologic features, diagnosis, and treatment. Archives of Internal Medicine 154: 524–528

Crook L D, Tempest B 1992 Plague. A clinical review of 27 cases. *Archives of Internal Medicine* 152: 1253–1256

Cross J T, Jacobs R F 1993 Tularemia: treatment failures with outpatient use of ceftriaxone. Clinical Infectious Diseases 17: 976–980

Cuadra C M 1956 Salmonellosis complication in human bartonellosis. *Texas Reports on Biological Medicine* 14: 97–113

Daly J S, Worthington M G, Brenner D J et al 1993 *Rochalimea elizabethae* spp. nov. isolated from a patient with endocarditis. *Journal of Clinical Microbiology* 31: 872–881

Dattwyler R J, Halperin J J, Volkman D J, Luft B J 1988 Treatment of late Lyme borreliosis randomized comparison of ceftriaxone and penicillin. *Lancet* i: 1191–1194

Dumler J S, Sutker W L, Walker D H 1993 Persistent infection with *Ehrlichia chaffeensis*. *Clinical Infectious Diseases* 17: 903–905

Eaton M, Cohen M T, Shlim D R, Ennis B 1989 Ciprofloxacin treatment of typhus. *Journal of the American Medical Association* 262: 772–773

Enria D A, Maiztegui J I 1994 Antiviral treatment of Argentine hemorrhagic fever. *Antiviral Research* 23: 23–31

Everett E D, Evans K A, Henry R B, McDonald G 1994 Human ehrlichiosis in adults after tick exposure. *Annals of Internal Medicine* 120: 730–735

Farrar W E 1995 *Leptospira* species (leptospirosis). In: Mandell G L, Bennett J E, Dolin R (eds) Mandell, Douglas and Bennett's principles and practice of infectious diseases, 4th edn. Churchill Livingstone, New York, p 2137–2141

Ferguson I R 1993 Leptospirosis surveillance: 1990–1992. *Communicable Diseases Report CDR Review* 3: R47–R48

Fernandez Guerrero M L 1993 Zoonotic endocarditis. *Infectious Diseases Clinics of North America* 7: 135–152

Fischer G W 1995 Cat scratch disease. In: Mandell G L, Bennett J E, Dolin R (eds) Mandell, Douglas and Bennett's principles and practice of infectious diseases, 4th edn. Churchill Livingstone, New York, p 1311–1312

Fishbein D B, Dawson J E, Robinson L E 1994 Human ehrlichiosis in the United States, 1985 to 1990. *Annals of Internal Medicine* 120: 736–743

Gilks C F, Lambert H P, Broughton E S, Baker C C 1988 Failure of penicillin prophylaxis in laboratory acquired leptospirosis. *Postgraduate Medical Journal* 64: 236–238

Goldstein E J C 1995 Bites. In: Mandell G L, Bennett J E, Dolin R (eds) Mandell, Douglas and Bennett's principles and practice of infectious diseases, 4th edn. Churchill Livingstone, New York, p 2765–2767

Green C R, Fishbein D, Gleiberman I 1990 Brill Zinsser: still with us. *Journal of American Medical Association* 264: 1811–1812

Gudiol F, Pallares R, Carratala J et al 1989 Randomized double blind evaluation of ciprofloxacin and doxycycline for Mediterranean spotted fever. *Antimicrobial Agents and Chemotherapy* 33: 987–988

Horton J M, Blaser M J 1985 The spectrum of relapsing fever in the Rocky Mountains. *Archives of Internal Medicine* 145: 871–875

Hall W H 1990 Modern chemotherapy for brucellosis in humans. *Reviews of Infectious Diseases* 12: 1060–1099

Huggins J W, Hsiang C M, Cosgriff T M et al 1991 Prospective, double blind, concurrent, placebo controlled trial of intravenous ribavirin therapy of hemorrhagic fever with renal syndrome. *Journal of Infectious Diseases* 164: 1119–1127

Hutton J P, Everett E D 1985 Response of tularemic meningitis to antimicrobial therapy. *Southern Medical Journal* 78: 189–190

Jacobs F, Abramowicz D, Vereerstraeten P et al 1990 *Brucella* endocarditis: the role of combined medical and surgical treatment. *Reviews of Infectious Diseases* 12: 740–744

Janbon F 1993 Aspects actuels des brucelloses. *Revue de Medecine Interne* 14: 307–312

John T J 1994 India: is it plague? *Lancet* 344: 1359–1360

Johnson W D 1985 *Borrelia* species (relapsing fever). In: Mandell G L, Douglas R G, Bennett R G (eds) Principles and practice of infectious diseases, 2nd edn. Wiley, New York, p 1341–1343

Kaplan R F, Meadows M E, Vincent L C et al 1992 Memory impairment and depression in patients with Lyme encephalopathy: comparison with fibromyalgia and nonpsychotically depressed patients. *Neurology* 42: 1263–1267

Kelly P J, Mason P R 1991 Tick bite fever in Zimbabwe. Survey of antibodies to *Rickettsia conorii* in man and dogs, and of rickettsia like organisms in dog ticks. *South African Medical Journal* 80: 233–236

Khuri Bulos N A, Daoud A H, Azab S M 1993 Treatment of childhood brucellosis: results of a prospective trial on 113 children. *Pediatric Infectious Diseases Journal* 12: 377–381

Knudson G B 1986 Treatment of anthrax in man: history and current concepts. *Military Medicine* 151: 71–77

Koehler J E, Glaser C A, Tappero J W 1994 *Rochalimea henselae* infection: new zoonosis with the domestic cat as reservoir. *Journal of the American Medical Association* 271: 531–535

Lang R, Dagan R, Potasman I, Einhorn M, Raz R 1992 Failure of ceftriaxone in the treatment of acute brucellosis. *Clinical Infectious Diseases* 14: 506–509

Langley J M, Marrie T J, Covert A et al 1988 Poker players pneumonia. An urban outbreak following exposure to a parturient cat. *New England Journal of Medicine* 319: 354–356

Lee H C, Horowitz E, Linder W 1991 Treatment of tularemia with imipenem–cilastatin sodium. *Southern Medical Journal* 84: 1277–1278

Levy P Y, Drancourt M, Etienne J et al 1991 Comparison of different antibiotic regimens for therapy of 32 cases of Q fever endocarditis. *Antimicrobial Agents and Chemotherapy* 35: 533–537

Lew D 1995 *Bacillus anthracis* (anthrax). In: Mandell G L, Bennett J E, Dolin R (eds) Mandell, Douglas and Bennett's principles and practice of infectious diseases, 4th edn. Churchill Livingstone, New York, p 1885–1890

Lucey D, Dolan M J, Moss C W et al 1992 Relapsing illness due to *Rochalimaea henselae* in immunocompetent hosts: implication for therapy and new epidemiological associations. *Clinical Infectious Diseases* 14: 683–688

Maeda K, Markowitz N, Hawley R C et al 1987 Human infection with *Ehrlichia canis*, a leukocytic *Rickettsia*. *New England Journal of Medicine* 316: 853–856

Magid D M, Schwartz B, Craft J, Schwartz J S 1992 Prevention of Lyme disease after tick bites. *New England Journal of Medicine* 327: 534–541

Mann J M 1982 Peripatetic plague. *Journal of American Medical Association* 247: 47–48

Marrie T J 1995 *Coxiella burnetii* (Q fever). In: Mandell G L, Bennett J E, Dolin R (eds) Mandell, Douglas and Bennett's principles and practice of infectious diseases, 4th edn. Churchill Livingstone, New York, p 1727–1735

Marshall J D Jr, Joy R J T, Ai N V, Gibson F L 1967 Plague in Vietnam 1965–1966. *American Journal of Epidemiology* 86: 603–616

Mason W L, Eigelsbach H T, Little S F, Bates J H 1980 Treatment of tularemia, including pulmonary tularemia, with gentamicin. *American Review of Respiratory Disease* 121: 39–45

McClain J B L, Ballou W R, Harrison S M, Steinweg D L 1984 Doxycycline therapy for leptospirosis. *Annals of Internal Medicine* 100: 696–698

McCormack R C, Kaye D, Hook E W 1967 Endocarditis due to *Streptobacillus moniliformis*. A report of two cases and review of the literature. *Journal of American Medical Association* 200: 77–79

McCormick J B, King I J, Webb P A et al 1986 Lassa fever: effective therapy with ribavirin. *New England Journal of Medicine* 314: 20–26

McEvoy M B, Noah N D, Pilsworth R 1987 Outbreak of fever caused by *Strep. moniliformis*. *Lancet* ii: 1361–1363

McLean D R, Russell N, Khan M Y 1992 Neurobrucellosis: clinical and therapeutic features. *Clinical Infectious Diseases* 15: 582–590

Meyer K F 1950 Modern therapy of plague. *Journal of the American Medical Association* 144: 982–985

Montejo J M, Alberola I, Glez Zarate P 1993 Open, randomized therapeutic trial of six antimicrobial regimens in the treatment of human brucellosis. *Clinical Infectious Diseases* 16: 671–676

Nadelman R B, Luger S W, Frank E, Wisniewski M, Collins J J, Wormser G P 1992 Comparison of cefuroxime axetil and doxycycline in the treatment of early Lyme disease. *Annals of Internal Medicine* 117: 273–280

Odendaal M W, Pieterson P M, de Vos V, Botha A D 1991 The antibiotic sensitivity patterns of *Bacillus anthracis* isolated from the Kruger National Park, Onderstepoort. *Journal of Veterinary Research* 58: 17–19

Olson J G, Bourgeois A L, Fang R C Y, Coolbaugh J C, Dennis D T 1980 Prevention of scrub typhus: prophylactic administration of doxycycline in a randomized double blind trial. *American Journal of Tropical Medicine and Hygiene* 29: 989–997

Penn R L 1995 *Francisella tularensis* tularemia. In: Mandell G L, Bennett J E, Dolin R (eds) Mandell, Douglas and Bennett's principles and practice of infectious diseases, 4th edn. Churchill Livingstone, New York, p 2060–2068

Penn R L, Kinasewicz G T 1987 Factors associated with a poor clinical outcome in tularemia. *Archives of Internal Medicine* 147: 265–268

Perine P L, Awoke S, Krause D W, McDade J E 1974 Single dose doxycycline treatment of louse borne relapsing fever and epidemic typhus. *Lancet* ii: 742–744

Perine P L, Teklu B 1983 Antibiotic treatment of louse borne relapsing fever in Ethiopia: a report of 377 cases. *American Journal of Tropical Medicine and Hygiene* 32: 1096–1100

Peters C L, Johnson K M 1995 Lymphocytic choriomeningitis, Lassa virus, and other arenaviruses. In: Mandell G L, Bennett J E, Dolin R (eds) Mandell, Douglas and Bennett's principles and practice of infectious diseases, 4th edn. Churchill Livingstone, New York, p 1572–1578

Pfister H W, Preac Mursic V, Wilske B, Schielke E, Sorgel F, Einhaupl K M 1991 Randomized comparison of ceftriaxone and cefotaxime in Lyme neuroborreliosis. Journal of Infectious Diseases 163: 311–318

Pratt D S, Tenney J H, Bjork C M, Reller L B 1978 Successful treatment of Brucella melitensis endocarditis. American Journal of Medicine 64: 897–900

Roberts N J 1995 Bartonella bacilliformis (bartonellosis). In: Mandell G L, Bennett J E, Dolin R (eds) Mandell, Douglas and Bennett's principles and practice of infectious diseases, 4th edn. Churchill Livingstone, New York, p 2209–2210

Ruiz B R, Herrero J I 1992 Evaluation of ciprofloxacin and doxycycline in the treatment of Mediterranean spotted fever. European Journal of Clinical Microbiology and Infectious Diseases 11: 427–431

Rygg M, Bruun C F 1992 Rat bite fever (Streptobacillus moniliformis) with septicemia in a child. Scandinavian Journal of Infectious Diseases 24: 535–540

Schultz M G 1968 A history of bartonellosis (Carrion's disease). American Journal of Tropical Medicine and Hygiene 17: 503–515

Shapiro E D, Gerber M A, Holabird N B, Berg A T, Feder H M, Bell G L, Rys P L, Persing D H 1992 A controlled trial of antimicrobial prophylaxis for Lyme disease after deer tick bites. New England Journal of Medicine 327: 1769–1773

Silpapojakul K, Chayakul P, Krisanapan S, Silpapojakul K 1993 Murine typhus in Thailand: clinical features, diagnosis and treatment. Quarterly Journal of Medicine 86: 43–47

Singh R S, Sridhar M S, Sekhar P C, Bhaskar C J 1992 Cutaneous anthrax: a report of ten cases. Journal of the Association of Physicians of India 40: 46–49

Slater L N, Welch D F 1995 Rochalimea species (recently renamed Bartonella). In: Mandell G L, Bennett J E, Dolin R (eds) Mandell, Douglas and Bennett's principles and practice of Infectious Diseases, 4th edn. Churchill Livingstone, New York, p 1741–1747

Sobradillo V, Zalacain R, Capelastegui A, Uresandi F, Corral J 1992 Antibiotic treatment in pneumonia due to Q fever. Thorax 47: 276–278

Solera J, Martinez Alfaro E, Saez L 1994 Metaanalisis sobre la eficacia de la combinacion de rifampicina y doxiciclina en el tratamiento de la brucelosis humana. Medicina Clinica Barcelona 102: 731–738

Spelman D W 1982 Q fever: a study of 111 consecutive cases. Medical Journal of Australia 1: 547–553

Steere A C 1989 Lyme disease. New England Journal of Medicine 321: 586–596

Steere A C, Malawista S E, Snydman D R et al 1977 Lyme arthritis: an epidemic of oligoarticular arthritis in children and adults in three Connecticut communities. Arthritis and Rheumatology 20: 7–17

Steere A C, Taylor E, McHugh G L et al 1993 The overdiagnosis of Lyme disease. Journal of the American Medical Association 269: 1812–1816

Sturchler D 1988 Endemic areas of tropical infections, 2nd edn. Hans Huber, Stuttgart

Syrjala H, Schildt R, Raisainen S 1991 In vitro susceptibility of Francisella tularensis to fluoroquinolones and treatment of tularemia with norfloxacin and ciprofloxacin. European Journal of Clinical Microbiology of Infectious Diseases 10: 68–70

Takafuji E T, Kirkpatrick J W, Miller R N et al 1984 An efficacy trial of doxycycline chemoprophylaxis against leptospirosis. New England Journal of Medicine 310: 497–500

Teklu B, Habte Michael A, Warrell D A, White N J, Wright D J M 1983 Meptazinol diminishes the Jarisch–Herxheimer reaction of relapsing fever. Lancet i: 835–839

Tigertt W D, Benenson A S, Shope R E 1956 Studies on Q fever in man. Transactions of the Association of American Physicians 69: 98–104

Urteaga O, Payne E H 1955 Treatment of the acute febrile phase of Carrion's disease with chloramphenicol. American Journal of Tropical Medicine and Hygiene 4: 507–511

Vaughan C, Cronin C C, Walsh E K, Whelton M 1994 The Jarisch–Herxheimer reaction in leptospirosis. Postgraduate Medical Journal 70: 118–121

Volkman D J, Kaell A T, Bosler E M, Benach J L 1993 Prevention of Lyme disease after tick bites. New England Journal of Medicine 328: 138–139

Walker D H, Dumler J S 1995 Ehrlichia chaffeensis (human ehrlichiosis) and other ehrlichiae In: Mandell G L, Bennett J E, Dolin R (eds) Mandell, Douglas and Bennett's principles and practice of infectious diseases, 4th edn. Churchill Livingstone, New York, p 1747–1752

Warrell D A, Perine P L, Krause D W, Bing D H, McDougal S J 1983 Pathophysiology and immunology of the Jarisch–Herxheimer like reaction in louse borne relapsing fever: comparison of tetracycline and slow release penicillin. Journal of Infectious Diseases 147: 898–909

Washburn R G 1995 Spirilium minus (rat bite fever) and Strep. moniliformis (rat bite fever). In: Mandell G L, Bennett J E,

Dolin R (eds) Mandell, Douglas and Bennett's principles and practice of infectious diseases, 4th edn. Churchill Livingstone, New York, p 2084–2086, 2155–2156

Watt G, Padre L P, Tuazon M L et al 1988 Placebo controlled trial of intravenous penicillin for severe and late leptospirosis. *Lancet* i: 433–435

Weber D J, Hansen A R 1991 Infections resulting from animal bites. *Infectious Diseases Clinics of North America* 5: 663–680

WHO 1986 Joint FAO/WHO Expert Committee on Brucellosis. WHO, Geneva

Woodward W E, Hornick R B 1985 *Rickettsia rickettsii* (Rocky Mountain spotted fever). In: Mandell G L, Douglas R G, Bennett J G (eds) Principles and practice of infectious diseases, 2nd edn. Wiley, New York, p 1082–1087

Yagupsky P, Wolach B 1993 Fatal Israeli spotted fever in children. *Clinical Infectious Diseases* 17: 850–853

Young E J 1995 *Brucella* species. In: Mandell G L, Bennett J E, Dolin R (eds) Mandell, Douglas and Bennett's principles and practice of infectious diseases, 4th edn. Churchill Livingstone, New York, p 2053–2060

62

Malaria

N. J. White

Introduction

Malaria is the most important parasitic disease of man. It is estimated to affect approximately 200 million people with an annual death toll from *Plasmodium falciparum* infections of between 1 and 2.5 million. Pregnant women, infants and those over 60 years old are at greatest risk. Most of the deaths are in African children, and most occur away from facilities where optimum antimalarial treatment can be given. Much antimalarial treatment is still administered for the empirical treatment of febrile illnesses in the tropics. The amounts used are enormous. Chloroquine is probably the second most widely used drug in the world. As malaria is one of the most common causes of fever in tropical countries it must be excluded in any febrile patient living in, or returning from the tropics. Ideally, antimalarial drugs should be given only for the treatment of microscopically confirmed malaria infections or for the prevention of malaria in pregnant women or travellers. In recent years the rapid development of resistance to most of the available antimalarial drugs by the potentially lethal parasite *Plasmodium falciparum* has compromised considerably recommendations for both prevention and treatment (White 1992). As with antibacterials, treatment recommendations must be under constant review, and will inevitably change as resistance progresses.

ANTIMALARIAL DRUG RESISTANCE

Although suspected for three centuries, the first documented cases of quinine resistance occurred 85 years ago. Fortunately, this has progressed slowly and quinine still remains a useful drug today. It is the mainstay of treatment for drug resistant *P. falciparum* infections. Shortly after the introduction of the dihydrofolate reductase inhibitors,

pyrimethamine and proguanil, in the late 1940s and early 1950s, resistance was noted in both *P. falciparum* and *Plasmodium vivax* (Covell et al 1955). These drugs remained useful in prophylaxis, but for treatment use of proguanil was discontinued, and pyrimethamine was prescribed in a fixed combination with long-acting sulphonamides – most commonly sulphadoxine. Meanwhile, chloroquine took over as the treatment of choice for all malaria. Chloroquine-resistance in *P. falciparum* was first recorded in the late 1950s, and by the early 1970s had become a significant problem in South America and South-East Asia. During the 1980s, chloroquine resistance spread remorselessly across southern Asia and the entire length and breadth of the African continent, such that few countries are now unaffected. Chloroquine resistance in *P. vivax* has been confirmed recently on the island of New Guinea (Baird et al 1991). Resistance to the combination of pyrimethamine and long-acting sulphonamides developed rapidly after their introduction for routine treatment in South-East Asia and South America, but they still remain highly efficacious in most parts of Africa. Mefloquine is effective against multi-drug-resistant strains of *P. falciparum*, but resistance has been an increasing problem in certain countries in South-East Asia over the past 5 years, and now there are some areas on the eastern and western borders of Thailand where mefloquine alone is no longer effective (Fontanet et al 1994, Nosten et al 1994). Although halofantrine is intrinsically more active than mefloquine, susceptibility to the two drugs is linked. Thus in highly mefloquine-resistant areas, resistance to halofantrine occurs too. Fortunately, resistance to quinine has remained low grade in South America and South-East Asia (although susceptibility is declining slowly) and has not been a problem in Africa. But compliance is poor with the 5–7 day courses of quinine necessary for cure, and in resistant areas failure rates up to 50% have been reported. Quinine is usually combined with either tetracycline or in some areas sulphadoxine-pyrimethamine or clindamycin to prevent recrudescences of falciparum malaria. Even in highly resistant areas the quinine–tetracycline combination, given for 7 days, retains cure rates over 85% (Watt et al 1992). The most important new additions to our limited antimalarial armamentarium are the antimalarial peroxides derived from qinghao or *Artemisia annua* (sweet wormood). These compounds were discovered in China and are the most rapidly effective and potent of all antimalarial drugs (Hien & White 1993). They have been used extensively in South-East Asia since 1992, as they retain excellent efficacy against multidrug-resistant parasites, and they are rapidly effective in severe malaria. To date, there have been no well-documented cases of resistance to artemisinin or its derivatives.

TYPES OF RESISTANCE

Low-grade resistance (R1 resistance) is usually manifest by recrudescences which tend to occur several weeks after primary treatment. Most recrudescences occur within 6 weeks of initial treatment. For quinine the median time to recrudescence is approximately 3 weeks, but for drugs which have long terminal half-lives, such as mefloquine, the recrudescences can occur up to 10 weeks, and possibly longer, after the primary treatment. Although the treatment is unable to eradicate the parasites in such cases, the multiplication rate is suppressed whilst therapeutic blood concentrations are still present in the blood. The more susceptible the parasites, the lower are the blood concentrations required to suppress parasite multiplication. As resistance worsens, the median time to recrudescence becomes shorter and an increasing portion of patients are seen in whom parasitaemia fails to clear by 7 days following treatment (R2 resistance). Eventually the situation deteriorates such that some patients fail to respond at all to antimalarial treatment (R3 resistance). Obviously, alternative treatment should be employed before this stage. In the individual patient long parasite clearance times (>4 days) are a common predictor of subsequent recrudescence.

Uncomplicated malaria

MANAGEMENT

Infections with *P. vivax*, *Plasmodium malariae*, or *P. ovale* are very rarely fatal, but *P. falciparum* malaria may progress rapidly to severe disease and death, particularly in the non-immune, or young children in endemic areas. If the clinician is in any doubt about the severity of the infection, the patient should remain in hospital under observation. Otherwise,

uncomplicated malaria can be treated on an outpatient basis. If there is any uncertainty over speciation of the parasites they should be considered as *P. falciparum*, and if there is any doubt over chloroquine sensitivity the infection should be considered as chloroquine resistant. A thorough history and examination should pay particular attention to likely origin of the infection, and any previous antimalarial treatment. Except in areas without facilities for microscopic examination of blood slides, antimalarial treatment should be given only for slide-confirmed malaria. In general, administration of the first dose should be observed, particularly for single-dose treatments such as mefloquine or sulfadoxine–pyrimethamine. Symptomatic measures are important. The incidence of vomiting, particularly in children, is proportional to fever. Young children with high fevers should be cooled, given paracetamol (15 mg/kg), and allowed to settle before receiving the first oral dose of antimalarial treatment. The patient should be observed for 1 h after drug administration, and if vomiting occurs within this period the drugs should be readministered (see below). Ideally, patients should be seen daily for a clinical examination and a blood smear until they are asymptomatic and parasite negative. They should be advised to return to the same hospital or clinic if fever recurs within 6 weeks.

SPECIFIC ANTIMALARIAL TREATMENT

P. vivax, *P. ovalae* and *P. malariae*

P. vivax is the most common cause of malaria in the Indian subcontinent, Central America, North Africa, and the Middle East. There is unequivocal evidence of chloroquine resistance in *P. vivax* from the island of New Guinea (Baird et al 1991), but elsewhere infections with this parasite, and the other two that cause the benign human malarias, remain uniformly sensitive to choloquine. Treatment is rapidly effective and usually well tolerated. The main adverse effect is troublesome pruritus in dark-skinned patients, which occurs in approximately 50% of cases. The quinoline antimalarials may all exacerbate the orthostatic hypotension that commonly complicates malaria, and symptomatic postural hypotension is common (Supararanond et al 1993). Rarely (less than 1 : 1000) chloroquine treatment is associated with transient neuropsychiatric abnormalities.

The total dose of chloroquine is 25 mg base/kg divided classically as 10, 10 and 5 mg/kg given on days 0, 1 and 2, respectively (adult dose 600 mg base followed by three doses of 300 mg). Recent studies confirm that this schedule may be compressed into a 36 h treatment regimen, giving 10, 5, 5 and 5 mg/kg at 12-hour intervals (Pussard et al 1991) (Table 62.1). Both *P. vivax* and *P. ovale* infections often have persistent dormant hepatic forms of the parasite (hypnozoites), which are resistant to chloroquine. These

Table 62.1 *Antimalarial drugs: recommended doses for treatment*

	Uncomplicated malaria: dose	Usual adult Dose	Severe malaria*
Chloroquine	10 mg base/kg followed by 10 mg/kg at 24 h and 5 mg/kg at 48 h or 5 mg/kg at 12, 24 and 36 h. Total dose 25 mg base/kg For *P. vivax* or *P. ovale* add primaquine 0.25 mg base/kg daily for 14 days[†] for radical cure.	4 × 150-mg tablets followed by 4 then 2 or 2, 2, 2	10 mg base/kg by constant-rate infusion over 8 h followed by 15 mg/kg over 24 h or 3.5 mg base/kg by intramuscular or subcutaneous injection every 6 h. Total dose 25 mg base/kg
Sulphadoxine–pyrimethamine	20/1 mg/kg single oral dose	3 tablets	Efficacy of the parenteral formulation in severe malaria unproven
Mefloquine	For semi-immunes: 15 mg base/kg single dose. In mefloquine resistant areas or for non-immunes: second 10 mg/kg dose 8–24 h later	3 × 250 mg tablets ± 2 × 250 mg	
Halofantrine	8 mg base/kg 3 times in one day[‡]	2 × 250 mg three times	
Quinine	10 mg salt/kg 8-hourly for 7 days. Often combined with tetracycline[§] (4 mg/kg) four times daily for 7 days	2 × 300 mg three times daily 1 × 250 mg four times daily	20 mg salt/kg by intravenous infusion over 4 h[//] followed by 10 mg/kg infused over 2–8 h every 8 h
Quinidine	Recommended *only* if alternatives unavailable. Dose as for quinine		10 mg base/kg infused at constant rate over 1 h followed by 0.02 mg/kg per minute, with electrocardiographic monitoring
Artesunate	In combination with 25 mg/kg mefloquine, 10–12 mg/kg is given in divided doses over 3–5 days. If used alone, the same dose is divided over 7 days	4 × 50 mg daily for 3 days 4 × 50 mg followed by 2 × 50 mg for 2 days then 50 mg/day × 4	2.4 mg/kg i.v. or i.m. immediately followed by 1.2 mg/kg at (12), 24 h and then daily
Artemether	Same oral dose regimen as artesunate	5 × 40 mg daily for 3 days	3.2 mg/kg i.m. immediately followed by 1.6 mg/kg daily

* Oral treatment should be substituted as soon as the patient can take tablets by mouth.
[†] In Oceania and South-East Asia the dose should be 0.33 mg base/kg.
[‡] In 'non-immunes' it is recommended that a repeat 3-dose treatment be given on day 7.
[§] Tetracycline should not be given to pregnant women or children <8 years old. Doxycycline 3 mg/kg/day is an alternative to tetracycline.
[//] Alternatively for the initial loading dose, 7 mg salt/kg can be infused over 30 min followed by 10 mg salt/kg over 4 h.

become activated between 3 weeks and 1 year after the primary infection, and cause the relapses so characteristic of these infections. (Note: A *relapse* is a recurrent infection caused by the development of persistent hypnozoites. The primary blood stage infection has cleared. A *recrudescence* is a blood stage infection which is not eradicated, but may decline below the level of microscopic detection, and then increases later causing patient parasitaemia and usually symptoms.) The hypnozoites are sensitive only to the 8-aminoquinoline compounds (WHO 1986). Primaquine, the only currently available compound of this class, is usually given in an adult daily dose of 15 mg base (0.25 mg/kg) for 14 days. The eradication of both the blood stage and the persistent liver stages of malaria is called a 'radical cure'. Strains of *P. vivax* from Oceania and some parts of South-

East Asia appear to be more resistant to the hypnozoitocidal effects of primaquine, and a daily dose of 22.5 mg base (0.375 mg/kg) should be given for 14 days for infections originating in these areas. Primaquine is an oxidant drug and causes haemolysis in patients with hereditary defects in the pentose–phosphate shunt, most commonly glucose-6-phosphate dehydrogenase (G6PD) deficiency. In patients with severe variants of G6PD deficiency primaquine is contraindicated, but for patients with mild variants primaquine should be given in a weekly dose of 45 mg base (0.75 mg/kg) for 6 weeks. Although chloroquine is considered safe, primaquine should not be used in pregnancy or given to newborns. Pyrimethamine and the pyrimethamine–sulphonamide combinations are relatively ineffective against *P. vivax*. All the other antimalarial drugs are active, and so for mixed infections requiring treatment for *P. falciparum* it is not necessary to add chloroquine. However, primaquine should be given as well to prevent relapses.

Uncomplicated chloroquine-sensitive *P. falciparum* malaria

In those areas such as central America or North Africa where *P. falciparum* remains sensitive, chloroquine should be used in a total treatment dose of 25 mg base/kg (adult dose 1500 mg). There is no significant difference between the phosphate, sulphate or hydrochloride salts. If there is any doubt about antimalarial sensitivity in the area where malaria was acquired, *P. falciparum* infections should be considered resistant.

Uncomplicated chloroquine-resistant, sulphadoxine–pyrimethamine-sensitive *P. falciparum* malaria

Amodiaquine is more effective than chloroquine against resistant strains of *P. falciparum*. In some countries amodiaquine in a total dose of 25–35 mg base/kg (adult dose 1.5–2.5 g), divided over 3 days, is given where there is low-level chloroquine resistance.

A single dose of sulphadoxine–pyrimethamine (20/1 mg/kg; corresponding to three tablets in an adult) is a well-tolerated and effective treatment for sensitive strains. This is now a first-line treatment for *P. falciparum* malaria in some countries in East Africa. The principal adverse effects result from sulphonamide allergy. When used in prophylaxis the incidence of serious adverse effects is approximately 1 : 7000, and fatal adverse effects occur in 1 : 18000 (Miller et al 1986). In single-dose treatment the incidence of serious adverse effects appears to be significantly lower. Pyrimethamine-induced blood dyscrasias, seen usually in patients with underlying folate deficiency, are most unusual. As an alternative, combinations of chlorproguanil and dapsone are currently under evaluation.

Chloroquine and sulphadoxine–pyrimethamine-resistant *P. falciparum* malaria

The choice now lies between three drugs: mefloquine, halofantrine and quinine. Quinine sulphate, the time-honoured remedy, at a dose of 10 mg salt/kg (adult dose 600 mg) three times daily is effective in a 7-day course. Shorter courses (3–5 days) may be used in combination with a 7-day course of tetracycline or doxycycline (Table 62.1) or, in areas where full sensitivity to all drugs is retained, a single dose of sulphadoxine–pyrimethamine (adult dose three tablets) may be added. Quinine is not well tolerated. The characteristic syndrome of 'cinchonism', comprising nausea, vomiting, dizziness, dysphoria and high-tone deafness is a predictable accompaniment of quinine

treatment. In addition, the drug is extremely bitter and many children find it unacceptable. However, serious adverse effects, principally blindness, deafness or cardiac dysrhythmia, are unusual. Hypoglycaemia is more common in severe malaria, although it may also develop in uncomplicated malaria treated by quinine, particularly in young children or pregnant women. Hypoglycaemia results from stimulation of the pancreatic β-cells and consequent hyperinsulinaemia.

Mefloquine (hydrochloride) has the advantage of a long terminal elimination half-life of 2–3 weeks and it may therefore be given in a single dose (Karbwang & White 1990). In semi-immune patients, 15 mg base/kg (adult dose three tablets of 250 mg) is effective, but in resistant areas and in non-immune patients (i.e. travellers) 25 mg base/kg (five tablets) should be given. Peak whole blood concentrations above 1000 ng/ml are effective. Recent studies suggest that absorption is augmented, but adverse effects are not increased, if the treatment dose is split, i.e. a 25 mg base/kg dose is given as 15 mg/kg initially, followed by 10 mg/kg at 8–24 h later. As with many antimalarial drugs, children tolerate mefloquine better than adults (ter Kuile et al 1993). The principal adverse effect is immediate vomiting, and this is of serious concern for a single-dose treatment. Therefore patients must be observed for 1 h after the drug has been given. If vomiting occurs within 30 min the full dose of mefloquine should be repeated. For vomiting 30–60 min later, half the dose should be given. Vomiting after 1 h does not require retreatment. Later adverse effects are all more common in adults and comprise nausea, dysphoria, dizziness or 'muzziness', poor concentration, sleeplessness, nightmares and postural hypotension. Adverse effects following mefloquine treatment are reported more frequently in women than in men. Serious, but reversible neuropsychiatric reactions occur in approximately 1 : 1300 Asians patients receiving high-dose mefloquine treatment. A higher incidence has been reported in European and African patients.

Halofantrine is intrinsically more active than mefloquine, and is better tolerated (ter Kuile et al 1993). It suffers the disadvantages of requiring multiple dose administration as it has erratic oral bioavailability. The current recommendation is to give 24 mg base/kg divided into three doses 8 h apart (adult dose 500 mg × 3), and to repeat this one week later in non-immune subjects. In mefloquine resistant areas, the single-day regimen has a failure rate of approximately 40%. Use of halofantrine has been associated with sudden death. Halofantrine, like quinidine, induces a predictable prolongation of the electrocardiograph QT interval (delayed ventricular repolarization) (Nosten et al 1993). This can be proarrhythmic. Atrioventricular conduction abnormalities first- and, rarely, second-degree block) have also been seen. These cardiac effects are augmented by previous treatment with mefloquine.

Halofantrine should not be given to patients who have received mefloquine in the previous month, or to patients with either known prolongation of the QT interval, or who are receiving other drugs known to prolong the QT interval. Ideally, an electrocardiogram should be performed before starting treatment to exclude a baseline long QTc interval. Halofantrine absorption is augmented considerably by co-administration with fats or fatty food. The other adverse effect reported with high-dose treatment is diarrhoea. Halofantrine does not have significant adverse central nervous system effects.

Multidrug-resistant *P. falciparum* malaria

In some parts of Thailand, Burma and Cambodia, *P. falciparum* malaria is resistant to all the drugs mentioned previously. Everywhere else in the world resistance is much less. Fortunately, the combination of artesunate in a total treatment dose of 10–12 mg/kg given over 3–5 days (adult dose 600 mg) in addition to 25 mg base/kg of mefloquine (adult dose 1500 mg) remains over 90% effective (Looareesuwan et al 1992, Nosten et al 1994) against multi-drug-resistant *P. falciparum* malaria. Artesunate is very well tolerated, with no evident adverse effects, and can be given once daily. The therapeutic response is more rapid than following other antimalarials, with faster fever and parasite clearance times, and an earlier return to school or work. Artesunate, or artemether in the same doses, may be used alone, but with treatment regimens of less than 7 days there is a significant recrudescence rate (>10%). As the artemisinin derivatives are effective in severe *P. falciparum* malaria, and as they are the last reserves for multidrug-resistant malaria, their use in uncomplicated disease should be limited only to those areas where they are essential. Unregulated use will inevitably lead to earlier development of resistance. These drugs are currently not available in Europe, the USA or Australasia. Travellers returning to these countries with multidrug-resistant *P. falciparum* malaria should be treated with quinine plus tetracycline or doxycycline.

Severe *P. falciparum* malaria

MANAGEMENT

Severe malaria is a multisystem disease requiring intensive-care management. Unfortunately, optimum treatment is usually not available in most of the areas of the world where severe malaria occurs. Severe malaria is defined as the presence of one or more of the following: unrousable coma (cerebral malaria), severe anaemia (haematocrit <15% plus parasitaemia >10 000/µl), renal failure (serum creatinine >265 µmol/l), pulmonary oedema, hypoglycaemia (glucose <2.2 mmol/l), shock, bleeding, repeated seizures, metabolic acidosis or haemoglobinuria. The clinician should not feel restricted by this definition (WHO 1990). Patients with hyperparasitaemia (>5%), any degree of impaired consciousness, acidotic breathing or prostration should also receive carefully supervised treatment. Any patient in whom there is doubt as to the severity of the infection should be managed as described below.

A rapid clinical appraisal should be made. This includes assessment of the level of consciousness or central nervous system dysfunction, measurement of vital signs (particularly respiratory rate), questioning of the patient or relatives concerning earlier antimalarial treatment, duration of impaired consciousness, convulsions and urine output. A malaria parasite count (thick and thin blood films), blood glucose, blood lactate and haematocrit should be measured immediately. The patient should be rehydrated with saline and, if there is any doubt about the jugular venous pressure, a central venous line should be inserted and central pressure monitored. If hypogylcaemia is suspected or confirmed, 0.3 g/kg (25 g) of glucose should be given by slow intravenous injection. A prophylactic intramuscular injection of phenobarbitone (7–20 mg/kg) should be given to unconscious patients, and prompt anticonvulsant therapy (intravenous lorazepam, midazolam or diazepam) given if there are convulsions. A lumbar puncture should be performed to exclude coincident meningitis. Dialysis should be started early in patients with acute renal failure, and blood (preferably fresh) should be transfused if the haematocrit falls below 20%. Antimalarial drugs should be given on a milligram per kilogram basis. The patient should be weighed and the parenteral quinoline antimalarials given by slow intravenous infusions. If, by 48 h after starting treatment, parasitaemia has not fallen by more than 75% (R3 resistance), then the treatment should be changed. Rises in parasitaemia in the first 6–12 h after antimalarial treatment has started should *not* be attributed to drug resistance. Conversely, a rapid decline in parasitaemia shortly after drug administration does not indicate a very sensitive infection. These changes result from natural fluctuations in parasitaemia related to synchronous schizogony and sequestration. Therapeutic responses are assessed in terms of clinical measures: times to recovery of consciousness, and in adults the times to reach Glasgow coma scores of 8, 11 and 15, and the time until fever falls below 37.5°C and remains below this for 24 h; and laboratory measures; which include the rate of fall in plasma lactate and the times to reduce parasitaemia by 50%, 90% and 100%. If the parasitaemia has not cleared by 7 days, treatment should be continued. Adult patients receiving quinine, artesunate or artemether should receive a 7-day course of doxycycline, which starts when the patient can take oral medicine.

SPECIFIC ANTIMALARIAL THERAPY

Chloroquine

In those few fully chloroquine-sensitive areas, intravenous chloroquine is still the treatment of choice. However, if there is any doubt then quinine, quinidine or, if available, one of the artemisinin derivatives should be given, as described below. Chloroquine has unusual pharmacokinetic properties characterized by an enormous total apparent volume of distribution and a very slow terminal elimination phase (half-life 1–2 months). As a consequence, blood concentrations in the treatment of acute malaria are determined by distribution rather than elimination processes. Provided chloroquine enters the circulation slowly, immediate toxicity (principally hypotension or cardiac dysfunction) will not occur. Intravenous chloroquine in 'normal' saline or 5% dextrose should be given by carefully rate controlled infusion in a dose of 10 mg base/kg over 8 h, followed by 15 mg base/kg infused over 24 h. Intramuscular and subcutaneous chloroquine are absorbed rapidly, even in the most severely ill patients. Doses higher than 3.5 mg/kg risk producing transiently toxic blood concentrations. Intramuscular or subcutaneous chloroquine should be given in a dose of 3.5 mg base/kg 6-hourly, or 2.5 mg base/kg 4-hourly, until the patient recovers sufficiently to complete the total dose (25 mg/kg) of treatment by mouth (World Health Organization 1990). The principal adverse effect of parenteral chloroquine is hypotension, but the risks may be reduced considerably by careful attention to dose and rate of administration. Although a parenteral (intramuscular) formulation of sulfadoxine-pyrimethamine is available (Winstanley et al 1992), it has not been assessed sufficiently in the treatment of severe malaria and should not be used. There are no generally available parenteral formulations of halofantrine or mefloquine.

SEVERE CHLOROQUINE-RESISTANT MALARIA

Quinine

Parenteral quinine should be given by slow rate-controlled intravenous infusion. Where this is not possible, intramuscular administration is an effective alternative. In order to achieve therapeutic concentrations as early as possible in the course of treatment, which may be life-saving, an initial loading dose is recommended. A variety of approaches have been described. The simplest is to give a loading dose of 20 mg quinine dihydrochloride salt/kg by constant rate infusion over 4 h, dissolved in 5% or 10% dextrose, or normal (0.9%) saline (White et al 1983). Alternatively, 7 mg salt/kg may be infused over 30 min, followed immediately by 10 mg/kg over 4 h (Davis et al 1990). It has been suggested that in East Africa, where *P. falciparum*

is considerably more susceptible to quinine than in South-East Asia or South America, a loading dose of 15 mg/kg would suffice (Winstanley et al 1994), but this is unproven and could lead to undertreatment in some patients. After the initial loading dose, maintenance doses of 10 mg salt/kg should be given every 8 h. For the treatment of children in sensitive areas 12-hourly administration suffices. Maintenance dose intravenous infusions can be given over 2–12 h. Quinine should never be given by intravenous injection. Intramuscular bioavailability is good even in severe malaria, although there is still uncertainty as to the optimum dilution. If undiluted quinine dihydrochloride (300 mg/ml) is given, then this is acidic (pH 2) and painful, and may occasionally result in sterile abscesses or tetanus. More dilute solutions are less painful, but risk more rapid absorption and the possibility of occasional transiently toxic concentrations. The therapeutic range for quinine has not been defined previously, but total plasma concentrations between 8 and 15 mg/l are safe and effective (White 1992b). There is an increased potential risk of toxicity with free (unbound) quinine levels over 2 mg/l (corresponding to total plasma concentrations of approximately 20 mg/l). To prevent accumulation to toxic levels the dose of quinine should be reduced by one third on the third day of treatment if there is no clinical improvement or the patient is in acute renal failure.

The principal adverse effect of quinine in the treatment of severe malaria is hypoglycaemia (White et al 1983b). This is a particular problem in children and pregnant women (occurring in 50% of the latter group) and tends to occur after 24 h of treatment in those patients who remain severely ill. Management is difficult as hypoglycaemia is often recurrent. A maintenance infusion of 10% glucose should be given after correction with a bolus of 0.3 g/kg (25 g) of glucose given by slow intravenous injection. Cinchonism is common in recovering patients, but does not limit dosage. Adverse cardiovascular or central nervous system effects (particularly retinal blindness or deafness) are very unusual and, in general, parenteral quinine is well tolerated in the treatment of severe malaria. Electrocardiographic monitoring is not necessary except in patients with previous heart disease. In the tropics there have been concerns over the use of a loading dose in areas where patients are commonly pretreated before admission to hospital and therefore may already have therapeutic blood concentrations of quinine on admission. Our practice is to give a loading dose of quinine unless the patient has definitely received 25 mg/kg of quinine or more in the preceding 48 h. We have not seen any serious complications using these guidelines.

Quinidine

In some countries, notably the USA, parenteral quinine is not available. In this case quinidine (the dextrorotatory diastereomer) may be used as an alternative. This is usually available as the gluconate salt. Quinidine is intrinsically more active than quinine as an antimalarial, but it also has an approximately four-fold greater effect on the heart, and electrocardiographic monitoring is necessary. The dose is 10 mg base/kg given by constant rate intravenous infusion over 1 h as a loading dose, followed by 0.02 mg/kg per minute (1.2 mg/kg per hour) thereafter until the patient can be safely switched to oral treatment (Miller et al 1989). If the QT interval is prolonged by more than 25% of the baseline value, or exceeds an absolute value of 0.6 s, the infusion should be stopped. Quinidine has the same propensity as quinine to induce hypoglycaemia. As with quinine, the therapeutic range has not been determined precisely, but total plasma concentrations of 5–8 mg/l are effective, and usually tolerated. This corresponds to free concentrations of approximately 1–1.6 mg/l. Plasma concentration monitoring is advisable. If it is not available then the dose of quinidine should be reduced by one third on the third day of treatment if there is no clinical improvement, or the patient is in renal failure.

Artemisinin, artemether and artesunate

Artemisinin and its derivatives have proved remarkably effective alternatives to quinine for the treatment of severe chloroquine-resistant *P. falciparum* malaria. In both uncomplicated and severe infections they have given consistently faster parasite and fever clearance times, and have proved rapidly effective in cerebral malaria (Hien & White 1993). Most experience to date concerns the use of artesunate (by intravenous or intramuscular injection), artemether (intramuscular injection) or artemisinin (suppository formulation). As reproducible methods for the assay of these compounds, or the biologically active metabolite dihydroartemisinin, in body fluids are not generally available, there is a paucity of reliable pharmacokinetic information. Indeed, there are no reliable data on the clinical pharmacokinetics of either artesunate or artemether in severe malaria. Dosage regimens are therefore empirical. These drugs are not available in Europe, the USA, the Indian subcontinent or many countries in Africa.

Artesunate (Guilin No. 2 Factory, People's Republic of China). This is provided for parenteral use as artesunic acid powder, which is dispensed together with an ampoule of 5% sodium bicarbonate. The two are mixed immediately before injection. The resulting sodium artesunate is hydrolysed rapidly in vivo to the biologically active metabolite dihydroartemisinin. Artesunate is usually diluted in 5–10 ml of 5% dextrose before intravenous or intramuscular injection. The currently recommended dose is an initial dose of 2.4 mg/kg followed at 12 and 24 h and then daily by single doses of 1.2 mg/kg.

Artemether (Kunming Pharmaceutical Company, Rhône-Poulenc-Rorer). This is dissolved in ground-nut oil and is given by intramuscular injection in an initial dose of 3.2 mg/kg, followed by daily injections of 1.6 mg/kg. Oral treatment is substituted as soon as possible. Mefloquine should not be used because the incidence of neurotoxicity is increased following severe malaria.

In two recent large randomised comparative studies in severe malaria intramuscular artemether shortened parasite clearance times, slightly prolonged coma recovery, but did not reduce mortality significantly compared with quinine (Hien et al 1996, Boele van Hensbroek et al 1996). This confirms that artemether is an effective alternative to quinine for the treatment of severe malaria. There are still a number of uncertainties over the artemisinin compounds. Although oral artesunate and oral artemether are equivalent there is some indirect evidence that parenteral artesunate is superior to artemether in severe disease, probably because therapeutic concentrations are reached earlier. However, artesunate is not widely available, and is not produced to the standards required for international regulatory approval. Artemether is likely to become much more widely available, and the World Health Organization is supporting the development of a very closely related compound, arteether. Suppository formulations of these drugs are likely to become available in the near future.

Use of the artemisinin derivatives has not been associated with any reported toxicity in the treatment of severe malaria. In animal models the oil-soluble ethers, artemether and arteether, have both produced selective toxicity to brain-stem nuclei. Similar neurotoxicity also followed administration of dihydroartemisinin, the common metabolite. To date there is no evidence that similar effects occur in man, but further studies are in progress.

Antimalarial treatment of children

Apart from early vomiting, children generally tolerate the antimalarial drugs better than adults. For oral treatment, particularly in younger children, care should be taken to cool and calm the patient before oral treatment is given. If the temperature is >38.5°C, tepid sponging and oral or rectal paracetamol (15 mg/kg) should be administered and the antimalarials given after the temperature has been lowered (usually 30–60 min). Tablets should be crushed and mixed with water or sweet drink or disguised in jam. The suspension may be drawn up into a syringe so that an accurate dose (on a milligram per kilogram basis) can be instilled into the mouth. Although the pharmacokinetic properties of some antimalarials differ in children, these differences are not great. Dose regimens on a milligram per kilogram basis are the same as in adults, except that: primaquine should not be given to neonates; tetracyclines should not be given to children <8 years old; and in resistant areas, the dose of quinine should be increased to 15 mg/kg three times daily after the fourth day.

Children with severe malaria are more likely than adults to have convulsions, or become severely anaemic or hypoglycaemic. They are less likely to develop renal failure, pulmonary oedema or jaundice. In general, children deteriorate more rapidly than adults, but they also recover more quickly.

Antimalarial treatment in pregnancy

Pregnant women should be treated in the same way as nonpregnant adults, except that tetracyclines (or doxycycline), long-acting sulphonamides near term and primaquine should not be used. Furthermore, oral artemisinin derivatives for uncomplicated malaria should be avoided in the first trimester unless there is no alternative.

There is no information available on halofantrine in pregnancy and it should therefore be avoided. Mefloquine appears to be safe, but more information is needed. Chloroquine, pyrimethamine, proguanil and quinine are all considered safe, although quinine-stimulated hyperinsulin-aemia is more problematic in late pregnancy. Pregnant women with symptomatic malaria should always be treated in hospital.

BREAST FEEDING

Primaquine should be avoided, but the other drugs can be used as the doses received by the suckling infant are very small.

Malaria prophylaxis

It is difficult to make generalized recommendations for antimalarial prophylaxis, as the risks of acquiring malaria and antimalarial drug sensitivity vary considerably over short geographic distances. Antimalarial prophylaxis is indicated in two circumstances: in non-immune travellers visiting areas where they may acquire malaria, and in pregnant women who live in endemic areas. Antimalarial prophylaxis is not generally recommended for the indigenous population in malaria endemic areas. Drugs are only one component of personal protection against malaria.

The risks of acquiring malaria can be reduced considerably by avoiding contact with malaria vectors, by use of appropriate protective clothing, window netting, insect repellents and sleeping under insecticide-impregnated bed-nets. Travellers should seek medical advice urgently if they develop a febrile illness. Stand-by treatment sufficient for one complete antimalarial course may be given to those who will be unable to reach medical services for extended periods. As the geographic distribution of drug resistance changes rapidly, the following general recommendations should be under constant scrutiny.

Except for those areas where *P. falciparum* malaria remains chloroquine sensitive (such as North Africa, the Middle East and Central America north of the Panama Canal), or where the combination of chloroquine plus proguanil is still effective, weekly mefloquine (3.5 mg base/kg equivalent to an adult dose of 250 mg) is the antimalarial prophylactic of choice (Figure 62.1). Mefloquine should be started at least 1 week, and preferably 2 weeks, before entering the malarious area, so that therapeutic levels are achieved before exposure and any adverse effects have declared themselves. Mefloquine is generally well tolerated, with an incidence of serious adverse (neuropsychiatric) effects similar to that with chloroquine prophylaxis (about 1 : 10 000 recipients). In 70% of cases these arise within the first 3 weeks of prophylaxis. Less serious central nervous system effects such as dizziness, muzziness, feelings of dissociation, difficulty concentrating, sleeplessness and nightmares are more common, but these are usually not sufficiently troublesome to limit prophylaxis. Because of inadequate data, rather than evidence of toxicity, mefloquine is considered 'not indicated' in the first trimester of pregnancy or in children <2 years old (Tables 62.2 and 62.3). Serious neuropsychiatric reactions (seizures, encephalopathy and psychosis) are more common if there is a previous history of seizures or psychiatric abnormalities, if quinine has been taken, and when mefloquine is used for treatment rather than prophylaxis. These reactions usually resolve spontaneously. Mefloquine should be continued for 1 month after leaving the endemic area. A maximum of 12 months continuous use is currently recommended.

The combination of chloroquine (5 mg base/kg per week) and proguanil (3 mg/kg daily) is still effective in many areas, and would be an alternative to mefloquine treatment if reliable data indicates sensitivity of *P. falciparum*. Chloroquine is also the prophylactic of choice in those rare situations where only *P. vivax* is encountered. Chloroquine should be given in a dose of 5 mg base/kg (adult 300 mg) weekly. It is generally well tolerated, although pruritus is common in dark-skinned patients and it may cause occasional skin eruptions or worsening of psoriasis. As chloroquine accumulates in the body, and may cause retinal damage, ophthalmological examinations are advisable for people who take continuous chloroquine for 5 years or more (total dose >100 g). Retinal toxicity is more common when chloroquine is taken daily for rheumatic diseases, and is probably very unusual with antimalarial prophylaxis. Proguanil is given in a daily dose of 3 mg/kg (adult 200 mg). It is very safe and well tolerated. The main adverse effects are mouth ulcers and, less commonly, alopecia. In renal failure proguanil and its principal metabolite cycloguanil accumulate, and blood dyscrasias have been reported.

The fixed-dose combination of pyrimethamine (12.5 mg) and dapsone (100 mg) once weekly has generally been superseded by mefloquine, but it remains a second-line treatment for Oceania and other areas where alternative drugs are not useable.

In those few areas where multi drug-resistant *P. falciparum* is also resistant to mefloquine (on the eastern and western borders of Thailand and adjacent Cambodia and Burma), daily doxycycline should be given. As with the other prophylactic drugs this should be continued for 4 weeks after leaving the transmission area. The main adverse effects are nausea, diarrhoea, photosensitivity and, in women, candida vaginitis. Doxycycline should be taken after meals with copious fluids to avoid oesophagitis. It should not be given to children under 8 years of age (in the UK a 12-year age limit is recommended as there are very limited data on prophylactic use in older children) (Bradley & Warhurst 1995) (Tables 62.2 and 62.3), to pregnant women or for more than 3 months. Chloroquine is certainly safe in all age groups and in pregnancy but, although there are no adverse effects reported with mefloquine in pregnancy, experience is still limited and this should remain under review. Neither the pyrimethamine–sulphadoxine combination nor amodiaquine are now recommended for prophylactic use because of toxicity. Travellers should obtain detailed information on the risks of malaria and the efficacy of antimalarial drugs in the area that they will visit. Most travellers visiting South-East Asia do not enter areas of risk

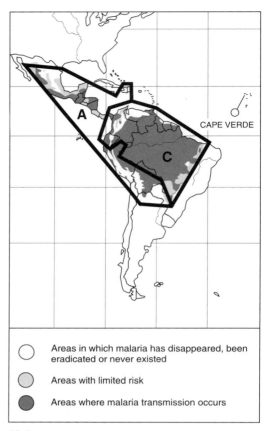

Fig. 62.1

◯	Areas in which malaria has disappeared, been eradicated or never existed
◐	Areas with limited risk
●	Areas where malaria transmission occurs

and do not need to take antimalarial drugs. For India and for South America the risks depend very much on the area to be visited, and for sub-Saharan Africa north of South Africa and Oceania, malaria risks are very high and prophylaxis is required.

Table 62.2 *The UK recommendations for prophylactic regimens against malaria in adults (Bradley & Warhurst 1995)**

Regimen	Dose for chemoprophylaxis	Usual amount per tablet (mg)
Areas of chloroquine-resistant *P. falciparum*		
Mefloquine[†]	I tablet weekly	250 (228 in the USA)
Proguanil + chloroquine	2 tablets daily + 2 tablets weekly	100 plus 150 (base)
Pyrimethamine–dapsone (Maloprim)[‡] + chloroquine	I tablet weekly + 2 tablets weekly	12.5 (P) plus 100 (D) plus 150 (base) (C)
Doxycycline[§]	I tablet daily	100
Areas without drug resistance		
Chloroquine	2 tablets weekly	150 (base)
Proguanil	2 tablets daily	100

* All antimalarials are to be avoided in severe hepatic and renal impairment. Chloroquine doses are given as the base. Folate supplements should be given to those taking proguanil or Maloprim when pregnant.
† Avoid during first trimester of pregnancy, during lactation and avoid pregnancy for 3 months after stopping the drug. Do not prescribe mefloquine if there is a history of epilepsy or of severe psychiatric disorder. Appropriate for up to I year abroad.
‡ Best avoided in the first trimester of pregnancy.
§ Contraindicated during pregnancy and lactation, and for children under 12 years.
P, pyrimethamine; D, dapsone; C, chloroquine.

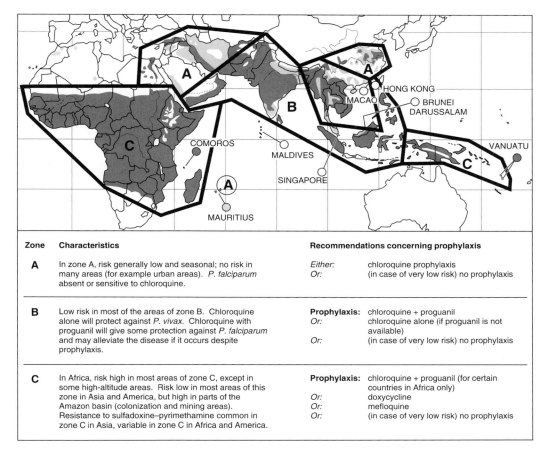

Zone	Characteristics	Recommendations concerning prophylaxis	
A	In zone A, risk generally low and seasonal; no risk in many areas (for example urban areas). *P. falciparum* absent or sensitive to chloroquine.	*Either:* *Or:*	chloroquine prophylaxis (in case of very low risk) no prophylaxis
B	Low risk in most of the areas of zone B. Chloroquine alone will protect against *P. vivax*. Chloroquine with proguanil will give some protection against *P. falciparum* and may alleviate the disease if it occurs despite prophylaxis.	**Prophylaxis:** *Or:* *Or:*	chloroquine + proguanil chloroquine alone (if proguanil is not available) (in case of very low risk) no prophylaxis
C	In Africa, risk high in most areas of zone C, except in some high-altitude areas. Risk low in most areas of this zone in Asia and America, but high in parts of the Amazon basin (colonization and mining areas). Resistance to sulfadoxine–pyrimethamine common in zone C in Asia, variable in zone C in Africa and America.	**Prophylaxis:** *Or:* *Or:* *Or:*	chloroquine + proguanil (for certain countries in Africa only) doxycycline mefloquine (in case of very low risk) no prophylaxis

Fig. 62.1 *Current World Health Organization recommendations for antimalarial prophylaxis by geographic area. C = chloroquine, P = proguanil, M = mefloquine.*

Table 62.3 *The UK recommendations for doses of prophylatic antimalarials for children (Bradley & Warhurst 1995)**

Age	Weight (kg)†	Fraction of adult dose		
		Chloroquine + proguanil	Maloprim (pyrimethamine–dapsone)	Mefloquine
0–5 weeks		$1/8$	Not recommended	Not recommended
6 weeks		$1/4$	$1/8$‡	Not recommended
1–5 years	10–19	$1/2$	$1/4$	Not recommended under age 2 years or 15 kg; $1/4$ (2–5 years)
6–11 years	20–39	$3/4$	$1/2$	$1/2$ (6–8 years), $3/4$ (9–11 years) up to 45 kg
≥12 years	40	Adult dose	Adult dose	Adult dose

* For children aged under 2 years in areas of chloroquine resistance the appropriate drug is chloroquine + proguanil. Chloroquine is available as a syrup, but the proguanil has to be powdered onto jam or food. Antimosquito bite measures are especially important. Doxycycline is considered unsuitable for children under 12 years.
† When both are available weight is a better guide than age for children over 6 months.
‡ Not feasible to prepare unless a paediatric formulation is available.

References

Baird J K, Basri H, Purnomo et al 1991 Resistance to chloroquine by *Plasmodium vivax* in Irian Jaya, Indonesia. *American Journal of Tropical Medicine and Hygiene* 44: 547–552

Boele van Hensbroek M, Onyiorah E, Jaffar S et al 1996 A comparison of the effect of artemether and quinine on survival from childhood cerebral malaria. *New England Journal of Medicine* 335: 69–75

Bradley D J, Warhurst D C 1995 Malaria prophylaxis: guidelines for travellers from Britain. *British Medical Journal* 310: 709–714

Covell G, Coatney G R, Field J W, Singh J 1955 Chemotherapy of malaria (WHO monograph series 27). WHO, Geneva

Davis T M E, Supanaranond W, Pukrittayakamee S et al 1990 A safe and effective consecutive-infusion regimen for rapid quinine loading in severe *falciparum* malaria. *Journal of Infectious Diseases* 161: 1305–1308

Fontanet A L, Johnston B D, Walker A M, Bergqvist Y, Hellgren U, Rooney W 1994 *Falciparum* malaria in eastern Thailand: a randomized trial of the efficacy of a single dose of mefloquine. *Bulletin of the World Health Organization* 72: 73–81

Hien T T, White N J 1993 Qinghaosu. *Lancet* 341: 603–608

Hien T T, Day N P J, Phu N H et al 1996 A comparison of intramuscular quinine and artemether in Vietnamese adults with severe falciparum malaria. *New England Journal of Medicine* 335: 76–83

Karbwang J, White N J 1990. Clinical pharmacokinetics of mefloquine. *Clinical Pharmacokinetics* 19: 264–279

Karbwang J, Davis T M E, Looareesuwan S, Molunto P, Bunnag D, White N J 1993 A comparison of the pharmacokinetic and pharmacodynamic properties of quinine and quinidine in healthy Thai males. *British Journal of Clinical Pharmacology* 35: 265–271

Looareesuwan S, Viravan C, Vanijanonta S et al 1992 A randomised trial of mefloquine, artesunate, and artesunate followed by mefloquine in acute uncomplicated *falciparum* malaria. *Lancet* 339: 821–824

Miller K D, Lobel H O, Satriale R F, Kuritsky J N, Stern R, Campbell C C 1986 Severe cutaneous reactions among American travellers using pyrimethamine-sulfadoxine (Fansidar®) for malaria prophylaxis. *American Journal of Tropical Medicine and Hygiene* 35: 451–458

Miller K D, Greenberg A E, Campbell C C 1989 Treatment of severe malaria in the United States with a continuous infusion of quinidine gluconate and exchange transfusion. *New England Journal of Medicine* 321: 65–70

Nosten F, ter Kuile F O, Luxemburger C et al 1993 Cardiac effects of antimalarial treatment with halofantrine. *Lancet* 341: 1054–1056

Nosten F, Luxemburger C, ter Kuile F O et al 1994 Optimum artesunate–mefloquine combination for the treatment of multi drug-resistant *P. falciparum* malaria. *Journal of Infectious Diseases* 170: 971–977

Pussard E, Lepers J P, Clavier F et al 1991 Efficacy of a loading dose of oral chloroquine in a 36-hour treatment schedule for uncomplicated *Plasmodium falciparum* malaria. *Antimicrobial Agents and Chemotherapy* 35: 406–409

Supanaranond W, Davis T M E, Pukrittayakamee S, Nagachinta B, White N J 1993 Abnormal circulatory control in *falciparum* malaria: the effects of antimalarial drugs. *European Journal of Clinical Pharmacology* 44: 325–330

ter Kuile F O, Dolan G, Nosten F et al 1993 Halofantrine versus mefloquine in the treatment of multidrug resistant *falciparum* malaria. *Lancet* 341: 1044–1049

Watt G, Loesuttivibool L, Shanks G D et al 1992 Quinine with tetracycline for the treatment of drug-resistant *falciparum* malaria in Thailand. *American Journal of Tropical Medicine and Hygiene* 47: 108–111

White N J 1992a Antimalarial drug resistance: the pace quickens. *Journal of Antimicrobial Chemotherapy* 30: 571–585

White N J 1992b Antimalarial phamacokinetics and treatment regimens. *British Journal of Clinical Pharmacology* 34: 1–10

White N J, Looareesuwan S, Warrell D A et al 1983a Quinine loading dose in cerebral malaria. *American Journal of Tropical Medicine and Hygiene* 32: 1–5

White N J, Warrell D A, Chanthavanich P et al 1983b Severe hypoglycemia and hyperinsulinemia in *falciparum* malaria. *New England Journal of Medicine* 309: 61–66

Winstanley P A, Watkins W M, Newton C R et al 1992 The disposition of oral and intramuscular pyrimethamine/sulphadoxine in Kenyan children with high parasitaemia but clinically non-severe *falciparum* malaria. *British Journal of Clinical Pharmacology* 33: 143–148

Winstanley P, Mberu E K, Watkins W M, Murphy S A, Lowe B, Marsh K 1994 Towards optimal regimens of parenteral quinine for young children with cerebral malaria: unbound quinine concentrations following a simple loading dose regimen. *Transactions of the Royal Society of Tropical Medicine and Hygiene* 87: 201–206

World Health Organization 1986 The chemotherapy of malaria. In: Bruce-Chwatt L J (ed) WHO Monograph Series 27, revised edn. WHO, Geneva

World Health Organization 1990 Control of tropical diseases. Severe and complicated malaria. *Transactions of the Royal Society of Tropical Medicine and Hygiene* 80 (suppl 2) : 1–85

Other protozoal infections

P. L. Chiodini

Toxoplasmosis

The regimen of choice is pyrimethamine plus sulphadiazine. The combination is synergistic against toxoplasma tachyzoites. Pyrimethamine is given at a dose of 25–50 mg/day, preceded by a loading dose of 100 mg twice daily for one day. Sulphadiazine is given as 2–8 g/day (in 4 divided doses). Some authors recommend a loading dose of 75 mg/kg up to 4 g. Alternatives to sulphadiazine are sulphatriad or sulphadimidine.

Therapy with pyrimethamine/sulphadiazine (or an alternative) should be accompanied by folinic acid 15 mg/day orally. Duration and dose of combination therapy is influenced by the variant of toxoplasmosis being treated and clinical progress on therapy.

Where sulphonamides are contraindicated or cannot be tolerated, clindamycin 2.4–4.8 g/day in 4 divided doses can be substituted and given in combination with pyrimethamine.

Spiramycin 2–3 g/day in 3 or 4 divided doses is less active than pyrimethamine/sulphadiazine (Nguyen & Stadtsbaeder 1983). Its main application lies in the management of toxoplasmosis in pregnancy (Ch. 57).

NON-PREGNANT IMMUNOLOGICALLY INTACT INDIVIDUALS

Many infections in the normal population are asymptomatic and thus not recognized. Most symptomatic cases resolve without treatment and thus do not require drug therapy, but severely ill patients should be treated. The regimen consists of pyrimethamine 25 mg/day plus sulphadiazine 2 g/day plus folinic acid, for 2–4 weeks. Cerebral, pulmonary, hepatic or cardiac involvement also constitute indications for giving antitoxoplasma drugs (Joss 1992).

OCULAR TOXOPLASMOSIS (Ch. 55)

Rothova et al (1989) examined the action of pyrimethamine 100 mg on the first day followed by 25 mg twice daily, plus sulphadiazine 1 g four times daily, plus folinic acid, plus corticosteroids, with the action of clindamycin 300 mg four times daily plus sulphadiazine (as above) with an untreated control group. Pyrimethamine/sulphadiazine/corticosteroids significantly reduced the size of the retinal lesion in 52% of patients and 25% of controls. Improvement on clindamycin/sulphadiazine/corticosteroids was borderline (retinal lesion reduced in size in 32% of patients). In contrast, Dutton (1989a) preferred clindamycin/sulphadiazine to pyrimethamine/sulphadiazine.

Antitoxoplasma drugs are indicated for ocular toxoplasmosis where there is a threat to vision, either from local posterior pole lesions, or from more general inflammation. Systemic corticosteroids are indicated in the presence of posterior pole lesions, if there is a possibility of large vessel involvement, or if the lesions are in the patient's only eye. Steroid therapy must be accompanied by antitoxoplasma drugs and is reserved for sight-threatening lesions.

Indications for surgical intervention include cataract, uncontrolled rise in intraocular pressure, vitreous membranes, epiretinal membranes and retinal detachment. Systemic steroid cover is given if operative surgery is undertaken for ocular toxoplasmosis. Peripheral retinal lesions representing no threat to vision are kept under observation and do not usually require specific antitoxoplasma drugs (Dutton 1989b).

TOXOPLASMOSIS IN THE IMMUNOCOMPROMISED PATIENT

Toxoplasmosis of the central nervous system is discussed in Chapter 46, page 671.

Cardiac transplantation

Cardiac transplantation is the organ donation most likely to lead to toxoplasmosis in the recipient. Most instances occur when the donor heart comes from a seropositive patient and the recipient is seronegative. The other possibility is reactivation of latent toxoplasmosis under the burden of immunosuppression, in an already seropositive recipient.

Luft et al (1983) reported a series of 50 heart or heart–lung transplant patients. Of 4 patients who were seronegative before receiving a heart from a seropositive donor, 3 developed life-threatening toxoplasmosis. None of 19 patients who were seropositive before transplantation developed illness attributable to toxoplasmosis, although 10 showed significant increases in toxoplasma antibody titres. Another series (Wreghitt et al 1989) studied 21 seronegative recipients of seropositive heart or heart–lung transplants. Four patients (2 of whom died) from the first 7 suffered clinical toxoplasmosis within 17–32 days of the transplant. The next 14 transplant patients deemed at risk of toxoplasmosis received pyrimethamine prophylaxis 25 mg/day plus folinic acid 15 mg three times daily for 6 weeks postoperatively, with only 2 cases of toxoplasmosis.

Treatment of acute toxoplasmosis after heart or heart–lung transplantation is with pyrimethamine/sulphadiazine/folinic acid, continuing until 4–6 weeks after all symptoms and signs have resolved.

Renal transplantation

The risk of the recipient developing toxoplasmosis after renal transplantation appears to be small (Derouin et al 1987). However, toxoplasma infection has been reported in a seronegative recipient of a kidney from a seropositive donor (Mason et al 1987).

Hepatic transplantation

It is unclear at present whether or not seronegative recipients of seropositive donors need prophylaxis.

Bone marrow transplantation

In contrast to solid organ transplants, toxoplasmosis in bone-marrow-graft recipients appears to be due largely to reactivation of latent infection in the recipient, rather than infection coming from the transplanted organ (Derouin et al 1992). Thus, there are likely to be more problems in countries with a higher toxoplasma seroprevalence rate (Ho-Yen 1992). It has been suggested that recipients seropositive before bone-marrow transplantation be given chemoprophylaxis from months 2 to 6 after grafting, but this has not been formally studied (McCabe & Chirurgi 1993).

AIDS

See cerebral toxoplasmosis (Ch. 46).

TOXOPLASMOSIS IN PREGNANCY

Berrebi et al (1994) reported a prospective study of conservative management of fetal toxoplasmosis which should have a major effect on treatment strategy for this condition. One-hundred and sixty-three mothers bearing 165 fetuses and who seroconverted to *Toxoplasma* between 8 and 26 weeks of pregnancy were enrolled. Each mother received spiramycin 2.8 g/day (Anon 1993) until the end of pregnancy. If umbilical cord blood (taken during gestation via ultrasound-guided cordocentesis) revealed evidence of fetal toxoplasma infection, pyrimethamine 25 mg and sulphadiazine 500 mg were given by mouth twice weekly, along with folinic acid 400 μg/day for 1 month, in addition to spiramycin therapy (23 mothers).

Three fetuses died in utero. One hundred and sixty-two live born babies, from 160 mothers, were followed-up for 15–71 (mean 36) months. One hundred and thirty-five had no evidence of congenital toxoplasmosis. Twenty-seven of the 162 babies (17%) were born with congenital toxoplasmosis, of whom 17 had no clinical or laboratory abnormalities at 15–71 months follow-up. Ten of 27 (37%) had one or more clinical signs of congenital toxoplasmosis, but 9 of the 10 had never exhibited symptoms attributed to toxoplasmosis. At their most recent paediatric visit, all the infants had normal neurological examination, and weight and height growth curves. On the basis of their study, Berrebi et al no longer recommend early termination of pregnancy in cases of fetal infection with toxoplasmosis before the 28th week. Instead, they offer treatment with spiramycin pyrimethamine and sulphadiazine, plus fetal ultrasonography every 2 weeks. Termination of pregnancy is advised only in the presence of intrauterine fetal death or sonographic evidence of hydrocephalus. For women who seroconvert after 26 weeks, treatment with spiramycin, pyrimethamine and sulphadiazine is usually given. Fetal infection in those patients is common but not severe, and Berrebi et al regard termination as not indicated.

Daffos et al (1994) regard the best predictor of severity of fetal infection as gestational age at the time of maternal infection. From their series, if infection took place before 16 weeks of amenorrhoea, 60% of fetuses had ultrasound evidence of infection and 48% had cerebral ventricular dilatation. Based on this, their policy is to accept parental requests for termination when infection occurs before 16 weeks.

Wallon et al (1994) reported on 540 acute toxoplasma infections in pregnant women, who received pyrimethamine–sulfadoxine or spiramycin therapy according to the stage of pregnancy at seroconversion. Monthly fetal ultrasonography was undertaken if maternal infection occurred after the second trimester or if fetal blood sampling or amniocentesis (offered if infection occurred after the 9th week of pregnancy) revealed evidence of toxoplasma infection. In 5 fetuses, neurological abnormalities were detected and termination of pregnancy was performed. Eight spontaneous abortions occurred, 3 mothers requested termination of pregnancy and 2 mothers miscarried after fetal blood sampling. None of 522 living children had abnormal morphology at birth and 490 (94%) were followed up for at least 1 year. Three-hundred and seventy-four of 490 (76%) had negative toxoplasma serology at 1 year of age. One-hundred and sixteen children were found to be infected, and their mothers had all contracted toxoplasmosis after the 13th week of gestation. The offspring were treated with pyrimethamine–sulfadoxine for an average of 14 months. At 1 year, 31 (27%) had cerebral calcifications or retinal lesions without severely impaired vision. Two had macular lesions causing some visual impairment. None had evidence of neurological or mental defect.

When acute maternal toxoplasmosis is diagnosed during pregnancy, tests for fetal toxoplasma infection should be undertaken. In expert hands, available techniques, including fetal blood sampling, gave a reported sensitivity of 92% for in utero diagnosis (Daffos et al 1988).

Once acute maternal infection has been confirmed, the mother should be treated with spiramycin 3 g/day in 3 or 4 divided doses. This regimen produces a 60% reduction in the frequency of transmission of *Toxoplasma* to the fetus (Wong & Remington 1994). Spiramycin levels in the placenta are 3–5 times higher than in maternal serum, but cord serum levels are only half those in maternal serum. This may explain why spiramycin does not modify the pattern of infection in the infected fetus (Wong & Remington 1994). Thus, in the presence of fetal infection, the mother should receive pyrimethamine 25 mg/day and sulphadiazine 4 g/day plus folinic acid. This regimen is given for 3 weeks, followed by spiramycin 3 g/day for 3 weeks, in alternating blocks until term. Pyrimethamine should not be used in the first trimester of pregnancy (Wong & Remington 1994).

Hohlfeld et al (1989) reported seven cases where maternal toxoplasmosis was contracted in the first trimester of pregnancy and therapeutic abortion was performed. Despite no lesions being detectable on ultrasonography, necropsy demonstrated severe brain damage with large areas of necrosis in each fetus. Thus, some authorities regard fetal infection in early pregnancy without demonstrable lesions on ultrasonography, as an indication for discussing therapeutic abortion.

In advising the mother on the options available for management of toxoplasmosis acquired during pregnancy, it is important to make a clear distinction between maternal infection and maternal plus fetal infection. The incidence of fetal infection depends upon the stage of pregnancy during which the mother acquires toxoplasmosis. Without specific therapy the incidence of fetal infection is 10–15% if the mother becomes infected in the first trimester, 30% in the second and 60% in the third trimester. Severity of fetal infection decreases the later the infection is acquired (Wong & Remington 1994). Thus, a policy of advising termination of pregnancy where maternal toxoplasmosis is acquired in the first trimester would abort a number of uninfected fetuses, but a policy of advising continuation of the pregnancy would produce some severely damaged infants. Wong & Remington (1994) advise that therapeutic abortion be offered to a pregnant woman only when fetal infection has been confirmed by prenatal testing. Berrebi et al (1994) concluded that in first- and second-trimester pregnancies with acute fetal toxoplasma infection, the pregnancy need not be interrupted if repeated fetal ultrasound is normal and antiparasitic treatment is given. However, only three of their 27 cases of congenital toxoplasmosis had first-trimester infection. If their encouraging results on first-trimester fetal toxoplasmosis prove to be typical, a conservative approach to this most difficult therapeutic problem would be justified.

Pregnant women infected with human immunodeficiency virus (HIV) who are seronegative for *Toxoplasma* remain susceptible to contracting acute toxoplasmosis in the same way as HIV-negative women. In addition, HIV-positive women, particularly those with acquired immune deficiency syndrome (AIDS), with serological evidence of past toxoplasma infection are at risk of reactivation of their latent toxoplasma from dormant tissue cysts. Thus, the mother may develop severe toxoplasmosis and may transmit the infection to her fetus. There is a need for further study of this problem. In the meantime, Wong & Remington (1994) suggest treating HIV-infected, toxoplasma seropositive women with CD4 lymphocyte counts below 200/mm^3 (0.2 × 10^9/l) with spiramycin 3 g/day during the first trimester of pregnancy. Pyrimethamine–sulphadiazine or trimethoprim–sulphamethoxazole therapy should be considered from the 17th week of gestation onwards.

NEONATAL TOXOPLASMOSIS

Most infants with congenital toxoplasma infection appear clinically normal at birth.

Guerina et al (1994) studied 52 babies with congenital toxoplasmosis, identified in a neonatal screening programme. Fifty had normal routine physical examinations, but on closer scrutiny 40% of them had central nervous system (CNS) or retinal abnormalities.

Koppe et al (1986) followed 12 congenitally infected children (5 treated, 7 untreated) annually from birth until 20 years of age. No new abnormalities appeared in the first 5 years, except for a squint in one child with chlorioretinitis. However, new lesions appeared in subsequent years, some in the teenage years, though the authors could not exclude relapses due to infection acquired after birth.

Neonates should be managed according to the degree of

evidence of infection. Chatterton (1992) has summarized the strategy. Infected neonates with clinical damage should receive pyrimethamine 1 mg/kg daily, sulphadiazine 85 mg/kg daily and folinic acid 5 mg every 3 days, for 6 months. For the following 6 months, this regimen should alternate monthly with spiramycin 100 mg/kg daily. In the presence of an inflammatory process (chorioretinitis, high cerebrospinal fluid (CSF) protein level, generalized infection or jaundice) corticosteroids should be added.

Where the neonate is subclinically infected, the management consists of pyrimethamine–sulphadiazine–folinic acid for 6 weeks, then spiramycin for 6 weeks, followed by alternating the regimens for 4- and 6-week periods respectively for 1 year.

If it is initially unclear whether or not congenital infection has occurred, treatment is determined according to the infection status of the mother. If the mother had proven *Toxoplasma* infection in pregnancy, the neonate should receive pyrimethamine–sulphadiazine–folinic acid for 4 weeks. If maternal infection was suspected rather than proven, the neonate should be treated with spiramycin for 4 weeks. In both instances the neonates are followed up. If congenital infection is confirmed, further therapy can be given.

Leishmaniasis

CUTANEOUS LEISHMANIASIS

Most lesions of Old World cutaneous leishmaniasis heal spontaneously. Treatment may produce more rapid healing and less severe scarring and is indicated for multiple sores, those at risk of causing disfigurement or disability, or those sited where healing is expected to be slow. Options for local drug treatment are topical aminosidine (paromomycin) ointment (Bryceson et al 1994) or infiltration of sodium stibogluconate into the edge and base of the sore (Harms et al 1991).

If *Leishmania brasiliensis* is suspected, the cutaneous lesion should be treated systemically to prevent the development of mucocutaneous leishmaniasis. Systemic therapy of cutaneous leishmaniasis is undertaken with pentavalent antimonials (sodium stibogluconate or meglumine antimoniate). Diffuse cutaneous leishmaniasis requires expert assessment and follow-up. In principle, *Leishmania aethiopica* is treated with aminosidine plus sodium stibogluconate daily (Teklemariam et al 1994). Therapy is continued until the parasite is felt to have been eliminated, which may take a few months. Weekly pentamidine is an alternative (Bryceson 1970). Mucosal leishmaniasis (*L. braziliensis*) is treated with antimonials at 20 mg antimony/kg daily for 6–8 weeks, provided the patient is previously untreated and does not have laryngeal involvement. For those previously treated, or in whom the larynx is involved, amphotericin B

1 mg/kg is given by intravenous infusion on alternate days for 6–8 weeks (Bryceson 1987).

VISCERAL LEISHMANIASIS

Pentavalent antimonials have until recently been the first choice for therapy of visceral leishmaniasis. Sodium stibogluconate solution contains 100 mg antimony/ml, while meglumine antimoniate solution contains 85 mg antimony/ml. Parasite resistance to pentavalent antimonials has now become a problem, notably in recent epidemics in India and the Sudan, where intermittent therapy or suboptimal dosage regimens can favour development and spread of resistant strains. Traditional dosage regimens as recommended by the World Health Organization (WHO 1990) advocate 20 mg/kg daily of antimony, subject to a maximum daily dose of 850 mg antimony, for a minimum of 20 days, until no parasites are found in consecutive splenic aspirates taken at 14-day intervals. Herwaldt & Berman (1992) advocated lifting of the 850 mg ceiling for antimony dosage, with close monitoring of the patient for drug-related reactions. An alternative and preferable regimen is to calculate dosage on the basis of body surface area (Anabwani & Bryceson 1982).

The emergence of antimony-resistant VL has led to the study of adjunctive immunotherapy. A controlled trial of combination therapy of Kenyan VL with alternate-day γ-interferon plus daily sodium stibogluconate, versus daily sodium stibogluconate alone, suggested that combination therapy may have accelerated the early clearance of parasites (Squires et al 1993). Sundar et al (1994) used sodium stibogluconate 20 mg/kg daily intravenously for 30 days, plus γ-interferon 25 μg/m^2 subcutaneously on day 1, 50 μg/m^2 on day 2 and 100 μg/m^2 daily for 28 days, to treat 15 Indian patients, all of whom had failed an initial course of 30 or more days of antimony treatment at 20 mg/kg daily. Eight of the patients had received two courses and seven had received three or four treatment courses. Combination therapy was discontinued in two patients, both of whom died. After 30 days of therapy, 9/13 (69%) of the patients were apparently cured. All nine had negative bone-marrow smears at 6 months and none relapsed after a mean follow-up of 15.9 ± 1.7 months. Combination therapy with antimonials plus γ-interferon may have a role in selected refractory cases, but its cost renders it unsuitable for widespread use in the tropics.

Secondary infection is an important cause of morbidity and mortality in VL. Granulocyte–macrophage colony-stimulating factor (GM-CSF) was compared to placebo as adjunctive therapy in Brazilian patients with VL and leucopenia due to *Leishmania chagasi*. Patients received antimony 10–20 mg/kg daily for 20 days plus GM-CSF 5 μg/kg daily or placebo, for 10 days. Neutrophil counts were significantly higher in the GM-CSF group at 5 and 10 days. Eosinophil and monocyte counts were significantly higher at 10 days in the patients who received GM-CSF. Significantly fewer secondary infections occurred in the GM-CSF group (Badaro et al 1994).

Aminosidine (paromomycin) is active against antimony-resistant strains causing VL (Olliaro & Bryceson 1993). Scott et al (1992) treated seven patients with Mediterranean VL with daily intravenous infusions of aminosidine 14–16 mg/kg for 21 days or for 1 week after demonstration of parasitological cure, whichever was the longer. Four of the seven patients (treated for between 22 and 54 days) were cured. One relapsed 4 months after an apparent cure, but was successfully retreated with a second course lasting 63 days. The remaining two patients showed a partial parasitological response.

Indian VL has become less responsive to pentavalent antimonials. For example, it has been estimated that 10% of VL patients in the state of Bihar are insensitive to sodium stibogluconate. By the early 1990s the regimen for VL treatment in that area was sodium stibogluconate 20 mg/kg daily for 40 or more days, a dosage regimen associated with increased toxicity and higher costs of hospitalization. Following reports of a study from Kenya, where aminosidine 12 mg/kg daily in combination with sodium stibogluconate 20 mg/kg daily for 20 days appeared more effective than sodium stibogluconate alone, Thakur et al (1992) undertook a pilot study of the activity of the combination on VL in Bihar, India. Twenty-four patients were assigned to receive aminosidine 12 mg/kg daily plus sodium stibogluconate, for 20 days. Two patients died before completing the course, one from haemorrhage following splenic puncture and one as a result of severe gastroenteritis. Of 22 patients who completed therapy, 18 (82%) were cured and did not relapse within a 6-month follow-up period. The remaining four patients improved clinically and parasitologically. Mishra et al (1994) compared conventional amphotericin B with sodium stibogluconate in the treatment of Indian visceral leishmaniasis. Eighty patients, none of them previously treated with antileishmanial agents, were randomized to receive either sodium stibogluconate 20 mg/kg in 2 divided doses intramuscularly daily for 40 days or amphotericin 0.5 mg/kg infused in 5% dextrose on alternate days for 14 doses. All 40 patients who received amphotericin showed initial cure (no fever and no amastigotes in a bone-marrow smear after 6 weeks) and definitive cure (well at the end of 12 months). In the stibogluconate-treated group 28/40 (70%) showed initial cure and 25/40 (62.5%) showed definitive cure. Patients who failed to respond to stibogluconate, or who relapsed after an initial cure, were treated with, and cured by, amphotericin.

The amastigotes of *Leishmania* are found in macrophages which also clear liposomes from the circulation. Thus, the sites of infection can be targeted by amphotericin, itself a more active antileishmanial drug than is sodium stibogluconate. Davidson et al (1994) reported a multicentre trial of liposomal amphotericin B in Mediterranean VL. Ten immunocompetent patients (6 of them children) received 1–1.38 mg/kg daily for 21 days and a further 10 (9 of them children) received 3 mg/kg daily for 10 days. All were clinically cured after a follow-up period of at least 12 months. Torre-Cisneros et al (1993) described two cases of VL in HIV-infected patients and summarized reports of three similar cases. Patients received liposomal amphotericin B to a total dose of 1.05–2.0 g each. All were reported cured at the end of therapy and no relapses were noted in a follow-up period lasting 2–12 months. Two patients, followed for 10 and 12 months, received bimonthly maintenance therapy with 1 mg liposomal amphotericin B. In contrast, Davidson & Russo (1994) described 7 HIV-infected adults (4 had AIDS) with VL treated with liposomal amphotericin B 100 mg (1.38–1.85 mg/kg) daily for 21 days (total dose 2.1 g). All 7 appeared cured at first, but 6 relapsed between 3 and 22 months after the end of treatment. A further 10 HIV-infected VL patients received liposomal amphotericin B 4 mg/kg on days 1–5, 10, 17, 24, 31 and 38, to a total dose of 40 mg/kg. Six relapsed within 6 months. Torre-Cisneros et al (1993) suggested a total dose of 1.0 g and, in the case of relapse, retreatment with a total dose of 2.0 g, followed by permanent bimonthly secondary prophylaxis. Comparative trials are certainly required in order to address the question of maintenance therapy.

Where resources permit, liposomal amphotericin B is now the treatment of choice for VL. The dosage schedule is 2–3 mg/kg per dose, equivalent to 21–24 mg/kg total dose for the course, given in 7–10 doses, the last on day 10 (Bryceson A D M 1995 Personal communication). This regimen produces individual doses in multiples of 50 mg, avoids splitting any 50 mg ampoules and reduces wastage of an expensive drug.

Amphotericin B cholesterol dispersion (Amphocil) consists of a 1:1 molar ratio of cholesterol sulphate and amphotericin B in disc-shaped particles, 115 nm in diameter and 4 nm thick. Dietze et al (1993) treated Brazilian patients with VL using two different regimens. Ten patients received amphotericin B cholesterol dispersion 2 mg/kg daily intravenously for 10 days, and another 10 patients received a 7-day course. The authors reported treatment success in all patients. One patient who received the 7-day course had scanty particles in the bone-marrow smear 15 days after treatment, but the remainder (95%) had negative bone-marrow smears. All patients were well after 6 months follow-up. Side-effects consisting of fever, chills and respiratory distress were noted in children under 3 years of age.

Trypanosomiasis

TRYPANOSOMA BRUCEI GAMBIENSE INFECTION

Haemolymphatic disease can be treated with eflornithine or

suramin or pentamidine. Eflornithine (α-difluoromethyl-ornithine, DFMO) has been evaluated for the treatment of established gambiense sleeping sickness (i.e. with CNS involvement) (McCann et al 1986, Pepin et al 1987, Milord et al 1992) but can also be used to treat haemolymphatic disease due to *T. b. gambiense*.

Suramin is used to attempt radical cure of the haemo-lymphatic stage of the disease or to clear trypanosomes from the blood and lymph prior to melarsoprol therapy. All doses are given by slow intravenous infusion of a 10% aqueous solution. A test dose of 200 mg is given first, then 20 mg/kg (maximum dose 1 g) on days 1, 3, 7, 14 and 21.

Pentamidine 4 mg/kg daily by intramuscular injection daily or on alternate days for 10 doses is an alternative, for *T. b. gambiense* only.

In the absence of treatment, late-stage infection, with meningoencephalitis, is uniformly fatal. Until recently the mainstay of therapy was melarsoprol, an arsenical compound with significant toxicity. The development of eflornithine has proved to be a major advance (McCann et al 1986). Pepin at al (1987) treated 26 patients with *T. b. gambiense* sleeping sickness resistant to arsenicals (melarsoprol or trimelarsan) with eflornithine, 100 mg/kg every 6 h (total daily dose 400 mg/kg) by intravenous infusion over 1 h for 14 days, followed by oral eflornithine 75 mg/kg every 6 h (300 mg/kg daily) for a further 30 or 21 days. Five patients died. Follow-up of the surviving 21 patients for a mean of 16 (range 6–30) months showed no relapses. Trypanosomes disappeared rapidly from the CSF, the CSF lymphocyte count gradually fell and there was improvement in symptoms after the first 2 weeks of treatment, such that most patients were asymp-tomatic by the time of hospital discharge. Giving 2 weeks intravenous eflornithine before commencing oral treatment appeared to give a lower relapse rate than did oral therapy reported from other studies. The authors felt that reducing the oral phase of therapy from 30 to 21 days may reduce the frequency of side-effects.

Milord et al (1992) examined the effect of three different eflornithine treatment regimens on a group of 207 patients with late-stage *T. b. gambiense* sleeping sickness. In some cases eflornithine was the first antitrypanosomal drug administered, while other patients had relapsed after melarsoprol or nifurtimox or pentamidine plus suramin. Of 152 patients followed for at least 1 year only 13 (9%) relapsed. Relapse after eflornithine was more frequent in children under 12 years of age and in previously untreated than in relapsing cases. Patients with a CSF leucocytosis of ≥100/µl were slightly though not significantly more likely to relapse than those with lower CSF white cell counts. Relapse rates in patients with trypanosomes seen in the CSF were not significantly different from those in patients in whom none were seen. Therapy with eflornithine 100 mg/kg intra-venously every 6 h for 14 days, followed by 75 mg/kg orally every 6 h for 21 days showed no relapses in 28 patients

followed for at least 1 year after treatment. In patients treated by the intravenous route only (200 mg/kg 12-hourly for 14 days) the relapse rate was 10/108 (9%), compared with 19% (3/16) in those treated by the oral route (75 mg/kg 6-hourly for 35 days).

Melarsoprol (Mel B) has been superseded by eflornithine for the therapy of late-stage *T. b. gambiense* sleeping sickness. Similarly, nifurtimox (Ch. 29, p. 400) is too toxic to be preferred to eflornithine. Pepin et al (1992) treated 30 patients suffering from arseno-resistant *T. b. gambiense* sleeping sickness, with high-dose nifurtimox (30 mg/kg daily for 30 days). Trypanosomes disappeared from the CSF of the 9 patients in whom they were shown before therapy, and the CSF white count fell in all but one patient. Nine of 25 (36%) patients relapsed after follow-up, 7 with trypanosomes in either CSF or blood. The relapse rate was lower than in the authors' previous study using nifurtimox 15 mg/kg daily for 60 days, when only 31% (6/19) were cured. However, high-dose nifurtimox produced serious toxicity; one patient died and another eight developed neurological problems, the most common being a cerebellar syndrome. Pepin et al (1992) advise restricting use of high-dose nifurtimox to patients who have relapsed after both melarsoprol and eflornithine, or for the treatment of arseno-resistant trypanosomiasis if eflornithine is not available.

TRYPANOSOMA BRUCEI RHODESIENSE INFECTION

Haemolymphatic disease is treated with suramin (see *T. b. gambiense*). Pentamidine is ineffective against *T. b. rhodesiense*.

For late-stage disease with CNS involvement, eflornithine is less effective than it is against *T. b. gambiense*, and the treatment of choice for late-stage *T. b. rhodesiense* infection remains melarsoprol (Mel B). Several different treatment regimens are currently advocated, though there is no clear evidence that one is superior (WHO 1990). The regimens usually consist of 3 or 4 daily injections, separated by 7- to 10-day periods off treatment (Table 63.1) (WHO 1990).

Therapy with melarsoprol can be followed by a Herxheimer reaction which may be very severe. Thus, melarsoprol therapy is usually preceded by suramin treatment in the case of *T. b. rhodesiense* (Table 63.1). As many as 1–5% of patients die during melarsoprol therapy, so it must be used only where there is clear evidence for CNS involvement in *T. b. rhodesiense* infection. Especially dangerous is reactive encephalopathy, with headache, tremor, slurred speech, convulsions and coma. The syndrome appears 3–10 days after the first dose of melarsoprol (WHO 1990). Pepin et al (1989) examined the effect of prednisolone on the incidence of melarsoprol-induced encephalopathy in *T. b. gambiense* (rather than *T. b. rhodesiense*) sleeping sickness. Three

Table 63.1 *Treatment schedules (adults and children) for African trypanosomiasis with meningoencephalitic involvement**

Day	Drug[†]	Dose (mg/kg)
For *T. b. rhodesiense* infection, as used in Kenya and Zambia		
1	Suramin	5.00
3	Suramin	10.00
5	Suramin	20.00
7	Melarsoprol	0.36
8	Melarsoprol	0.72
9	Melarsoprol	1.10
16	Melarsoprol	1.40
17	Melarsoprol	1.80
18	Melarsoprol	1.80
25	Melarsoprol	2.20
26	Melarsoprol	2.90
27	Melarsoprol	3.60
34	Melarsoprol	3.60
35	Melarsoprol	3.60
36	Melarsoprol	3.60
For *T. b. rhodesiense* infection, as used in Uganda and the United Republic of Tanzania		
1	Suramin	5.00
3	Suramin	10.00
5	Melarsoprol	1.80
6	Melarsoprol	2.20
7	Melarsoprol	2.56
14	Melarsoprol	2.56
15	Melarsoprol	2.90
16	Melarsoprol	3.26
23	Melarsoprol	3.60
24	Melarsoprol	3.60
25	Melarsoprol	3.60
For *T. b. gambiense* infection, as used in Côte d'Ivoire		
1	Pentamidine i.m.	4.00
2	Pentamidine i.m.	4.00
4	Melarsoprol	1.20
5	Melarsoprol	2.40
6	Melarsoprol	3.60
17	Melarsoprol	1.20
18	Melarsoprol	2.40
19	Melarsoprol	3.60
20	Melarsoprol	3.60
30	Melarsoprol	1.20
31	Melarsoprol	2.40
32	Melarsoprol	3.60
33	Melarsoprol	3.60

* Reproduced with permission from WHO (1990).
† All given intravenously unless otherwise stated.

hundred and eight control patients received melarsoprol, preceded by a single dose of suramin to decrease peripheral parasitaemia, while 290 patients received the same drugs plus prednisolone 1 mg/kg (maximum 40 mg) daily by mouth. The prednisolone group showed a significant ($p = 0.002$) reduction in the incidence of encephalopathy compared to controls. However, there was no significant difference in case fatality rate for encephalopathy between the two groups (66.7% in the prednisolone group, 54.3% in the control

group). The presence of fever during an episode of encephalopathy was associated with an adverse outcome; 0/10 patients with fever and 20/37 without fever survived. Thus, reduction in encephalopathy-associated death was due to a lower incidence of encephalopathy rather than a lower case-fatality rate. Reduction of the encephalopathy rate by prednisolone supports an autoimmune aetiology for this complication, since steroids seem unlikely to decrease direct toxicity of arsenicals. In contrast, the incidence of poly-neuropathy, thought to be due to a direct toxic effect of arsenic, was not reduced by prednisolone (Pepin et al 1989). The authors rightly advise exclusion of strongyloidiasis and amoebiasis before giving prednisolone, in view of the propensity of these infections to fulminate in steroid-treated individuals. Although the study was undertaken in *T. b. gambiense* sleeping sickness, the authors feel that prednisolone should also be given to patients with *T. b. rhodesiense* sleeping sickness receiving melarsoprol.

TRYPANOSOMA CRUZI INFECTION

There have been few advances in the chemotherapy of this infection for many years. Both the standard drugs, nifurtimox and benznidazole, are toxic, with adverse reaction rates of 30–55% (Gallerano et al 1990). Despite the toxicity, patients in the acute stage of the disease should receive drug therapy. Tanowitz et al (1992), reviewing Chagas' disease, drew attention to studies in which 42% of rabbits receiving benznidazole and 33% of rabbits receiving nifurtimox developed widely invasive lymphomas, yet none of the control animals did so. They also point out that both agents have been widely used in Latin America for several decades, without reports of an increased frequency of lymphomas in treated patients.

Nifurtimox acts against trypomastigotes and amastigotes. The treatment regimen is 10 mg/kg, divided into three equal doses, daily by mouth, for 60–90 days. The paediatric dose is 15 mg/kg daily (WHO 1991).

Patients in whom Chagas' disease is complicated by acute meningoencephalitis can be given up to 25 mg/kg daily of nifurtimox. Side-effects of nifurtimox are common and dose related. Recognized side-effects include headache, vertigo, excitability, myalgia, arthralgia, convulsions and peripheral polyneuritis (WHO 1990).

Benznidazole is also active against trypomastigotes and amastigotes. The dosage regimen is 5–10 mg/kg daily orally in two divided doses for 60 days; children receive 10 mg/kg daily. Side-effects commonly occur, including rashes, fever, purpura, peripheral polyneuritis, leucopenia and agranulocytosis (WHO 1990, 1991). Response to therapy is variable; for example, some central Brazilian strains are less sensitive. Andrade et al (1992) isolated 11 strains of *Trypanosoma cruzi* from patients with Chagas' disease in central Brazil and characterized them biologically and by isoenzyme analysis. Patients received benznidazole or benznidazole plus nifurtimox. Mice infected with the corresponding strain were treated with the drug or drugs corresponding to the regimen received by the patient. Mice underwent a test of cure 3–6 months after the end of treatment. Patients were tested by xenodiagnosis monthly on at least 25 occasions. Mice infected with type II (zymodeme 2) strains showed 66–100% cure rates, but those infected with type III (zymodeme 1) strains showed 0–9% cure rates. In humans, 5/6 patients with type II strains but only 2/5 patients with type III strains were cured. There was correlation between treatment outcome in patients and mice in 9/11 (81.8%) cases.

Allopurinol 600 mg daily for 30–60 days has trypanosomicidal action (WHO 1991). Gallerano et al (1990), working in Argentina, compared allopurinol 600 or 900 mg/day for 60 days with benznidazole or nifurtimox therapy and with an untreated group, in a study on patients with chronic Chagas' disease. Follow-up was based on objective laboratory criteria: serology and xenodiagnosis. Significantly more patients from the four treatment groups, whether analysed separately or together, were rendered seronegative, compared to the untreated patients. There was no significant difference between the treatment regimens in seronegativity rates after therapy. The parasitaemia cleared in 63–88% of treated patients, but in only 10% of those untreated ($p <$ 0.01%). There was no difference in efficacy between treatment regimens. Adverse reaction rates were significantly higher in the nifurtimox or benznidazole groups than in the allopurinol groups; toxic hepatitis and CNS disturbances occurred with benznidazole and with nifurtimox; skin reactions were as frequent as with allopurinol. Further work is needed to define the role of allopurinol in chronic Chagas' disease. It is unclear whether or not it will have a role in treating acute cases.

Congenital Chagas' disease can be treated with nifurtimox 8–25 mg/kg daily for 30 days or more, or with benznidazole 5–10 mg/kg daily for 30–60 days (WHO 1991).

Solari et al (1993) reported a patient with haemophilia and AIDS complicated by multifocal necrotic encephalitis due to *Trypanosoma cruzi*. Two weeks' therapy with benznidazole 400 mg per day failed to improve the condition, but itraconazole 200 mg/day, later changed to fluconazole 400 mg/day in an attempt to achieve better CNS penetration, was associated with resolution of fever and stabilization of the neurological symptoms. Further evaluation of triazole antifungal agents against *T. cruzi* infections should be undertaken.

Additional studies are required to determine whether or not specific chemotherapy is worthwhile in the indeterminate stage of Chagas' disease. In established chronic disease, symptomatic treatment is the most appropriate management strategy.

Entamoeba histolytica

Choice of treatment regimen depends upon the particular clinical presentation of amoebic infection.

AMOEBIC DYSENTERY

The treatment of choice is metronidazole followed by diloxanide furoate. Metronidazole 800 mg three times daily for 5 days produced a cure rate in excess of 90% (Powell et al 1967). Tinidazole is an alternative agent (Scragg et al 1976), the adult dose being 2 g/day for 3–5 days. Using the above regimens, neither metronidazole nor tinidazole achieves adequate clearance of amoebic cysts from the intestinal lumen. It is thus necessary to follow them with a luminal amoebicide. Diloxanide furoate 500 mg by mouth three times daily for 10 days is first choice, alternatives being paromomycin (aminosidine) 500 mg by mouth three times daily for 10 days, or iodoquinol (diiodohydroxyquin) 650 mg three times daily for 20 days (Reed 1992). However, diiodohydroxyquin therapy, albeit in longer courses, has been associated with the development of blindness (Fleisher et al 1974) and, since there are good alternative agents available, the use of diiodohydroxyquin for the therapy of amoebiasis is not recommended.

AMOEBIC LIVER ABSCESS

The dose of metronidazole required in amoebic liver abscess is lower than in amoebic dysentery. Amoebic liver abscess is treated with metronidazole 400 mg by mouth three times daily for 5 days (Powell et al 1967) followed by diloxanide furoate (as above). Tinidazole is an alternative to metronidazole. Initial work used a dosage regimen of 800 mg three times daily for 5 days (Hatchuel 1975), but 2 g/day by mouth for 3–5 days is currently used. Scragg & Proctor (1977) achieved a 92% cure rate in children with amoebic liver abscess, using tinidazole in a mean dose of 55 mg/kg daily for 3–5 days, in combination with therapeutic aspiration.

Rarely, when nitroimidazoles do not seem to be effective despite therapeutic aspiration of the abscess (see below), dehydroemetine or emetine can be considered. However, both have serious side-effects, notably cardiotoxicity. Where it is essential to use one of them, dehydroemetine is preferred as it is less toxic than emetine. The dosage regimen is dehydroemetine 1.25 mg/kg (maximum daily dose 90 mg) intramuscularly or deep subcutaneously for 10 days. Emetine dosage is 1 mg/kg (maximum daily dose 60 mg) intramuscularly or deep subcutaneously for 10 days (Knight 1980, Du Pont 1994).

Chloroquine is another alternative, where nitroimidazoles

fail or cannot be used. However, it is only moderately effective in amoebic liver abscess and ineffective in amoebic dysentery (Powell et al 1967). The regimen is chloroquine 150 mg base four times daily for 2 days, then 150 mg base twice daily for 19 days (Du Pont 1994).

Aspiration of an amoebic liver abscess is occasionally necessary. Reed (1992) gives the following indications:

1. To rule out a pyogenic abscess, particularly with multiple lesions. We consider that aspiration for diagnostic purposes should only rarely be required, provided good-quality amoebic serology is available and if appropriate antibacterial and antiamoebic therapy can be given from the outset pending the outcome of blood cultures and amoebic serology. Scragg (1975) felt there was no place for diagnostic aspiration and that aspiration should be considered as part of treatment.
2. As an adjunct to medical treatment, if a patient fails to respond to therapy within 3–5 days and if rupture is believed to be imminent.
3. To decrease the risk of rupture of an abscess of the left lobe of the liver into the pericardium.

ASYMPTOMATIC CYST PASSAGE

The decision whether or not to treat asymptomatic cyst passage depends on several factors. If the patient is ordinarily resident in an area highly endemic for *Entamoeba histolytica* and thus likely to become reinfected fairly quickly, the benefit of eradicating cyst carriage has to be weighed against the cost of treatment and likely benefit to the individual, bearing in mind the fact that most strains of '*E. histolytica*' are non-pathogenic. (*Entamoeba histolytica* has now been split into *E. histolytica* which is always regarded as pathogenic, and *E. dispar* (formerly non-pathogenic *E. histolytica*) which had originally been proposed by Brumpt in 1925 and was confirmed by Sargeaunt (1993).) However, where asymptomatic cyst passage persists following therapy of amoebic dysentery or amoebic liver abscess, further treatment with a luminal amoebicide is mandatory, otherwise relapse is frequent (Knight 1980).

In areas where indigenous amoebiasis is very uncommon, most *E. histolytica/E. dispar* infections are imported, and good luminal amoebicides are readily available, so the decision is more in favour of treatment. Ideally, treatment strategy should be based on the results of isoenzyme or monoclonal antibody typing (after initial culture of tropho-zoites from the amoebic cysts) to separate *E. histolytica* from *E. dispar* (since they are morphologically identical), but the technique is time-consuming and available in only a few centres. Some population groups appear to harbour only non-pathogenic strains. For example, Allason-Jones et al (1988) studied '*E. histolytica*' cysts from male homosexuals

in London and all strains had a non-pathogenic zymodeme pattern. They concluded that asymptomatic '*E. histolytica*', cyst passage in homosexual men did not require treatment.

Giardiasis

The treatment of choice is tinidazole 2 g as a single dose, a regimen effective in approximately 90% of cases. Metroni-dazole 2 g/day for 3 days gives a similar cure rate. Low dose, longer duration metronidazole regimens (200 mg three times daily for 7–10 days) give reported cure rates of 60–87% (Mendelson 1980). Failure of therapy with nitro-imidazole therapy may be due to variety of possible factors: reinfection, underlying immunodeficiency, or drug resis-tance. Where nitroimidazole resistance is thought to be the explanation, there are few alternative agents.

Mepacrine (quinacrine, atebrin) is active against *Giardia* (Thomas 1952) and is given as 100 mg three times daily for 5–7 days with reported cure rates of 90–95% (Wolfe 1992, Hill 1993). It should be used with caution in view of its known side-effects. Wolfe (1978) reported toxic psychosis in 1.5% of adult patients treated with this agent. Other side-effects include CNS stimulation and (on prolonged therapy) yellow discoloration of the skin.

Furazolidone provides another option (Farthing 1992) and is given at 100 mg four times daily for 7 days, with reported cure rates of 75–90% (Wolfe 1992). Side-effects, though usually mild, occur in approximately 20% of patients (Mendelson 1980) and patients with glucose-6-phosphate dehydrogenase(G-6-PD) deficiency may develop haemolysis on furazolidone.

Hall & Nahar (1993) compared the efficacy of albendazole with that of metronidazole against *Giardia* infection of children in Bangladesh. Albendazole, 400 mg/day for 5 days produced a 94.8% cure rate, no different from the 97.4% cure rate produced in children receiving metronidazole 375 mg/day for 5 days.

Paromomycin (aminosidine) (25–30 mg/kg daily in 3 divided doses for 5–10 days) is effective in 60 to 70% of cases (Hill 1993). As it is excreted nearly 100% unchanged in the faeces, it is used by some practitioners when nitroimidazoles cannot be used in pregnancy.

Trichomonas vaginalis

Metronidazole 2 g as a single oral dose has produced cure rates as high as 97% (Lossick 1980). An alternative regimen is 400 mg twice daily for 7 days. Tidwell et al (1994) compared a single 2 g oral dose of metronidazole with a single 2 g intravaginal dose: 88% of the oral group but only 50% of the intravaginal group were microbiologically cured ($p = 0.0037$).

Tinidazole 2 g as a single dose, repeated if the first dose fails to produce clinical benefit, is an alternative to metronidazole.

Secnidazole, another nitroimidazole, is also effective against *Trichomonas* when given as a single 2 g dose (Bagnoli 1994).

The commonest causes of treatment failure are reinfection or non-compliance with therapy, but metronidazole-resistant strains of *Trichomonas vaginalis* are well documented (Lossick et al 1986). Higher doses of metronidazole have been used in an attempt to clear the infection, e.g. 2 g/day by mouth plus 500 mg intravaginally in women, for 7–14 days, and some clinicians have used high-dose intravenous therapy (Dombrowski et al 1987). However, side-effects can reduce compliance with high-dose therapy. As the alternative agents to metronidazole are also nitroimidazoles, there is an urgent need for new antitrichomonal agents.

Cryptosporidium parvum

Diarrhoea due to this organism is usually self-limiting in those with normal immunity, but can be devastating in the immunocompromised, notably in patients suffering from AIDS. There is no highly effective treatment, but paromomycin has been reported effective in a double-blind placebo-controlled trial (White et al 1994). Vargas et al (1993) reported successful use of azithromycin in two cases in immunocompromised children. Hyperimmune bovine colostrum has also been used (Plettenberg et al 1993, Shield et al 1993).

Isospora belli

The treatment of choice is co-trimoxazole (De Hovitz et al 1986). Furazolidone is an alternative.

Cyclospora cayetanensis

Cyclospora infection may be self-limiting, so antimicrobial therapy is not required in every case. Where specific treatment is deemed necessary, the agent of choice is co-trimoxazole (Pape et al 1994, Hoge et al 1995).

Microsporidiosis

Intestinal microsporidiosis in AIDS patients is caused by *Enterocytozoon bieneusi* or *Septata intestinalis* (renamed *Encephalitozoon intestinalis*). Both can be treated with albendazole, but this agent appears to be less effective on *E. bieneusi* (Weber & Bryan 1994, Molina et al 1995).

Babesiosis

BABESIA BOVIS/BABESIA DIVERGENS

This is usually encountered in splenectomized humans, leading to fulminant illness and death. There are no controlled trials of treatment. Diminazene (Berenil) is active against animal babesiosis and was used in a case of human infection with *B. divergens*, but the patient did not survive (Raoult et al 1987). The same authors reported successful treatment of a splenectomized patient infected with this parasite using pentamidine plus co-trimoxazole. Successful treatment of three cases with massive exchange blood transfusion (2–3 blood volumes) followed by intravenous clindamycin and oral quinine was reported by Brasseur & Gorenflot (1992).

BABESIA MICROTI INFECTION

In most cases patients suffer a mild illness and recover spontaneously. Where illness is severe enough to merit treatment, quinine plus clindamycin is the treatment of choice (Telford et al 1993). Whole blood or red cell exchange transfusion has produced a rapid and substantial fall in parasitaemia (Jacoby et al 1980). Azithromycin (Weiss et al 1993) and atovaquone (Hughes & Oz 1995) have shown encouraging activity against *B. microti* in a hamster model.

References

Allason-Jones E, Mindel A, Sargeaunt P, Katz D 1988 Outcome of untreated infection with *Entamoeba histolytica* in homosexual men with and without HIV antibody. *British Medical Journal* 297: 654–657

Anabwani G M, Bryceson A D M 1982 Visceral leishmaniasis in Kenyan children. *Indian Paediatrics* 19: 819–822

Andrade S G, Rassi A, Magalhaes J B, Ferriolli-Filho F, Luquetti A O 1992 Specific chemotherapy of Chagas' disease: a comparison between the response in patients and experimental animals inoculated with the same strains. *Transactions of the Royal Society of Tropical Medicine and Hygiene* 86: 624–626

Anon 1993 Spiramycin. In: Reynolds J E F (ed) Martindale, the extra pharmacopoeia, 30th edn. Pharmaceutical Press, London, p 202.3–203.2

Badaro R, Nascimento C, Carvalho J S et al 1994 Recombinant human granulocyte–macrophage colony-stimulating factor reverses neutropenia and reduces secondary infections in visceral leishmaniasis. *Journal of Infectious Diseases* 170: 413–418

Bagnoli V R 1994 An overview of the clinical experience with secnidazole in bacterial vaginosis and trichomoniasis. *Drugs under Investigation* 8 (suppl 1): 53–60

Berrebi A, Kobuch W E, Bessieres M H et al 1994 Termination of pregnancy for maternal toxoplasmosis. *Lancet* 344: 36–39

Brasseur P, Gorenflot A 1992 Human babesiosis in Europe. *Memorias do Instituto Oswaldo Cruz* 87: 131–132

Bryceson A D M 1970 Diffuse cutaneous leishmaniasis in Ethiopia: II treatment. *Transactions of the Royal Society of Tropical Medicine and Hygiene* 64: 369–379

Bryceson A D M 1987 Therapy in man. In: Peters W, Killick-Kendrick R E (eds) The leishmaniases in biology and medicine. Academic Press, London, vol 2, p 848–907

Bryceson A D M, Murphy A, Moody A 1994 treatment of 'Old World' cutaneous leishmaniasis with aminosidine ointment: results of an open study in London. *Transactions of the Royal Society of Tropical Medicine and Hygiene* 88: 226–228

Chatterton J M W 1992 Pregnancy. In: Ho-Yen D O, Joss A W L (eds) Human toxoplasmosis. Oxford University Press, Oxford, p 144–183

Daffos F, Forestier F, Capella-Pavlovsky M et al 1988 Prenatal management of 746 pregnancies at risk for congenital toxoplasmosis. *New England Journal of Medicine* 318: 271–275

Daffos F, Mirlesse V, Hohlfeld P, Jacquemard F, Thulliez P, Forestier F 1994 Toxoplasmosis in pregnancy [letter]. *Lancet* 344: 541

Davidson R N, Russo R 1994 Relapse of visceral leishmaniasis in patients who were coinfected with human immunodeficiency virus and who received treatment with liposomal amphotericin B. *Clinical Infectious Diseases* 19: 560

Davidson R N, DiMartino L, Gradoni L et al 1994 Liposomal amphotericin B (AmBisome) in Mediterranean visceral leishmaniasis: a multi-centre trial. *Quarterly Journal of Medicine* 87: 75–81

De Hovitz J A, Pape J W, Boncy M, Johnson W D 1986 Clinical manifestations and therapy of *Isospora belli* infection in patients with the acquired immunodeficiency syndrome. *New England Journal of Medicine* 315: 87–90

Derouin F, Debure A, Godeaut E, Lariviere M, Kreis H 1987 *Toxoplasma* antibody titres in renal transplant recipients. *Transplantation* 44: 515–518

Derouin F, Devergie A, Auber P et al 1992 Toxoplasmosis in bone marrow transplant recipients: report of seven cases and review. *Clinical Infectious Diseases* 15: 267–270

Dietze R, Milan E P, Berman J D et al 1993 Treatment of Brazilian Kala-Azar with a short course of Amphocil (amphotericin B cholesterol dispersion). *Clinical Infectious Diseases* 17: 981–986

Dombrowski M P, Sokol R J, Brown W J, Bronsteeen R A 1987 Intravenous therapy of metronidazole-resistant *Trichomonas vaginalis*. *Obstetrics and Gynecology* 69: 524–525

Du Pont H L 1994 Prevention and treatment strategies in giardiasis and amoebiasis. *Drugs under Investigation* 8 (suppl 1): 19–25

Dutton G N 1989a Toxoplasmic retinochoroiditis – a historical review and current concepts. *Annals of the Academy of Medicine Singapore* 18: 214–221

Dutton G N 1989b Recent developments in the prevention and treatment of congenital toxoplasmosis. *International Ophthalmology* 13: 407–413

Farthing M J G 1992 *Giardia* comes of age: progress in epidemiology, immunology and chemotherapy. *Journal of Antimicrobial Chemotherapy* 30: 563–566

Fleisher D I, Hepler R S, Landau J W 1974 Blindness during diiodohydroxyquin (Diodoquin®) therapy: a case report. *Pediatrics* 54: 106–108

Gallerano R H, Marr J J, Sosa R R 1990 Therapeutic efficacy of allopurinol in patients with chronic Chagas' disease. *American Journal of Tropical Medicine and Hygiene* 43: 159–166

Guerina N G, Ho-Wen H, Meissner H C et al 1994 Neonatal serologic screening and early treatment for congenital *Toxoplasma gondii* infection. *New England Journal of Medicine* 330: 1858–1863

Hall A, Nahar Q 1993 Albendazole as a treatment for infections with *Giardia duodenalis* in children in Bangladesh. *Transactions of the Royal Society of Tropical Medicine and Hygiene* 87: 84–86

Harms G, Chehade A K, Douba M et al 1991 A randomized trial comparing a pentavalent antimonial drug and recombinant interferon-gamma in the local treatment of cutaneous leishmaniasis. *Transactions of the Royal Society of Tropical Medicine and Hygiene* 85: 214–216

Hatchuel W 1975 Tinidazole for the treatment of amoebic liver abscess. *South African Medical Journal* 49: 1879–1881

Herwaldt B L, Berman J D 1992 Recommendations for treating leishmaniasis with sodium stibogluconate (pentostam) and review of pertinent clinical studies. *American Journal of Tropical Medicine and Hygiene* 46: 296–306

Hill D R 1993 Giardiasis. *Infectious Disease Clinics of North America* 7: 503–526

Hoge C W, Shlim D R, Ghimire M et al 1995 Placebo-controlled trial of co-trimoxazole for cyclospora infections among travellers and foreign residents in Nepal. *Lancet* 345: 691–693

Hohlfeld P, Daffos F, Thulliez P et al 1989 Fetal toxoplasmosis: outcome of pregnancy and infant follow-up after in utero treatment. *Journal of Paediatrics* 115: 765–769

Ho-Yen D O 1992 Immunocompromised patients. In: Ho-Yen D O, Joss A W L (eds) Human toxoplasmosis. Oxford University Press, Oxford, p 184–203

Hughes W T, Oz H S 1995 Successful prevention and treatment of babesiosis with atovaquone. *Journal of Infectious Diseases* 172: 1042–1046

Jacoby G A, Hunt J V, Kosinski K S et al 1980 Treatment of transfusion-transmitted babesiosis by exchange transfusion. *New England Journal of Medicine* 303: 1098–1100

Joss A W L 1992 Treatment. In: Ho-Yen D O, Joss A W L (eds) Human toxoplasmosis. Oxford University Press, Oxford, p 119–143

Knight R 1980 The chemotherapy of amoebiasis. *Journal of Antimicrobial Chemotherapy* 6: 577–593

Koppe J G, Loewer-Sieger D H, De Roever-Bonnet H 1986 Results of 20-year follow-up of congenital toxoplasmosis. *Lancet* i: 254–256

Luft B J, Noat Y, Araujo F G, Stinson E B, Remington J S 1983 Primary and reactivated toxoplasma infection in patients with cardiac transplants. Clinical spectrum and problems in diagnosis in a defined population. *Annals of Internal Medicine* 99: 27–31

Lossick J G 1980 Single-dose metronidazole treatment for vaginal trichomonas. *Obstetrics and Gynaecology* 56: 508–510

Lossick J G, Muller M, Gorrell T E 1986 In vitro drug susceptibility and doses of metronidazole required for cure in cases of refractory vaginal trichomoniasis. *Journal of Infectious Diseases* 153: 948–955

McCabe R, Chirurgi V 1993 Issues in toxoplasmosis. *Infectious Disease Clinics of North America* 7: 587–604

McCann P P, Bacchi C J, Clarkson A B et al 1986 Inhibition of polyamine biosynthesis by α-difluoromethylornithine in African trypanosomes and *Pneumocystis carinii* as a basis of chemotherapy: biochemical and clinical aspects. *American Journal of Tropical Medicine and Hygiene* 35: 1153–1156

Mason J C, Ordelheide K S, Grames G M et al 1987 Toxoplasmosis in two renal transplant recipients from a single donor. *Transplantation* 44: 588–591

Mendelson R M 1980 The treatment of giardiasis. *Transactions of the Royal Society of Tropical Medicine and Hygiene* 74: 438–439

Milord F, Pepin J, Loko L, Ethier L, Mpia B 1992 Efficacy and toxicity of eflornithine for treatment of *Trypanosoma brucei gambiense* sleeping sickness. *Lancet* 340: 652–655

Mishra M, Biswas U K, Jha A M, Khan A B 1994 Amphotericin versus sodium stibogluconate in first-line treatment of Indian kala-azar. *Lancet* 344: 1599–1600

Molina J-M, Oksenhendler E, Beauvais B et al 1995 Disseminated microsporidiosis due to *Septata intestinalis* in patients with AIDS: clinical features and response to albendazole therapy. *Journal of Infectious Diseases* 171: 245–249

Nguyen B T, Stadtsbaeder S 1983 Comparative effects of cotrimoxazole (trimethoprim–sulphamethoxazole), pyrimethamine–sulphadiazine and spiramycin during avirulent infection with *Toxoplasma gondii* (Beverley strain) in mice. *British Journal of Pharmacology* 79: 923–928

Olliaro P L, Bryceson A D M 1993 Practical progress and new drugs for changing patterns of leishmaniasis. *Parasitology Today* 9: 323–328

Pape J W, Verdier R I, Boncy M, Bincy J, Johnson W D Jr 1994 *Cyclospora* infection in adults infected with HIV. Clinical manifestations, treatment, and prophylaxis. *Annals of Internal Medicine* 121: 654–657

Pepin J, Milord F, Guern C, Schechter P J 1987 Difluoromethylornithine for arseno-resistant *Trypanosoma brucei gambiense* sleeping sickness. *Lancet* ii: 1431–1433

Pepin J, Milord F, Guern C, Mpia B, Ethier L, Mansinsa D 1989 Trial of prednisolone for prevention of melarsoprol-induced encephalopathy in Gambiense sleeping sickness. *Lancet* i: 1246–1250

Pepin J, Milord F, Meurice F, Ethier L, Loko L, Mpia B 1992 High dose nifurtimox for arseno-resistant *Trypanosoma brucei gambiense* sleeping sickness: an open trial in Central Zaire. *Transactions of the Royal Society of Tropical Medicine and Hygiene* 86: 254–256

Plettenberg A, Stoehr A, Stellbrink H-J, Albrecht H, Meigel W 1993 A preparation from bovine colostrum in the treatment of HIV-positive patients with chronic diarrhoea. *Clinical Investigator* 71: 42–45

Powell S J, Wilmott A J, Elsdon-Dew R 1967 Further trials of metronidazole in amoebic dysentery and amoebic liver abscess. *Annals of Tropical Medicine and Parasitology* 61: 511–514

Raoult D, Soulayrol L, Toga B, Dumon H, Casanovna P 1987 Babesiosis, pentamidine and cotrimoxazole. *Annals of Internal Medicine* 107: 944

Reed S L 1992 Amoebiasis: an update. *Clinical Infectious Diseases* 14: 385–393

Rothova A, Buitenhuis H J, Meenken C et al 1989 Therapy of ocular toxoplasmosis. *International Ophthalmology* 13: 415–419

Sargeaunt P G 1993 *Entamoeba histolytica*: a question answered. *Tropical Disease Bulletin* 90: R1–R2

Scott J A G, Davidson R N, Moody A H et al 1992 Aminosidine (paromomycin) in the treatment of leishmaniasis imported into the United Kingdom. *Transactions of the Royal Society of Tropical Medicine and Hygiene* 86: 617–619

Scragg J N 1975 Hepatic amoebiasis in childhood. *Tropical Doctor* 5: 132–134

Scragg J N, Proctor E M 1977 Tinidazole in treatment of amoebic liver abscess in children. *Archives of Diseases of Childhood* 52: 408–410

Scragg J N, Rubidge C J, Proctor E M 1976 Tinidazole in treatment of acute amoebic dysentery in children. *Archives of Diseases of Childhood* 51: 385–387

Shield J, Melville C, Novelli V et al 1993 Bovine colostrum immunoglobulin concentrate for cryptosporidiosis in AIDS. *Archives of Diseases of Childhood* 69: 451–453

Solari A, Saavedra H, Sepulveda C et al 1993 Successful treatment of *Trypanosoma cruzi* encephalitis in a patient with haemophilia and AIDS. *Clinical Infectious Diseases* 16: 255–259

Squires K E, Rosenkaimer F, Sherwood J A, Forni A L, Were J B O, Murray H W 1993 Immunochemotherapy for visceral leishmaniasis: a controlled pilot trial of antimony versus antimony plus interferon-gamma. *American Journal of Tropical Medicine and Hygiene* 48: 666–669

Sundar S, Rosenkaimer F, Murray H W 1994 Successful treatment of refractory visceral leishmaniasis in India using antimony plus interferon-gamma. *Journal of Infectious Diseases* 170: 659–662

Tanowitz H B, Kirchhoff L V, Simon D, Morris S A, Weiss L M, Wittner M 1992 Chagas' disease. *Clinical Microbiology Reviews* 5: 400–419

Teklemariam S, Hiwot A G, Frommel D, Miko T L, Ganlov G, Bryceson A 1994 Aminosidine and its combination with sodium stibogluconate in the treatment of diffuse cutaneous leishmaniasis caused by *Leishmania aethiopica*. *Transactions of the Royal Society of Medicine and Hygiene* 88: 334–339

Telford S R III, Gorenflot A, Brasseur P, Spielman A 1993 Babesial infections in humans and wildlife. In: Krier J P, Baker J R (eds) Parasitic protozoa, 2nd edn. Academic Press, San Diego, vol 5, p 1–47

Thakur C P, Olliaro P, Gothoskar S et al 1992 Treatment of visceral leishmaniasis (kala-azar) with aminosidine (=paromomycin)–antimonial combinations, a pilot study in Bihar, India. *Transactions of the Royal Society of Tropical Medicine and Hygiene* 86: 615–616

Thomas M E M 1952 Observations upon the effects of mepacrine and other substances on *Giardia intestinalis*. *Parasitology* 42: 262–268

Tidwell B H, Lushbaugh W B, Laughlin M D, Cleary J D, Finley R W 1994 A double-blind placebo-controlled trial of single-dose intravaginal versus single-dose oral metronidazole in the treatment of trichomonal vaginitis. *Journal of Infectious Diseases* 170: 242–246

Torre-Cisneros J, Villanueva J L, Kindelan J M, Jurado R, Sanchez-Guijo P 1993 Successful treatment of antimony-resistant visceral leishmaniasis with liposomal amphotericin B in patients infected with human immunodeficiency virus. *Clinical Infectious Diseases* 17: 625–627

Vargas S L, Shenep J L, Flynn P M, Pui C-H, Santana V M, Hughes W T 1993 Azithromycin for treatment of severe *Cryptosporidium* diarrhoea in two children with cancer. *Journal of Pediatrics* 123: 154–156

Wallon M, Gandilhon F, Peyron F, Mojon M 1994 Toxoplasmosis in pregnancy [letter]. *Lancet* 344: 541

Weber R, Bryan R T 1994 Microsporidial infections in immunodeficient and immunocompetent patients. *Clinical Infectious Diseases* 19: 517–521

Weiss L M, Wittner M, Wasserman S, Oz H S, Retsema J, Tanowitz H B 1993 Efficacy of azithromycin for treating *Babesia microti* infection in the hamster model. *Journal of Infectious Diseases* 168: 1289–1292

White A C Jr, Chappel C L, Hayat C S, Kimball K T, Flanigan T P, Goodgame R W 1994 Paromomycin for cryptosporidiosis in AIDS: a prospective, double-blind trial. *Journal of Infectious Diseases* 170: 419–424

WHO 1990 Drugs used in parasitic diseases. WHO, Geneva

WHO 1991 Control of Chagas' disease. WHO technical report series 811. WHO, Geneva

Wolfe M S 1978 Giardiasis. *New England Journal of Medicine* 298: 319–321

Wolfe M S 1992 Giardiasis. *Clinical Microbiology Reviews* 5: 93–100

Wong S-Y, Remington J S 1994 Toxoplasmosis in pregnancy. *Clinical Infectious Diseases* 18: 853–862

Wreghitt T G, Hakim M, Gray J J et al 1989 Toxoplasmosis in heart and heart and lung transplant recipients. *Journal of Clinical Pathology* 42: 194–199

Helminthic infections

G. C. Cook

Nematodes, trematodes, and cestodes can all account for significant human pathology (Tables 64.1 and 64.2) (Leech et al 1988, Cook 1990, 1991, 1996, Blaser 1995, Mandell et al 1995). Whilst serious manifestations are unusual, when they do occur disastrous consequences may ensue (see below). Serodiagnostic and imaging techniques have, in recent years, made diagnosis far more straightforward; however, the need for a careful geographical history (precise whereabouts of overseas travel should not be neglected) in addition to careful parasitological investigation remains of paramount importance. From a chemotherapeutic viewpoint, introduction of the benzimidazole compounds (now dominated by albendazole) for nematode, and praziquantel for trematode and cestode infections, has revolutionized management (Cook 1990, Mandell et al 1995) (Ch. 38).

Table 64.1 Taxonomic classification of the more common helminthic infections affecting man

Group or class	Organism	Mode of transmission to man
Nematodes (roundworms)	Ascaris lumbricoides	Ingestion of embryonated eggs
	Ancylostoma duodenale, Necator americanus	Skin penetration by larvae
	Strongyloides stercoralis	Larval penetration of skin or colorectum
	Trichuris trichiura	Ingestion of embryonated eggs
	Enterobius vermicularis	Ingestion of eggs
	Trichinella spiralis	Ingestion of muscle larvae
	Wuchereria bancrofti, Brugia malayi	Injection of larvae during mosquito bite
	Onchocerca volvulus, Loa loa, Dracunculus medinensis	Injection of larvae during black fly bite
Trematodes (flukes)	Schistosoma haematobium, Schis. mansoni, Schis. japonicum, Schis. intercalatum, Schis. mekongi	Penetration of intact human skin by cercariae
	Clonorchis sinensis, Opisthorchis viverrini	Ingestion of metacercariae in freshwater fish
	Fasciola hepatica	Ingestion of metacercariae on aquatic plants
Cestodes (tapeworms)	Taenia solium	Ingestion of cysticerci in pork
	Taenia solium	Ingestion of eggs from infected person
	Taenia saginata	Ingestion of cysticerci in beef
	Echinococcus granulosus, E. multilocularis	Ingestion of eggs in faecally contaminated food/water

Table 64.2   *Less common helminthic infections (and resultant clinical manifestations) affecting man*

Group or class	Organism	Mode of transmission to man
Nematodes (roundworms)	Eosinophilic meningitis: *Angiostrongylus cantonensis*	Ingestion of larvae in undercooked snail, crab, prawn, or slug-contaminated vegetables
	Gnathostoma spinigerum	Ingestion of encysted larvae in flesh of intermediate host(s)
	Toxocara canis	Ingestion of larvae in canine faeces
	Other causes of visceral larva migrans	
Trematodes (flukes)	*Paragonimus westermani*	Ingestion of metacercariae in crayfish or freshwater crabs
Cestodes (tapeworms)	Coenuriasis: *Diphyllobothrium latum*	Ingestion of eggs in freshwater fish

Nematode infections

GEOHELMINTHS

The intestinal helminths (geohelminths) account for literally millions of human infections throughout tropical and subtropical countries (Cook 1990, Mandell et al 1995). *Ascaris lumbricoides* and hookworm (*Ancylostoma duodenale* and *Necator americanus*) infections account for the majority. The former is acquired via contaminated food or water, but the latter by larval invasion of intact skin. Both are easily diagnosed by identification of characteristic eggs in a faecal sample. Chemotherapy is with one of the benzimidazole compounds (which should preferably be avoided during pregnancy); when available, albendazole (400 mg twice daily for 3 days) gives a very high success rate. Other agents are now rarely used in a temperate (developed) country, but in those where funding is unsatisfactory, one or the other of the older preparations continues to be used. Side-effects from benzimidazole compounds when used at low dosage are very unusual.

STRONGYLOIDES STERCORALIS INFECTION

Strongyloides stercoralis is a small nematode that occurs world-wide, but more commonly in certain parts of the tropics than others – notably west Africa, the Caribbean and South-East Asia (Cook 1990, Mandell et al 1995). It is by no means uncommon in some temperate areas also, including much of Europe and northern America. As with hookworm, infection usually occurs when intact skin is penetrated by *S. stercoralis* larvae (which can survive in moist soil contaminated with human faeces for many weeks); faecal–oral transmission is also possible. The human life-cycle (as with the other geohelminths, see above) consists of migration through the lungs, trachea and pharynx, and thence to the small intestine where maturation to egg-laying adults occurs. After hatching, the eggs produce rhabditiform larvae; although usually excreted in faeces (from which a parasitological diagnosis can be readily made), they can also reinfect their host (autoinfection) by re-entering at ileal, colorectal and/or anal sites. This cycle (which is not present with either *A. lumbricoides* or hookworm infection) can persist for ≥40 years. During migration, numerous systemic sequelae can present clinically, the most spectacular of which consists of a serpiginous urticarial rash (larva currens) over the trunk, buttocks and groins (Cook 1990).

The major importance of this particular nematode, however, is that in the presence of severe immunosuppression such as corticosteroid administration, HTLV-1-associated lymphoma, acute leukaemia or renal transplant, an overwhelming infection ('hyperinfection syndrome') in which all organs can be invaded by *S. stercoralis* larvae may occur (Igra-Siegman et al 1981, Vishwanath et al 1982, Cook 1987), although HIV-positive subjects do not appear to be at particular risk. This syndrome frequently presents with paralytic ileus and is followed by Gram-negative septicaemia caused by faecal organisms (which include *Escherichia coli*), and meningitis (see below); the condition is frequently fatal if chemotherapy is not immediately instituted. A mortality rate up to 77% has been recorded; however, the condition is frequently superimposed on a serious underlying disease, often neoplastic. Rarely, this syndrome occurs in the immunocompetent individual. When central nervous system (CNS) invasion occurs, the usual sequel is meningitis, which is caused by *Esch. coli* and/or larvae of *S. stercoralis*; both organisms are often detected in cerebrospinal fluid (CSF) (Smallman et al 1986). This condition can masquerade as cerebral vasculitis. Larvae are deposited throughout the CNS via haematogenous spread (resulting in small infarcts) and perivascular spaces (leading to involvement of dura, subarachnoid space, and meninges).

In addition to the CNS findings, peripheral blood eosinophilia (sometimes also reflected in CSF) is usually, but not always present. An enzyme-linked immunosorbent assay (ELISA) is of value, and serological tests for filariasis often give false-positive results.

Thiabendazole is of value, whether or not the hyper-infection syndrome is present (see below) (Igra-Siegman et al 1981, Vishwanath et al 1982, Cook 1987); in a straightforward infection, a standard 3-day course (25 mg/kg daily) has been recommended for many years. Recently, albendazole (400 mg twice daily for 7 days) has been used with encouraging results. Like albendazole, thiabendazole is well absorbed, and dizziness and gastro-intestinal disturbances (especially anorexia, nausea and vomiting) are common; other symptoms include: pruritus, skin rashes, headache, fatigue, drowsiness, drying of mucous membranes, hyperglycaemia, visual disturbances (especially with colour vision), leucopenia, tinnitus, cholestasis (and parenchymal liver damage). Crystalluria, bradycardia and hypotension have been recorded; Stevens–Johnson syndrome, toxic epidermal necrolysis, convulsions and mental disturbances are rare. Fever, chills, angioedema and lymphadenopathy are probably the result of an allergic response to dead parasites. A case can be made for prophylactic benzimidazole chemotherapy in immunosuppressed patients if there is doubt as to whether the infection has been eradicated (Cook 1987).

In the immunosuppressed individual, with the 'hyper-infection syndrome', the benzimidazole compounds also form the basis of effective chemotherapy; however, dose regimens are, of necessity, longer, and even then the eradication rate is certainly <100% (Igra-Siegman et al 1981, Vishwanath et al 1982, Cook 1987). Albendazole 400 mg twice daily for 14 days is usually adequate; however, prolonged (repeated) courses are often necessary and limited evidence indicates that thiabendazole (a compound which produces far more side-effects) (Igra-Siegman et al 1981) gives a superior result.

COLORECTAL INFECTIONS

Two colorectal nematode infections, *Trichuris trichiura* (whipworm) and *Enterobius vermicularis* (threadworm), are easily treated with one of the benzimidazole compounds (Cook 1990, 1996); both mebendazole and albendazole give a satisfactory cure result.

TRICHINELLA SPIRALIS INFECTION

Trichinellosis (or trichinosis) results from infection by the nematode *T. spiralis* (Gay et al 1982, Murrell 1991, Cook 1985a) acquired in man by ingestion of muscles of infected

wild animals or domestic pigs. Arctic polar bears also carry infection. The infection is a major clinical problem in the USA, Mexico, Chile and some other South American countries; among tropical countries, Thailand, Kenya, Tanzania and Senegal encounter the disease. Following an initial intestinal phase, the invasive stage begins 7–9 days later, and involvement of skeletal muscles usually dominates the clinical picture. Other organ (including myocardial and CNS) involvement is rarely prominent; in the latter, meningeal irritation may simulate meningitis, and intra-cranial haemorrhage is an occasional accompaniment (Gay et al 1982, Murrell 1991). Dizziness, ataxia, hysteria and psychoses may be present; in a severe infection, seizures, monoparesis and coma may ensue. Rarely, CNS involvement proves fatal. Peripheral blood and/or CSF eosinophilia is usually present. CSF may be xanthochromic. An ELISA is of diagnostic value. Muscle biopsy frequently confirms the diagnosis; relevant enzymes may be elevated. Cortico-steroids are indicated if cerebral oedema is present. Thiabendazole and other benzimidazoles have shown a high degree of efficacy (Murrell 1991).

HUMAN FILARIASES

The human filariases comprise several systemic nematode infections: *Wuchereria bancrofti* and *Brugia malayi* (lymphatic filariases) (Cook 1990, 1996), onchocerciasis (river blindness) (Cook 1990, 1996), loaiasis (Duke 1991, Negesse et al 1985) and dracontiasis (Muller 1971). Diethylcarbamazine (DEC) has formed the major chemothe-rapeutic weapon for several decades. Recently, ivermectin has been widely introduced for *Onchocerca volvulus* infection (Cook 1996).

Management of the lymphatic filariases is usually straightforward; a 21-day course of DEC (2–3 mg/kg three times daily) is the standard chemotherapeutic regimen.

Filarial infections do not usually involve the CNS. However, *Loa loa* (Duke 1991, Negesse et al 1985) and *Dracunculus medinensis* (Muller 1971) occasionally produce problems. *O. volvulus* has a profound effect on the eye, but brain and spinal cord pathology has not been well documented; however, microfilariae have rarely been demonstrated in CSF.

Loa loa infection

Loaiasis is a human nematode infection (confined to west and central Africa) which is transmitted by tabanid flies belonging to the genus *Chrysops*. Clinical sequelae include: subcutaneous (Calabar) swellings, and migration of the adult worm conjunctivally (Negesse et al 1985, Duke 1991). Microfilariae are present in peripheral blood during the middle part of the day (unlike the lymphatic filariases, when microfilaraemia usually occurs at night). However, visceral lesions can occur, the most serious of which is meningo-encephalitis (the subarachnoid space contains many micro-filariae, and they may be present in CSF). Encephalitis (often accompanied by retinal haemorrhages) results from an allergic reaction to dead and dying microfilariae which obstruct the cerebral capillaries; this rarely proves fatal. The mechanism by which occlusive thrombi form around *L. loa* microfilariae is unclear, but the syndrome has usually been associated with treatment (and killing of microfilariae) with DEC. Diagnosis is by detection of microfilariae in peripheral blood (a concentration technique may be necessary); an ELISA is usually positive. Loaiasis tends to be considered the least important of the human filariases, but its potential seriousness must be emphasized. DEC (see above) is the most effective chemotherapeutic agent, but a corticosteroid 'cover' is advisable, especially in a severe infection. Prophylactic regimens using DEC are now being applied in affected areas (Nutman et al 1988).

Dracunculus medinensis infection

Guinea worm infection causes lesions, usually superficial, in connective tissue and subcutaneous tissue(s) (Muller 1971); these result from perforation of the skin by the female worm with larval release into the surrounding water (tetanus is an occasional added complication). The larvae infect *Cyclops* spp., which are subsequently ingested in contaminated drinking water, to complete the life-cycle. The disease is present in west and central Africa, western parts of the Indian subcontinent and the Arabian peninsula. In some cases, instead of bursting through subcutaneous tissue, the worm penetrates a joint(s); this rarely affects the vertebral column, in which case a spinal extradural abscess with neurological damage may result; paraplegia, with subse-quent mortality, has been recorded. Serology is of value in diagnosis, and peripheral blood eosinophilia may be present. The benzimidazole compounds (thiabendazole), metronidazole and niridazole have all been used in chemotherapy (Muller 1971). However, surgical intervention and antibiotics are frequently necessary to deal with complications. The World Health Organization (WHO) has instituted a campaign for global eradication.

LESS COMMON NEMATODE INFECTIONS

Table 64.2 summarizes some less common nematode infections (with resultant clinical manifestations) affecting man (Cook 1990, 1996).

Animal nematodes, i.e. those 'foreign' to man – which have not achieved a significant degree of adaptation to this species, occasionally produce severe disease involving the CNS: *Angiostrongylus cantonensis*, *Gnathostoma spinigerum*,

Toxocara canis, *Capillaria hepatica* and *T. spiralis* (see above) fall into this category. The most dramatic illness of all can be caused by *S. stercoralis* (see above), but virtually always in the presence of severe immunosuppression. In addition to the infections covered in this section, two cases of *Micronema deletrix*, a saprophagous nematode infection causing fatal meningoencephalitis, have been recorded.

Eosinophilic meningoencephalitis

This term usually refers to infection by the rat lungworm *A. cantonensis* (Punyagupta et al 1975, Cook 1991). However, a rare condition – eosinophilic myeloencephalitis – which results from *G. spinigerum* infection (Bunnag et al 1970), presents in a similar way. Other infections which should be considered in differential diagnosis include: acute cysticercosis, paragonimiasis and toxocariasis; rarely, *Ascaris lumbricoides* and *S. stercoralis* (during their migratory cycles), and *Fasciola hepatica* also produce eosinophilic meningitis. Another example, albeit a rare one, is the trematode infection schistosomiasis (see below). Escargots have also been implicated (Editorial 1988). The diagnosis of this group of infections is unsatisfactory; unless larvae are demonstrated – occasionally in the brain or meninges (at biopsy or post-mortem examination) – the diagnosis is essentially a clinical one. Treatment of CNS nematode infections remains unsatisfactory; albendazole, not yet adequately evaluated, will probably prove the best available chemotherapeutic agent.

Angiostrongylus cantonensis infection

Although widely spread throughout the tropics, human infection most commonly occurs in South-East Asia, Papua New Guinea, the Pacific and Australia (Bunnag 1984, Cook 1990, 1996). The adult helminth is a delicate filariform nematode measuring 17–25 mm in length; it is neurotropic and requires a period of development in the brain of its definitive host, despite the fact that adults inhabit the pulmonary arteries of a wide range of rodents. Eggs are laid in the pulmonary capillaries, where they lodge and hatch; resultant larvae enter alveolar spaces, migrate into the trachea and subsequently enter the gastro-intestinal tract. Following excretion in faeces, they infect intermediate hosts (snails and slugs). When ingested by the rat, larvae migrate to the brain and thence to pulmonary arteries, thus completing the life cycle; at this latter point in the cycle, man may become an incidental host by accidentally ingesting larvae in raw or undercooked dishes containing snails, crabs, prawns or slug-contaminated vegetables. Cerebral congestion and small haemorrhages may be present; larvae of *A. cantonensis* can be recovered from meninges, blood vessels, or perivascular space(s) on the surface of the brain and spinal cord, and rarely eyes.

The incubation period is 6–15 days; most cases occur during the rainy season (Bunnag 1984). Severe occipital and bitemporal headache, nausea, vomiting, neck stiffness and sensory impairment may be present. Fever is uncommon. There may be evidence of meningitis, radiculitis and/or encephalitis. Motor weakness, localized paraesthesiae and cranial nerve involvement have been recorded; haemorrhage(s) and retinal detachment may be present.

CSF pressure is usually raised, and the fluid is turbid (>500 leucocytes/cm^3); in most cases eosinophils are present, and larvae are sometimes visualized. Peripheral eosinophilia is inconstant. An ELISA has been developed, but its availability in routine practice is limited.

Analgesics and corticosteroids may relieve symptoms, but specific therapy remains unsatisfactory (thiabendazole is ineffective, but albendazole seems promising); disease is usually self-limiting in 4–6 weeks and fatalities are rare (Bunnag 1991). Prevention depends on proper cooking of edible snails, especially the giant African snail *Achaina fulica,* and thorough washing of salad vegetables.

Gnathostoma spinigerum infection

Although most reports of this infection have been made in Asia (notably Thailand and Japan), sporadic cases occur in the Middle East, Europe, Africa and the Americas (Bunnag et al 1970, Cook 1990, 1996). Human infection is acquired by consumption of raw or undercooked flesh of intermediate hosts containing encysted larvae; it is possible that drinking water infected with *Cyclops* can convey infection.

Adults (males 11–25 and females 25–50 mm in length) lie coiled in a mass in the stomach wall of domestic and wild cats and dogs; eggs are extruded and excreted in faeces. In freshwater, the larvae hatch and infect *Cyclops*; here, they undergo development and are ingested by a fish, frog, snake or bird; when these animals are eaten by the definitive host, the parasites localize to the stomach, and mature in 3–12 months. Man is an incidental host in whom the life cycle is not completed; the worms are migratory and can involve any organ with production of necroses, haemorrhage(s) and an eosinophilic infiltration. The brain, spinal cord, choroid plexuses and eye may all be affected; in the latter, subconjunctival oedema, haemorrhage(s) and retinal damage can occur.

Clinically, a creeping eruption, migratory swellings (which are intensely itchy), low-grade fever, abdominal pain, tender hepatomegaly, pneumonitis and peripheral eosinophilia may be present (Bunnag et al 1970); other signs and symptoms depend on the system(s) involved. Neurologically, agonizing nerve root pain with paralysis of extremities and sensory impairment may be present; cerebral haemorrhage (sometimes massive) may occur. Ophthalmic involvement is unusual. The fatality rate is relatively high. Diagnosis is frequently difficult, and other helminthic infections (see above) should be considered; the myeloencephalitis should be distinguishable clinically from that caused by *A. cantonensis* (see above).

CSF is often xanthochromic or frankly bloody with an eosinophilic pleocytosis (leucocyte count >500 cells/mm^3). Serological studies are rarely conclusive. Definitive diagnosis depends on identifying the worm(s) at biopsy or post-mortem examination.

Antihistamines and corticosteroids are valuable in symptomatic relief of cutaneous swellings; surgical excision of a subcutaneous worm (for confirmation of the diagnosis) is occasionally feasible. Recent evidence indicates that albendazole produces a satisfactory chemotherapeutic response. Prevention consists of avoiding uncooked or poorly cooked freshwater fish, chicken, birds, snakes and other intermediate hosts; untreated drinking water should also be avoided.

Toxocariasis (visceral larva migrans)

Toxocara canis is a common and important canine zoonosis, occurring world-wide (Cook 1989, 1990, 1996). Although *T. canis* has been recognized in dogs since 1782, larval disease in man was not recognized until 1952 (Glickman & Schantz 1981). Its major importance in human disease is that it occasionally causes a retinal lesion (almost always unilateral) (ocular larva migrans) in children who have contact with pet dogs, which leads to blindness. CNS involvement occasionally occurs as part of the migratory cycle – visceral larva migrans; eosinophilic meningitis (Gould et al 1985) and convulsions have occasionally been reported.

Human infection is by accidental ingestion of embryonated eggs in food (from soil contaminated by dog faeces), or by sucking contaminated fingers (in children) (Gillespie 1987). Adult nematodes live in the dog small intestine, and infection usually occurs in utero or perinatally. Human infection takes place when embryonated ova (85 μm × 75 μm), which hatch into larvae (350 μm × 20 μm) in the lumen of the proximal small intestine, are ingested; following penetration of the mucosa the larvae enter the portal circulation and/or lymphatics and are transmitted to the liver; here, they are either halted (producing a granulomatous hepatitis) or pass into the lungs or another organ (brain and eye included) where granulomas are also formed.

Clinically, initial infection may be accompanied by fever, cough and malaise; this constitutes the host's immune response to migrating larvae (Taylor et al 1988). Abdominal pain, hepatomegaly, transient pneumonitis (with cough and wheeze) and lymphadenopathy may also be present (Schantz & Glickman 1978). In the CNS (Hill et al 1985), transient encephalitis can occur; in addition to Jacksonian or generalized seizures, ataxia, paresis and diabetes insipidus have been recorded. In fully developed disease choroidoretinitis (which must be differentiated from retinoblastoma) may be the sole evidence of infection. The possibility that *T. canis* (and possibly other migratory nematodes) can introduce pathogenic viruses (which include poliomyelitis and Japanese B encephalitis) to the brain by mechanical means has not been discounted.

Investigation reveals peripheral blood eosinophilia during the invasive stage. Descriptions of investigations when CNS involvement is present are scanty; however, eosinophilic pleocytosis in CSF is to be expected. Immunoglobulin G (IgG) and, to a lesser extent, immunoglobulins M and E (IgM and IgE) are elevated. An ELISA gives a high degree of sensitivity and specificity. Chest radiography may reveal generalized transient, peribronchial infiltrates. Myocardial involvement occasionally produces electrocardiographic changes. Liver histology frequently reveals *T. canis* ova surrounded by granulomas; the serum alkaline phosphatase concentration is usually elevated.

Although several chemotherapeutic agents, including diethylcarbamazine, albendazole, thiabendazole, fenbendazole and mebendazole, have been used, none has been adequately evaluated (Gillespie 1987). When CNS and/or ophthalmic involvement is present (or suspected), a corticosteroid 'cover' seems advisable. Prevention is by deworming pet dogs and by discontinuing (by legal means if possible) canine defaecation in public places, including pleasure parks.

Other causes of visceral larva migrans

This syndrome is caused rarely by *Capillaria hepatica*, a parasite which is confined to South-East Asia. Occasionally granulomata are discovered incidentally in brain at operation or post-mortem examination. *A. lumbricoides* and various dog ascarids have occasionally been identified. Any human small-intestinal nematode that undergoes a migratory cycle can produce a cerebral lesion(s).

Trematode infections

Table 64.1 and 64.2 summarize the more common trematode infections affecting man (Cook 1990, 1996).

SCHISTOSOMIASIS

Schistosoma mansoni and *S. haematobium* infection

S. mansoni is present throughout much of tropical Africa, the Middle East (including Saudi Arabia) and South America (Cook 1990, 1996). Human infection occurs by exposure of intact skin to freshwater containing cercariae of this trematode. Initial infection is occasionally followed by a local itchy eruption (swimmers' itch). Following this, schistosomulae are produced; following migration throughout most organs some localize to the portal venous system.

Between infection and maturation to adult worms (usually some 4–6 weeks) a clinical syndrome (acute schistosomiasis; Katayama fever) sometimes occurs in the previously unexposed individual (Cook 1990, 1996). The immunopathology of this disease is ill-understood; migratory schistosomulae, the beginning of egg laying by newly matured adults and an immune complex basis have all been postulated in aetiopathogenesis. Clinically, a febrile illness with diarrhoea, hepatosplenomegaly, bronchospasm, a giant urticarial rash and, rarely, CNS involvement (with an eosinophilia) are present with varying degrees of severity in acute infection. Although usually a self-limiting illness, significant mortality may result when infection is heavy. Specific antischistosomal chemotherapy (when given at this stage) should be accompanied by a corticosteroid 'cover'.

Following the initial illness, adult worm pairs settle into an 'ideal environment' in the inferior mesenteric venules, where they produce up to 3000 eggs daily (which become deposited in any organ – principally the colorectum and liver or in the case of *S. haematobium*, the lower urinary tract – with granuloma formation and fibrosis) for 30 years or more. Eggs are deposited in faeces or urine, and miracidia are produced when they reach freshwater; they infect freshwater snails to complete the life cycle. It is estimated that world-wide 100 million individuals suffer from hepatosplenic schistosomiasis.

The most common CNS complication of *S. mansoni* infection is transverse myelitis (Marcial-Rojas & Fiol 1963, Siddorn 1978); in addition to an eosinophilia in peripheral blood, the CSF shows a pleocytosis, often without eosinophils, and an elevated protein concentration. Anterior spinal artery occlusion (Efthimiou & Denning 1984, Bosnett & Dellen 1986), a granulomatous multiple root syndrome, intrathecal granuloma formation and myelitis have also been recorded. Although eggs are frequently deposited in the brain (especially when cardiopulmonary involvement is present), they rarely produce symptoms except in a very heavy infection. However, one study (from Egypt) using computed tomography (CT) scanning documented cortical atrophy in a high percentage (36%) of patients with chronic *Schis. mansoni* infection.

Diagnosis depends on detection of characteristic eggs in a faecal sample, rectal or liver biopsy (urine or bladder wall in the case of *S. haematobium* infection); a highly sensitive and specific ELISA is now available, but does not differentiate between various species of schistosome. CSF serology is usually positive. Myelography is of value diagnostically.

Chemotherapy consists of praziquantel (50 mg/kg given

as a single dose, or 40 mg/kg in two divided doses 4–6 h apart) for all species (Strickland & Abdel-Wahab 1991) or oxamniquine (15 mg/kg as a single dose or 20 mg daily for 3 days, depending on the geographical region) for *S. mansoni* (Efthimiou & Denning 1984). As an alternative, metriphonate (10 mg/kg body weight in three alternate weeks), can be used in a *Schis. haematobium* infection. When CNS involvement is proved or suspected, a corticosteroid cover is recommended; successful outcome after the chemo-therapy of CNS disease is well documented, but surgical decompression is occasionally necessary. Most campaigns designed to prevent transmission of this disease have failed.

Schistosoma japonicum infection

Endemic areas for this trematode exist in China, the Philippines, Indonesia, Laos, Thailand and Cambodia. The life cycle and clinical presentation are similar to those in *S. mansoni* infection. However, brain involvement is more common; the reason for this is unclear. In a study from the Philippines, generalized and Jacksonian seizures and psychomotor epilepsy were common, and in one study electroencephalographic abnormalities were present in 68% of 75 infected patients. Treatment is with praziquantel (60 mg/kg in three divided doses on a single day); oxamniquine is ineffective.

CLONORCHIS SINENSIS AND OPISTHORCHIS VIVERRINI

These food-borne trematode infections are confined to South-East Asia (Cook 1990, 1996). Metacercariae are ingested in freshwater fish. Infection involves the biliary tract; chronic cholangitis (which may be suppurative) ensues and a long-term complication is adenocarcinoma of the biliary system. Chemotherapy is straightforward; praziquantel (25 mg/kg after meals three times daily for 1–2 days) is highly effective.

FASCIOLA HEPATICA

This ubiquitous liver fluke occurs world-wide. Whilst praziquantel would, on a priori grounds, seem likely to eradicate infection, in practice it is an unsatisfactory chemotherapeutic agent and bithionol (1 g three times daily on alternate days to a total dose of 45 g) remains in use, although triclabendazole has provided encouraging results (Cook 1996).

LESS COMMON TREMATODE INFECTIONS

Table 64.2 includes a less common trematode infection (with resultant clinical manifestations) which affects man (Cook 1990, 1996).

Paragonimiasis

The genus *Paragonimus* comprises several species of lung fluke (Goldsmith et al 1991). The most common is *Paragonimus westermani*, which has a reservoir in fresh-water crayfish and crabs (as well as several mammalian species including tigers and cattle) in South-East Asia, the Indian subcontinent, the Philippines, Indonesia and Papua New Guinea. Other species, which produce similar clinical manifestations, exist in parts of Africa (especially the west) and South and Central America. (Another trematode, *Alaria*, has been reported to produce CNS involvement (with petechiae in the cortex and white matter), subarachnoid haemorrhage and spinal cord involvement.)

Ingestion of crayfish and crabs (which contain encysted metacercariae) is the usual method of infection; after excysting in the small intestine they mature to adult worms in 5–6 weeks in the lungs; they live for at least 6–7 years in the form of cysts in the respiratory tree. The life cycle is completed when they are coughed up or swallowed and excreted in faeces; after deposition in freshwater free-swimming miracidia are liberated, which in turn infect a suitable snail host; cercariae (which invade the viscera of crayfish and crabs) are produced.

Most human infections are asymptomatic, but a cough with rusty sputum, chronic pulmonary disease (including chronic bronchitis, bronchiectasis, pleural effusion and fibrosis) may occur; pleural adhesions and calcification are late events. Pulmonary tuberculosis is often simulated. Flukes can develop in ectopic sites, two being the brain and spinal cord (children are especially vulnerable) (Goldsmith et al 1991). Invasion seems to take place via the soft tissues of the neck and through the large foramina, including the jugular foramen. Clinically, cysts are usually present in the temporal and occipital (but also parietal) lobes; signs of a space-occupying lesion with epilepsy and paresis may result; optic atrophy with papilloedema is less usual. Headache, visual disturbances, hemiplegia, mental deterioration and nausea and vomiting may also occur. Invasion of the vertebral canal is a rare event, but spinal cord compression, with resultant paralysis, is a possible sequel. Other syndromes include: meningitis, subacute or chronic progressive encephalopathy, a 'tumour-like' presentation, and cerebral infarction; cerebral haemorrhage has been recorded. Transverse myelitis has also been documented.

P. westermani eggs may be present in sputum, faeces, pleural fluid or cutaneous lesions (Goldsmith et al 1991); adults can be removed surgically and identified. Serology is also of value. When CNS involvement is present, CSF usually shows an elevated protein concentration with mononuclear pleocytosis. In a minority of cases eosinophils are present, and there may be evidence of haemorrhage. A wide spectrum of CT findings has been documented, including ventricular dilatation. Cerebral involvement may be accompanied by intracranial calcification.

Treatment was formerly with bithionol. A high success rate has now been reported with praziquantel (25 mg/kg after meals three times daily for 3 days) (Goldsmith et al 1991). Cerebral lesions may require drainage or surgical removal.

Cestode infections

TAENIA SOLIUM INFECTION

Throughout the world, the larval stage of *Taenia solium* infects man via human faecal contamination. Any organ can be involved; the most common clinical presentation is with subcutaneous nodules. It is also the most common helminth to produce CNS infection in man (Cook 1988).

Infection is endemic in all continents, with the exception of Australia (Earnest et al 1987); however, even there, cases in immigrants are now being identified. It is very common in Latin America; in Mexico, evidence of cysticercosis is found in 1.4–3.6% of post-mortem examinations in the general population. Foci also exist in the USSR, China, India, Pakistan, the Philippines and Indonesia (an epidemic occurred in Irian Jaya following a donation of infected pigs from Bali); it occurs sporadically throughout Africa. In Europe it is unusual, but exists in the Iberian peninsula and Slavic countries. It is a significant problem in immigrant populations in North America. Cysticercosis is unusual in non-pork-eating communities, e.g. Jews and Muslims.

Infection is caused by the larval stage (*Cysticercus cellulosae*) of the pig tapeworm *T. solium*; it has been recognized in pigs for more than two millennia. Highest infection rates exist where hygienic standards and practices are low; infection results from contamination of food by *T. solium* eggs, and not by ingestion of 'measly' pork. Man is the only definitive host for *T. solium*, and therefore is the sole source of eggs. Following ingestion (in infected pork), the scolex emerges from the cyst and attaches to the human small-intestinal wall; here it grows into a mature *T. solium* (which may live for up to 25 years) in 5–12 weeks. A solitary worm is present in most human infection. The scolex remains anchored to the small-intestinal mucosa, while the remainder of the worm (the strobila consists of up to 1000 proglotids and varies from 2 to 10 m in length) may extend into the ileum. Gravid segments detach themselves and are either expressed in faeces or liberate thick-walled eggs in the colon; these remain viable in contaminated soil for several weeks. Ingestion of eggs (which eventually produce cysticerci in muscle masses) by pigs (the intermediate host) completes the life cycle. Treatment of a human *T. solium* infection is with praziquantel, niclosamide, dichlorophen or mepacrine.

Neurocysticercosis

Human cysticercosis arises when man becomes an incidental intermediate host; this occurs when eggs are ingested in food or water contaminated with human faeces. The egg wall is dissolved in the upper gastro-intestinal tract, and resultant oncospheres penetrate the intestinal mucosa to enter local lymphatics and mesenteric vessels; they are transmitted to many organs, including subcutaneous tissues, skeletal muscle and most importantly, the CNS. Within 2–3 months the oncospheres lose their hooks and develop into cysticerci. External autoinfection (i.e. ingestion of faecal eggs by the infected individual) is possible; internal autoinfection has never been satisfactorily demonstrated, and if it does occur is a rare event. Cysticerci evoke a local chronic lymphocytic and granulomatous reaction. The capsule ultimately fibroses and is surrounded by neutrophils, eosinophils and round cells. In the brain, the cyst(s) lie within a wall of neuroglia, which later undergoes degenerative change and appears as a discoloured ring walled off from normal tissue. These space-occupying cysts may persist for at least 20 years, eventually becoming calcified; they can be demonstrated radiographically as spindle- or oat-shaped lesions in skeletal muscles and as oval or spherical lesions in the CNS.

Presentation of disease occurs between 2 months and 30 years after infection (Kalra & Sethi 1992). Initially, one or more small subcutaneous nodules are noticed by the infected patient; there may be a myositis. Every organ can be affected; in the absence of CNS involvement it remains a 'benign' disease. Any part of the CNS can be affected (Shanley & Jordan 1980). About 50% of infected individuals develop symptoms, the most common of which are seizures, increased intracranial pressure and stroke. In an endemic area, neurocysticercosis is the most common cause of epilepsy in young adults. CNS involvement can be divided into four groups depending on the site of the cyst: parenchymal, meningeal, ventricular or in the spinal cord.

In addition, numerous other clinical syndromes have been described, and many CNS lesions (including those produced by several other parasitic infections) mimicked. In children, in particular, clinical presentation may be as an acute encephalitis. Severe and aggressive disease results from a racemose meningeal form. Status epilepticus and sequelae of intracranial hypertension are the most common causes of death; they are directly attributable to the presence of cysts.

Definitive diagnosis is dependent on histological examination of a cysticercal cyst; if subcutaneous nodules (present in about 50% of cases of neurocysticercosis) are present, they can be easily excised. However, CNS involvement may be present in the absence of a cyst(s) easily accessible to removal or biopsy. Radiologically, intracranial elliptiform calcifications are sometimes visualized. A central scolex surrounded by a cyst wall – both calcified – is pathogenic. However, calcification rarely occurs before 3 years and usually much later. CT and magnetic resonance image (MRI) scanning may reveal non-calcified cysts and is the most valuable radiological procedure (Jena et al 1992, Colli et al 1993); this has largely supplanted invasive diagnostic techniques. Peripheral blood eosinophilia is of limited diagnostic value; detection of *T. solium* eggs in a faecal sample is unusual.

CSF pressure may be elevated. A pleocytosis of 5–500 cells with an eosinophil or lymphocyte preponderance is inconstant. Total protein and IgG concentration may be elevated, and glucose concentration reduced. Immuno-diagnosis (formerly unreliable) has recently improved, but cross-reaction with other helminths remains a problem. Using an ELISA, sensitivity and specificity rates of around 90% have been reported in active neurocysticercosis, from centres in Colombia, Mexico and South Africa. Serological evidence in CSF is probably preferable to that in serum. Antigen derived from cysticercal fluid possesses reactivity which is undoubtedly greater than that from the cyst wall.

Before 1979, the only means of management was surgical (Jena et al 1992, Zee et al 1993); long-term chemotherapy has now produced results that are generally encouraging. There are many reports on the use of praziquantel (Del Brutto et al 1993), but most have involved small numbers of patients; furthermore, some, but not all, have combined this agent with a corticosteroid cover. Several relatively large series (using praziquantel) have now been reported from several centres in South and Central America. An inflammatory reaction (characterized by fever, headache, meningismus and exacerbation of the neurological symptoms) to dead and dying larvae, possibly analogous to the Jarisch–Herxheimer reaction, has been documented when corticosteroids are not administered simultaneously; this can occasionally prove fatal. Therefore, corticosteroid cover should always be added. The following presentations seem well suited to praziquantel therapy:

1. Active cerebral disease with cysts located in the parenchyma or subarachnoid space
2. Cysts in brain parenchyma, subarachnoid space, and ventricular system
3. Miliary cysticercosis – numerous cysts are present but are too small for detection by CT scanning.

When the cysts are solely within the ventricular system, including some of those in group (2), or when they involve the spinal cord, early (but sometimes later) surgery is usually indicated. When the intracranial pressure is raised, cysts are localized to the chiasma (with an inflammatory

reaction and adhesive arachnoiditis), and when there is failure of response to chemotherapy, surgery is also indicated. Albendazole (Del Brutto et al 1993, Botera et al 1993), flubendazole and metriphonate have been used in small series of cases, but all these agents require further evaluation in larger studies (Sotelo et al 1990); albendazole has given results comparable with praziquantel. Long courses of these agents are not without side-effects (Cook 1995). Prevention depends on improving standards of hygiene and sanitation; man is the sole definitive host, and elimination of human infection would result in total disappearance of the disease. Husbandry practices must be improved; cysticerci can be killed by freezing pork at −20°C for 12 h, or by cooking at 50°C.

Prognosis depends largely upon the site of the cyst(s). While most cases now respond satisfactorily to chemotherapy, disease involving the ventricular system and the racemose meningobasal form of the disease continue to carry a poor prognosis. The invasive racemose variety can cause occlusion of the right internal carotid artery. Sudden death may occur when obstructive hydrocephalus develops rapidly.

ECHINOCOCCOSIS (HYDATID DISEASE)

This infection is frequently considered to be 'tropical'; however, this is not strictly the case, and *Echinococcus granulosus* infection can occur whenever man lives in close proximity to sheep and dogs. Infection occurs in Wales, western England and much of the Middle East. Several other mammalian species also harbour hydatid cysts. *E. granulosus* is one of the smallest cestodes. The dog (and other canids) acts as the definitive host, becoming infected by ingesting a hydatid cyst present in uncooked offal from sheep, goat or other herbivore. The adult worm (consisting of 2–5 segments 3–8 mm long) attaches to small-intestinal mucosa. Up to 70 000 worms have been recovered from a dog fed a single hydatid cyst.

Human infection results from the ingestion of food contaminated with dog faeces; frequent and intimate contact with dogs, together with poor personal hygiene, contribute to the likelihood of infection. Eggs hatch in the small intestine where the liberated oncosphere penetrates the mucosa, from whence it is transported by mesenteric blood and lymphatics to the liver, lungs and other organs. A related species *Echinococcus multilocularis* produces a more serious disease. It maintains a proliferative stage in man; masses of small cysts (which can occasionally metastasize) may be present, and the brain occasionally becomes the site of metastatic spread.

Clinically, the vast majority of human infections are asymptomatic and discovered during routine examination or investigation (including chest radiography), or at post-mortem examination. A significant number of infections are associated with morbidity and occasional mortality. The liver is most often affected (60%) followed by the lungs (25%) and other organs including the brain (<1%) and, rarely, the spinal cord; 80% of cysts are solitary. Cerebral (together with spinal cord and ocular) cysts sometimes produce symptoms in children, but clinical presentation is usually in young adults. Presenting symptoms and signs depend on the site of the cyst(s); the disease should always be suspected in the presence of a space-occupying lesion within the CNS or elsewhere, in one who has lived in an area where the disease exists. Vertebral involvement (a high proportion of bone lesions affects this site) can result in spinal cord compression. An important differential diagnosis is neurocysticercosis (see above); however, in that infection cysts are usually more numerous.

Until recently, serological methods were unreliable, lacking both sensitivity and specificity; an ELISA has now proved of value, especially when antibody against Arc-5 (a genus-specific antigen isolated from unilocular hydatid cyst fluid) is used. Eosinophilia in peripheral blood is an inconstant feature. Parasite identification can be made from a cyst removed either at surgery or post-mortem examination; a single fluid-filled cavity is surrounded by a translucent white membrane containing opaque dots (representing scolices), brood capsules and hydatid 'sand'. The scolex has four spherical suckers, a rostellum and two rows of hooks. A novel approach to diagnosis has been reported; fine-needle aspiration of hydatid cysts (Hira et al 1988) in 11 patients yielded fluid containing characteristic hooklets. Although no complications arose from the procedure, confirmation of its safety is necessary; aspiration of a hydatid cyst has been considered potentially hazardous, due to the possibility of spillage and/or an anaphylactoid response to leaking fluid. CT scanning is an invaluable technique for localization in all forms of the disease.

Treatment was until recently surgical. Cysts in most organs were initially injected with silver nitrate, formalin or cetrimide in order to kill the protoscolices, while those in the brain and spinal cord were dissected out with great care (usually without prior treatment) thus avoiding damage to neural tissue. Over the last decade the benzimidazole compounds have been introduced; they continue to undergo evaluation (Davis et al 1986, Morris et al 1987, Wilson et al 1987, Todorov et al 1988, Singounas et al 1992, Moskopp & Lotterer 1993, Teggi et al 1993, Yue-Han et al 1993).

The most effective therapeutic agent is presently albendazole (Benger et al 1981, Moskopp & Lotterer 1993, Teggi et al 1993, Yue-Han et al 1993); this compound is very rapidly absorbed from the small intestine. There is excellent evidence that an adequate concentration of this agent (or another benzimidazole compound) within the cyst is scolicidal. Viability is assessed by ELISA, specific IgG, and CT scanning. Praziquantel has also been shown to possess protoscolicidal properties, and clinical evaluation continues. Results of large multicentre, controlled trials of albendazole and praziquantel, or both, are keenly awaited; side-effects should be monitored (Cook 1995). Some intracranial and spinal cord cysts will presumably always require surgery, but only after prior albendazole and/or praziquantel chemotherapy. Prognosis in CNS disease obviously depends to a considerable extent on the site of the cyst(s). Prevention is by deworming dogs and eliminating access to infected offal and carcasses of diseased animals.

LESS COMMON CESTODE INFECTIONS

Table 64.2 shows two less common cestode infections of man. Diphylobothriasis is widely spread geographically and rarely produces problems apart from the rare sequel of vitamin B_{12} deficiency megaloblastic anaemia.

Coenuriasis

This zoonotic disease of man is caused by the larval stage of *Taenia* (*Multiceps*) species (Benger et al 1981). Of major importance is the fact that in neurocoenuriasis clinical manifestations are very similar to those of neurocysticercosis (see above). Although a rare disease overall, cases have been reported from the UK, France, Africa, North America and Brazil. The adult worms are present in the small intestine of dogs and cats and other canids; proglottids, which are excreted in faeces, disintegrate with the production of numerous free eggs which, when ingested by man, develop into coeneuri in the CNS and skeletal muscles. The sheep is the major intermediate host.

In man, a single intracranial space-occupying lesion (2–6 cm in diameter) may be present in the cerebrum, ventricle(s), posterior horn of the lateral ventricle, brain stem or spinal cord. Alternatively, there may be involvement of the cranial nerves. Ophthalmic involvement has been reported. Subcutaneous cysts may be present, as in cysticercosis. The value of serology is limited; cross-reaction occurs with cysticercosis and hydatid disease. CT scanning is of value in delineating intracranial cyst(s). Definitive diagnosis depends on surgical removal and confirmation. No chemotherapeutic agent is of proven efficacy. Prevention should be aimed at treating dogs with praziquantel (or niclosamide), thus reducing environmental contamination with eggs.

References

Benger A, Rennie R P, Roberts J T et al 1981 A human *Coenurus* infection in Canada. *American Journal of Tropical Medicine and Hygiene* 30: 638–644

Blaser M J, Smith P D, Ravdin J I, Greenberg H B, Guerrant R L (eds) 1995 Infections of the gastrointestinal tract. Raven, New York, p 1155–1222

Botero D, Uribe C S, Sanchez J L et al 1993 Short course albendazole treatment for neurocysticercosis in Columbia. *Transactions of the Royal Society of Tropical Medicine and Hygiene* 87: 576–577

Bunnag T 1991 Angiostrongyliasis. In: Strickland G T (ed) *Hunter's tropical medicine*, 7th edn. W B Saunders, Philadelphia, p 767–773

Bunnag T, Comer D S, Punyagupta S 1970 Eosinophilic myeloencephalitis caused by *Gnathostoma spinigerum*: neuropathology of nine cases. *J Neurol Sci* 10: 419–434

Colli B O, Pereira C U, Assirati J A, Machado H R 1993 Isolated fourth ventricle in neurocysticercosis: pathophysiology, diagnosis, and treatment. *Surgical Neurology* 39: 305–310

Cook G C 1987 *Strongyloides stercoralis* hyperinfection syndrome: how often is it missed? *Quarterly Journal of Medicine* 64: 625–629

Cook G C 1988 Neurocysticercosis: parasitology, clinical presentation, diagnosis and recent advances in management. *Quarterly Journal of Medicine* 68: 575–583

Cook G C 1989 Canine-associated zoonoses: an unacceptable hazard to human health. *Quarterly Journal of Medicine* 70: 5–26

Cook G C 1990 Parasitic disease in clinical practice. Springer-Verlag, London, p 272

Cook G C 1991 Protozoan and helminthic infections. In: Lambert H P (ed) Infections of the central nervous system. Edward Arnold, London, p 264–282

Cook G C 1995 Adverse effects of chemotherapeutic agents used in tropical medicine. *Drug Safety* 13: 31–45

Cook G C (ed) 1996 Manson's tropical diseases, 20th edn. W B Saunders, London p 1779

Cosnett J E, Dellen J R van 1986 Schistosomiasis (bilharzia) of the spinal cord: case reports and clinical profile. *Quarterly Journal of Medicine* 61: 1131–1139

Davis A, Pawlowski Z S, Dixon H 1986 Multicentre clinical trials of benzimidazolecarbamates in human echinococcosis. *Bulletin of the World Health Organization* 64: 383–388

Del Brutto O H, Sotelo J, Roman G C 1993 Therapy for neurocysticercosis: a reappraisal. *Clinical Infectious Diseases* 17: 730–735

Earnest M P, Reller L B, Filley C M, Grek A J 1987 Neurocysticercosis in the United States: 35 cases and a review. *Reviews of Infectious Diseases* 9: 961–979

Editorial 1988 Escargots and eosinophilic meningitis. *Lancet* ii: 320

Efthimiou J, Denning D 1984 Spinal cord disease due to *Schistosoma mansoni* successfully treated with oxamniquine. *British Medical Journal* 288: 1343–1344

Gay T, Pankey G A, Beckman E N et al 1982 Fatal CNS trichinosis. *Journal of the American Medical Association* 247: 1024–1025

Gillespie S H 1987 Human toxocariasis. *Journal of Applied Bacteriology* 63: 473–479

Glickman L T, Schantz P M 1981 Epidemiology and pathogenesis of zoonotic toxocariasis. *Epidemiology Reviews* 3: 230–250

Goldsmith R, Bunnag D, Bunnag T 1991 Lung fluke infections: paragonimiasis. In: Strickland G T (ed) *Hunter's tropical medicine*, 7th edn. W B Saunders, Philadelphia, p 827–831

Gould I M, Newell S, Green S H, George R H 1985 Toxocariasis and eosinophilic meningitis. *British Medical Journal* 291: 1239–1240

Hill I R, Denham D A, Scholtz C L 1985 *Toxocara canis* larvae in the brain of a British child. *Transactions of the Royal Society of Tropical Medicine and Hygiene* 79: 351–354

Hira P R, Shweiki H, Lindberg L G et al 1988 Diagnosis of cystic hydatid disease: role of aspiration cytology. *Lancet* ii: 655–657

Igra-Siegman Y, Kapila R, Sen P et al 1981 Syndrome of hyperinfection with *Strongyloides stercoralis*. *Reviews of Infectious Diseases* 3: 397–407

Jena A, Sanchetee P C, Tripathi R, Jain R K, Gupta A K, Sapra M L 1992 MR observations on the effects of praziquantel in neurocysticercosis. *Magnetic Resonance Imaging* 10: 77–80

Kalra V, Sethi A 1992 Childhood neurocysticercosis – epidemiology, diagnosis and course. *Acta Paediatrica Japonica* 34: 365–370

Strickland G T, Abdel-Wahab M F 1991 Schistosomiasis. In: Strickland G T (ed) *Hunter's tropical medicine*, 7th edn. W B Saunders, Philadelphia, p 781–809

Leech J H, Sande M A, Root R K (eds) 1988 Parasitic infections. Churchill Livingstone, New York, p 364

Mandell G L, Bennett J E, Dolin R (eds) 1995 Diseases of helminths. In: Mandell G L, Bennett J E, Dolin R (eds) Mandell, Douglas and Bennett's principles and practice of infectious diseases. 4th edn. Churchill Livingstone, New York, p 2525–2557

Marcial-Rojas R A, Fiol R E 1963 Neurologic complications of schistosomiasis: review of the literature and report of two cases of transverse myelitis due to *S. mansoni*. *Annals of Internal Medicine* 59: 215–230

Morris D L, Chinnery J B, Georgiou G et al 1987 Penetration of albendazole sulphoxide into hydatid cysts. Gut 28: 75–80

Moskopp D, Lotterer E 1993 Concentrations of albendazole in serum, cerebrospinal fluid and hydatidous brain cyst. Neurosurgical Review 16: 35–37

Muller R 1971 Dracunculus and dracunculiasis. Advances in Parasitology 9: 73–151

Duke Boh 1991 Loiasis. In: Strickland G T (ed) Hunter's tropical medicine, 7th edn. W B Saunders, Philadelphia, p 727–729

Murrell K D 1991 Trichinosis. In: Strickland G T (ed) Hunter's tropical medicine, 7th edn. W B Saunders, Philadelphia, p 756–761

Negesse Y, Lanoie L O, Neafie R C, Connor D H 1985 Loiasis: 'Calabar' swellings and involvement of deep organs. American Journal of Tropical Medicine and Hygiene 34: 537–546

Nutman T B, Miller K D, Mulligan M et al 1988 Diethylcarbamazine prophylaxis for human loiasis. New England Journal of Medicine 319: 752–756

Punyagupta S, Juttijudata P, Bunnag T 1975 Eosinophilic meningitis in Thailand: clinical studies of 484 typical cases probably caused by Angiostrongylus cantonensis. American Journal of Tropical Medicine and Hygiene 24: 921–931

Schantz P M, Glickman L T 1978 Toxocaral visceral larva migrans. New England Journal of Medicine 298: 436–439

Shanley J D, Jordan M C 1980 Clinical aspects of CNS cysticercosis. Archives of Internal Medicine 140: 1309–1313

Siddorn J A 1978 Schistosomiasis and anterior spinal artery occlusion. American Journal of Tropical Medicine and Hygiene 27: 532–534

Singounas E G, Leventis A S, Sakas D E, Hadley D M, Lampadarios D A, Karvounis P C 1992 Successful treatment of intracerebral hydatid cysts with albendazole: case report and review of the literature. Neurosurgery 31: 571–574

Smallman L A, Young J A, Shortland-Webb W R et al 1986 Strongyloides stercoralis hyperinfestation syndrome with Escherichia coli meningitis: report of two cases. Journal of Clinical Pathology 39: 366–370

Sotelo J, del Brutto O H, Penagos P et al 1990 Comparison of therapeutic regimen of anticysticercal drugs for parenchymal brain cysticercosis. Journal of Neurology 237: 69–72

Taylor M R H, Keane C T, O'Connor P et al 1988 The expanded spectrum of toxocaral disease. Lancet i: 692–695

Teggi A, Lastilla M G, Rosa F de 1993 Therapy of human hydatid disease with mebendazole and albendazole. Antimicrobial Agents and Chemotherapy 37: 1679–1684

Todorov T, Vutova K, Petkov D, Balkanski G 1988 Albendazole treatment of multiple cerebral hydatid cysts: case report. Transactions of the Royal Society of Tropical Medicine and Hygiene 82: 150–152

Vishwanath S, Baker R A, Mansheim B J 1982 Strongyloides infection and meningitis in an immunocompromised host. American Journal of Tropical Medicine and Hygiene 31: 857–858

Wilson J F, Rausch R L, McMahon B J et al 1987 Albendazole therapy in alveolar hydatid disease: a report of favorable results in two patients after short-term therapy. American Journal of Tropical Medicine and Hygiene 37: 162–168

Yue-Han L, Xiao-Gen W, Deng-Gao Y 1993 Cerebral alveolar echinococcosis treated with albendazole. Transactions of the Royal Society of Tropical Medicine and Hygiene 87: 481

Zee C S, Segall H D, Destian S, Ahmadi J, Apuzzo M L J 1993 MRI of intraventricular cysticercosis: surgical implications. Journal of Computer Assisted Tomography 17: 932–939

Index